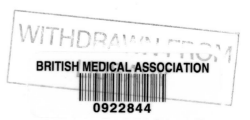

Orell & Sterrett's Fine Needle Aspiration Cytology

Commissioning Editor: *Michael Houston*
Development Editor: *Sharon Nash*
Project Manager: *Mahalakshmi Nithyanand*
Design: *Charles Gray*
Illustration Manager: *Gillian Richards*
Illustrator: *Samantha Elmhurst*
Marketing Manager(s) (UK): *Gaynor Jones;* **(US):** *Tracie Pasker*

Orell & Sterrett's Fine Needle Aspiration Cytology

FIFTH EDITION

Svante R Orell
ML(Stockholm) FRCPA FIAC

Consultant Pathologist
Clinpath Laboratories
Kent Town, South Australia
Formerly Director of Cytology and Associate Professor of Pathology
Flinders Medical Centre
Flinders University of South Australia
Australia

Gregory F Sterrett
MBBS FRCPA FIAC

Pathologist, PathWest Laboratory Medicine
Clinical Professor, School of Pathology and Laboratory Medicine
University of Western Australia
QE II Medical Centre
Nedlands, Perth, Western Australia

For additional online content visit expertconsult.com

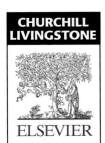

CHURCHILL
LIVINGSTONE

ELSEVIER

Edinburgh   London   New York   Oxford   Philadelphia   St Louis   Sydney   Toronto   2012

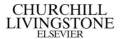

CHURCHILL
LIVINGSTONE
ELSEVIER

Churchill Livingstone an imprint of Elsevier Limited

First edition 1986
Second edition 1992
Third edition 1999
Fourth edition 2005

Notices
Knowledge and best practice in this field are constantly changing. As new research and experience broaden our understanding, changes in research methods, professional practices, or medical treatment may become necessary.

Practitioners and researchers must always rely on their own experience and knowledge in evaluating and using any information, methods, compounds, or experiments described herein. In using such information or methods they should be mindful of their own safety and the safety of others, including parties for whom they have a professional responsibility.

With respect to any drug or pharmaceutical products identified, readers are advised to check the most current information provided (i) on procedures featured or (ii) by the manufacturer of each product to be administered, to verify the recommended dose or formula, the method and duration of administration, and contraindications. It is the responsibility of practitioners, relying on their own experience and knowledge of their patients, to make diagnoses, to determine dosages and the best treatment for each individual patient, and to take all appropriate safety precautions.

To the fullest extent of the law, neither the Publisher nor the authors, contributors, or editors, assume any liability for any injury and/or damage to persons or property as a matter of products liability, negligence or otherwise, or from any use or operation of any methods, products, instructions, or ideas contained in the material herein.

ISBN: 978-0-7020-3151-9

British Library Cataloguing in Publication Data

Orell, Svante R.
  Orell and Sterrett's fine needle aspiration cytology. – 5th ed.
  1. Cytodiagnosis – Handbooks, manuals, etc. 2. Needle biopsy – Handbooks, manuals, etc. 3. Pathology, Surgical – Handbooks, manuals, etc.
  I. Title II. Fine needle aspiration cytology III. Sterrett, Gregory F. IV. Orell, Svante R. Fine needle aspiration cytology.
  616'.07582 – dc22

Printed in China
Last digit is the print number: 9 8 7 6 5 4 3 2 1

Contents

Preface

When we began work on the first edition of this book in 1983, our plan was to put together a practical handbook focusing mainly on the kind of lesions and conditions that a hospital pathologist was likely to face in routine practice. We wanted to provide short checklists and carefully selected illustrations, which would be useful in the diagnostic work at the microscope, in the compact format of a handbook. Hence the title Manual and Atlas of Fine Needle Aspiration Cytology.

The second and third editions were the result of an irresistible incentive to cover an increasing number of pathological entities including less common conditions, to try to illustrate the variability of patterns seen in some entities and to reflect the extraordinary proliferation of the literature on fine needle aspiration cytology. In the fourth edition we sought to illustrate the cytological features of most entities as seen both in air-dried MGG-stained and in alcohol-fixed Pap-stained smears in parallel, and to include the main immunocytochemical findings in the lists of cytological diagnostic criteria. All this inevitably led to an expansion of text, illustrations and references, and thus the format of the book departed, to a degree, from the original concept.

The text of all chapters has been updated for the current edition. Many illustrations have been exchanged or improved, and some new photos have been added. In this process, every effort was made to avoid a major increase in the overall volume of both text and pictures. Several new co-authors have joined the team and have made invaluable contributions. Dr Steve Chryssidis has revised and updated Chapter 3, Dr John Miliauskas Chapter 5, Dr Gita Jayaram Chapter 6, Drs Joan Cangiarella and Aylin Simsin Chapter 7, Drs Amanda Segal and Felicity Frost Chapters 8 and 9, Dr Bastiaan de Boer Chapters 10 and 11, Dr Miguel Perez-Guillermo Chapter 13, Dr Henryk Domanski Chapters 14, 15 and 16 and Drs Reda Saad and Harsharan Singh Chapter 17. A new chapter specifically on the cytological findings in infectious diseases has been added by Dr Andrew Field. As a result, the book has taken on the format of a textbook on Fine Needle Aspiration Cytology. Some readers may regret the departure from the convenient compact handbook format, but we hope that the changes have resulted in worthwhile increased coverage and usefulness.

S Orell, G Sterrett

List of contributors

Måns Åkerman MD PhD FIAC
Former Associate Professor and Senior Cytopathologist
Department of Pathology and Cytology
University Hospital
Lund, Sweden

Joan Cangiarella MD
Vice-Chair of Clinical Operations
Associate Professor of Pathology
Department of Pathology
New York University School of Medicine
New York, NY, USA

Steve Chryssidis MBBS FRANZCR
Consultant Radiologist
Dr Jones and Partners Medical Imaging
Stepney, Australia

Bastiaan de Boer MBBS FRCPA MIAC
Clinical Associate Professor
School of Pathology and Laboratory Medicine
University of Western Australia
Consultant Pathologist
PathWest Laboratory Medicine
QE II Medical Centre
Nedlands, WA, Australia

Henryk Domanski MD PhD
Associate Professor of Pathology
Coordinator of the Cytology Service
Department of Pathology
University and Regional Laboratories Region Skåne
Lund, Sweden

**Andrew S Field MBBS(Hons) FRCPA FIAC
DipCytopath(RCPA)**
Deputy Director and Senior Consultant
Department of Anatomical Pathology
St Vincent's Hospital
Associate Professor
Notre Dame Medical School Sydney
Conjoint Senior Lecturer
University of New South Wales Sydney
New South Wales, Australia

Felicity A. Frost MBBS FRCPA FIAC Dip Cytopathol (RCPA)
Head, Cytopathology
PathWest Laboratory Medicine WA
QEII Medical Centre
Nedlands WA Australia

Kim R Geisinger MD
Professor and Director of Surgical Pathology and
of Cytology
Professor of Internal Medicine (Gastroenterology)
Department of Pathology
Wake Forest University School of Medicine
Winston-Salem, NC, USA

Gita Jayaram MDPath MIAC FRCPath AMM FICPath
Consultant Pathologist
Ramakrishna Diagnostic Center
Ootacamund, India

Jerzy Klijanienko MD PhD MIAC
Senior Consulting Pathologist
Cytopathology Unit
Institut Curie
Paris, France

**Suzanne Le P Langlois MB BS FRANZCR DDU MRACMA
Grad Dip Gast (LCB)**
Consultant Radiologist
Former Director of Radiology and Associate Professor,
Royal Adelaide Hospital, South Australia,
and The Townsville Hospital
Queensland, Australia

John R Miliauskas MBBS FRCPA FIAC FASCP
Associate Professor of Pathology
Flinders Medical Centre, Flinders University and
Queen Elizabeth Hospital
Consultant Pathologist, Healthscope Pathology
Adelaide, SA, Australia

Svante R Orell ML(Stockholm) FRCPA FIAC
Consultant Pathologist
Clinpath Laboratories
Kent Town, South Australia
Formerly Director of Cytology and Associate Professor of
Pathology
Flinders Medical Centre
Flinders University of South Australia
Australia

Miguel Perez-Guillermo MD PhD FIAC
Head of Pathology Department
Department of Pathology
Hospital Universitario Santa María del Rosell
Cartagena, Spain

Reda S Saad MD PhD FRCPC
Associate Professor of Pathology
Department of Laboratory Medicine and Pathobiology/
University of Toronto
Staff Pathologist at Sunnybrook Health Sciences Center
Toronto, Canada

Amanda Segal MBBS FRCPA
Consultant Pathologist
PathWest Laboratory Medicine WA
QEII Medical Centre
Nedlands, WA, Australia

Jan F Silverman MD
Professor, Temple University School of Medicine and
Drexel University College of Medicine
System Chair of Pathology, West Penn Allegheny
Health System
Chairman and Director of Anatomic Pathology,
Allegheny General Hospital
Pittsburgh, PA, USA

Aylin Simsir MD
Associate Professor
Director of Cytopathology Laboratories
Department of Pathology
New York University School of Medicine
New York, NY, USA

Harsharan K Singh MD
Professor of Pathology and Laboratory Medicine
Director, Electron Microscopy Services, UNC Hospitals
Associate Director, UNC Nephropathology Laboratory
The University of North Carolina School of Medicine
Chapel Hill, NC, USA

Gregory F Sterrett MBBS FRCPA FIAC
Pathologist, PathWest Laboratory Medicine
Clinical Professor, School of Pathology and
Laboratory Medicine,
University of Western Australia
QE II Medical Centre
Nedlands, Perth, Western Australia

Philippe Vielh MD PhD MIAC
Head of Cytopathology
Department of Pathology
Institut de Cancérologie Gustave Roussy
Villejuif, France

Acknowledgements

As with the previous editions, we have been most indebted to our working colleagues, who have taken on the task of preparing the next generation of Cytologists and Cytopathologists for practice, who provide us with our second opinions, and who give cautionary advice. The ease with which they absorbed what for us was a sometimes painful process of learning about FNA cytology is daunting but gratifying for the discipline. We would like to single out Drs Felicity Frost, Bastiaan de Boer, Amanda Segal and Dominic Spagnolo from PathWest QE II Medical Centre, Drs Jonathan Allin and Suchitra Somers from Clinpath Laboratories and Drs John Miliauskas and David Ellis from Flinders Medical Centre for their help and support.

We wish to express our thanks to all the co-authors and contributors to the current edition. Without their generous support this new edition would not have been accomplished. They are represented both by the newer, most promising and the most experienced practitioners of the art of FNA today. Their expertise has markedly extended the range of information that we could bring to this edition.

Our thanks are due to the Elsevier team which has guided and managed the project from its conception to its completion with great expertise and remarkable patience: Michael Houston, Sharon Nash, Mahalakshmi Nithyanand, Charles Gray, Gillian Richards and also to Lee Bowers for copyediting.

We pay tribute to Dr Darrel Whitaker, now deceased, who began the project with us now 3 decades ago and was part of the editorial team for the first 4 editions. Darrel was an outstanding Cytologist and Scientist and a friend and colleague to many of the contributors to the book. He was one of the foremost practitioners and developers of the field of Diagnostic Cytology and provided encouragement, inspiration and support to all of us. Darrel would be very pleased with our aim to hand on the project to new authors and especially those from the younger generation.

S Orell
G Sterrett

CHAPTER 1

Introduction

Svante R. Orell and Gregory F. Sterrett

Historical perspective

Fine needle aspiration cytology as we know it today dates back to around 1950. However, the idea to obtain cells and tissue fragments through a needle introduced into the abnormal tissue was by no means new. In the mid-nineteenth century, Kün[1] (1847), Lebert[2] (1851) and Menetrier[3] (1886) employed needles to obtain cells and tissue fragments to diagnose cancer. Leyden[4] (1883) used the same method to isolate pneumonic microorganisms. Few early pathologists were, however, involved in this pioneering work, and the development of needle aspiration cytology along with exfoliative cytology was, to a large extent, performed by 'professional hybrids',[5] clinicians who used these simple techniques as aids to rapid diagnosis. For example, the common use of needling the bone marrow as an integral part of the investigation of hematological problems continued to serve as a reminder that almost every tissue could be sampled by a simple technique requiring neither anesthesia nor the expensive intervention of surgeons.[6] In the UK in 1927, Dudgeon and Patrick[7] proposed the needling of tumors as a means of rapid microscopic diagnosis. About the same time, Martin and Ellis[8] at the Memorial Hospital in the USA were also advocates of needle aspiration, although the pathologists working with them initially insisted on sectioning as well as smearing the samples and would only make a confident diagnosis if tissue fragments were obtained. Consequently, Martin and Ellis used needles of a thicker caliber (18 gauge) than those commonly in use today. The pathologists at Memorial continued to use the technique, but it took nearly another 40 years for a general interest in 'aspiration biopsy' to develop in the USA.[9,10]

It was in Europe that 'fine needle aspiration cytology' (FNAC), as the technique was usually called, began to flourish in the 1950s and 1960s. Söderström[11] and Franzén[12] in Sweden, Lopes Cardozo[13,14] in Holland (all clinician/ hematologists by training), Zajdela[15] in France, and others became major proponents, studying thousands of cases each year. Zajicek,[16,17] among the first of pathologists to embrace FNAC in collaboration with Franzén at the oncologic center (Radiumhemmet) of the Karolinska Hospital, applied the requisite scientific rigor to define precise diagnostic criteria and to determine diagnostic accuracy in a variety of conditions. FNAC soon became accepted and integrated in the diagnostic routines by the team of pathologists and clinicians at the Radiumhemmet. In the following years, experience accumulated rapidly and pathologists and oncologists from Sweden and many other countries came to study the technique, which subsequently spread to the rest of Europe, the Americas, Asia and Australia. FNAC is now part of the service of all sophisticated departments of pathology.

The history of clinical cytology by Grunze and Spriggs,[18] and a comprehensive review of the development of cytopathology in the twentieth century by Naylor,[19] are highly recommended reading. A very recent historical overview of fine needle aspiration biopsy by M. Rosa in *Diagnostic Cytopathology*[20] should also be mentioned.

FNAC as a tool in clinical investigation

Fine needle aspiration cytology was initially conceived as a means to confirm a clinical suspicion of local recurrence or metastasis of known cancer without subjecting the patient to further surgical intervention. This remains one of the most important contributions of the technique from a practical point of view. Following success in this area, the interest focused on preliminary preoperative diagnosis of all kinds of neoplastic processes, benign or malignant, in any organ or tissue of the body and on definitive, specific diagnosis in inoperable cases as a guide to rational treatment. The expansion of FNAC in primary diagnosis of tumors in the last 30 years or so has been impressive and generally successful. This development is to a large degree the result of consistent, continuous and critical correlation between cytological assessment and histopathological diagnosis facilitated by the organisational coordination of laboratory resources.[21]

The clinical value of FNAC is not limited to neoplastic conditions. It is also valuable in the diagnosis of inflammatory, infectious and degenerative conditions, in which samples can be used for microbiological and biochemical analysis in addition to cytological preparations. This is of particular importance in patients with acquired immunodeficiency syndrome (AIDS) and in other immunocompromised patients.[22] FNAC has proven useful in the diagnosis and monitoring

DOI: 10.1016/B978-0-7020-3151-9.00001-3

of graft rejection in transplantation surgery,[23,24] an area that is beyond the scope of this book.

Intraoperative cytology is another application using similar techniques and diagnostic criteria as in FNAC. It is a valuable alternative or complement to frozen section examination with a comparable level of accuracy.[25–29]

Advantages and limitations

Fine needle aspiration cytology offers clear advantages to patients, doctors and taxpayers. The technique is minimally invasive, produces a speedy result and is inexpensive. Its accuracy in many situations, when applied by experienced and well-trained practitioners, can approach that of histopathology in providing an unequivocal diagnosis. We should stress, however, that aspiration cytology is not a substitute for conventional surgical histopathology. It should be regarded as an essential component of the preoperative/pretreatment investigation of pathological processes, in combination with clinical, radiological and other laboratory data. A definitive specific diagnosis may not be possible by cytology in a proportion of cases, but a categorisation of disease and a differential diagnosis with an estimate of probability can usually be provided to suggest the most efficient further investigations, saving time and resources. Applied in this manner, it has become just as indispensable as surgical histopathology.

The method is applicable to superficial lesions that are easily palpable, in the skin, subcutis and soft tissues, thyroid, breast, salivary glands and superficial lymph nodes. Fine needle biopsy (FNB) is less demanding technologically than surgical biopsy, has a low risk of complications and can be performed as an office procedure, in outpatient departments and in radiology theaters, saving expensive days in hospital. It is also highly suitable in debilitated patients, is readily repeatable and allows biopsy of multiple lesions in one session. Modern imaging techniques, mainly ultrasonography (US) and computed tomography (CT), make percutaneous, transthoracic and transperitoneal fine needle biopsy of deeper structures possible and safe.[30] Samples may be obtained from the lung and mediastinum, the abdominal, retroperitoneal and pelvic organs and tissues, deep sites in the head and neck, the skeleton and the soft tissues. US-directed FNB can also be performed through an endoscope, mainly of lesions in the pancreas or adjacent tissues.[31–33] A tissue diagnosis, preliminary or differential, can be provided within minutes rather than days to guide further investigation and management.

Instances of serious complications have been reported in relation to different sites and organs, such as major hemorrhage, septicemia, bile peritonitis, acute pancreatitis, pneumothorax, etc.[34] However, such complications are extremely rare in view of the vast numbers of uncomplicated FNBs performed in major centers where close monitoring of patients is the rule. Complications have also been reduced by advances in endoscopic ultrasound guidance techniques, allowing safer sampling of intra-abdominal organs such as pancreas or lesions previously relatively inaccessible such as paraoesophageal and paratracheal nodes and tumors. The possibility of cancer cells being disseminated along the needle track,[35] as has been reported at the site of incisional

biopsy or of core needle biopsy, initially caused a great deal of concern. Reviews of the literature by Roussel et al.[36] in 1989 and by Powers[37] in 1996 showed the risk of needle track seeding to be extremely low when truly fine needles of 22 gauge or less are used. Multiple passes, larger needles and absence of normal parenchyma covering the lesion appear to increase the risk. The question is further discussed in relation to specific organs and sites in several of the following chapters. The rare severe complications do not diminish the clinical value and wide applications of FNAC, but awareness of their existence should be a reminder always to consider the indications for any invasive procedure, including FNB.

Another concern is that preoperative FNB may cause local tissue changes, which could render subsequent histological diagnosis difficult. Such changes, including hematoma, infarction, capsular pseudoinvasion and pseudomalignant reparative reactions, have indeed been reported.[38] They rarely cause real diagnostic difficulties except where fine needle aspiration (FNA) sampling technique has been unduly aggressive. The biopsy technique should always be careful and gentle with a view to minimising tissue damage.

Practitioners of FNAC must be aware that the technique has certain inherent limitations. Firstly, results and accuracy are highly dependent on the quality of samples and smears. Appropriate training and experience is essential to consistently achieve optimal material for diagnosis. Secondly, many pathological processes are heterogeneous, and the tiny samples obtained with a fine needle may not be representative even when the biopsy is guided by imaging. Multiple biopsies help, but the number of passes is limited by the need to minimise trauma. Thirdly, some lesions are recognised mainly on the specific microarchitectural pattern, which may not be sufficiently represented in cytological preparations. Fourthly, the small FNB sample may not allow the full armamentarium of ancillary techniques to be drawn upon, for example batteries of immune markers. Finally, precise cytological criteria have not yet been defined in some rare conditions. In particularly difficult areas of diagnosis, such as soft tissue tumors,[39] paediatric tumors,[40] malignant lymphoma, etc., patients are best referred to major centers with specialised oncological expertise. Continuous frequent exposure to a particular category of tumors has been clearly shown to be a major factor deciding diagnostic accuracy. On the other hand, because such cases will be seen initially in general medical practices and surgical clinics, all cytopathologists must be able to at least categorise the condition and suggest the appropriate referral. This requires a wide knowledge of the range of possible conditions in any given site.

The numerous case reports of all kinds of rare and exotic tumors and other pathological processes diagnosed by FNAC published in the cytology journals create the impression that nothing is impossible for this technique. However, by studying the literature we can also appreciate the wide range of diagnostic pitfalls, which is a warning against overconfidence in cytodiagnosis.[41] The cytological diagnosis is in many cases preliminary, and the report should therefore include an estimate of the level of probability of the diagnosis and suggest possible differentials. A level of diagnostic accuracy high enough to constitute a sufficient basis for major therapeutic decisions can only be reached through the analysis of large series of cases with histological follow-up. In 1989, the value and limitations of aspiration cytology in the diagnosis of primary tumors was debated at an international symposium moderated by Hajdu and attended by a number of international experts.[42] A continuing debate of this type and an ongoing evaluation and interchange of the increasing experience is important since all parties involved must fully understand the limitations of the technique.

In recent years, there has been a swing back to core needle biopsy and to histological sectioning of tissue fragments in the preoperative investigation of some tumors. Core needle biopsy has virtually replaced FNAC in the diagnosis of prostate cancer and in some institutions also of non-palpable, screen-detected breast lesions.[43,44] There are several reasons for this trend. One is the increasing pressure on pathologists to make definitive and specific preoperative diagnoses on FNB samples in all kinds of disease processes in all sites. The demand for a definitive diagnosis is particularly strong in the investigation of tumors in deep sites, in which needle biopsy guided by radiological imaging is the only alternative to explorative laparotomy or thoracotomy. In addition, oncologists increasingly expect various prognostic parameters to be included in the preoperative assessment of tumors, for which FNB may not provide sufficient material. Another important reason is the high dependency on, and the shortage of, pathologists with sufficient training and experience to successfully practice FNAC. Supervision of sampling and specimen handling by a competent pathologist is crucial to achieving a high diagnostic accuracy,[45] and this may prove logistically unattainable. Core needle biopsy specimens, on the other hand, are handled in theaters and received in laboratories in the same way as any other surgical biopsy.

Although core biopsy needles used today are usually of a lesser caliber than those of the pre-FNAC era, the procedure is more traumatic and carries a slightly greater risk of complications than FNB, including the possibility of tumor seeding in the needle track. Cost effectiveness is an important consideration in practices that involve large numbers of patients such as breast cancer screening. There is also emerging evidence that core needle biopsy may not necessarily improve diagnostic accuracy.[46-48] We therefore feel that it is not a question of choosing one method to the exclusion of the other, but that the two techniques should be seen as complementary, each with its own specific indications.[49,50] In our opinion, FNB should be the first line approach to the investigation of suspected malignant disease and is able to resolve the problem in a variable proportion of cases depending on location and type. Core needle biopsy should be used selectively when the information provided by cytology is, or is likely to be, insufficient, incomplete or indecisive. In order to make optimal use of the simple, fast and inexpensive method of FNB, every effort should be made to improve the sampling and preparation techniques, to establish diagnostic criteria and to identify and record possible causes of diagnostic error in all sites.

The practice of FNAC

The success of FNAC depends on four fundamental requirements:

- Samples must be representative of the lesion investigated.
- Samples must be adequate in terms of cells and other tissue components.
- Samples must be correctly smeared and processed.
- The biopsy must be accompanied by sufficient and correct clinical/radiological information.

Definite diagnostic conclusions cannot possibly be drawn if these requirements are not filled. We agree with Rollins[51] that '9/10 of making a correct cytological diagnosis depends upon the information gained from the history and physical examination and the quality of the specimen submitted'. It is true that ancillary techniques such as immunocytochemistry, electron microscopy, cytogenetics and molecular biology can significantly enhance the potential to make precise, type-specific diagnoses.[52] Nevertheless, the requirements listed above will always remain a sine qua non, no matter how sophisticated the supplementary techniques. Any information obtained by FNAC must always be correlated with clinical judgment, radiological imaging and other investigations.

The aims, and therefore the practice, of FNAC are different in the community (referrals from general practitioners, general physicians and surgeons, community health centers and general hospital outpatient clinics) and in major hospitals or oncology centers.[53] At the community level, FNB should be regarded as a simple screening test or triage for serious disease that needs further investigation and specialist referral, in a population of patients most of whom have conditions that can be followed and treated conservatively. For example, lymphadenopathy is a common cause of concern to both patients and doctors, but is most often non-specific, reactive and likely to regress in due course. The relatively small number of cases caused by malignant disease or by a specific infection that requires treatment can be identified by FNB at an early stage, and these patients can be promptly referred to the appropriate specialist.[54] Another example is the categorisation of soft tissue tumors by FNA to prevent incisional biopsy or inadequate surgical excision in cases of unexpected sarcoma.[55] A precise, type-specific and definitive diagnosis is not essential at this stage since further investigations will be undertaken at the specialist center anyway. At the community level, costly ancillary laboratory tests are therefore not often indicated, and should be used selectively and with constraint.

In the major hospital, on the other hand, FNB is an essential component of the preoperative/pretreatment investigations on which clinical management is based. The aim is to establish a precise and, if possible, type-specific diagnosis, and prognostic indicators if required. The full armamentarium of laboratory techniques may be called upon to achieve this goal and the supplementary use of core needle biopsy may also be considered. The information obtained by FNB may be of decisive importance in the planning of surgery, radiotherapy, chemotherapy, etc.

Who should actually perform the procedure of FNB for palpable lesions has been much debated. In the past, it was our opinion that the pathologist should be the main protagonist, particularly at the community level, and the service should be offered by community-based laboratories equipped with an FNAC clinic.[56,57] To achieve a high standard of proficiency, constant daily experience, practice and feedback are essential,[58,59] and we still need a cadre of pathologists experienced in all of the technical aspects of sampling to provide such a service. Material collected by untrained and inexperienced medical staff is often unsatisfactory and impossible to interpret. In the major hospital/specialist clinic situation, a team approach is the ideal. However, a dedicated and expert image-guided sampling service is now usually assumed to be the first point of patient referral, rather than the pathologist. This may be the most efficient method for community-based practice, to the advantage of patients in terms of convenience. It allows a decision as to the need for FNAC sampling as well as on-the-spot biopsy and slide preparation, including the collection of material for ancillary tests when appropriate. Imaging provides increasingly accurate assessment of the nature of the lesion and its relations to other structures. Ultrasound needle guidance may also help representative sampling of palpable superficial lesions. However, the laboratory has a crucial role in teaching radiologists a standard approach to sampling and specimen preparation. The US-guided procedure of placing the needle may increase bleeding at the biopsy site and compromise the quality of samples, particularly in the thyroid and lymph nodes. There is clearly a need for pathologists to provide education and feedback to radiologists about FNB techniques and smear preparation.

In deeply sited lesions requiring radiological guidance, the radiologist directs the needle to the target, but even then the presence of a pathologist or a specially trained clinician is required. The quality of the preparations is assured, samples can be checked immediately for adequacy reducing the number of passes, and material can be secured for appropriate ancillary testing.[60,61] This practice has been shown to considerably reduce the rate of unsatisfactory biopsies, resulting in significant cost savings.[62]

Before attempting diagnosis by FNB, the pathologist must have full knowledge of the clinical history, physical examination, imaging and other laboratory tests. Clinical data serve as a safeguard in the interpretation of the cytology and should not bias the pathologist. Any discordance calls for reevaluation of results. In reporting results, the pathologist must make it clear if the diagnosis is conclusive or indeterminate, requiring further sampling or other investigations.[63] Standard reporting formats have been recommended to facilitate the communication of results to the clinician.[64-66]

FNB smears must first be studied in low power to assess overall cellularity, microarchitectural features, stromal components and any secretory products, inflammatory cells or necrosis in the background, any heterogeneity of the cell population and the proportions between different constituents. The overall pattern is of crucial importance to diagnosis. The next step is the study of single cells in high power. The approach to the interpretation of a FNB smear is therefore closer to histopathology than to exfoliative cytology. It is the pathologist who examines the entire slide, not the cyto-screener. If only a few abnormal cells can be found in a population of cells normal for the site, the sample in most cases should be reported as unsatisfactory and the procedure repeated.

There has been a great deal of controversy regarding the advantages and disadvantages of using air-dried May-Grunwald-Giemsa (MGG) or Diff-Quik-stained smears as against wet-fixed Papanicolaou (Pap) and hematoxylin and eosin (H&E) preparations. We believe that the methods are complementary and that both should be employed in parallel whenever possible. Certain features are particularly distinctive in each and familiarity with both stains is indispensable in many situations (see Chapter 2). The subject is elaborated further in the text in which we have tried to demonstrate the advantage of using both techniques in parallel.

Nomenclature

The nomenclature applied to the discipline has been the subject of some discussion. Most Scandinavian and North American workers use the designation 'fine needle aspiration biopsy' or 'aspiration biopsy cytology' for both the art as a whole and for the operative procedure. Zajdela,[67] who first introduced the non-aspiration technique, calls it 'fine needle sampling'. We believe that 'fine needle aspiration cytology' (FNAC) is still an acceptable description of the whole of the art even if aspiration is often not used. We refer to the material expressed from the needle as samples or aspirates and use the terminology 'fine needle biopsy' (FNB) for the operative procedure.

The aims of the book

We acknowledge the debt owed to clinicians in the development of FNAC, but the discipline now lies squarely in the realm of diagnostic pathology, along with surgical pathology and exfoliative cytology. In most countries, it is now taught as an integral part of specialist training programs in pathology. However, since many hospital pathologists see only a limited number of FNBs in their routine work, there is a need for continuing education and refresher courses as well as for easily accessible references. Checklists of diagnostic criteria and of common problems and pitfalls can provide valuable assistance when reporting FNB specimens.

This book is therefore directed towards the practicing diagnostic pathologist working in community-based laboratories and general hospitals. The range of conditions that can be expected to constitute the main workload in a busy general hospital is treated in some depth, whereas uncommon lesions are described in less detail, supplemented by references. In this respect we have been guided by our own experience, which may well differ from that of other centers. The enormous expansion of the literature on cytopathology in recent year has also created a dilemma to keep the number of references within reasonable limits by selecting those considered most relevant to clinical practice.

The aim of the book is to provide guidelines and criteria for diagnosis and differential diagnosis based on routinely prepared processed and stained FNB samples generated in a busy outpatient clinic and easily handled by a standard equipped laboratory. Common, basic immune markers are included with diagnostic criteria for most entities. Sophisticated ancillary techniques, such as advanced immunohistochemistry, flow cytometry, DNA quantitation and cell proliferation, molecular biology and cytogenetics, are reviewed by Dr Philippe Vielh in Chapter 2. Indications for the use of ancillary techniques and their contribution to diagnosis and prognosis in malignant disease are discussed, and selected references are provided for readers who seek more detailed information on methodology and interpretation of results. Chapter 3, on radiological tumor imaging and guidance of needle biopsy, has been updated by Dr Stephen Chryssidis. The refinements of roentgenological techniques may appear beyond the scope of this book, but we wish to emphasise the importance of close cooperation and mutual understanding between radiologist and pathologist to the success of FNAC.

The enormous expansion in recent years has made it increasingly difficult to adequately cover the whole discipline of FNAC. Several new contributors have joined the team of eminent cytopathologists from the fourth edition and have reviewed, updated and expanded the chapters in their respective areas of expertise, for which we are sincerely grateful. A new chapter has been added, dedicated to the application of FNAC in infectious diseases, contributed by Dr Andrew Field.

We have chosen to present FNAC within the framework of anatomical regions rather than on the basis of histopathological classifications. Although this inevitably leads to some repetition, it conforms to the way problems present in clinical practice. Each of the descriptive chapters is subdivided into two parts: a text division in which indications, accuracy, techniques and complications are discussed, and an atlas division in which the cytological patterns are described and illustrated. The text and illustrations are designed to be simple and to relate to daily diagnostic decisions. The magnification used for the microphotographs is simply recorded as low power (LP), intermediate power (IP), high power (HP) and high power/oil immersion (HP oil), which correspond approximately to × 100, × 250, × 400 and × 1000, respectively. Cropping and resizing of some of the reproductions inevitably causes deviations from the original magnification. Red blood cells or lymphocytes have therefore been included in most photos to provide a baseline for the appreciation of size.

Obviously, no book can ever compensate for lack of experience but we hope that this updated version can offer some help in the daily diagnostic work and will be useful as a practical atlas kept close at hand beside the microscope.

The challenge ahead

Fine needle aspiration cytology, from being a technique mastered only by specialist cytopathologists, has become an expected part of the skills of all anatomical pathologists. Education and examinations in FNAC techniques are now an essential part of training in anatomical pathology. The skepticism of some histopathologists about the technique has largely abated, along with fears about FNAC claiming to be a replacement for tissue diagnosis.

The aim and the ambition level of FNAC to be applied in a particular setting must be clearly defined, understood and agreed to by pathologists and clinicians. It decides the way available techniques are utilised, how results are reported and how results are used in patient management. Is FNAC to be used simply as a triage/screening method, or to obtain a maximum of pretreatment information regardless of effort and cost? The rapid and cost-effective screening of a large population of patients to identify the small proportion with potentially significant disease that requires further investigation is very different from the diagnostic and prognostic work-up of individual patients, in which much time and laboratory resources have to be invested. The distinction of these two separate levels of FNAC needs to be clarified and recognized. One is centered in the community; the other should ideally be sited in specialised multi-disciplinary units dealing with a defined area such as lymphoproliferative diseases, soft tissue and bone tumors, head and neck, etc.

The task of convincing clinicians of the value of the technique has been extremely successful. For superficial lesions, the diffusion of the technique into general medical practice has led to unique responsibilities for the pathologist in the education of clinicians about the limitations of the technique and the protection of clinicians who may not always be aware of the need for, or the nature of, further investigations. This is crucial in an increasingly unforgiving medico-legal climate. Standardisation of report formats, as referred to above, will promote communication between pathologists and clinicians and allow comparisons between laboratories, for quality assurance purposes. For commonly performed tests such as FNB of breast, expected levels of accuracy will be specified and audited through professional bodies. For deep-sited lesions, definitive diagnosis and typing of tumors of all sites is expected and low error rates are assumed. The pathologist must therefore be prepared to apply any appropriate ancillary diagnostic techniques to cytological material and to advise the use of other techniques such as fine core biopsy, large core biopsy or open biopsy when these are more appropriate. The innovations relating to the ease, accuracy, efficiency and low complication rates for core biopsy sampling, including almost painless sampling in many sites, should not be minimised. In many situations, core sampling can be just as easily performed as FNB and may provide more diagnostic material and better diagnostic results. However, the cost and the time factors can not be ignored. Accurate and safe diagnosis is always the aim, and the cytopathologist is best placed to advise the clinician on the choice of biopsy method in the individual case, based on current literature and with full knowledge of the needs of the clinician in particular sites and cases.

Although the use of FNAC has widened, there are pressures for specialisation in this discipline, as there are in other areas of anatomical pathology, and a balance between focused expertise and the availability of the test must be achieved. A certain minimum ongoing experience is necessary and this will become further defined. Clinicians, in particular surgeons, will become more aware of the advantages of concentration of sampling expertise with cytopathologists who work in a clinic setting offering rapid diagnosis. An important question is how the pathologist can best liaise with and educate local medical practitioners in remote areas about optimising sampling and specimen preparation. These developments will ensure a dynamic and challenging discipline, which continues to occupy a unique place straddling clinical and tissue diagnosis.

References

1. Kün M. A new instrument for the diagnosis of tumours. Monthly J Med Sci 1846;7:853.

2. Lebert H. Traité pratique des maladies cancéreuses et des affections curables confondues avec le cancer. Paris: J B Baillière; 1851.

3. Menetrier P. Cancer primitif du poumon. Bull Soc Anat (Paris) 1886;11:643.

4. Leyden OO. Ueber infectiöse Pneumonie. Dtsch Med Wschr 1883;9:52–4.

5. Söderström N. Thin needle aspiration biopsy. Letter. Acta Cytol 1980;24:468.

6. Hirschfeldt H. Bericht über einige histologisch-mikroskopische und experimentelle Arbeiten bei den bösartigen Geschwulsten. Krebsforsch 1919;16:33.

7. Dudgeon LS, Patrick CV. A new method for the rapid microscopical diagnosis of tumours. Br J Surg 1927;15:250–61.

8. Martin HE, Ellis EB. Aspiration biopsy. Surg Gynecol Obstet 1934;59:578–89.

9. Kline TS. Fine needle aspiration biopsy. Past, present and future. Arch Pathol Lab Med 1980;104:117.

10. Frable WJ. Needle aspiration biopsy: past, present and future. Human Pathol 1989;20:504–17.

11. Söderström N. Fine needle aspiration biopsy. Stockholm: Almqvist and Wiksell; 1966.

12. Franzén S, Giertz G, Zajicek J. Cytological diagnosis of prostatic tumours by transrectal aspiration biopsy: a preliminary report. Br J Urol 1960;32:193–6.

13. Lopes Cardozo P. Clinical cytology. Leiden: Safleu; 1954.

14. Lopes Cardozo P. Atlas of clinical cytology. Leiden: 1978.

15. Zajdela A. Valeur et intérêt du diagnostic dans les tumeurs du sein par ponction. Etude de 600 cas confrontés cytologiquement et histologiquement. Arch Anat Pathol 1963;11:85–7.

16. Zajicek J. Aspiration biopsy cytology. Part 1. Cytology of supra-diaphragmatic organs. Monographs in clinical cytology, Vol. 4. Basel: Karger; 1974.

17. Zajicek J. Aspiration biopsy cytology. Part 2. Cytology of infra-diaphragmatic organs. Monographs in clinical cytology, Vol. 7. Basel: Karger; 1979.

18. Grunze H, Spriggs AI. History of clinical cytology – a selection of documents. Darmstadt: E. Giebeler; 1980.

19. Naylor B. The century for cytopathology. Acta Cytol 2000;44:709–25.

20. Rosa M. Fine-Needle Aspiration Biopsy: A Historical Overview. Diagn Cytopathol 2008;36:773–5.

21. Bedrossian CWM. Bridging the gap between cytopathology and surgical pathology. Diagn Cytopathol 1995; 12:1–2.

22. Strigle SM, Rarick MU, Cosgrove MM, et al. A review of the fine-needle aspiration cytology findings in human immunodeficiency virus infection. Diagn Cytopathol 1992;8:41–52.

23. Häyry P, Lautenschlager I. Fine needle aspiration biopsy in transplantation pathology. Semin Diagn Pathol 1992;9:232–7.

24. Sariya D, Kluskens L, Assad L, et al. Diagnostic role of fine-needle aspiration of pancreatic allograft to detect rejection. Diagn Cytopathol 2002;27:266–70.

25. Philips J. Intraoperative cytological diagnosis. In: Russell P, Farnsworth A, editors. Surgical pathology of the ovaries. 2nd ed. Edinburgh: Churchill Livingstone; 1997. p. 643–56.

26. Shidham V, Gupta D, Galindo LM, et al. Intraoperative scrape cytology: comparison with frozen sections, using receiver operating characteristics (ROC) curve. Diagn Cytopathol 2000;23:134–9.

27. Bleggi-Torres LF, de Noronha L, Schneider Gugelmin E, et al. Accuracy of the smear technique in the cytological diagnosis of 650 lesions of the central nervous system. Diagn Cytopathol 2001;24:293–5.

28. Liu Y, Silverman JF, Sturgis CD, et al. Utility of intraoperative consultation touch preparations. Diagn Cytopathol 2002;26:329–33.

29. Scucchi LF, Di Stefano D, Cosentino L, et al. Value of cytology as an adjunctive intraoperative diagnostic method. An audit of 2,250 consecutive cases. Acta Cytol 1997;41:1489–96.

30. Silverman JF, Geisinger KR. Fine needle aspiration cytology of the thorax and abdomen. Edinburgh: Churchill Livingstone; 1996.

31. Erickson RA, Sayage-Rabie L, Avots-Avotins A. Clinical utility of endoscopic ultrasound-guided fine needle aspiration. Acta Cytol 1997;41:1647–53.

32. Bentz JS, Kochman ML, Faigel DO, et al. Endoscopic ultrasound-guided real-time fine-needle aspiration: clinicopathologic features of 60 patients. Diagn Cytopathol 1998;18:98–109.

33. Ballo MS, Guy CD. Percutaneous fine-needle aspiration of gastrointestinal wall lesions with image guidance. Diagn Cytopathol 2001;24:16–20.

34. Smith EH: complications of percutaneous abdominal fine-needle biopsy. Review. Radiology 1991; 178:253–8.

35. Mighell AJ, High AS. Histologic identification of carcinoma in 21 gauge needle tracks after fine needle aspiration biopsy of head and neck carcinoma. J Clin Pathol 1998;51:241–3.

36. Roussel F, Dalion J, Benozio M: The risk of tumoral seeding in needle biopsies. Acta Cytol 1989;33:936–9.

37. Powers CN. Complications of fine needle aspiration biopsy: the reality behind the myths. In: Schmidt WA, editor. Cytopathology. Chicago: ASCP Press; 1996. p. 69–91.

38. Chan JKC, Tang SK, Tsang WYW, et al. Histologic changes induced by fine needle aspiration. Advances Anat Pathol 1996;3:71–90.

39. Akerman M, Domanski HA. The cytology of soft tissue tumours. Monographs in Clinical Cytology, vol. 16. Basel: Karger; 2003.

40. Wakely PE, Kardos TF, Frable WJ. Application of fine needle aspiration biopsy to paediatrics. Human Pathol 1988;19:1383–6.

41. Orell SR. Pitfalls in fine needle aspiration cytology. Cytopathol 2003;14:173–82.

42. Hajdu SI, Ehya H, Frable WJ, et al. The value and limitations of aspiration cytology in the diagnosis of primary tumors. A symposium. Acta Cytol 1989;33:741–90.

43. Britton PD. Fine needle aspiration or core biopsy. The Breast 1999;8:1–4.

44. Cobb CJ, Raza AS. Obituary: Alas poor FNA of breast – we knew thee well. Diagn Cytopathol 2005;32:1–4.

45. Stanley MW, Löwhagen T. Fine needle aspiration of palpable masses. Boston: Butterworth-Heinemann; 1993.

46. Greif J, Marmur S, Schwarz Y, et al. Percutaneous core cutting needle biopsy compared with fine-needle aspiration in the diagnosis of peripheral lung malignant lesions. Results in 156 patients. Cancer (Cancer Cytopathol) 1998;84:144–7.

47. Masood S. Core needle biopsy versus fine-needle aspiration biopsy: are there similar sampling and diagnostic issues? The Breast Journal 2003;9: 145–6.

48. Epstein JL, Walsh PC, Sanfilippo F. Clinical and cost impact of second-opinion pathology. Review of prostate biopsies prior to radical prostatectomy. Am J Surg Pathol 1996;20:851–7.

49. Masood S. Fine-needle aspiration biopsy of nonpalpable breast lesions. Challenges and promises. Cancer (Cancer Cytopathol) 1998;84:197–9. FNB vs CNB, advocat combin.

50. Koscick RL, Petersilge CA, Makley JT, et al. CT-guided fine needle aspiration and needle core biopsy of skeletal lesions. Complementary diagnostic techniques. Acta Cytol 1998;42:697–702.

51. Rollins SD. Editorial comments. Diagn Cytopathol 1994;10:172–3.

52. Saleh H, Masood S. Value of ancillary studies in fine-needle aspiration biopsy. Diagn Cytopathol 1995;13:310–5.

53. Orell SR. The two faces of fine-needle biopsy: its role in the teaching hospital

and in the community. Diagn Cytopathol 1992;8:557–8.

54. Thomas JO, Adeyi D, Amanguno H. Fine-needle aspiration in the management of peripheral lymphadenopathy in a developing country. Diagn Cytopathol 1999;21:159–62.

55. Maitra A, Ashfaq R, Saboorian MH, et al. The role of fine-needle aspiration biopsy in the primary diagnosis of mesenchymal lesions. A community hospital-based experience. Cancer (Cancer Cytopathol) 2000;90:178–85.

56. Carson HJ, Saint Martin GA, Castelli MJ, et al. Unsatisfactory aspirates from fine needle aspiration biopsies: a review. Diagn Cytopathol 1995;12:280–4.

57. Rollins SD. The breast and aspirate – outside the ivory tower. Diagn Cytopathol 1996;16:197–9.

58. Coghill SB, Brown LA. Why pathologists should take needle aspiration specimens. Editorial. Cytopathol 1994;6:1–4.

59. Ljung B-M, Drejet A, Chiampi N, et al. Diagnostic accuracy of fine-needle aspiration biopsy is determined by physician training in sampling technique. Cancer (Cancer Cytopathol) 2001;93:263–8.

60. Austin JH, Cohen MB. Value of having a cytopathologist present during percutaneous fine needle aspiration biopsy of lung: report of 55 cancer patients and metaanalysis of the literature. AJR 1993;160:175–7.

61. Saleh HA, Khatib G. Positive economic and diagnostic accuracy impacts of on-site evaluation of fine needle aspiration biopsies by pathologists. Acta Cytol 1996;40:1227–30.

62. Nasuti JF, Gupta PK, Baloch ZW. Diagnostic value and cost-effectiveness of on-site evaluation of fine-needle aspiration specimens: review of 5,688 cases. Diagn Cytopathol 2002;27:1–4.

63. Kline TS, Bedrossian CWM. Communication and cytopathology: part V: the term 'suspicious'. Diagn Cytopathol 1996;14:viii–ix.

64. The Papanicolaou Society of Cytopathology Task Force on Standards of Practice. Guidelines of the Papanicolaou Society of Cytopathology for fine-needle aspiration procedure and reporting. Diagn Cytopathol 1997;17:239–47.

65. Abati A, Abele J, Bacus SS, et al. The uniform approach to breast fine-needle aspiration biopsy. Diagn Cytopathol 1997;16:295–311.

66. Yang J, Schnadig V, Logrono R, et al. Fine-needle aspiration of thyroid nodules: A study of 4703 patients with histologic and clinical correlations. Cancer Cytopathol 2007;111:306–15.

67. Zajdela A, Zillhardt P, Voillemot N. Cytological diagnosis by fine needle sampling without aspiration. Cancer 1987;59:1201–5.

CHAPTER 2

The techniques of FNA cytology

Svante R. Orell and Philippe Vielh

Basic techniques

Svante R. Orell

The success of fine needle aspiration cytology (FNAC) depends to a high degree on perfecting the technique of sampling and preparation of samples. Palpation skills learnt through practice and experience, judiciously complemented by radiological image guidance when appropriate, are essential to obtain *representative samples*. The choice of needles, the use or not of aspiration, and the manipulation of the needle within the target relative to the type of tissue decide the *adequacy of samples*. Finally, correct *smearing, fixation and staining* of samples is critical to assure optimal preservation and presentation of cells and non-cellular components on which a confident diagnosis can be based.

Consequently, the cytopathologist should be in a position to control and give advice on sampling and preparation techniques, directly or indirectly, to achieve a high proportion of satisfactory and diagnostic biopsies. Close cooperation with the referring clinician and radiologist is essential.

Indications for fine needle biopsy (FNB) of various organs and tissues are explained in detail in the following chapters. Meanwhile, some general principles apply. To be suitable for FNB, the disease process must be localized and clearly defined by clinical examination or radiological imaging. FNB may be tried in some diffuse processes with the understanding that a negative result has little value. The principles of screening by exfoliative cytology are obviously completely different.

Although severe complications are rare[1,2] the possible benefits of a cytological diagnosis should be weighed against risks and patient discomfort. Risk factors such as age, coagulation disorders, respiratory failure, etc. should be taken into account. FNB of superficial lesions can safely be carried out as an office procedure. Biopsies of most deep sites (transpleural, transperitoneal, etc.) are better performed in hospital so that patients can be sedated if necessary and kept under observation for a few hours after the procedure. The pathologist should be consulted before the procedure to give advice on feasibility, the likely informative value of the test, the need for and choice of ancillary techniques, etc.

Preparation for biopsy

Equipment

Needles

Standard disposable 27–22-gauge (0.4–0.7 mm), 30–50 mm long needles are suitable for superficial, palpable lesions. We use 25-gauge needles for most lesions, but increasingly 27 gauge for cell-rich and vascular tissues such as lymph nodes and thyroids, in children and in sensitive sites such as orbit, eyelids, genitals and intracutaneous lesions. Although the yield is a little less, samples are usually adequate and smear quality tends to be better due to less admixture with blood. The yield from fibrotic lesions in the breast and soft tissues is less predictable. Needles of 23–22 gauge are most often used, but thinner needles can sometimes be more efficient. Larger-bore needles may be required to obtain sufficient material for ancillary tests.

Twenty-two-gauge, 90-mm disposable lumbar puncture needles with trocar, or 22-gauge 150 or 250 mm Chiba needles are used for deep biopsies. They are sufficiently rigid and the trocar prevents contamination during the passage through surrounding tissues. Special long 23-gauge needles are supplied with the Franzén instrumentarium for biopsy of pelvic organs (Unimed, Lausanne, Switzerland).

If the purpose of the biopsy is to obtain a core of tissue for paraffin embedding and sectioning, a cutting core needle is used. A range of small-gauge cutting core needles is commercially available. Core needle biopsy (CNB) fragments allow the study of tissue architecture and provide more tissue for ancillary tests. However, CNB is more traumatic and more costly, has a slightly greater risk of complications, and must be processed in a laboratory, precluding an immediate, on-site assessment of adequacy or a preliminary diagnosis.[3,4]

Syringes and syringe holder

Standard disposable plastic syringes mounted in a syringe holder/pistol grip are suitable for conventional aspiration

©2011 Elsevier Ltd
DOI: 10.1016/B978-0-7020-3151-9.00002-5

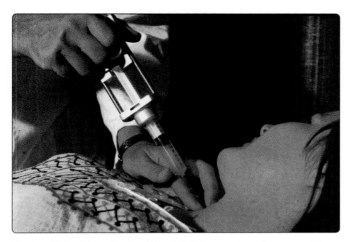

Fig. 2.1 FNB with aspiration (thyroid) Syringe and needle mounted in a pistol grip is operated by one hand, leaving the other free to feel and fix the target. Note the thumb supporting the syringe.

biopsy. The Cameco Syringe Pistol (Cameco AB, Taby, Sweden) is made to fit 10-cc plastic syringes. The holder leaves one hand free to fix and to feel the target, which allows better precision in placing the needle (Fig. 2.1).

Containers and slides

Small sterile containers with tight lids containing physiological saline or a transport medium such as Hank's balanced salt solution should be at hand if a cell suspension or a cell block is needed, or to rinse needles and syringes. Special culture media may be required in certain instances.

Glass slides must be clean, dry and free of grease. Slides with frosted ends are convenient for immediate labeling. Coated or charged slides for better adhesion are recommended if smears are to be used for immunostaining.

Fixatives and stains

Smears are air-dried or wet-fixed. Routine wet fixation is either in 70–90% ethanol or using a commercial spray fixative. Carnoy's fixative has the advantage of lysing red blood cells. Glutaraldehyde and 10% buffered formalin should be available if tissue fragments for EM or for paraffin embedding are obtained. Note that formalin must be kept in an airtight container since formalin fumes may adversely affect air-dried smears if stored together.

A set of Diff-Quik stains in suitable containers, and a lightweight portable microscope should be available at all times to allow immediate checking of smears for adequacy and an immediate preliminary diagnosis if required. Some pathologists may prefer rapid Papanicolaou staining.

Other

Skin disinfectant (pre-injection swabs), sterile dressings, local anesthetic, tongue depressors, a small electric torch and sterile scalpel blades (scrape smears from skin or mucus membranes) should also be available on the biopsy tray, tool box or trolley. Latex gloves and face masks may be required for safety reasons. A small hair dryer is a useful tool to dry smears rapidly for MGG/Diff-Quik staining.

Patient preparation

The procedure should be clearly explained to the patient to assure his/her consent and cooperation.[5] A formal written consent may be required, at least for deep biopsies. The procedure is usually carried out with the patient supine on an examination couch with easy access from either side. A couch with stirrups is preferable for transrectal and transvaginal biopsy, and an examination chair with adjustable headrest for biopsy of lesions in the head and neck.

Simple skin disinfectant using prepacked swabs for injections is adequate for biopsy of superficial lesions. Preparations as for minor surgical procedures (surgical skin disinfectant, fenestrated sterile cloth, sterile gloves) are recommended for transpleural, transperitoneal and bone biopsies.

Anesthesia

Pre-biopsy sedation is rarely necessary. Atropine is recommended in preparation for transpleural biopsy to prevent the unlikely risk of vasovagal reflex. The biopsy may be coordinated with other procedures that require general anesthesia.

Local anesthesia is not often warranted in superficial biopsies. However, we recommend the injection of a local anesthetic in transpleural, transperitoneal and transperiosteal biopsies to prevent uncontrolled movements or jerks by the patient during the procedure and to make multiple passes more acceptable. A spray anesthetic can be used in biopsies of targets in the mouth, pharynx or other mucosal sites. An anesthetic ointment applied at least half an hour before the procedure is useful in children.

The biopsy procedure

Insertion of the needle

With frequent practice and growing experience, the operator acquires the ability to feel the consistency of the tissue through the needle. This helps considerably to position the needle accurately without technical aids. The 'fingertip sensitivity' is much greater when the needle is held directly without the interposition of a syringe and holder, as in the non-aspiration technique. A near vertical pathway tends to be less painful and allows better appreciation of depth; a tangential path is preferable in superficial skin lesions and for lesions in the chest wall.

The use of radiological imaging techniques to guide deep biopsies is described in Chapter 3. Ultrasonographic (US) guidance may be of value even in palpable lesions. It defines the lesion exactly, gives the optimal depth for biopsy, guides the needle to a solid portion of a complex lesion, and shows the relationship to other anatomical structures such as major vessels, pleura, etc.

FNB with aspiration (Figs. 2.1 and 2.2)

The aspiration technique is illustrated diagrammatically in Figure 2.2. The negative pressure does not tear cells from the tissue but merely holds the tissue against the sharp cutting edge of the needle, which scrapes or cuts softer tissue components along the track as the needle advances through the

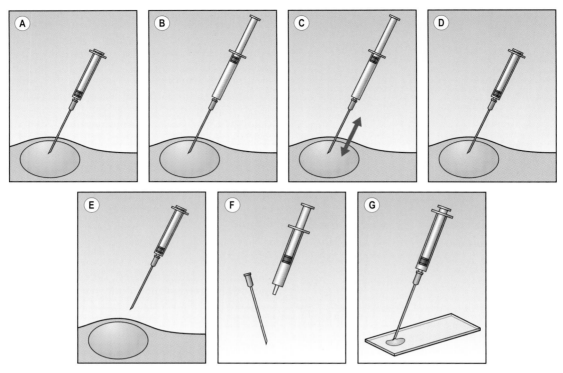

Fig. 2.2 FNB with aspiration Diagrammatic stepwise illustration of biopsy procedure: (**A**) needle positioned within the target tissue; (**B**) plunger pulled to apply negative pressure; (**C**) needle moved back and forth inside target; (**D**) negative pressure released while needle remains in target tissue; (**E**) needle withdrawn; (**F**) needle detached and air drawn into syringe; (**G**) sample blown onto microscopy slide.

tissue.[6] Highly cellular tissue components are softer and more friable than the supporting stroma and are selectively sampled. Fibrous stromal components are poorly represented, whereas myxoid stroma is more easily sampled. To increase the yield, the needle should be moved back and forth within the lesion with the negative pressure maintained, more vigorously in fibrous tissues with low cell content. Several passes may be necessary to sample a sufficient number of cells. In highly cellular and vascular tissues such as spleen, lymph nodes, liver and thyroid, a few rapid passes usually suffice. Additional passes mainly increase the amount of blood aspirated, causing dilution of the cellular component. Admixture with blood tends to be less if the needle is moved along the same track rather than in multiple directions. One should never wait to see material enter the hub of the needle, except when evacuating a cyst or an abscess. The ideal aspirate has a creamy consistency due to high cell content in a small amount of fluid and remains inside the needle.

The negative pressure must be released before the needle is withdrawn. Even so, part of the aspirate is often drawn up into the hub of the needle (see below). A maintained negative pressure may draw the aspirate into the syringe, which must then be rinsed with fluid to recover the specimen. It can also cause contamination by material aspirated along the track during withdrawal of the needle. Aspiration of US gel in guided FNB of breast lesions (Chapter 7) is a good example.

Fine needle sampling without aspiration
(Figs 2.3 and 2.4)

As mentioned, the negative pressure plays a relatively minor role compared to the scraping or cutting effect of the advanc-

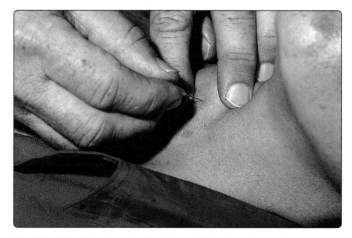

Fig. 2.3 FNB without aspiration (thyroid) Needle held with finger tips, other hand feels and fixes the target.

ing oblique needle tip. Fine needle biopsy without aspiration was introduced by Zajdela in 1987.[7] This technique is based on the observation that the capillary pressure in a fine needle is sufficient to keep the detached cells inside its lumen. A 27–23-gauge standard needle is held directly with the fingers, inserted into the target tissue, moved back and forth in several directions for a few seconds depending on the cellularity and the vascularity of the tissue, and is then withdrawn. Using this technique, the operator gets an excellent feel of the consistency of the tissues. This is a valuable piece of diagnostic information and improves precision when sampling small lesions. Admixture with blood is

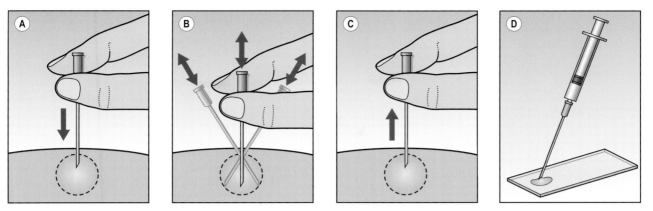

Fig. 2.4 FNB without aspiration Diagrammatic stepwise illustration of biopsy procedure: (**A**) needle inserted into target tissue; (**B**) needle moved back and forth, varying the angle; (**C**) needle withdrawn; (**D**) needle attached to syringe and sample blown onto microscopy slide.

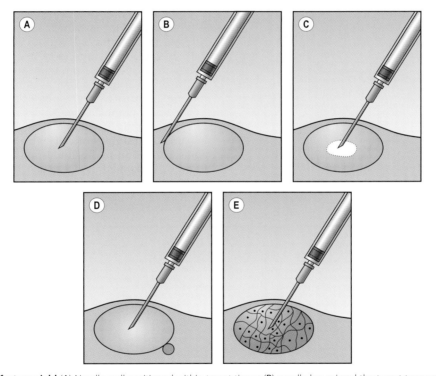

Fig. 2.5 Causes of unsatisfactory yield (**A**) Needle well positioned within target tissue; (**B**) needle has missed the target tangentially; (**C**) needle in central cystic/necrotic/hemorrhagic area devoid of diagnostic cells; (**D**) needle sampling a dominant benign mass but missing a small adjacent malignant lesion; (**E**) fibrotic/desmoplastic target tissue giving a scant cell yield.

generally less than with aspiration. The technique is particularly well suited for biopsy of the thyroid and other vascular tissues. The cell yield may be smaller than with aspiration but not significantly so.[8,9] We use sampling without aspiration routinely in superficial biopsies except in cystic lesions and in fibrotic paucicellular tumors in the breast and soft tissues. Aspiration with 22-gauge needles is used in most deep biopsies in order to obtain a maximum volume of cells with a minimum number of passes, in view of the frequent demand for ancillary tests. However, non-aspiration biopsy sometimes produces better samples in highly vascular lesions, for example in renal tumors.

After biopsy of superficial lesions, pressure should be applied over the biopsy site to minimize bruising or post-

biopsy hematoma. Patients should be kept under observation for a couple of hours after biopsy of deep sited lesions.

Failure to obtain a representative sample

Possible causes of failure to obtain a representative sample are illustrated diagrammatically in Figure 2.5. If the needle narrowly misses the target (Fig. 2.5B), only the adjacent tissues are sampled. An inflammatory reaction around the tumor may lead to an erroneous diagnosis. If the sample is derived from a central focus of necrosis, hemorrhage or cystic change (Fig. 2.5C), no diagnostic elements may be included. A dominant benign lesion like a cyst or lipoma can hide a small adjacent malignancy (Fig. 2.5D), for example in the breast or thyroid. Repeat biopsy of any remaining palpable abnormality after evacuation of a cyst is important. Finally, adequate samples may be difficult to obtain from desmoplastic tumor tissue in which cells are firmly held in a dense collagenous framework (Fig. 2.5E).

Processing the sample

The sample contained in the needle is expelled on to a clean and dry microscopy slide using air in a syringe. Care must be taken to avoid splashing. Not infrequently, the best part of the sample is found in the hub of the needle and is not easily expelled. In this case, the sample can be aspirated from the hub using another needle (Fig. 2.6).

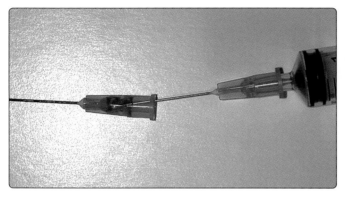

Fig. 2.6 Collecting a sample trapped in the hub of the biopsy needle
The sample is aspirated with another needle mounted on a syringe.

Direct smearing (Figs 2.7–2.12)

Smear quality is highly dependent on the smear being thin and evenly spread, ideally as a monolayer of cells. Perfect smearing is not easily learned. This is one of the reasons why FNB generally has a higher success rate when the biopsy procedure is attended by laboratory staff. Nuclear detail is poorly shown and confusing artifacts are common if smears are thick, uneven and dry slowly (Figs 2.9–2.11). Sometimes, even well prepared smears, particularly of lymphoid cells, may show a peculiar raisin-like distortion of the nuclei probably caused by moisture on the slide (Fig. 2.12). Exposure of air-dried smears to formalin vapor, which can occur during transport of material to the laboratory, can affect nuclear staining and cause loss of morphologic detail.[10]

The optimal sample, obtainable from cell-rich tissues, has a creamy consistency due to high cellularity with little or no blood or fluid ('dry' sample). A 'dry' sample is best smeared with the flat of a second slide exerting a light pressure as it is moved along the specimen slide (Fig. 2.7, top). The pressure must be carefully adjusted to achieve a thin, even spread without causing disruption of tissue fragments with loss of micro-architecture, or smudging artifacts as in Figure 2.11A. Optimal smearing is a fine balance between too thick and too thin. Smears of 'dry' aspirates dry quickly, resulting in a milky, finely granular film on the slide.

A 'wet' aspirate consists mainly of blood or fluid containing smaller numbers of cells. The cells can be concentrated and separated from the fluid using a two-step smearing technique as illustrated in Figure 2.7. The smearing slide is held against the specimen slide at a blunt angle near one end of the slide, allowing the fluid to accumulate in the angle. The

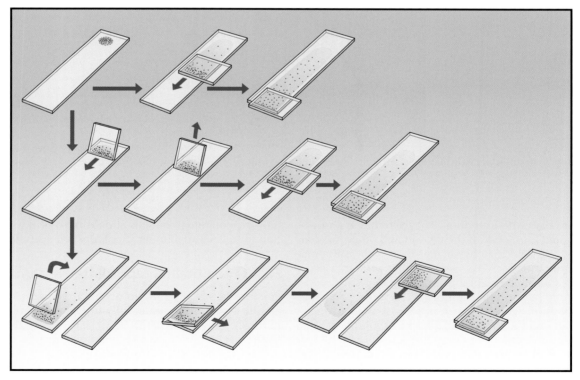

Fig. 2.7 Direct smearing Diagrammatic illustration of smearing of 'dry' and 'wet' samples. *Top line*: a 'dry' sample is smeared with the flat of a slide exerting a well-balanced pressure; *middle line*: two-step smearing of a 'wet' sample on one slide; *bottom line*: two-step smearing of a 'wet' sample with plenty of fluid moving the concentrated cells to a second slide. For details see text.

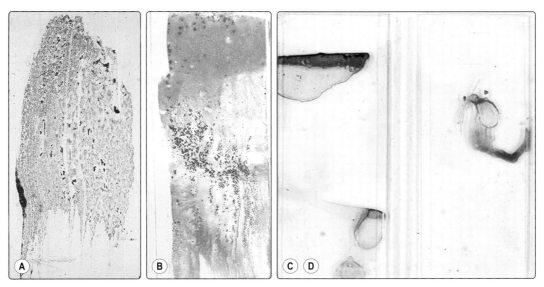

Fig. 2.8 Macro appearance of air-dried smears (A) Optimal smear of 'dry' sample (carcinoma of prostate); cell clusters seen as blue dots, evenly spread; (B) Smear of 'wet' sample by two-step smearing; mainly blood at top end, cell clusters concentrated and evenly spread in the thin mid portion; (C, D) Examples of poorly prepared smears of bloody material, partly dried or clotted before smearing.

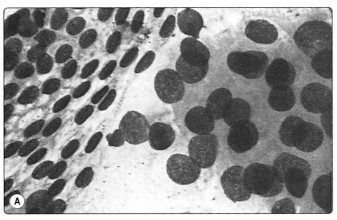

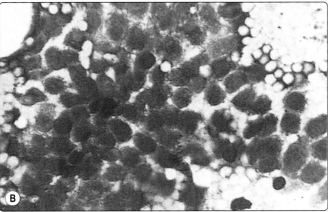

Fig. 2.9 Optimal and suboptimal air-dried smears (A) Optimal spread and fixation of 'dry' sample (carcinoma prostate); (B) Artifacts caused by slow drying of thick bloody smear (prostatic hyperplasia) render diagnosis impossible in spite of good cell yield (MGG, HP).

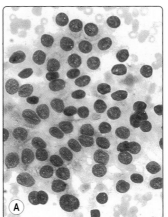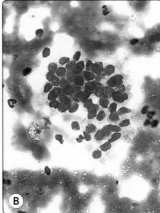

Fig. 2.10 Optimal and suboptimal air-dried smears (A) Thinly spread, well-fixed smear of papillary carcinoma of thyroid. Typical nuclear morphology well demonstrated; (B) Cells in a thick, bloody part of the same smear. Nuclei show shrinking artifacts: small and dark, structural detail not visible (MGG, IP).

smeared with the flat of the slide as for a 'dry' aspirate, either on the same specimen slide, or swiped to another slide.

If a larger volume of blood or fluid is obtained, it can be spread on a slide or watch glass using the needle, or by tilting the slide. With a suitable background, tiny tissue fragments become visible and can be picked up with a needle or a slide, moved to another slide and smeared. Or fragments can be placed in a drop of blood, thrombin added, to form a clot for processing as a cell block. It is critical that bloody samples are processed quickly before coagulation occurs as clotting blood makes it nearly impossible to produce optimal smears.

Examples of the macroscopical appearances of smears are shown in Figure 2.8. Figure 2.8A is an optimal smear of carcinoma showing numerous cell aggregates seen as granules spread evenly over the slide. Figure 2.8B is a two-step smear of carcinoma showing a film of blood at the top and concentrated cells at the middle, seen as a granular material.

smearing slide is then rapidly moved along the specimen slide, half way or all the way depending on the amount of fluid. Most of the fluid is left behind while the cells tend to follow the smearing slide. The concentrated cells are then

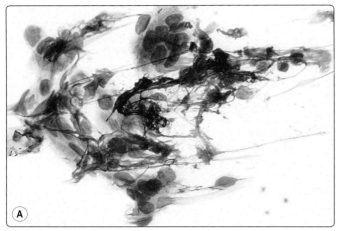

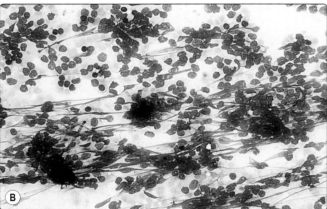

Fig. 2.11 Artifacts caused by smearing (A) Smudging artifacts at tail of smear caused by heavy pressure; fibroadenoma of breast (MGG, HP); (B) Clumping of cells and shrinkage artifacts due to slow drying/fixation of thick and bloody smear; lymphoid tissue (MGG, IP); Interpretation difficult or impossible in both in spite of good cell yield.

Figure 2.8C and 2.8D are examples of unsatisfactory smears from external sources.

Indirect smearing

Thin watery samples are processed by centrifugation in a cyto-centrifuge. Millipore or Nucleopore filtration is an alternative but has been less satisfactory in our hands. Some laboratories prefer to rinse needles and syringes routinely with saline or with a fixative, which is then centrifuged or filtered onto slides.[11,12] More recently, the ThinPrep technique developed for gynecological cytology has been increasingly applied also to FNB specimens.[13-16] These techniques offer alternative solutions to the frequent problem of suboptimal samples received from distant sources, when the laboratory has no control over the biopsy procedure. However, the ThinPrep technique has its specific problems, and established diagnostic criteria may have to be redefined for FNB samples.[17,18] In our opinion, direct smears expertly prepared by an experienced cytopathologist remain the optimal basis for FNAC diagnosis available today, and our first priority is to perfect this technique. ThinPrep preparations are a valuable supplement, particularly for immunocytochemical staining (see below).

Monolayered smears with optimal cell preservation are particularly important in the diagnosis of malignant lym-

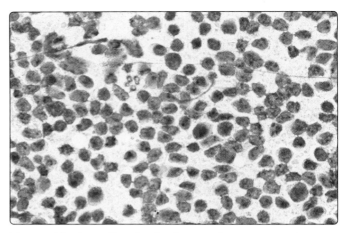

Fig. 2.12 Fixation artifacts Peculiar fixation artifacts in a smear of lymphoma. Raisinoid nuclei with a 'prickly' contour, nuclear chromatin appears irregular (MGG, HP).

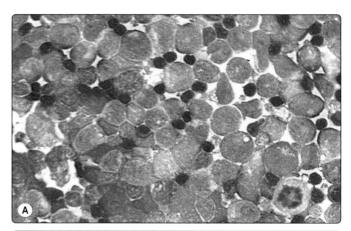

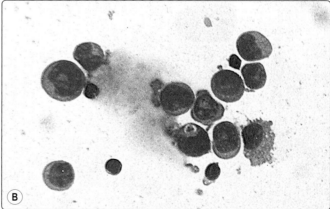

Fig. 2.13 Cytocentrifuge smears of lymphoid cells Cell suspension in Hank's balanced salt solution of FNB sample of cells from lymphoma; cytocentrifugation smears. (A) Undiluted specimen; (B) Optimal dilution (MGG, HP).

phoma. For lymph node aspirates, we recommend that a cell suspension be prepared in addition to direct smears. Hank's balanced salt solution with the addition of 10–20% fetal calf serum is ideal for this purpose. The suspension is spun on the cytocentrifuge at low r.p.m. Dilution may be necessary to achieve optimal dispersion of cells on the slide and to avoid clumping (Fig. 2.13). A number of slides can usually be made from one aspirate to allow immunocytochemical studies. Further details on techniques suitable for lymph node samples are given in Chapter 5.

Tissue fragments and cell blocks

Sometimes, a thin core or fragments of tissue may be obtained with a standard 22-gauge needle (Fig. 2.14). Tissue fragments are fixed in 5–10% buffered isotonic formalin and processed as for routine histology.

Some laboratories recommend the routine preparation of cell blocks for paraffin embedding of FNB samples. Cell blocks may give a better idea of tissue architecture and allow multiple sections for panels of immune markers with controls.[19-21] However, they are relatively time consuming and costly compared to routine smears.[22] We use cell blocks selectively, mainly if a need for immunocytochemistry is anticipated. Cell blocks are helpful if samples are heavily admixed with blood. Surprisingly good tissue fragments are often found in a cell block even when smears show only blood.

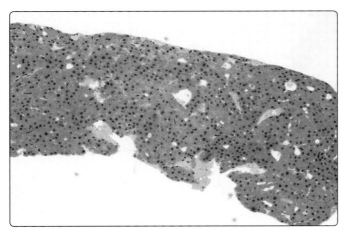

Fig. 2.14 Tissue core by 22-gauge lumbar puncture needle Tissue section of a 22-gauge lumbar puncture needle core from a well-differentiated hepatocellular carcinoma (H&E, LP).

More recently, we have developed a simplified technique for cell blocks that we call 'cell buttons', shown diagrammatically in Figure 2.15. It is applicable to cell-rich tissues such as lymph nodes and cellular neoplasms. A drop of thick, creamy material obtainable from such tissues using a 27–25-gauge needle without aspiration is gently expelled onto a glass slide as usual, but is not spread or smeared. After a few seconds to allow the drop to adhere to the slide, the slide is carefully immersed in 90% ethanol. The sample remains stuck to the slide as a drop ('button'). Alcohol-fixation, unlike formalin, holds the sample together. After fixation, the 'button' is gently detached with a scalpel blade and processed like a small biopsy. The amount of tissue obtained in this way can be substantial, cell preservation and fixation is excellent, and the material is well suited to immunocytochemical studies (Fig. 2.16). An advantage over a conventional cell block is that the cell material is concentrated, whereas multiple sections may be necessary to find scanty tissue fragments in a cell block.

Fixation and staining

Two fundamentally different methods of fixation and staining are used in FNAC: air-drying followed by a Romanowsky-type stain such as MGG, Jenner-Giemsa, Wright's stain or Diff-Quik (Harleco, Philadelphia); and alcohol-fixation followed by Papanicolaou (Pap) or hematoxylin and eosin (H&E) staining. Both methods have their advantages and deficiencies. The effect produced on cells by air-drying and wet-fixation is easily understood if one compares the three-dimensional shape of a fried egg with that of a boiled egg (Fig. 2.17). Air-drying causes the cell, both cytoplasm and nucleus, to flatten on the slide just like an egg flattens in the frying pan. It therefore appears larger than a cell fixed in ethanol, which maintains its three-dimensional rounded shape. Nuclear enlargement and variation in nuclear size are exaggerated in air-dried smears. This enhances the difference between normal and abnormal cells (see Fig. 2.9A).

Optimal fixation of air-dried smears depends on rapid drying. This can be enhanced by using a hair dryer with

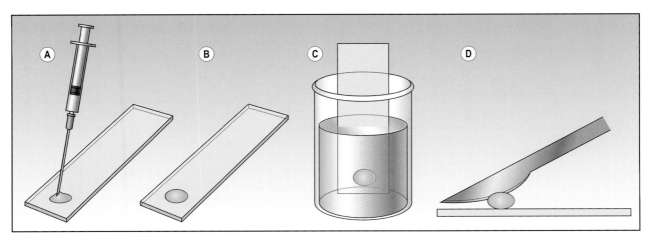

Fig. 2.15 Preparation of a 'cell button' (A) The FNB sample is blown onto a clean and dry microscopy slide; (B) The sample/drop is left untouched on the slide a few seconds to adhere without drying; (C) The slide with the sample is immersed in 95% ethanol and left to fix; (D) The solidified fixed 'cell button' is carefully removed from the slide with a scalpel and processed routinely like any small biopsy.

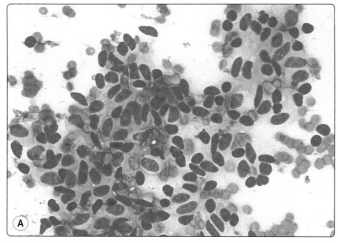

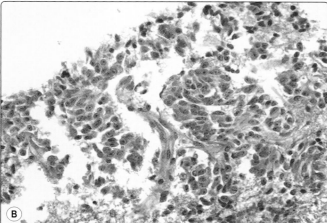

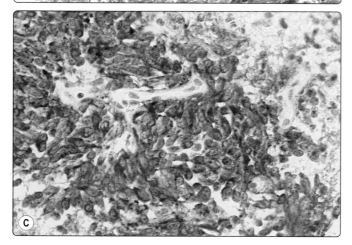

Fig. 2.16 FNB with 'cell button' FNB of peripheral lung tumor: (**A**) Air-dried direct smear (Diff-Quik, HP); (**B, C**) Tissue section of 'cell button'; solid islands/cords of tumor tissue with a prominently vascular stroma (H&E, HP); positive synaptophysin (HP). Diagnosis of peripheral carcinoid tumor.

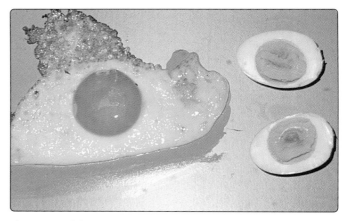

Fig. 2.17 'Cell fixation' Two eggs of similar weight, one fried, the other boiled and bisected. Compare sizes of the whole egg and of the yolk. Air-drying and alcohol-fixation of cells produce a similar result on cells and nuclei.

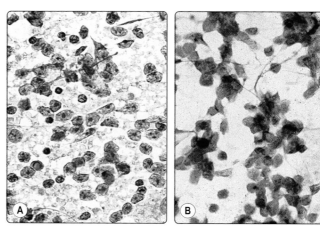

Fig. 2.18 Drying artifacts, alcohol-fixed smear FNB of large-cell non-Hodgkin's lymphoma: (**A**) Well-fixed smear, nuclear detail well demonstrated; (**B**) Severe drying artifacts, nuclei blurred, interpretation impossible (H&E, HP)

moderate heat. Slow drying of thick bloody smears tends to produce artifacts, in particular shrinkage of cells and nuclei, which may render diagnosis impossible (see Fig. 2.10). The main problem with wet-fixed smears is that highly cellular smears dry so quickly that drying artifacts can be difficult to avoid (Fig. 2.18).

Pathologists trained in gynecological cytology usually prefer alcohol-fixation and Pap staining also for FNB smears while those trained in hematology choose air-dried MGG-stained smears. If sufficient material is available, the two methods should be used in parallel since some features of cells, cell products and stroma are better demonstrated by one than by the other. The differences between air-dried MGG smears and alcohol-fixed Pap smears and the features highlighted by each method are listed in Tables 2.1 and 2.2. The two methods obviously provide complementary diagnostic information. If only air-dried smears are available, some can later be rehydrated and stained with Pap or H&E.[23] However, additional material processed as a cell block may be required to allow special stains, multiple immune markers or other ancillary tests.

Many pathologists feel that nuclear chromatin structure is not well shown in air-dried Giemsa smears. However, hematologists examining blood films and bone marrow smears

Table 2.1 Comparison of airdried and wet-fixed smears – general properties

	Airdried MGG	Wet-fixed Pap
Dependence on smearing technique	Strong	Moderate
The 'dry' smear	Good fixation	Drying artefacts common
The 'wet' smear	Arifacts common	Good fixation
Tissue fragments	Cells poorly seen due to heavily stained ground substance	Individual cells usually clearly seen
Cell and nuclear size	Exaggerated, differences enhanced	Comparable to tissue sections
Cytoplasmic detail	Well demonstrated	Poorly demonstrated
Nuclear detail	Pattern different from the familiar Pap stain	Excellently demonstrated
Nucleoli	Not always discernible	Well demonstrated
Stromal components	Well shown and often differentially stained	Poorly demonstrated
Partially necrotic tissue	Poor definition of cell details	Good definition of single intact cells

Table 2.2 Comparison of airdried and wet-fixed smears – tissues-specific properties

Tissue	Feature emphasized by MGG	Feature emphasized by Pap
Epithelial tissues	Mucin, intra- or extracellular Colloid (thyroid) Secretory granules (prostate) Lipofuscin granules (seminal vesicle) Lipid vacuoles Bare bipolar nuclei (benign breast) Bile plugs Stromal globules (e.g. adenoid cystic carcinoma) Amyloid	Squamous differentiation/keratinization Oncocytes (salivary gland tumors) Nuclear chromatin patterns Nucleoli Nuclear grooves
Lymphoid tissue	Cytoplasmic basophilia Lymphoid globules (lymphoglandular bodies) Hemopoietic cells Lipid vacuoles	Nuclear outline Nuclear chromatin pattern Nucleoli
Mesenchymal tissues	Fibromyxoid/chondromyxoid ground substance (pleomorphic adenoma, chondroid hamartoma, fibroadenoma, chondroid tissue, chordoma) Osteoid Basement membrane Amyloid Intracytoplasmic lipid vacuoles	Nuclear detail in solid tissue fragments
Neuroendocrine tissues	Cytoplasmic granularity (medullary carcinoma of thyroid, paraganglioma, carcinoid, islet cell tumors)	Speckled nuclear chromatin
Inflammatory tissue	Eosinophils	Macrophages (xanthogranulomatous pyelonephritis, old haematoma, fat necrosis)

traditionally rely mainly on this technique diagnosing megaloblastic anemia, leukemia, metastatic malignancy, etc. Nuclear chromatin pattern is well shown also in high-quality Romanowsky-stained smears, but appearances are different from Pap smears and have to be learned.

Diff-Quik is a rapid Romanowsky-type stain (2–3 minutes), handy to use in theater or in the radiology department, to check immediately if the sample is satisfactory and if additional tests are needed. The technique was originally designed for blood films, and the staining time must be adjusted to the thickness of FNB smears. In most cases we increase the time in solution 3 to about twice that recommended for blood films. In this way, the staining does not differ signifi-

cantly from MGG. Rapid modifications of H&E, Pap and other stains have also been developed.[24–26]

Air-dried smears should be sterilized by fixation in methanol soon after drying to prevent cross-infection, if a significant infective process is suspected.

Special stains

Special stains commonly used in histopathology are also applicable to cytological smears without major modifications.[27] Examples are PAS/diastase or Alcian blue for mucins, Prussian blue for iron, Masson-Fontana for melanin, Grimelius for argyrophilic granules and Congo red for

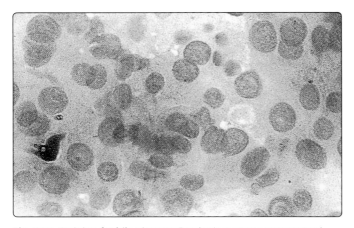

Fig. 2.19 Staining for bile pigment Fouchet's reagent counterstained with Sirius red applied to smear from hepatocellular carcinoma (HP).

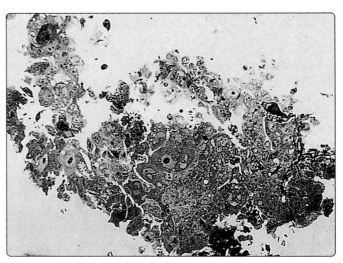

Fig. 2.20 Resin-embedded tissue fragment for EM Fragment of sarcoma obtained with a standard 22-gauge needle, fixed in glutaraldehyde and processed on the slide, 1 μm section (Toluidin blue, HP).

amyloid. Microorganisms are identified by Gram, PAS, Ziehl-Neelsen or Gomori's silver stain. Stains for the demonstration of *Pneumocystis*, *Nocardia* and *Actinomyces* in smears have been developed. [28,29] Glycogen is stained by PAS and fat by oil-red-O in air-dried smears. Fouchet's reagent counterstained with Sirius red demonstrates bile pigment beautifully (Fig. 2.19).

The reader is referred to handbooks on histological techniques for descriptions of the staining methods mentioned. Minor adjustments to suit the variable quality of cytological material may be necessary.

Phase contrast microscopy

Phase contrast microscopy of unstained smears has been used in cytological diagnosis. We do not see it as a substitute for routine stains but it is a useful tool to check the adequacy of smears to be used for immunocytochemical staining or for EM, so that time and reagents are not wasted on unsatisfactory samples. [30]

Other investigations

Microbiology (see also Chapter 18)

Fine needle biopsy samples can be used for microbiological culture in cases of suspected infectious disease. Frank pus is best transported to the microbiology department in the aspirating needle and syringe, as rapidly as possible. Very small amounts of pus are washed into a sterile container with a few milliliters of sterile normal saline to prevent drying and desiccation of organisms. This may not provide for anaerobic or unusual organisms; however, dividing very small amounts of material into several types of media is singularly unprofitable. The use of needle washings, after most of the aspirate has been expelled onto slides for microscopy, also seldom yields results. The single most important determinant of whether an organism can be cultured seems to be the amount of aspirated material. Repeated biopsies, using all the contents of the needle for culture, are most valuable. [31]

In FNB of deep infectious lesions, optimal results are achieved if a microbiologist can be present at the biopsy to process material, particularly in the case of immunosuppressed patients where unusual infections are likely.

Electron microscopy [32–38]

Although immunocytochemistry has become the most important ancillary method for tumor subtyping, we still find EM necessary for some cases. EM is particularly useful in unusual lung or mediastinal lesions. In Silverman's experience, FNB samples are the most frequent non-renal samples sent for EM.

We decide on cases to be further studied after an initial evaluation of material in the radiology theater. The most commonly used method of fixation is to eject the aspirate into a small test tube containing glutaraldehyde. Many methods of processing tissue are suggested, mainly with the aim of separating tumor tissue from contaminating red cells. We use Lazaro's method of cell concentration. The small pellet produced by centrifugation is carefully removed and processed. [39] For highly cellular aspirates, the material can be ejected as a semisolid droplet onto a carefully cleaned slide, which is then immersed in glutaraldehyde (compare cell 'buttons' as described above). The droplet can be processed on the slide or popped off for further handling. A report can be given in 24–48 hours if necessary.

There is evidence for representative sampling and superior fixation of FNB material compared with surgically excised material (Figs 2.20–2.22). [24] In a review of 150 of our cases from various sites, 100 contained adequate well-preserved material for assessment. In 60% of these cases EM only confirmed the LM diagnosis, but in 40% the findings were diagnostic per se. The common applications of EM in FNAC are summarized in Table 2.3. In our experience, most value is obtained in recognizing *neuroendocrine tumors* and in the specific diagnosis of *melanoma*, *mesothelioma* and some *carcinomas*, including metastases, where immunocytochemistry often cannot provide such positive diagnostic features. An expanding literature about techniques and applications is available.

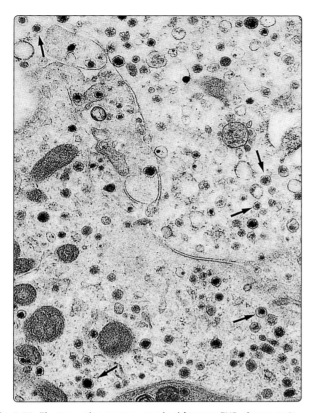

Fig. 2.21 Electron microscopy – carcinoid tumor FNB of metastatic neoplasm in the liver. Numerous intracytoplasmic rounded neurosecretory granules averaging 155 nm in diameter. In some, a submembranous lucent halo is seen (*arrows*) (EM × 13 650).

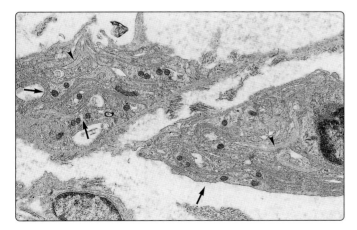

Fig. 2.22 Electron microscopy – schwannoma Screw needle biopsy (Rotex II) of an atypical soft tissue tumor in the neck of a 20-year-old man. The complex intertwining cytoplasmic processes (*arrows*) and the associated external (basal) lamina (*arrowheads*) indicate schwannian differentiation. The abundance of the lucent proteoglycan-containing extracellular matrix is in keeping with Antoni B tissue (EM × 9940).

Immunocytochemistry[37,40–43]

The increasing commercial availability of monoclonal antisera to a variety of proteins and other cell products, which are more or less specific to different cell lines, is probably the most important recent development in diagnostic cytol-

Table 2.3 Electron microscopy and fine needle aspiration

Value	Tumor type

Unequivocal identification of cell type or differentiation (where available immune markers may not be specific enough for definitive diagnosis)	Melanoma
	Neuroendocrine differentiation
	Mesothelioma
	Small round cell tumors
	  Ewing's sarcoma
	  Rhabdomyosarcoma
	  Neuroblastoma
	  Primitive neuroectodermal tumor
	  Wilms' tumor
	Well-differentiated spindle cell tumors
	  Schwann cell tumors
	  Smooth muscle tumors
	  Fibrohistiocytic tumors

Supports cytologic diagnosis or aids in subclassification (where immune marker studies are unlikely to be helpful)	Neuroendocrine malignancies
	  Carcinoid tumor
	  Well-differentiated neuroendocrine carcinoma (atypical carcinoid)
	  Small cell carcinoma
	Adenocarcinoma subtyping
	  Acinic cell carcinoma
	  Hepatocellular carcinoma
	  Bronchiolo-alveolar carcinoma
	  Colonic carcinoma
	  Renal cell carcinoma
	  Adrenal carcinoma

Answers general questions of cell type (where immune markers have not been diagnostic or where material is insufficient for a panel of markers)	Small cell malignancies
	  Lymphoma
	  Small cell carcinoma
	Large cell malignancies
	  Lymphoma
	  Anaplastic carcinoma
	  Melanoma
	  Germ cell tumors
	  Pleomorphic spindle cell tumors
	  Sarcoma
	  Sarcomatoid carcinoma
	  Melanoma
	Other tumors
	  Thymoma/thymic carcinoma

ogy. The demonstration and identification of such cell products in smears and cell blocks is of immense value as it offers a means of objectively recognizing the line of differentiation shown by the cells. Immunostaining may allow a confident specific diagnosis even on relatively scanty material (e.g. medullary carcinoma of thyroid, Fig. 2.23). Immune markers are extremely useful in the differentiation between anaplastic carcinoma, neuroendocrine tumors, malignant lymphoma and amelanotic melanoma (cytokeratin, EMA, chromogranin, NSE, LCA, S-100, etc.), in the search for a primary in metastatic malignancies (e.g. differential staining for a number of cytokeratins), and in the histogenetic typing of mesenchymal tumors (see Chapter 15). Markers for B and T cells, immunoglobulins and light chains are indispensable in the typing of lymphoma (see Chapter 5). Monoclonal antibodies to certain tumor antigens have been found to be useful in the distinction between malignant and benign epithelial cells.[44] A list of the most

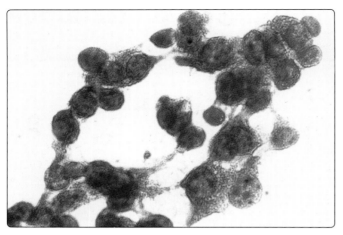

Fig. 2.23 Immunoperoxidase staining Strongly positive cytoplasmic staining for calcitonin in a direct FNB smear from medullary carcinoma of thyroid (HP).

Table 2.4 Immunoperoxidase (IPOX) studies and fine needle aspiration

Tumor type or differential diagnosis	Useful tumor markers
Small cell malignancies	
Lymphoma	Leukocyte common antigen (LCA)/CD45
Small cell carcinoma	Cytokeratin (AE1/AE3, CAM 5.2, CK 20); neuroendocrine markers
Small round cell tumors	Cytokeratin; CD 99; Wilms' tumor gene product (WT-1); neurofilaments; myogenin
Large cell malignancies	
Lymphoma	LCA/CD 45, CD 30
Anaplastic carcinoma	Cytokeratins, carcinoembryonic antigen (CEA)
Melanoma	S-100; HMB-45, Melan A
Germ cell tumors	Human chorionic gonadotrophin (HCG); alpha fetoprotein (AFP); placental alkaline phosphatase (PLAP), CD 30, CD 117
Pleomorphic spindle cell tumors	
Sarcoma	Cytokeratin; vimentin; desmin; muscle actins; CD 34; S-100
Sarcomatoid carcinoma	Cytokeratin and vimentin coexpression; epithelial membrane antigen (EMA)
Melanoma	S-100; HMB-45; Melan A
Tubulo-glandular malignancies	
Mesothelioma	Calretinin, CK 5/6, EMA
Adenocarcinoma	CEA; CD 15; Ber EP 4; B 72.3; CK 7, CK 20
Lymphoma typing	CD 20; CD 3; CD 5; CD 43; CD 15; CD 30; CD 10, Alk-1, cyclin D1; kappa and lambda light chains
Specific tumors	
Prostatic carcinoma	Prostate-specific antigen (PSA); prostatic acid phosphatase (PAP)
Thyroid carcinoma	Thyroid transcription factor-1 (TTF-1); thyroglobulin; calcitonin
Breast carcinoma	Gross cystic disease fluid protein-15 (GCDFP-15); Estrogen receptor/progesteron receptor
Lung carcinoma	TTF-1
Neuroendocrine tumors (carcinoid; neuroendocrine carcinomas)	Synaptophysin; bombesin; chromogranin; ACTH; serotonin
Metastatic malignancies	CK7, CK20, Cam5.2, AE1/AE3, CEA, TTF-1, CDX2, CA-19,9, CA120

common immune markers used in FNAC is presented in Table 2.4. Immunoprofiles are also included with other diagnostic criteria for most entities in the following chapters.

Sections of cell blocks fixed in 10% formalin and transferred to TBS for immunoperoxidase staining, or tissue fragments obtained by core needle biopsy, in general provide the best material for immunocytochemistry. Cell blocks and core biopsies offer the great advantage of a large number of sections, sufficient for a panel of markers and for the indispensable negative controls. On the other hand, some antigens are not well preserved in formalin-fixed material, but are demonstrable in air-dried smears. In stroma-rich tumors, FNB selectively samples the abnormal cells detached from the stroma, which sometimes facilitates interpretation.

If tissue fragments are not available, immunostaining can be performed on direct smears, or on smears derived from a cell suspension using the cytocentrifuge (Fig. 2.24). Alcohol-fixed smears are usually preferable to air-dried smears. Thin-Prep slides of FNAC material have been found highly suitable for immunocytochemical staining.[45,46] This technique has the advantage of eliminating background interference by blood and debris (see *liquid-based cytology* below). The limited number of tests possible when only smears are available can be increased by circling areas 3 mm apart on the same slide with a diamond pencil and wiping the smear between. This allows 2–3 different tests per slide. De-stained previously Pap-stained smears can be used, although poor attachment of the cells to the slide can be a problem.[47] Sections of alcohol-fixed and paraffin-embedded cell 'buttons' are a good alternative to tissue cores and cell blocks (Fig. 2.25 and see Fig. 2.16).

The avidin–biotin complex method is the most commonly used with both monoclonal and polyclonal primary antibodies. Diaminobenzidine is used as the marker dye. Immunoalkaline phosphatase staining appears to offer several advantages in cytological preparations. Commercially produced kits have made immunohistochemistry a relatively simple method available to any cytology laboratory, and an ever-increasing number of antisera are being marketed in this form. Appropriate controls are crucial to achieving diagnostic accuracy.[48] A review of immunostaining techniques adapted to cytological preparations can be found in *Diagnostic Cytopathology*.[44]

Interpretation of immunohistochemical staining is often more difficult in smears than in histological sections because the cytoplasm of neoplastic cells detached from the stroma is often fragile and dispersed in the

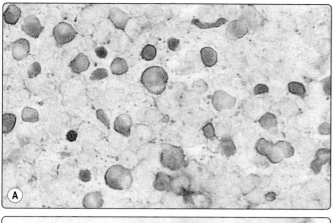

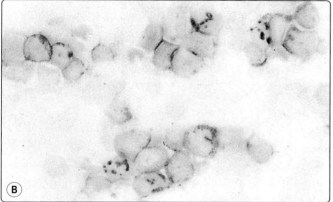

Fig. 2.24 Immunoperoxidase staining Smears of non-Hodgkin's lymphoma. (**A**) Direct smear; interpretation difficult due to background staining caused by fragmentation of cytoplasm; (**B**) Cytocentrifuge preparation; positive staining distinctly related to individual cells (HP).

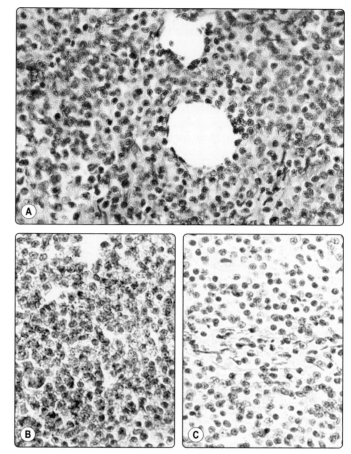

Fig. 2.25 Immunoperoxidase staining 'Cell button' of FNB sample of non-Hodgkin's B-cell lymphoma; (**A**) Tissue section, H&E; (**B**) Positive staining with a pan-B marker; (**C**) negative staining with a pan-T marker (IP).

background. Blood, serum or secretory products are often superimposed on the cells. All this makes it difficult to ascribe any positive staining to specific, identifiable cells. Ways to overcome the difficulties are discussed in the paper by Suthipintawong and Leong referred to above.[44] When examining the smears, it is best to focus on tissue fragments, in which the cells are protected leaving cell membranes and cytoplasm intact. Background staining is a lesser problem in cytospin preparations if the cells are washed, in ThinPrep smears, and in paraffin sections from a cell 'button'. The results of immunocytochemistry must

be interpreted with caution and in the context of conventional cytomorphology and clinical data.[49]

Standardized/simplified approaches to FNB for radiologists

The challenges facing laboratories include how to standardize the approach to sampling by radiologists in case pathology staff is not available. This includes guidelines for setting aside material for ancillary techniques, and the transport of cytological material to laboratories from radiology practices.

Miscellaneous techniques

Philippe Vielh

Depending on the type of question asked, the (cyto)pathologist may have to triage specimens according to the type of technique needed to solve a specific problem. From that point of view, on-site examination of a given specimen using rapid stainings will help tremendsously. Table 2.5 summarizes the possibilities and limitations of using different techniques according to the type of cellular specimen.

Liquid-based cytology

New cytopreparatory techniques include the so-called liquid-based cytology technology. Various systems are commercially available. They are mostly used for cervical cancer screening but are also adapted for FNAC samples. The basic principle is to collect cell samples into a liquid fixative solution and then create a monolayer of cells ready for microscopic observation after staining. The presence of the liquid helps collecting cells remaining in the needle, whereas immediate fixation due to the presence of methanol or ethanol in the fixative optimizes cell preservation and usually reduces dramatically the bloody background. This potentially may: (1) help in the visual and automatic detection of cells of interest, (2) improve the quality and reproducibility of immunocytochemical methods (but antibodies used should be selected considering the fact that fixation is made using coagulant compounds), and (3) preserve nucleic acids, specially DNA. However, flow cytometric methods, cytogenetic analysis, as well as more sophisticated molecular techniques such as gene expression studies based on quantification of RNA still need fresh material.

Image analysis

Image analysis deals with three different areas, namely morphometry, object counting and cytometry, which are not mutually exclusive.[50]

Morphometry is the quantitative description of geometric features of structures such as tissues, cells, nuclei or nucleoli.[51,52] It includes (1) stereology techniques estimating the fraction of different tissue components, inner and outer surface density, as well as shape and volume by means of a test system of lower dimension (i.e. point or line grids) than the structure itself, and (2) measurement of geometric features of structures in the two-dimensional microscopical image, also called planimetry.[53] Currently, the microscopical image is recorded by a video camera and displayed on a computer screen which makes it possible to trace the outlines of nuclei on the screen and then compute nuclear areas as well as nuclear shape using dedicated software able to produce quantitative data in the form of cytograms and histograms.[54]

Object counting mainly concerns quantitation of mitoses or measurement of the proliferation fraction of a cell population using antibodies raised against incorporated nonisotopic labels during S-phase fraction, for example, 5-bromodeoxyuridin (BrdU) or proliferation-associated molecules such as the molecule recognized by the Ki-67 or the MIB-1 antibody and the proliferating cell nuclear antigen.[55] It also makes it possible to quantitate apoptotic figures by means of the TUNEL assay.[56]

Cytometry depends on the ability to detect a substance of interest by a specific dye and to measure the concentration of that dye by computing optical density.[57] Its main application, based on the discovery of the Feulgen reaction, is DNA cytometry by means of a specific stoichiometric stain for DNA, permitting quantitative evaluation of nuclear DNA by absorbance cytometry since the amount of stain is proportional to the amount of DNA present. This can also be done using various fluorochromes, which also bind stoichiometrically, i.e. in a proportional way, such as Hoechst 4,6-dimanidino-2-phenylindole (DAPI) and propidium iodide dyes.[58–60] Powerful computers also have stimulated the development of systems for automatic cell classification based on pattern recognition for diagnostic,[61,62] prognostic,[63–65] and predictive[66] purposes. Quantitation of nuclear immunostain of estrogen and progesterone receptors,[67] proliferation markers[68–70] and tumor suppressor genes such as p53[71] stresses the need for standardization of

Table 2.5 Technical possibilities according to the type of cellular material

Techniques					
Cellular material	**ICC**	**FISH**	**FCM**	**GE**	**Cytogenetics**
Fixed	preferred	preferred	not recommended	not recommended	impossible
Frozen	need to be post fixed	need to be post fixed	possible	preferred (−80°C)	impossible
Fresh	need to be post fixed	need to be post fixed	need to be put in appropriate liquid culture medium	need to be put in appropriate preservative	required

ICC, immunocytochemistry; FISH, fluorescent in situ hybridization; FCM, flow cytometry; GE, gene expression studied by reverse polymerase chain reaction or on micro-arrays using specific oligonucleotides.

immunocytochemical techniques and quality control networks since immunocytochemical staining of antigens is not stoichiometric and therefore requires calibration with known external and internal controls as for DNA image cytometry.[72] Finally, a new device named the laser scanning cytometer has recently been developed.[73] It is supposed to bridge the gap between an image analyser machine and a flow cytometer, since it makes it possible to perform multiparameter analyses.[74,75]

Flow cytometry

Also based on the fundamental work showing that DNA content, measured by ultraviolet and visible light in unstained cells, doubled during the cell cycle,[76] followed by the improved detection of antigens using fluorescence methods[77] and the development of an apparatus capable of counting[78] and sizing[79] blood cells, flow cytometry has mainly been applied to the measurement of DNA content in human cancer and quantitation of cell surface antigens in hematopathology.[80] Current flow cytometers provide rapid, sensitive and quantitative measurements of any cell component that can be specifically stained using appropriate fluorochromes for DNA or RNA and monoclonal antibodies raised against cytoplasmic, nuclear and membrane antigens. They permit the acquisition of monoparametric and multiparametric data characterizing heterogeneous populations in a cell suspension obtained, for example, by fine needle sampling of human cancer.[81,82] Again, quality controls are mandatory[83–85] for estimating the usefulness of flow cytometry measurements in a clinical setting and for comparing data published by various teams around the world. This is particularly critical when dealing with data which may influence diagnosis and which have prognostic and therapeutic implications such as flow immunophenotyping of hematologic malignancies,[86,87] evaluation of proliferation by measurement of S-phase fraction[88–90] and assessment of spontaneous or drug-induced human cancer apoptosis.[91] However, since flow cytometry and image analysis are complementary, it is likely that the combination of both methods will contribute to better estimation of relevant pathological processes.[92]

The practical application of flow cytometry to the diagnosis and typing of lymphoma is discussed in Chapter 5.

Molecular cytopathology (Table 2.6)

The application of molecular probes to cytologic samples of human malignancies has refined the diagnostic and prognostic armamentarium.[93–96] The use of genotypic rather than phenotypic diagnostic criteria also makes it possible to measure and combine information from both morphologic and molecular observations by means of digital image analysis.[97] Current diagnostic and potential prognostic applications in pathology have improved tremendously using in situ hybridization, in situ amplification techniques and other recently developed nucleic acid-based methods of analysis.

In situ hybridization is a technique for the localization of specific nucleic acid (endogenous DNA, messenger RNA,

Table 2.6 Examples of current and potential useful diagnostic and prognostic molecular markers according to tissue-derived tumours (see text for details)

Tissue-derived tumors	Useful diagnostic molecular markers	Useful prognostic molecular markers
Epithelial	Gain or loss of DNA (potential) RNA-specific transcripts (thyroid)	DNA flow cytometric-derived S-phase fraction (breast) In situ detection of HER-2/neu amplification (breast)
Lymphoid	DNA translocations and amplifications	Gain or loss of DNA (potential)
Mesenchymal	DNA translocations	Gain or loss of DNA and RNA-specific transcripts (potential)
Neuroectodermal	RNA-specific transcripts	

viral or bacterial) sequences within individual cells based on the complementary binding of a nucleotide probe (usually oligomers), labeled with nonisotopic (for example, fluorochromes) reporter molecules, to a specific target sequence of DNA or RNA.[98] Given optimal preparation of cytologic specimens,[99] applications of in situ hybridisation techniques in cytopathology are numerous, including detection of bacterial and viral infections and detection of messenger RNA of genes coding for oncoproteins, growth factors and growth factor receptors, cytokines, adhesion and multidrug resistance molecules as well as cycle proteins.[98] Using probes to chromosome-specific (centromeric or telomeric) sequences, it is possible to detect aneuploidy in interphase nuclei[100,101] and losses, gains or amplifications of chromosome regions with known prognostic value.[102,103] Using sequence-specific probes, recurrent chromosomal rearrangements[104,105] of great diagnostic value can easily be identified and documented. Finally, comparative genomic hybridization[106] is a newly developed and global approach to detecting and defining the specific combination of genetic changes in individual tumors. All these molecular approaches based on in situ hybridization need the development of digital imaging analyzers for optimal quantitation.

In situ amplification techniques are based on the polymerase chain reaction (PCR) which allows recovery of large amounts of DNA from minute quantities of starting material.[107] Various adaptations of the PCR have been developed for cytological preparations[108] such as PCR in situ hybridization, in situ PCR, reverse transcriptase in situ PCR,[109] methylation-specific PCR[110] and primed in situ synthesis.[111] Fixation and preparation of cells are critical steps for optimal in situ amplification with oligonucleotide primers followed by detection of the amplified product using nonisotopic reporter molecules. Appropriate controls including reference control genes, known negative samples for the target sequence, together with irrelevant primers and probes, are mandatory for specificity and quantitation of the reaction.[111] This is also the case for detection of gene fusions encoding chimeric messenger RNA used as specific diagnostic genetic markers in several lymphoid and myeloid malignancies and in some solid tumors.[112] In the same way, DNA or RNA amplification by means of in vitro PCR or reverse tranziptase PCR have recently been successfully performed using cytologic material laser-dissected[113] or directly scraped from routinely stained, archival slides.[114–117]

Other nucleic acid-based methods such as microsatellite analysis,[118] quantitation of telomerase activity,[119] methodologies using DNA[120] and cDNA[121,122] chip arrays and serial analysis of gene expression [118] in small clinical samples, and the proton magnetic resonance technique[123,124] are currently under evaluation.

Future prospects

Coordinating driving forces coming from the development of robust protocols using new versatile fluorochromes and automated digital optical imaging will undoubtedly help the pathologist in quantifying in situ amplification and hybridization techniques and in applying new technologies such as in situ hybridization techniques and micro-arrays for the study of DNA and RNA.[125] It is also anticipated that proteomic evaluation of cytologic material may help the cytopathologist in better evaluating the diagnosis of a particular tumor and the prognosis of a given patient.[126]

These very promising perspectives reinforce the central role, responsibility and future implications of the (cyto) pathologist in helping the clinician to tailor and adapt the treatment of patients.[127,128]

References

1. Smith EH. Complications of percutaneous abdominal fine-needle biopsy. Review. Radiology 1991;178: 253–8.
2. Powers CN. Complications of fine needle aspiration biopsy: the reality behind the myths. In: Schmidt WA, editor. Cytopathology. Chicago: ASCP Press; 1996. p. 69–91.
3. Logan-Young W, Dawson AE, Wilbur DC, et al. The cost effectiveness of fine-needle aspiration cytology and 14-gauge core needle biopsy compared with open surgical biopsy in the diagnosis of breast carcinoma. Cancer 1998;82:1867–73.
4. Liberman L. Percutaneous image-guided core breast biopsy. Radiol Clin N Am 2002;40:483–500.
5. Haack LA, Meier JS, Gluth J, et al. The other side of the needle: a patient's perspective. Diagn Cytopathol 2006;34: 303–6.
6. Thompson P. Thin needle aspiration biopsy. Letter. Acta Cytol 1982;26: 262–3.
7. Zajdela A, Zillhardt P, Voillemot N. Cytological diagnosis by fine needle sampling without aspiration. Cancer 1987;59:1201–5.
8. Akhtar SS, Imran-Ul-Huq, Faiz-U-Din M, et al. Efficacy of fine-needle capillary biopsy in the assessment of patients with superficial lymphadenopathy. Cancer (Cancer Cytopathol) 1997;81:277–80.
9. Kate MS, Kamal MM, Bobhate SK, et al. Evaluation of fine needle capillary sampling in superficial and deep-seated lesions. An analysis of 670 cases. Acta Cytol 1998;42:679–84.
10. Choo C, Frost F. Blue smears: a new artifact in FNA smears due to formalin vapour. Cytoletter 2002;20: 4–6.
11. Boon ME, Lykles C. Imaginative approach to fine needle aspiration cytology. Lancet 1980;2:1031–2.

12. Sirkin W, Auger M, Donat E, et al. Cytospin – an alternative method for fine needle aspiration cytology of the breast: a study of 148 cases. Diagn Cytopathol 1995;13:266–9.
13. Bédard YC, Pollett AF. Breast fine-needle aspiration. A comparison of ThinPrep and conventional smears. Am J Clin Pathol 1999;111:523–7.
14. Nasuti JF. Utility of the ThinPrep technique in thyroid fine needle aspiration: optimal vs. practical approaches. Acta Cytol 2006;50:3–4.
15. Saleh H, Bassily N, Hammoud J. Utility of a liquid-based, monolayer preparation in the evaluation of thyroid lesions by fine needle aspiration biopsy. Comparison with the conventional smear method. Acta Cytol 2009;53: 130–6.
16. Hoda RS. Non-gynecological cytology on liquid-based preparations. A morphologic review of facts and artifacts. Diagn Cytopathol 2007;35: 621–34.
17. Michael CW, Hunter B. Interpretation of fine-needle aspirates processed by the ThinPrep technique: cytologic artifacts and diagnostic pitfalls. Diagn Cytopathol 2000;23:6–13.
18. Nasuti JF, Tam D, Gupta PK. Diagnostic value of liquid-based (ThinPrep) preparations in nongynecologic cases. Diagn Cytopathol 2001;24:137–41.
19. Bell DA, Carr CP, Szyfelbein WM. Fine needle aspiration cytology of focal liver lesions. Results obtained with examination of both cytologic and histologic preparations. Acta Cytol 1986;30:397–402.
20. De Boer WB, Segal A, Frost FA, et al. Can CD34 discriminate between benign and malignant hepatocytic lesions in fine-needle aspirates and thin core biopsies? Cancer (Cancer Cytopathol) 2000;90:273–8.
21. Nathan NA, Narayan E, Smith MM, et al. Cell block cytology. Improved

preparation and its efficacy in diagnostic cytology. Am J Clin Pathol 2000;114:599–606.
22. Liu K, Dodge R, Glasgow BJ, et al. Fine-needle aspiration: comparison of smear, cytospin, and cell block preparations in diagnostic and cost effectiveness. Diagn Cytopathol 1998; 19:70–4.
23. Shidham VB, Kampalath B, England J. Routine air drying of all smears prepared during fine needle aspiration and intraoperative cytologic studies. An opportunity to practice a unified protocol offering the flexibility of choosing a variety of staining methods. Acta Cytol 2001;45:60–8.
24. Pak HY, Yokota S, Teplitz RL, et al. Rapid staining techniques employed in fine needle aspiration of the lung. Acta Cytol 1981;25:178–84.
25. Pak HY, Yokota SB, Teplitz RL. Rapid staining techniques employed in fine needle aspirations. Acta Cytol 1983;27: 81–2.
26. Yang GCH, Alvarez II. Ultrafast Papanicolaou stain: an alternative preparation for fine needle aspiration cytology. Acta Cytol 1995;39:55–60.
27. Sachdeva R, Kline TS. Aspiration biopsy cytology and special stains. Acta Cytol 1981;25:678–83.
28. Pintozzi RL, Blecka LJ, Nanon S. The morphologic identification of *Pneumocystis carinii*. Acta Cytol 1979;23:35–9.
29. Pollock PG, Valicenti JF, Meyers DS, et al. The use of fluorescent and special staining techniques in the aspiration of nocardiosis and actinomycosis. Acta Cytol 1978;22:575–9.
30. Boccato P, Briani G, Bizzaro N, et al. Cytology in 'black and white'. Acta Cytol 1987;31:643–5.
31. Krane JF, Renshaw AA. Relative value and cost-effectiveness of culture and special stains in fine needle aspirates of the lung. Acta Cytol 1998;42:305–11.

32. Dabbs DJ, Silverman JF. Selective use of electron microscopy in fine needle aspiration cytology. Acta Cytol 1988;32:880–4.

33. Dardick I, Yazdi HM, Brosko C, et al. A quantitative comparison of light and electron microscopic diagnoses in specimens obtained by fine needle aspiration biopsy. Ultrastruct Pathol 1991;15:105–29.

34. Akhtar M, Bakry M, Al-Jeaid AS, et al. Electron microscopy of fine needle aspiration biopsy specimens: a brief review. Diagn Cytopathol 1992;8: 278–82.

35. Kurtz SM. Rapid ultrastructural examination of FNAs in the diagnosis of intrathoracic tumours. Diagn Cytopathol 1992;8:289–92.

36. Yazdi HM, Dardick I. Diagnostic immunocytochemistry and electron microscopy. Guides to clinical aspiration biopsy. New York: Igaku-Shoin; 1992.

37. Davidson DD, Goheen MP. Preparation of fine needle aspiration biopsies for electron microscopy. In: Schmidt WA, editor. Cytopathology annual. Baltimore: Williams and Wilkins; 1993. p. 255–64.

38. Qiononez GE, Ravinsky E, Paraskevas M, et al. Contribution of transmission electron microscopy to fine-needle aspiration biopsy diagnosis: comparison of cytology and combined cytology and transmission electron microscopy with final histological diagnosis. Diagn Cytopathol 1996;15: 282–7.

39. Lazaro AV. Technical note: improved preparation of fine needle aspiration biopsies for transmission electron microscopy. Pathology 1983;15:399–402.

40. Van Hoeven KH, Fitzpatrick BT, Bibbo M. Update of immunocytochemistry in cytopathology. In: Rosen PP, Fechner RE, editors. Pathology annual, vol.30, part 2. Stanford: Appleton and Lange; 1995.

41. Osborn M, Domagala W. Immunocytochemistry. In: Bibbo M, editor. Comprehensive cytopathology, 2nd ed. Philadelphia: Saunders; 1997.

42. Polak J, van Noorden S. Introduction to immunocytochemistry. Current techniques and problems. 2nd ed. Berlin: Springer-Verlag; 1997.

43. Suthipintawong C, Leong AS-Y. Immunostaining of cell preparations: a comparative evaluation of common fixatives and protocols. Diagn Cytopathol 1996;15:167–74.

44. Campbell F, Herrington CS. Application of cytokeratin 7 and 20 immunohistochemistry to diagnostic pathology. Current Diagn Pathol 2001;7:113–22.

45. Leung SW, Bedard YC. Immunocytochemical staining on ThinPrep processed smears. Mod Pathol 1996;9:304–6.

46. Dabbs DJ, Abendroth CS, Grenko RT, et al. Immunocytochemistry on the ThinPrep processor. Diagn Cytopathol 1997;17:388–92.

47. Abendroth CS, Dabbs DJ. Immunocytochemical staining of unstained versus previously stained cytologic preparations. Acta Cytol 1995;39:379–86.

48. Kurtycz DFI, Logrono R, Leopando M, et al. Immunocytochemistry controls using cell cultures. Diagn Cytopathol 1997;17:74–9.

49. Holmes GF, Eisele DW, Rosenthal D. PSA immunoreactivity in a parotid oncocytoma: a diagnostic pitfall in discriminating primary parotid neoplasms from metastatic prostate cancer. Diagn Cytopathol 1998;19: 221–5.

50. Meijer GA, Beliën JAM, van Diest PJ, et al. Image analysis in clinical pathology. J Clin Pathol 1997;50: 365–70.

51. Baak JPA. Manual of quantitative pathology in cancer diagnosis and prognosis. Berlin: Springer-Verlag; 1991.

52. Hamilton PW, Allen DC. Quantitative clinical pathology. Oxford: Blackwell Scientific; 1995.

53. Zajdela A, de la Riva L, Ghossein N. The relation of prognosis to the nuclear diameter of breast cancer obtained by cytologic aspiration. Acta Cytol 1984;23:75–80.

54. True LD. Morphometric applications in anatomic pathology. Human Pathol 1996;27:450–67.

55. Hall PA, Coates PJ. Assessment of cell proliferation in pathology – what next? Histopathology 1995;26:105–12.

56. Maciorowski Z, Klijanienko J, Padoy, et al. Comparative image and flow cytometric TUNEL analysis of fine needle samples of breast carcinoma. Cytometry 2001;46:150–6.

57. Caspersson TO. History of the development of cytophotometry from 1935 to the present. Anal Quant Cytol Histol 1987;9:2–6.

58. Mikel UV. Quantitative staining techniques for image cytometry. In: Mikel UV, editor. Advanced laboratory methods in histology and pathology. Washington DC: Armed Forces Institute of Pathology; 1994. p. 131–60.

59. Maciorowski Z, Veilleux C, Gibaud A, et al. Comparison of fixation procedures for fluorescent quantitation of DNA content using image cytometry. Cytometry 1997;26:123–9.

60. Truong K, Vielh P, Malfoy B, et al. Fluorescence-based analysis of DNA ploidy and cell proliferation within fine needle samplings of breast tumors; a new approach using automated image cytometry. Cancer 1998;84:309–16.

61. Cross SS, Bury JP, Stephenson TJ, et al. Image analysis of low magnification images of fine needle aspirates of the breast produces useful discrimination between benign and malignant cases. Cytopathol 1997;8:265–73.

62. Teague MW, Wolberg WH, Street WN, et al. Indeterminate fine needle aspiration of the breast: image analysis-assisted diagnosis. Cancer (Cancer Cytopathol) 1997;81:129–35.

63. Briffod M, Le Doussal V, Spyratos F. Cytologic nuclear grading of fine-needle cytopunctures of breast carcinoma. Comparison with histologic nuclear grading and image cytometric data. Anal Quant Cytol Histol 1997;19: 114–22.

64. Cohen C. Image cytometric analysis in pathology. Human Pathol 1996;27: 482–93.

65. Wolberg WH, Street WN, Mangasarian OL. Computer-derived nuclear features compared with axillary lymph node status for breast carcinoma prognosis. Cancer (Cancer Cytopathol) 1997;81: 172–9.

66. Briffod M, Spyratos F, Hacène K, et al. Evaluation of breast carcinoma chemosensitivity by flow cytometric DNA analysis and computer-assisted image analysis. Cytometry 1992;13:250–8.

67. Auger M, Katz RL, Johnston DA, et al. Quantitation of immunocytochemical estrogen and progesterone receptor content in fine needle aspirates of breast carcinoma using the SAMBA 4000 image analysis system. Anal Quant Cytol Histol 1993;15: 274–80.

68. Bozzetti C, Nizzoli R, Camisa R, et al. Comparison between Ki-67 index and S-phase fraction on fine needle aspiration samples from breast carcinoma. Cancer (Cancer Cytopathol) 1997;81:287–92.

69. Katz RL, Wojcik EM, El-Naggar AK, et al. Proliferation markers in non-Hodgkin's lymphoma: a comparative study between cytophotometric quantitation of Ki-67 and flow cytometric proliferation index on fine needle aspirates. Anal Quant Cytol Histol 1993;15:179–86.

70. Oud PS, Bauwens A, Nauwelaers FA. Multiparameter absorption measurements in automated microscopy: simultaneous quantitative determination of DNA and nuclear antigen. Acta Cytol 1997;41:188–96.

71. Friedrich K, Thieme B, Haroske G, et al. Nuclear image analysis of p53-positive and -negative cells in breast carcinoma. Anal Quant Cytol Histol 1997;19: 285–93.

72. Marchevsky A. Quality assurance issues in DNA image cytometry. Cytometry (Commun Clin Cytometry) 1996; 26:101–7.

73. Kamentsky LA, Burger DE, Gershamn RJ, et al. Slide-based laser scanning cytometry. Acta Cytol 1997;41:123–43.

74. Clatch RJ, Walloch JL. Multiparameter immunophenotypic analysis of fine needle aspiration biopsies and other hematologic specimens by laser scanning cytometry. Acta Cytol 1997;41:109–22.

75. Gorczyca W, Darzynkiewicz Z, Melamed MR. Laser scanning cytometry in pathology of solid tumors. Acta Cytol 1997;41:98–108.

76. Caspersson TO, Schultz J. Nucleic acid metabolism of the chromosomes in relation to gene reproduction. Nature 1938;142:294–7.

77. Coons AH, Kaplan MH. Localization of antigen in tissue cells. II. Improvements in a method for the detection of antigen by means of fluorescent antibody. J Exp Med 1950;91:1–4.

78. Crosland-Taylor PJ. A device for counting small particles suspended in a fluid through a tube. Nature 1953;171:37–8.

79. Coulter WH. High speed automatic blood cell counter and cell size analyser. Proc Natl Electronics Conf 1956;12:1034–42.

80. Giaretti W. Flow cytometry and applications in oncology. J Clin Pathol 1997;50:275–7.

81. Robins DB, Katz RL, Swan F Jr, et al. Immunotyping of lymphoma by fine needle aspiration. A comparative study of cytospin preparations and flow cytometry. Am J Clin Pathol 1994;101:569–76.

82. Vielh P. Flow cytometry. Guides to clinical aspiration biopsy. New York: Igaku-Shoin; 1991.

83. Braylan RC, Borowitz MJ, Davis BH, et al. U.S. –Canadian consensus recommendations on the immunophenotypic analysis of hematologic neoplasia by flow cytometry. Cytometry (Commun Clin Cytometry) 1997;30:213.

84. Duque RE, Andreeff M, Braylan RC, et al. Consensus review of the clinical utility of DNA flow cytometry in neoplastic hematopathology. Cytometry 1993;14:492–6.

85. Hiddemann W, Schumann J, Andreeff M, et al. Convention on nomenclature for DNA cytometry. Cancer Genet Cytogenet 1984;13:181–3.

86. Jennings CD, Foon KA. Recent advances in flow cytometry: application to the diagnosis of hematologic malignancy. Blood 1997;90:2863–92.

87. Zeppa P, Marino G, Troncone G, et al. Fine-needle cytology and flow cytometry immunophenotyping and subclassification of non-Hodgkin lymphoma. Cancer 2004;102:55–65.

88. Vielh P, Carton M, Padoy E, et al. S-phase fraction as an independent prognostic factor of long-term overall survival in patients with early-stage or locally advanced invasive carcinoma. Cancer 2005;105:476–82.

89. D'Hautcourt JL, Spyratos F, Chassevent A. Quality control study by the French Cytometry Association on flow cytometric DNA content and S-phase fraction (S%). Cytometry (Commun Clin Cytometry) 1996;26:32–9.

90. Silvestrini R. Quality control for evaluation of the S-phase fraction by flow cytometry: a multicentric study. Cytometry (Commun Clin Cytometry) 1994;18:11–6.

91. Darzynkiewicz A, Juan G, Li X, et al. Cytometry in cell necrobiology: analysis of apoptosis and accidental cell death (necrosis). Cytometry 1997;27:1–20

92. Maciorowski Z, Klijanienko J, Padoy E, et al. Differential expression of Bax and Bcl2 in the assessment of cellular dynamics in fine-needle samples of primary breast carcinomas. Cytometry 2000;42:264–9.

93. Krishnamurthy S, Applications of molecular techniques to fine-needle aspiration biopsy. Cancer 2007;11:106–22.

94. Schmitt F, Loghatto-Filho A, Valent A, et al. Molecular techniques in cytopathology practice. J Clin Pathol 2008;61:258–67.

95. Chevillard S, Pouillart P, Beldjord C, et al. Sequential assessment of multidrug resistance phenotype and measurement of S-phase fraction as predictive markers of breast cancer response to neoadjuvant chemotherapy. Cancer 1996;77:292–300.

96. Chevillard S, Lebeau J, Pouillart P, et al. Biological and clinical significance of concurrent p53 gene alterations, MDR1 gene expression, and S-phase fraction analyses in breast cancer patients treated with primary chemotherapy or radiotherapy. Clin Cancer Res 1997;3:2471–8.

97. Waldman FM, Sauter G, Sudar D, et al. Molecular cytometry of cancer. Human Pathol 1996;27:441–9.

98. McNicol AM, Farquharson MA. In: situ hybridization and its diagnostic applications in pathology. J Pathol 1997;182:250–61.

99. Abati A, Sanford JS, Fetsch P, et al. Fluorescence in situ hybridization (FISH): a user's guide to optimal preparation of cytologic specimens. Diagn Cytopathol 1995;13:485–92.

100. Sauer T, Beraki K, Jebsen PW, et al. Ploidy analysis by in situ hybridization of interphase cell nuclei in fine needle aspirates from breast carcinomas: correlation with cytologic grading. Diagn Cytopathol 1997;17:267–71.

101. Truong K, Guilly MN, Gerbault-Seureau M, et al. Quantitative FISH by image cytometry for the detection of chromosome 1 imbalances in breast cancer: a novel approach analyzing chromosome rearrangements within interphase nuclei. Lab Invest 1998;78:1607–13.

102. Wolman S. Applications of fluorescence in situ hybridization techniques in cytopathol. Cancer (Cancer Cytopathol) 1997;81:193–7.

103. Klijanienko J, Couturier J, Galut M, et al. Detection and quantitation by FISH and image analysis of HER-2/neu gene amplification in breast cancer fine-needle samples. Cancer 1999;87:312–8.

104. Mitelman F, Johansson B, Mandahl N, et al. Clinical significance of cytogenetic findings in solid tumors. Cancer Genet Cytogenet 1997;95:1–8.

105. Gong Y, Caraway N, Gu J, et al. Evaluation of interphase fluorescence in situ hybridization for the t(14;18)(q32;q21) translocation in the diagnosis of follicular lymphoma on fine-needle aspirates. Cancer 2003;99:385–93.

106. Forozan F, Karhu R, Kononen J, et al. Genome screening by comparative genomic hybridization. Trends Genet 1997;13:405–9.

107. O'Leary JJ, Engels K, Dada MA. The polymerase chain reaction in pathology. J Clin Pathol 1997;50:805–10.

108. Tisserand P, Fouquet C, Marck V, et al. ThinPrep-processed fine-needle samples of breast are effective material for RNA- and DNA-based molecular diagnosis. Cancer 2003;99:223–32.

109. Gazagne A, Claret E, Wijdenes J, et al. A fluorospot assay to detect single T lymphocytes simultaneously producing multiple cytokines. J Immunol Methods 2003;283:91–8.

110. Pu RT, Laitala LE, Alli PM, et al. Methylation profiling of benign and malignant breast lesions and its application to cytopathology. Mod Pathol 2003;16:1095–101.

111. O'Leary JJ, Landers RJ, Chetty R. In: situ amplification in cytological preparations. Cytopathology 1997;8:148–60.

112. Sheer D, Squire J. Clinical applications of genetic rearrangements in cancer. Semin Cancer Biol 1996;7:25–32.

113. Orba Y, Tanaka S, Nishihara H, et al. Application of laser capture microdissection to cytologic specimens for the detection of immunoglobulin heavy chain rearrangement in patients with malignant lymphoma. Cancer 2003;99:198–204.

114. Chen J-T, Lane MA, Clark DP. Inhibitors of the polymerase chain reaction in Papanicolaou stain: removal with a simple destaining procedure. Acta Cytol 1996;40:873–7.

115. Lovchik J, Lane MA, Clark DP. Polymerase chain reaction-based detection of B-cell clonality in the fine

needle aspiration biopsy of a thyroid mucosa-associated lymphoid tissue (MALT) lymphoma. Human Pathol 1997;28:989–92.

116. Schlott T, Nagel H, Ruschenburg I, et al. Reverse transcriptase polymerase chain reaction for detecting Ewing's sarcoma in archival fine needle aspiration biopsies. Acta Cytol 1997;41:795–801.

117. Mittledorf CA, Leite KR, Darini E, et al. Optimal recovery of DNA for polymerase chain reaction-based assays from fine-needle aspirates. Acta Cytol 2002;46:1117–22.

118. Sidransky D. Nucleic acid-based methods for the detection of cancer. Science 1997;278:1054–8.

119. Iwao T, Hiyama E, Yokoyama T, et al. Telomerase activity for the preoperative diagnosis of pancreatic cancer. J Natl Cancer Inst 1997;89:1621–3.

120. Heselmeyer-Haddad K, Chaudri N, Stoltzfus P, et al. Detection of chromosomal aneuploidies and gene copy number changes in fine-needle aspirates is a specific, sensitive, and objective genetic test for the diagnosis of breast cancer. Cancer Res 2002;62:2365–9.

121. Staudt LM. Molecular diagnosis of the hematologic cancers. N Engl J Med 2003;348:1777–85.

122. Symmans WF, Ayers M, Clark EA, et al. Total RNA yield and microarray gene expression from fine-needle aspiration biopsy and core-needle biopsy samples of breast carcinoma. Cancer 2003;97:2960–71.

123. Mountford CE, Lean CL, MacKinnon WB, et al. The use of proton MR in cancer pathology. In: Webb GA, editor. Annual reports on NMR spectroscopy, vol. 27. London: Academic Press; 1993. p. 173–216.

124. Russel P, Lean CL, Delbridge L, et al. Proton magnetic resonance and human thyroid neoplasia I. Discrimination between benign and malignant neoplasms. Am J Med 1994;96:383–8.

125. Lansdorp PM, Verwoerd NP, van de Riijke FM, et al. Heterogeneity in telomere length of human chromosomes. Human Mol Genet 1996;5:685–91.

126. Fetsch PA, Simone NL, Bryant-Greenwood PK, et al. Proteomic evaluation of archival cytologic material using SELDI affinity mass spectrometry. Am J Clin Pathol 2002;118:870–6.

127. Bibbo M. How technology is reshaping the practice of nongynecologic cytology: frontiers of cytology symposium. Acta Cytol 2007;51:123–52.

128. Clark DP. Seize the opportunity: underutilization of fine-needle aspiration biopsy to inform targeted cancer therapy decisions. Cancer 2009;117:289–97.

CHAPTER 3

Imaging methods for guidance of aspiration cytology

Suzanne Le P Langlois and Steve Chryssidis

Percutaneous biopsy is a well-established and routine practice in imaging departments,[1,2] and is a frequently performed interventional radiographic procedure, either as an inpatient or outpatient examination, by most trained radiologists. The technique, indications and complications are extensively described in basic imaging textbooks.[3] Development of expertise often occurs by 'apprenticeship' during undergraduate training for radiologists and for many other clinicians. The procedure is safe, inexpensive and minimally invasive. An understanding of the imaging modalities, the lesion to be biopsied and overall experience of the proceduralist contribute to the success of the procedure.

Fine needle aspiration biopsy (FNAB) typically yields a small sample for cytological assessment, with limited or no architectural information. The decision to proceed to larger-diameter needles (core biopsy) may be determined either by the results of the fine needle aspirate or, in some instances, due to the cytologist being unavailable to interpret the findings at the time of the biopsy.

Fine needle aspiration biopsy and core biopsy often complement each other in facilitating and assisting in the diagnostic process.

There have been continuous improvements in needles, biopsy guides and mechanical biopsy devices, together with technological advances in the major imaging methods of computed tomography (CT) and ultrasonography (US). The use of magnetic resonance imaging (MRI), and the development of stereotactic guidance, particularly for brain and breast biopsies, is now more readily available. Previously inaccessible lesions can be safely sampled and many more areas of the body are now routinely biopsied under guidance. Radiological guidance has allowed the development of more invasive procedures such as catheter drainage, villus biopsy, fetal blood and tissue sampling and core biopsy.[4] This leads to a reduction in open biopsy and two-stage surgical procedures by providing a definitive diagnosis prior to primary surgical treatment.

More than one imaging modality may be required, first to localize the lesion and then to obtain biopsy material. The radiologist performing the procedure should determine the method used and will be influenced by availability of equipment, difficulty in scheduling, urgency of the procedure and perhaps operator preference and experience.

Ultrasound guidance offers flexibility and speed, whereas CT often provides safer access for deeper tissue biopsy. Ultimately, the imaging modality which offers the best lesion visualization and safest route will dictate the biopsy pathway. Fluoroscopy is an alternative which may be utilized for pulmonary and bone lesions, although not as widely used as CT guidance.

All the imaging techniques have advantages and disadvantages in various parts of the body.

The portability, ease of use and relative speed of ultrasound make it a favourable modality for guided biopsy procedures, particularly for superficial and moderately deep lesions. The utility of ultrasound guided biopsy has also been recognized by specialties outside of radiology, particularly for intraoperative guided lesion assessments and biopsy.

Where practical, ultrasound is the preferred biopsy option, particularly given there is no ionizing radiation. In many instances, however, the nature and position of a lesion may mandate the use of CT guidance. Modern CT equipment allows for real-time assessment of the needle position using CT fluoroscopy, streamlining the biopsy process. This pathway involves ionizing radiation, exposing both the patient and the interventional team. The increasing body mass index of the patient population, particularly within the Western world, has led to a progressive increase in the imaging dose required to visualize relevant structures and organs. The end result is an increased radiation dose to the patient and to the interventional team members. An elevated awareness of this issue has motivated the implementation of dose minimization strategies where practicable.

Ultimately, however, the modality used will be dictated by the availability of equipment, staff and site of the lesion.

The presence of a pathologist at the biopsy generally facilitates a more efficient process. Optimal results can only be obtained by meticulous localization before biopsy and this may occupy most of the procedural time; fortunately, this can be performed prior to the arrival of the pathologist (Fig. 3.1). The pathologist may direct the radiologist to a different area of the lesion, for example to the viable periphery rather than the central necrotic area of a solid lesion, and may request additional tissue for ancillary tests, such as special stains, electron microscopy or culture, or to determine the need for a core biopsy.[5]

©2012 Elsevier Ltd
DOI: 10.1016/B978-0-7020-3151-9.00003-7

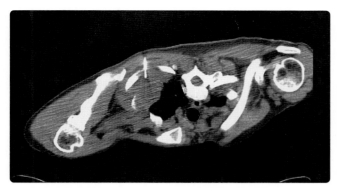

Fig. 3.1 Pancoast tumour biopsy Care is required in positioning the patient for maximum comfort and access to the lesion to avoid ribs and scapula.

It matters little whether the radiologist or pathologist performs the actual aspiration. In many cases, however, the radiologist is more skilled in interpreting the images and is better able to manipulate the needle in three dimensions while viewing a two-dimensional image.

Fluoroscopy

Fluoroscopy is the traditional method for guidance of biopsies to most parts of the body. With the advent of highly technical guidance methods such as CT and US, it is used less and is often considered less accurate. However, it provides a quick alternative for those radiologists not experienced in US guidance and is most useful in guidance for small, very mobile lesions, such as focal lower zone lung lesions. In this instance, the real-time fluoroscopy may be the only method of accurately placing the needle tip within a small lesion. It also offers efficient sampling options for cortical bony lesions. Fluoroscopy is a reasonable biopsy alternative because of its low cost and general availability.

Although fluoroscopic guided biopsy may be easier with a biplane system, a single-plane system with tube tilting to provide a stereotactic type of view of the lesion and needle can also be used.

Ultrasound

Ultrasound (US) is the only real-time guidance which allows imaging in any plane and is the only suitable guidance for biopsy of fetal tissues. Its use is limited in certain areas, as ultrasound is not transmitted through air or bone. Some parts of the body,[6] such as the chest wall and musculoskeletal system, though neglected in the past, have undergone an increase in interest for both diagnostic and interventional studies. Developments such as operative probes and vaginal and rectal transducers are now combined with portable, handheld (as compared to mobile) US units, for use in intensive care areas and operating theaters, wards and clinics, and to regional and remote areas.[7]

Real-time monitoring is a major advantage as the exact location of the needle tip can be seen during biopsy and adjustments to its position can be performed to increase the accuracy of sampling. Visibility of needles can be a problem and needles should be tested for echogenicity prior to use. Many manufacturers also provide fine needle aspiration biopsy needles with etched tips to aid in ultrasound visualization. Stylets within needles, and particularly movement of the stylet within the needle, will improve visibility. The gauge of the needle does not necessarily relate to echogenicity and in many instances a fine needle may be more highly echogenic than a subsequent core biopsy needle. Using color Doppler may enhance visibility during movement of the needle.

The choice of transducer and frequency is dictated by the area of the body to be biopsied and depth of the lesion. Intracavitary probes and developments with intravascular and intraluminal transducers allow biopsy and intervention into virtually every part of the body.

While freehand guidance is usually preferred, if a biopsy attachment is used there should be easy separation of the needle to reduce the risk of tearing tissues, particularly in areas of the body where respiratory movement may occur, for example liver and kidney. The shortest puncture route is normally chosen, though as with hepatic biopsies it is advisable that the needle traverses at least a rim of normal parenchyma to reduce the risk of hemorrhage.

While sterile water can be used as a coupling medium, there appears to be no real risk of reaction from use of sterile coupling medium, but it must not contaminate the aspirate. Sterilization of the transducer and attachment is routine, including universal precautions against infection.

Technique of ultrasound guided biopsy

The longest part of the examination is preparation – identifying the lesion, positioning the patient, and identifying the site of puncture and direction of the needle. The depth of the lesion from the skin surface is measured to determine the length of the needle required; the biopsy route is typically oblique and thus measurements need to reflect this. Continuous real-time ultrasound is used to visualize the tip of the needle entering the lesion. Scanning continues during aspiration to ensure that the needle stays within the lesion, and the aspirate may be seen moving within the needle lumen.

Maintaining sterility

Sterility of the transducer can be achieved by wiping the transducer with skin preparation, placing a layer of gel onto the end of the transducer, and carefully placing it into a sterile bag (sterilized plastic wrap, specially manufactured covers held there by a sterile rubber band), maintaining sterility at all times. Care must be taken with the transducer cord to prevent it draping over the sterile area. If coupling gel is used it should be sterile, but an alternative to gel is to use sterile saline or skin disinfectant, although these require occasional replenishment as the alcohol or water rapidly dries on the skin. The tip of the transducer merely needs to be dipped into the fluid, and enough will usually adhere to provide adequate transmission of sound waves. Coupling agents such as betadine or chlorhexidine solution may be preferred over sterile gel in some instances, as this may contaminate samples and compromise sample quality.

Biopsy procedure

The transducer is ideally held in the optimal longitudinal position to visualize the lesion. Prior to insertion of the needle, it is imperative that the alignment of the transducer is checked, so that the image on the screen is aligned with the correct orientation. Optimally, this is done by tilting the transducer slightly up and down, and assessing the areas brought into view, but should be confirmed by pressing lightly on the point of proposed skin puncture by the needle, so that the visible disturbance of the soft tissues confirms correct orientation.

Some operators have an assistant holding the transducer, maintaining its position exactly parallel to the long axis of the lesion, and ensuring that it does not slip away from the puncture site. This allows the operator to concentrate on introducing the needle exactly parallel to the transducer, and is a useful technique particularly in complex biopsy cases. Some prefer to hold both and relinquish the transducer once the needle has punctured the lesion. Only practice will determine which method is more comfortable for each individual.

Under real-time guidance the needle is introduced through the skin, 1–2 cm proximal to the transducer, and at the midpoint of the narrow side of the transducer. The needle is then advanced along the line of the transducer. The length of the needle should become visible, and the tip is seen to puncture the front wall of the lesion, then inserted a few more millimeters. If the needle does not become visible on the screen, the transducer can be used to find it, or alternatively the needle alignment can be adjusted. The angle of the needle should be changed to lie parallel to the transducer, as it is only when the lesion and the needle are in line that a successful puncture can occur.

Some operators prefer to use the transducer in an axis transverse to the lesion, once again located just distal to the proposed point of entry. This is less accurate, and does not necessarily locate the tip of the needle, merely showing a portion of the shaft.

CT scanning

There are very few areas of the body which cannot be biopsied under CT control, and extremely small lesions can be sampled. Focal masses of several millimeters within the lung and skull base (Fig. 3.2) can be biopsied and retroperitoneal biopsies are limited only by availability of needles long enough to traverse the abdomen of large patients. Traversing with fine needles offers fewer risks compared with the larger-caliber needles.[7] CT gantry tilt also further facilitates lesion access where appropriate.

Localization of the needle tip within a lesion is very accurate with CT (Fig. 3.3). It provides detailed cross-sectional images of the body which are not limited by the same physical properties as are ultrasound images, such as interference from bowel gas and bone.

Many of the CT scanners in modern imaging departments have biopsy software packages, allowing for real-time and relatively fast visualization of the target lesion and its relationship to the biopsy needle.

Successful biopsy of lung lesions is often dependent on the coordination of patient breath holding, CT fluoroscopic

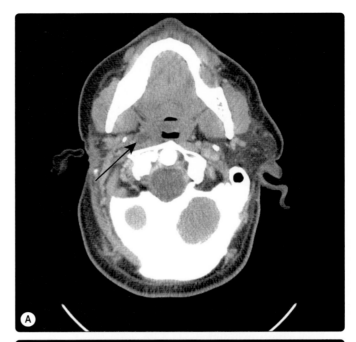

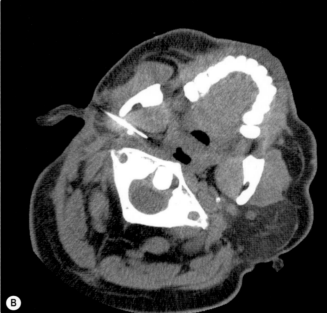

Fig. 3.2 (**A**) Circular low dense lesion right retropharyngeal node in a patient post right parotidectomy and radiotherapy for parotid squamous cell carcinoma. (**B**) Coaxial fine needle aspiration biopsy technique under CT control confirmed nodal recurrence. The utility of CT biopsy techniques and fine needle aspiration biopsy helped direct this patient's management.

imaging and needle positioning. Confirmation of the location of the needle tip should be obtained prior to sampling. Extrapleural approaches to medially situated lesions, particularly lesions in the anterior mediastinal, subcarinal or paraspinal regions, avoids the traversing of aerated lung, thereby negating the potential for pneumothorax or air leak after transthoracic needle biopsy.[8] When a paraspinal

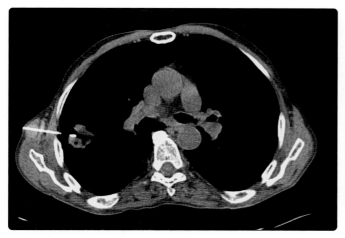

Fig. 3.3 Inflammatory lesion of the lung Tissue is obtained for culture and other appropriate tests. Local anaesthetic is visible in the subcutaneous tissues.

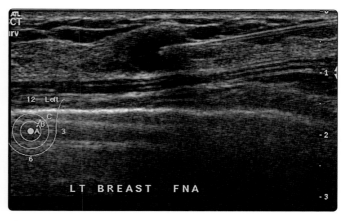

Fig. 3.4 Fine needle biopsy of a suspicious tumour mass in a small breast Continuous visualization of the needle tip prevents the risk of pneumothorax.

extrapleural approach is used, successive 10-ml aliquots of a mixture of equal saline and 1% lidocaine (lignocaine) are injected and intermittent scanning is performed to assess the needle route. Once a safe extrapleural route to the lesion has developed, a coaxial needle system or biopsy gun is advanced into the lesion for sampling.

The CT scans allow cross-sectional localization of needle placement.

The needle tip should be localized as accurately as possible to a position a few millimeters short of the area to be biopsied and the needle advanced the last few millimeters only during the biopsy. This prevents blood from accumulating around the needle tip and degrading the cytology specimen during the time required for scanning. Various techniques are available, including the use of guide or tandem needles and also stereotaxis. Artifacts from metallic needles and respiratory movement are rarely significant, particularly with the latest generation of CT scanners.

Magnetic resonance imaging (MRI)

It was initially predicted that MRI would never be suitable for guidance of biopsy and interventional procedures. However, the sensitivity of this new imaging technique is generally greater than that of other imaging methods and shows lesions which would not otherwise be detected. This is particularly evident in the brain, liver and breast.[9] Biopsy needles with low ferromagnetic properties have been developed to allow biopsy under MRI control.

MRI guided biopsy has offered particular utility in the evaluation of breast lesions, particularly where they are not well visualized by other imaging techniques, or if the biopsy is technically difficult. It has extended the evaluation options for the ill-defined and subcentimeter mass, as well as those not well demonstrated by mammography or sonography.[10] While MRI guided biopsy offers some logistical challenges, progress in devices and techniques are positioning this option more in the realm of mainstream lesion biopsy algorithms. Very fast scan times are also available, overcoming one of the earlier problems with MRI.

Dedicated interventional scanners are available, with easy access to the patient and lower field strengths to overcome anaesthetic and needle problems, yet still providing adequate resolution. Unfortunately, the expense of such dedicated scanners and their complex installation needs to restrict its availability to major clinical and research centers.

Breast biopsy and carbon marking for localization of clinically occult lesions

Mammographic screening has led to developments in biopsy and localisation of the small, clinically occult lesions detected by these programs. The most useful and common methods are ultrasound with and without a transducer attachment, a stereotactic attachment for upright mammographic X-ray units (Fig. 3.4) or a dedicated prone stereotactic mammographic biopsy table. When combined with FNAB and localization, either with a hookwire or preferably with carbon marking of the track,[11] these techniques efficiently provide maximal information for the clinician with the minimum of inconvenience to the patient (Table 3.1).[11] There is then the option to proceed to core biopsy if indicated by the FNAB result.

Digital stereotactic localization, with either the upright or prone units, shortens the time of the procedure in comparison with a film-screen radiographic technique and gives rapid accurate localization. There are disadvantages to the prone units, particularly in cost and inability to utilize them for other mammographic purposes, and there is some restriction in positioning and access to deep lesions in the breast. These are overcome with some modern upright mammographic units which allow gantry tilt and, with a digital stereotactic attachment, can localize a breast lesion from any projection, including from the inferior aspect, with the patient lying on her side. This mitigates the problem of vasovagal attacks, one of the criticisms of the upright biopsy method. There is also much greater access to the breast with this method.

Many operators prefer US guidance for its speed, flexibility and real-time facilities. The patient is also able to lie comfortably during the procedure. The method is limited by the

Table 3.1 Advantages of carbon marking compared to hookwire localization

Carbon marking	Hookwire
Accurate	Position less accurate
Permanent	May pull out or migrate
Comfortable for patient	Less comfortable for patient
Safe	Known risks, e.g. pneumothorax
Can be inserted at any time	Must be inserted immediately prior to surgery
Results of FNAB/core available prior to surgery	
Reduces two-stage surgical procedures	
Easily visible	Surgeons more familiar with technique
Radiologists easily trained	Surgeons require familiarization
Very inexpensive	Significant expense for hookwires

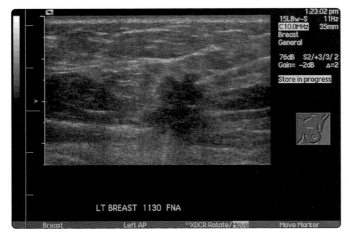

Fig. 3.5 FNA biopsy of a breast lesion with aggressive features Several passes may be necessary to yield sufficient cells.

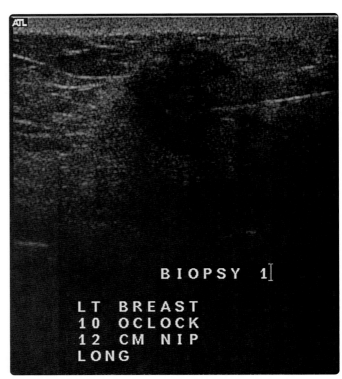

Fig. 3.6 Nonpalpable primary breast carcinoma Ultrasound-guided fine needle biopsy and carbon marking of the needle track.

type of lesion; many microcalcifications are not visible on ultrasound examination. There is also the slight risk of pleural puncture or pneumothorax if used by inexperienced operators. The needle should run parallel to the chest wall and never be introduced perpendicular to the ribcage (see Fig. 3.4). By positioning the patient and compressing the breast, the depth of the lesion can be reduced. Breast lesions often require multiple sampling, typically best achieved using ultrasound guidance (Fig. 3.5).

If core biopsy is performed for a suspected malignant lesion, it is recommended that the needle track be resected during subsequent surgery to avoid the potential of tumor seeding the track. This surgery can best be guided by injection of carbon along a line parallel to and a few millimeters from the core biopsy track. The surgeon is then able to follow this to the lesion, without further localization being required.

Carbon localization of nonpalpable breast lesions

The introduction of breast screening programs in many parts of the world has been an impetus for more extensive use of aspiration biopsy, and the expertise and experience gained has increased the use of aspiration biopsy in all areas of the body. Until the introduction of carbon localization of occult breast lesions, hookwire localization under either mammographic (grid or stereotactic) or ultrasound localization was required. The use of carbon marking of the track from skin to lesion has many advantages[11] (see Table 3.1) and and can almost always replace hookwire localization (Fig. 3.6).

Carbon marking consists of injecting 1–2 mL of a sterile solution of 4% medical grade charcoal in normal saline through a 20G or 22G needle from the lesion to the skin surface, after the needle tip is localized exactly at the lesion, while gradually withdrawing the needle. A small skin tattoo remains to indicate to the surgeon the site for resection. The carbon solution is a suspension, not a solution, and occasionally the needle may block during injection due to a large particle of carbon. It is useful to draw the solution into a syringe at the start of the procedure, then leave the syringe lying flat, so that large particles will precipitate to the bottom of the barrel. The syringe should lie in that position during transport and injection, without agitation – sterile tubing allows this to occur for any localizing route. Heating or refrigeration of the suspension does not decrease the chance of a needle blocking with large particles of carbon, nor does limited or excessive agitation, although regular users of the technique may advocate these. A major advantage of carbon localization is that it can be performed routinely at the same

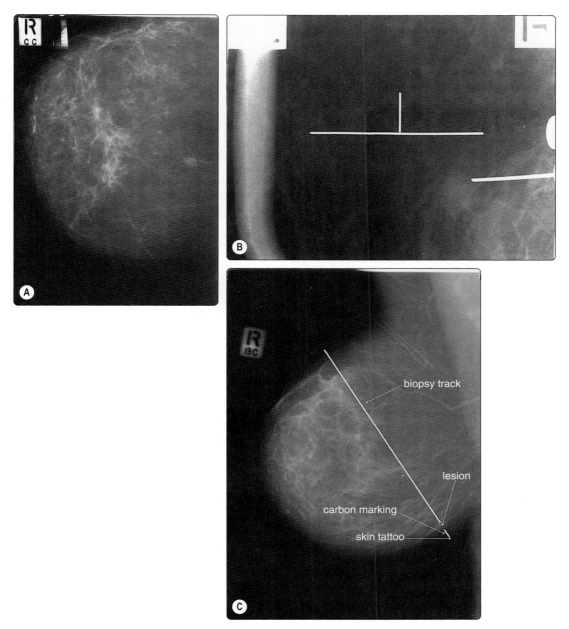

Fig. 3.7 'Push through technique' of carbon localization of a clinically occult breast lesion. (**A**) C–C view of an inferior breast lesion (proven to be a primary carcinoma, <1 cm), biopsied and carbon localized by the 'push through technique'. (**B**) Stereotactic confirmation of the tip of the needle adjacent to the lesion is essential prior to aspiration and carbon track marking. (**C**) Diagrammatic representation of 'push through technique'. Stereotactic biopsy in a C–C projection is performed, then a track is marked from the lesion to the inferior skin surface, producing a skin tattoo marking the site for surgical resection.

time as aspiration biopsy, if there is any likelihood of surgical biopsy being required. The track of the biopsy is then marked for resection, decreasing the risk of implantation of malignant cells. The results of fine needle biopsy (and, if indicated, core biopsy), are known prior to a decision on surgery, and if the lesion is considered benign the carbon track can remain indefinitely, unlike hookwire localization where surgery is required to remove the hookwire. When core biopsy is performed, the carbon track is placed several millimeters to the side of the biopsy track, so that it persists after the hematoma due to the biopsy has subsided. If surgery is performed soon after a core biopsy, the surgeon may not

need to visualise the carbon track, as extensive hemorrhage caused by a core biopsy will guide the resection. If the decision is made that surgery is not required, the skin tattoo and track marking can remain permanently with no ill effects.

One of the many advantages of carbon localization is that lesions which are only visible in the cranio-caudal view on mammography, but which lie in the inferior part of the breast, can be marked by carbon injection from the lesion to the inferior skin ('push through technique'), avoiding a wire traversing the bulk of the breast, and preventing a long dissection or a cut-down to the wire (Fig. 3.7)

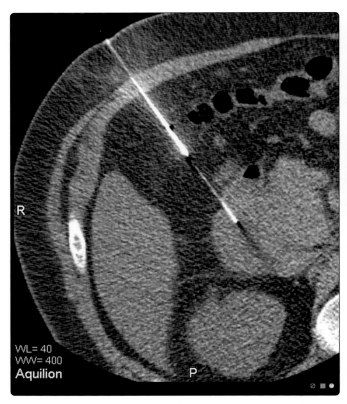

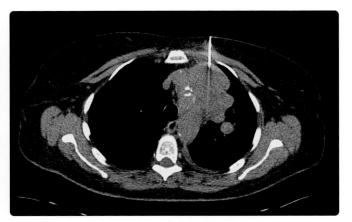

Fig. 3.9 Mediastinal mass An extrapleural approach reduces the risk of complications.

Fig. 3.8 Use of the coaxial technique delivers the FNA biopsy needle to the target lesion.

Use of guide needles

A guide needle may range from a short 2–3-cm needle to 12-cm needle, through which a fine-gauge needle is passed in a coaxial method (Fig. 3.8). The gauges of the needle combinations are usually 18/22 or 22/26. Use of these needles has been advocated during guided techniques for the following reasons:[6]

1. Needle stability is increased.
2. Multiple passes can be made through the guide needle and the biopsy repeated several times in various directions and depths to obtain material from several areas of the lesion.
3. Any risk of spread of tumour or infection is minimized by reducing the path length of the contaminated biopsy needle.
4. Only one skin puncture is required, thus lessening the discomfort of the procedure for the patient.
5. Deviation of the fine needle, due to resistance to its passage through firm skin, subcutaneous tissues and muscle wall, is avoided.
6. Microbubbles in local anaesthetic infiltrated into the tissues may obscure the scan field. This is prevented by using a focal area of anesthesia for a single guide needle.

Risks and complications

Complications depend on the site of the lesion.

The main complications for CT guided lung biopsy include hemoptysis and pneumothorax.[6,12] In particular, the rate of pneumothorax following lung biopsy with CT guidance reported in the literature ranges from 10% to 60%.[2,12,13] The various items which may influence this rate include patient factors (age, sex, lung function, and presence of emphysema), lesion variables (size, depth, location, and pleural contact), and procedure related factors (experience of the operator, degree of difficulty, and type of needle used) (Fig. 3.9). Where possible, an extrapleural route for biopsy is preferred. The reported incidence depends on the method used to detect such a pneumothorax. Radiographs are routinely taken 4 hours after the procedure with expiratory films if there is any doubt. Patients with chronic lung disease are at much greater risk of pneumothorax complications.

The procedure can be safely performed on outpatients, but there should be adequate counseling to return if pain, dyspnea or significant hemoptysis occurs.

Soft tissue and solid organ biopsy risks may include hemorrhage, infection,[7] tumor implantation,[14] and occasionally major disability or death. In addition, liver interventions may develop a bile leak, and contribute to a bile peritonitis, typically mild. Skull base biopsy procedures may cause neuropraxia or vascular trauma. Nevertheless, the benefits of fine needle biopsy, and the low risk compared to other diagnostic investigations including interventional imaging procedures and surgery, make it an invaluable tool in the investigation of any indeterminate lesion (Fig. 3.9).

There is always a risk of false-positive results (<1%) and false-negatives (>10% in lung lesions).[3] This is especially important in benign lesions where the tissues may be nonspecific and the biopsy result nondiagnostic. In these patients it is imperative radiographically to confirm that the needle tip is in the lesion during the actual aspiration. There can then be appropriate assessment of the cells obtained during discussion with the treating clinician. The importance of imaging and recording the position of the tip of the needle at aspiration is critical in certain situations, such as during adrenal mass biopsy, as the pathologist is unable to distinguish between cells from a cortical adenoma and normal adrenal cortical cells. This may also apply to other benign neoplasms which are of small size and composed of cells similar to the normal tissue of origin.

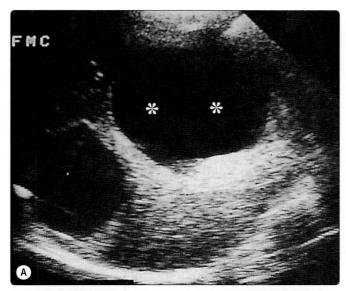

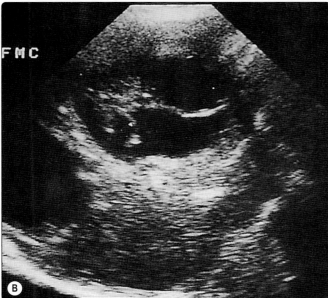

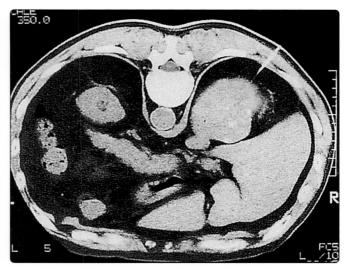

Fig. 3.11 Adrenal mass biopsy in a hemophiliac patient The patient was a severe haemophiliac with only 2% of normal levels of factor VIII. As he was experiencing discomfort in the right upper quadrant, a cytological diagnosis was sought for the mass within the right adrenal. Biopsy was performed during several days of infusion of factor VIII. No complications occurred and the cytological diagnosis indicated old organising haemorrhage.

Fig. 3.10 Aspiration biopsy of hydatid disease without complication (A) Two clearly defined anechoic cysts within the liver. The more anterior cyst (**) was completely aspirated without complication. (B) Five months later the patient was rescanned and multiple loculi within the cyst provided the diagnosis of hydatid disease. This was confirmed at surgery.

Seriously unwell patients have greater morbidity and mortality from biopsy, and decreased ability to cope with complications.[3] However, the alternatives to making a diagnosis often pose a greater risk. Communication with the clinicians is imperative to determine the need, relative risk and type of investigation required.

Fine needle biopsies of liver lesions, including hydatids and hemangiomata, are safe provided the needle passes through normal liver tissue to act as a seal (Fig. 3.10).

Fine needle biopsies in patients with very low platelets or poor bleeding and clotting studies are relatively safe, but are best done under real-time ultrasound control, preferably with minimal number of passes, and front wall puncture only, allowing for focal compression after the biopsy. The length of observation required after biopsy to determine possible complications varies with the site of biopsy, the patient's clinical condition, prior risk factors (for example bleeding and clotting studies) and whether a responsible adult will be available at home to assist in return to the hospital should a complication occur. This should also be considered in rural and remote areas where the distance to hospital can be significant. All factors should be considered before determining if the procedure is safely performed as an outpatient examination, and a period of observation of 1–4 hours is usually adequate after most internal organ biopsies. These procedures should always be scheduled during the morning so that if complications arise, staff are available to treat them, and the period of observation is during normal working hours.

The overall mortality and morbidity related to FNAB have been estimated in many studies and the risk of death is approximately 1 : 15 000. This compares favorably with the more invasive studies which the technique replaces. Experience and the use of certain guidelines will reduce the risk of hemorrhage and spread of infection or tumor, especially in liver biopsies.

Ultrasound has considerable advantage in the upper abdomen because of the ability to guide biopsies in oblique planes. CT guidance is usually used in the axial plane to image the needle perpendicular to that plane, gantry tilt provides a practical and simple means of avoiding bone, pleura and other organs. It is particularly useful for spine and disc aspirates and in the upper abdomen.

Various contraindications to FNAB have been given in the literature. These include the risk of biopsy of pheochromocytomas, hydatid cysts (Fig. 3.11)[15] and hemangiomas and of biopsy in the presence of ascites. The risks are considerably less than previously stated[15] and ascites does not affect the risk of biopsy.

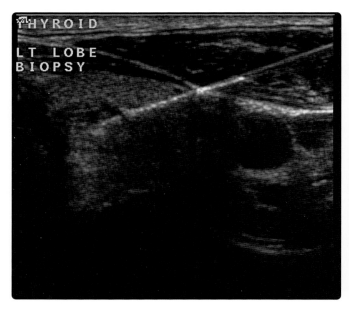

Fig. 3.12 Thyroid biopsy Aspirate is visible in the needle, and is seen to move during aspiration.

Regular audit of the results of FNAB will indicate the risk from all procedures performed in a department,[2] and will indicate individual operators who may require review of their technique or indications in relation to excessive complications or nondiagnostic yield. This is an important part of quality assurance.

Pitfalls in aspiration biopsy technique

Occasional errors may include:

1. Forgetting to remove the stilette from the needle when using the 'French technique' where no aspiration is used. The cells enter the needle during manipulation by capillary and mechanical action. The aspirate is usually more cellular and less bloody than with aspiration.
2. Maintaining negative suction while withdrawing the needle; aspirated tissue is then sucked into the syringe.[3]
3. Using anesthesia inappropriately. Anesthesia must be used sparingly with ultrasound-guided biopsies, as the microbubbles in the fluid prevent transmission of sound, and a clearly visible lesion will disappear into 'clouds' after local anesthetic has been liberally instilled into the tissues. Also, bubbles within the syringe are best cleared prior to injecting.
4. The CT and ultrasound modalities can be used to administer the targeted pleural or peritoneal anesthesia as well as assist in delineating the biopsy needle path. A needle guide, perhaps an 18G needle, may assist the biopsy process, making it more comfortable for the patient. It may also reduce the risk of pneumothorax, and, when placed through the pleura and into the lesion, allows both aspiration and core tissue biopsies to be obtained after a single pleural puncture.[16]
5. Obtaining bloody aspirates. To avoid bloody aspirates, especially if this occurs on the first pass, use the

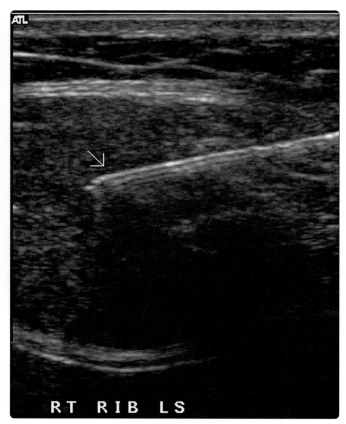

Fig. 3.13 Liver biopsy Metastatic lesion in liver, biopsied under real-time ultrasound control. Care is required to prevent a 'fixed system' which may cause tearing of tissues.

'French technique' (no aspiration).[17] The use of a longer coaxial needle, e.g. 9 cm, may prevent hemorrhagic aspirates. In pancreatic biopsies, the outer needle can be sited and confirmed in position by CT, with its tip a few centimeters from the lesion. The biopsy needle is then advanced to the required depth and only enters the lesion during the actual aspirate, rather than during confirmatory CT scans, etc. This prevents continuous trauma and local bleeding.

6. Excessive suction. Only 1–2 cc of suction via a 10-mL syringe is required to provide adequate tissue,[17] and greater aspiration pressures increase blood aspirate and may traumatize the tissue. Some radiologists continue to aspirate until they see blood in the needle hub or syringe. This always indicates an excessive aspirate of poor quality; cells should be aspirated gently and only into the needle (Fig. 3.12).
7. Maintaining a fixed system which can tear tissues. It is important not to hold the needle while the patient is breathing or moving. The correct sequence is: ask patient to breath-hold (not necessarily a full breath in, just to stop breathing, which is more comfortable for patient), oscillate needle, remove hand and release needle, allow patient to breathe, then repeat needle manipulation during breath-holding. The use of plastic tubing between the needle and syringe helps to avoid a fixed system (Fig. 3.13).

8. Changing imaging modalities. While complementary methods of imaging can be used, such as ultrasound, CT or even MRI, to further characterize a lesion prior to biopsy, the selected imaging method for biopsy should be the one which best and most readily visualizes the lesion. This is particularly important in breast biopsies, when a lesion seen on mammography may not be the lesion seen on ultrasound. Specimen radiography (mammographic quality only) and ultrasound of the breast specimen are also essential to ensure that the surgeon has removed the lesion(s). Ultrasound examination of the surgical specimen does not delay reporting to the surgeon in the operating theater as it can be performed while the mammographic X-rays are processed, and often provides further information on margins around the lesion.

9. Deviation of needles. This may be due to tissue planes or tough capsules on lesions, e.g. fibroadenoma, which causes the tip to deviate around the mass. There is a tendency to increase the size of the needle to overcome this, but it is better to decrease the diameter of the needle, as there is a greater chance that the sharp tip will penetrate the capsule (e.g. 18–20G instead of 14–16G). If the lesion can be penetrated by a fine needle, adequate tissue may be obtained, and sometimes the path of the fine needle can be seen within the lesion on ultrasound, and the puncture hole entered with a larger or core biopsy needle.

10. Poor aspiration technique. Needle manipulation must be practiced – it should be oscillated 1–2 cm, depending on the size of the lesion. It is usually possible to 'feel' the lesion. The texture of a lesion may give a guide to the possible histology, for example the gritty feel of a carcinoma (like an unripe pear), the sharp 'pop' when entering a cyst, or the rubbery texture of a fibroadenoma.

11. Poor smearing technique. Smearing the aspirate on slides should only be performed when a trained cytologist is not available, but should be practised; direct pathologist feedback may assist in improving technique.

References

1. Nordenstrom B. A new technique for transthoracic biopsy of lung changes. Br J Radiol 1965;38:550–3.

2. Cardella JF, Curtis WB, Bertino RE, et al. Quality improvement guidelines for image-guided percutaneous biopsy in adults. J Vasc Interv Radiol 2003;14:S227–30.

3. Grainger RG, Allison DJ, editors. Diagnostic Radiology – a textbook of medical imaging. 4th ed. vol. 2. London: Churchill Livingstone; 2001. p. 1272.

4. Langlois S, Le P, Henderson DW, et al. Antenatal diagnosis of lamellar ichthyosis by ultrasonically guided needle biopsy of foetal skin. In: Gill RW, Dadd MJ, editors. Proceedings of 4th Meeting of the World Federation for Ultrasound in Medicine and Biology. Oxford: Pergamon Press; 1985. p. 305.

5. VanSonnenberg E, Goodacre BW, Wittich GR, et al. Image-guided 25-gauge needle biopsy for thoracic lesions: diagnostic feasibility and safety. Radiology 2003;227:414–18.

6. Ho LM, Thomas J, Fine SA, et al. Usefulness of sonographic guidance during percutaneous biopsy of mesenteric masses. AJR 2003;180:1563–6.

7. Langlois S, Le P. Portable ultrasound on deployment. ADF Health 2003;4(2):77–80.

8. Langen Hi, Jochims M, Schneider W, et al. Distension of extrapleural spaces with contrast medium or air: value in creating safe percutaneous access to the mediastinum in cadavers. AJR 1995;164:843–9.

9. Morris EA, Liberman L, Ballon DJ, et al. MR of occult breast carcinoma in a high-risk population. AJR 2003;181:619–26.

10. Han B-K, Schnall MD, Orel SG, et al. Outcome of MRI-guided breast biopsy. AJR 2008;191:1798–804.

11. Langlois S, Le P, Carter ML. Carbon localisation of impalpable mammographic abnormalities. Australasian Radiol 1991;35(3):237–41.

12. Geraghty PR, Kee ST, McFarlane G, et al. CT-guided transthoracic needle aspiration biopsy of pulmonary nodules: needle size and pneumothorax rate. Radiology 2003;229(2):475–81.

13. Saji H, Nakamura H, Tsuchida T, et al. The incidence and risk of pneumothorax and chest tube placement after percutaneous CT-guided lung biopsy: the angle of the needle trajectory is a novel predictor. Chest 2002;121:1521–6.

14. Logan PM, Connell DG, O'Connell JX, et al. Image guided percutaneous biopsy of musculoskeletal tumours:an algorithm for selection of specific biopsy techniques. AJR 1996;166:137–41.

15. Langlois S, Le P. Fine-needle biopsy of hepatic hydatids and haemangiomas: an overstated hazard. Australasian Radiol 1989;33:144–9.

16. Moulton JS, Moore PT. Coaxial percutaneous biopsy technique with automated biopsy devices:value in improving accuracy and negative predictive value. Radiology 1993;186:515–22.

17. Titton RL, Gervais DA, Boland GW, et al. Sonography and sonographically guided fine-needle aspiration biopsy of the thyroid gland: indications and techniques, pearls and pitfalls. AJR 2003;181:267–71.

CHAPTER 4

Head and neck; salivary glands

Svante R. Orell and Jerzy Klijanienko

CLINICAL ASPECTS

The proximity of tissues of various types and the wide range of primary and metastatic neoplasms are responsible for this site being among the most interesting and challenging in FNAC diagnosis. Close cooperation with the clinician and the radiologist is necessary to clarify the anatomical relations of the target lesion, the nature of any previous lesion, and the details of any prior therapy.

FNB, as a minimally invasive technique, is particularly suitable in this sensitive area where an incisional biopsy can cause problems. A cytological diagnosis of a non-neoplastic lesion, or confirming suspected metastatic or recurrent tumor can obviate the need for surgery. In other cases, categorisation of disease to guide clinical management including further investigation, appropriate referral or rational planning of surgery can be offered. A type-specific cytological diagnosis is often possible but may require special experience and the use of ancillary laboratory techniques, and is often better deferred to the histological examination of paraffin blocks.

A discussion and review of the usefulness, indications and techniques of FNAC of tumors in the head and neck, with general guidelines for the UK, appeared recently in *Cytopathology*.[1]

Head and neck

Lesions of the salivary glands are presented in a separate section of this chapter, cervical lymph nodes in Chapter 5 and lesions of the thyroid in Chapter 6.

The place of FNA in the investigative sequence

The investigation of suspected local recurrence or nodal metastasis of previously diagnosed cancer is a common indication for FNB in the head and neck. It is of considerable clinical value in the management of these patients since therapeutic decisions can be made without delay and without the need for further diagnostic surgery. It is usually not difficult to distinguish between tumor recurrence, on the one hand, and inflammation or scarring, on the other. However,

it may be difficult to locate a small recurrence in an area of post-radiation edema and fibrosis and to obtain a representative sample. The difficulties in distinguishing radiation-induced cellular atypia from recurrent tumor are well known.

The most common primary tumors in the head and neck are squamous cell carcinoma of the lip, tongue, oral cavity, larynx, etc. Adenoma, adenocarcinoma, lymphoma and sarcoma are also encountered in many of these sites. Tumors involving a mucous membrane of the upper digestive or respiratory tracts are usually diagnosed by conventional surgical or endoscopic biopsy or by cytological examination of brush or scrape smears. Lesions that do not involve a mucous membrane are accessible to preoperative FNB, which can be performed directly under visual control or with radiological guidance. This applies to numerous different sites: scalp, eyelids, pinna of ear, nose, oral cavity, nasal sinuses, floor of mouth, tongue, palate, tonsils, nasopharynx, pharynx and parapharyngeal space.[2] Branchial and thyroglossal cysts are easily sampled. A variety of orbital and intraocular tumors, e.g. lacrimal gland tumors, lymphoma, retinoblastoma and melanoma, have been successfully diagnosed by FNB.

FNAC has been shown to be helpful also in intraoperative assessment of head and neck masses.[3] The application of FNAC in the investigation of head and neck tumors in children has been studied by Rapkiewicz et al.[4]

Single examples of serious complications have been reported following FNB of carotid body and glomus jugulare tumors.[5] Confirmation by radiological investigation is therefore preferable to needle biopsy. However, since the diagnosis may not be suspected clinically and paragangliomas can occur in unexpected sites, the pathologist must be familiar with the cytological features of these tumors.

Accuracy of diagnosis

The diagnostic accuracy of FNAC in suspected recurrent or metastatic tumors is generally high. Small nodal metastases can be missed and very well-differentiated squamous cell carcinoma can be misinterpreted as benign. Diagnosis can be difficult in irradiated tissues, with some risk of a false-positive cytological diagnosis. Samples must be quantitatively and qualitatively satisfactory, and unequivocal criteria of malignancy must be met for a positive diagnosis.

©2012 Elsevier Ltd
DOI: 10.1016/B978-0-7020-3151-9.00004-9

In primary diagnosis, accuracy varies with the size and site of the lesion, the tissue of origin and the nature of the process.[6-8] The potential for cytological diagnosis of all kinds of lesions in the head and neck has been confirmed by numerous case reports and small series of cases, but relatively few large series of specific entities have been analyzed statistically. In any case, even if a definitive, type-specific diagnosis is not possible, FNB can provide cytological categorization of the disease process with a list of differential diagnoses to guide further investigations.

Cystic lesions in the neck are common and constitute an important problem in FNAC. For example, the distinction between inflamed branchial cyst and nodal metastasis of well-differentiated squamous cell carcinoma with liquefactive necrosis can be quite difficult. False-negative diagnoses are common and false-positive diagnoses have also been reported. This problem is discussed below.

Technical considerations

Non-aspiration sampling with a 27–25-gauge needle is recommended for superficial, easily accessible lesions. Careful and gentle needling is minimally traumatic, admixture with blood is less and the operator gets a better feel of the consistency of the tissues than with the conventional technique. A syringe in a pistol grip can be used for lesions in the oral cavity or pharynx to provide sufficient operating length to reach the target. A spray surface anesthetic is useful in transmucosal biopsies. CT or US guidance is needed for non-palpable and deep-sited targets, and to obtain representative samples from small, heterogeneous or partly cystic lesions. Both air-dried and alcohol-fixed smears should be made routinely, and spare slides kept for special stains or immune markers. Cell blocks or liquid-based preparations can be very useful for voluminous aspirates of mainly fluid or blood. Selective, cost-effective use of ancillary techniques is best achieved if the pathologist is present at the biopsy and can assess samples immediately. In lesions of a suspected infectious nature, material should be collected specifically for microbiological investigation.

Salivary glands

Salivary gland tumors are generally not subjected to incisional or core needle biopsy because of the possible risk of causing a fistula or disruption of the capsule with seeding of tumor cells and subsequent recurrence. There is no evidence that FNB causes either of these complications.

The place of FNA in the investigative sequence

The 1991 WHO classification of salivary gland tumors lists nine types of primary benign tumors (adenomas) and 18 types of malignant tumors (carcinomas), some with subtypes. In addition, there are non-epithelial tumors, malignant lymphoma, secondary tumors and a number of tumor-like conditions.[9] Faced with this extraordinary variety of entities, a precise diagnosis by FNAC may seem an impossible task. However, the aim of FNAC combined with clinical and radiological findings is to provide a preliminary assessment on which management decisions can be based, not necessarily a definitive, type-specific diagnosis. Is surgery indicated or can the lesion be watched? How urgent is the surgery and how extensive is it likely to be?

We recommend a stepwise approach to the cytological diagnosis of salivary gland lesions:

1. Is the lesion arising from the salivary gland or from adjacent tissues?
2. If of salivary gland origin, is it non-neoplastic or neoplastic?
3. If neoplastic, is it benign, low-grade or high-grade malignant?
4. The exact tumor type can be predicted in many cases but this is often best left to histology.

   ad1 This is not always easy to decide. Metastasis to intraparotid lymph nodes and mesenchymal tumors arising from the salivary gland stroma can cause confusion. Lesions arising from lymph nodes, soft tissue or skin adjacent to the gland can mimic salivary gland tumors,[10] and ectopic salivary gland tissue can occur in other sites.

   ad2 The choice between surgical or conservative treatment often depends on the outcome of FNB. Over 50% of patients referred to our clinics for FNB of an enlarged salivary gland had a non-neoplastic disorder such as sialadenosis, sialadenitis, sialolithiasis or retention cyst. Less than 10% of these patients had surgery.[11] However, diagnostic difficulties occur already at this level. Is inflammation and mucus retention seen in the samples due to sialadenitis or a consequence of underlying neoplasia? A cystic tumor can be misinterpreted as a simple cyst if the solid component is not sampled. Florid regenerative hyperplasia, metaplasia and atypia of duct epithelium in chronic sialadenitis can be mistaken for neoplasia. Necrotizing sialometaplasia caused by infarction of minor salivary glands of the palate is the most drastic example. Low-grade mucoepidermoid carcinoma can mimic chronic sialadenitis and vice versa. Inflammation and subsequent fibrosis can be focal, appearing as a palpable nodule clinically suggestive of a neoplasm, mainly in the submandibular gland (Küttner's tumor).

   ad3 It could be argued that all salivary gland tumors should be completely excised and that the distinction between benign, low grade and high grade is of little importance. However, a cytological suspicion of malignancy ensures immediate surgery, whereas surgery may be wait-listed and delayed if the tumor is thought to be benign. If the tumor is benign, surgery can be avoided in elderly patients and patients of poor surgical risk. A suggestion of high-grade malignancy alerts the surgeon to the possible need for more extensive surgery. Intraoperative confirmation by frozen section may be advisable if there is a risk of sacrificing the facial nerve, or if neck dissection is considered. In case of inoperable malignancy, a cytological diagnosis may allow the choice of palliative treatment without a need for diagnostic surgery.

ad4 A type-specific preoperative diagnosis by FNB is not often essential. Although cytological criteria are well defined and the diagnosis is relatively easy for the commonest salivary gland tumors, the heterogeneity of many tumors and the overlap of cytomorphologic features limit the accuracy of subtyping. FNB samples are tiny and may not be representative of the whole lesion, a limitation that is to a variable extent shared by core needle biopsies and small incisional biopsies. It may be preferable to report the FNB as a shortlist of differential diagnoses with a preference rather than as a type-specific diagnosis.

The potential cost-savings achievable by preoperative FNB of salivary gland tumors have been analyzed by Layfield et al.[12]

Accuracy of diagnosis

A number of papers documenting the diagnostic accuracy of FNB in large numbers of cases of salivary gland neoplasms of several types were published from the Karolinska Hospital in Sweden in the 1960s.[13-17] Over 90% of neoplasms were recognized, over 90% of pleomorphic adenomas were correctly typed, and most malignant tumors were diagnosed as such. The accuracy increased with increasing experience. Many other studies of large series of cases have since followed.[18-20] A review of the literature in 1994 found that the diagnostic sensitivity varied between 81% and 100%, specificity was 94–100% and the accuracy of tumor typing was 61–80%.[21] In a more recent study by Klijanienko et al. the sensitivity was 94%, specificity was 97% and the accuracy was 95%.[22]

Using the criteria developed by the Karolinska group reinforced by later authors, the diagnosis of pleomorphic adenoma and of Warthin's tumor is reliable in most cases. Adenoid cystic and acinic cell carcinomas also have distinctive cytological features. However, there are many pitfalls. These may be due to sampling problems, for example false-negative diagnoses in cystic tumors. Pleomorphic adenoma, Warthin's tumor, low-grade mucoepidermoid carcinoma and acinic cell carcinoma can all occasionally be predominantly cystic. The limitation to accuracy due to the small size and selective character of FNB samples has been mentioned. Other examples of diagnostic difficulties are regenerative epithelial hyperplasia and squamous metaplasia in sialadenitis or Warthin's tumor, and epithelial atypia and high cellularity in pleomorphic adenoma. Overlapping cytological features between different tumor types are common, for example hyaline stromal globules initially regarded as distinctive of adenoid cystic carcinoma can occur in other tumors. The distinction between primary and metastatic cancer may be very difficult in poorly differentiated malignancies.

Problems and pitfalls in FNAC diagnosis of salivary gland lesions have attracted considerable interest and a number of papers on this topic can be found in the literature.[23-27]

Complications

Needling of non-neoplastic lesions, particularly in the submandibular gland, is often moderately painful and may cause local bleeding. Blood may seep into the mouth causing patient concern, and may cause some post-biopsy swelling. Tumor implantation in the needle track has not been reported post-FNB, nor has serious damage to adjacent structures such as the facial nerve.

Infarction or hemorrhage of salivary gland tumors post-FNB occasionally occurs.[28] Necrosis and subsequent reactive changes and repair can cause difficulties in histological diagnosis.[29,30] A gentle biopsy technique using thin needles reduces the incidence of this complication.

Technical considerations

Biopsy without aspiration using a 27–25-gauge needle is recommended. Heavily bloodstained samples may contain tissue fragments, which can be recovered in a cell block. Liquid-based preparations can be useful as a supplement to conventional smears.[31] Fluid aspirated from both non-neoplastic and neoplastic cystic lesions is often very poor in cells. Material obtained from the cyst wall is more likely to be diagnostic. If this is not possible, follow-up should be recommended and the biopsy repeated with US guidance. Most cystic lesions are multilocular so that complete emptying is not possible except in the rare simple cysts.

We recommend the use of both air-dried (MGG, Diff-Quik) and wet-fixed (Pap, H&E) smears in parallel. A mucin stain can be helpful, and cell blocks in selected cases.

FNB material can be used for various ancillary techniques for which cell blocks or liquid-based preparations are particularly suitable. Immunocytochemistry has a limited role in FNAC of salivary gland lesions. Antibodies directed against S-100 protein, keratins, GFAP, smooth muscle actin, desmin and p63 may be useful to differentiate pleomorphic adenoma, myoepithelioma, myoepithelial carcinoma, rhabdomyosarcoma, sarcoma and epithelial-myoepithelial carcinoma. Cytogenetic rearrangements have been found in pleomorphic adenoma and mucoepidermoid carcinoma. Loss of heterozygosity has been described in pleomorphic adenoma, adenoid cystic carcinoma, carcinoma ex pleomorphic adenoma and mucoepidermoid carcinoma. HPV DNA is commonly seen in head and neck squamous carcinomas and its identification by molecular techniques is a valuable guide to diagnosis in some cases (see below cystic squamous lesions, p. 41).

CYTOLOGICAL FINDINGS

Head and neck

Non-neoplastic lesions

Branchial cyst (Fig. 4.1)[32,33]

CRITERIA FOR DIAGNOSIS

- Variably thick, gray–yellow, pus-like fluid,
- Anuclear, keratinized cells,
- Squamous epithelial cells, mainly mature, some metaplastic,
- A background of amorphous debris, and often inflammatory cells,
- Appropriate anatomical site.

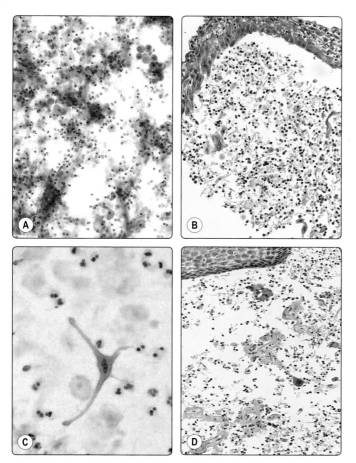

Fig. 4.1 Branchial cyst (A) FNB smear. Neutrophils, debris and mature squamous cells including degenerate forms; (B) Corresponding tissue (C, D) Other case Single highly atypical squamous cells in FNB smear (C) and in tissue section (D).

Nodal metastasis of well-differentiated SCC with liquefactive necrosis is a common, important and often difficult differential diagnosis (Figs. 4.2 and 4.3).[34,35] Although 75% of branchial cysts occur in the age group 20–40 and metastatic squamous carcinoma mainly in patients over 40, there is a considerable overlap in the age group 40–60.[32] We have seen several patients in whom a branchial cyst first presented clinically at the age of 60 or even later, and on the other hand, metastatic SCC can occur in young adults. The sensitivity of FNB in diagnosing malignancy in lateral cervical cysts varies widely (35–75%). In a review of the literature by Sheahan et al.[36] 4–24% of cases initially diagnosed as branchial cysts had unsuspected squamous cell carcinoma on histological examination. Many therefore recommend biopsy for histology even when FNB is negative, especially in patients over 40.

The diagnostic difficulties are due to the fact that squamous epithelial cells aspirated from a cystic metastasis of well-differentiated SCC are often anucleate or of parakeratotic type with a mature cytoplasm and a small pyknotic nucleus appearing cytologically bland, while inflammation of a benign cyst can result in immature squamous metaplasia and worrying cytological atypia. Figures 4.1 and 4.2 compare cells exfoliating from the lining of inflamed branchial cysts with those from cystic SCCs seen in histological sections. Helpful clues are that material sampled from a cystic SCC is more obviously necrotic than inflammatory, and a careful search usually reveals a few squamous epithelial cells with malignant nuclear features or abnormal keratinised cells with bizarre, globoid shapes and dense orangeophilic (Pap) cytoplasm. The nuclear atypia and hyperchromasia seen in squamous cells from a benign cyst is of degenerative type. But the distinction is not always easy (see Figs 4.1C and D). In some cases, the FNB can only be reported as indeterminate. The only ancillary test we have found useful in this setting is HPV DNA sequencing. Occult tonsillar carcinomas and other oral cavity carcinomas with cystic lymph node metastases are a common clinical problem. Many such carcinomas contain HPV DNA as evaluated by PCR or other molecular testing and a positive result in an FNA sample is strong evidence that a lesion is metastatic carcinoma rather than a branchial cleft cyst or other benign cyst.

A branchial cyst can develop relatively rapidly as a firm mass of significant size in the lateral neck. It is most often seen in young adults but may become clinically apparent at any age. The sudden appearance of a mass may cause both the patient and the doctor considerable anxiety. A malignant cervical lymph node or a thyroid tumor may be suspected, or it may result in a useless course of antibiotics. An instant diagnosis by FNB is therefore of clinical value.

The aspiration of fluid causes the mass to decrease in size but it rarely disappears completely. The aspirate resembles pus also in non-inflamed cysts but the fluid is usually sterile. Sometimes the fluid contains large numbers of acute inflammatory cells. Multinucleate giant cells representing a granulomatous reaction in the wall of the cyst are sometimes seen. Lymphoid tissue, although evident in tissue sections, is not often represented in smears.

PROBLEMS AND DIFFERENTIAL DIAGNOSIS

- ◆ Well-differentiated squamous cell carcinoma with cystic degeneration,
- ◆ Thyroglossal cyst.

Other non-neoplastic cysts

The content of a *thyroglossal cyst* can be cytologically indistinguishable from that of a branchial cyst. The differential diagnosis is mainly based on the anatomical site of the lesion. The content is sometimes mucinous and mucin-secreting and/or ciliated columnar epithelial cells may be found in the smears. Thyroid epithelial cells are rarely present (see p. 122).[37]

Mucocele of the lips, oral mucosa, tongue,[38] and occasionally of the paranasal sinuses may be referred to FNB to exclude neoplasia or infection. The aspirated mucinous material contains mainly mucinophages and some inflammatory cells. Mucinophages sometimes appear atypical, especially in MGG-stained smears, and a suspicion of well-differentiated mucinous adenocarcinoma can arise (see Fig. 4.23).

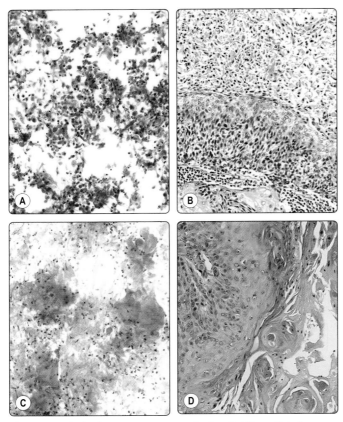

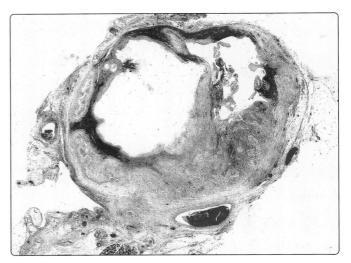

Fig. 4.3 Cystic metastasis of squamous carcinoma Whole section of cervical lymph node containing metastatic deposit of squamous carcinoma with central cystic degeneration. Note similarity to branchial cyst (HE).

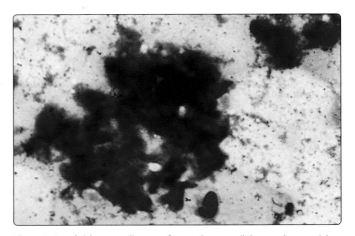

Fig. 4.4 Amyloid tumor Clumps of amorphous acellular purple material (MGG, HP).

Fig. 4.2 Cystically degenerate metastasis of well-differentiated squamous carcinoma (A, B) Exfoliating atypical cells of 'parakeratotic' type in FNB smear and corresponding tissue section; (C, D) Other example with predominance of anucleate keratinized cells and clumps of keratin in the cyst lumen.

Amyloid tumor (Fig. 4.4)

CRITERIA FOR DIAGNOSIS

◆ Clumps of amorphous acellular material,
◆ Apple-green birefringence with Congo red stain.

Solitary deposits of amyloid, so-called amyloid tumors, are occasionally found submucosally in the hypopharynx, the larynx and other parts of the upper respiratory tract. Amyloid stains an intense magenta color with MGG, less specific yellowish-green with Papanicolaou. It has a fairly dense amorphous texture with a finely fibrillar rather than hyaline structure discernible in high power. In FNB smears, the amyloid may be associated with histiocytic giant cells, lymphocytes or epithelial and/or mesenchymal cells from surrounding tissues (see also Chapter 14).

PROBLEMS AND DIFFERENTIAL DIAGNOSIS

The appearances of amyloid in cytological smears are not always characteristic enough to be diagnostic. It can be confused with dense thyroid colloid or hyalinised fibrous stroma.[39] Its nature should therefore be confirmed by staining with Congo red and polarisation. In the head and neck, the possibility of origin from medullary thyroid carcinoma, primary or metastatic, must always be considered, and immunostaining for calcitonin performed.

Inflammatory conditions

The cytology of *lymphadenitis* is described in Chapter 5. Special attention has been given to the diagnosis of *sarcoid* and of *tuberculous lymphadenitis* in the head and neck region.[40] We have seen examples of *actinomycosis* of the parotid region and of the pharynx, clinically suspected of neoplasia due to the induration of the tissues. Sulphur granules were not seen macroscopically but microscopically a few clumps of finely filamentous microorganisms surrounded by polymorphs suggested the correct diagnosis, subsequently confirmed by culture of the aspirate (Fig. 4.5). (See also Chapter 18.)

Neoplasms

Squamous cell carcinoma (Figs 4.2 and 4.6)

Squamous cell carcinoma (SCC) is by far the commonest type of carcinoma encountered in the head and neck. Diagnostic criteria are listed in Chapter 8. Lymph node metastases of well-differentiated squamous carcinoma, particularly those arising in the Waldeyer's ring, have a

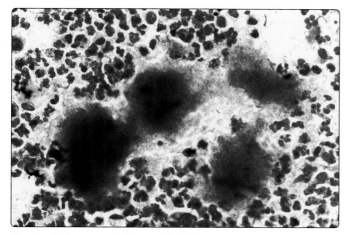

Fig. 4.5 Actinomycosis Clumps of finely fibrillar organisms in a background of neutrophils (MGG, HP).

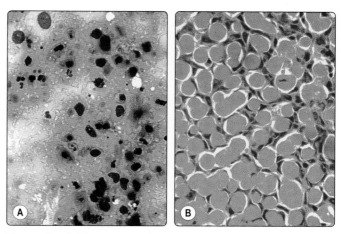

Fig. 4.7 Basaloid squamous cell carcinoma of head and neck (A) Poorly differentiated cells with squamous features (MGG, HP; (B) Tissue section mimicking adenoid cystic carcinoma (H&E, IP).

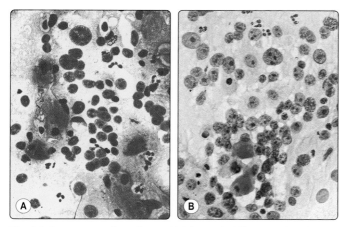

Fig. 4.6 Squamous cell carcinoma Mainly poorly differentiated malignant cells with large vesicular nuclei and large nucleoli; a few squamous and keratinized cells. FNB smears of cervical lymph node metastasis from squamous carcinoma of larynx (A, MGG; B, Pap, HP).

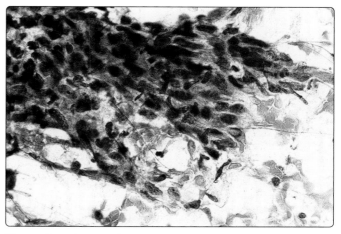

Fig. 4.8 Nasopharyngeal carcinoma (squamous cell carcinoma, WHO type II) Epithelial fragment of spindly and basaloid squamous epithelial cells with no evidence of keratinization (Pap, HP).

tendency to undergo liquefactive degeneration (see Fig. 4.3).[41] The existence of primary SCC arising in a pre-existing branchial cyst has been doubted and is, in any case, an extremely rare event.[42] The distinction from non-neoplastic cysts, mainly branchial cysts has been discussed above. Non-keratinizing squamous cell carcinoma may be represented in smears mainly by small basaloid cells in which case the differential diagnosis includes basal cell carcinoma, pilomatrixoma, poorly differentiated adenoid cystic carcinoma and other small cell tumors. Cells from a poorly differentiated squamous cell carcinoma have large vesicular nuclei and macronucleoli and resemble other anaplastic tumors such as melanoma and large cell lymphoma (Fig. 4.6).

Basaloid squamous carcinoma (Fig. 4.7) is a rare distinct variant of squamous cell carcinoma of the head and neck, which is clinically aggressive and has a predilection for the hypopharynx and the tongue. The smear findings are of squamous cell carcinoma without specific features, but a predominance of basal cells may make the distinction from the solid variant of adenoid cystic carcinoma difficult.[43]

Nasopharyngeal carcinoma (NPC) (Figs 4.8, 4.9, and 5.59)[44–47]

CRITERIA FOR DIAGNOSIS (UNDIFFERENTIATED CARCINOMA NASOPHARYNGEAL TYPE (UCNT)/WHO TYPE III/LYMPHOEPITHELIAL CARCINOMA)

◆ Undifferentiated malignant cells, single and in clusters,
◆ Variable amount of pale, fragile cytoplasm,
◆ Large vesicular nuclei with prominent central nucleoli,
◆ Admixture with, and background of, lymphoid cells, often with prominent plasma cells,
◆ Ancillary tests: neoplastic cells positive for cytokeratin, negative for lymphocyte markers. EBV-associated nuclear antigen.

Nasopharyngeal carcinoma (NPC) is a clinicopathologic entity different from other squamous cell carcinomata of the head and neck. It is distinguished by its particular histology, geographic distribution, relationship to Epstein-Barr virus, and the absence of an alcohol or tobacco etiological relationship. A proportion of NPCs show squamous differentiation

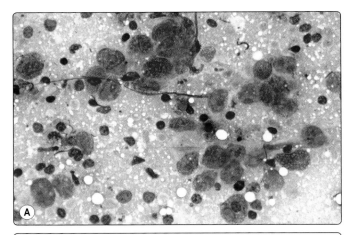

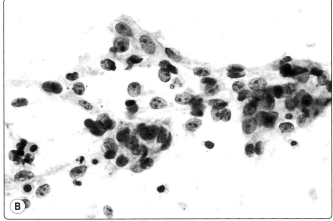

Fig. 4.9 Nasopharyngeal carcinoma (undifferentiated, lymphoepithelial type, WHO type III) Loose clusters of undifferentiated epithelial cells with vesicular nuclei, prominent nucleoli and pale fragile cytoplasm. Background of lymphocytes. (**A**, MGG, HP; **B**, H&E, HP).

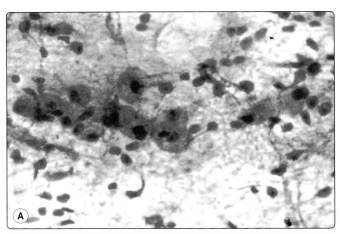

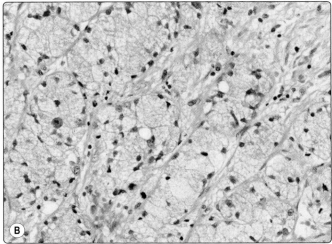

Fig. 4.10 Mucinous adenocarcinoma of maxillary sinus (**A**) Poorly cohesive round cells with abundant vacuolated cytoplasm and relatively bland nuclei resembling mucinophages in a background of mucus; FNB of cervical lymph node metastasis (Diff-Quik, HP); (**B**) Corresponding tissue section of primary tumor (H&E; IP).

and the cytological pattern of non-keratinizing squamous cell carcinoma (squamous cell carcinoma/WHO type II) (Fig. 4.8). Keratinized cells (WHO type I) are uncommonly found. The majority of NPC are poorly differentiated or undifferentiated. Cells from undifferentiated NPC (UCNT, WHO type III) form loose clusters with no specific microarchitectural pattern, and are usually mixed with lymphoid cells. In the 'lymphoepitheliomatous' type (Schmincke-Regaud) the cells tend to be less cohesive, resembling Hodgkin's disease or large cell non-Hodgkin lymphoma. However, in NPC, the malignant cells are still clustered and have more abundant pale cytoplasm contrasting with the lymphoid cells in the background (Fig. 4.9). Plasma cells are frequently found among the lymphoid cells. Immunostaining for cytokeratin and a pan-lymphocyte marker is helpful. Epstein-Barr virus-associated nuclear antigen is demonstrable by anticomplement immunofluorescence in undifferentiated tumors. Other patterns of growth may occur and may cause diagnostic problems; for example, spindle cell forms may be difficult to recognize as carcinoma.

NPC frequently presents to the cytologist as a lymph node metastasis in the neck without a known primary. Cytological recognition is important since the primary is often clinically occult.

Carcinoma of sinonasal tract

Primary or secondary sinonasal tract malignancies are rare and demonstrate a wide range of cytologic patterns. An accurate and definitive diagnosis can be made in many tumors, especially in carcinomas similar to transitional and squamous cell carcinoma, carcinoma with specific differentiation, sarcoma or melanoma.[48] Poorly differentiated nasal sinus carcinomas of transitional cell type yield clusters of tightly packed cells and single cells with obvious malignant nuclear features and scanty cytoplasm.[49] Smears of the intestinal type of adenocarcinoma of paranasal sinuses show aggregates of well-differentiated adenocarcinoma cells, including columnar cells and goblet cells, with a background of abundant mucus. In a case of mucinous adenocarcinoma of maxillary sinus, FNB smears from a regional lymph node metastasis showed dispersed cells with abundant cytoplasm distended by mucus and small relatively bland nuclei. A background of abundant mucus contributes to a close resemblance to a mucocele (Fig. 4.10).

Paraganglioma (carotid body and glomus jugulare tumors) (Figs 4.11–4.13)[5,50–52]

CRITERIA FOR DIAGNOSIS

- ◆ Neoplastic cells single and loosely clustered, often forming curved rows or a vaguely follicular pattern; bloody background,
- ◆ Abundant pale cytoplasm with indistinct cell borders,
- ◆ A fine red cytoplasmic granulation (MGG) may be seen in some cells,
- ◆ Nuclei rounded to spindle with granular or speckled, evenly distributed chromatin,
- ◆ Variable anisokaryosis; scattered single cells with considerably enlarged nuclei, some bi-nucleate, in a background of generally uniform nuclei is characteristic,
- ◆ Positive staining with neuroendocrine markers.

PROBLEMS AND DIFFERENTIAL DIAGNOSIS

The cytological pattern is suggestive of an endocrine neoplasm and, given the anatomical site, the main differential diagnosis is a thyroid tumor. A follicular arrangement of the tumor cells may suggest a follicular carcinoma, but the fine red cytoplasmic granulation, the characteristic anisokaryosis and the presence of spindle cells closely resemble medullary carcinoma, and this is the main differential diagnosis (Fig. 4.12). Immune markers are helpful. Cells of paraganglioma stain positively for neuroendocrine markers. Staining for calcitonin is negative in most cases, but can occasionally be positive. Cytokeratin, thyroglobulin and TTF1 are negative. Intranuclear cytoplasmic inclusions as in papillary and some other carcinomas of the thyroid can be found in some paragangliomas.[50] Knowledge of the exact anatomical site is obviously important. However, paraganglioma can occur in atypical locations including, although rarely, the thyroid. For example, one of our cases diagnosed by FNB had a tumor in the tonsillar region, clinically thought to be a deep parotid tumor (Fig. 4.11); another had a supraclavicular mass diagnosed clinically as lymphadenopathy. Both were histologically confirmed as paragangliomas.

Paraganglioma with a spindle cell pattern can mimic other spindle cell tumors in the neck such as spindle cell medullary carcinoma of thyroid and soft tissue tumors. Nuclear pleomorphism can sometimes be prominent enough to suggest malignancy (Fig. 4.13).[5] As in other endocrine tumors, pleomorphism is not a reliable indicator of malignancy, mitotic rate and evidence of necrosis are better related to clinical behavior, and metastasis is the only definitive proof.

Paragangliomas are extremely vascular lesions and the aspirate often appears to be pure blood. If this is the case, smears may be non-diagnostic but diagnostic tissue fragments can sometimes be found in a cell block.
- ◆ Thyroid neoplasms
- ◆ Paraganglioma in atypical sites
- ◆ Spindle cell pattern
- ◆ Nuclear pleomorphism

Malignant lymphoma

Malignant lymphoma can involve several sites in the head and neck including tonsils, salivary glands, orbit, scalp and cervical lymph nodes. Cytological criteria are given in Chapter 5. The distinction from reactive lymphoproliferative lesions can be difficult. A mixed population of lymphoid cells dominated by lymphocytes and including germinal center material favors a reactive process. Immune marker studies by flow cytometry to demonstrate monoclonality versus polyclonality is generally indispensable in this situation.

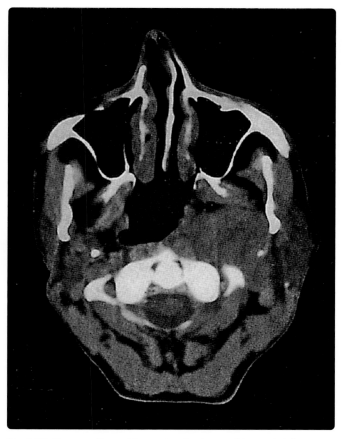

Fig. 4.11 Paraganglioma CT scan showing large solid mass in left oropharynx; paraganglioma diagnosed by FNB.

Meningioma (Fig. 4.14)[53–55]

CRITERIA FOR DIAGNOSIS

- ◆ Fibroblast-like spindle cells in loose clusters, cell balls and whorls,
- ◆ Small, tight whorls of cells; occasional psammoma bodies,
- ◆ Pale cytoplasm, indistinct cell borders,
- ◆ Pale ovoid or elongated nuclei with finely granular, evenly distributed chromatin,
- ◆ Immunostaining: vimentin, CK and S-100 positive, smooth muscle actin negative.

Extracranial meningiomas occur in relation to the base of the skull, the scalp, the orbit, the nasal cavity, the paranasal sinuses and the middle ear. In one of our cases, a meningioma extended from the base of the skull to present as a maxillary gingival lump which was correctly diagnosed by FNB. Although uncommon, meningioma should be remembered in the differential diagnosis of any tumor in the head and neck. The exact anatomical location shown by CT, the presence of characteristic whorls and the bland nuclear morphology are pointers to the correct diagnosis.

Olfactory neuroblastoma (Fig. 4.15)[49,56,57]

This rare tumor occurs in the upper nasal cavity and may cause nasal obstruction. It may also present as lymph node

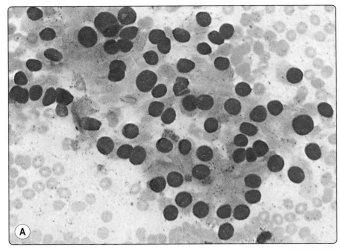

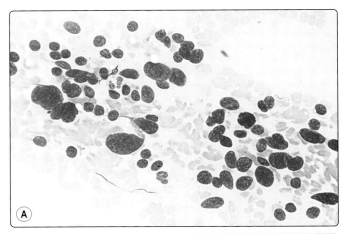

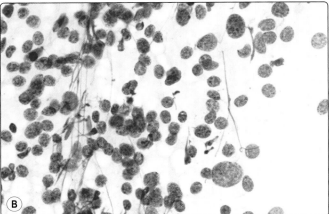

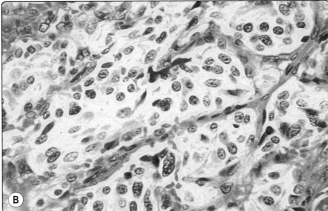

Fig. 4.13 Paraganglioma (atypical) (A) Smear showing prominent anisokaryosis but a uniformly bland chromatin pattern (MGG, HP); (B) Tissue section of the same case (H&E, IP).

Fig. 4.12 Paraganglioma Loosely clustered cells; suggestion of follicular arrangement resembling thyroid epithelium; anisokaryosis and 'speckled' chromatin (Pap) typical of neuroendocrine tumors. Very fine eosinophilic cytoplasmic granules visible under the microscope but not in photograph; (**A**, MGG, HP; **B**, Pap, HP).

secondaries in the neck. Several cases diagnosed by FNB have been reported. The pseudorosettes formed by the tumor cells may be mistaken for microacini of an adenocarcinoma, but the nuclear morphology is relatively bland, and finely fibrillar material may be seen in the center of the rosettes, similar to the common neuroblastoma. Immunostaining for neuroendocrine and epithelial markers is helpful in the differential diagnosis.

Tumors of the orbit

The orbital region contains a variety of anatomical structures including eyelid, conjunctiva, caruncle, uvea, retina, lacrimal gland, lacrimal drainage system, skin, skin adnexa and soft tissues, and is surrounded by bone and cartilage. This complexity of adjacent, highly specialized tissues may give rise to a variety of inflammatory, benign and malignant conditions. Furthermore, the rich vascularity of the orbital region is responsible for the common occurrence of metastases from various organs, mainly from the breast and the lung.

Palpable orbital tumors can be successfully diagnosed using the FNB technique. A comparative cytological/

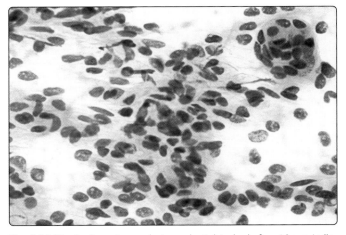

Fig. 4.14 Meningioma Loose cluster and a tight whorl of ovoid or spindle cells with a bland, finely granular nuclear chromatin (H&E, HP).

histological study of 286 aspirates of palpable orbital and eyelid tumors showed that a concordant diagnosis of malignancy and of tumor type was achieved in 87% of cases. A false-positive diagnosis was made in 1.6% and a false-negative diagnosis in 1.8% of cases.[58] Image-guided FNB is recommended for non-palpable lesions.[59]

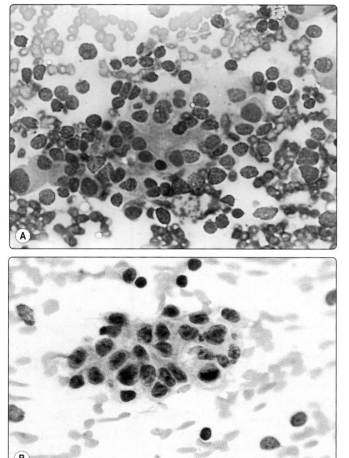

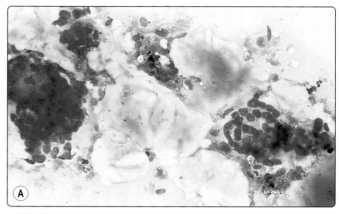

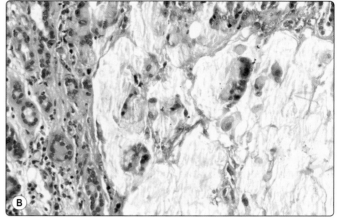

Fig. 4.16 Mucinous adenocarcinoma, lacrimal gland Clusters of small, relatively bland glandular epithelial cells, some columnar or goblet cells, background of abundant mucin (**A**, smear, MGG, IP; **B**, tissue section, H&E, IP).

Fig. 4.15 Olfactory neuroblastoma Clustered and single neoplastic cells with irregular nuclei and vaguely microacinar groups resembling adenocarcinoma; rosettes not obvious in this example (**A**, MGG, HP; **B**, Pap, HP).

Lymphoproliferative processes constitute the main problem in the orbit. A cytological diagnosis can be difficult, but FNB is useful and is a valuable addition to ultrasound, CT and MRI. The technique is reliable and safe. The combination with ancillary techniques, mainly immunocytochemistry, flow cytometry and genomic techniques, provides a reliable basis for accurate typing,[60–64] and this tool may help to avoid a traumatic surgical intervention.

Extramedullary erythropoiesis/myeloid metaplasia can also give rise to an orbital mass, for example in patients with myelofibrosis. Erythroblasts, megakaryocytes and granulocytic precursors are found in the aspirate, usually easily recognized in MGG-stained smears (see p. 286). As mentioned above, *metastatic malignancy* is also relatively common in this site. Orbital tumors such as retinoblastoma, melanoma and metastases usually exhibit specific cytologic morphology allowing an accurate diagnosis.

Tumors of the lacrimal gland are mainly similar to primary salivary gland tumors and the same diagnostic criteria (see below) apply.[65] The question whether the tumor is primary or metastatic in this site should be investigated.[66] The commonest lacrimal gland tumors are pleomorphic adenoma,

carcinoma ex pleomorphic adenoma and salivary duct carcinoma. An example of FNB of a well-differentiated mucinous adenocarcinoma primary in the lacrimal gland is illustrated in Figure 4.16. Malignant lymphoma of lacrimal gland has been reported.

A variety of inflammatory conditions of the orbit can also be diagnosed by FNB. These may present as masses, cysts, abscesses, discharging sinuses and dermal plaques and nodules. Granulomatous inflammations are most common, such as chalazion, tuberculosis, *Cysticercus cellulosae* and ruptured epidermal cysts.[67]

Intraocular tumors

Fine needle biopsy of intraocular tumors, performed in theater, has not gained wide acceptance among ophthalmologists because of the (negligible) risk of tumor cell dissemination, intraocular complications and unfamiliarity with the technique. It offers a means of distinguishing – in the exceptional case when this is a problem for clinical diagnosis and management – between a primary and a metastatic intraocular malignancy. In our experience, the only complication has been vitreous hematoma. Indications for

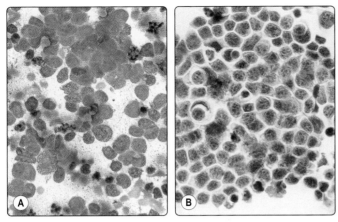
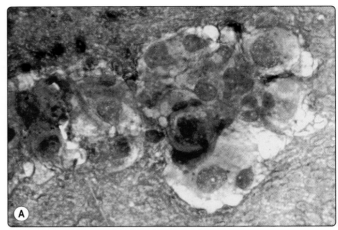

Fig. 4.17 Retinoblastoma Smear pattern of a malignant small round cell tumor, some clustering but no distinctive microarchitectural features (**A**, MGG, HP; **B**, Pap, HP).

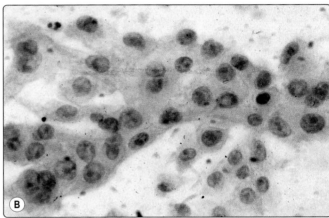

Fig. 4.18 Chordoma Physalipherous cells embedded in chondromyxoid stroma. The characteristic vacuolated cytoplasm and the chondromyxoid stroma are much less obvious in the Pap-stained smear. This tumor presented clinically as a retropharyngeal mass (**A**, MGG, HP; **B**, Pap, HP).

intraocular FNB are: (1) the patient refuses enucleation, (2) a definitive diagnosis cannot be made by conventional and ancillary ophthalmologic techniques, (3) metastatic tumor is suspected in the absence of a known primary site, and (4) genomic analysis of intraocular melanoma.[68] Malignant melanoma, retinoblastoma, medulloepithelioma and metastatic tumors are the commonest intraocular tumors.

FNB smears of *intraocular melanoma* are similar to those of melanomas from other sites. Uveal melanomas are usually rich in pigment. The cells are often relatively bland, monomorphous spindle cells. Immunostaining for S-100 and HMB-45 provides a means of confirmation if melanin is not visible.[69] For a detailed description of the cytology of melanoma, see Chapter 14.

Retinoblastoma has a characteristic age distribution, family history, radiologic findings and fundus semiology. Cells of retinoblastoma may be found in fluid aspirated from the anterior chamber of the eye. The cytology is similar to other malignant small round cell tumors (Fig. 4.17).[70,71] The cells are small with hyperchromatic nuclei and scant basophilic cytoplasm. Rosette-like structures, nuclear molding and necrosis are frequently seen.

Metastatic intraocular tumors can derive from any organ but are most commonly from the lungs and breast.

Malignant lymphoma may rarely involve the uveal tract and can be diagnosed by cytological examination of fluid aspirated from the vitreous.[72]

Intracranial tumors

We have little experience of FNB of intracranial tumors and the reader is referred to the literature, for example the review by Willems.[73] The cytology of intracranial tumors applied to intraoperative diagnosis was beautifully described 60 years ago by Russel.[74] This application is of great clinical value in view of the technical difficulties with frozen sections.[75–77] Rarely, intracranial tumors involve extracranial sites in the head and neck. Meningioma is the most common example. FNB of extracranial metastasis of glioblastoma multiforme has been reported.[78] Tumors of the base of the skull such as pituitary tumors are accessible to FNB through the nose.

Tumors of soft tissues and bone

Soft tissue tumors such as *spindle cell lipoma, nerve sheath tumors* and *malignant fibrous histiocytoma* are not uncommon in the head and neck and can occur in sites where they may be clinically mistaken for lymphadenopathy, salivary gland tumor, etc. The tongue is a site of predilection for *granular cell tumor*.[79] Distinction between this tumor elsewhere in the neck and *adult rhabdomyoma* may be difficult.[80] A not infrequent pitfall is proliferative non-neoplastic lesions in the neck, mainly nodular and proliferative fasciitis, which can be mistaken for a malignant soft tissue tumor. *Rhabdomyosarcoma*, usually of the embryonal type, is among the most common malignant head and neck tumors in children. Cytological criteria and differential diagnosis for soft tissue tumors are presented in Chapter 15.

Chordoma may present as an orbital, nasal or posterior pharyngeal mass accessible to FNB through the oral cavity

(Fig. 4.18). Of bone tumors affecting the skull, *eosinophilic granuloma*, *multiple myeloma* and *metastatic carcinoma* lend themselves to cytological diagnosis. Cytomorphological criteria for bone tumors are given in Chapter 16.

FNB has not been extensively applied to odontogenic tumors and cysts. A few reports of FNB of lesions in the jawbones[81,82] and of *ameloblastoma*[83,84] and ameloblastic carcinoma[85] have appeared in the literature. Cells of ameloblastoma are basaloid, often spindle or rounded, and occur in clusters or pseudopapillary projections. Squamoid and keratinized cells without prominent atypia are usually present (Fig. 4.19).

Metastatic tumors

Metastatic tumors are common in this region. For example, tumors of the scalp have been shown to be predominantly metastatic.[86] Guidelines for the identification of the primary tumor are given elsewhere.

Salivary glands

Normal structures (Fig. 4.20)

- Acinar cells (serous or mucinous),
- Ductal epithelial cells,
- Scant fibrovascular stroma

Smears from normal or near-normal glands are usually poor in cells and heavily blood stained. Sometimes a surprisingly large number of acinar cells and tissue fragments are obtained, which can occasionally raise a suspicion of neoplasia (well-differentiated acinic cell carcinoma). The acinar cells form cohesive tissue fragments of regular spherical acini delineated by their basement membrane, often joined by small ductular structures and held together by a small amount of fibrovascular stroma, resembling a bunch of grapes. Serous acinar cells have abundant, finely vacuolated bubbly cytoplasm, an eccentric small round, dark nucleus at the base of the cell, and a small nucleolus. Scattered, stripped acinar cell nuclei may be present in the background. These must not be mistaken for lymphocytes. Ductal epithelial cells may also be found forming small cohesive flat sheets or tubules. The cells are smaller, the cytoplasm is dense, sometimes squamoid, and the nuclei are round or oval. Other common findings are adipose and loose fibrous tissue and strands of endothelial cells. Lymphoid cells may be present, derived from adjacent or intraglandular lymph nodes.

Non-neoplastic lesions

Sialadenosis (Fig. 4.21)[87,88]

Sialadenosis is a non-neoplastic, non-inflammatory enlargement of salivary glands, mainly the parotid. It presents clinically as soft, often bilateral and recurrent mumps-like swelling of the gland. It is usually associated with certain systemic disorders. FNB yields plenty of acinar epithelial cells, which appear normal or slightly increased in size. The microarchitectural pattern of regular acini joined by small ducts and fibrovascular stroma is the same as of normal salivary gland tissue. Smears are therefore unlikely to be

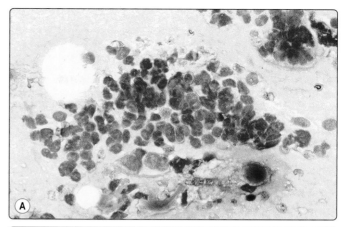
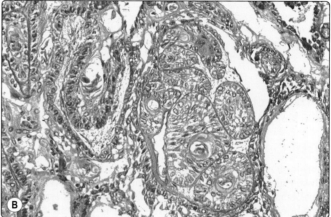

Fig. 4.19 Ameloblastoma (**A**) Cell-rich smear composed of basaloid cells with a suggestion of peripheral palisading. A few larger and paler cells are also seen and a single cell with squamous features (*lower right*) (MGG, HP); (**B**) tissue section, same case (H&E, IP).

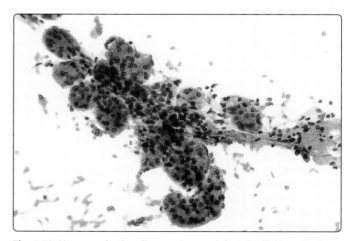

Fig. 4.20 Non-neoplastic salivary acinar and ductal cells Normal salivary gland tissue in a FNB smear. Tissue fragment of uniform, well-formed acini along a small duct (Pap, IP).

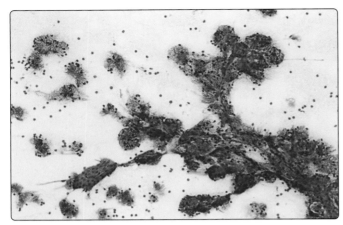

Fig. 4.21 Sialadenosis Abundant material of normal or hyperplastic salivary gland acini adherent to a thin fibrovascular stroma. Note large number of naked nuclei of epithelial cell origin in the background (MGG, LP).

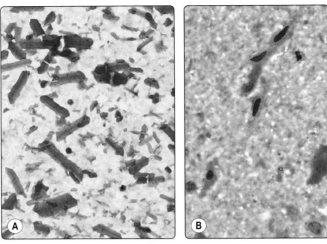

Fig. 4.22 Non-neoplastic salivary gland cysts (A) Cyst fluid containing numerous non-tyrosine crystalloids and a few inflammatory cells (MGG, IP); (B) Fluid from a lymphoepithelial cyst with a few degenerate spindle squamous metaplastic cells, resembling cystically degenerate squamous cell carcinoma (MGG, HP).

mistaken for low-grade acinic cell carcinoma in spite of the cellular yield. There are no inflammatory cells.

Cysts (Figs 4.22–4.24)

Non-neoplastic cysts are relatively uncommon in the major salivary glands. There are several types: retention cysts, which may be associated with sialolithiasis; salivary duct cysts; and lymphoepithelial cysts. Aspirated fluid is poor in cells but there may be a variable number of histiocytes and inflammatory cells, and a few degenerate epithelial cells.[89] Sometimes, the fluid contains numerous crystalloids (non-tyrosine, Fig. 4.22A).[90–92] These have been linked with an oncocytic epithelial lining and can be found also in neoplastic cysts but their presence favors a benign lesion. *Lymphoepithelial cysts* are most commonly seen in HIV-infected patients.[93,94] Cytological findings are similar to other non-neoplastic cysts, but lymphoid cells from subepithelial lymphoid tissue are often present. Fluid from *retention cysts* tends to be mucinous with a more prominent inflammatory component. Metaplastic squamous epithelial cells derived from duct epithelium in a mucous background may cause a suspicion of cystic, low-grade mucoepidermoid tumor. If the background is non-specific acellular debris, atypical metaplastic squamous epithelial cells could raise a suspicion of cystically degenerate squamous cell carcinoma (Fig 4.22B).

Mucocele is a pseudocyst of extravasated mucinous secretion, which commonly develops in minor salivary glands, particularly on the lips but also in other sites of the oral cavity and tongue. FNB yields mucus with a variable number of mucinophages and inflammatory cells. Well-preserved epithelial cells are not seen, but mucinophages may cluster and may appear atypical, particularly in MGG smears, resembling mucinous adenocarcinoma (Fig. 4.23).

Cystic neoplasm is the most important differential diagnosis of non-neoplastic salivary gland cyst. The majority of cysts occurring in the major salivary glands are, in fact, associated with neoplasms, which may be benign or malignant. Warthin's tumor and low-grade mucoepidermoid carcinoma are the commonest, but pleomorphic adenoma, cystadenoma,

acinic cell carcinoma and other tumors may also be predominantly or partly cystic (Fig. 4.24). Aspirated fluid from a cystic neoplasm is often poor in cells and indistinguishable from fluid from a non-neoplastic cyst. If the lesion disappears completely after evacuation of the fluid, it is most likely of non-neoplastic nature. However, any remaining solid part must be biopsied. US guidance is helpful in this situation, particularly because the cyst may refill with blood following the initial FNB, rendering the solid portion impalpable. Clinical follow-up of cystic salivary gland lesions is essential if a specific diagnosis cannot be made.

Sialadenitis (Figs 4.25, 4.26)

> **CRITERIA FOR DIAGNOSIS**
>
> - Purulent aspirate in acute, infective sialadenitis,
> - Scanty material of mainly ductal epithelial cells, few acinar cells in chronic sialadenitis,
> - Sheets of ductal epithelium showing regenerative atypia and/or squamous metaplasia,
> - Variable numbers of inflammatory cells, usually few in chronic sialadenitis,
> - Fragments of fibrous stroma.

Purulent material aspirated from a tender, swollen gland suggests *infective sialadenitis*. Smears contain a mixed population of numerous neutrophils, foamy degenerate cells and endothelial cells. The swelling should subside after antiinflammatory treatment.

Most cases of *chronic sialadenitis* referred for FNB are in a late stage when interstitial fibrosis and atrophy of acinar tissue have taken place. The inflammatory cell infiltration

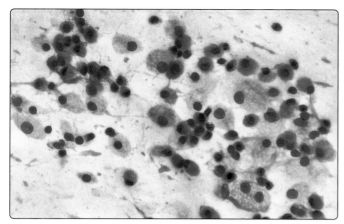

Fig. 4.23 Non-neoplastic salivary gland cyst Numerous mucinophages, some clustered, in aspirate from mucocele of lip; compare Fig. 4.10 (MGG, HP).

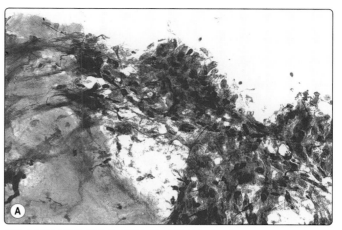

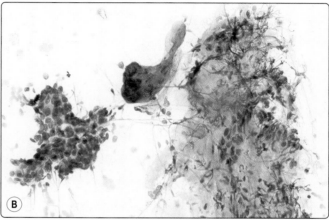

Fig. 4.25 Chronic sialadenitis Fragments of epithelium mainly of ductal origin showing mild reactive atypia and some squamous metaplasia; fragments of fibrous stroma; relatively few chronic inflammatory cells. (**A**, MGG, IP; (**B**, Pap, IP).

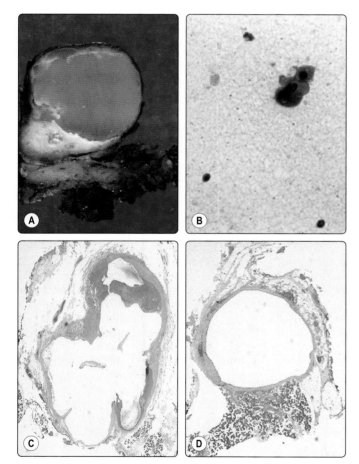

Fig. 4.24 Cystic salivary gland neoplasms (A) Cystic Warthin's tumor (macro); (B) Cyst fluid from same lesion with a single small group of bland oncocytic epithelial cells (Pap, IP); (C) Predominantly cystic pleomorphic adenoma (tissue section, H&E); (D) Cystic mucoepidermoid carcinoma with small tumor nodules in the cyst wall (tissue section, H&E). The fluids aspirated from (C) and (D) were practically acellular.

may have subsided and may be sparse and patchy. FNB smears are therefore often scanty, mainly of ductal epithelial cells associated with only few acinar cells and inconspicuous inflammatory cells. Fragments of fibrous stroma are often present (Fig. 4.25). Crystalloids may be present in the aspirate.[95] Regenerating ductal epithelium in chronic sialadenitis may undergo squamous metaplasia and may appear atypical (Fig. 4.26). Mucus-like material from dilated ducts may be present. This may be suggestive of a neoplastic lesion or even of malignancy, mainly low-grade mucoepidermoid tumor. Multiple sampling and clinical correlation usually solves the problem.

FNB diagnosis of sialadenitis and other salilvary gland lesions in patients infected with HIV has been reported by several authors.[93,94,96,97]

Granulomatous inflammation in FNB samples from major salivary glands most likely represents granulomatous lymphadenitis related to intraparenchymal lymph nodes. The usual range of differential diagnoses must be considered (see Chapter 5). Granulomatous clusters of epithelioid cells and multinucleated giant cells without evidence of necrosis, associated with normal salivary gland components, suggest *sarcoidosis* involving the salivary gland directly.

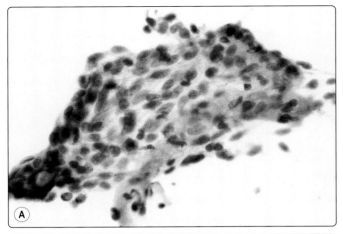

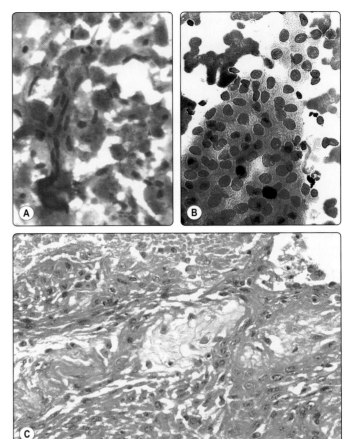

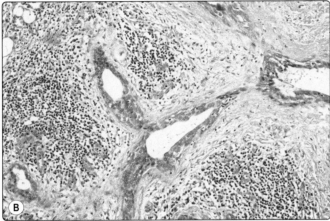

Fig. 4.26 Chronic sialadenitis (A) Sheet of ductal epithelium showing squamous metaplasia. This could be mistaken for low-grade mucoepidermoid carcinoma or other low-grade neoplasm (Pap, HP); (B) Corresponding histology, most acinar epithelium replaced by fibrous tissue with patchy inflammatory cell infiltration, and prominent ducts showing mild reactive atypia and squamous metaplasia (H&E, IP).

Fig. 4.27 Necrotising sialometaplasia (A) Seminecrotic material including degenerate squamous epithelial cells with pyknotic spindle nuclei resembling cells of cystic squamous carcinoma; (B) Metaplastic squamous epithelial cells showing mild reactive atypia (MGG, HP); (C) Corresponding tissue section (H&E, IP).

PROBLEMS AND DIFFERENTIAL DIAGNOSIS

◆ Stripped nuclei of dispersed normal acinar epithelial cells resembling lymphocytes,
◆ Necrotizing sialometaplasia and other lesions with an atypical squamous epithelial component,
◆ Küttner's tumor,
◆ Adenomatoid hyperplasia,
◆ Low-grade mucoepidermoid carcinoma.

Stripped nuclei of dispersed non-neoplastic acinar epithelial cells in smears of normal salivary gland tissue are of similar size and shape as lymphocytes. This must not be misinterpreted as chronic sialadenitis.

Epithelial atypia and squamous metaplasia are particularly prominent in *necrotising sialometaplasia*. This is a self-healing inflammatory condition of unknown etiology, possibly related to previous surgery, radiotherapy or infarction, which mainly affects minor salivary glands.[98] Cellular smears of squamous metaplastic cells showing regenerative atypia and degenerative changes with necrotic material in the background can closely mimic well-differentiated squamous cell carcinoma (Fig. 4.27). Worrysome squamous epithelial cell atypia can be found in a wide spectrum of salivary gland lesions, causing diagnostic difficulties in FNB.[99]

Chronic sialadenitis can involve a gland focally and produce a firm nodule, which may be clinically mistaken for neoplasm. Such 'pseudotumors' are most common in the submandibular gland (Küttner's tumor)[100,101] and may be either the result of obstruction or a manifestation of the immunopathic so-called 'IgG4 disease' in cases where calculus can be reasonably excluded. Histologically, the nodule shows similar features as described in chronic sialadenitis: acinar cell atrophy, ductal and ductular hyperplasia often with squamous metaplasia and a fibrous or myxoid stroma. Chronic inflammatory cell infiltration is of variable degree and may be mild. The aggregates of ductal epithelial cells associated with myxoid stromal fragments can be mistaken for pleomorphic adenoma, low-grade mucoepidermoid carcinoma or other neoplasms in FNB smears.

Inflammatory *pseudotumor* caused by a proliferation of myofibrohistiocytic cells can occur in several sites such as

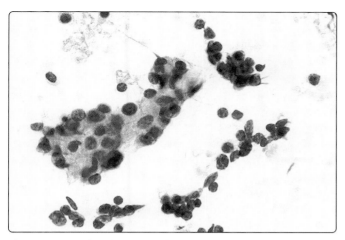

Fig. 4.28 Benign lymphoepithelial lesion Aggregate of ductal epithelial cells associated with many lymphoid cells (Pap, HP).

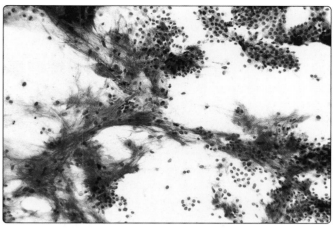

Fig. 4.29 Pleomorphic adenoma Typical low-power pattern of poorly cohesive epithelial-like cells associated with fibrillar fibromyxoid stroma staining brightly red/magenta (MGG, LP).

lung, liver and soft tissues and have also been described in major salivary glands.[102] Another non-neoplastic lesion that can clinically mimic a neoplasm is *adenomatoid hyperplasia* of the small glands of the palate.[103] This lesion is of simple hyperplastic nature, forming a focal increase in the amount of acinar tissue.

Benign lymphoepithelial lesion/ myoepithelial sialadenitis

Benign lymphoepithelial lesions are swellings of salivary glands caused by a reactive lymphoid infiltrate with follicular hyperplasia, which obliterates the acinar glandular tissue and causes proliferation and disruption of ductal epithelium. It may clinically manifest as Sjögren's syndrome. Smears from a benign lymphoepithelial lesion are characterized by small clusters of ductal epithelial cells associated with lymphocytes and with a background of lymphoid cells (Fig. 4.28). The smear pattern is reminiscent of autoimmune thyroiditis. The condition is associated with HIV infection.[97]

The most important differential diagnosis is lymphoma, mainly MALT lymphoma. This often requires immunological studies, most conveniently by flow cytometry of aspirated material. Branchial cyst in which only the lymphoid component has been sampled should also be considered.

Benign neoplasms

Pleomorphic adenoma (PA) (Figs 4.29–4.35)[14,104,105]

CRITERIA FOR DIAGNOSIS

- Fibrillary chondromyxoid ground substance,
- Variable cellularity of single cells and poorly cohesive clusters and sheets,
- Mainly myoepithelial cells, ovoid, plasmacytoid or spindle, with abundant well-defined cytoplasm, abundant well-defind cytoplasm,
- Regular ovoid nuclei with bland finely granular nuclear chromatin and smooth nuclear membrane,
- Spindle-shaped myoepithelial cells embedded in stromal matrix,
- Sometimes, metaplastic cells (oncocytic, sebaceous, squamous).

The chondromyxoid matrix is particularly characteristic in MGG smears, distinctly fibrillar and staining intensely red to purple (Figs. 4.29 and 4.30A). Staining may be so intense that it obscures the cellular component in tissue fragments. Cell detail is therefore better seen in alcohol-fixed Pap smears. With Pap staining, the ground substance is gray–green to orange in color and appears relatively amorphous or finely fibrillar (Fig. 4.30B). Spindle or rounded cells are present within the stromal fragments. The cellular component consists of relatively uniform oval, plasmacytoid or spindle cells. Nuclei are round or oval, eccentric, and have a bland, finely granular chromatin and inconspicuous nucleoli. Moderate anisokaryosis is a common feature. The cytoplasm is pale but well defined with distinct cell borders. Stripped, naked nuclei are not a feature. Often, the cells are strikingly plasmacytoid with abundant cytoplasm and eccentric nuclei (Fig. 4.31). They are generally poorly cohesive and dispersed but also form aggregates with no specific microarchitectural pattern. Red-staining intercellular material (MGG) is present within the aggregates. Tyrosine crystals have been noted in some cases.[106]

The majority of cells of PA are myoepithelial but a proportion of the cells may be epithelial of basaloid type. If present, they are not clearly distinguishable from the myoepithelial cells in routine stained smears. A study using immune markers for epithelial cells showed them to be present in 9 of 20 Pas, so examined.[107]

PROBLEMS AND DIFFERENTIAL DIAGNOSIS

- Selective sampling,
- Well-differentiated adenoid cystic carcinoma,
- Basal cell adenoma,
- Pleomorphic adenoma with cytological atypia versus carcinoma ex pleomorphic adenoma.
- Metaplastic cells – squamous, sebaceous, oncocytic, goblet cells,
- Background mucus,
- Inflammatory 'pseudotumor' and intraparotid schwannoma.

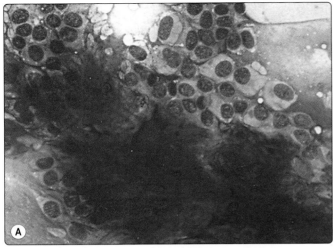

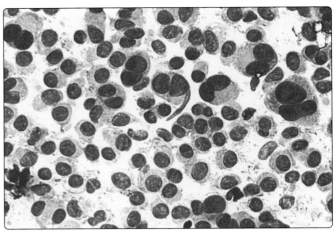

Fig. 4.32 **Pleomorphic adenoma** Epithelial cell predominance, cellular smear; prominent anisokaryosis should not suggest malignancy (MGG, HP).

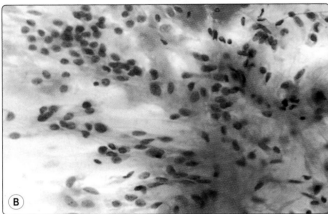

Fig. 4.30 **Pleomorphic adenoma** High-power view showing myoepithelial cells with abundant pale cytoplasm and bland nuclei; fibrillar fibromyxoid stroma including single oval and spindle cells (**A**, MGG, HP; **B**, Pap, IP).

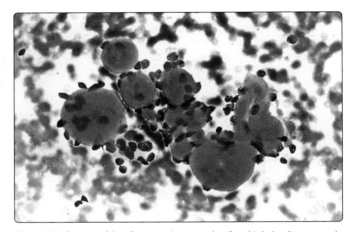

Fig. 4.33 **Pleomorphic adenoma** An example of multiple hyaline stromal globules in pleomorphic adenoma. Note bland appearance of epithelial cell nuclei (MGG, IP).

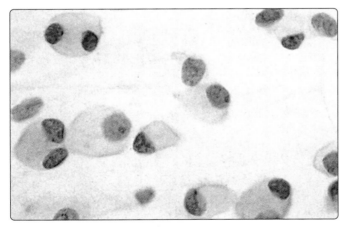

Fig. 4.31 **Pleomorphic adenoma** Plasma cell-like (hyaline-cell) pattern (Pap, HP).

The cytological diagnosis of PA is not difficult in typical cases. However, the pattern can vary considerably between different parts of the same tumor. This can cause diagnostic difficulties due to the limited and often selective sampling by the thin needle.[108,109] One particular feature present only focally in tissue sections may dominate the smears to the extent that the true nature of the tumor is not recognised. For example, samples of chondromyxoid matrix with few or no cells can mimic cartilage, whereas highly cellular areas with scant stroma can be mistaken for basal cell adenoma or adenoid cystic carcinoma. Aspiration of mucoid paucicellular fluid may suggest low-grade mucoepidermoid carcinoma or mucoepidermoid carcinoma arising in pleomorphic adenoma.[110] PA can be predominantly cystic (see Fig. 4.24C).[111] Multiple sampling is important to overcome the problems due to selective sampling.

The distinction of PA from well-differentiated adenoid cystic carcinoma is clinically important. Both tumors have relatively uniform epithelial-like cells and both may have a fibrillar myxoid stromal component. Hyaline stromal globules resembling those characteristic of adenoid cystic carcinoma, or a beaded hyaline stroma, sometimes occur also in PA (Fig. 4.33).[25,112] The differential diagnosis must not be based solely on the stromal component, but cytological detail must also be closley studied. A well-defined cytoplasm, no or few stripped nuclei, and a bland, finely granular nuclear chromatin favor PA; scanty cytoplasm, a high N:C ratio, naked nuclei, nuclear molding, and nuclear

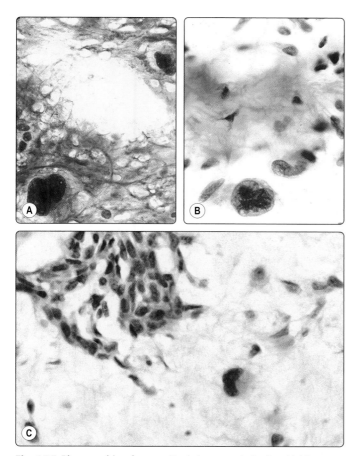

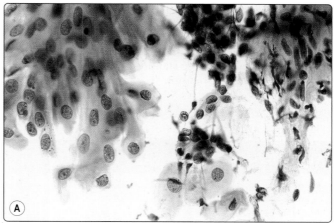

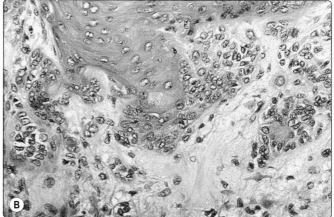

Fig. 4.34 Pleomorphic adenoma Single large atypical cells with bizarre nuclei and a background of usual elements of pleomorphic adenoma; no histological evidence of malignancy (**A**, MGG HP; **B**, H&E, HP; **C**, tissue section, H&E, IP).

Fig. 4.35 Pleomorphic adenoma Prominent component of squamous epithelial cells (*left and center*); some myoepithelial cells and myxoid stroma at upper right reveal the nature of the lesion (**A**, Pap, HP; **B**, tissue section, H&E, IP).

hyperchromasia and coarseness favor adenoid cystic carcinoma. Multiple sampling and well-prepared smears, both MGG and Pap, reduce the likelihood of error.

If a stromal component is scanty or missing and smears are highly cellular, the distinction from basal cell adenoma and myoepithelial adenoma can be difficult or impossible. However, the distinction is not of clinical significance since these tumors are managed in the same way.

Worrisome cytological atypia can occur in PA in several forms. The myoepithelial cells of a common benign PA occasionally display prominent anisokaryosis that may cause suspicion of malignancy (Fig. 4.32). However, if the nuclear chromatin is bland, if there is no mitotic activity or necrosis, and if the anisokaryosis is randomly distributed, the pattern is consistent with a benign PA. In other cases, one may find single scattered stromal cells with considerably enlarged, irregular and multilobated, even bizarre nuclei, seen both in smears and in tissue sections of histologically benign tumors (Fig. 4.34).[25] Such atypical cells are probably degenerative in nature and may be equivalent to the nuclear atypia seen in ancient schwannoma.[113] Aggregates of atypical epithelial cells showing nuclear enlargement, abnormal nuclear chromatin and nucleolar prominence, coexistent with bland epithelial cells and fibromyxoid stroma typical of PA, suggest *carcinoma arising in pleomorphic adenoma* (see Figs 4.69,

4.70).[25,114] This entity is further discussed in relation to malignant tumors.

Epithelial metaplasia, mainly squamous and oncocytic, is often seen in PA. Goblet cells are sometimes present and squamous metaplasia can be a prominent feature. If a squamous component is selectively sampled by FNB and if the metaplastic cells appear atypical, the possibility of low-grade mucoepidermoid tumor may be considered (Fig. 4.35). Sebaceous metaplasia is less frequent. The presence of groups of bland epithelial cells typical of PA and a few fragments of myxoid stroma suggest the correct diagnosis.

Tumor-like nodules caused by focal chronic inflammation have been mentioned in the section on chronic sialadenitis. The presence of epithelial cell aggregates associated with fibrillar fibrous stroma could be mistaken for PA, but the fragments of ductal epithelium – with or without squamous metaplasia – are cohesive and the stroma is not chondromyxoid. FNB samples of intraparotid schwannoma can also include tissue fragments resembling the fibromyxoid stroma of PA, but the cellular component is clearly different from the myoepithelial cells of PA.[115]

In summary, the hallmark of PA is the combination of bland, mainly myoepithelial cells and fragments of chondromyxoid stroma with spindle cells. In the presence of any such stromal fragments and bland epithelium, pleomorphic adenoma should be included in the differential diagnosis even when other features dominate the smears. In difficult cases, positive immunostaining for intermediate filaments such as GFAP and negative staining of the majority of cells for cytokeratin can be helpful.[116]

Basal cell and canalicular adenoma
(Figs 4.36–4.40)[117,118]

CRITERIA FOR DIAGNOSIS

◆ Numerous small basaloid epithelial cells, both single and multilayered clusters with occasional peripheral palisading,
◆ Scanty cytoplasm, many naked nuclei,
◆ Regular round or oval nuclei, may appear dark but with bland, granular chromatin,
◆ Scanty fibrous stroma, hyaline material probably of basement membrane origin in some tumors,
◆ Frequent squamous metaplasia

Basal cell adenoma (BCA) and canalicular adenoma have overlapping cytomorphologic features. Several subtypes of BCA are distinguished by the architectural patterns: solid, trabecular, tubular and membranous. These subtypes cannot always be distinguished in cytological smears. BCA is mainly seen in the major salivary glands and usually in elderly patients; canalicular adenoma mainly occur in small glands of the oral cavity.[119]

The cells of BCA are of basaloid epithelial type and lack the abundant cytoplasm and distinct cell borders of myoepithelial cells. Many cells present as naked nuclei. Stromal material is scanty and non-characteristic in most tumors, but basement membrane material may be prominent, delineating groups of cells or forming a background to the cells (membranous variant).

PROBLEMS AND DIFFERENTIAL DIAGNOSIS

◆ Hyaline stromal globules resembling adenoid cystic carcinoma,
◆ Membranous variant and its distinction from some cutaneous tumors,
◆ Pleomorphic adenoma,
◆ Basal cell adenocarcinoma

Adenoid cystic carcinoma is the most important differential diagnosis, given its malignant nature. Smears from the trabecular variant of BCA and from canalicular adenoma may contain hyaline globules resembling those seen in adenoid cystic carcinoma (Figs 4.38, 4.39).[25,118] However, the globules of monomorphic adenoma are smaller, of more uniform size and have a less hyaline texture. Other tumors in which hyaline globules occur such as polymorphous low-grade adenocarcinoma, epithelial-myoepithelial carcinoma and pleomorphic adenoma may also enter the differential diagnosis. The epithelial cells of basal cell adenoma are small with scanty cytoplasm. On close scrutiny in high magnification, the nuclear chromatin is finely and evenly granular and nucleoli are inconspicuous. The cells of adenoid cystic carcinoma are similarly small with a high N : C ratio,

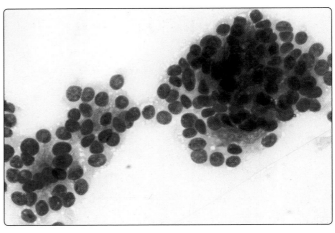

Fig. 4.36 Basal cell adenoma, solid variant Clusters of small basaloid epithelial cells with scanty fragile cytoplasm and bland rounded nuclei; inconspicuous stroma (MGG, HP).

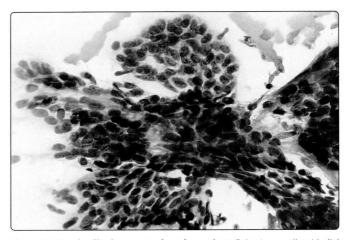

Fig. 4.37 Basal cell adenoma trabecular variant Cohesive small epithelial cells forming a trabecular microarchitectural pattern (Pap, HP).

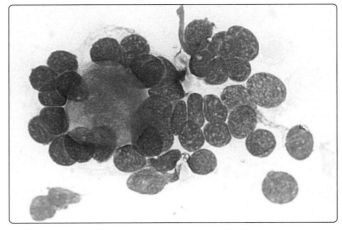

Fig. 4.38 Basal cell adenoma trabecular variant Hyaline stromal globule surrounded by small epithelial cells with bland granular nuclear chromatin (MGG, HP oil). *(Courtesy Dr K. Lindholm, Malmö General Hospital).*

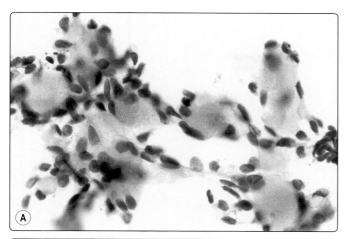

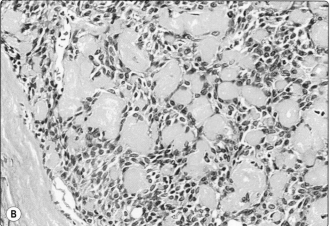

Fig. 4.39 Basal cell adenoma trabecular variant (A) Multiple small rounded hyaline stromal globules surrounded by small bland epithelial cells (Pap, HP); (B) Corresponding tissue section (H&E, IP).

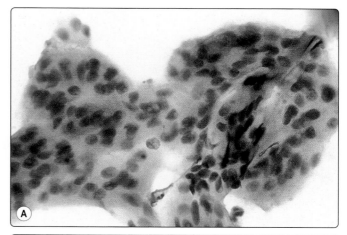

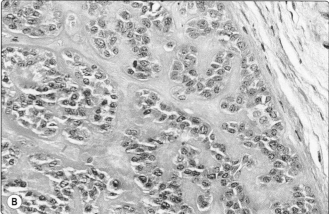

Fig. 4.40 Basal cell adenoma, membranous type (A) Tissue fragment of small, uniform epithelial cells adherent to a background sheet of hyaline basement membrane material (Pap, HP); (B) Corresponding tissue section (H&E, IP).

but nuclei are less regular, hyperchromatic, with a coarsely granular chromatin, and nucleoli are more prominent. Nuclear molding is a common finding in adenoid cystic carcinoma but is not seen in BCA.

The *membranous variant* (dermal analogue tumor) resembles cutaneous cylindroma. Smears may show large aggregates or cohesive sheets of small basaloid cells enveloped in a rim of hyaline basement membrane material or stuck to a sheet of such material. It stains variably with both Papanicolaou and MGG (Fig. 4.40) and may or may not be metachromatic.[120] The microarchitectural pattern is most striking at low magnification and is unlike that seen in either adenoid cystic carcinoma or pleomorphic adenoma. Nevertheless, hyaline basement membrane globules, as mentioned above, can cause diagnostic difficulties also in this tumor.

Distinction from cellular pleomorphic adenoma with scanty stroma is not always possible. Spindle-shaped or plasmacytoid cells with well-defined cytoplasm is against basal cell adenoma, a high N:C ratio and naked nuclei in favor. There is some overlap between these two tumors but the distinction is not of great significance clinically.

The distinction from *basal cell adenocarcinoma* is obviously more important and can be equally difficult. However, a review of the literature showed that FNB was accurate in all

reported cases. Mitotic figures, nuclear atypia, and evidence of necrosis indicate malignancy.[118]

Warthin's tumor (Figs 4.41–4.44)[1,13]

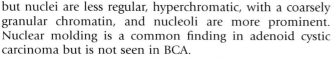

CRITERIA FOR DIAGNOSIS

◆ Aspirate of mucoid, murky fluid,
◆ Background of amorphous and granular debris,
◆ Bland oncocytic cells in cohesive, monolayered sheets,
◆ Many lymphoid cells,
◆ Mast cells commonly associated with the oncocytic cells.

The amorphous and granular debris representing cyst contents aspirated from Warthin's tumor (WT) has a mucoid appearance and stains blue with MGG. The oncocytes form flat, monolayered sheets with an irregular outline. They have plentiful cytoplasm and uniformly small, round, central nuclei with a bland chromatin and inconspicuous nucleoli. With Pap staining, the cytoplasm is dense, green to orangeophilic and may be finely granular; with MGG it is gray–blue and appears more homogeneous (Fig. 4.41). In MGG smears, oncocytes can be mistaken for other types of cells

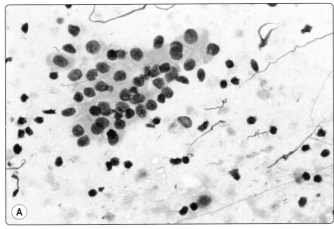

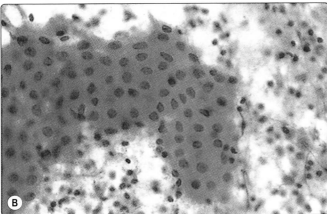

Fig. 4.41 **Warthin's tumor** Diagnostic triad of monolayered sheets of uniform oncocytic epithelial cells with small bland nuclei, lymphocytes and proteinaceous material representing cyst fluid (**A**, MGG, HP; **B**, Pap, HP).

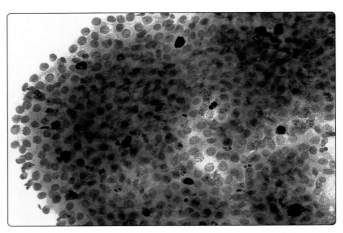

Fig. 4.42 **Warthin's tumor** Large sheet of bland oncocytic epithelium; note scattered single mast cells staining dark blue (MGG, HP).

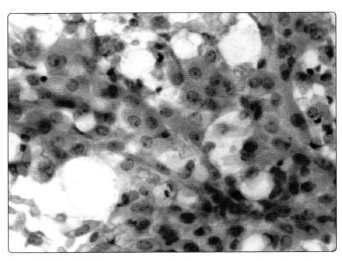

Fig. 4.43 **Warthin's tumor** Aggregates of squamous metaplastic cells showing mild atypia and a few cells with intracytoplasmic vacuoles. This could be mistaken for low-grade mucoepidermoid tumor but there were typical features of Warthin's tumor in other parts of the smear (Pap, HP).

such as ductal epithelial cells or metaplastic squamous cells. They are more easily identified in Pap preparations. Mast cells are often seen scattered among the oncocytes (Fig. 4.42).

PROBLEMS IN DIAGNOSIS

◆ Distinction from other cystic lesions, benign and malignant,
◆ Solid oncocytoma,
◆ Squamous metaplasia and degeneration producing worrisome atypia,
◆ Acinic cell carcinoma,
◆ Rare malignant variant.

Obtaining diagnostic material may be difficult in a predominantly cystic WT. Both oncocytic and lymphoid cells must be identified for a definitive diagnosis, but either component may be sparse, absent or obscured by mucoid debris. The mucoid fluid from a WT with flakes of homogeneous and granular debris is characteristic but not specific. Similar hypocellular material may be obtained from low-grade mucoepidermoid carcinoma and other tumors. If the overall smear pattern is suggestive of WT but the cells appear atypical and lack a distinctly oxyphil cytoplasm, the alternative of a mucoepidermoid tumor should be considered. The problem is enhanced by the occasional finding of goblet cells in WT, and special staining for mucin may not be helpful (Fig. 4.43).

If oncocytes dominate the smears and the lymphoid and cystic component is inconspicuous, distinction from oncocytoma is difficult. The oncocytic cells of oncocytoma form multilayered aggregates rather than flat sheets as in WT.

WT may become inflamed or infarcted, spontaneously or post previous FNB. Repair results in more or less extensive squamous metaplasia. Smears contain metaplastic squamous cells showing regenerative atypia and degenerating cells, which may closely resemble malignant squamous epithelial cells of 'fiber-cell' type (Fig. 4.44). False-positive or suspicious diagnosis of squamous cell carcinoma with liquefaction necrosis is not uncommon.[89,121,122] However, the glassy refractile nature of true keratinization is absent in degenerate metaplastic squamous cells or oncocytes. As

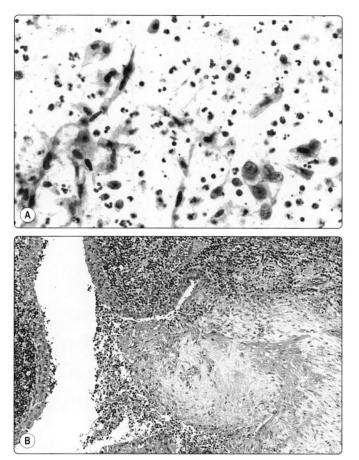

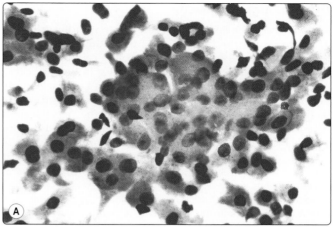

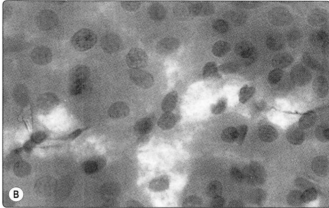

Fig. 4.44 Warthin's tumor (A) Degenerating spindle metaplastic squamous epithelial cells with nuclear pyknosis and cells showing regenerative atypia mimic cystic well-differentiated squamous carcinoma (Pap, HP); (B) The corresponding tissue section shows infarction, repair and squamous metaplasia in a Warthin's tumor (H&E, IP).

Fig. 4.45 Oncocytoma Multilayered aggregates of cohesive oxyphil cells showing some nuclear enlargement and anisokaryosis but bland nuclear chromatin (A, MGG, HP; B, Pap, HP).

mentioned above, mucin-secreting goblet cells can be present in the metaplastic epithelium and may suggest a low-grade mucoepidermoid tumor.

In some acinic cell tumors the cytoplasm of tumor cells may be oncocyte-like, dense and relatively homogeneous and not pale and vacuolated/bubbly or granular as in typical acinic cell carcinoma (see Fig. 4.49). Acinic cell nuclei are generally larger and more variable in size than those of oncocytes and the cells are more fragile, as shown by large numbers of bare nuclei. A microacinar architectural pattern is usually discernible in smears of acinic cell tumors. The not uncommon presence of a lymphoid stroma in acinic cell tumors can make the distinction from WT very difficult at times.

Malignant Warthin's tumor is extremely rare and has not yet been defined cytologically.

Oncocytoma (Fig. 4.45)[13,22,123]

Clear cell and eosinophilic variants of oncocytoma have been described.[124]

Cells with abundant cytoplasm from non-oncocytic tumors can resemble oncocytes in MGG-stained preparations. Acinic cell carcinoma has been mentioned above. Cells from mucoepidermoid tumors and from adenocarcinoma sometimes also have this appearance.

Oncocytomas may be cystic and their relationship to Warthin's tumors is then uncertain. In general, cyst fluid with debris, oncocytes and lymphoid cells indicate a Warthin's tumor, especially if the oncocytes lie in flat sheets.

Multifocal oncocytic hyperplasia of salivary gland may suggest oncocytoma in FNB smears.[125]

The cytologic findings in malignant oncocytic neoplasms have been described in a small number of cases.[22] See also Oncocytic salivary duct carcinoma, page 70.

Other benign neoplasms

Myoepithelial adenoma[22,126,127] may be of spindle cell (Fig. 4.46A), plasmacytoid (Fig. 4.46B) or epithelioid type. This tumor may not be distinguishable from a cellular pleomorphic adenoma in which a solid focus of spindle or plasmacytoid cells without specific stroma has been selectively sampled. The spindle cell type can also be confused with a benign soft tissue tumor. Distinction of the plasmacytoid type from malignant myoepithelioma can be difficult since anisokaryosis and mild nuclear atypia can occur. Mitotic figures and necrosis suggest malignancy. Positive nuclear staining for p63 supports a diagnosis of myoepithelial adenoma (Fig. 4.46C).

Sebaceous adenoma, *ductal papilloma* and *cystadenoma* are rare and few cases with cytology have been reported.[22]

Benign *mesenchymal tumors*, most commonly lipoma and schwannoma, occur in or adjacent to salivary glands, particularly the parotid. Schwannoma can be mistaken for pleomorphic adenoma or basal cell adenoma if smears are suboptimal (Fig. 4.47).[128]

Malignant neoplasms

Acinic cell carcinoma (Figs 4.48–4.50)[129,130]

> **CRITERIA FOR DIAGNOSIS**
>
> ◆ Abundant cell material with a clean background,
> ◆ Cells mainly in clusters, scanty inconspicuous fibrovascular stroma,
> ◆ Microacinar groupings,
> ◆ Abundant, fragile, finely vacuolated, occasionally dense oncocyte-like cytoplasm,
> ◆ Rounded, medium-sized nuclei, mild to moderate anisokaryosis, bland chromatin,
> ◆ Many stripped nuclei.

Acinic cell carcinoma (AcCC) is relatively common in our population. It not infrequently occurs in children and adolescents. The cells of well-differentiated AcCC resemble normal acinar epithelial cells but do not form discrete round acini defined by a basement membrane and are not associated with small ducts as in non-neoplastic salivary gland tissue (Fig. 4.48). The cells are relatively uniform, cohesive, with abundant vacuolated, foamy or bubbly cytoplasm of variable density. A clear cell appearance is sometimes seen and in some tumors the cells have a dense grayish (MGG) oncocyte-like cytoplasm (Fig. 4.49). The cytoplasm is fragile, leaving many nuclei stripped. Nuclei are round with a bland chromatin. The cells are less uniform and the nuclei are larger and less evenly distributed than those of normal acinar cells. The nuclear:cytoplasmic ratio is higher, particularly in less well-differentiated tumors. Stroma is overall scant and inconspicuous. The adherence of tumor cells to thin strands of fibrovascular stroma occasionally produces a pseudopapillary appearance. In some acinic cell tumors, the stroma contains a prominent lymphoid component.

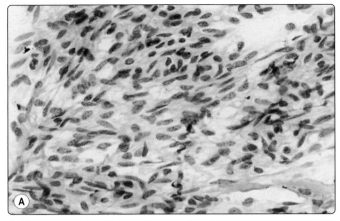
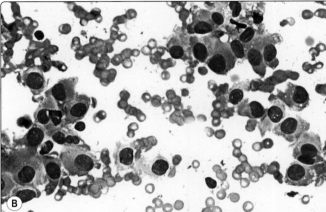
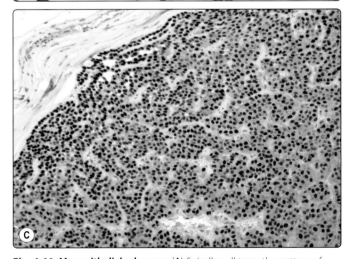

Fig. 4.46 Myoepithelial adenoma (A) Spindle cell type; the pattern of bland spindle cells could be mistaken for a benign soft tissue tumor (Pap, HP); (B) Plasmacytoid type; poorly cohesive cells with abundant cytoplasm and eccentric nuclei. The nuclear atypica in this case caused some concern (MGG, HP); (C) Tissue section corresponding to (B), immunostaining for p63 (IP).

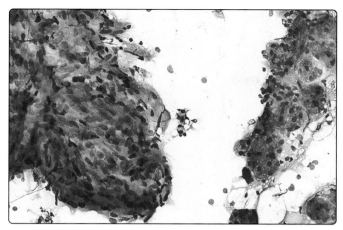

Fig. 4.47 Intraparotid Schwannoma Tissue fragment of cohesive bland spindle cells and fibrillar fibrous stroma, normal salivary gland acini to the right (MGG, LP).

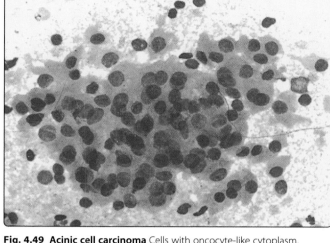

Fig. 4.49 Acinic cell carcinoma Cells with oncocyte-like cytoplasm, distinction from oncocytoma difficult (MGG, HP).

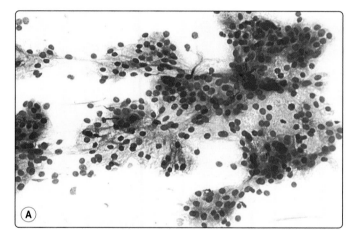

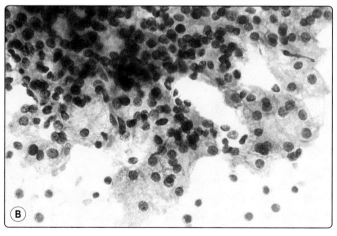

Fig. 4.48 Acinic cell carcinoma Epithelial fragments composed of cells with abundant vacuolated cytoplasm and relatively bland nuclei, resembling normal acinar cells; many naked nuclei; scanty, thin fibrovascular stroma. Note absence of well-formed acinar structures (A, MGG, IP; B, Pap, HP).

PROBLEMS AND DIFFERENTIAL DIAGNOSIS

◆ Resemblance to non-neoplastic salivary gland tissue,
◆ Distinction from other tumors with a clear cell component,
◆ Oncocytic tumors,
◆ Specific diagnosis of less well-differentiated acinic cell carcinoma,
◆ Cystic tumors.

The similarity between cells of low-grade AcCC and non-neoplastic acinar cells has been mentioned. Smears from sialadenosis can be quite cellular, but less so than samples from an acinic cell tumor. The microarchitectural patterns are distinctly different.

A clear cell pattern of large cells with abundant fragile and vacuolated cytoplasm may be seen in several other tumors, for example epithelial-myoepithelial carcinoma and low-grade mucoepidermoid carcinoma. The cytology of these tumors is described in detail below. Intracellular mucin vacuoles are not found in AcCC. Renal cell carcinoma can metastasize to the parotid gland and must be remembered in the differential diagnosis. The characteristic vascular pattern of renal cell carcinoma is a clue, and nuclear atypia is usually more prominent.

As mentioned above in relation to WT and oncocytoma, the distinction from oncocytic tumors can sometimes be difficult. This is due to the resemblance of the neoplastic cells to oncocytes in some AcCC and to the not infrequent presence of infiltrates of lymphoid cells in the stroma. Cells with vacuolated cytoplasm and many naked nuclei favor AcCC.

Less well-differentiated AcCC has a less characteristic cytological appearance which merges with adenocarcinoma of no special type (Fig. 4.50). A type-specific diagnosis may not be possible without ancillary tests such as EM.

AcCC, particularly the papillary cystic variant, can be predominantly cystic and FNB may yield only hypocellular fluid with no diagnostic cells.[131,132] A false-negative diagnosis of simple cyst is possible. US guidance may solve the problem.

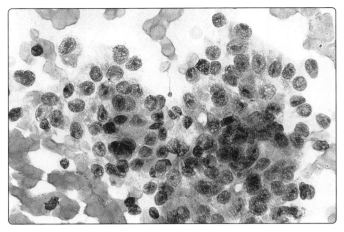

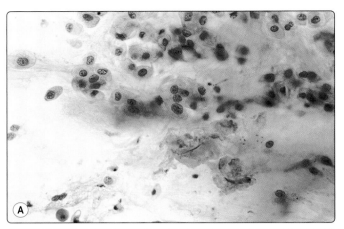

Fig. 4.50 Acinic cell carcinoma A less well-differentiated tumor may be difficult to type as acinic cell carcinoma. Ancillary techniques such as EM may help (MGG. HP).

Mucoepidermoid carcinoma (Figs 4.51–4.56)[17,133–135]

CRITERIA FOR DIAGNOSIS (LOW-GRADE TUMORS)

◆ Smears usually of low cellularity, a 'dirty' background of mucus and debris,
◆ Cohesive clusters and sheets of epithelial cells and small streams of cells within mucus,
◆ Predominantly intermediate cells resembling squamous metaplastic cells; some mucin-secreting cells; infrequently differentiated squamous epithelial cells,
◆ Relatively bland nuclei; prominent nucleoli in some cells.

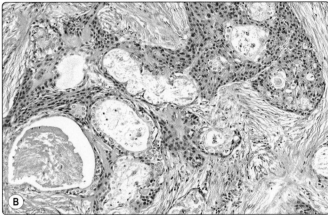

Fig. 4.51 Low-grade mucoepidermoid carcinoma (A) Moderately cellular smear of scattered intermediate cells resembling squamous metaplasia with a 'dirty' background of mucus and some inflammatory cells (Pap, HP); (B) Corresponding tissue section (H&E, IP).

Low-grade mucoepidermoid carcinoma (MEC) is one of the commoner malignant salivary gland tumors, occurring in all age groups including children and adolescents. The clinical presentation may be innocuous. In FNB smears, the background mucus and debris stain blue–violet with MGG and may obscure the cellular component, resembling Warthin's tumor. Cell detail is more evident in alcohol-fixed material. Scattered small clusters of intermediate cells in a mucoid background are suggestive of MEC (Figs 4.51, 4.52). The intermediate cells resemble the squamous metaplastic cells seen in cervical Pap smears. They are relatively cohesive, have a well-defined cytoplasm and mainly bland nuclei. True squamous differentiation and keratinization are uncommon in low-grade tumors. Some of the cells have abundant, finely vacuolated cytoplasm and are difficult to distinguish from macrophages. Other cells contain intracellular mucin vacuoles staining metachromatically with MGG and may have the appearance of goblet cells (Figs 4.53B–4.54). Nucleoli may be prominent, but nuclear chromatin is generally bland in low-grade tumors. Lymphoid cells are sometimes present.

A definitive diagnosis of MEC requires the coexistence in smears of cells showing squamous differentiation and of mucin-secreting cells (Fig. 4.55). Unequivocal evidence of both is not always found, particularly in cystic tumors. In such cases, only a tentative or differential diagnosis can be offered, prompting further investigation.

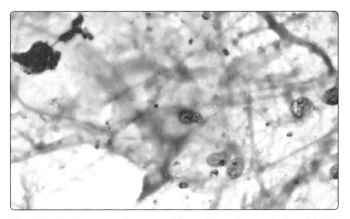

Fig. 4.52 Cystic low-grade mucoepidermoid carcinoma Aspirated fluid typically has a 'dirty' appearance of mucus, debris, inflammatory cells and macrophages; a couple of small aggregates of small bland epithelial cells upper left (MGG, IP).

Smears of *high-grade mucoepidermoid carcinoma* contain obviously malignant squamous epithelial cells (Fig. 4.56). Mucin-secreting cells can be difficult to find, and it may be difficult or impossible to distinguish primary high-grade MEC from metastatic squamous cell carcinoma.

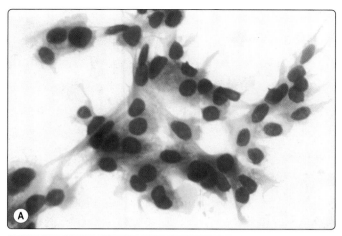

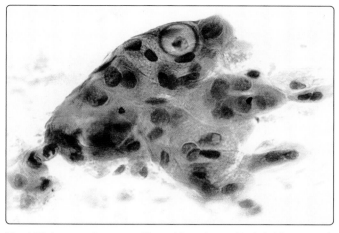

Fig. 4.55 **Low-grade mucoepidermoid carcinoma** Epithelial fragment of intermediate cells, squamoid cells and a cell with an intracytoplasmic mucin vacuole, diagnostic of mucoepidermoid carcinoma (Pap, HP).

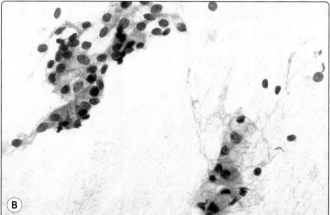

Fig. 4.53 **Low-grade mucoepidermoid carcinoma** (A) Poorly cohesive non-characteristic bland epithelial cells resembling squamous metaplasia represent intermediate cells (MGG, HP); (B) In this example, the group of cells at upper left has a similar non-characteristic metaplastic appearance, the group at lower right show cytoplasmic vacuolation and a goblet cell (Pap, IP).

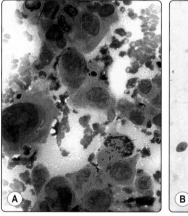
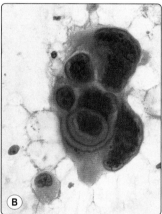

Fig. 4.56 **High-grade mucoepidermoid carcinoma** Pleomorphic, clearly malignant cells, some with squamous differentiation; mitotic figures; distinction from squamous carcinoma not possible (**A**, MGG, HP; **B**, Pap, HP).

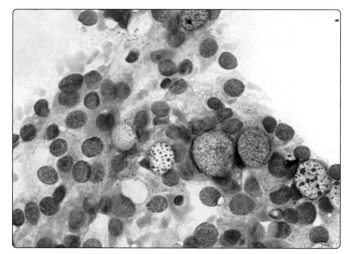

Fig. 4.54 **Low-grade mucoepidermoid carcinoma** Intermediate cells with pale vacuolated cytoplasm and relatively bland nuclei; several intracytoplasmic mucin vacuoles highlighted by the Giemsa staining (MGG, HP).

PROBLEMS AND DIFFERENTIAL DIAGNOSIS

◆ Cystic tumors,
◆ Smears of low cellularity,
◆ Chronic sialadenitis and Küttner's tumor,
◆ Warthin's tumor
◆ Specific typing of high-grade tumors.

Contrary to the high-grade variant, low-grade MEC is difficult to diagnose as malignant cytologically and is one of the most common sources of false-negative FNB diagnoses. The main reason is that many tumors are partly or predominantly cystic (Fig. 4.24D). The aspirated material is often hypocellular and non-characteristic, consisting mainly of mucoid secretion, debris and some inflammatory cells. Cohesive epithelial cell clusters in such a background should raise a suspicion of low-grade MEC even if the cells appear bland, and should cause a diligent search for more diagnostic elements.[25,136] Occasional goblet cells support the suspicion. Smears from

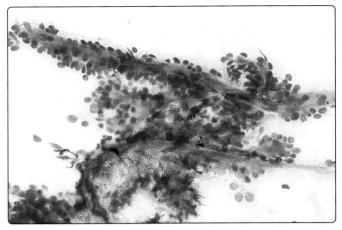

Fig. 4.57 Polymorphous low-grade adenocarcinoma Tissue fragment with a trabecular ('pseudopapillary') microarchitectural pattern; small basaloid cells adhere to anastomosing strands of fibrovascular stroma (MGG, IP).

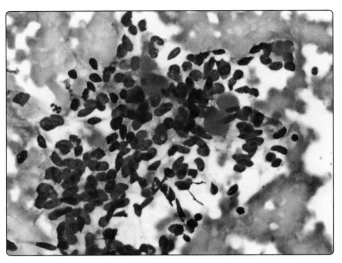

Fig. 4.58 Polymorphous low-grade adenocarcinoma Cluster of small cells with oval, mildly irregular nuclei; bland nuclear chromatin; a few small hyaline stromal globules; some resemblance to adenoid cystic carcinoma (MGG, HP).

non-neoplastic cysts such as retention cysts and lymphoepithelial cysts may also show mucus, debris, metaplastic squamous cells and glandular cells in combination, mimicking low-grade MEC. Warthin's tumor is another benign cystic lesion that can cause differential diagnostic difficulty.[136,137] Multiple sampling with US guidance is often rewarding.

The mucinous background with macrophages and inflammatory cells and the similarity of the intermediate cells of MEC to regenerating, metaplastic ductal epithelial cells in chronic sialadenitis may cause an erroneous diagnosis either way. A clinical suspicion of neoplasia (Küttner's tumor) may add to the difficulty, but history and clinical findings are more often helpful. Similar difficulties can occur in relation to Warthin's tumor. Cells of uniformly oncocytic type and a lymphoid cell population rather than inflammatory cells favor Warthin's tumor.

High-grade, poorly differentiated MEC may not be distinguishable from primary or metastatic squamous carcinoma unless an obvious mucinous component is demonstrated, although obvious keratinization identified cytologically effectively excludes MEC.

Polymorphous low-grade adenocarcinoma (Figs 4.57–4.59)[138–140]

USUAL FINDINGS

◆ Cells in clusters, tissue fragments and single cells,
◆ Cells adhering to strands of fibrovascular stroma in a trabecular (pseudopapillary) pattern,
◆ Hyaline stromal globules often present,
◆ Small basaloid epithelial cells, or slightly larger cells resembling ductal epithelium or metaplastic squamous cells,
◆ Mildly enlarged, pale, ovoid, homogenous nuclei.

Polymorphous low-grade (terminal duct) adenocarcinoma is an uncommon tumor of low-grade malignancy occurring in minor salivary glands, mainly the palate. It is extremely rare in the parotid. Not many cases with FNB findings have been reported. The cells are mainly clustered or in epithelial fragments, which often have a trabecular/pseudopapillary

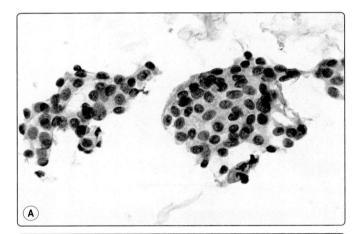

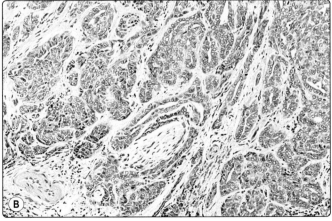

Fig. 4.59 Polymorphous low-grade adenocarcinoma (A) Smears from this tumor of the palate were relatively scanty of small sheets of bland epithelial cells resembling squamous metaplasia (Pap, IP); (B) The corresponding tissue section shows a malignant infiltrative pattern with prominent perineural invasion (H&E, IP).

structure with a fibrous stromal core (Fig. 4.57). The pattern may resemble adenoid cystic carcinoma, especially since small hyaline stromal globules are commonly seen (Fig. 4.58). The nuclei may appear deceptively bland even in tumors showing locally aggressive growth (Fig. 4.59), and false-negative reports are not uncommon.[139]

Epithelial-myoepithelial carcinoma

(Figs 4.60–4.62)[113,141–144]

> ### USUAL FINDINGS
>
> ◆ Cells in tissue fragments, clusters and single,
> ◆ Fragments have a trabecular/pseudopapillary pattern with strands of fibrous stroma,
> ◆ Hyaline stromal globules may be prominent,
> ◆ A distinctly biphasic population is seen only in some tumors,
> ◆ Myoepithelial (clear) cells less cohesive with pale, fragile cytoplasm, moderate nuclear enlargement and atypia; naked nuclei common,
> ◆ Epithelial cells smaller, uniform, mainly in tight clusters.

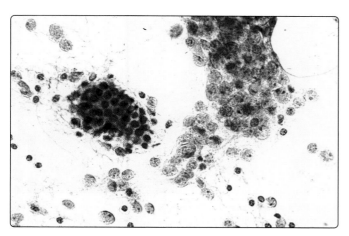

Fig. 4.60 Epithelial-myoepithelial carcinoma Obvious biphasic pattern of clustered small epithelial cells (*left*), and less cohesive cells with pale fragile cytoplasm and large vesicular nuclei; no distinctly 'clear' cells (Pap, HP).

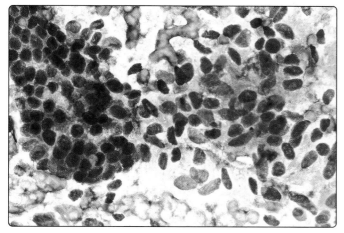

Fig. 4.61 Epithelial-myoepithelial carcinoma Vaguely biphasic pattern of cohesive epithelial cells with rounded nuclei (*left*) and larger cells with indistinct cytoplasm and oval, mildly atypical nuclei. This case presented with pulmonary metastases (MGG, HP).

Epithelial-myoepithelial carcinoma is an uncommon tumor of low to intermediate malignancy, which mainly occurs in the parotid gland. The tumor has a metastatic potential. One of our cases initially presented with multiple tumor metastases in the lung from an unknown primary, another as a carcinoma ex pleomorphic adenoma.[145] The cytological

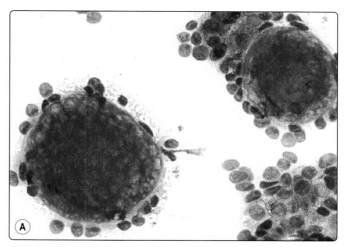

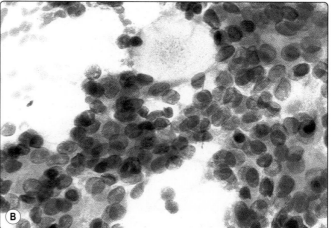

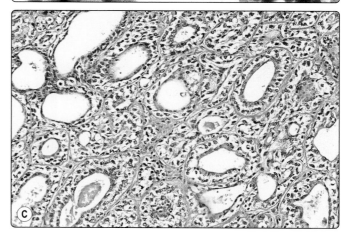

Fig. 4.62 Epithelial-myoepithelial carcinoma In this case there were numerous hyaline stromal globules suggestive of adenoid cystic carcinoma. Note, however, fragile pale cytoplasm and bland nuclear chromatin; (A, MGG, IP; B, Pap, HP), (C) Tissue section, hyaline globules present only focally (H&E, IP) (*Courtesy Dr. J. Wright, Gribbles Pathology, Adelaide*).

diagnosis is difficult for two reasons: a biphasic pattern is not often discernible, and the myoepithelial cells are not easily recognized as clear cells in cytological smears. The pale and indistinct cytoplasm is so fragile that it disperses in the background and most of the cells appear as naked nuclei, dispersed or clustered. The nuclei are mildly atypical, showing moderate enlargement and variation in size and shape, but have a pale chromatin and discrete central nucleoli. If present, epithelial cells are small and uniform and form tight cohesive clusters. Hyaline stromal material is often present, sometimes in the form of hyaline stromal globules similar to those of adenoid cystic carcinoma (Fig. 4.62). The composite population of both epithelial and myoepithelial cells can be confirmed by immunostaining.

A number of different neoplasms occurring in the salivary glands have a prominent *clear cell component*,[146] clear cell carcinoma NOS, mainly epithelial-myoepithelial carcinoma, clear cell carcinoma NOS, sebaceous adenoma and metastatic renal cell carcinoma. A clear cell pattern can be present focally or uniformly in acinic cell and low-grade mucoepidermoid carcinoma and occasionally in oncocytoma, pleomorphic adenoma and basal cell adenoma. Although the clear cell pattern is striking in tissue sections, it is generally not well reproduced in cytological smears. The cytoplasm is never truly clear. At best it is abundant, pale and vacuolated with visible cell membranes, but it is often fragile and disperses in the background leaving the nuclei bare. *Renal cell carcinoma* not uncommonly metastasises to the parotid. The cells of renal cell carcinoma have abundant vacuolated pale cytoplasm with visible cell membranes. Nuclei vary in size and show variable but obvious atypia and often prominent nucleoli. Typically, the tumor cells adhere to strands of endothelial cells or vascular basement membrane material (see Fig. 4.77 and Chapter 12).

Adenoid cystic carcinoma (Figs 4.63–4.68)[15,147,148]

CRITERIA FOR DIAGNOSIS
◆ Cellular smears, cells both single and clustered,
◆ Hyaline spherical globules of varying size with adherent tumor cells,
◆ Cellular tissue fragments with finger-like or beaded cords or strands of hyaline stroma,
◆ Multilayered dense cell clusters and cup-shaped fragments composed of tumor cells,
◆ Scanty cytoplasm, high nuclear:cytoplasmic ratio, nuclear molding, naked nuclei,
◆ Relatively uniform, round or oval hyperchromatic nuclei; coarse nuclear chromatin; nucleoli,
◆ Hyaline stromal material may be absent in poorly differentiated tumors.

Adenoid cystic carcinoma (AdCC) is a common malignancy in the minor salivary glands and occasionally occurs in unusual sites such as the airways, lacrimal glands and external auditory canal.[149] The hyaline stromal globules are the most striking feature of this neoplasm, but are not diagnostic thereof. They occur in several other entities (basal cell adenoma, canalicular adenoma, basal cell adenocarcinoma

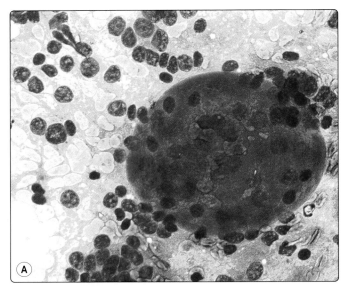

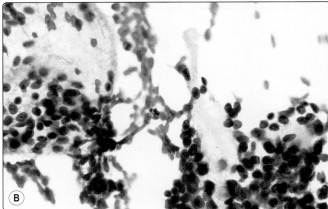

Fig. 4.63 Adenoid cystic carcinoma (A) Small uniform epithelial cells with hyperchromatic nuclei and coarse chromatin, dispersed and adhering to a large, hyaline stromal globule (MGG, HP); (B) The hyaline stromal globules are less striking in Pap-stained smears and are pale, almost transparent (Pap, HP).

pleomorphic adenoma, polymorphous low-grade adenocarcinoma, epithelial-myoepithelial carcinoma). The globules vary considerably in size, stain bright red or purple and appear dense and homogeneous in MGG-stained smears. With Pap or H&E, the globules are pale, semi-translucent and less conspicuous (Fig. 4.63A,B). Finger-like or beaded strands or cords of stromal material have similar staining properties and hyaline texture (Fig. 4.66). They are characteristic but again not specific to AdCC. The tumor cells are both in multilayered, dense aggregates and dispersed as single cells and often adhere to the stromal material. The nuclei are rather uniform in size but have an irregular shape. They are hyperchromatic with coarsely granular chromatin and visible nucleoli. The cytoplasm is scanty, the N:C ratio is high and more nuclear molding is common. The tumor cells often form cup-shaped epithelial fragments with an open end reproducing the typical histology (Fig. 4.64).[147] Malignant nuclear features are more obvious in poorly differentiated tumors with tight clusters of basaloid cells and little or no stroma (Fig. 4.68).

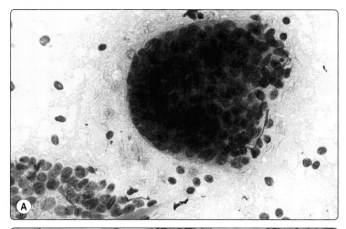

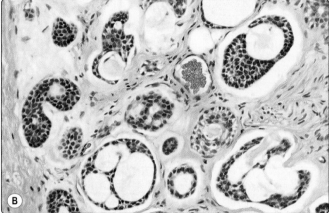

Fig. 4.64 Adenoid cystic carcinoma Cellular epithelial tissue fragments with a characteristic cup shape open at one end; (**A**, MGG, IP; **B**, corresponding tissue section, H&E, IP).

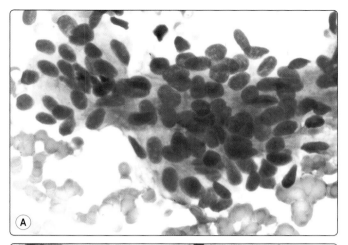

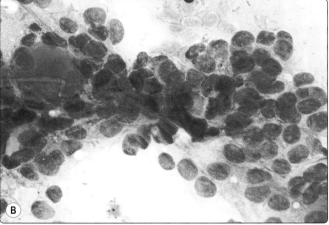

Fig. 4.65 Adenoid cystic carcinoma vs pleomorphic adenoma (A) Pleomorphic adenoma; (**B**) Adenoid cystic carcinoma. Note bland nuclei of pleomorphic adenoma, coarse irregular chromatin and some nuclear molding in adenoid cystic carcinoma (MGG, HP).

Not infrequently, FNB of an AdCC may cause intense pain, perhaps in some way related to the tendency for this tumor to infiltrate along nerve fibers. This can be a useful hint to the nature of the lesion.

PROBLEMS AND DIFFERENTIAL DIAGNOSIS

- ◆ Distinction from other tumors with hyaline stromal globules,
- ◆ Dermal sweat gland, solid tumors and basal cell carcinoma,
- ◆ Poorly differentiated, solid tumors.

Distinction from basal cell adenoma can be a problem (see basal cell adenoma). This mainly concerns the membranous and trabecular variants, which can contain prominent hyaline stromal globules.[25,117,118] Marked variation in size and a dense, truly hyaline texture of the globules suggest AdCC. The nuclear morphology is an important distinguishing feature. The nuclei of AdCC are similarly small and relatively monomorphic but are hyperchromatic with a coarse chromatin, best seen in Pap-stained smears. Nucleoli may be prominent and nuclear membranes irregular and thickened. Other tumors that may contain hyaline stromal globules are pleomorphic adenoma, epithelial-myoepithelial carcinoma and polymorphous low-grade adenocarcinoma. Distinction from highly cellular pleomorphic adenoma is not always easy. Hyaline stromal globules may be seen in pleomorphic adenoma and, conversely, the stroma may focally appear fibromyxoid in AdCC (Figs 4.65–4.67). However, truly chondromyxoid matrix with spindle cells is specific to pleomorphic adenoma. In summary, a diagnosis of AdCC must not be based solely on the presence of hyaline globules, but requires a close scrutiny of cellular and nuclear features.

Some dermal neoplasms can closely resemble AdCC cytologically, and this may cause a problem if the tumor is situated superficially in the parotid region. For example, distinction from cutaneous cylindroma and basal cell carcinoma may be difficult.[150,151] In a case from our files of recurrent cutaneous basal cell carcinoma deeply invading the parotid gland, smears were indistinguishable from poorly differentiated AdCC. Similar cases have been reported.[152]

A specific diagnosis of AdCC may be difficult in poorly differentiated tumors with a solid growth pattern due to the absence of characteristic stroma.[153] Basaloid squamous carcinoma of the head and neck (see p. 43) is a rare tumor that should also be considered. The differential diagnosis depends on the identification of cells with obvious squamous differentiation. Neuroendocrine carcinoma and poorly differentiated metastatic carcinoma also enter the differential diagnosis.

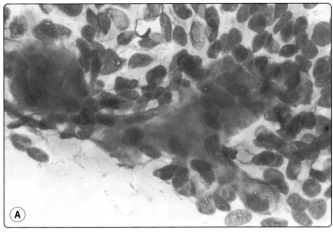

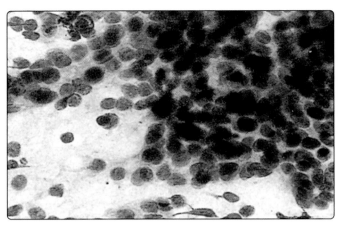

Fig. 4.68 Adenoid cystic carcinoma, poorly differentiated Numerous small epithelial cells, single and in dense clusters; hyperchromatic nuclei with coarse chromatin, stromal elements absent (Pap, HP).

Carcinoma ex pleomorphic adenoma
(Figs 4.69, 4.70)[110,114,154]

CRITERIA FOR DIAGNOSIS

◆ A history of recent increase in size of a longstanding tumor,
◆ A dual population of malignant epithelial cells and benign cells and stromal components of pleomorphic adenoma.

This is an uncommon event said to occur in 3–4% of pleomorphic adenomas.[98] Clinically, a sudden increase in size of a tumor present for years signals the possibility of a malignant change. Most often, carcinoma ex pleomorphic adenoma is a salivary duct carcinoma or a poorly differentiated carcinoma of no specific type, but mucoepidermoid and squamous cell carcinoma, epithelial-myoepithelial carcinoma and acinic cell carcinoma have also been observed arising in PA.[110,155,156]

The main problem is to obtain representative samples from this type of tumor. The malignant component can be missed or overlooked. The occasional finding of worrying cytological atypia in benign pleomorphic adenoma has been mentioned. Carcinoma ex pleomorphic adenoma has the highest false-negative rate (35.3%) for FNB of all malignant salivary gland tumors.[114] On the other hand, if no benign components are found in the sample, an unqualified diagnosis of malignancy is likely given. Since the prognosis and management of carcinoma ex pleomorphic adenoma are the same as for benign pleomorphic adenoma as long as the cancer remains confined within the capsule, an unqualified malignant diagnosis may result in unnecessarily extensive surgery. Clinical correlation is therefore essential.

Salivary duct carcinoma (Figs 4.71–4.73)[157–161]

CRITERIA FOR DIAGNOSIS

◆ Clearly malignant epithelial cells, single and in clusters,
◆ Abundant cytoplasm, squamoid, sometimes oncocyte-like,
◆ No typical stromal component,
◆ Background of necrotic debris,
◆ Low-grade tumors with a cribriform pattern and uniform cells have been reported.

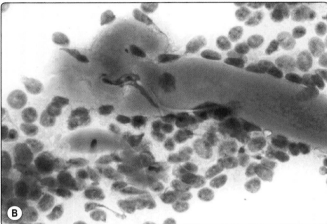

Fig. 4.66 Adenoid cystic carcinoma vs pleomorphic adenoma (A) Pleomorphic adenoma; (B) Adenoid cystic carcinoma. Similar finger-like cords of hyaline stroma in both (MGG, HP).

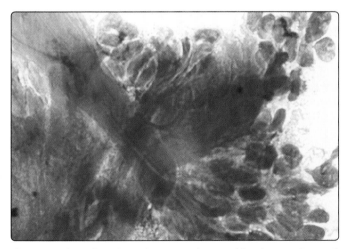

Fig. 4.67 Adenoid cystic carcinoma vs pleomorphic adenoma Smear of adenoid cystic carcinoma showing a fibrillar fibromyxoid stroma similar to pleomorphic adenoma, but atypical nuclear chromatin (MGG, HP).

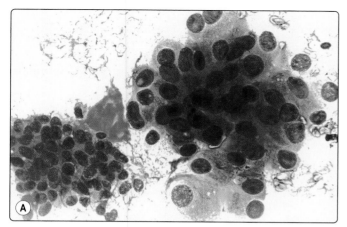

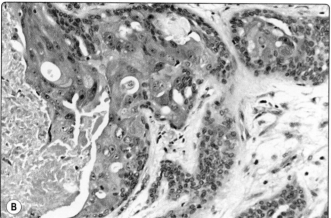

Fig. 4.69 Carcinoma ex pleomorphic adenoma (A) The epithelial cell cluster to the right shows prominent nuclear enlargement and atypia; the cluster to the left is of benign cells associated with a fragment of myxoid stroma (MGG, HP); (B) Corresponding tissue section showing high-grade carcinoma of salivary duct carcinoma type (H&E, IP).

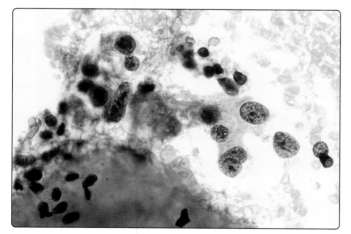

Fig. 4.70 Carcinoma ex pleomorphic adenoma Poorly cohesive malignant epithelial cells in a bloody background; the cells at lower left appear bland with uniform oval nuclei. Histology showed a poorly differentiated carcinoma and some foci of residual benign pleomorphic adenoma (Pap, HP).

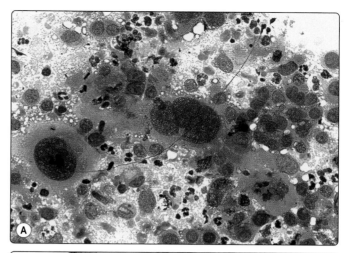

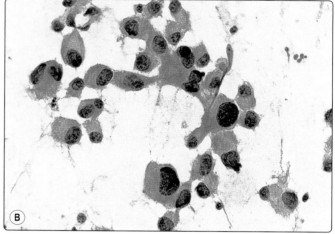

Fig. 4.71 Salivary duct carcinoma Poorly cohesive, obviously malignant epithelial cells; large pleomorphic and hyperchromatic nuclei, abundant cytoplasm, no microarchitectural pattern, necrotic debris and inflammatory cells (A, MGG, HP; B, Pap, HP).

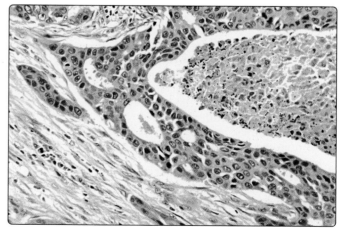

Fig. 4.72 Salivary duct carcinoma Tissue section from similar case as Fig. 4.70. Note resemblance to high-grade ductal carcinoma in situ of breast (H&E, IP).

Most salivary duct carcinomas are of high malignancy grade. They resemble high-grade ductal carcinoma in situ (comedocarcinoma) of the breast both histologically and cytologically. The neoplastic cells are obviously malignant with abundant cytoplasm and large, pleomorphic nuclei. Necrotic

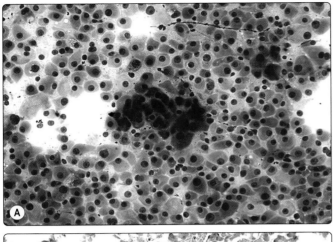

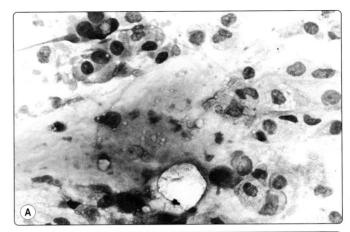

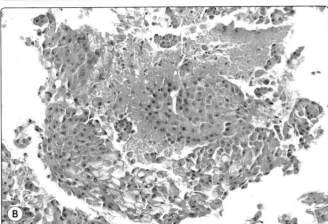

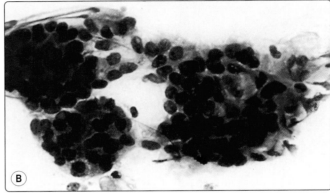

Fig. 4.73 Salivary duct carcinoma oncocytic type (A) Smear showing numerous dispersed strikingly plasmacytoid cells with abundant dense cytoplasm, eccentric nuclei, anisokaryosis and prominent nucleoli (Diff-Quik, HP); (B) Cell button of same sample showing obvious tumor necrosis (H&E, IP).

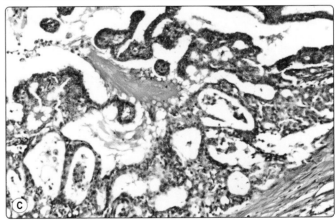

Fig. 4.74 Mucus-secreting 'adenopapillary' carcinoma (A) Poorly cohesive, moderately atypical epithelial cells with a background of mucus. (B) Papillary clusters of similar epithelial cells, some with intracytoplasmic mucus (MGG, HP), (C) Corresponding tissue section (H&E, IP).

debris is usually present as in comedocarcinoma. The differential diagnosis is with other high-grade carcinomas such as high-grade mucoepidermoid and squamous carcinoma, and also includes metastatic breast carcinoma. In some cases, the cells are predominantly of or oncocytic type, suggesting malignant oncocytoma. Smears from one of our cases initially diagnosed as myoepithelial or oncocytic carcinoma showed prominently plasmacytoid cells with abundant dense cytoplasm and eccentric nuclei. The presence of focal tumor necrosis in a cell block pointed to salivary duct carcinoma, subsequently confirmed (Fig. 4.73).

Immune markers may be helpful in the distinction from other tumors with squamoid cells.[162]

Adenocarcinoma of no special type

(Figs 4.74, 4.75)[163]

> **USUAL FINDINGS**
>
> - Nuclear features of malignancy,
> - Some glandular differentiation (microglandular pattern),
> - Intracellular and/or extracellular mucin,
> - Absence of features to suggest a specific entity.

Primary adenocarcinoma of no special type is rare, mainly seen in minor salivary glands, or arising in pre-existing pleomorphic adenoma. There is a spectrum of patterns from relatively well-differentiated papillary cystadenocarcinoma, mucinous adenocarcinoma and 'adenopapillary' carcinoma (Fig. 4.74) to pleomorphic poorly differentiated carcinoma. It may represent a poorly differentiated component of a specific type such as acinic cell carcinoma. Metastatic origin can be difficult to exclude. Clinical examination and history are therefore essential and definitive

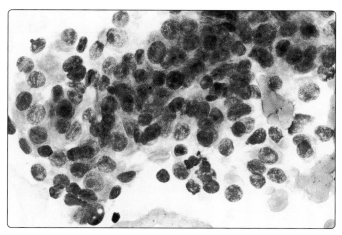

Fig. 4.75 Adenocarcinoma NOS Poorly differentiated adenocarcinoma without specific features (MGG, HP).

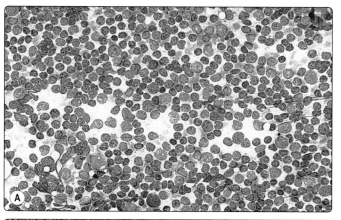

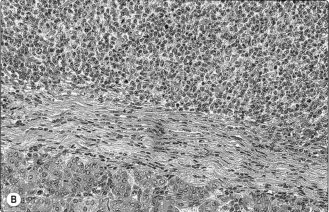

Fig. 4.76 Small cell carcinoma Small cell neuroendocrine carcinoma primary in the parotid. Dispersed population of small cells with round nuclei and scanty cytoplasm resembling malignant lymphoma; neuroendocrine markers positive (**A**, MGG, HP; **B**, tissue section, H&E, IP).

type-specific diagnosis may have to await histological examination.

Squamous cell carcinoma[164]

The criteria for diagnosis are as for other sites. The common presence of lymph nodes within the parotid gland and adjacent to other salivary glands makes it difficult to decide if a squamous carcinoma is primary or metastatic by FNB. Distinction from poorly differentiated mucoepidermoid carcinoma may also be impossible.

Atypical metaplastic and degenerate squamous epithelial cells in some benign conditions such as necrotizing sialometaplasia, Warthin's tumor and pleomorphic adenoma with squamous metaplasia can occasionally be mistaken for well-differentiated squamous cell carcinoma. Multiple sampling and clinical correlation are essential.

Other malignant neoplasms

Small cell anaplastic (neuroendocrine) carcinoma (Fig. 4.76) rarely occurs as a primary tumor in the salivary glands. The cytological pattern is the same as for neuroendocrine carcinomas in other sites, and a primary elsewhere, particularly in the lung, must be excluded before making this diagnosis.[165] The smear pattern can be mistaken for malignant lymphoma, but there is usually a greater tendency to clustering of cells and nuclear molding. The diagnosis should be supported by immunostaining for neuroendocrine and pan-lymphocyte markers or by ultrastructural examination.

Malignant myoepithelioma,[166–168] *malignant oncocytoma,*[169,170] *carcinoma ex Warthin's tumor,*[22,171] and *sebaceous carcinoma*[172] are rare malignant tumors of the salivary glands, which have not yet been well characterized cytologically. The reader is referred to single case reports and small series for descriptions of these entities. *Undifferentiated carcinoma* of the parotid gland has been reported in elderly patients. *Lymphoepithelial carcinoma* of nasopharyngeal type has also been described in the salivary glands.[173,174]

Metastatic carcinoma, melanoma and lymphoma[175–177] may involve either the salivary glands or lymph nodes

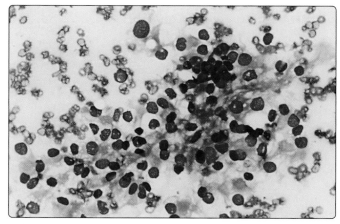

Fig. 4.77 Renal cell carcinoma metastatic to parotid Aggregate of epithelial cells with abundant pale vacuolated ('clear') cytoplasm adherent to strands of vascular basement membrane (MGG, HP).

adjacent to or within the gland. The commonest primary tumor is cutaneous squamous cell carcinoma of the head and neck. Metastatic renal cell carcinoma (Fig. 4.77) is to be distinguished from primary clear cell tumors, as mentioned above. The possibility of metastatic origin must be kept in mind when examining salivary gland aspirates.

References

1. Kocjan G, Ramsay A, Beale T, O'Flynn P. Head and neck cancer in the UK. What is expected of cytopathology Cytopathol 2009;20:69–95.

2. Oliai BR, Sheth S, Burroughs FH, Ali SZ. 'Parapharyngeal space' tumors. A cytopathologic study of 24 cases on fine-needle aspiration. Diagn Cytopathol 2005;32:11–5.

3. Arabi H, Yousef N, Bandyopadhyay S, et al. Fine needle aspiration of head and neck masses in the operating room: accuracy and potential benefits. Diagn Cytopathol 2008;36:369–74.

4. Rapkiewicz A, Le BT, Simsir A, et al. Spectrum of H & N lesions diagnosed by F-NAC in the paediatric population. Cancer Cytopathol 2007;111:242–51.

5. Engzell U, Franzen S, Zajicek J. Aspiration biopsy of tumours of the neck. II. Cytologic findings in 13 cases of carotid body tumour. Acta Cytol 1971;15:25–30.

6. Daskalopoulou D, Rapidis AD, Maounis N, Markidou S. Fine-needle aspiration cytology in tumors and tumor-like conditions of the oral and maxillofacial region. Diagnostic reliability and limitations. Cancer (Cancer Cytopathol) 1997;81: 238–52.

7. Bardales RH, Baker SJ, Mukunyadzi P. Fine-needle aspiration cytology findings in 214 cases of nonparotid lesions in the head. Diagn Cytopathol 2000;22: 211–7.

8. Layfield L. Fine-needle aspiration in the diagnosis of head and neck lesions: a review and discussion of problems in differential diagnosis. Diagn Cytopathol 2007;35:798–805.

9. Seifert G, Sobin LH. The World Health Organization's histological classification of salivary gland tumors. A commentary on the second edition. Cancer 1992;70: 379–85.

10. Chan M, McGuire L. Cytodiagnosis of lesions presenting as salivary gland swellings. A report of seven cases. Diagn Cytopathol 1992;8:439–43.

11. Nettle WJ, Orell SR. Fine needle aspiration in the diagnosis of salivary gland lesions. Aust NZ J Surg 1989;59:47–51.

12. Layfield L, Gopez E, Hirschowitz S. Cost efficiency analysis for fine-needle aspiration in the workup of parotid and submandibular gland nodules. Diagn Cytopathol 2006;34:734–8.

13. Eneroth CM, Zajicek J. Aspiration biopsy of salivary gland tumours. II. Morphologic studies on smears and histologic sections from oncocytic tumours. Acta Cytol 1965;9:355–61.

14. Eneroth CM, Zajicek J. Aspiration biopsy of salivary gland tumours. III. Morphologic studies on smears and histologic sections from 368 mixed tumours. Acta Cytol 1966;10:440–54.

15. Eneroth CM, Zajicek J. Aspiration biopsy of salivary gland tumours. IV. Morphologic studies on smears and histologic sections from 45 cases of adenoid cystic carcinoma. Acta Cytol 1969;13:59–63.

16. Zajicek J, Eneroth CM. Cytological diagnosis of salivary gland carcinomata from aspiration biopsy smears. Acta Otolaryng 1970;263(Suppl.):183–5.

17. Zajicek J., Eneroth CM, Jakobson P. Aspiration biopsy of salivary gland tumors. VI. Morphologic studies on smears and histologic sections from mucoepidermoid carcinoma. Acta Cytol. 1976;20:35–41.

18. Atuta T, Grenman R, Laippala P, Klemi P-J. Fine-needle aspiration biopsy in the diagnosis of parotid gland lesions: evaluation of 438 biopsies. Diagn Cytopathol 1996;15:185–90.

19. Al-Khafaji B, Nestok BR, Katz RL. Fine-needle aspiration of 154 parotid masses with histologic correlation. Ten-year experience at the University of Texas M.D.Anderson Cancer Center. Cancer (Cancer Cytopathol) 1998;84:153–9.

20. Stewart CJR, MacKenzie K, McGarry GW, Mowat A. Fine-needle aspiration cytology of salivary gland: a review of 341 cases. Diagn Cytopathol 2000;22: 139–46.

21. Young JA. Diagnostic problems in fine needle aspiration cytopathology of the salivary glands. J Clin Pathol 1994;47:193–8.

22. Klijanienko J, Vielh P, Batsakis JD, et al. Monographs in Clinical Cytology. Volume 15. Salivary Gland Tumours. Basel, Switzerland: Karger; 2000.

23. Cramer H, Layfield L, Lampe H. Fine needle aspiration of salivary gland lesions. In: Schmidt WA, editor. Cytopathology annual. Baltimore: Williams and Wilkins; 1993. p. 181–206.

24. MacLeod CB, Frable WJ. Fine needle aspiration biopsy cytology of the salivary glands: problem cases. Diagn Cytopathol 1993;9:216–25.

25. Orell SR. Diagnostic difficulties in the interpretation of fine needle aspirates of salivary gland lesions: the problem revisited. Cytopathol 1995;6:285–300.

26. Raywanshi A, Gupta K, Gupta N, et al. Fine needle aspiration cytology of salivary glands. Diagnostic pitfalls revisited. Diagn Cytopathol 2006;34:580–4.

27. Daneshbod Y, Daneshbod K, Khaderi B. Diagnostic difficulties in the interpretation of fine needle aspirate samples in salivary lesions. Diagnostic pitfalls revisited. Acta Cytol 2009;53:53–70.

28. Mukunyadzi P, Bardales RH, Palmer HE, Stanley MW. Tissue effects of salivary gland fine-needle aspiration. Does this procedure preclude accurate histologic diagnosis? Am J Clin Pathol 2000;114:741–5

29. Batsakis JG, Sneige N, El-Naggar AK. Fine-needle aspiration of salivary glands: its utility and tissue effects. Ann Otol Rhinol Laryngol 1992;101:185–8.

30. Li S, Baloch ZW, Tomaszewski JE, LiVolsi VA. Worrisome histologic alterations following fine-needle aspiration of benign parotid lesions. Arch Pathol Lab Med 2000;124:87–91.

31. Parfitt JR, McLachlin M, Weir MM. Comparison of Thin Prep and conventional smears in salivary gland fine-needle aspiration biopsies. Cancer 2007;111:123–9.

32. Engzell U, Zajicek J. Aspiration biopsy of tumours of the neck. I. Aspiration biopsy and cytologic findings in 100 cases of congenital cysts. Acta Cytol 1970;14:51–7.

33. Frable WJ, Frable MAS. Thin-needle aspiration biopsy: the diagnosis of head and neck tumours revisited. Cancer 1979;43:1541–8.

34. Burgess KL, Hartwick RWJ, Bedard YC. Metastatic squamous carcinoma presenting as a neck cyst. Differential diagnosis from inflamed branchial cleft cyst in fine needle aspirates. Acta Cytol 1993;37:494–8.

35. Üstün M, Risberg B, Davidson B, Berner A. Cystic change in metastatic lymph nodes: a common diagnostic pitfall in fine-needle aspiration cytology. Diagn Cytopathol 2002;27:387–92.

36. Sheahan P, O'Leary G, Lee G, Fitzgibbon J. Cystic cervical metastases: incidence and diagnosis using FNAB. Otolaryngol Head Neck Surg 2002;127:294–8.

37. Shakin A, Burroughs FH, Kirby JP, Ali SZ. Thyroglossal duct cyst: a cytopathologic study of 26 cases. Diagn Cytopathol 2005;33:365–9.

38. De Las Casas L, Bardales RH. Fine-needle aspiration cytology of mucous retention cyst of the tongue: distinction from other cystic lesions of the tongue. Diagn Cytopathol 2000;22:308–12.

39. Michael CW, Naylor B. Amyloid in cytologic specimens. Differential diagnosis and diagnostic pitfalls. Acta Cytol 1999;43:746–55.

40. Frable MA, Frable WJ. Fine needle aspiration biopsy in the diagnosis of sarcoid of the head and neck. Acta Cytol 1984;28:175–7.

41. Micheau C, Klijanienko J, Luboinski B, Richard J. So-called branchiogenic

carcinoma is actually cystic metastases in the neck from a tonsillar primary. Laryngoscope 1990;100:878–83.

42. Bhanote M, Yang GCH. Malignant first branchial cleft cysts presenting as submandibular abscesses in fine-needle aspiration: report of three cases and review of the literature. Diagn Cytopathol 2008;36:876–81.

43. Klijanienko J, El-Naggar A, Ponzio-Prion A, et al. Basaloid squamous carcinoma of head and neck. Immunohistochemical comparison with adenoid cystic carcinoma and squamous cell carcinoma. Arch Otolaryngol Head Neck Surg 1993;119:887–90.

44. Micheau C. What's new in histological classification and recognition of naso-pharyngeal carcinoma (N.P.C.). Path Res Pract 1986;181:249–53.

45. Jayaram G, Swain M, Khanijow V, Jalaludin MA. Fine-needle aspiration cytology of metastatic nasopharyngeal carcinoma. Diagn Cytopathol 1998;19:168–72.

46. Kollur SM, El Hag IA. Fine-needle aspiration cytology of metastatic nasopharyngeal carcinoma in cervical lymph nodes: comparison with metastatic squamous cell carcinoma, and Hodgkin's and non-Hodgkin's lymphoma. Diagn Cytopathol 2003;28:18–22.

47. Viguer JM, Jimenez-Hefferman JA, Lopez-Ferrer P, et al. Fine-needle aspiration cytology of metastatic nasopharyngeal carcinoma. Diagn Cytopathol 2005;32:233–7.

48. Helsel JC, Bardales RH, Mukunyadzi P. Fine-needle aspiration biopsy cytology of malignant neoplasms of the sinonasal tract. A review of 22 primary and metastatic tumors. Cancer (Cancer Cytopathol) 2003;99:105–12.

49. Bellizzi AM, Bourne TD, Mills SE, Stelow EB. The cytologic features of sinonasal undifferentiated carcinoma and olfactory neuroblastoma. Am J Clin Pathol 2008;129:367–76.

50. Lack EE, Cubilla AL, Woodruff JM. Paragangliomas of the head and neck region. A pathologic study of tumours from 71 patients. Human Pathol 1979;10:191–218.

51. Fleming MV, Oertel YC, Rodrigues ER. Fine-needle aspiration of six carotid body paragangliomas. Diagn Cytopathol 1993;9:510–5.

52. Verma K, et al. Cytomorphological spectrum in paraganglioma. Acta Cytol 2008;52:549–56

53. Solares J, Lacruz C. Fine needle aspiration cytology diagnosis of an extracranial meningioma presenting as a cervical mass. Acta Cytol 1987;31:502–4.

54. Tan LHC. Meningioma presenting as a parapharyngeal tumor. Report of a case with fine needle aspiration cytology. Acta Cytol 2001;45:1053–9.

55. Hameed A, Gokden M, Hanna EY. Fine-needle aspiration cytology of a primary ectopic meningioma. Diagn Cytopathol 2002;26:297–300.

56. Collins BT, Cramer HM, Hearn SA. Fine needle aspiration cytology of metastatic olfactory neuroblastoma. Acta Cytol 1997;41:802–10.

57. Logrono R, Futoran RM, Hartig G, Inhorn SL. Olfactory neuroblastoma (esthesioneuroblastoma): appearance on fine-needle aspiration: report of a case. Diagn Cytopathol 1997;17:205–8.

58. Zajdela A, Vielh P, Schlinger P, Haye C. Fine-needle cytology of 292 palpable orbital and eyelid tumors. Am J Clin Pathol 1990;93:100–4.

59. Gupta S, Sood B, Gulati M, et al. Orbital mass lesions: US-guided fine-needle aspiration biopsy – experience in 37 patients. Radiology 1999;213:568–72.

60. Krzystolik Z, Roslawska A, Bedner E. The cytological, immunocytochemical and molecular genetic analysis in diagnosis of the neoplasms of the eye, eye adnexa and orbit. Doc Ophthalmol 1994;88:155–63.

61. Nassar DL, Raab SS, Silverman JF, et al. Fine-needle aspiration for the diagnosis of orbital hematolymphoid lesions. Diagn Cytopathol 2000;23:314–7.

62. Rastogi A, Jain S. Fine needle aspiration biopsy in orbital lesions. Orbit 2001; 20:11–23.

63. Wolska-Szmidt E, Jakkubowska A, et al. Fine needle aspiration biopsy and molecular analysis in differential diagnosis of lymphoproliferative diseases of the orbit and eye adnexa. Pol J Pathol 2004;55:51–7.

64. Tani E, Seregard S, Rupp G, et al. Fine-needle aspiration cytology and immunocytochemistry of orbital masses. Diagn Cytopathol 2006;34:1–5.

65. Sturgis CD, Silverman JF, Kennerdell JS, Raab SS. Fine-needle aspiration for the diagnosis of primary epithelial tumors of the lacrymal gland and ocular adnexa. Diagn Cytopathol 2001;24: 86–9.

66. Klijanienko J, El-Naggar AK, Servois V, et al. Histologically similar synchronous or metachronous lacrimal salivary-type and parotid gland tumors: A series of 11 cases. Head Neck 1999;21:512–6.

67. Dhaliwal U, Arora VK, Singh N, Bhatia A. Clinical and cytopathologic correlation in chronic inflammations of the orbit and ocular adnexa: a review of 55 cases. Orbit 2004;23:219–25.

68. Trolet J, Hupé P, Huon I, et al. Genomic profiling and identification of high-risk uveal melanoma by array CGH analysis of primary tumors and liver metastases. Invest Ophthalmol Vis Sci 2009;50:2572–80. Epub 2009 Jan 17.

69. Chan DH, Miller TR, Ljung BM, et al. Fine needle aspiration biopsy in uveal melanoma. Acta Cytol 1989;33: 599–605.

70. Sen S, Singha U, Kumar H, et al. Diagnostic intraocular fine-needle aspiration biopsy – an experience in three cases of retinoblastoma. Diagn Cytopathol 1999;21:331–4.

71. Karcioglu ZA. Fine needle aspiration biopsy (FNAB) for retinoblastoma. Retina 2002;22:707–10.

72. Ljung B-M, Chan D, Miller TR, et al. Intraocular lymphoma. Cytologic diagnosis and the role of immunologic markers. Acta Cytol 1988;32:840–7.

73. Willems J. Aspiration biopsy cytology of tumors of the central nervous system and the base of the skull. In: Linsk JA, Franzen S, editors. Clinical aspiration cytology. Philadelphia: Lippincott; 1983. p. 361–70.

74. Russel D. The wet-film technique in neurosurgery. In: Recent advances in clinical pathology. London: Churchill; 1947.

75. Smith AR, Elsheik TM, Silverman JF. Intraoperative cytologic diagnosis of suprasellar and sellar cystic lesions. Diagn Cytopathol 1999;20:137–47.

76. Bleggi-Torres LF, de Noronha L, Schneider Gugelmin E, et al. Accuracy of the smear technique in the cytological diagnosis of 650 lesions of the central nervous system. Diagn Cytopathol 2001;24:293–5.

77. Roessler K, Dietrich W, Kitz K. High diagnostic accuracy of cytologic smears of central nervous system tumors. A 15-year experience based on 4,172 patients. Acta Cytol 2002;46:667–74.

78. Vural G, Hagmar B, Walaas L. Extracranial metastasis of glioblastoma multiforme diagnosed by fine needle aspiration: a report of two cases and a review of the literature. Diagn Cytopathol 1996;15:60–5.

79. Domanski H, Akerman M. Fine-needle aspiration cytology of tongue swellings. A study of 75 cases. Diagn Cytopathol 1998;18:387–92.

80. Jin B, Saleh H. Pitfalls in the diagnosis of adult rhabdomyoma by fine needle aspiration: report of a case and a brief literature review. Diagn Cytopathol 2009;37:483–6.

81. Günhan Ö, Dogan N, Celasun B, et al. Fine needle aspiration cytology of oral cavity and jaw bone lesions. A report of 102 cases. Acta Cytol 1993;37: 135–41.

82. Vargas PA, da Cruz-Perez DE, Mata GM, et al. Fine needle aspiration cytology as an additional tool in the diagnosis of odontogenic keratocyst. Cytopathol 2007;18:361–6.

83. Ramzy I, Aufdemorte TB, Duncan OL. Diagnosis of radiolucent lesions of the jaw by fine needle aspiration biopsy. Acta Cytol 1985;29:419–24.

84. Mathew S, Rappaport K, Ali SZ, et al. Ameloblastoma. Cytologic findings and

literature review. Acta Cytol 1997;41:955–60.

85. Ingram EA, Evans ML, Zitsch RP. Fine needle aspiration cytology of ameloblastic carcinoma of the maxilla: a rare tumor. Diagn Cytopathol 1996;14:249–52.

86. Spitz DJ, Reddy V, Selvaggi SM, et al. Fine-needle aspiration of scalp lesions. Diagn Cytopathol 2000;23:35–8.

87. Henry-Stanley MJ, Bencke J, Bardales RH, Stanley MW. Fine-needle aspiration of normal tissue from enlarged salivary glands: sialosis or missed target? Diagn Cytopathol 1995;13:300–3.

88. Gupta S., Sodhani P. Sialadenosis of parotid gland. A cytomorphologic and morphometric study of four cases. Analyt. Quant. Cytol. Histol 1998;20:225–8.

89. Layfield LJ, Gopez EV. Cystic lesions of the salivary glands: cytologic features in fine-needle aspiration biopsies. Diagn Cytopathol 2002;27:197–204.

90. Jayaram G, Khurana N, Basu S. Crystalloids in a cystic lesion of parotid salivary gland. Diagn Cytopathol 1993;9:70–1.

91. Nasuti JF, Gupta PK, Fleisher SR, LiVolsi VA. Nontyrosine crystalloids in salivary gland lesions: report of seven cases with fine-needle aspiration cytology and follow-up surgical pathology. Diagn Cytopathol 2000;22:167–71.

92. Pantanowitz L, Goulart RA, Cao QJ. Salivary gland crystalloids. Diagn Cytopathol 2006;34:749.

93. Elliott JN, Oertel YC. Lymphoepithelial cysts of the salivary glands. Histological and cytologic features. Am J Clin Pathol 1990;93:39–43

94. Chhieng DC, Argosino R, McKenna B, et al. Utility of fine-needle aspiration in the diagnosis of salivary gland lesions in patients infected with human immunodeficiency virus. Diagn Cytopathol 1999;21:260–4.

95. Johnson FB, Oertel YC, Ammann K. Sialadenitis with crystalloid formation: a report of six cases diagnosed by fine-needle aspiration. Diagn Cytopathol 1995;12:76–80.

96. Wax TD, Layfield LJ, Zaleski S, et al. Cytomegalovirus sialadenitis in patients with the acquired immunodeficiency syndrome: a potential diagnostic pitfall with fine-needle aspiration cytology. Diagn Cytopathol 1994;10:169–74.

97. Casiano RR, Cooper JD, Gould E, et al. Value of needle biopsy in directing management of parotid lesions in HIV-positive patients. Head Neck 1991;13:411–4.

98. Ellis GL, Auclair PL, Gnepp DR. Surgical pathology of the salivary glands. Philadelphia: Saunders; 1991.

99. Mooney EE, Dodd LG, Layfield LJ. Squamous cells in fine-needle aspiration biopsies of salivary gland lesions: Potential pitfalls in cytologic diagnosis. Diagn Cytopathol 1996;15:447–52.

100. Cheuk W, Chan JKC. Kuttner tumor of the submandibular gland. Fine-needle aspiration cytologic findings of seven cases. Am J Clin Pathol 2002;117:103–8.

101. Kaba S, Kojima M, Matsuda H, et al. Kuttner's tumor of the submandibular glands: report of five cases with fine-needle aspiration cytology. Diagn Cytopathol 2006;34:631–5.

102. Williams SB, Foss RD, Ellis GL. Inflammatory pseudotumors of the major salivary glands. Clinicopathologic and immunohistochemical analysis of six cases. Am J Surg Pathol 1992;16:896–902.

103. Aufdemorte TB, Ramzy I, Holt GR, et al. Focal adenomatoid hyperplasia of salivary glands. A differential diagnostic problem in fine needle aspiration biopsy. Acta Cytol 1985;29:23–8.

104. Klijanienko J, Vielh P. Fine-needle sampling of salivary gland lesions I. Cytology and histology correlation of 412 cases of pleomorphic adenoma. Diagn Cytopathol 1996;14:195–200.

105. Viguer JM, Vicandi B, Jiménez-Hefferman JA, et al. Fine needle aspiration cytology of pleomorphic adenoma. An anlysis of 212 cases. Acta Cytol 1997;41:786–94.

106. Bottles K, Ferrell LD, Miller TR. Tyrosine crystals in fine needle aspirates of a pleomorphic adenoma of the parotid gland. Acta Cytol 1984;28:490–2.

107. Kawahara A, Harada H, Kage M, et al. Characterization of the epithelial components in pleomorphic adenoma of salivary gland. Acta Cytol 2002;46:1095–100.

108. Stanley MW. Selected problems in fine needle aspiration of head and neck masses. Mod Pathol 2002;15:342–50.

109. Handa U, Dhingra N, Chopra R, Mohan H. Pleomorphic adenoma: cytologic variants and potential diagnostic pitfalls. Diagn Cytopathol 2009;37:11–5.

110. Klijanienko J, El-Naggar AK, Servois V, et al. Mucoepidermoid carcinoma ex pleomorphic adenoma. Nonspecific preoperative cytologic findings in six cases. Cancer 1998;84:231–4.

111. Siddaraju N, Murugam P, Basu D, Verma SK. Preoperative diagnosis of cystic pleomorphic adenoma with squamous metaplasia and cholesterol crystals. Acta Cytol 2009;53:101.

112. Layfield LJ, Glasgow BJ. Aspiration cytology of clear-cell lesions of the parotid gland: morphologic features and differential diagnosis. Diagn. Cytopathol 1993;9:705–12.

113. Wax T, Layfield L. Epithelial-myoepithelial cell carcinoma of the parotid gland: a case report and comparison of cytologic features with other stromal, epithelial, and myoepithelial cell containing lesions of the salivary glands. Diagn Cytopathol 1996;14:298–304.

114. Klijanienko J, El-Naggar AK, Vielh P.Fine-needle findings in 26 carcinoma ex pleomorphic adenomas: diagnostic pitfalls and clinical considerations. Diagn Cytopathol 1999;21:163–6.

115. Kapila K, Mathur S, Verma K. Schwannomas: a pitfall in the diagnosis of pleomorphic adenomas on fine-needle aspiration cytology. Diagn Cytopathol 2002;27:53–9.

116. Domagala W, Halczy-Kowalik L, Welen K, Osborn M. Coexpression of glial fibrillary acid protein, keratin and vimentin. A unique feature useful in the diagnosis of pleomorphic adenoma in the salivary gland in fine needle aspiration biopsy smears. Acta Cytol 1988;32:403–8.

117. Stanley MW, Horwitz CA, Rollins SD, et al. Basal cell (monomorphic) and minimally pleomorphic adenomas of the salivary glands. Distinction from the solid (anaplastic) type of adenoid cystic carcinoma in fine-needle aspiration. Am. J. Clin. Pathol 1996;106:35–41.

118. Klijanienko J, El-Naggar AK, Vielh P. Comparative cytological and histological study of 15 salivary basal cell tumors; diagnostic and differential diagnostic considerations. Diagn Cytopathol 1999;21:30–4.

119. Fregnani ER, Gerhard R, da Cruz-Perez DE, et al. Cytological features of intraoral tumors. Cytopathol 2006;17:205–7.

120. Sparrow SA, Frost FA. Salivary monomorphic adenoma of dermal analogue type: report of two cases. Diagn Cytopathol 1993;9:300–3.

121. Klijanienko J, Vielh P. Fine needle sampling of salivary gland lesions II. Cytology and histology correlation of 71 cases of Warthin's tumor (adenolymphoma). Diagn Cytopathol 1997;16:221–5.

122. Ballo MS, Shin HJC, Sneige N. Sources of diagnostic error in the fine needle aspiration diagnosis of Warthin's tumor and clues to a correct diagnosis. Diagn Cytopathol 1997;17:230–4.

123. Parwani AV, Ali SZ. Diagnostic accuracy and pitfalls in fine-needle aspiration interpretation of Warthin's tumor. Cancer (Cancer Cytopathol) 2003;99:166–71.

124. O'Dwyer P, Farrar WB, James AG, et al. Needle aspiration biopsy of major salivary gland tumors: Its value. Cancer 1986;57:554–7.

125. Sagi A, Giorgadze TA, Eleazar J, et al. Clear cell and eosinophilic oncocytomas of salivary gland: cytological variants or parallels? Diagn Cytopathol 2007;35:158–63.

126. Goyal R, Ahuja A, Gupta N, et al. Multifocal nodular oncocytic hyperplasia in parotid gland. A case report. Acta Cytol 2007;51: 621–3.

127. Dodd LG, Caraway NP, Luna MA, Byers RM. Myoepithelioma of the parotid. Report of a case initially examined by fine needle aspiration biopsy. Acta Cytol 1994;38:417–21.

128. Siddaraju N, Badhe BA, Goneppanavar M, Mishra MM. Preoperative fine needle aspiration cytologic diagnosis of spindle cell myoepithelioma of the parotid gland. A case report. Acta Cytol 2008;52:495–9.

129. Chhieng DC, Cohen J-M, Cangiarella JF. Fine-needle aspiration of spindle cell and mesenchymal lesions of the salivary glands. Diagn Cytopathol 2000;23:253–9.

130. Klijanienko J, Vielh P. Fine needle sampling of salivary gland lesions V. Cytology of 22 cases of acinic cell carcinoma with histologic correlation. Diagn Cytopathol 1997;17:347–52.

131. Nagel H, Laskawi R, Büter JJ, et al. Cytologic diagnosis of acinic-cell carcinoma of salivary glands. Diagn Cytopathol 1997;16:402–12.

132. Shet T, Ghodke R, Kane S, Chinoy R. Cytomorphologic patterns in papillary cystic variant of acinic cell carcinoma of the salivary gland. Acta Cytol 2006; 50:388–92.

133. Mosunjac MB, Siddiqui MT, Tadros T. Acinic cell carcinoma – papillary cystic variant. Pitfalls of fine needle aspiration diagnosis: study of five cases and review of literature. Cytopathol 2009;20: 96–102.

134. Cohen MB, Fisher PE, Holly EA, et al. Fine needle aspiration biopsy diagnosis of mucoepidermoid carcinoma. Acta Cytol 1990;34:43–9.

135. Kumar N, Kapila K, Verma K. Fine needle aspiration cytology of mucoepidermoid carcinoma: a diagnostic problem. Acta Cytol 1991; 35:357–9.

136. Klijanienko J, Vielh P. Fine needle sampling of salivary gland lesions IV. Review of 50 cases of mucoepidermoid carcinoma with histologic correlation. Diagn Cytopathol 1997;17:92–8.

137. Goonewardene SA, Nasuti JF. Value of mucin detection in distinguishing MEC from Warthin's tumor on fine needle aspiration. Acta Cytol 2002; 46:704–8.

138. Edwards PC, Wasserman P. Evaluation of cystic salivary gland lesions by FNA. Acta Cytol 2005;49:489–94.

139. Frierson Jr HF, Covell JL, Mills SE. Fine needle aspiration cytology of terminal duct carcinoma of minor salivary gland. Diagn Cytopathol 1987;3:159–62.

140. Klijanienko J, Vielh P. Salivary carcinomas with papillae: cytology and histology analysis of polymorphous low-grade adenocarcinoma and papillary cystadenocarcinoma. Diagnostic Cytopathology 1998; 19:244–9.

141. Gibbons D, Saboorian MH, Vuitch F, et al. Fine-needle aspiration findings in patients with polymorphous low grade adenocarcinoma of the salivary glands. Cancer (Cancer Cytopathology) 1999;87:31–6.

142. Kocjan G, Milroy C, Fisher EW, Eveson JW. Cytologic features of epithelial-myoepithelial carcinoma of salivary gland: potential pitfalls in diagnosis. Cytopathol 1993;4:173–80.

143. Klijanienko J, Vielh P. Fine needle sampling of salivary gland lesions VII. Cytology and histology correlation of 5 cases of epithelial-myoepithelial carcinoma. Diagn Cytopathol 1998;19:405–9.

144. Ng WK, Choy C, Ip P, et al. Fine aspiration cytology of epithelial-myoepithelial carcinoma of salivary glands. A report of three cases. Acta Cytol 1999;43:675–80.

145. Miliauskas J, Orell SR. Fine-needle aspiration cytological findings in five cases of epithelial/myoepithelial carcinoma of salivary glands. Diagn Cytopathol 2003;28:163–7.

146. Seifert G. Classification and differential diagnosis of clear and basal cell tumors of the salivary glands. Semin Diagn Pathol 1996;13:95–103.

147. Klijanienko J, Vielh P. Fine needle sampling of salivary gland lesions III. Cytology and histology correlation of 75 cases of adenoid cystic carcinoma. Review and experience at the Institut Curie with emphasis on cytologic pitfalls. Diagn Cytopathol 1997; 17:36–41.

148. Nagel H, Hotze HJ, Laskawi R, et al. Cytologic diagnosis of adenoid cystic carcinoma of salivary glands. Diagn Cytopathol 1999;20:358–66.

149. Mohan H, Handa U, Amanjit, et al. Adenoid cystic carcinoma of the external auditory canal. A case report with diagnosis by fine needle aspiration. Acta Cytol 2003;47:792–4.

150. Bondeson L, Lindholm K, Thorstenson S. Benign dermal eccrine cylindroma. A pitfall in the cytologic diagnosis of adenoid cystic carcinoma. Acta Cytol 1983;27:326–8.

151. Yang GCH, Waisman J. Distinguishing adenoid cystic carcinoma from cylindromatous adenomas in salivary gland fine-needle aspirates: the cytologic clues and their ultrastructural basis. Diagn Cytopathol 2006;34: 284–8.

152. Stanley MW, Hurwitz CA, Bardales RH, et al. Basal cell carcinoma metastatic to the salivary glands: differential diagnosis in fine-needle aspiration cytology. Diagn Cytopathol 1997;16:247–52.

153. Yu GH, Caraway NP. Poorly-differentiated adenoid cystic carcinoma: cytologic appearance in fine-needle aspirates of distant metastases. Diagn Cytopathol 1996;15:296–300.

154. Smith-Frable MA, Frable WJ. Fine-needle aspiration biopsy of salivary glands. Laryngoscope 1991;101:245–9.

155. Jacobs JC. Low grade mucoepidermoid carcinoma ex pleomorphic adenoma. A diagnostic problem in fine needle aspiration biopsy. Acta Cytol 1994;38:93–7.

156. Miliauskas J, Orell SR. Acinic cell carcinoma arising in pleomorphic adenoma of parotid gland. Cytopathology 2000;11:356–9.

157. Elsheikh TM, Bernachi EG, Pisharodi L. Fine needle aspiration cytology of salivary duct carcinoma. Diagn Cytopathol 1994;11:47–51.

158. Fyrat P, Cramer H, Feczko J, et al. Fine needle aspiration biopsy of salivary duct carcinoma: report of five cases. Diagn Cytopathol 1997;16:526–30.

159. Khurana KK, Pitman MB, Powers CN, et al. Diagnostic pitfalls of aspiration cytology of salivary duct carcinoma. Cancer (Cancer Cytopathol) 1997;81:373–8.

160. Klijanienko J, Vielh P. Cytologic characteristics and histomorphologic correlations of 21 salivary duct carcinomas. Diagn Cytopathol 1998;19:333–7.

161. Garcia-Bonafé M, Catala I, Tarragona J, Tallada N. Cytologic diagnosis of salivary duct carcinoma: a review of seven cases. Diagn Cytopathol 1998;19:120–3.

162. Kawakara A, Harada H, Akiba J, Kage M. Salivary duct carcinoma cytologically diagnosed distinctly from salivary gland carcinomas with squamous differentiation. Diagn Cytopathol 2008;36:485–93.

163. Batsakis JG, El-Naggar AK, Luna MA. 'Adenocarcinoma, not otherwise specified': a diminishing group of salivary carcinomas. Ann. Otol Rhinol Laryngol 1992;101:102–4.

164. Klijanienko J, Vielh P. Fine needle sampling of salivary gland lesions VI. Cytological review of 44 cases of primary salivary squamous-cell carcinoma with histologic correlation. Diagn Cytopathol 1998;18:174–8.

165. Klijanienko J, Lagacé R, Servois V, et al. Fine-needle sampling of primary neuroendocrine carcinomas of salivary glands: cyto-histological correlations and clinical analysis. Diagn Cytopathol 2001;24:163–6.

166. Torlakovic E, Ames ED, Manivel JC, Stanley MW. Benign and malignant neoplasms of myoepithelial cells: cytologic findings. Diagn. Cytopathol 1993;9:655–60.

167. Dipalma S, Alasio L, Pilotti S. Fine needle aspiration appearances of

malignant myoepithelioma of the parotid gland. Cytopathology 1996;7:357–65.

168. Chhieng DC, Paulino AF. Cytology of myoepithelial carcinoma of the salivary gland. A study of four cases. Cancer (Cancer Cytopathol) 2002;96:32–6.

169. Harrison RF, Smallman LA, Young JA, Watkinson JC. Oncocytic carcinoma of the parotid gland: a problem in fine needle aspiration diagnosis. Cytopathology 1995;6:54–8.

170. Wu HHJ, Silvernagel SW. Fine-needle aspiration cytology of an oncocytic carcinoma of the submandibular gland. Diagn. Cytopathol 1998;19:186–9.

171. Croce A, Moretti A, Bianchedi M, et al. Carcinoma in ectopic Warthin's tumor: a case study and review of the literature. Acta Otorhinolaryngol Ital 1996;16:543–9.

172. Mandreker S, Pinto RW, Usgaonkar U. Sebaceous carcinoma of the eyelid with metastasis to the parotid region. Diagnosis by fine needle aspiration cytology. Acta Cytol 1997;41:1636–7.

173. Moore JG, Bocklage T. Fine-needle aspiration biopsy of large-cell undifferentiated carcinoma of the salivary glands: presentation of two cases, literature review, and differential cytodiagnosis of high-grade salivary gland malignancies. Diagn Cytopathol 1998;19:44–50.

174. Safneck JR, Ravinsky E, Yadzi HM, et al. Fine needle aspiration biopsy findings in lymphoepithelial carcinoma of salivary gland. Acta Cytol 1997;41:1023–30.

175. Lussier C, Klijanienko J, Vielh P. Fine-needle sampling of metastatic non-lymphomatous tumors to the major salivary glands. A clinico-pathologic study of 40 cases cytologically diagnosed and histologically correlated. Cancer 2000;90:350–6.

176. Zhang C, Cohen J-M, Cangiarella JF, et al. Fine-needle aspiration of secondary neoplasms involving the salivary glands. A report of 36 cases. Am J Clin Pathol 2000;113:21–8.

177. Chhieng DC, Cangiarella JF, Cohen J-M. Fine-needle aspiration cytology of lymphoproliferative lesions involving the major salivary glands. Am J Clin Pathol 2000;13:563–71.

CHAPTER 5

Lymph nodes

John Miliauskas

CLINICAL ASPECTS

Lymphadenopathy is a commonly encountered clinical problem which has a multitude of causes. The commonest cause of peripheral lymphadenopathy is a non-specific reactive hyperplasia in which the underlying etiology is infrequently found (probably an asymptomatic inflammatory process). In general practice, less than 1% of patients with peripheral lymphadenopathy have a malignant process.[1] In comparison, retroperitoneal or intra-abdominal lymphadenopathy is usually malignant. In contrast, in young patients, intrathoracic lymphadenopathy is often associated with infectious mononucleosis, sarcoidosis and tuberculosis. The likelihood of malignant disease as a cause of peripheral lymphadenopathy increases over the age of 40 years, nodes over 2 cm in size, firm or matted nodes and non-tender/non-painful nodes.[2] Ultrasound is also used in the assessment of lymphadenopathy, from the point of view of a reactive versus a pathological process.[3] The bounds of the 'triple test' are being expanded beyond breast pathology.

Although surgical excision of a palpable peripheral node is relatively simple, vicinity to other anatomical structures in the neck sometimes causes problems. The procedure does require anesthesia, strict sterility and theater time, and it may leave a scar. To avoid surgery, patients are usually watched for some time before a decision of open biopsy is taken, unless the clinical suspicion of malignancy is strong. Fine needle biopsy (FNB) offers the alternative of an immediate, preliminary, although not always specific diagnosis with little trauma and cost, thus providing ample information for further management.[4–8]

The plethora of monoclonal antibodies available has proven invaluable in lymph node cytology.[9] In particular, it assists in identifying the source of metastatic tumor to lymph nodes, and in distinguishing between various small and large cell neoplasms and malignant lymphoma. The role of cytology in the diagnosis and typing of lymphoma has become better defined in recent years, principally due to immunophenotyping supplementation of routine cytologic preparations. Flow cytometry (FCM) has revolutionized lymphoma diagnosis and typing by FNB and plays a pivotal role.[10,11] Immunophenotyping can also be accomplished by immune studies on cytocentrifuge preparations (cytospins) or cell blocks of lymph node aspirates, or core needle biopsy (CNB) specimens.[9,12–20] In many cases, definitive diagnosis and typing of lymphoma is possible if cytomorphology is combined with analysis of immunophenotype, and/or cytogenetics and molecular studies.[21–32]

The place of FNA in the investigative sequence

As a rule, cytological examination of FNB smears can determine whether lymphadenopathy is due to reactive hyperplasia, infection, metastatic malignancy or malignant lymphoma. In order to make the most rational use of fine needle aspiration cytology (FNAC), clinicians and pathologists alike must understand and accept that the aims and purpose of FNB of peripheral lymph nodes at the 'primary' or 'community' level are different from those at the 'secondary' or 'specialist' level. At the primary level, FNAC is used as a triage to distinguish between cases of lymphadenopathy with a high or a low level of suspicion of significant disease by the simplest, least invasive and least costly method. This preliminary assessment is based on routine cytologic smears only. Depending on the result, an immediate decision can be made whether to simply observe the node, to recommend a course of antibiotics, or to refer the patient to a specialist for further investigations. Reactive lymphadenopathy is likely to resolve spontaneously in due course. Since the great majority of lymphadenopathy cases seen at the primary level are reactive, this approach has obvious practical, economical and psychological advantages.

In case of reactive hyperplasia, surgical excision is not indicated, unless the subsequent course is atypical or there is significant discrepancy with the clinical or imaging findings. Follow-up is still recommended, since there is a small but significant risk that lymphoma or other malignancy could be missed or undercalled by FNB. A specific diagnosis can be made in some cases in this category, for example of an infectious process, but most often the etiology remains obscure. If appropriate, and depending on the clinical presentation, part of the biopsy material may be used for microbiological investigation, which can be supplemented by serology.

At the specialist/secondary level, the role of FNB is to provide material for further cytomorphologic analysis and

DOI: 10.1016/B978-0-7020-3151-9.00005-0

for ancillary studies. The aim is to arrive at a definitive diagnosis and lymphoma typing making full use of the armamentarium of ancillary laboratory techniques. This also applies to most abnormal lymph nodes in deep sites. In some centers, this strategy has been very successful and has virtually replaced surgical removal of nodes. This requires readily available expertise in FCM, cytogenetics, immunostaining, molecular analysis (e.g. PCR), haematopathology and cytopathology. Others, including the author, feel that a tissue sample obtained by CNB or surgical biopsy is often still needed. Lymphoma diagnosis and typing relies not only on cytology but also on altered tissue and immmuno-architecture,[33] which requires a tissue sample, although a small fragment obtained by CNB or occasionally a cell block may suffice. Tissue samples can also help to overcome deviations from classical immunophenotypes on FCM. They also enable spatial recognition, assisting in the diagnosis of various reactive lymphadenopathies. Close correlation of cytological, immunological and clinical features is essential when using FCM to make a diagnosis of lymphoma and in its classification. At times, additional correlation with the cytogenetic and molecular studies will be necessary.

Lymph nodes clinically suspected of metastatic malignancy constitute one of the commonest indications for FNB. In patients with known, histologically proven malignancy, who subsequently present with lymphadenopathy, a cytological diagnosis may obviate further surgery, merely to confirm metastasis. In patients without a previous malignant diagnosis, not only can metastatic malignancy be confirmed by FNB, but clues to the nature and site of the primary can also be given in most cases. Cytocentrifuge preparations or cell blocks, or multiple smears when used for histochemical and immunohistochemical staining, are of great value in this situation. Only when FNB and supplementary investigations do not provide clues to the origin of the metastasis, and when this information is of importance to clinical management, is a diagnostic surgical excision or CNB of the node indicated. The distinction between anaplastic carcinoma and lymphoma is obviously of clinical importance. In addition, a specific diagnosis by FNB of disseminated carcinoma of the prostate, breast, ovary and thyroid, germ cell tumors and neuroendocrine carcinoma should be pursued since treatment is available.

The value of FNB in the investigation of suspected lymphoma can be summarized as follows:

1. At the community/general practitioner level, a preliminary cytological diagnosis suggests appropriate management/referral and further investigations without delay.
2. A representative node can be selected for surgical biopsy by FNB sampling of multiple nodes. The biggest or the most easily accessible node is not always the most suitable and may show only reactive change.
3. If a suspicion of lymphoma is known beforehand, any surgical tissue specimen will be used to ensure a complete immunologic investigation and the preparation of imprint smears to provide additional cytonuclear detail.
4. Other biopsies – bone marrow, liver, spleen – can be coordinated with node excision, saving time and additional anesthesia.

5. In patients with advanced intra-abdominal or mediastinal lymphoma without involvement of superficial nodes, FNB combined with FCM and clinical and radiological assessment of the extent of disease may be a sufficient basis for therapeutic decisions. Alternatively, a CNB, with or without FNB, can be used to obtain more tissue for ancillary studies, a greatly expanded immunopanel and to give some idea of tissue and immunoarchitecture.[34,35] Surgical intervention, with its risk of morbidity, to obtain tissue for histologic examination can be avoided.
6. Suspected recurrent or residual disease in patients with previously confirmed lymphoma can be substantiated by FNB alone.[21,36] Any change in the type or grade of lymphoma will also usually be recognized. Since the recurrent tumor may be the only sign of disease by which the response to systemic therapy can be monitored, it is best left intact.
7. At the secondary/specialist level, an accurate lymphoma subtype may be provided when supported by a range of ancillary studies and by appropriate expertise.

Accuracy of diagnosis

The accuracy of FNAC of lymph nodes in the diagnosis of metastatic malignancy is influenced by many factors such as the size and site of the node, fibrosis, necrosis, previous irradiation and the number of punctures made. Small mobile nodes high up in the axilla are difficult to sample, while adequate material can easily be obtained from nodes only a few millimeters in diameter in a cervical or supraclavicular position.[37] Deep nodes are accessible to FNB by means of radiological imaging and guidance.[38,39] Fibrosis sometimes makes it difficult to obtain sufficient material for diagnosis from reactive inguinal nodes. It can also be a problem in nodular sclerosis Hodgkin lymphoma[40] and in some mediastinal and retroperitoneal non-Hodgkin lymphomas (NHL).[9]

Diagnostic sensitivity is occasionally limited by the fact that small metastatic deposits, metastases confined to the subcapsular sinus and single-cell metastases can be missed. However, early micrometastases rarely produce significant lymph node enlargement and if a lymph node is palpable it is likely to contain enough tumor tissue to be detectable by FNB. The diagnostic sensitivity of metastatic and recurring malignancy reported in the literature is usually above 95%.[23,41–53] Failure to obtain a representative sample is responsible for most false-negative diagnoses. Interpretation of a representative sample can be problematic, more often with lymphoma than with metastatic malignancy. For example, without immunophenotyping low-grade follicular lymphoma can easily be mistaken for reactive follicular hyperplasia.[54] Thus, although a negative cytological report makes malignancy unlikely, it is not singularly diagnostic,[37] and if the lymphadenopathy does not show signs of regression within a month or two, FNB should be repeated or a node should be excised for histology.

Diagnostic specificity for malignancy, on the other hand, is high. False-positive diagnoses are rare[23,42,48,52–57] if particular caution is observed in the interpretation of smears from nodes in fields of previous irradiation and in the presence of necrosis. The existence of benign epithelial inclusions in lymph nodes (see p. 89) should be kept in mind. Again, the main problem is in relation to lymphoma, particularly the distinction between reactive follicular hyperplasia and follicular lymphoma. Most false-positive diagnoses are cases of reactive lymphadenopathy reported as suspicious of lymphoma.

Diagnostic accuracy not only depends on the aspirate being representative, but also very much on the quality of the cytological preparations. This is particularly the case in the diagnosis of some reactive lymphadenopathies and in the diagnosis and classification of lymphoma, which depends on the study of fine cytological detail in high magnification, and on an estimate of proportions of various cell types in the smear.[54,55,58–60] It is essential that the aspirates are handled and smears prepared by staff with experience in cytology to achieve satisfactory results.

There are conflicting opinions regarding the accuracy of cytological diagnosis and typing of malignant lymphoma.[19–26,30,55,60–65] It is difficult to extract exact figures for several reasons. Most series include relatively small numbers of cases, with histologic correlation and/or consistent follow-up. Early series are based on cytomorphology (in FNB smears) alone, later series combine cytomorphology and immunophenotyping by flow cytometry and/or immunostaining of smears. The case mix (types of lymphoma; primary diagnosis or recurrent disease) is variable and often is not specified. With these reservations, it appears that the accuracy of diagnosing NHL by cytomorphology alone is in the range 60–80%, significantly lower for low-grade than for high-grade lymphomas.[26,37,45,48,51,66]

Diagnostic sensitivity has generally been found to be lower for lymphoma than for metastatic malignancy.[23,48,67,68] For a diagnosis of lymphoma to be of clinically practical value, it must identify good and bad prognosis subgroups and therefore must specify the subtype. In an extensive review of the literature, two-thirds of the 30 studies reviewed, in which FNB was supplemented by immunophenotyping, diagnostic sensitivity was over 80% and specificity over 90%. However, only three of eight studies achieved a correct and precise subtyping in the primary diagnosis of NHL in more than 80% of cases.[22] Difficulties in correlating cytology and histology of lymphoma have been enhanced by the parallel use and frequent modifications of different systems of classification over the years. The advent of the World Health Organization (WHO) lymphoma classification based on clinical, cytologic, immunophenotypic and genetic features has improved both the detection rate and classification of NHL, due to diminished importance placed on architectural features in subtyping NHL.[22,26,30,32] However, the accuracy of cytologic diagnosis is still limited in some forms of NHL, notably lymphomas with predominantly small cells, mainly marginal zone lymphoma, and in peripheral T-cell lymphoma, T-cell/histiocyte rich B-cell lymphoma and nodular lymphocyte predominant Hodgkin lymphoma. This is also the case with the diagnosis of composite lymphoma and in the grading of follicular lymphoma.

The wide variation in the reported accuracy of diagnosis and typing of NHL probably reflects the environment in which the studies were carried out. A high accuracy has been achieved in a few highly specialized centers equipped with the full armamentarium and expertise related to ancillary laboratory techniques, but many hospitals have limited resources, and most pathologists still consider histology necessary in the primary diagnosis of lymphoma. This enables determination of any altered tissue and immunoarchitecture, and also reveals the cellular compartments and their composition in the tissue section, which is not reflected per se in the aspirated cell sample.

As a rule, FNB samples from malignant lymphoma are very cellular and can be used for ancillary studies.[9,31,54,69–72] However, more material to allow a wider range of immune markers, assessment of tissue and immunoarchitecture as well as storage of material for ancillary studies and research can be obtained by supplementary CNB of the node, principally in intra-abdominal or intrathoracic nodal disease. With deep-seated masses, CNB is a useful adjunct to FNB. The FNB provides superior cytomorphology and is an excellent source for flow cytometry cell suspensions. This combined approach can increase diagnostic accuracy, assist in classification and reduce the number of insufficient samples.[73,74]

The accuracy of cytological diagnosis of Hodgkin lymphoma (HL) is quite variable, frequently high, and in some studies greater than 85%.[22,23,75–77] The main problems in cytodiagnosis are in relation to the nodular lymphocyte predominant and lymphocyte-rich variants as well as separation from HL mimics. The accuracy of subtyping HL in FNB smears is relatively poor.[22–24] Performing immunocytochemistry on cell block preparations, cytospins or NCB may help to a degree but a formal node biopsy is still necessary to provide reliable subtyping in most cases.

Complications

Significant complications do not occur. Post-aspiration hematoma or necrosis is rare.[78,79] To date, septic complications or tumor implantation in the needle track have not been reported following FNB of lymph nodes.

Technical considerations

Both reactive nodes and nodes involved by metastatic malignancy or lymphoma are highly cellular and moderately vascular tissues. Sufficient material is therefore easily obtained using 23–27-gauge needles, except sometimes in the presence of fibrosis or necrosis. FNB without aspiration has been used routinely for several years in some institutions. It has the advantage over the traditional aspiration of giving the operator a more direct and sensitive feeling of the consistency of tissues through the needle. This is helpful when small or deep nodes are biopsied. Non-aspiration also results in less admixture with blood. An abundance of blood adversely affects cell fixation and tends to cause shrinkage and distortion of cells. If aspiration is used, multiple rapid biopsies from different points of entry are preferable to multiple passes in different directions, in order to obtain a representative and adequate sample without too much blood.

Local anesthetic is not used and simple skin disinfection as for an injection is adequate. Two or more samples may be necessary to secure enough material for both routine smears and for special investigations and to reduce sampling error in focal disease. The use of gloves and extreme care in handling used needles are important safety precautions. The techniques involved in the biopsy of deep nodes using radiological guidance are described in Chapter 3. If the standard technique does not yield sufficient material, for example due to fibrosis (nodular sclerosis Hodgkin lymphoma and some sclerosing NHLs), a cutting core needle can be tried.[34,35] In general, large-caliber core needles of 14–18 gauge are recommended in the definitive diagnosis and typing of NHL, as they allow a more accurate assessment of tissue and immunoarchitecture as mentioned above. Artifactual change is less than with a 20-gauge needle.

It is not easy to make perfect direct smears from samples of lymphoid tissue and this takes considerable practice. An air-dried smear has to dry quickly for optimal fixation and has to be made thin and even. The smearing pressure must be well balanced to obtain a thin smear and at the same time avoiding crush artifacts. If the aspirate is bloody or thinned by a large amount of lymph fluid, cells need to be concentrated and separated as much as possible from the fluid. This can be achieved by using the two-step technique illustrated in Figure 2.7. A wet-fixed smear must be fixed immediately to minimize drying artifacts. Only those parts of the smears where the cells are evenly dispersed, well fixed and not distorted by the trauma of smearing should be chosen for diagnostic evaluation.

While air-dried MGG or Diff-Quik-stained smears are essential for the evaluation of cytoplasm and background elements, alcohol fixation and staining with H&E or Pap is helpful in assessing nucleoli and chromatin pattern. Whenever possible, both air-dried and wet-fixed smears should be made of each FNB sample as they may provide complementary information. Extra smears to allow cytochemical stains are often of great value. Staining for microorganisms (Ziehl-Neelsen, PAS, Gomori's silver stain), mucin (PAS/diastase, Alcian blue), melanin (Masson-Fontana), and immunocytochemical studies are those most commonly used.

Heavy reliance is placed on ancillary techniques in FNB of nodes. A cell suspension made by gently dispersing the sample in Hank's balanced salt solution with 10–20% fetal calf serum or by rinsing the needle with the fluid is a suitable preparation for this purpose. The suspension is spun in a cytocentrifuge at 300–700 rpm for 3–5 minutes. Processing should be done as soon as possible after biopsy since cell fragility increases rapidly with time. Cytospin preparations and cell blocks/cell buttons (see Chapter 2) allow assessment by a panel of immune markers by immunocytochemical staining as illustrated in the section on lymphoma. An elementary NHL screening panel could consist of CD20, CD3, CD5, kappa and lambda light chains, and this can be extended as appropriate. Background staining due to serum proteins and fragmented cells can be reduced by resuspending the cells in Hank's fluid after initial centrifugation. Direct smears may be unsuitable due to the dispersal of cytoplasm and proteins in the background (see Chapter 2). However, immunostaining of FNB smear specimens can be utilized with the use of formal saline fixation. It eliminates background staining while allowing preservation of cellular antigenicity and morphology.[80] Immunocytochemistry is helpful in tracing the origin of metastatic malignancy, in the differentiation of lymphoma from reactive processes and from anaplastic carcinoma or melanoma, and in the classification of lymphoma.[13–16,18] FCM analysis of aspirated cells is vital in immunophenotyping lymphoid populations, determining clonality and aberrant antigen expression. FNB material can be rinsed in a buffered balanced salt solution or RPMI

solution to provide material for analysis. In addition , aspirated material can be used in conventional cytogenetics or fluorescence in situ hybridization (FISH) to assess for chromosomal translocations as well as in molecular studies/PCR to assess gene rearrangements.

If there is any suspicion of an infective process, the needle can be rinsed with sterile saline after the smears have been prepared, but preferably the biopsy should be repeated to provide sufficient material for culture for microorganisms (see p. 18 and Chapter 18).

Liquid-based preparations have been used minimally for nodal FNB samples. If used, they must be interpreted with caution as there are many cytomorphologic alterations.[81]

CYTOLOGICAL FINDINGS

Fine needle biopsy samples of lymphoid tissue, nodal or extranodal, benign or malignant, as a rule have a very high cell content. This is obvious to the naked eye as the aspirate is smeared. It looks like a film of slimy material which turns gray on drying. The cytoplasm of lymphoid cells is fragile. Many cells are represented by naked nuclei or have only a small rim of cytoplasm. A variable number of rounded cytoplasmic fragments measuring up to 8 microns in diameter are scattered in the background (Fig. 5.1). The cytoplasmic fragments were named 'lymphoglandular bodies' by Söderström. The term 'lymphoid globules' is prefered since they are present in smears from any lymphoid infiltration, not only from lymph nodes. The fragments stain an uniform pale blue, identical to the cytoplasm of intact cells, with Giemsa stain. They differ from necrotic debris by their regular round shape and their uniform staining. Necrotic debris and nuclear fragments (karyorrhexis and apoptotic bodies) are characteristic of smears of small cell undifferentiated carcinoma (Fig. 5.2). The recognition of 'lymphoid globules' is of diagnostic value in the distinction of lymphoma from anaplastic carcinoma and some other tumors.

Most of the lymphoid cells are dispersed as single cells but some may form clumps or aggregates, especially in smears of bloody samples. Cell detail is obscured in dense clusters, which are of no diagnostic value as they can be found in

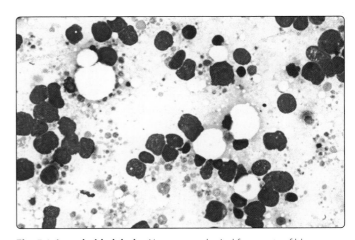

Fig. 5.1 Lymphoid globules Numerous spherical fragments of blue cytoplasm of variable sizes dispersed between the lymphoid cells; some nuclear fragments. Large cell lymphoma of tonsil (MGG, HP).

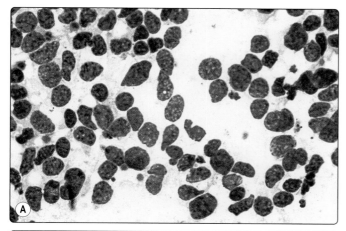

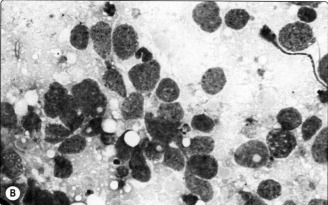

Fig. 5.2 Small cell anaplastic carcinoma Dispersed malignant cells with dense chromatin, irregular nuclear contour, nuclear molding, inconspicuous nucleoli and cytoplasm; note irregular cytoplasmic (**B**) and nuclear fragments in the background representing tumor necrosis (**A** and **B**) (MGG, HP).

both reactive and malignant nodes. However, a tendency for neoplastic follicular center cells to form aggregates resembling neuroendocrine carcinoma is commonly seen in follicular lymphoma,[82,83] and cells of anaplastic large cell lymphoma can also form carcinoma-like aggregates.[84–86] Tissue fragments consisting of a vascular core of endothelial cells with adherent lymphoid cells and histiocytes are sometimes present in smears from reactive nodes (Fig. 5.3).

The reactive node (Figs 5.4–5.16)

CRITERIA FOR DIAGNOSIS

◆ A mixed population of lymphoid cells,
◆ Numerical predominance of small lymphocytes,
◆ Centroblasts, centrocytes, immunoblasts and plasma cells in variable but 'logical' proportions,
◆ Dendritic reticulum cells associated with centroblasts and centrocytes (derived from germinal centers),
◆ Scattered histiocytes with intracytoplasmic nuclear debris (tingible body macrophages),
◆ Pale histiocytes, interdigitating cells, endothelial cells, eosinophils, neutrophils (variable).

The reactive pattern is variable depending on the degree of stimulation, the number and size of germinal centers and on whether the sample derives mainly from a germinal center or from interfollicular or paracortical tissue. Germinal center material is represented by poorly defined tissue fragments composed of centroblasts, centrocytes, 'tingible body' macrophages (Figs 5.4, 5.5), and a number of lymphocytes which adhere to the syncytial cytoplasm (pale gray/violet in MGG) of dendritic reticulum cells (Fig. 5.6A). Dendritic reticulum cells have oval or round nuclei with a smooth nuclear membrane, a coarsely granular, uniformly distributed chromatin and small distinct nucleoli (Fig. 5.6B). The cytoplasm is dispersed in the background. A smear, which derives mainly from interfollicular tissue, consists predominantly of lymphocytes with a variable but much smaller number of scattered immunoblasts, plasma cells, nonspecific histiocytes and endothelial cells (Fig. 5.7). Multiple biopsies diminish the bias caused by selective sampling.

The main features which distinguish a reactive process from lymphoma are:

1. a mixed population of lymphoid cells representing the whole range of lymphocyte transformation from small lymphocytes to immunoblasts and plasma cells,
2. a predominance of small, sometimes slightly larger 'stimulated' lymphocytes, which have small round nuclei and a characteristic chromatin pattern of large, ill-defined condensations,
3. centroblasts and centrocytes associated with dendritic reticulum cells and tingible body macrophages derived from germinal centres.[87,88]

Axillary nodes undergoing fat involution are sometimes sampled as they may become quite large, although of soft consistency. Smears of such nodes show fat droplets, fragments of adipose tissue, a number of small lymphocytes and a few blasts. The predominance of small lymphocytes may cause a suspicion of CLL (see section on small cell lymphoma). Fibrotic but otherwise normal inguinal nodes also give a scanty yield.

PROBLEMS AND DIFFERENTIAL DIAGNOSIS

◆ Follicular hyperplasia with large germinal centers,
◆ Follicular lymphoma,
◆ Paracortical hyperplasia with a prominent immunoblastic and plasmacellular reaction,
◆ Prominent histiocytic component,
◆ Prominent eosinophilic component,
◆ Prominent neutrophilic component,
◆ Multinucleate giant cells.

Morphologically similar to reactive lymphoid hyperplasia and rarely distinguishable are HIV-associated lymphadenitis, progressive transformation of germinal centers and Castleman's disease. When germinal centers are very large, as in some cases of reactive follicular hyperplasia, the proportion of large cells (centroblasts, dendritic reticulum cells) and the number of mitoses, in a FNB sample, may be impressive enough to suggest malignant lymphoma. However, the full range of lymphocyte transformation is still preserved,

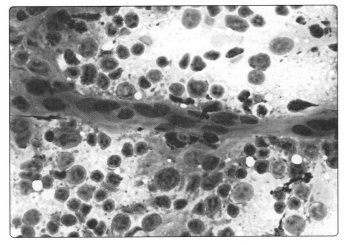

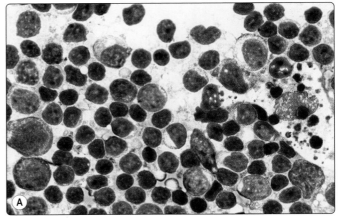

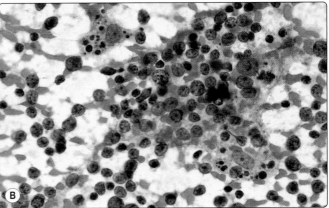

Fig. 5.3 Fragment of lymphoid tissue Lymphoid cells and histiocytes adhering to a strand of endothelial cells representing a small blood vessel (MGG, HP).

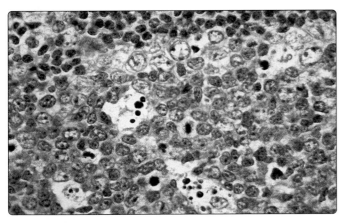

Fig. 5.5 Reactive lymphadenopathy, follicular Smear derived from reactive follicle. Centroblasts, centrocytes, small lymphocytes and tingible body macrophages with nuclear fragments (**A**, MGG; **B**, Pap; HP).

Fig. 5.4 Reactive lymphadenopathy, follicular Tissue section showing detail of germinal center with centroblasts, centrocytes and tingible body macrophages. Outer rim of small lymphocytes. The corresponding cytological pattern is shown in Figure 5.5 (H&E, HP). (Reproduced with permission from van Heerde et al.[9])

including small lymphocytes, and the various cell types occur in logical proportions. Small or slightly enlarged lymphocytes are still numerically predominant. A variable number of plasma cells can usually be found. The presence of macrophages with tingible bodies favors reactive hyperplasia but does not rule out lymphoma. Especially in high-grade lymphomas with a high turnover of cells, a considerable number of 'starry sky' macrophages may be present (see Figs 5.48 and 5.51A). A cytological pattern of reactive hyperplasia with a large number of plasma cells but no other distinguishing features can be seen, for example, in cases of secondary syphilis, rheumatoid arthritis, autoimmune syndromes, IgG4-related lymphadenopathy, HIV infection and the plasma cell variant of Castleman's disease.

The differential diagnosis between prominent follicular hyperplasia and follicular lymphoma grade 1–2 can be very difficult in FNB smears even for experienced cytopathologists. The smear patterns of follicular hyperplasia have been described. In follicular lymphoma, the predominant cell type may appear small, but the nucleus is of intermediate size and has an irregular shape and a more granular chromatin

similar to a centrocyte. Immunoblasts, plasma cells and tingible body macrophages are usually absent or few in numbers. The difficulty in distinguishing between the two conditions is largely due to the fact that dendritic reticulum cells associated with centroblasts and centrocytes are seen in both conditions, and that interfollicular areas in follicular lymphoma may contain large numbers of lymphocytes. Immunological demonstration usually by FCM of poly- or monoclonality may be necessary to solve the problem.

A prominent immunoblastic and plasmacellular reaction is found in several conditions. In viral lymphadenitis, particularly in infectious mononucleosis,[89,90] immunoblasts, plasmacytoid cells, mature plasma cells and atypical lymphocytes can be numerous but the range of cells is still in logical proportions (Figs 5.7, 5.8 and 5.9). The atypical lymphocytes have an abundant basophilic cytoplasm, an enlarged, often eccentric, nucleus and a paler nuclear chromatin than a normal lymphocyte. Immunoblastic cells can cause differential diagnostic problems. The main differential diagnoses are large cell lymphoma (with numerous immunoblasts) and HL. Atypical binucleate immunoblasts closely resembling Reed-Sternberg cells are rarely seen (see Fig. 5.69).[91] Occasionally, immunoblasts are mistaken for mononuclear Hodgkin cells; however, they are smaller with smaller nucleoli and greater basophilic cytoplasm than Hodgkin cells. Mononucleosis is usually suggested by the clinical presentation and can be confirmed by serological tests.

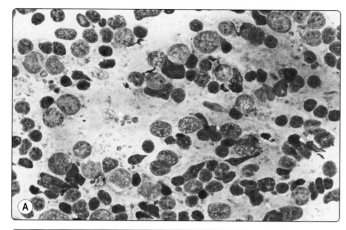

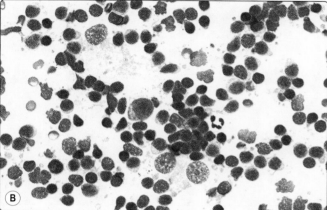

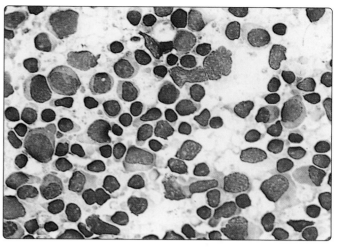

Fig. 5.8 Infectious mononucleosis Many transforming lymphocytes, plasmacytoid cells and immunoblasts (MGG, HP).

Fig. 5.6 Reactive lymphadenopathy (A) Smear derived from germinal center; loose tissue fragment of dendritic reticulum cells with ovoid nuclei and granular chromatin, centroblasts, centrocytes and some lymphocytes; syncytial background of pale cytoplasm; (B) Mixed population of lymphoid cells; two nuclei of dendritic reticulum cells with granular chromatin and small distinct nucleoli lower mid (MGG; HP).

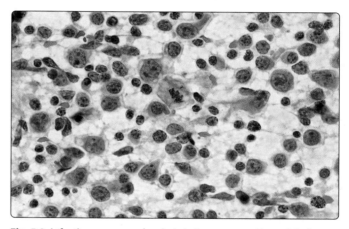

Fig. 5.9 Infectious mononucleosis A similar pattern to Figure 5.8 of a high proportion of transformed lymphocytes and a mitotic figure (Pap, HP).

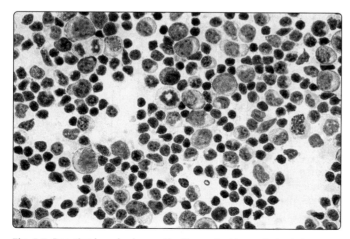

Fig. 5.7 Reactive lymphadenopathy Paracortical hyperplasia, viral induced. Spectrum of basophilic cells, ranging from mature plasma cells to immunoblasts with a background of many small lymphocytes, favors a reactive lesion (MGG, HP).

Abnormal immunoblastic reactions with prominent immunoblasts and sometimes Reed-Sternberg-like cells can at times be difficult to distinguish from large cell lymphoma. This pattern may be seen, for example, in postvaccinial lymphadenitis and Dilantin hypersensitivity lymphadenitis (Fig. 5.10). The clinical history may provide a clue in such cases (e.g. patients taking Dilantin usually develop adenopathy in the first 6 months of therapy). A definitive diagnosis would require either further ancillary investigation or a formal histological examination. Immunologic studies can help to confirm the polyclonal nature of the immunoblasts.

Histiocytes, which have an abundant, pale or sometimes eosinophilic cytoplasm, may be prominent in smears of lymph node aspirates. The histiocytes occur singly or in small groups. The cytoplasm is often vacuolated or granular and may contain phagocytosed debris or pigment. An increased number of histiocytes without specific features can be seen in smears from non-specific reactive nodes, and are suggestive of sinus histiocytosis (Fig. 5.11). The cytological findings in sinus histiocytosis with massive lymphadenopathy (Rosai-Dorfman disease) have been described by van Heerde and others.[9,92–94] In this condition, smears contain many large histiocytes showing lymphophagocytosis (Fig. 5.12). Prominent histiocytes and multinucleated giant cells

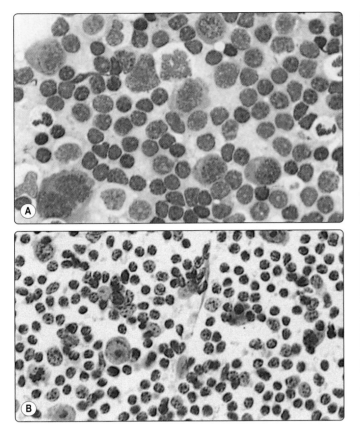

Fig. 5.10 **Immunoblastic reaction** Several immunoblasts including a binucleate form; case of Dilantin lymphadenopathy (A, MGG, HP; **B**, H & E, HP).

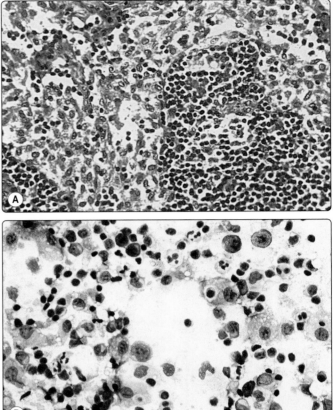

Fig. 5.11 **Sinus histiocytosis** (A) Tissue section. Marginal sinus filled with large pink-stained histiocytes (H&E, IP); (**B**) Smear showing histiocytes with abundant pale blue vacuolated cytoplasm and phagocytosis of a lymphocyte near the centre right (MGG, IP).

as a reaction to foreign material can occasionally be seen in axillary nodes of women with silicone breast prostheses[95] (Fig. 5.13) or inguinal lymphadenopathy associated with artificial hip joint replacement.[96]

Scattered small clusters of a few histiocytes with ovoid, pale nuclei and abundant cytoplasm resembling epithelioid cells in a smear consistent overall with follicular hyperplasia are suggestive of toxoplasmosis (Fig. 5.14A). Well-formed histiocytic granulomata resembling sarcoid granulomata are unusual but occur occasionally. Lymphoid cells with relatively large, ovoid, pale nuclei may also be seen (Fig. 5.14B). These cells probably correspond to the pale monocytoid B cells observed in histological sections. Occasionally, the presence of many of these large cells can raise a suspicion of malignancy. The cytological pattern is not diagnostic by itself and needs confirmation by serological tests. Microcysts and toxoplasma organisms are rarely found in smears of toxoplasma lymphadenitis (see Chapter 18).[97–100]

Numerous noncohesive, pale, histiocyte-like cells (interdigitating cells) with typical folded nuclei (Fig. 5.15) are present in dermatopathic lymphadenopathy. Some macrophages containing pigment, either hemosiderin or melanin, are usually found. These have smaller and more consistently oval, nonfolded nuclei different from interdigitating cells, and have a better-defined cytoplasm. There may be a variable number of eosinophils. The background is predominantly of lymphocytes, which may appear slightly 'atypical' with small pale, central nucleoli (stimulated T cells) and blast forms are less common.

The histiocytes of Langerhans cell histiocytosis (histiocytosis X) have characteristically large nuclei of irregular shape. They may be folded, convoluted, lobulated and grooved (Fig. 5.16 and Fig. 16.10). Mitotic activity may be seen and sometimes necrosis. Such cells seen in a lymph node aspirate, especially in the absence of eosinophils, may raise a suspicion of metastatic malignancy such as melanoma. However, the nuclear chromatin of Langerhans histiocytes is bland and finely granular. If suspected, the diagnosis may be confirmed by immunocytochemistry (CD1a, S-100, langerin)[69,101] and/ or by electronmicroscopy (Birbeck granules).[9,101–104] Histiocytic sarcoma is described on page 111 (see Fig. 5.76).[105]

A prominent component of eosinophils may be seen in reactive and neoplastic processes. The reactive conditions are hypersensitivity lymphadenitis, parasitic infestations with granulomas, Churg-Strauss disease and Kimura's disease. The neoplasms associated with eosinophilia are HL, peripheral T-cell lymphoma, Langerhans cell histiocytosis, mast cell disease, eosinophilic myeloid disorders and some metastatic carcinomas (mainly nasopharyngeal carcinoma).

A prominent component of neutrophils may also be seen in reactive and neoplastic processes. The reactive conditions are acute lymphadenitis, abscess and suppurative granulomas. The neoplasms associated with neutrophilia are HL, anaplastic large cell lymphoma, histiocytic sarcoma and metastatic squamous carcinoma.

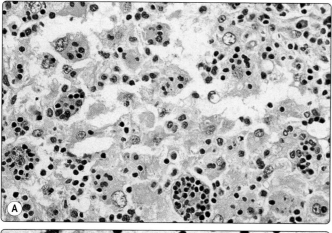

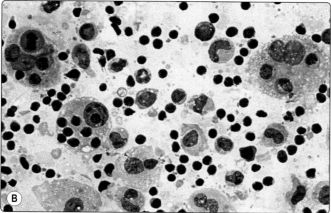

Fig. 5.12 Sinus histiocytosis with massive lymphadenopathy (Rosai-Dorfman disease) (A) Tissue section showing very large histiocytes harboring many lymphocytes (and some plasma cells) in their cytoplasm, (H&E, IP); (B) Smear showing large histiocytes with intracytoplasmic lymphocytes and plasma cells (MGG, IP). (Reproduced with permission from van Heerde et al.[9])

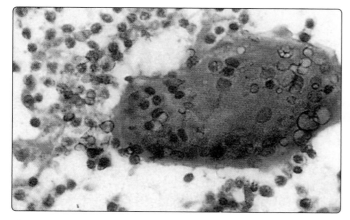

Fig. 5.13 Silicone adenopathy Histiocytes and large multinucleated foreign body-type giant cell with cytoplasmic vacuoles (Pap, IP).

Multinucleate giant cells are usually of histocytic origin and frequently associated with granulomas; however, Warthin-Finkeldey multinucleate giant cells (polykaryocytes) are T cells. They can occasionally be seen in reactive lymphadenitis associated with measles, HIV and Kimura's disease. Additionally, they may be seen with various lymphomas.[106]

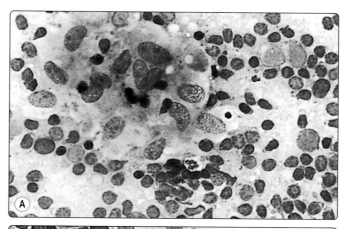

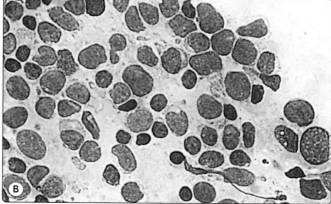

Fig. 5.14 Toxoplasmosis (A) Granuloma-like cluster of histiocytes with epithelioid features; (B) Activated lymphoid cells possibly including some monocytoid B-cell forms. (MGG, HP).

Descriptions of the cytology of angiofollicular lymphoid hyperplasia can also be found in the literature,[9,107–109] as well as of Kimura's disease.[110,111] Follicular dendritic sarcoma may arise in association with Castleman's disease or de novo.[112,113] Rare descriptions of interdigitating dendritic cell sarcoma are also in the literature.[114]

Granulomatous lymphadenitis (Figs 5.17–5.20)

CRITERIA FOR DIAGNOSIS

- ◆ Histiocytes of epithelioid type forming cohesive clusters are characteristic,
- ◆ Multinucleated giant cells usually of Langhans type.

Epithelioid cells are quite distinctive in FNB smears. They have elongated nuclei the shape of which resembles the sole of a shoe or boomerang. The nuclear chromatin is finely granular and pale and the cytoplasm is pale without distinct cell borders (Fig. 5.17). Epithelioid cells of granulomatous lymphadenitis form clusters; large clusters resemble granulomas in tissue sections. Multinucleated Langhans giant cells may be few in numbers and are sometimes absent. Granulomatous lymphadenitis may or may not show necrosis or suppuration. Necrosis may be of fibrinoid or caseous types.

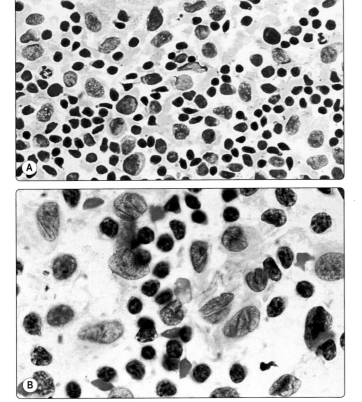

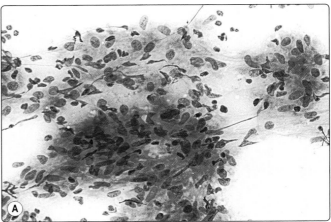

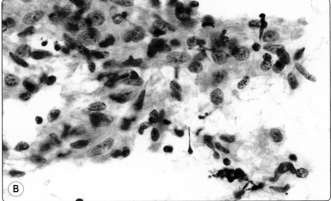

Fig. 5.15 Dermatopathic lymphadenopathy (A) Numerous pale histiocytes/interdigitating cells in a background of predominantly small lymphocytes. Intracytoplasmic pigment was sparse in this case (MGG, IP). (B) Interdigitating cells with conspicuous nuclear folding due to long channel-like invaginations of the nuclear membrane (H&E, HP).

Fig. 5.17 Granulomatous lymphadenitis (sarcoidosis) Clusters of loosely cohesive epithelioid histiocytes with characteristically pale, elongated sole-shaped nuclei; few lymphocytes; no necrosis; no giant cells seen in this example (A, MGG, IP; B, Pap, HP).

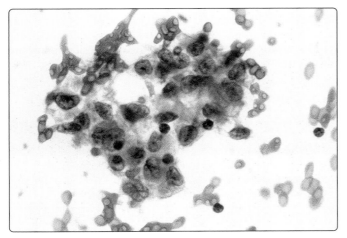

Fig. 5.16 Langerhans histiocytosis Loose cluster of large histiocytic cells with large, vesicular, irregularly folded, lobated or convoluted nuclei; no eosinophils seen in this example (Pap, HP).

Caseous material appears granular and eosinophilic in smears and usually lacks recognizable cell remnants (Fig. 5.18).

Granulomata with caseous necrosis is the hallmark of tuberculous lymphadenitis. However, necrotizing granulo-mata may also be seen with fungal infections. Granuloma-like clusters of epithelioid cells, in the absence of necrosis, are more suggestive of sarcoidosis, but tuberculosis and fungal infections cannot be ruled out and staining for acid-fast bacilli and fungi is imperative in all cases of granuloma-tous lymphadenitis. Smears from a tuberculous lymph node may sometimes show only polymorphs and necrotic debris without histiocytes, particularly in immunocompromised patients. Acid-fast bacilli should, of course, be looked for both in direct smears and in culture from the aspirate. PCR is a sensitive way to detect mycobacterial organisms.[115–120]

Non-necrotizing sarcoidal type granulomata may also be seen with foreign body reactions, brucellosis, Crohn's disease, leishmaniasis and leprosy. Leprosy in lymph nodes has also been diagnosed by FNAC.[121] Conspicuous neu-trophils in a smear showing epithelioid granulomas and necrosis – suppurative granuloma (Fig. 5.19) – suggest atypi-cal mycobacterial infection if the aspirate is from a cervical node in a child, cat scratch disease if from an axillary node,[122–124] and lymphogranuloma venereum if it is from an inguinal node. Fungal and corynebacterial infections may produce a similar reaction, as can chronic granulomatous disease of childhood, leishmaniasis, *Yersinia enterocolitica* and tularemia. Occasionally, groups of epithelioid histio-cytes in toxoplasmosis may be large enough to mimic true

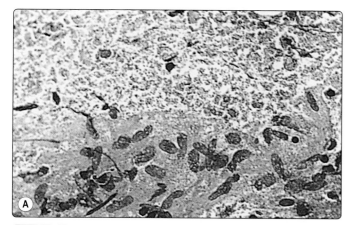

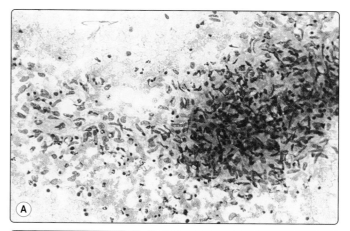

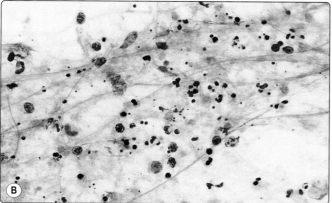

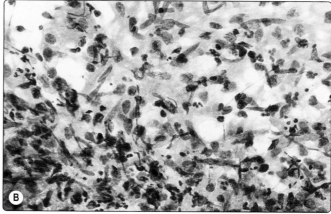

Fig. 5.18 Granulomatous lymphadenitis (tuberculosis) (A) Granuloma-like group of epithelioid histiocytes in a background of granular caseous necrosis (MGG, HP); (B) Granular material of caseous necrosis with degenerating and fragmented nuclei. Note presence of polymorphs, a not uncommon feature, particularly in AIDS patients (Pap, HP).

Fig. 5.19 Granulomatous lymphadenitis (A) Lymphogranuloma venereum. Tissue fragment of epithelioid histiocytes, neutrophils and debris (MGG, LP); (B) Cat scratch disease. Epithelioid histiocytes, lymphocytes and debris with polymorphs (*lower*), probably corresponding to a 'stellate abscess' (Pap, HP).

granulomatous lymphadenitis. Inclusions within histiocytes and giant cells such as birefringent particles, asteroid bodies, Schaumann bodies, etc. are not particularly helpful in making a specific diagnosis. If no etiological agent is found, one can only report the case as granulomatous lymphadenitis with or without necrosis and/or suppuration, and the etiology must be pursued by other means.

PROBLEMS AND DIFFERENTIAL DIAGNOSIS

◆ Tumor necrosis,

◆ Other cell types resembling epithelioid cells (e.g. endothelial cells/Kaposi's sarcoma),

◆ Granuloma in malignant lymphoma and in nodes regional to carcinoma with or without metastatic deposits.

If an aspirate consists entirely of necrotic material, it may be difficult to decide whether it represents caseous necrosis or tumor necrosis (see Figs 8.6). Sampling should be repeated if no bacilli, epithelioid cells or tumor cells are found on careful examination of the smears.

Sometimes, only a few epithelioid cells are found in small groups or as single cells or the histiocytes may not quite have the typical appearance of epithelioid cells. The pattern then approaches that of non-specific, reactive lymphadenitis with prominent histiocytes. This may be the case in toxoplasma lymphadenitis and in the early stages of sarcoidosis. Endothelial cells can sometimes also be mistaken for epithelioid histiocytes. One such example is Kaposi's sarcoma in which tissue fragments may resemble a granuloma, but the nuclei are more elongated and spindly and usually are hyperchromatic. They lack the 'sand shoe' indentations of epithelioid histiocytes and multinucleated giant cells are not seen (Fig. 5.20) (See also Chapter 18).[125–127] In Kaposi's sarcoma the cells are HHV-8, CD31, CD34 and D2-40 positive.

Clusters of epithelioid cells are sometimes found in cases of malignant lymphoma, particularly in HL and in peripheral T-cell (Lennert's) lymphoma. They can also occur in metastatic seminoma and in lymph nodes regional to a carcinoma. A florid granulomatous reaction may occasionally be seen in NHL (e.g. Burkitt and lymphoplasmacytic lymphomas) and this may impair diagnosis. At times, an exuberant granulomatous reaction may also obscure an underlying metastatic carcinoma. One must therefore look carefully for abnormal lymphoid cells and for nonlymphoid cells in smears containing epithelioid histiocytes. Full knowledge of the clinical presentation is obviously essential.

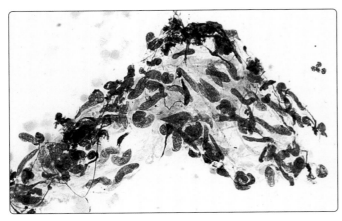

Fig. 5.20 Kaposi's sarcoma Cluster of spindle cells resembling epithelioid granuloma but nuclei are more elongated, irregular and hyperchromatic (MGG, HP).

Lymph node necrosis

Focal, extensive or total necrosis/infarction of lymph nodes occurs in some inflammatory processes (e.g. viral and bacterial infections), in metastatic malignancy, in malignant lymphoma and rarely in relation to vasculitis (e.g. Kawasaki's disease) and to trauma. If necrosis is extensive, FNB smears may not include any well-preserved cells necessary for diagnosis.

Amorphous, granular material without identifiable cell remnants suggests caseous necrosis and smears should be searched for acid-fast bacilli and other microorganisms. In acute inflammatory necrosis, the aspirate and smears have a purulent character.

Necrotising lymphadenitis (Kikuchi-Fujimoto disease) is a condition of unknown etiology, seen mainly in young women, in which there is focal necrosis with a proliferation of histiocytes, lymphocytes and plasmacytoid dendritic cells, usually in cervical lymph nodes.[128–130] The presence of large mononuclear cells in such nodes may cause a suspicion of malignant lymphoma. In FNB smears, the characteristic findings are of large numbers of pale, phagocytosing histiocytes with eccentric, crescentic nuclei, debris with nuclear fragments, absence of neutrophils and a reactive background of lymphoid cells (Fig. 5.21). The histiocytic cells are CD68, CD163 and myeloperoxidase positive.

Necrosis in lymph nodes may also occur in systemic lupus erythematosus. In systemic lupus there may be significant numbers of plasma cells and/or hematoxylin bodies, which may help to distinguish it from Kikuchi-Fujimoto disease. If these features are absent, then serology would be necessary to make this distinction.[131]

Smears from areas of coagulation necrosis in lymph nodes show numerous cell shadows, some with preserved but pyknotic nuclei. Unless there is a clear history of trauma, such findings raise a strong suspicion of either metastatic carcinoma or malignant lymphoma. Nodal metastases of small cell anaplastic carcinoma of lung, melanoma and breast carcinoma are prone to necrosis and the necrotic cells with pyknotic nuclei can be indistinguishable from necrotic lymphoid cells. Extensive necrosis/infarction is common in malignant lymphoma, both non-Hodgkin and Hodgkin.

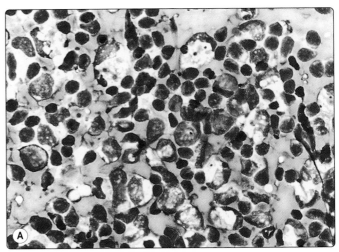
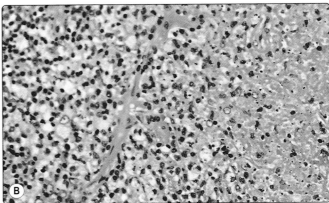

Fig. 5.21 Kikuchi-Fujimoto disease Many large pale histiocytes with crescentic nuclei and phagocytosed debris with background of reactive lymphocytes; necrosis obvious in the tissue section (**A**, smear, MGG, HP; **B**, tissue section H&E, IP).

Total infarction of a lymph node can sometimes precede manifest lymphoma. It has been shown that the demonstration of clonal immunoglobulin or T-cell gene rearrangement in the infarcted node can suggest a diagnosis of lymphoma.[132]

Lymphadenopathy in immune compromised states

The reader is referred to Chapter 18.

Metastatic malignancy

Metastatic malignancy is a more common etiology of peripheral lymphadenopathy than lymphoma, especially in patients over 40 years of age.

CRITERIA FOR DIAGNOSIS

◆ Abnormal nonlymphoid cells amongst normal/reactive lymphoid cells,
◆ Cytological criteria of malignancy.

Micrometastases, either in the subcapsular sinus or as scattered single cells, are unlikely to be sampled even by repeated aspirations. Small metastatic deposits can be missed also by histological examination of an excised node. Partial lymph node involvement is the main cause of false-negative cytological reports.

Benign epithelial inclusions of salivary gland or thyroid origin have been observed in cervical nodes, inclusions of Müllerian origin in pelvic nodes. Mediastinal nodes rarely have mesothelial inclusions while neval cells may be found in axillary nodes. Such inclusions are usually very small. Although a rare occurrence, this possibility should be kept in mind when only a few epithelial cells without obvious malignant characteristics are found in lymph node aspirates in the appropriate context. Groups of glandular epithelial cells of apocrine type are commonly found in FNB smears from axillary nodes. The presence of such cells could give rise to a suspicion of metastasis from breast cancer if the benign characteristics of the cells are not appreciated. The cells most likely represent contaminants from adjacent sweat glands (see Chapter 7).

The common problem of differentiating between necrotising granulomatous lymphadenitis and necrotic tumor has already been mentioned. Squamous cell carcinoma is particularly prone to undergo liquefactive necrosis. An aspirate from such a node consists of thin, mucoid, yellow fluid. Well-preserved neoplastic squamous cells may be few in number and are often very well differentiated (see Fig. 4.2). There is therefore a risk of mistaking a cystic metastasis of well-differentiated squamous carcinoma in a cervical gland for a branchial cyst (see Chapter 4).[83,133] Cystic nodes in the neck may also represent metastases of papillary carcinoma of the thyroid. This possibility should be remembered, particularly in cases of unexplained cervical lymphadenopathy in a young patient (see Chapter 6).

Follicular lymphoma (grade 1–2) may mimic metastatic small cell anaplastic carcinoma or Merkel cell carcinoma in FNB smears.[134,135] This is because of the tendency for neoplastic cells of centrocytic type to form cohesive clusters, sometimes with nuclear molding. This problem will be further discussed in the section on lymphoma as will the differentiation of large cell lymphomas (centroblastic, immunoblastic) from other large cell malignancies by immunocytochemistry[12,105] and pseudoepithelial clustering of lymphoid cells.

Indicators of the primary site

A stepwise approach to the investigation of nodal metastasis is suggested. This should include:

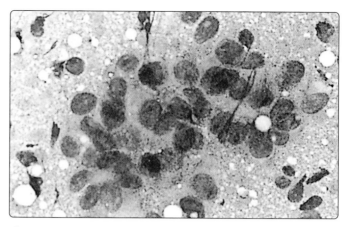

Fig. 5.22 Prostatic carcinoma Supraclavicular node aspirate containing malignant cells from a metastatic adenocarcinoma (MGG, HP).

1. patient's age and sex,
2. anatomical site of the involved node,
3. tumor cytomorphology,
4. cytochemical stains and immunoprofile.

The patient's age is an important consideration when assessing metastatic disease as certain tumors are more common in younger age groups, for example the small round blue cell group of tumors and nasopharyngeal carcinoma.

The anatomical site of the node may give some indication to the possible location of the primary tumor. For example, the axilla commonly harbors metastatic deposits from the breast, lungs or ovaries in middle-aged females. Nodes in the left supraclavicular fossa may be the site of presentation of pelvic malignancies, for example from the prostate, testis or ovaries as well as abdominal malignancies from the gastrointestinal tract.

The cytological patterns seen in routinely stained smears often give clues to the site of the primary tumor. Columnar cells with elongated nuclei arranged in palisades, stringy mucus and necrosis suggest a primary in the large bowel (see Fig 10.32), while mucin-containing signet ring cells suggest the stomach as the most likely primary site among several other possibilities. Glandular cells, moderately pleomorphic, arranged in a gland-in-gland or a cribriform pattern suggest prostatic carcinoma (Fig. 5.22). Large cells with abundant pale, granular or finely vacuolated cytoplasm and a low N:C ratio suggest a renal cell carcinoma. Very large central nucleoli are typical of less well-differentiated forms of this tumor and are also seen in large cell anaplastic carcinoma of lung and nasopharynx (see Fig. 5.55) and in hepatocellular carcinoma. Pulmonary and pancreatic adenocarcinoma can have a variety of patterns. They usually show a moderate degree of glandular differentiation, prominent nuclear pleomorphism and obvious mucin secretion. As a rule, the presence of intracytoplasmic mucin excludes renal, adrenal, hepatocellular and thyroid carcinoma. Breast cancer usually displays poor glandular differentiation while cell balls and single files of cells are more common. Nuclear pleomorphism is often relatively mild. Cells with intracytoplasmic neolumina containing 'bull's-eye' inclusions are also suggestive of breast carcinoma.

The nuclei of a small cell anaplastic carcinoma of lung may appear large in air-dried smears but the amount of

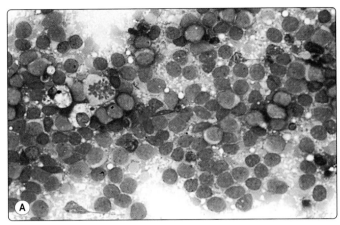

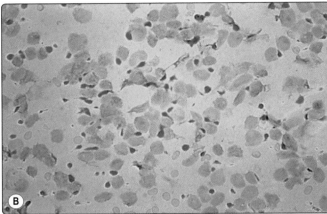

Fig. 5.23 Merkel cell carcinoma (**A**) FNB lymph node with predominantly dissociated undifferentiated tumor cells, superficially resembling NHL. However, lymphoid globules absent and lymphoid markers negative (MGG, HP). (**B**) Immunostaining of same case showing characteristic dot-like positivity of Merkel cell carcinoma with CAM 5.2 (HP).

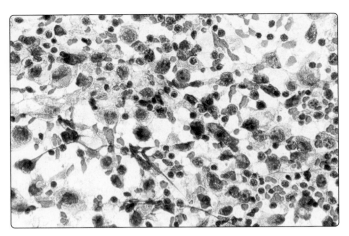

Fig. 5.24 Lymph node metastasis of testicular seminoma Smear from enlarged left supraclavicular lymph node. Mainly dispersed population of malignant cells with fragile nuclei, prominent nucleoli, and dispersed cytoplasm, intermingled with many lymphocytes (Pap, HP).

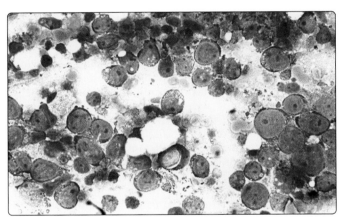

Fig. 5.25 Transitional carcinoma mimicking lymphoma Dispersed malignant cells with large rounded nuclei, prominent nucleoli and scant blue cytoplasm. Irregular cytoplasmic fragments represent tumor necrosis, not lymphoid globules (MGG, HP).

cytoplasm is minimal. Nucleoli are very small and indistinct in typical cases. The cells are closely packed together in aggregates or as single files with prominent nuclear molding. Pyknotic nuclei and nuclear debris are commonly seen between preserved cells (see Fig. 5.2), in the absence of massive necrosis. 'Tear-drop' nuclear artifacts caused by smearing are characteristic (see Figs 8.25 and 8.27). Merkel cell carcinoma (neuroendocrine carcinoma of skin) is characterized by mainly solitary undifferentiated small cells mimicking NHL. However, lymphoid globules are absent while CAM 5.2 and cytokeratin 20 staining is positive with a characteristic dot-like distribution (Fig. 5.23). Neuroendocrine markers (synaptophysin, chromogranin, CD56) are often positive. Features suggesting a neuroendocrine primary are: dispersal, 'neuroendocrine anisonucleosis', bland chromatin that may be speckled, cells in curved rows and poorly formed follicles (see Chapters 8 and 10).

Malignant melanoma is the great mimicker. Smears usually show total dissociation of cells, well-defined cytoplasm, eccentric nuclei, prominent anisokaryosis, a uniformly dense chromatin which does not vary much from nucleus to nucleus, often large nucleoli, binucleate cells, intranuclear vacuoles and often some cells with intracytoplasmic pigment (see Chapter 14). Malignant cells with abundant cytoplasm and a dark-staining paranuclear area are a clue in amelanotic

melanoma. It can occasionally mimic lymphoma in smears (see Fig. 5.60), carcinoma when cellular groups are present, sarcomas with prominent numbers of spindle cells and even pleomorphic malignancies. Testicular tumors may be clinically occult and present with metastases to pelvic, para-aortic or supraclavicular nodes. The cytological pattern of seminoma is characteristic. The tumor cells are mainly dissociated and are mixed with lymphocytes and often with epithelioid cells. They have large, rounded, vesicular nuclei and an evenly distributed nuclear chromatin. Nucleoli are prominent but not very large in wet-fixed smears. The cytoplasm is pale and both cytoplasm and nuclei are very fragile, the dispersed cytoplasm forming a 'tigroid' background to the nuclei (Fig. 5.24, see also Fig. 5.27).[9,136] A tigroid background can, on occasions, also be seen in other glycogen-rich tumors: clear cell sarcoma, clear cell adenocarcinoma of the cervix and clear cell squamous carcinoma. Cells from a transitional cell carcinoma (TCC) may also be dispersed, resembling a large cell lymphoma (Fig. 5.25), or may form solid and sometimes papillary groups. The cells have abundant, relatively dense cytoplasm with distinct borders and

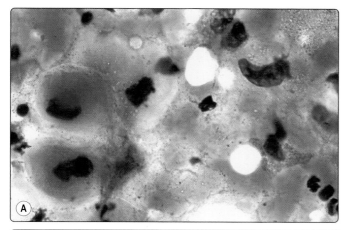

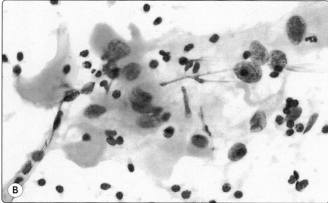

Fig. 5.26 Squamous cell carcinoma (A) Characteristic clear blue cytoplasmic staining, indicating squamous differentiation (MGG, HP). (B) Abundant dense cytoplasm and an occasional orangeophilic keratinised cell (Pap, HP).

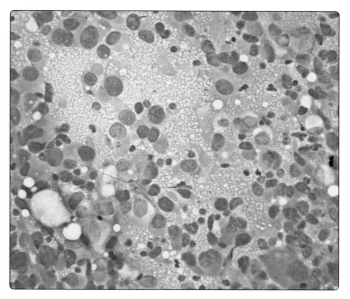

Fig. 5.27 Nodal metastatic clear cell sarcoma Tigroid background with round tumor nuclei and moderate cytoplasm.

pleomorphic, often eccentric, nuclei. A tendency to squamous differentiation or a spindle cell pattern (cercariform cells) may be seen, whereas papillary structures are uncommon in metastatic TCC.

Cytochemical stains and immune markers are often helpful. Squamous differentiation is most obvious in alcohol-fixed Pap-stained smears but can also be distinguished in MGG-stained preparations (Fig. 5.26A). Histochemical demonstration of intracytoplasmic mucin droplets confirms a diagnosis of adenocarcinoma. Positive immunocytochemical staining for prostatic acid phosphatase and/or prostate-specific antigen in an adenocarcinoma supports a prostatic origin.[137] This staining should be performed in all metastatic adenocarcinomas of unknown origin in male patients in view of the palliative treatment available for disseminated prostatic carcinoma.

Immunocytochemical staining for S-100, Melan A and HMB-45 is of great value in diagnosing melanoma. Immune markers with some 'relative tumor specificity' can be very helpful, e.g. PSA (prostate), TTF-1 (lung and thyroid), GCDFP-15 (breast and sweat gland, salivary gland) and PAX-2 (renal and mullerian). Other useful tumor markers are chromogranin, CD56 and synaptophysin in neuroendocrine tumors, a variety of hormones and polypeptides in endocrine tumors, glypican-3, Hep-Par1 and alpha-fetoprotein in hepatocellular carcinoma. Similarly, OCT4

and placental alkaline phosphatase (PLAP) are useful in some germ cell tumors, with CD117 in seminoma. Also, calcitonin and CEA in thyroid medullary carcinoma, and FLI-1 in primitive neuroectodermal tumor (see Table 2.4). CDX-2 is a colorectal carcinoma marker; however, it also reacts with some gastric and pancreatobiliary adenocarcinomas. Differential cytokeratins (CK7, CK20) may be helpful in suggesting the origin of metastatic carcinoma.[138,139] In some cases, electron microscopical examination of the aspirate and cytogenetic studies are extremely helpful, particularly in small round cell tumors and in some mesenchymal tumors (see Table 2.3).

Metastatic sarcomas are uncommon findings in lymph nodes.[140] Sarcomas other than Kaposi's, which have a tendency to involve regional nodes, are rhabdomyosarcoma, epithelioid sarcoma, clear cell sarcoma, angiosarcoma, Ewing's sarcoma and synovial sarcoma (Fig. 5.27)

Non-Hodgkin lymphoma[9,10,11,38,41,54,55,58,60,68–70,84,141–145]

Today, most pathologists use the WHO classification of lymphomas (Table 5.1) which is based on a combination of cytomorphology, immunophenotype, genetic characteristics and clinical findings.[69] Lymphoma cell types, including Hodgkin lymphoma, are diagramatically illustrated in Figure 5.28. This classification allowed a greater role for FNAC with FCM in lymphoma diagnosis and subclassification. Cytological subtyping of NHL in FNB smears can be difficult and needs extensive experience and ancillary support. It requires a complete comprehension of the WHO classification of lymphomas (and/or hematopathology experience), a working knowledge of FCM and immunoperoxidase use and interpretation as well as cytogenetic and molecular studies in order to make the appropriate correlation with clinical information so that a classification can be made. There should also be close collaboration with

Table 5.1 Entities of WHO classification of lymphoid tumours

B-cell lymphomas	T/NK-cell lymphoma
B-lymphoblastic lymphoma/ leukaemia	T-lymphoblastic lymphoma/ leukaemia
Chronic lymphocytic leukaemia/ small lymphocytic	T-cell prolymphocytic leukaemia
Prolymphocytic leukaemia	Chronic lymphoproliferative disorder of NK-cells
Lymphoplasmacytic lymphoma	T-cell large granular lymphocytic leukaemia
Splenic marginal zone lymphoma	Aggressive NK-cell leukaemia
Plasmacytoma/myeloma	Systemic EBV+ T-cell
Heavy chain disease	lymphoproliferative disease of childhood
Extranodal marginal zone (MALT) lymphoma	Hydroa vacciniform-like lymphoma
Nodal marginal zone lymphoma	Adult T-cell leukaemia/ lymphoma
Follicular lymphoma	Extranodal NK/T-cell lymphoma (nasal type)
Mantle cell lymphoma	Enteropathy-type T-cell lymphoma
Diffuse large B-cell lymphoma, NOS	
T-cell/histiocyte rich large B-cell lymphoma	Hepatosplenic T-cell lymphoma
Primary DLBCL of CNS	Subcutaneous panniculitis-like T-cell lymphoma
Primary cutaneous DLBCL, leg type	Mycosis fungoides/Sezary's syndrome
EBV+ DLBCL of elderly	Primary cutaneous CD30+ T-cell lymphoproliferative disorder
DLBCL associated with chronic inflammation	Primary cutaneous aggressive epidermotropic CD8-positive cytotoxic T-cell lymphoma
Mediastinal (thymic) large B-cell lymphoma	Primary cutaneous gamma-delta T-cell lymphoma
Intravascular large B-cell lymphoma	Primary cutaneous small/ medium CD4-positive T-cell lymphoma
Primary effusion lymphoma	
Plasmablastic lymphoma	Angioimmunoblastic T-cell lymphoma
ALK positive large B-cell lymphoma	Peripheral T-cell lymphoma, NOS
Large B-cell lymphoma arising in HHV-8 multicentric Castleman disease	Anaplastic large cell lymphoma, ALK positive
Lymphomatoid granulomatosis	Anaplastic large cell lymphoma, ALK negative
Burkitt lymphoma	
B-cell lymphoma, unclassifiable with features intermediate between diffuse large B-cell and Burkitt lymphoma	
B-cell lymphoma, unclassifiable with features intermediate between diffuse large B-cell and classical Hodgkin lymphoma	

hematopathologists/hematologists and senior people in the molecular, FCM and genetic laboratories.

FCM is the mainstay in the diagnosis and classification of NHL using FNB. FCM immunophenotyping provides quantitative evidence of cell lineage, B-cell clonality and T-cell aberrancies, and facilitates subclassification. FCM is not infallible and has pitfalls which may lead to misclassification or incorrect diagnosis. It is essential to correlate morphology with FCM data and the clinical situation.

The original 2001 WHO classification was revised in late 2008. It contains additions of new entities and subtypes (e.g. in the large cell lymphoma group), recognition of specific gray-zone areas and more degrees of acceptable uncertainty. More uncertainty has been recognized even within well-established entities, e.g. distinguishing lymphoplasmacytic lymphoma from other B-cell lymphomas with plasmacytic differentiation. These and other changes will add greater complexity to cytological subtyping of NHL. The number of possible diagnoses has more than doubled since the 2001 edition.

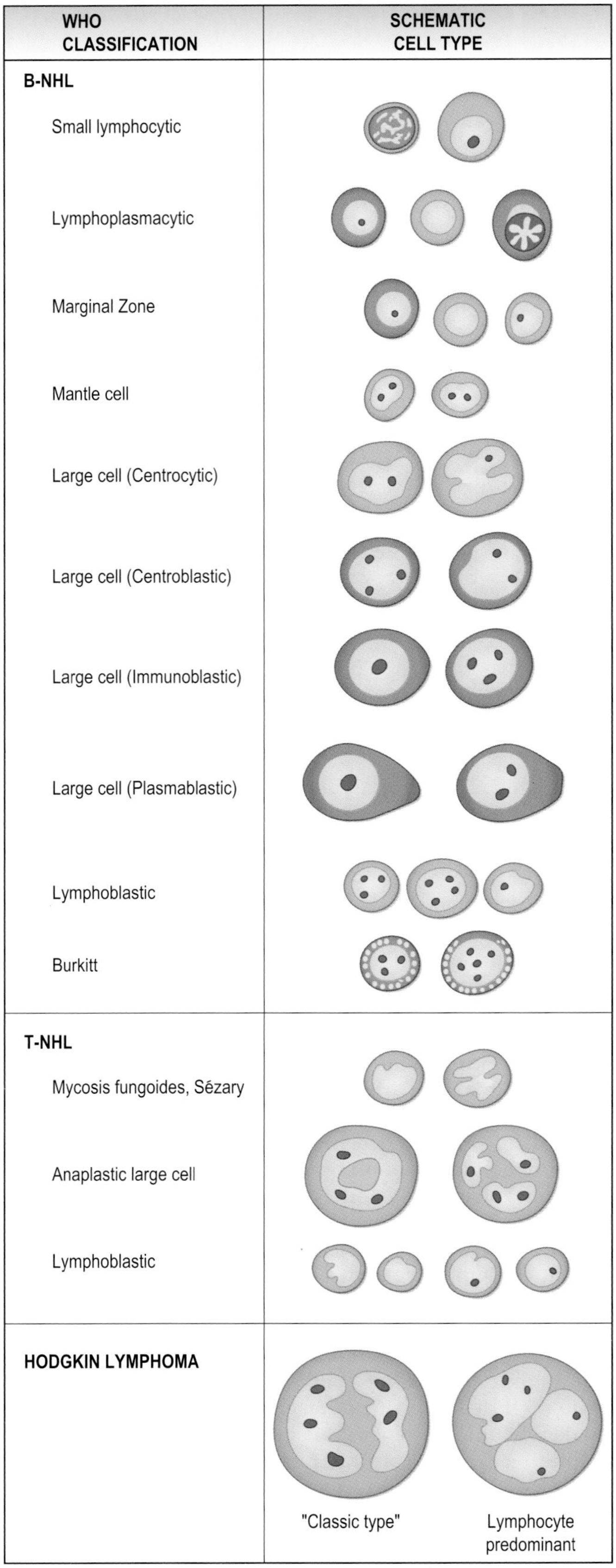

WHO CLASSIFICATION	SCHEMATIC CELL TYPE
B-NHL	
Small lymphocytic	
Lymphoplasmacytic	
Marginal Zone	
Mantle cell	
Large cell (Centrocytic)	
Large cell (Centroblastic)	
Large cell (Immunoblastic)	
Large cell (Plasmablastic)	
Lymphoblastic	
Burkitt	
T-NHL	
Mycosis fungoides, Sézary	
Anaplastic large cell	
Lymphoblastic	
HODGKIN LYMPHOMA	
"Classic type"	Lymphocyte predominant

Fig. 5.28 Diagrammatic representation of the most common cell types of malignant lymphomas.

Over 90% of NHL are B-cell neoplasms, with diffuse large B-cell lymphoma and follicular lymphoma accounting for 65% of these. Less than 10% of NHL are T- and NK-cell neoplasms. As the B-cell lymphomas are commonly seen in daily practice, these will be highlighted, but not all of those listed in the WHO classification will be discussed. Some of the T-cell lymphomas also will be briefly discussed.

FNAC diagnosis of NHL is based largely on monomorphism of smear populations or disproportionate representation of cell types, often with features similar to their benign counterparts, which contrasts to most neoplasms diagnosed on the basis of cellular atypia. Assessment of cell size and nuclear features aid in subtyping. Small cells are less than 1.5 × the size of a normal lymphocyte. Medium sized cells are 1.5–2 × the size of a normal lymphocyte or no larger than a histiocyte nucleus. Large cells are more than 2–3 × the size of normal lymphocytes or larger than a histiocyte nucleus. The various cellular populations and cell size group entities are illustrated in Figure 5.29. The morphologic findings are then integrated with the immunophenotyping.

B-Cell neoplasms

Small cell lymphoid proliferations may have morphologic similarities and at times may be difficult to differentiate from reactive nodes. FCM is essential in distinguishing reactive from neoplastic small cell lymphoid populations as it demonstrates monoclonality in the neoplastic B cells, and

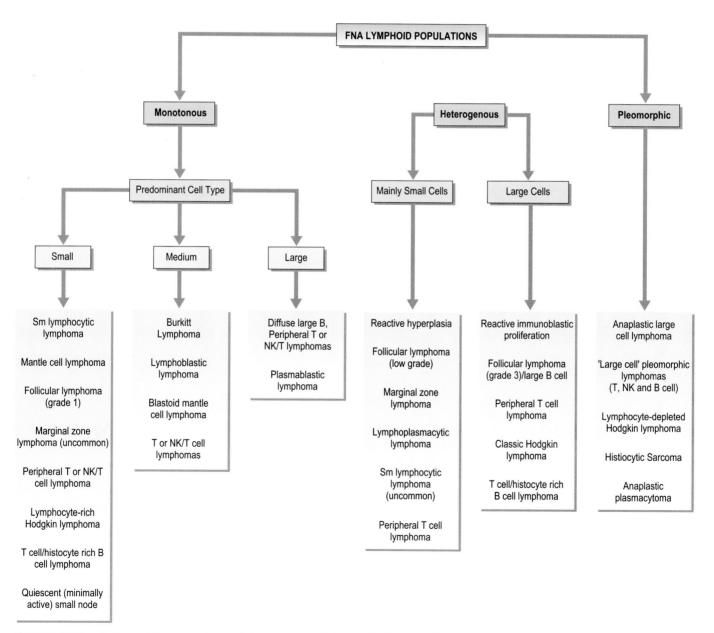

Fig. 5.29 FNA lymphoid populations: monotonous, heterogeneous and pleomorphic (Sm = small).

Table 5.2 Small B-cell lymphomas

Lymphoma type	CD5	CD10	CD23	Cyclin-D1	Cytogenetics
Small lymphocytic	+	−	+	−	Trisomy 12
Mantle cell	+	−	−**	+	t(11;14)
Follicular (low grade)	−	+/(−)*	−/(+)	−	t(14;18)
Lymphoplasmacytic	−**	−	−**	−	non-specific
Marginal zone (nodal)	−**	−	−	−	Trisomies 3,7,18

* 10–40% negative; ** rarely positive; + positive; − negative.

aids in subtyping by assessing CD5, CD10, CD23 and FMC7 expression on the neoplastic B cells. This distinction can be difficult based on morphology alone (Table 5.2). Cytogenetics can also aid in subtyping.

SMALL LYMPHOCYTIC LYMPHOMA/CHRONIC LYMPHOCYTIC LEUKAEMIA (SLL/CLL) (FIGS 5.30–5.33)

Patients are mostly middle aged and elderly.

1. a monotonous population of small lymphoid cells,
2. mainly round nuclei slightly larger than those of normal small lymphocytes,
3. characteristically coarse granular nuclear chromatin ('grumelé', highlighted by Pap staining); nucleoli absent,
4. a varying number of prolymphocytes: larger size, more cytoplasm, pale chromatin, single central nucleolus,
5. large paraimmunoblasts with prominent nucleolus and gray-blue cytoplasm,
6. Rare tingible-body macrophages,
7. immunophenotype: CD19, CD20, faint SIg, CD5, CD23 (CD10 and FMC7 negative) (Fig. 5.30),
8. aberrant immunophenotype: CD5 or CD23 negative[69] (rarely CD10 positive),
9. genetics: trisomy 12 (20%), deletion 13q (50%).

Recognition of the subtle morphological differences between small lymphocytes and the small cells of lymphocytic lymphoma requires optimal cytological preparations. The typical SLL/CLL is readily recognized by the monotonous population of cells resembling small lymphocytes (Fig. 5.31). Difficulties can arise if the process contains numerous proliferation centers with many large and intermediate size cells – paraimmunoblasts and prolymphocytes (Fig. 5.32). A large B cell lymphoma may develop in 2–8% of patients with B-CLL, the so-called Richter syndrome (Fig. 5.33) or rarely HL.[9,69,145]

Lymphoplasmacytic lymphoma (LPL) (Fig. 5.34)

Most patients are elderly and the majority of cases have a serum monoclonal IgM paraprotein.

CRITERIA FOR DIAGNOSIS

1. a mixed population of lymphocytes, plasma cells and occasionally some blasts,
2. a variable number of lymphocytes with plasmacytoid features and Dutcher bodies,
3. may occasionally have amyloid,
4. immunophenotype: strong SIg and CIg, CD19, CD20, CD79a (CD5 and CD23 negative),
5. aberrant immunophenotype: occasionally CD5 and/or CD23 positive (rarely CD10),
6. genetics: no specific abnormality in node.

Occasional cases have a large number of immunoblasts. This may indicate a worse prognosis. Transformation to a large cell lymphoma is rare.[69] Other small cell lymphomas with plasmacytic features need to be excluded. At times marginal zone lymphoma may not be clearly separated from LPL.

Plasmacytoma (Figs 5.35, 5.36)[9,69,146,147]

Usually in middle aged or elderly patients. Commonly involve bones, upper airways and only rarely lymph nodes.[9,71]

CRITERIA FOR DIAGNOSIS

1. cells resembling mature or immature (nucleoli-containing) plasma cells,
2. eccentric nuclei, condensed chromatin or blastic-like, condensed cytoplasm,
3. immunophenotype: CD38, CD79a, CD138, OCT-2, CIg; CD 20 and Pax 5 very often negative,
4. aberrant immunophenotype: CD56, CD10, CD117, cyclin D1.

Be wary of unusual cellular morphology, e.g. occasional cases dominated by pleomorphic, signet ring, clear and sarcomatoid cells, which may be difficult to recognize as plasma cells. The rare variant with a small lymphocyte-like morphology may mimic a B-cell lymphoma.

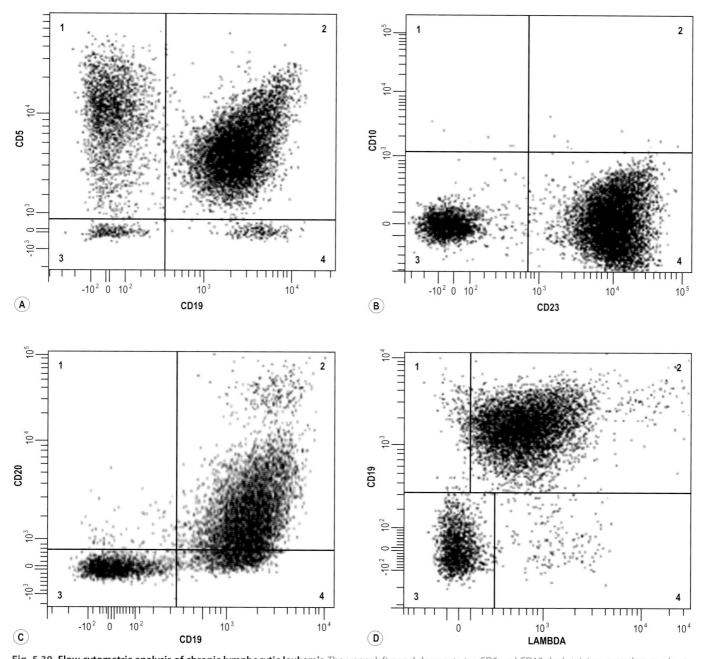

Fig. 5.30 Flow cytometric analysis of chronic lymphocytic leukemia The upper left panel demonstrates CD5 and CD19 dual staining; note that quadrant 2 contains cells positive for both CD19 and CD5. Quadrant 1 contains the remaining CD5-positive T cells. The upper right panel demonstrates that the CLL cells are positive for CD23 (quadrant 4) and negative for CD10. The lower left panel demonstrates dual staining with CD19 and CD20. Note the typical weak CD20 staining on CLL cells. The lower right quadrant demonstrates the lambda light chain restriction, in that virtually all of the CD19-positive cells express (weak) lambda light chain. (Courtesy A/Prof P. Macardle, Flinders Medical Center).

Follicular lymphoma (FL) (Figs 5.37–5.39)[69]

Follicular lymphoma constitutes about 30% of NHL and is composed of a mixture of centrocytic and centroblastic cells. In the WHO classification, follicular lymphomas are divided into three histologic grades based on the number of large centroblasts present: grade 1 – predominantly centrocytes (0–5 centroblasts/HPF), grade 2 – a mixture of centrocytes and centroblasts, (6–15 centroblasts/HPF) and grade 3 – predominantly centroblasts (> 15 centroblasts/HPF).

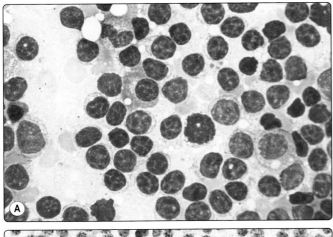

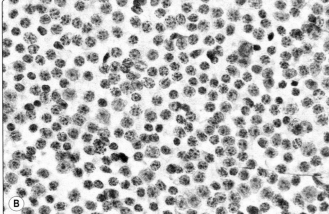

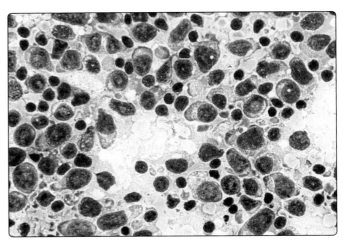

Fig. 5.33 Richter syndrome in B-CLL large B-cell lymphoma developing in terminal stage of B-CLL (MGG, HP).

Fig. 5.31 Small lymphocytic lymphoma (B-CLL) Monotonous population of slightly enlarged lymphocytes with coarsely granular chromatin (grumelé pattern) particularly obvious in Pap-stained smears; (**A**) MGG, HP; (**B**) Pap, HP.

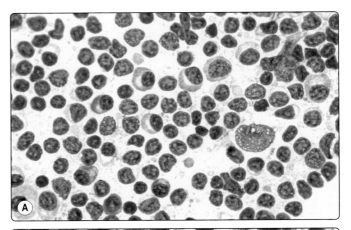

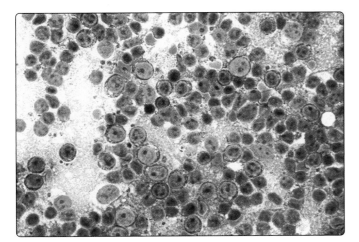

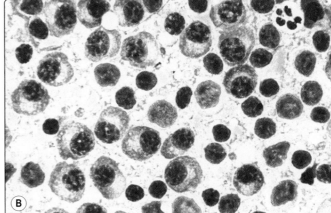

Fig. 5.32 Small lymphocytic lymphoma (B-CLL) Note the presence of many large cells with a single nucleolus (polymphocytes) representing proliferation center, especially in slightly understained cells (MGG, HP).

Fig. 5.34 Lymphoplasmacytic lymphoma (**A**) Predominantly small lymphocytes, some with plasmacytoid cytoplasm, and a single large blastic cell (MGG, HP) (Reproduced with permission from van Heerde et al.[9]); (**B**) Lymphoplasmacytic lymphoma with obvious plasma cell component (MGG, HP).

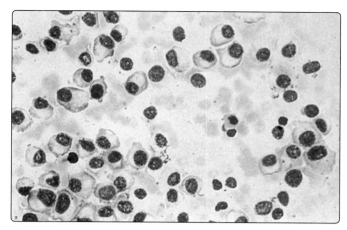

Fig. 5.35 **Plasmacytoma** Pure population of well-differentiated plasma cells (MGG, HP).

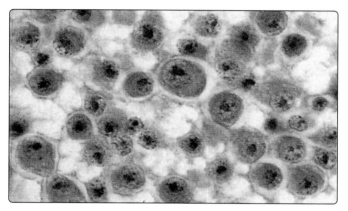

Fig. 5.36 **Myeloma in lymph node** Poorly differentiated plasma cells. This patient had multiple myeloma (Pap, HP).

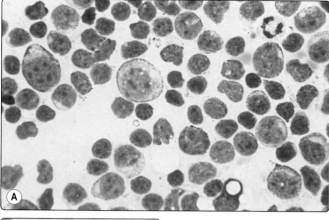

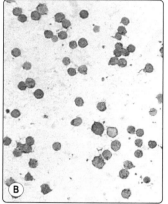

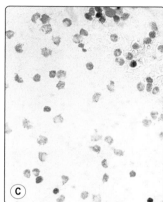

Fig. 5.37 **Follicular (grade 1) lymphoma** (A) Predominance of medium-sized cells with irregular, sometimes cleaved nuclei; a few centroblasts with multiple nucleoli. Relatively few small lymphocytes; (MGG, HP). (B,C) Kappa/lambda staining in cytospin preparation showing lambda monoclonality (B) (immunostain, alkaline phosphatase method, IP).

CRITERIA FOR DIAGNOSIS

1. lymphoid population composed of a mixture of centrocytes and centroblasts,
2. centroblasts with large round or slightly irregular nuclei, small nucleoli and basophilic cytoplasm,
3. centrocytes, small to medium-sized, with irregular or cleaved nuclei, inconspicuous nucleoli and little cytoplasm with a tendency to form clusters,
4. usually a relatively low number of small lymphocytes (Fig. 5.37A),
5. immunophenotype: monotypic SIg (Fig. 5.37B,C), CD19, CD20, CD10 (in 60–90% of cases), Bcl-2, Bcl-6, CD23 sometimes,
6. aberrant immunophenotype: CD5 (floral variant),
7. genetics: t(14;18) in over 90%.

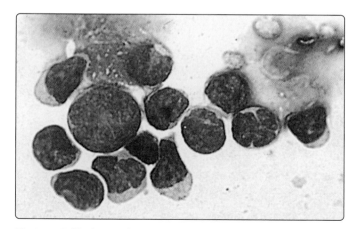

Fig. 5.38 **Follicular (grade 1) lymphoma** Cytocentrifuge preparation; centrocytes showing cleaved nuclei; one centroblast (MGG, HP oil).

It is not possible in FNB smears to reliably predict the architectural pattern of a follicular lymphoma (FL). However, some authors have greater success in identifying aggregates of follicle center cells.[142] A follicular pattern in cell blocks or NCB can be inferred by staining of dendritic cells with CD21/35. It is also difficult to assess the relative proportions of small and large centrocytes and centroblasts, as these are influenced by sampling bias. This makes grading difficult. Also, a clear distinction between FL grade 3B and DLBCL (mainly centroblastic) is often not possible. However, this distinction may not be critical for therapeutic management.

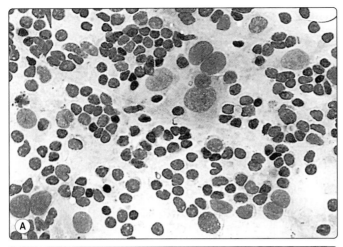

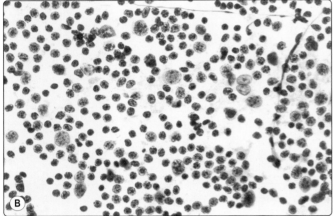

Fig. 5.39 Follicular (grade 1) lymphoma Dendritic reticulum cells may be prominent in follicular lymphomas; predominance of centrocytes; (A, MGG, B, Pap, HP).

There are no well-established criteria for grading FL in FNB smears. FL grade 3 has been variably defined,[21,29,145] for example, greater than 20%, or 50% centroblasts in the smear population, or there is sheeting of large cells. Grading has also been based on centroblast count with an associated proliferative index or proliferative index alone.[148,149] As a rule, this author favors FL grade 3 if half or more of the cell population, as assessed subjectively, are centroblasts.

In FL grade 1, the majority of cells are centrocytes. The characteristic cleaved nuclear morphology of centrocytes is well demonstrated in cytocentrifuge preparations of cell suspensions (Fig. 5.38). The irregular nuclear shape is often less obvious in direct smears and centrocytes are then identified by the intermediate size of the nuclei and by the nuclear chromatin, paler and more granular than that of lymphocytes. Starry-sky macrophages are usually absent. Dendritic reticulum cells are commonly seen (Fig. 5.39). FCM and/or immunohistochemistry are often necessary to distinguish follicular lymphoma from follicular hyperplasia in FNB smears. In 25–35% of FL there is transformation to a large cell lymphoma or high-grade Burkitt-resembling lymphoma. Rarely, they 'transdifferentiate' into various histiocytic and dendritic neoplasms.[69]

Mantle cell lymphoma (MCL) (Fig. 5.40)[143,150,151]
Usually in adults over 50 years of age

CRITERIA FOR DIAGNOSIS

1. monotonous population of small centrocyte-like cells with occasional histiocytes,
2. blastoid variant cells resemble lymphoblasts,
3. immunophenotype: CD19, CD20, SIg, CD5, FMC7, Cyclin-D1 (cell block or CNB); CD10 and CD23 negative,
4. aberrant immunophenotype: CD5 negative, CD5 and CD10 positive, CD23 weakly positive,[19,20,69]
5. genetics: t(11;14) almost all cases.

Mantle cell lymphomas are generally clinically aggressive neoplasms, usually high stage at the time of presentation: generalized lymphadenopathy, splenomegaly, bone marrow and blood involvement. One must be wary of some uncommon variants (pleomorphic, small round cell, marginal zone-like) which may overlap with other lymphoma subtypes.[69] The small cell variant appears to have a more indolent course. Immunostaining for Cyclin D1 on cytospin preparations can be unreliable.

Marginal zone lymphoma (MZL)

Marginal zone lymphoma accounts for approximately 10% of B-cell lymphomas. It has two major clinical presentations, extranodal (mucosal-associated lymphoid tissue) and nodal.

CRITERIA FOR DIAGNOSIS

1. heterogeneous population of cells (uncommonly monomorphous population),
2. small up to medium atypical cells with irregular nuclei,
3. mature small lymphocytes, plasma cells, large transformed cells,
4. variable numbers of monocytoid cells with clear cytoplasm; difficult to identify,
5. immunophenotype: CD19, CD20, CD79a, FMC7 (CD5, CD10, CD23 negative),
6. aberrant immunophenotype: CD5 or CD10 (rarely),
7. genetics: nodal – trisomies 3,7,18; extranodal – t(11;18), t(3;14), t(14;18).

MZL is one of the most difficult types to recognize in smears as it can have morphologic features which overlap with a reactive process.[25] It usually has a heterogeneous population and lacks specific cytologic and immunologic markers, apart from occasional cases having many monocytoid cells. In some of these latter cases, the cell population may be monotonous.[69,152,153] The high content of reactive cells may impair detection of B-cell clonality.

Diffuse large B-cell lymphoma, not otherwise specified (DLBCL, NOS)[69]

Diffuse large B-cell lymphoma (DLBCL) is a heterogeneous group. Those that do not belong to specific subtypes or disease entities are classified as diffuse large B-cell lymphoma, not otherwise specified (NOS). These make up 25–30% of NHL. There are three common variants:

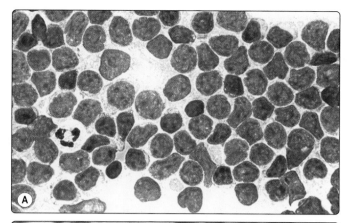

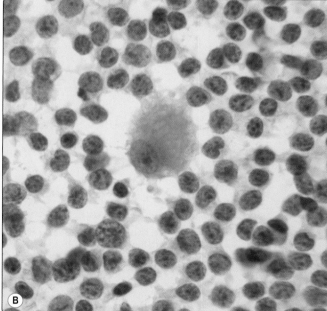

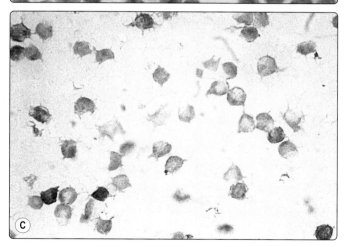

Fig. 5.40 Mantle cell lymphoma (**A**) Nuclei a little larger than those of lymphocytes irregular shape, finely granular chromatin without distinct nucleoli. A few normal lymphocytes present. (**B**) Central histiocyte for size comparison (**C**) Immunostaining with CD5: strongly positive reactive T cells and moderate positivity in malignant lymphoma cells (**A**, MGG, HP; **B**,Pap HP; **C** immunostain CD5, IP).

centroblastic, immunoblastic and anaplastic (pleomorphic). Not infrequently, the distinction between centroblastic and immunoblastic lymphoma is not clear, on morphologic grounds, due to a mixed population of large cells of different type.

CRITERIA FOR DIAGNOSIS

A. Centroblastic variant (Figs 5.41–5.43)
1. a population of mainly centroblasts,
2. characteristically round nuclei with multiple small nucleoli (Fig. 5.41),
3. a variable proportion of indented/cleaved or even multilobated nuclei often present (Fig. 5.42–5.43),
4. immunoblasts with abundant basophilic cytoplasm and large central nucleoli may be present in the 'polymorphous subtype' (Fig. 5.43A).

B. Immunoblastic variant (Figs 5.44–5.45)
1. a pleomorphic cell population dominated by large blasts; sometimes extreme pleomorphism and multinucleated cells,
2. unevenly distributed nuclear chromatin; prominent, usually single central nucleoli; occasionally multiple nucleoli; frequent mitoses,
3. abundant blue cytoplasm (MGG); perinuclear pale zone (Fig. 5.44A),
4. tingible body macrophages.

C. Anaplastic variant
1. cells resemble Hodgkin and/or Reed-Sternberg cells,
2. may resemble cells of anaplastic large cell lymphoma.

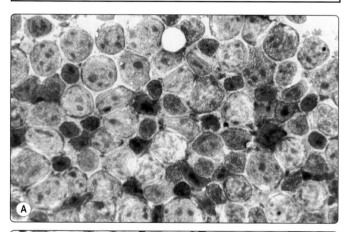

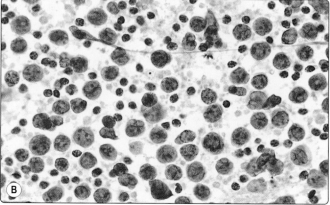

Fig. 5.41 Diffuse large B-cell lymphoma, NOS Predominance of large centroblastic lymphoid cells with pale nuclei, scanty cytoplasm and multiple, often peripheral, nucleoli (**A**, MGG, **B**, Pap, HP).

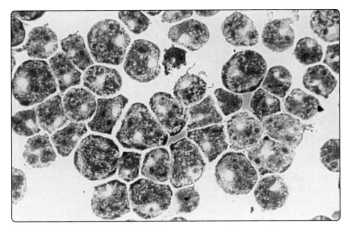

Fig. 5.42 Diffuse large B-cell lymphoma, NOS Cytocentrifuge preparation of cerebrospinal fluid showing pronounced irregularity of nuclear contour (MGG, HP).

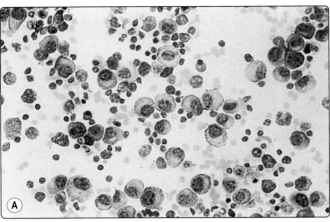

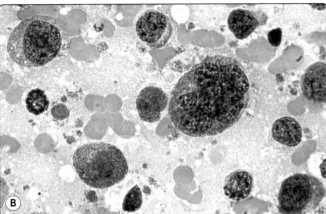

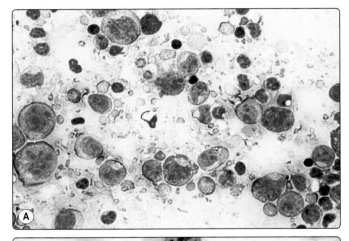

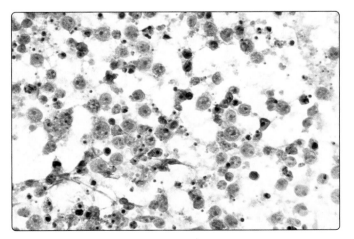

Fig. 5.44 Diffuse large cell lymphoma, NOS (immunoblastic B cells) Predominantly large lymphoid cells with large round nuclei, large nucleoli and abundant basophilic cytoplasm (A, MGG, IP; B, MGG, HP oil). (Reproduced with permission from van Heerde et al.[9])

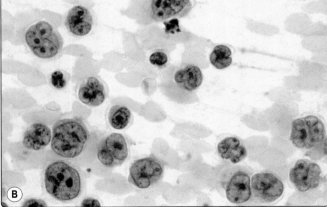

Fig. 5.43 Diffuse large B-cell lymphoma, NOS. Polymorphous. Centroblasts, immunoblasts and large centrocytic cells, particularly distinct in Pap-stained preparations (A, MGG, HP; B, Pap, HP oil).

Fig. 5.45 Diffuse large cell lymphoma, NOS (immunoblastic B cells) Predominance of large lymphoid cells with large vesicular round nuclei and large central nucleoli (Pap, HP).

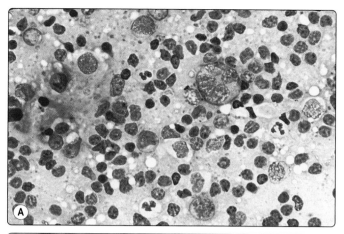

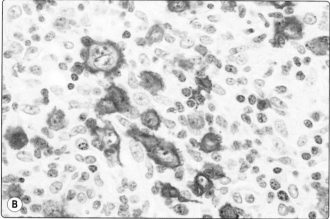

Fig. 5.46 T-cell/histiocyte rich B-cell lymphoma (A) Scattered large abnormal lymphoid cells with a background of reactive lymphocytes (MGG, HP); (B) The neoplastic B cell highlighted by immunostaining for CD20 (immunostain CD20, HP).

Diffuse large B-cell lymphoma, NOS, (groups A, B, C as above)

1. immunophenotype: CD19, CD20; often SIg, sometimes CIg; variable expression CD10, BCL6, BCL2 and MUM1; CD 30 most likely in anaplastic variant,
2. aberrant immunophenotype: CD5positve (10%); rarely cyclin D1 focal positivity,
3. genetics: t(14;18) in 30%, MYC rearrangement up to 10%,

T-cell/histiocyte-rich large B-cell lymphoma
(Fig. 5.46)

Affects mainly middle-aged men.

CRITERIA FOR DIAGNOSIS

1. smears dominated by small mature lymphocytes, over 90%,
2. variable numbers of epithelioid histiocytes,
3. scattered large cells mimicking Hodgkin or Reed-Sternberg cells, centroblasts, immunoblasts and 'popcorn cells',
4. immunophenotype: small cells, CD3, CD5, CD8; large cells, CD20, CD79a, BCL6 (CD15, CD30 negative),
5. genetics: non-specific.

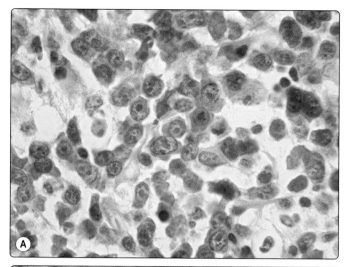

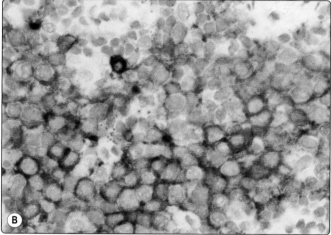

Fig. 5.47 Plasmablastic lymphoma (A) Uniform large cells with vesicular nucleus, prominent nucleoli and moderate cytoplasm-resembling immunoblasts (cell button. H&E, HP); (B) CD138 positive (immunostain CD138, HP).

It is difficult to diagnose on FNB smears and to distinguish from HL and reactive adenopathy[154-157] FCM is usually non-diagnostic. Usually a tissue biopsy with immune marker studies is essential to establish the diagnosis.

Primary mediastinal (thymic) large B-cell lymphoma (see chapter 9)

Plasmablastic lymphoma (Fig. 5.47)[69,158]

Plasmablastic lymphoma is uncommon and may be associated with immunodeficiency.

CRITERIA FOR DIAGNOSIS

1. monotonous cellular smear with cells resembling immunoblasts or a mixture of large nuclei, coarse chromatin, small nucleoli and smaller plasmacytic cells,
2. immunophenotype: CD138, CD38, MUM1, CD79a (positive 50–85%),
3. genetics: frequent IG/MYC translocations and gains in multiple chromosomal loci.

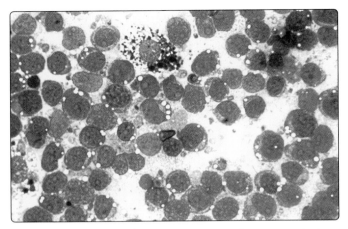

Fig. 5.48 Burkitt lymphoma Rounded lymphoid cells; some variation in nuclear size; distinct nucleoli; granular chromatin; dense blue cytoplasm with lipid vacuoles and some starry-sky macrophages (MGG, HP). (Reproduced with permission from van Heerde et al.[9])

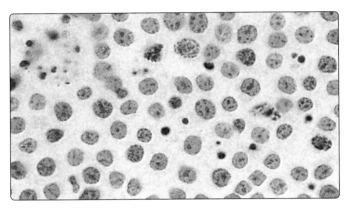

Fig. 5.49 Burkitt lymphoma Blastic cells with round nuclei of varying size and small amount of cytoplasm; occasional starry-sky macrophages (Pap, HP).

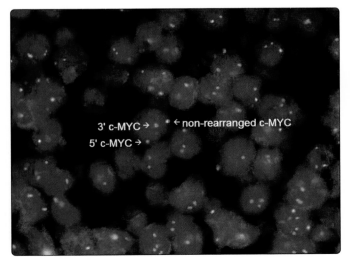

3' c-MYC →   ← non-rearranged c-MYC
5' c-MYC →

Fig. 5.50 Burkitt lymphoma Dual-color FISH with break-apart c-MYC probes (5'c-MYC probe orange and 3'c-MYC probe green) showing nuclei in which one pair of probe signals (*yellow*) is split apart due to a c-MYC region rearrangement. (Courtesy Sarah Moore, Institute of Medical and Veterinary Science).

It has an immunophenotype of plasma cells and needs to be distinguished from myeloma, principally on clinical and radiological findings.

Burkitt lymphoma (Figs 5.48–5.50)[159–161]

Burkitt lymphoma in African children is endemic and associated with Epstein-Barr virus. The jaws often being involved. In non-African cases, most patients present with abdominal localization.

CRITERIA FOR DIAGNOSIS

1. usually a relatively uniform cell population with a high mitotic rate,
2. rounded nuclei of variable but predominantly intermediate size,
3. granular or speckled chromatin pattern, multiple (2–5) small but prominent nucleoli,
4. variable, mostly thin rim of dense blue cytoplasm with small lipid vacuoles (MGG),
5. starry-sky macrophages often prominent with a 'dirty' background,
6. immunophenotype: SIgM, CD19, CD20, CD10, BCL6 (negative for BCL2, TdT); proliferative index (MIB1) nearly 100%,
7. genetics: t(8;14) in 80%, t(2;8) and t(8;22) (Fig. 5.50).

The diagnosis of Burkitt lymphoma requires a combination of ancillary techniques as there is no single diagnostic gold standard, e.g. the c-myc rearrangement is highly characteristic but not specific.[69] In addition, there may be cases with greater nuclear pleomorphism with fewer and more prominent nucleoli.

B-lymphoblastic leukemia/ lymphoma
(Fig. 5.51)[9,69,145,162]

The majority of patients are under 18 years of age and the lymphoma often involves nodes, skin and bones. It comprises 10% of lymphoblastic lymphomas.

CRITERIA FOR DIAGNOSIS

1. a homogeneous population of cells of similar type.
2. round nuclei mainly of intermediate size, occasionally showing considerable variation in size,
3. finely granular or 'speckled' nuclear chromatin with multiple small nucleoli,
4. moderately basophilic, fragile cytoplasm,
5. starry-sky macrophages may be present (Fig. 5.51A),
6. immunophenotype: CD19, CD79a, CD10, PAX5, TdT (CD34, CD20 variable expression),
7. genetics: many with variable genetic abnormalities having prognostic significance.

This lymphoblastic morphology may be seen with T-cell lymphoblastic lymphomas

T-lymphoblastic leukemia/lymphoma

(Figs 5.52, 5.53)

The lymphoma is frequently associated with a mediastinal mass and it comprises 90% of lymphoblastic lymphomas.

CRITERIA FOR DIAGNOSIS

1. a relatively uniform cell population with a high mitotic rate,
2. intermediate-sized nuclei, often prominent anisonucleosis,
3. variable number of convoluted (unipolar deeply indented) nuclei,
4. dense, finely granular chromatin; mostly inconspicuous nucleoli,
5. scanty, pale, fragile cytoplasm,
6. immunophenotype: TdT, most often CD3 (cytoplasmic) and CD7; often CD4 and CD8 double positive or double negative; variable positivity with CD1a, CD34, CD10,
7. genetics: 50–70% abnornal karyotype.

The convoluted, lobulated or segmented (cerebriform) shape is most striking in cytocentrifuge preparations of cell suspensions (Fig. 5.53A). It seems to be related to the mode of preparation to some extent and appears to be exaggerated by centrifugation. Lymphoblasts with convoluted nuclei often have markers for T cells but a similar morphology can be seen with some B-cell lymphoblastic lymphomas. Also, a similar nuclear complexity can be seen in several B-cell lymphomas after treatment. The cytomorphology alone is thus insufficient to classify the lymphoma as T-cell type and needs to be supported by immune marker typing.

Mature T and NK-Cell neoplasms

These lymphomas are more difficult to diagnose on FNAC than B-cell lymphomas as they do not have a specific immunophenotype, apart from anaplastic large cell lymphoma, ALK positive. In addition, FCM does not clearly demonstrate monoclonality as seen with B-cell lymphomas. However, immunophenotyping is essential to recognize T-cell lineage and aberrant T-cell phenotype, which is strong presumptive evidence of a monoclonal T-cell population. The loss of one or more of the pan-T-cell markers (CD2, CD3, CD5, CD7) is the most useful criterion in helping to make the diagnosis of T-cell neoplasia. Also suggestive are loss of both CD4 and CD8 or coexpression of both.[12,163] PCR for rearrangement of the T-cell receptor gene is often necessary to demonstrate clonality. Frequently tissue biopsy is necessary for initial diagnosis.

The cytology of peripheral T-cell lymphomas (PTCL) not otherwise specified (NOS) and NK/T lymphomas has been

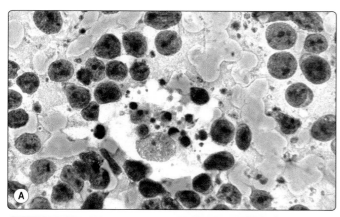

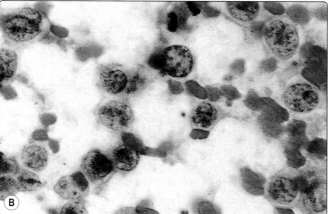

Fig. 5.51 B-lymphoblastic lymphoma Rounded nuclei of variable, mainly intermediate size; speckled nuclear chromatin; small but distinct nucleoli. Starry sky macrophages may be present (**A**, MGG, HP; **B**, Pap, HP).

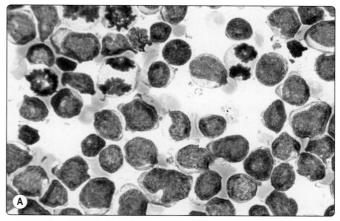

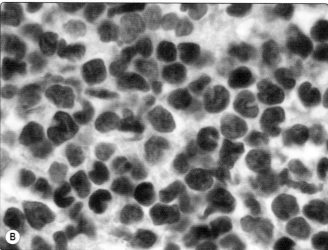

Fig. 5.52 T-lymphoblastic lymphoma Note unipolar indentation (convolution) in some cells. Anisokaryosis, dense chromatin without distinct nucleoli, many mitoses. TdT positivity. (**A**, MGG, HP; **B**, immunostain,TdT, HP).

reported.[164–168] PTCL NOS have a varied morphologic appearance, commonly heterogeneous, with atypical medium to large lymphocytes (some Reed Sternberg-like cells (see Fig. 5.71) and an exuberant benign host inflammatory reaction, producing difficulty in its separation from reactive lymphadenopathy. Occasionally, there is a monomorphous proliferation of small, medium or large atypical cells. The nuclei are often indented, grooved or knobbly.

Angioimmunoblastic T-cell lymphoma (Fig. 5.54 and see Fig. 5.70A)[69,169,170]

Typically seen with generalized lymphadenopathy, systemic symptoms and peripheral hypergammaglobulinaemia.

CRITERIA FOR DIAGNOSIS

1. heterogeneous cell population,
2. small to medium irregular lymphocytes,
3. variable number of large cells – including immunoblasts and at times pleomorphic cells (resembling Reed-Sternberg cells),
4. reactive background of small round lymphocytes, eosinophils, plasma cells, epithelioid and nonepithelioid histiocytes, dendritic cells,
5. immunophenotype: CD3, CD4, BCL6, CD10 , CXCL13, PD1,
6. PCR: T-cell gene rearrangement detectable in 75–90% of cases; clonal immunoglobulin gene rearrangement in 25–30% of cases,
7. genetics: trisomy 3 or 5 most common.

Anaplastic large cell lymphoma (ALCL), ALK positive (Fig. 5.55)[69,85,86,171–173]

Most frequent in childhood and young adults, presenting with lymphadenopathy.

CRITERIA FOR DIAGNOSIS

1. large cells with pleomorphic nuclei,
2. some Reed-Sternberg-like large cells,
3. irregular nuclei; horseshoe shaped (hallmark cells), donut, multinucleated with one or more prominent nucleoli,
4. cytoplasm abundant and may be vacuolated,
5. few lymphoglandular bodies,
6. cell clustering at times,
7. immunophenotype: CD30, ALK, EMA, one pan T-cell marker usually positive (null cell at times), perforin; variably positive for CD45 (CD15 and PAX5 negative),
8. genetics: t(2;5) in 84% of cases.

Several cytomorphologic variants exist, e.g. small cell, Hodgkin-like, sarcomatoid and lymphohistiocytic.[69] The ALK negative, anaplastic large cell lymphoma (ALCL) is seen in older adults and needs to be distinguished from HL (PAX 5 and cytotoxic markers being most helpful in making the distinction).

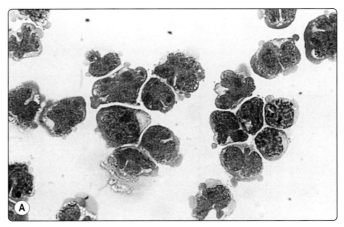

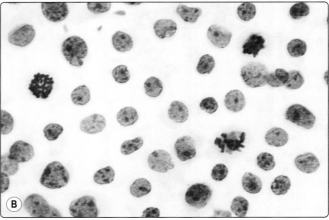

Fig. 5.53 T-lymphoblastic lymphoma (A) Cerebrospinal fluid. In cytocentrifuge preparations the convolutions are very pronounced (MGG, HP oil); (B) Lymph node smear. Note mitotic figures (Pap, HP).

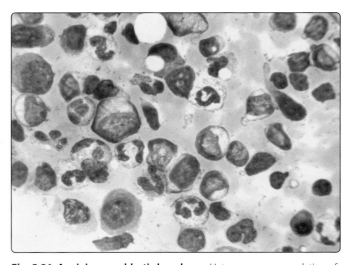

Fig. 5.54 Angioimmunoblastic lymphoma Heterogeneous population of cells with small, medium and large lymphocytes, neutrophils, eosinophils and plasmacytoid cells (Diff-Quik, HP).

PROBLEMS AND DIFFERENTIAL DIAGNOSIS (GENERAL)

1. suboptimal cytological preparations,
2. variable pattern in one node,
3. distinction from reactive lymphadenopathy,
4. NHL with few neoplastic cells in a dominant population of reactive lymphoid cells, e.g. T-cell/histiocyte rich B lymphoma,[155–157]
5. small cell anaplastic carcinoma and other small cell tumors, particularly versus low-grade follicular (centrocyte dominant), lymphoblastic and Burkitt lymphomas,
6. large cell malignancies, undifferentiated carcinoma, melanoma, seminoma, myeloid sarcoma versus large cell lymphoma, including anaplastic large cell lymphoma,[85,86,171–173]
7. limitations of ancillary techniques (PCR and FCM),
8. post-transplant lymphoproliferative disorders (PTLD),
9. gray zone (unclassifiable) lymphomas[69]

Direct smears must be made expertly, since poor preparation makes accurate diagnosis impossible. Suboptimal smears are the commonest cause of diagnostic difficulties and misinterpretations.

Sampling bias cannot always be avoided and may lead to an erroneous diagnosis. An aspirate from a node which is only partially involved with lymphoma may not be representative. Due to several mechanisms, the number of centroblasts and centrocytes does not always reflect the real composition within the lymph node. Thus, malignancy grading on cytological grounds is not reliable in follicular lymphomas.

The difference between normal lymphocytes and the neoplastic cells of small lymphocytic lymphoma is relatively subtle and the most obvious diagnostic feature is the monotony of the cell population. However, a sample including proliferation centers does not appear monotonous since there can be many cells of intermediate and large size (prolymphocytes and paraimmunoblasts[9,69] mixed with the typical cells of CLL type (see Figs 5.31 and 5.32). Such a case can be mistaken for reactive lymphadenopathy unless close attention is paid to fine cytological detail of the lymphocytes and to the result of immunocytology and FCM. Smears from small quiescent axillary and groin nodes may show a monotonous population of small lymphocytes. This can mimic small lymphocytic lymphoma, therefore this diagnosis should be avoided in small nodes unless there is immunologic proof of clonality.

Lymphoplasmacytic lymphoma (LPL) can also be mistaken for reactive lymphadenopathy in view of the sometimes heterogeneous character of the smear population. Again, a close study of cell detail usually reveals atypical lymphoid cells with plasmacytoid features. LPL is a diagnosis of exclusion, as other small cell lymphomas may have a mixture of relatively similar cells. At times, LPL cannot be separated from marginal zone lymphoma (MZL), as neither has a specific immunophenotype. MZL, with its mixed cell population, can mimic reactive hyperplasia. FCM, immunocytochemical, clinical and biochemical data are of utmost diagnostic importance.

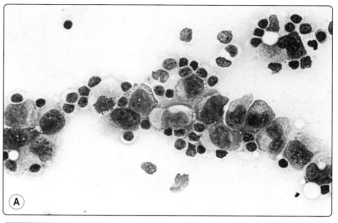

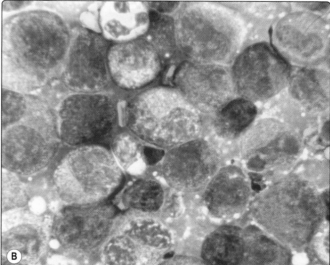

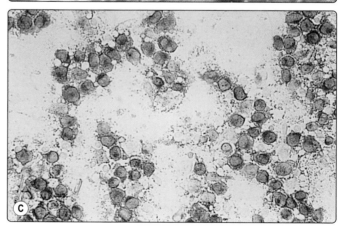

Fig. 5.55 Anaplastic large cell lymphoma (A), Large polymorphous cells with abundant cytoplasm; pseudoepithelial arrangement; multinucleation; distinct nucleoli. (B), Occasional 'hallmark' cells with horseshoe/boomerang nuclear forms. (C), CD30 (Ki-1) positive (A, MGG, IP; B, Diff-Quik, oil HP, C, immunostain CD30, IP).

In follicular lymphoma grade 1 there may be a high proportion of small lymphocytes to suggest a benign, reactive process. Also, the small centrocytes of some follicular lymphomas can be difficult to distinguish from lymphocytes in a reactive process, particularly if smears are not technically optimal. Nuclei must be studied carefully at high power to

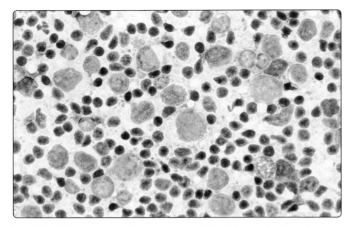

Fig. 5.56 Diffuse large cell lymphoma, NOS, with reactive lymphocytes
Scattered neoplastic cells with very large nuclei with a dominant background population of reactive lymphocytes (MGG, HP).

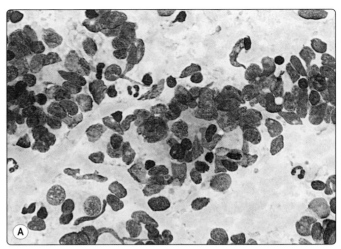

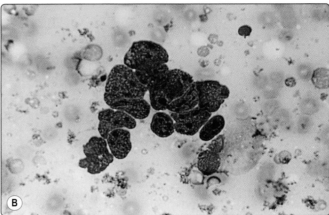

Fig. 5.57 Pseudoglandular clusters in lymphoma Such clusters may simulate small cell anaplastic carcinoma or adenocarcinoma; this problem mainly occurs in follicular lymphomas and large cell anaplastic lymphomas (A and B, MGG, HP).

appreciate the slightly larger size, irregular shape and granular chromatin. Follicular lymphoma grade 1 with a predominance of small centrocytes is the type of lymphoma which is most likely to be missed cytologically and misinterpreted as reactive lymphadenopathy. FCM demonstrating B-cell clonality with CD10 positivity is important in making this distinction.

At times, separating T-cell lymphomas with a polymorphous cell population from reactive hyperplasia can be difficult. In the evaluation, it is important to have the clinical history and presentation and to correlate it with the ancillary studies. Even then, a tissue biopsy is usually necessary to make a firm diagnosis.

In some cases of large cell lymphoma, the neoplastic cells may be relatively few in numbers, and the smears may be dominated by a background of reactive lymphocytes (Fig. 5.56). T-cell/histiocyte rich B-cell lymphoma is one important example (see Fig. 5.46).[155] Results of FCM may be difficult to interpret in such cases. Occasionally, distinction from reactive lymphadenopathy with scattered large, atypical-looking immunoblasts can be difficult.

In FNB smears from follicular lymphoma grade 1 and 2, the large centrocytic cells may have a tendency to clump together into aggregates showing some moulding of the nuclei. Rows and palisades of closely apposed, ovoid nuclei which appear columnar through moulding may simulate small cell anaplastic carcinoma or even adenocarcinoma (Fig. 5.57). However, the proportion of isolated cells is usually larger in lymphoma and many of these have the typical appearance of lymphoid cells with a rim of basophilic cytoplasm and a nuclear chromatin pattern which is different from that of carcinoma cells. Importantly, nuclei of lymphoma cells of a similar size to those of small cell anaplastic carcinoma usually have prominent nucleoli. This is a helpful but not infallible feature: nuclei of large centrocytes and of small cell carcinoma of intermediate type may be very similar in size and may have similar nucleoli. Nuclear molding and well-formed single files of tumor cells are more obvious in small cell carcinoma and other metastatic small cell tumors. The pale-blue, uniformly rounded cytoplasmic fragments characteristic of lymphoid tissue (lymphoid globules) are different from the cytoplasmic and nuclear fragments of tumor necrosis in smears of

carcinomas (compare Figs 5.1 and 5.2). Immunocytochemical staining for cytokeratin, EMA and CD45 can usually solve the problem of distinguishing between small cell carcinoma and lymphoma in difficult cases. Additionally, FCM can help as small cell carcinomas are CD 56 positive and CD 45 negative.

Burkitt and lymphoblastic lymphomas occur commonly in childhood and need to be differentiated from small round blue cell tumors of childhood via morphologic, immunologic and cytogenetic means (see Chapter 17).

Smears of undifferentiated carcinoma (Figs 5.58 and 5.59, and see Fig. 5.25) and melanoma (Fig. 5.60) may show total dissociation of the tumor cells, nuclei may be large, with fine chromatin, prominent nucleoli and abundant basophilic cytoplasm. This pattern can be indistinguishable from DLBCL (particularly immunoblastic rich type) or ALCL, and at times even HL. Also, a dissociated seminoma may similarly be difficult to distinguish from a lymphoma. Myeloid sarcomas may be mistaken for DLBCL. They have dissociated large cells with pale chromatin, prominent nucleoli and rarely cytoplasmic granules. The presence of lymphoid globules in lymphoma and lobulated nuclei is helpful. Well-formed, sharply delineated aggregates of tumor cells, not just clumping of cells, are not seen in lymphoma. Again, in difficult cases, immunological staining for cytokeratin, Melan-A, S-100, OCT4, myeloperoxidase and lymphoid associated markers is usually decisive (Table 5.3).[85,86,171–174]

FCM results may be unreliable or noninformative if the aspirated material is necrotic or heavily admixed with blood.

It must be remembered that B-cell clonality does not always equate with malignancy and its absence does not necessarily indicate a benign process. Polyclonality on flow cytometry may be seen in T-cell lymphoma, HL, partial involvement of a node by lymphoma, absence of immunoglobulin expression in some DLBCL NOS, occasionally marginal zone

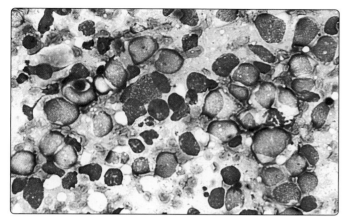

Fig. 5.58 Small cell anaplastic (neuroendocrine) carcinoma This example of a FNB smear from a lung tumor closely mimics anaplastic large cell lymphoma: dispersed cells with large eccentric nuclei and a thin rim of blue cytoplasm (MGG, HP).

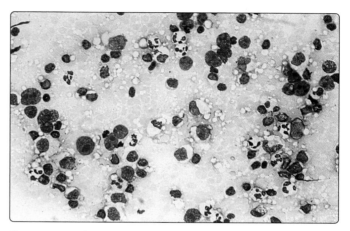

Fig. 5.59 Nasopharyngeal carcinoma Metastatic large cell undifferentiated carcinoma with solitary tumor cells may mimic large cell lymphoma (MGG, IP).

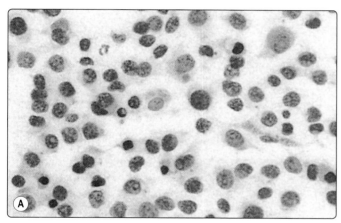

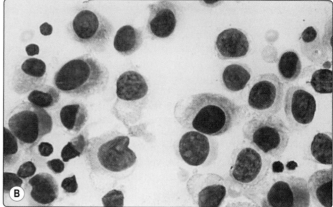

Fig. 5.60 Metastatic melanoma mimicking lymphoma (A) Dispersed malignant cells with eccentric nuclei and pale cytoplasm; lymphoid globules absent (Pap, HP). (B) Amelanotic melanoma showing dense smooth chromatin and characteristic paranuclear dark area in tumor cells (MGG, HP).

Table 5.3 Large cell malignancies

Tumor	Cytokeratin	Melan-A	S-100	CD45	CD15	CD30	ALK	CD20	OCT4	MPO
DLBCL	−	−	−	+	−	−/+	−	+	−	−
Carcinoma	+	−	−/(+)	−	−/(+)	−/(+)	−	−	−	−
Melanoma	−	+	+	−	−	−	−	−	−	−
Seminoma	−	−	−	−	−	−	−	−	+	−
CHL	−	−	−	−/(+)	+/(−)	+	−	−/(+)	−	−
ALCL	−	−	−	+/−	−	+	+/−	−	−	−
Myeloid sarcoma	−	−	−	+/−	+/−	−	−	−	−	+

ALCL, anaplastic large cell lymphoma; CHL, classical Hodgkin lymphoma; DLBCL, diffuse, large B-cell lymphoma, NOS; MPO, myelopeoxidase; + positive; − negative; (+) occasionally positive ; (−) occasionally negative.

lymphoma as well as in a reactive lymph node.[10] Close correlation of FNAC, immunologic and clinical findings is always essential. One must also be aware of aberrant immunophenotypes in B-cell NHL (see NHL overveiw) and also false-positive B-cell clones. An unusual, infrequent immunophenotype is the B-cell lymphoma coexpressing CD5 and CD10, such as follicular lymphoma, mantle cell lymphoma and DLBCL, NOS.[170] Rarely, with follicular hyperplasia in children and young adults there may be clonality.[175,176] The author has also seen similar false B-cell clonality in lymph nodes with metastatic melanoma and adenocarcinoma. Infrequently, in progressive transfomation of germinal centers, there may be coexpression of CD4 and CD8, causing confusion with a T-cell neoplasm.

PCR false-negative results may occur with follicular, marginal zone and DLBCL NOS.[177,178] In contrast, small lymphocytic lymphoma and mantle-cell lymphoma have a much lower rate of false-negative clonal detection.[179,180] False-positive results may occur with some benign conditions, for example autoimmune diseases and some infectious processes.[10]

PTLD are more often extranodal in presentation, and there is a spectrum ranging from plasma cell hyperplasia/infectious mononucleosis-like reaction to diffuse lymphoma (predominantly B cell), however T/NK-cell and Hodgkin lymphomas also occur. FNB may provide a rapid diagnosis of monomorphic PTLD as it usually resembles B-cell neoplasms: DLBCL, Burkitt lymphoma and plasma cell neoplasms.[69,181–183] In polymorphic PTLD there is a mixture of small and large lymphocytes with plasma cells, which may resemble a lymphoma with plasmacytic differentiation or infectious mononucleosis. In this category, the diagnosis requires flow cytometry, PCR and usually histologic assessment.[181]

There are two main groups in the gray-zone (unclassifiable) lymphomas. Firstly, cases from a morphological and phenotypical perspective resemble Burkitt lymphoma; however, some feature(s) prevent the diagnosis. Secondly, cases may morphologically resemble DLBCL; however, the phenotype is that of HL or vice versa. These cases cause difficulty in subtyping with histologic specimens, and equally cause problems with cytologic samples.

Hodgkin lymphoma (HL)
(Figs 5.61–5.68)[40,75–77,184,185]

Hodgkin lymphoma accounts for approximately 30% of all lymphomas.[69] It is comprised of two entities: nodular lymphocyte predominant HL and classic HL. The subtypes of classic HL are nodular sclerosis, mixed cellularity, lymphocyte-rich and lymphocyte depleted. These account for up to 95% of cases of HL.

Classic HL, in nearly all cases, is derived from B cells. In nodular lymphocyte predominant HL, the Reed-Sternberg ('popcorn') cells are B cells reacting with CD20, OCT-2, BOB.1 and CD79a, and the small background lymphocytes are predominantly B cells but there are also many T cells. In classic HL the background lymphocytes are usually predominantly T cells, except in the nodular lymphocyte-rich variant where they are usually predominantly B cells. The Reed-Sternberg cells in these classic variants are often but not always negative for B-cell markers CD20 and CD79a. When positive for these markers, only a minority of these cells

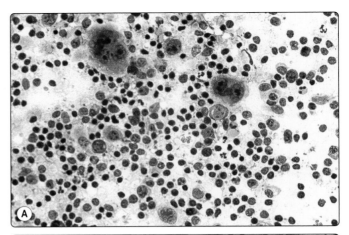
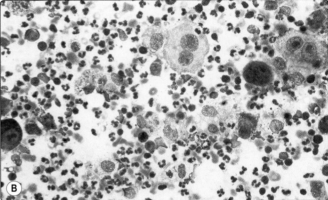

Fig. 5.61 Hodgkin lymphoma Binuclear Reed-Sternberg cells and mononuclear Hodgkin cells in a background of mainly small lymphocytes (**A**) and/or granulocytes (**B**). Varying basophilia (**A** and **B**, MGG, IP).

usually stains, and the staining intensity is varied. They are also weakly positive for PAX5.[69]

CRITERIA FOR DIAGNOSIS

1. atypical mononuclear cells ('Hodgkin cells'); nucleus is 3–4 × the size of a small lymphocyte,
2. Reed-Sternberg cells,
3. a variable number of eosinophils, plasma cells and histiocytes,
4. a background population of lymphocytes,
5. immunophenotype: classic Hodgkin lymphoma, Reed-Sternberg cells CD30, CD15, MUM1, weak PAX5; small lymphocytes usually predominantly CD3,
6. nodular lymphocyte predominant type, Reed-Sternberg cells CD20, CD79a, BCL6, OCT-2, BOB1, CD45, EMA; small lymphocytes usually predominantly CD20.[9,69]

A confident diagnosis of classic HL can only be made in the presence of typical Reed-Sternberg cells with a background of lymphocytes and reactive cells, as listed above, with its typical immunophenotype (Figs 5.61–5.65). Reed-Sternberg cells have large, lobulated nuclei which may appear symmetrically double (mirror nuclei) or complex and multiple. The nuclear chromatin is coarse and irregularly distributed in a reticular fashion with clear areas in between which give the nucleus an overall pale appearance. Nucleoli are large, often huge, eosinophilic in H&E preparations, pale

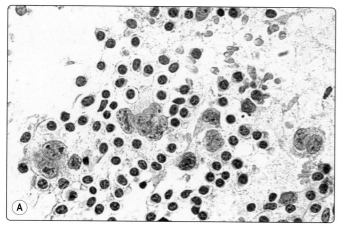

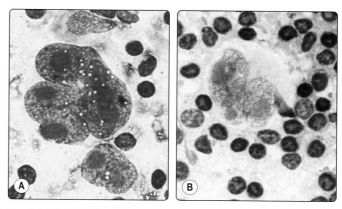

Fig. 5.64 Hodgkin lymphoma Examples of Reed-Sternberg cells from different cases; multiple or multilobated large nuclei with very large nucleoli; reticulate chromatin; pale cytoplasm (A and B, MGG, HP).

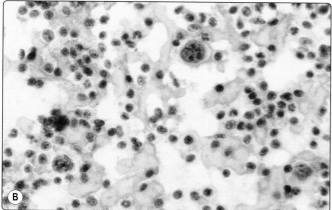

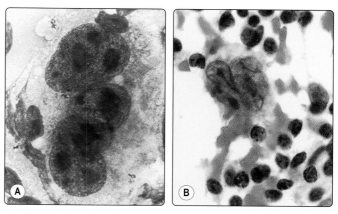

Fig. 5.62 Hodgkin lymphoma Many scattered binuclear or multilobated Reed-Sternberg cells with a background of lymphocytes (A and B Pap, HP).

Fig. 5.65 Hodgkin lymphoma Other examples of Reed-Sternberg giant cells (A, MGG; B, H&E, HP).

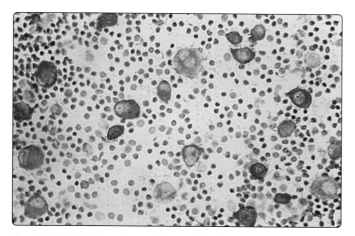

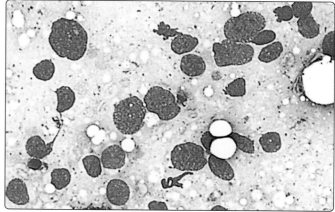

Fig. 5.63 Hodgkin lymphoma Characteristic CD30 positivity (immunostain CD30, IP).

Fig. 5.66 Hodgkin lymphoma Recurrent Hodgkin lymphoma; atypical mononuclear cell forms only (MGG, HP).

grayish to dark magenta in MGG-stained smears. The cytoplasm is abundant, but pale and fragile so that the nucleus often appears to be surrounded by an empty space (see Fig. 5.64). Sometimes the characteristic nucleoli are not well demonstrated. Frequently only mononuclear cells which have a nuclear structure similar to the typical Reed-Sternberg cells (mononuclear Hodgkin cells, Fig. 5.66) along with their bare nuclear forms are present. In such cases, the definitive diagnosis must await histological examination, except in

recurrent disease when classic Reed-Sternberg cells are not essential for diagnosis. The background cell population is mainly lymphocytes of reactive type, but polymorphs may be predominant in some cases (see Fig. 5.61B). The term 'suppurative variant of HL' has been proposed.[185]

Histological examination is also necessary to distinguish confidently the five subtypes of HL. The two extremes, lymphocyte predominant and lymphocyte depleted, are, of

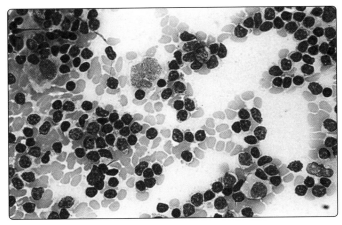

Fig. 5.67 Lymphocyte predominant Hodgkin lymphoma Multinucleated 'popcorn' cell in a background of small B lymphocytes and some histiocytes (MGG, IP).

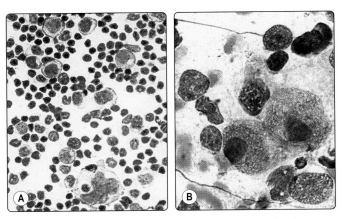

Fig. 5.69 Reed-Sternberg-like cells in infectious mononucleosis (A) Multilobated giant cell (MGG, IP); (B) Binucleate cell with very large nucleoli (MGG, HP), from two different cases of infectious mononucleosis.

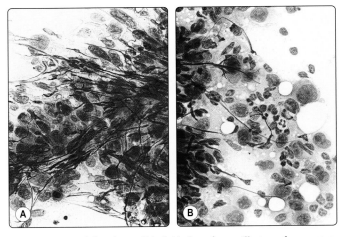

Fig. 5.68 Syncytial variant of Hodgkin lymphoma Clusters of numerous large atypical lymphoid cells dominate smears focally; some are of Reed-Sternberg type (**A** and **B**, MGG, HP).

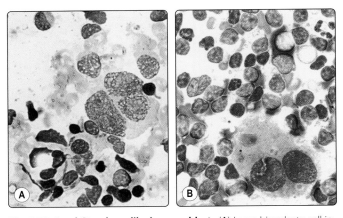

Fig. 5.70 Reed-Sternberg-like immunoblasts (A) Large binucleate cell in case of angioimmunoblastic T-cell lymphoma; (B) Binucleate cell in toxoplasma lymphadenitis (MGG, HP).

course, reflected in the smears by the number of lymphocytes relative to the number of Reed-Sternberg and mononuclear Hodgkin cells. A suggestion of the presence of the lacunar type of Reed-Sternberg cell, characteristic of nodular sclerosis Hodgkin lymphoma in histological sections, is occasionally present in FNB smears. The tough consistency of the node felt with the needle, a scanty aspirate and the presence of fibroblasts and collagen fragments in the smear are features suggestive of the nodular sclerosis type. In the mixed cellularity type, typical Reed-Sternberg cells are usually easy to find and there are many plasma cells and eosinophils as well as histiocytes in the background cell population.[186]

The nodular lymphocyte-predominant subtype is characterized by a monotonous population of slightly irregular small lymphocytes with relatively few scattered large pale multinucleated giant cells, corresponding to the 'popcorn' cells in histology, usually without distinct nucleoli (Fig. 5.67). In contrast to the other (classic) variants of HL, the bulk of the small cells and also the giant cells exhibit a B-cell phenotype.[9,69] This is a difficult diagnosis to make on FNB smears as there are usually few atypical cells in a sea of reactive small lymphoid cells and the architecture cannot be assessed.

PROBLEMS AND DIFFERENTIAL DIAGNOSIS

1. poor biopsy yield,
2. Reed-Sternberg look-alike cells in other conditions,
3. syncytial variant nodular sclerosis HL,
4. epithelioid histiocytes suggestive of granulomatous lymphadenitis,
5. small lymphocyte-rich smears, e.g. T-cell/histiocyte rich B-cell lymphoma,
6. gray-zone (unclassifiable) lymphomas.[69]
7. flow cytometry limitations

Poor biopsy yield is a problem mainly in the nodular sclerosis subtype. Not infrequently, smears show only a few lymphocytes, fibroblasts and fragments of collagen, which may suggest a chronic inflammatory process. Multiple biopsies or the use of a cutting core needle may be necessary to obtain sufficient material.

Large, multilobated nuclei resembling Reed-Sternberg cells can be seen in a variety of conditions (Figs 5.69–5.74). Atypical immunoblasts in non-neoplastic reactive lymphadenopathy, for example in mononucleosis (Fig. 5.69), toxoplasmosis (Fig. 5.70B), rheumatoid arthritis-associated and drug-induced lymphadenopathy, may have

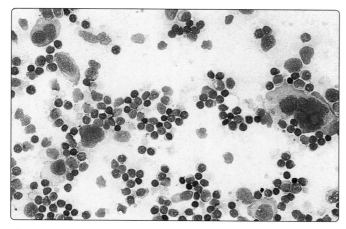

Fig. 5.71 Reed-Sternberg-like cells in peripheral T-cell lymphoma Pleomorphic T-cell lymphoma with Reed-Sternberg-like cells (MGG, IP). (Reproduced with permission from van Heerde et al.[9])

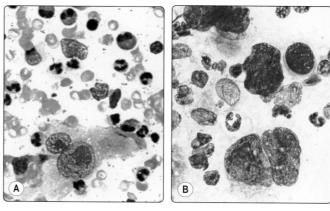

Fig. 5.73 Reed-Sternberg-like cells in metastatic carcinoma (A) Large binucleate cells with large nucleoli in metastatic nasopharyngeal carcinoma; note eosinophils in the background; (B) Large binucleate cell in lymph node metastasis from squamous cell carcinoma of floor of mouth (MGG, HP).

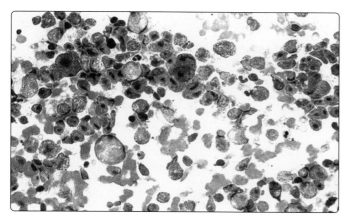

Fig. 5.72 Anaplastic large cell lymphoma Large cell anaplastic lymphoma, CD30 positive; differential diagnosis of Hodgkin lymphoma is a common problem in ALK negative cases (MGG, LP).

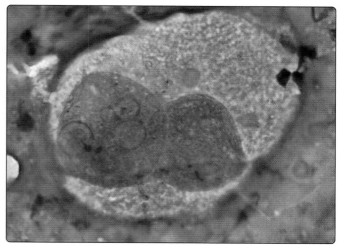

Fig. 5.74 Reed Sternberg-like cell in dendritic follicular cell sarcoma Large binucleate cell with large nucleoli (Diff-Quik, HP oil).

nuclei of this type. They usually differ from the typical Reed-Sternberg cells by having smaller and darker nucleoli, a denser chromatin and a basophilic cytoplasm. Multinucleated giant cells in small or large cell non-Hodgkin lymphoma, e.g. lymphoplasmacytic lymphoma, PTCL NOS (Fig. 5.71) and especially ALCL (Fig. 5.72), can also have large nucleoli similar to Reed-Sternberg cells.[9,187] The distinction is particularly difficult in the presence of eosinophils, plasma cells and epithelioid cells, which is not unusual in T-cell lymphoma. Immunological studies may be necessary to solve the problem. There are some examples of large malignant cells with very large nucleoli and with many eosinophils and reactive lymphoid cells in the background, representing single malignant cells of metastatic – especially nasopharyngeal – carcinoma (Fig. 5.73), which were misdiagnosed as HL. In addition, megakaryocytes can be mistaken for Reed-Sternberg cells, e.g. in nodal myeloid metaplasia/extramedullary hematopoiesis. Also rarely with follicular dendritic cell sarcoma, Reed-Sternberg-like cells may also be seen in an inflammatory background (Fig. 5.74).

The syncytial variant of HL, an uncommon form of nodular sclerosis HL, can be difficult to distinguish from NHL, carcinoma, melanoma, germ cell tumor and at times even sarcoma on FNB smears. Smears show cohesive sheets and clusters of large malignant cells with vesicular nuclei, prominent nucleoli and pale cytoplasm, and sometimes necrotic debris (see Fig. 5.68). Giant cells and multinucleated cells of Reed-Sternberg type can be recognized and may be numerous.[188] An immunologic panel can help in the diagnosis (see Table 5.3).

Clusters of epithelioid histiocytes are sometimes seen in smears of HL – as in some NHL – which could suggest granulomatous lymphadenitis (Fig. 5.75). The lymphoid cells must therefore always be carefully scrutinized in lymph node smears containing epithelioid cells.

Lymphocyte-rich smears may hide scanty numbers of large lymphoid neoplastic cells, resembling reactive lymphoid hyperplasia. Lymphocyte-rich classic HL may have a prominent small lymphocytic population with a few scattered Reed-Sternberg cells and variants. This may be difficult to distinguish from lymphocyte-predominant HL or T-cell/histiocyte rich B-cell lymphoma (see Fig. 5.46). Both of these may also have a paucity of large neoplastic cells in a rich reactive background. FNB is limited in making a distinction between nodular lymphocyte-predominant HL and T-cell/histiocyte rich B-cell lymphoma as the vital architecture

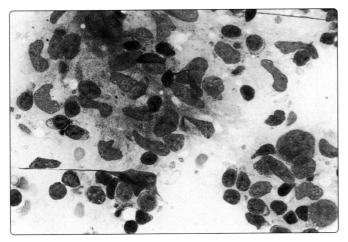

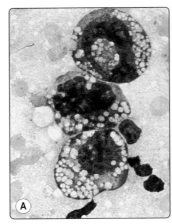
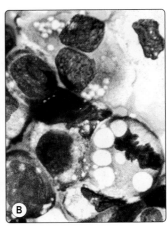

Fig. 5.75 Hodgkin lymphoma Clusters of epithelioid histiocytes resembling granulomatous lymphadenitis; note large abnormal cells lower right (MGG, HP).

Fig. 5.76 True histiocytic lymphoma Very polymorphous large cells, abundant basophilic cytoplasm, small vacuoles, ring-shaped nucleus in upper left corner, phagocytosis of erythrocytes in lower right corner; diagnosis confirmed by immunocytochemistry and EM (**A** and **B**, MGG, HP oil).

cannot be assessed. To make the distinction between these entities, immunologic studies need to be carried out on a formal node biopsy.

Falling into the gray-zone lymphoma group are cases morphologically resembling classic HL; however, their immunophenotype is that of DLBCL, NOS. A composite lymphoma needs to be excluded in biopsy specimens before making this classification.

FCM is of minimal value in the diagnosis of HL. An excess of CD4-positive T cells can be seen and a CD4/CD8 ratio greater than 4 should make one consider the diagnosis, even though it is not diagnostic. In nodular lymphocyte-predominant HL, not infrequently it may have a considerable proportion of CD4+CD8+(double-positive) T cells, a pointer to its diagnosis.[69]

Histiocytic and dendritic cell neoplasms

Histiocytic and dendritic cell neoplasms are rare and represent less than 1% of nodal tumors.[69] They comprise: Langerhans cell histiocytosis (see page 84) and sarcoma, histiocytic sarcoma,[9,105] follicular/interdigitating dendritic sarcoma,[112–114] and dendritic cell sarcoma, NOS. There are a few case reports of most of these in the cytologic literature.

Histiocytic sarcoma (Fig. 5.76)[9,105]

Formerly known as true histiocytic lymphoma, it is difficult to recognize this rare type of neoplasm correctly in routine cytological smears. A very pleomorphic cell population with multilobed nuclei and multinucleated cells which may resemble Reed-Sternberg cells should make one think of this possibility. The main differential diagnosis includes large cell non-Hodgkin lymphomas (especially ALCL), HL, pleomorphic carcinoma and melanoma (see Table 5.3). At times, it is morphologically indistinguishable from DLBCL, NOS.

1. immunophenotype: monocyte/macrophage markers like CD68, CD163, CD14 and lysozyme; absence of T- and B-cell characteristics; myeloperoxidase, CD33 and CD34 negativity,
2. PCR: lacks IgH or TCR rearrangement,
3. genetics: non-specific.

Acknowledgement

I would like to thank Anna Miliauskas for technological support.

References

1. Australian Cancer Network Diagnosis and Management of Lymphoma Guidelines Working Party. Guidelines for the Diagnosis and Management of Lymphoma. Sydney: The Cancer Council Australia and Australian Cancer Network; 2005. p. 136.
2. Ferrer R. Lymphadenopathy: differential diagnosis and evaluation. Am Fam Physician 1998;58:1313–20.
3. Dragoni F, Cartoni C, Pescarmona E, et al. The role of high resolution pulsed and colour Doppler ultrasound in the differential diagnosis of benign and malignant lymphadenopathy: results of multivariate analysis. Cancer 1999;85:2485–90.
4. Gupta AK, Nayar M, Chandra M. Reliability and limitations of fine needle aspiration cytology of lymphadenopathies: an analysis of 1,261 cases. Acta Cytol 1991;35:777–83.
5. Perkins SL, Segal GH, Kjoldsberg CR. Work-up of lymphadenopathy in children. Sem Diagn Pathology 1995;12:284.
6. Leong A SY, Stevens M. Fine-needle aspiration biopsy for the diagnosis of lymphoma: a perspective. Diagn Cytopathol 1996;15:352–7.
7. Daskalopoulou D, Harhalakis N, Maouni N, et al. Institution fine needle aspiration cytology of non-Hodgkin lymphomas: a morphologic and immunophenotypic study. Acta Cytol 1994;39:180–6.

8. Geisinger KR, Rainer RO, Field AS. Lymph nodes. In: Geisinger KR, Silverman JF, editors. Fine needle aspiration cytology of superficial organs and body sites. New York: Churchill-Livingstone; 1999. p. 1–49.

9. van Heerde P, Meyer CJLM, Noorduyn LA, et al. An atlas and textbook of malignant lymphomas. Cytology, histopathology and immunochemistry. USA: Oxford University Press; 1996.

10. Jorgensen JL. State of the Art Symposium: flow cytometry in the diagnosis of lymphoproliferative disorders by fine-needle aspiration. Cancer (Cancer Cytopathol) 2005;105:443–51.

11. Caraway NP. State of the Art Symposuim: strategies to diagnose lymphoproliferative disorders by fine-needle aspiration using ancillary studies. Cancer (Cancer Cytopathol) 2005;105:432–42.

12. Knowles DM. Neoplastic hematopathology. Philadelphia: Lippincott, Williams and Wilkins; 2001.

13. Aratake Y, Tamura K, Kotani T, et al. Application of the avidin-biotin complex method for the light microscopic analysis of lymphocyte subsets with monoclonal antibodies on air-dried smears. Acta Cytol 1988;32:117–22.

14. Levitt S, Cheng L, DuPuis MH, et al. Fine needle aspiration diagnosis of malignant lymphoma with confirmation by immunoperoxidase staining. Acta Cytol 1985;29:895–902.

15. Robey SS, Cafferty LL, Beschozner WE, et al. Value of lymphocyte marker studies in diagnostic cytopathology. Acta Cytol 1987;31:453–9.

16. Sneige N, Dekmezian RH, Katz RL, et al. Morphologic and immunocytochemical evaluation of 220 fine needle aspirates of malignant lymphoma and lymphoid hyperplasia. Acta Cytol 1990;34:311–22.

17. Tani EM, Christensson B, Porwit A, et al. Immunocytochemical analysis and cytomorphologic diagnosis on fine needle aspirates of lymphoproliferative disease. Acta Cytol 1988;32:209–15.

18. Robins DB, Katz RL, Swan F, et al. Immunotyping of lymphoma by fine-needle aspiration. A comparative study of cytospin preparations and flow-cytometry. Am J Clin Pathol 1994;101:569–76.

19. Meda BA, Buss DH, Woodruff RD, et al. Diagnosis and subclassification of primary and recurrent lymphoma. The usefulness and limitations of combined fine-needle aspiration cytomorphology and flow cytometry. Am J Clin Pathol 2000; 113:688–99.

20. Liu K, Stern RC, Rogers RT, et al. Diagnosis of hematopoetic processes by fine-needle aspiration in conjunction with flow cytometry: a review of 127 cases. Diagn Cytopathol 2001;24:1–10.

21. Young NA, Al-Saleem TI, Ehya H, et al. Utilization of fine-needle aspiration cytology and flow cytometry in the diagnosis and subclassification of primary and recurrent lymphoma. Cancer (Cancer Cytopathol) 1998;84:252–61.

22. Wakeley PE. Fine-needle aspiration cytopathology in diagnosis and classification of malignant lymphoma: accurate and reliable? Diagn Cytopathol 2000;22:120–5.

23. Prasad RRA, Narasimkan R, Sankarou V, et al. Fine-needle aspiration cytology in the diagnosis of superficial lymphadenopathy: and analysis of 2,418 cases. Diagn Cytopathol 1996;15:382–6.

24. Das DK. Value and limitations of fine-needle aspiration cytology in diagnosis and classification of lymphomas: a review. Diagn Cytopathol 1999;21:240–9.

25. Dong HY, Harris NL, Preffer FJ, et al. Fine needle aspiration in the diagnosis and classification of primary and recurrent lymphoma: a retrospective analysis of the utility of cytomorphology and flow cytometry. Mod Pathol 2001;14:472–81.

26. Zeppa P, Matrino G, Troncone G, et al. Fine-needle cytology and flow cytometry immunophenotyping and subclassification of non-Hodgkin lymphoma: a critical review of 307 cases with technical suggestions. Cancer 2004;102:55–65.

27. Sigstad E, Dong HP, Davidson B, et al. The role of flow cytometric immunophenotyping in improving the diagnostic accuracy in referred fine-needle aspiration specimens. Diagn Cytopathol 2004;31:159–613.

28. Nicol TL, Silberman M, Berner A, et al. The accuracy of combined cytopathologic and flow cytometric analysis of fine-needle aspirates of lymph nodes. Am Clin Pathol 2000;114:18–28.

29. Ravinsky E, Morales C, Kutryk E, et al. Cytodiagnosis of lymphoid proliferations by fine needle aspiration biopsy. Adjunctive value of flow cytometry. Acta Cytol 1999;43:1070–8.

30. Mourad WA, Tulbah A, Shoukri M, et al. Primary diagnosis and REAL/WHO classification of non-Hodgkin lymphoma by fine-needle aspiration: cytomorphologic and immunophenotypic approach. Diagn Cytopathol 2003;28:191–5.

31. Safley AM, Buckley PJ, Creager AJ, et al: The value of fluorescence in situ hybridization and polymerase chain reaction in the diagnosis of B-cell non-Hodgkin lymphoma by fine-needle aspiration. Arch Pathol Lab Med 2004;128:1395–403.

32. Bangerter M, Brudler O, Heinrich B, et al. Fine needle aspiration cytology and flow cytometry in the diagnosis and subclassification of non-Hodgkin lymphoma. Acta Cytol 2007;51:390–8.

33. Gascoyne RD. Establishing the diagnosis of lymphoma: from initial biopsy to clinical staging. Oncology 1998;12:11–16.

34. DeKerviler E, Guermazi A, Zagdanski AM, et al. Image-guided core-needle biopsy in patients with suspected or recurrent lymphoma. Cancer 2000;89:647–52.

35. Screaton NJ, Berman LH, Grant JW. Head and neck lymphadenopathy: evaluation with US-guided cutting needle biopsy. Radiology 2002;224: 75–81.

36. Surbone A, Longo DL, DeVita Jr VT, et al. Residual abdominal masses in aggressive non-Hodgkin lymphoma after combination chemotherapy: significance and management. J Clin Oncol 1988;6:1832–7.

37. Zajdela A, Ennuyer A, Bataini P, et al. Valeur du diagnostic cytologique des adenopathies par ponction aspiration. Confrontation cyto-histologique de 1756 cas. Bull Cancer (Paris) 1976;63:327–40.

38. Silverman SG, Lee BY, Mueller PR, et al. Impact of positive findings at image-guided biopsy of lymphoma on patient care: evaluation of clinical history, needle size, and pathologic findings on biopsy performance. Radiology 1994;190: 759–64.

39. Zornoza J, Cabanillas FF, Althoff TM, et al. Percutaneous needle biopsy in abdominal lymphoma. AJR 1981;136:97–103.

40. Friedman M, Kim U, Shimaoka K, et al. Appraisal of aspiration cytology in management of Hodgkin's disease. Cancer 1980;45:1653–63.

41. Lopes Cardozo P. The cytologic diagnosis of lymph node punctures. Acta Cytol 1964;8:194–205.

42. Betsill WL, Hajdu SI. Percutaneous aspiration biopsy of lymph nodes. Am J Clin Pathol 1980;73:471–9.

43. Cardillo MR. Fine needle aspiration cytology of superficial lymph nodes. Diagn Cytopathol 1989;5:166–73.

44. Engzell U, Jakobsson PA, Sigurdson A, et al. Aspiration biopsy of metastatic carcinoma in lymph nodes of the neck: a review of 1101 consecutive cases. Acta Otolaryngol 1971;72:138–47.

45. Kline TS, Kannan V, Kline IK. Lymphadenopathy and aspiration biopsy cytology. Review of 376 superficial nodes. Cancer 1984;54:1076–81.

46. Kline TS, Neal HS. Needle aspiration biopsy: a critical appraisal. Eight years and 3,267 specimens later. JAMA 1978;239:36–9.

47. Lee RE, Valaitis J, Kalis O, et al. Lymph node examination by fine needle aspiration in patients with known or suspected malignancy. Acta Cytol 1987;31:563–72.

48. Pilotti S, Di Palma S, Alasio L, et al. Diagnostic assessment of enlarged superficial lymph nodes by fine needle aspirate. Acta Cytol 1993;37:853–64.

49. Hsu C, Leung BS, Lau SK, et al. Efficacy of fine needle aspiration and sampling of lymph nodes in 1484 Chinese patients. Diagn Cytopathol 1990;6:154–9.

50. Shaha A, Webber C, Marti J. Fine needle aspiration in the diagnosis of cervical lymphadenopathy. Am J Surg 1986;152:420–3.

51. Steel B, Schwartz MR, Ramzy I. Fine needle aspiration biopsy in the diagnosis of lymphadenopathy in 1,103 patients. Acta Cytol 1995;39:76–81.

52. Gupta RK, Naran S, Lallu S, et al. Diagnostic value of needle aspiration cytology in the assessment of palpable inguinal lymph nodes. A study of 210 cases. Diagn Cytopathol 2003;28:175–80.

53. Jaffer S, Zakowski M. Fine-needle aspiration biopsy of axillary lymph nodes. Diagn Cytopathol 2002;26:69–74.

54. Cartagena N, Katz RL, Hirsch-Ginsberg C, et al. Accuracy of diagnosis of malignant lymphoma by combining fine needle aspiration cytomorphology with immunocytochemistry and in selected cases, southern blotting of aspirated cells: a tissue-controlled study of 86 patients. Diagn Cytopathol 1992;8:456–64.

55. van Heerde P, Go DMDS, Koolman-Schellekens MA, et al. Cytodiagnosis of non-Hodgkin lymphoma. A morphological analysis of 215 biopsy proven cases. Virchows Arch (Pathol Anat) 1984;403:213–33.

56. Cafferty LL, Katz RL, Ordonez NG, et al. Fine needle aspiration diagnosis of intraabdominal and retroperitoneal lymphomas by a morphologic and immunocytochemical approach. Cancer 1990;65:72–7.

57. Frable W. Fine needle aspiration biopsy. Philadelphia: Saunders; 1983.

58. Orell SR, Skinner JM. The typing of non-Hodgkin lymphoma using fine needle aspiration cytology. Pathology 1982;14:389–94.

59. Pitts WC, Weiss LM. Fine needle aspiration biopsy of lymph nodes. Pathol Annu 1988;23(pt 2):329–60.

60. Spieler P, Schmid U. How exact are the diagnosis and classification of malignant lymphomas from aspiration biopsy smears? Path Res Pract 1978;163:232–50.

61. Carter TR, Feldman PS, Innes Jr DJ, et al. The role of fine needle aspiration cytology in the diagnosis of lymphoma. Acta Cytol 1988;32:848–53.

62. Erwin BC, Brynes BK, Chan WC, et al. Percutaneous needle biopsy in the diagnosis and classification of lymphoma. Cancer 1986;57:1074–8.

63. Lopes Cardozo P. The significance of fine needle aspiration cytology for the diagnosis and treatment of malignant lymphomas. Folia Haematol (Leipzig) 1980;107:601–20.

64. Sandhaus LM. Fine-needle aspiration cytology in the diagnosis of lymphoma. The next step (edit). Am J Clin Pathol 2000;113:623–7.

65. Chhieng DC, Cohen JM, Cangiarella JF. Cytology and immunophenotyping of low and intermediate grade B-cell non-Hodgkin lymphomas with a prominent small cell component. Diagn Cytopathol 2001;24:90–7.

66. Russell J, Orell S, Skinner J, et al. Fine needle aspiration cytology in the management of lymphoma. Aust NZ J Med 1983;13:365–8.

67. Egea AS, González MAM, Barrios AP, et al. Usefulness of light microscopy in lymph node fine needle aspiration biopsy. Acta Cytol 2002;46:364–8.

68. Thomas JO, Adeyi D, Amanguno H. Fine-needle aspiration in the management of peripheral lymphadenopathy in a developing country. Diagn Cytopathol 1999;21:159–62.

69. Swerdlow SH, Campo E, Harris NL, et al. editors. WHO classification of tumours of haematopoietic and lymphoid tissues. Lyon: IARC; 2008.

70. Hu E, Horning S, Flynn S, et al. Diagnosis of B cell lymphoma by analysis of immunoglobulin gene rearrangements in biopsy specimens obtained by fine needle aspiration. J Clin Oncol 1986;4:278–83.

71. Jeffers MD, McCorriston J, Farquharson MA, et al. Analysis of clonality in cytologic material using the polymerase chain reaction (PCR). Cytopathology 1997;8:114–21.

72. Lubinski J, Chosia M, Kotanska K, et al. Genotypic analysis of DNA isolated from fine needle aspiration biopsies. Anal Quant Cytol Histol 1988;10:383–90.

73. Rovinsky E, Morales C. Diagnosis of lymphoma by image-guided needle biopsies: fine needle aspiration biopsy, core biopsy or both? Acta Cytol 2005;49:51–7.

74. Gong JZ, Synder MJ, Lagoo AS, et al. Diagnostic impact of core needle biopsy on fine needle aspiration of non-Hodgkin lymphoma. Diagn Cytopathol 2004;31:23–30.

75. Fulciniti F, Vetrani A, Zeppa P, et al. Hodgkin's disease: diagnostic accuracy of fine needle aspiration; a report based on 62 consecutive cases. Cytopathol 1994;5:226–33.

76. Jiménez-Hefferman JA, Vicandi B, López-Ferrer P, et al. Value of fine needle aspiration cytology in the initial diagnosis of Hodgkin disease. Analysis of 188 cases with an emphasis on diagnostic pitfalls. Acta Cytol 2001;45:300–6.

77. Chhieng DC, Cangiarella JF, Symmans WF, et al. Fine-needle aspiration cytology of Hodgkin disease. A study of 89 cases with emphasis on false-negative cases. Cancer (Cancer Cytopathol) 2001;93:52–9.

78. Behm FG, O'Dowd CJ, Frable WJ. Fine needle aspiration effects on benign lymph node histology. Am J Clin Pathol 1984;82:195–8.

79. Davies JD, Webb AJ. Segmental lymph-node infarction after fine needle aspiration. J Clin Pathol 1982;35:855–7.

80. Suthipintawong C, Leong AS-Y, Vinyuvat S. Immunostaining of cell preparations. A comparative evaluation of common fixatives and protocols. Diagn Cytopathol 1997;17:127–33.

81. Michael CW, Hunter B. Interpretation of fine-needle aspirates processed by ThinPrep techniques: cytologic artifacts and diagnostic pitfalls. Diagn Cytopathol 2000;23:6–13.

82. Söderström N. Fine needle aspiration biopsy. Stockholm: Almqvist and Wiksell; 1966.

83. Zajicek J. Aspiration biopsy cytology. Part I. Cytology of supradiaphragmatic organs. Basel: Karger; 1974.

84. Noorduyn LA, van Heerde P, Meyer CJLM. Cytology of Ki-1 (CD-30) positive large cell lymphoma. Cytopathol 1990;1:297–304.

85. Ng W-K, Ip P, Choy C, et al. Cytologic and immunocytochemical findings of anaplastic large cell lymphoma. Analysis of ten fine-needle aspiration specimens over 9-year period. Cancer (Cancer Cytopathol) 2003;99:33–43.

86. Zakowski MF, Feiner H, Finfer M, et al. Cytology of extranodal Ki-1 anaplastic large cell lymphoma. Diagn Cytopathol 1996;14:155–61.

87. Stani J. Cytologic diagnosis of reactive lymphadenopathy in fine needle aspiration biopsy specimens. Acta Cytol 1987;31:8–13.

88. O'Dowd GJ, Frable WJ, Behm FG. Fine needle aspiration cytology of benign lymph node hyperplasias. Diagnostic significance of lymphohistiocytic aggregates. Acta Cytol 1985;29:554–8.

89. Kardos TF, Kornstein MJ, Frable WJ. Cytology and immunocytology of infectious mononucleosis in fine needle aspirates of lymph nodes. Acta Cytol 1988;32:722–6.

90. Stanley MW, Steeper TA, Horwitz CA, et al. Fine-needle aspiration of lymph nodes in patients with acute infectious

mononucleosis. Diagn Cytopathol 1990;6:323–9.

91. Iacobuzio-Donahue CA, Clark DP, Ali SZ. Reed-Sternberg-like cells in lymph node aspirates in the absence of Hodgkin's disease: pathologic significance and differential diagnosis. Diagn Cytopathol 2002;27:335–9.

92. Kumar B, Karki, S, Paudgal P. Diagnosis of sinus histiocytosis with massive lymphadenopathy (Rosai-Dorfman disease) by fine needle aspiration cytology. Diagn Cytopathol 2008;36:691–5.

93. Alegret RA, Tello AM, Ramirez T, et al. Sinus histiocytosis with massive lymphadenopathy (Rosai-Dorfman disease): diagnosis with fine-needle aspiration in a case with nodal and nasal involvement. Diagn Cytopathol 1995;13:333–5.

94. Stastny JF, Wilkerson ML, Hamati HF, et al. Cytologic features of sinus histiocytosis with massive lymphadenopathy. A report of three cases. Acta Cytol 1997;41:871–6.

95. Santos-Briz A, López-Ríos F, Santos-Briz A, et al. Granulomatous reaction to silicone in axillary lymph nodes. A case report with cytologic findings. Acta Cytol 1999;43:1163–5.

96. Munichor M, Cohen H, Volpin G, et al. Chromium-induced lymph node histiocytic proliferation after hip replacement. Acta Cytol 2003;47:270–4.

97. Argyle JC, Schumann GB, Kjeldsberg CR, et al. Identification of a toxoplasma cyst by fine needle aspiration. Am J Clin Pathol 1983;80:256–8.

98. Christ ML, Feltes-Kennedy M. Fine needle aspiration cytology of toxoplasmic lymphadenitis. Acta Cytol 1982;26:425–8.

99. Jayaram N, Ramaprasad AV, Chethan M, et al. Toxoplasma lymphadenitis. Analysis of cytologic and histopathologic criteria and correlation with serologic tests. Acta Cytol 1997;41:653–8.

100. Zaharopoulos P. Demonstration of parasites in toxoplasma lymphadenitis by fine-needle aspiration cytology. Report of two cases. Diagn Cytopathol 2000;22:11–15.

101. van Heerde P, Egeler RM. The cytology of Langerhans cell histiocytosis (histiocytosis X). Cytopathol 1991;2:149–58.

102. Layfield LJ, Bhuta S. Fine needle aspiration cytology of histiocytosis X: a case report. Diagn Cytopathol 1988;4:140–3.

103. Kakkar S, Kapila K, Verma K. Langerhans cell histiocytosis in lymph nodes. Cytomorphologic diagnosis and pitfalls. Acta Cytol 2001;45:327–32.

104. Kumar PV, Mousavi A, Karimi M, et al. Fine needle aspiration of Langerhans cell histiocytosis of the lymph nodes. A

105. Miliauskas JR. Fine needle aspiration cytology of true histiocytic lymphoma/histiocytic sarcoma. Diagn Cytopathol 2003;29:233–5.

106. Desol G, Pradere M, Voigt JJ, et al. Warthin-Finkeldey-like cells in benign and malignant lymphoid proliferations. Histopathology 1982;6:451–65.

107. Hidvegi DF, Sorensen K, Lawrence JB, et al. Castleman's disease. Cytomorphologic and cytochemical features of a case. Acta Cytol 1982;26:243–6.

108. Meyer L, Gibbons D, Ashfaq R, et al. Fine-needle aspiration findings in Castleman's disease. Diagn Cytopathol 1999;21:57–60.

109. Deschenes M, Michel R, Tabah R, et al. Fine needle aspiration cytology of Castelman disease: Case report with review of the literature. Diagn Cytopathol 2008;36:904–8.

110. Jayaram G, Peh KB. Fine-needle aspiration cytology in Kimura's disease. Diagn Cytopathol 1995;13:295–9.

111. Deshpande AH, Nayak S, Munshi MM, et al. Kimura's disease. Diagnosis by aspiration cytology. Acta Cytol 2002;46:357–63.

112. Herceg RJ, Nayar R, De Frias DVS. Cytomorphologic appearance of follicular dendritic-cell tumor: a case report. Diagn Cytopathol 1999;20:237–40.

113. Loo CKC, Henderson C, Rogan K. Intraabdominal follicular dendritic cell sarcoma. Report of a case with fine needle aspiration findings. Acta Cytol 2001;45:999–1004.

114. Jayaram G, Mun KS, Elsayed EM, et al. Interdigitating dendritic reticulum cell sarcoma: cytologic, histologic and immunocytochemical features. Diagn Cytopathol 2005;33:43–8.

115. Bailey TM, Akhtar M, Ali MA. Fine needle aspiration biopsy in the diagnosis of tuberculosis. Acta Cytol 1985;29:732–6.

116. Klemi PJ, Elo JJ, Joensuu H. Fine needle aspiration biopsy of granulomatous disorders. Sarcoidosis 1987;4:38–41.

117. Radhika S, Gupta SK, Chakrabarti A, et al. Role of culture for mycobacteria in fine needle aspiration diagnosis of tuberculous lymphadenitis. Diagn Cytopathol 1989;5:260–2.

118. Gupta AK, Nayar M, Chandra M. Clinical appraisal of fine needle aspiration cytology in tuberculosis lymphadenitis. Acta Cytol 1992;36:391–4.

119. Ellison E, Lapuerta P, Martin SE. Fine needle aspiration diagnosis of mycobacterial lymphadenitis. Sensitivity and predictive value in the United States. Acta Cytol 1999;43:153–7.

120. Singh KK, Muralidhar M, Kumar A, et al. Comparison of in-house polymerase chain reaction with conventional techniques for the detection of Mycobacterium tuberculosis DNA in granulomatous lymphadenopathy. J. Clin. Pathol 2000;53:355–61.

121. Cavett III JR, McAfee R, Ramzy I. Hansen's disease (leprosy). Diagnosis by aspiration biopsy of lymph nodes. Acta Cytol 1986;30:189–93.

122. Silverman JF. Fine needle aspiration cytology of cat scratch disease. Acta Cytol 1985;29:542–7.

123. Donnelly A, Hendricks G, Martens S, et al. Cytologic diagnosis of cat scratch disease (CSD) by fine-needle aspiration. Diagn Cytopathol 1995;13:103–6.

124. Stastny JF, Wakeley PE, Frable WJ. Cytologic features of necrotizing granulomatous inflammation consistent with cat-scratch disease. Diagn Cytopathol 1996;15:108–15.

125. Gamborino E, Carrilho C, Ferro J, et al. FNA diagnosis of Kaposi's sarcoma in a developing country. Diagn Cytopathol 2000:23:322–5.

126. Gaglioano EF. Fine needle aspiration cytology of Kaposi's sarcoma in lymph nodes. A case report. Acta Cytol 1987;31:25–8.

127. Hales M, Bottles K, Miller T, et al. Diagnosis of Kaposi's sarcoma by fine needle aspiration biopsy. Am J Clin Pathol 1987;88:20–5.

128. Viguer JM, Jiménez-Heffernan JA, Pérez P, et al. Fine-needle aspiration cytology of Kikuchi's lymphadenitis: a report of ten cases. Diagn Cytopathol 2001;25:220–4.

129. Tswang WY, Chan JK. Fine needle aspiration cytologic findings of Kikuchi's lymphadenitis: an analysis of 27 cases. Am J Clin Pathol 1994;102:454–8.

130. Tong TRS, Chan OW, Lee K. Diagnosing Kikuchi disease on fine needle aspiration biopsy. A retrospective study of 44 cases diagnosed by cytology and 8 by histopathology. Acta Cytol 2001;45:953–7.

131. Pai MR, Adhikari P, Coimbatore RVR, et al. Fine needle aspiration cytology in systemic lupus erythematosus lymphadenopathy. A case report. Acta Cytol 2000;44:67–9.

132. Laszewski MJ, Belding PJ, Feddersen RM, et al. Clonal immunoglobulin gene rearrangement in the infracted lymph node syndrome. Am J Clin Pathol 1991;96:116–20.

133. Üstün M, Risberg B, Davidson B, et al. Cystic change in metastatic lymph nodes: a common diagnostic pitfall in fine-needle aspiration cytology. Diagn Cytopathol 2002;27:387–92.

134. Shin HJ, Caraway NP. Fine-needle aspiration biopsy of metastatic small

cell carcinoma from extrapulmonary sites. Diagn Cytopathol 1998;19:177–81.

135. Nicholson SA, Ryan MR. A review of cytologic findings in neuroendocrine carcinomas including carcinoid tumors with histologic correlation. Cancer (Cancer Cytopathol) 2000;90:48–61.

136. Highman J, Oliver RT. Diagnosis of metastases from testicular germ cell tumours using fine needle aspiration cytology. J Clin Pathol 1987;40:1324–33.

137. Allhoff EP, Proppe KH, Chapman CM, et al. Evaluation of prostatic specific acid phosphatase and prostatic specific antigen in identification of prostatic cancer. J Urol 1983;129:315–18.

138. Campbell F, Herrington CS. Application of cytokeratin 7 and 20 immunohistochemistry to diagnostic pathology. Current Diagn Pathol 2001;7:113–22.

139. Chu PG, Weiss LM. Keratin expression in human tissues and neoplasms. Histopathol 2002;40:403–39.

140. Fong Y, Coit DG, Woodruff JM, et al. Lymph node metastases from soft tissue sarcoma in adults: analysis of data from a prospective database of 1772 sarcoma patients. Ann Surg 1993;217:72–7.

141. Bizjak-Schwarzbartl M. Cytomorphologic characteristics of non-Hodgkin lymphoma. Acta Cytol 1988;32:216–20.

142. Frable WJ, Kardos TF. Fine needle aspiration biopsy. Applications in the diagnosis of lymphoproliferative diseases. Am J Surg Pathol 1988;12(Suppl. 1):62–72.

143. Gagneten D, Hijazi YM, Jaffe ES, et al. Mantle cell lymphoma. A cytopathological and immunocytochemical study. Diagn Cytopathol 1996;14:32–7.

144. Katz RL. Cytologic diagnosis of leukemia and lymphoma. Values and limitations. Clin Lab Med 1991;11:469–99.

145. Young NA, Al-Saleem TI. Diagnosis of lymphoma by fine-needle aspiration cytology using the revised European-American classification of lymphoid neoplasms. Cancer (Cancer Cytopathol) 1999;87:325–45.

146. Tani E, Santos GC, Svedmyr E, et al. Fine-needle aspiration cytology and immunocytochemistry of soft-tissue extramedullary plasma-cell neoplasms. Diagn Cytopathol 1999;20:120–4.

147. Bangerter M, Hildebrand A, Waidman O, et al. Fine needle aspiration cytology in extramedullary plasmacytoma. Acta Cytol 2000;44:287–91.

148. Sun W, Caraway NP, Zhang HZ, et al. Grading follicular lymphoma or fine needle aspiration specimens: Comparison with proliferative index of DNA image analysis and Ki-67 labelling indeed. Acta Cytol 2004;48:119–26.

149. Skoog L, Tani E. FNA cytology in the diagnosis of lymphoma. In: Orell SR, editor. Monographs in Clinical Cytology. Vol. 18. Basel: Karger; 2008. p. 26.

150. Rassidakis GZ, Tani E, Svedmyr E, et al. Diagnosis and subclassification of follicle center and mantle cell lymphomas on fine-needle aspirates. A cytologic and immunocytochemical approach based on the revised European–American Lymphoma (REAL) classification. Cancer (Cancer Cytopathol) 1999;87:216–23.

151. Hughes JH, Caraway NP, Katz RL. Blastic variant of mantle cell lymphoma: cytomorphologic, immunocytochemical and molecular genetic features of tissue obtained by fine needle aspiration biopsy. Diagn Cytopathol 1998;19:59–62.

152. Matsushima AY, Hamele-Bena D, Osborne BM. Fine-needle aspiration biopsy findings in marginal zone B cell lymphoma. Diagn Cytopathol 1999;20:190–8.

153. Murphy BA, Meda BA, Buss BH, et al. Marginal zone and mantle cell lymphomas: assessment of cytomorphology in subtyping small B-cell lymphomas. Diagn Cytopathol 2003;28:126–30.

154. De Jong D, van Gorp J, Sie-Go D, et al. T-cell rich B-cell non-Hodgkin lymphoma: a progressed form of follicle centre cell lymphoma and lymphocyte predominance Hodgkin's disease. Histopathology 1996;28:15–24.

155. Galindo LM, Havlioglu N, Grosso LE. Cytologic findings in a case of T-cell rich B-cell lymphoma: potential diagnostic pitfall in fine needle aspiration of lymph nodes. Diagn Cytopathol 1996;14:253–8.

156. Tani E, Johansson B, Skoog L. T-cell rich B-cell lymphoma: fine-needle aspiration cytology and immunocytochemistry. Diagn Cytopathol 1998;18:1–4.

157. Tong TR, Lee KC, Chow TC, et al. T-cell/histiocyte-rich diffuse large B-cell lymphoma. Report of a case diagnosed by fine needle aspiration biopsy with immunohistochemical and molecular pathologic correlation. Acta Cytol 2002;46:893–8.

158. Lin O, Gerhard R, Zerbini M, et al. Cytologic features of plasmablastic lymphoma. Diagn Cytopathol 2005;105:139–44.

159. Das DK, Gupta SK, Pathak IC, et al. Burkitt-type lymphoma. Diagnosis by fine needle aspiration cytology. Acta Cytol 1987;31:1–7.

160. Stastny JF, Almeida MM, Wakely PE, et al. Fine-needle aspiration biopsy and imprint cytology of small non-cleaved cell (Burkitt's) lymphoma. Diagn Cytopathol 1995;12:201–7.

161. Troxell ML, Bangs CD, Cherry AM, et al. Cytologic diagnosis of Burkitt lymphoma. Cancer 2005;105:310–18.

162. Dunphy CH, Katz RL, Fanning CV, et al. Leukemic lymphadenopathy: diagnosis by fine needle aspiration. Hematol Pathol 1989;3:35–44.

163. Frizzera G, Wu D, Inghiremi G. The usefulness of immunophenotypic and genotypic studies in the diagnosis and classification of hematopoietic and lymphoid neoplasms. Am J Clin Pathol 1999;111(Suppl. 1):S13–39.

164. Al Shanqeety O, Mourad WA. Diagnosis of peripheral T-cell lymphoma by fine-needle aspiration biopsy: a cytomorphologic and immunophenotypic approach. Diagn Cytopathol 2000;23:375–9.

165. Yao JL, Cangiarella JF, Cohen J-M, et al. Fine-needle aspiration biopsy of peripheral T-cell lymphomas. A cytologic and immunophenotypic study of 33 cases. Cancer (Cancer Cytopathol) 2001;93:151–9.

166. Oertel J, Oertel B, Lobeck KH, et al. Cytologic and immunocytologic studies of peripheral T-cell lymphoma. Acta Cytol 1991;35:285–93.

167. Chan ABW, Chan WY, Chow JHS. Cytologic features of NK/T-cell lymphoma. Acta Cytol 2003;47:595–601.

168. Wai-Kuen Ng, Lee CYK, Li ASM, et al. Nodal presentation of nasal-type NK/T-cell lymphoma: report of two cases with fine needle aspiration cytology findings. Acta Cytol 2003;47:1063–8.

169. Ng W-k, Ip P, Choy C, et al. Cytologic findings of angioimmunoblastic T-cell lymphoma. Analysis of 16 fine-needle aspirates over a 9-year period. Cancer (Cancer Cytopathol) 2002;96:166–73.

170. Attygalle A, Al-Jehani R, Diss TC, et al. Neoplastic T cells in angioimmunoblastic T-cell lymphoma express CD10. Blood 2002;99:627–33.

171. Tani E, Löwhagen T, Nasiell K, et al. Fine needle aspiration cytology and immunocytochemistry of large cell lymphomas expressing the Ki-1 antigen. Acta Cytol 1989;33:359–62.

172. Mourad WA, Nazer M, Tulbah A. Cytomorphologic differetiation of Hodgkin lymphoma and Ki-1+ anaplastic large cell lymphoma in fine needle aspirates. Acta Cytol 2003;47:744–8.

173. Rapkiewicz A, Wen H, Sen F, et al. Cytomorphologic examination of anaplastic large cell lymphoma by fine needle aspiration cytology. Cancer Cytopathol 2007;111:499–507.

174. Katz RL, Caraway NP. Lymph nodes. In: Koss LG, Melamed MR, editors. Koss Diagnostic cytology and its histopathologic bases. Vol. 2. 5th ed. 2006. p. 1205–8.

175. Gorczyca W, Liu Z, Tsang P, et al. B-cell lymphomas with coexpression of CD5

and CD10. Am J Clin Pathol 2003:119:218–30.

176. Kussick SJ, Kalnoski M, Braziel RM, et al. Prominent clonal B-cell populations identified by flow cytometry in histologically reactive lymphoid proliferations. Am. J Clin Pathol 2004;121:464–72.

177. Derksen PW, Langerak AW, Kerkhof E, et al. Comparison of different polymerase chain reaction-based approaches for clonality assessment of immunoglobulin heavy-chain gene rearrangements in B-cell neoplasia. Mod Pathol 1999;12:794–805.

178. Diss TC, Peng H, Wotherspoon AC, et al. Detection of monoclonality in low-grade B-cell lymphomas using the polymerase chain reaction is dependent on primer selection and lymphoma type. J Pathol 1993;169:291–195.

179. Achille A, Scarpa A, Montresor M, et al. Routine application of polymerase chain reaction in the diagnosis of monoclonality of B-cell lymphoid proliferations. Diag Mol Pathol 1995;4:14–24.

180. Segal GH, Jorgensen T, Masih AS, et al. Optimal primer selection for clonality assessment by polymerase chain reaction analysis: low-grade B-cell lymphoproliferative disorders of nonfollicular centre cell type. Hum Pathol 1994;25:1269–75.

181. Gattuso P, Castelli MJ, Peng Y, et al. Post transplant lymphoproliferative disorders: a fine needle aspiration biopsy study. Diagn Cytopathol 1997;16:392–5.

182. Hecht JL, Cibas ES, Kutok JL. Fine-needle aspiration cytology of lymphoproliferative disorders in the immunosuppressed patient: The diagnostic utility of in situ hybridization for Epstein-Barr virus. Diagn Cytopathol 2002;26:360–5.

183. Harris NL, Ferry JA, Swerdlow SH. Post transplant lymphoproliferative disorders: Summary of Society for Hematopathology Workshop. Sem Diagn Pathol 1997;14:8–14.

184. Dmitrovsky E, Martin SE, Krudy AG, et al. Lymph node aspiration in the management of Hodgkin's disease. J Clin Oncol 1986;4:306–10.

185. Kardos TF, Vinson JH, Behm FG, et al. Hodgkin's disease: diagnosis by fine needle aspiration biopsy. Analysis of cytologic criteria from a selected series. Am J Clin Pathol 1986;86:286–91.

186. Moriarty AT, Banks ER, Bloch T. Cytologic criteria for subclassification of Hodgkin's disease using fine needle aspiration. Diagn Cytopathol 1989;5:122–5.

187. Strum SB, Park JK, Rappaport H. Observation of cells resembling Sternberg-Reed cells in conditions other than Hodgkin's disease. Cancer 1970;26:176–90.

188. Stanley MW, Powers CN. Syncytial variant of nodular sclerosing Hodgkin's disease: fine-needle aspiration findings in two cases. Diagn Cytopathol 1997;17:477–9.

CHAPTER 6

Thyroid

Gita Jayaram and Svante R. Orell

CLINICAL ASPECTS

In the past five or six decades, fine needle aspiration (FNA) cytology of the thyroid has been increasingly utilized for the investigation of thyroid lesions.[1-5] The prevalence of thyroid nodules is 4–8% in Western populations.[6] Since cancer is more common in solitary cold nodules, they are conventionally viewed with suspicion. While most thyroid cancers are cold on scintiscanning, the converse is not true. The prevalence of malignancy in solitary cold nodules ranges from 10% to 44.7%.[7] Besides, non-palpable thyroid nodules are being increasingly detected by scanning techniques.[8] Preoperative distinction of benign lesions is of paramount importance to avoid unnecessary surgery. Simplicity, diagnostic accuracy and most of all cost effectiveness[4,9,10] have given FNA the status of the first-line diagnostic test in the preoperative evaluation of thyroid lesions. With increasing experience, FNA has been shown to be able to categorise many benign and malignant lesions and thereby guide therapeutic protocols. It is also useful in the diagnosis and monitoring of autoimmune thyroid lesions, especially in clinically equivocal cases and cases where biochemical and immunological parameters are normal or marginally abnormal.

The main indications of FNA in thyroid lesions are the following:

1. evaluation of solitary thyroid nodules (with a view to distinguish benign from malignant),
2. evaluation of diffuse thyroid lesions (with a view to distinguish inflammatory/autoimmune lesions from nodular goiter),
3. confirmation and categorization of clinically obvious thyroid malignancy (especially anaplastic carcinomas that may require preoperative palliative treatment, and lymphoma and metastatic malignancy where surgery is usually not indicated),
4. to obtain material for ancillary tests/prognostic parameters,
5. evaluation of lesions detected initially by imaging, measuring 1–1.5 cm in diameter with features suspicious of malignancy.[8]

FNA has been shown to be the safest and most accurate of diagnostic tools in thyroid lesions[11,12] with a sensitivity as high as 93.4%, a positive predictive value of malignancy of 98.6%, and a specificity of 74.9%; its use has simultaneously diminished the number of surgeries done for benign lesions and increased the proportion of malignancies in surgically resected thyroids. Cytological reports can and have been used to plan definitive surgery, although some surgeons still demand frozen section or paraffin-section confirmation to overcome cytological error. Frozen section has little to offer over cytology in the assessment of follicular neoplasms (FNs), as these require extensive sampling to identify capsular and/or vascular invasion. Imprints during frozen section could be very useful in the identification of follicular variant of papillary carcinoma (FV-PC)[13] as the characteristic nuclear morphology is brought out to advantage in cytologic smears and is easier to identify than in frozen sections.

The accuracy of FNA is distinctly higher in centers where not only the interpretation but the needling too is carried out by the pathologist.[12] Ultrasonography (US), thyroid function tests, antibody profiles and FNA, used in conjunction in selected cases, complement one another. US-guided FNA of thyroid is useful, especially in cystic and multinodular lesions harboring malignancy.[14] Its value in clinically impalpable nodules has been questioned (see Chapter 2 and 3) due to the insignificant percentage of cancers in this setting.[15] Recent guidelines recommending US examination in patients with palpable nodules[16] have led to an emerging trend in US-guided FNA. Published data indicate reduced non-diagnostic and false-negative rates with US evaluation and US guidance.[17,18]

Several studies have compared the accuracy and complications of core needle biopsy with that of FNA[19] that has increased adequacy rate but reduced sensitivity, especially for PC.[20] Combination of core needle biopsy with FNA increases diagnostic accuracy but the problem of distinguishing benign and malignant FNs remains. In general, safety and ease of use of FNA outweigh the slight increase in accuracy achieved by core needle biopsy.

The inability of FNA to distinguish follicular adenoma (FA) from follicular carcinoma (FC) has been debated at length[21-23] and in turn has led to the use of ancillary techniques to resolve this problem. Marked reduction in the incidence of FC (from 20% of thyroid cancers to less than 2%) since the practice of iodide supplementation of food supplies[22,24] has, however, shifted the focus to other follicular lesions such as cellular nodular goiter (NG) and FV-PC.[12]

©2012 Elsevier Ltd
DOI: 10.1016/B978-0-7020-3151-9.00006-2

Nomenclature used in reporting

Reporting of thyroid FNA specimens should follow a standard format that is clinically relevant in order to direct management. At the National Cancer Institute sponsored thyroid state of the science conference in Bethesda in October, 2007, consensus was reached regarding indications, pre-FNA requirements, FNA techniques, diagnostic terminology, etc.[25] The Bethesda System reporting terminology includes six categories: non-diagnostic, benign, atypia of undetermined origin, FN/suspicious of FN, suspicious for malignancy and malignant.[26] Every category carries with it the implied risk for malignancy. Each category should be further qualified as to the possible pathological entity.

If an indeterminate diagnosis is being made due to features suspicious but not diagnostic of a neoplasm, it should be so qualified, since repeat FNA may enable definitive diagnosis. If, on the other hand, it is being made for FN, qualifying it as such will clarify that distinction of benign from malignant cannot be achieved by repeat FNA, and either ancillary techniques or histological study are required. To simplify the issue, we suggest that in the former, a diagnosis of 'indeterminate (suspicious)' be given and in the latter 'indeterminate (FN)'. We suggest the revised Papanicolaou system of reporting[10] which is simple and easily reproducible with the following six categories that are useful in triaging patients for either clinical follow-up or surgery:

- unsatisfactory,
- benign,
- atypical cellular lesion,
- follicular neoplasm,
- suspicious for malignancy,
- positive for malignancy.

Accuracy and limitations of cytodiagnosis

In experienced hands, and in situations where the pathologist performs the needling, cytology can be a very sensitive tool with sensitivity and specificity of up to 94% and 98% for the diagnosis of malignant lesions[10] and nearly 90% accuracy rates for the identification of malignancy if follicular lesions are excluded.[27,28] Cytologic diagnosis is generally accurate in thyroiditis, usual type of PC, medullary carcinoma (MC), anaplastic carcinoma (AC) and high-grade lymphoma. False negatives generally occur in cystic lesions harboring malignancy, in low-grade or intermediate-grade lymphomas occurring in a background of Hashimoto's thyroiditis (HT), in AC with necrosis, in focal involvement of the gland by thyroiditis and in cases with dual pathology where the dominant non-neoplastic lesion overlies or obscures a small carcinoma.[29-31] False negatives have been shown to be minimized by using US-guided FNA. The false-positive rate can be reduced further by excluding indeterminate follicular lesions.

Complications

There are no contraindications to thyroid FNA. Local hemorrhage may be caused by needling, occasionally causing a hematoma in the anterior neck[32] that in turn may cause airway compression.[33] Carotid hematoma is an extremely rare complication.[34] Transient vocal cord paralysis,[35] acute transient goiter,[36] acute suppurative thyroiditis[37] and chemical neuritis[38] have been noted occasionally. Puncture of the trachea during needling usually causes coughing. Small amounts of blood may be coughed up but recovery is rapid. Needling may convert a hot nodule to a cold one and vice versa, therefore scans (and in general, all noninvasive investigations) should be done before FNA. Post-FNA infarction is an uncommon complication and most reported cases have been Hurthle cell nodules, followed by PC and FNs.[39] Hemorrhage, necrosis or infarction caused by needling may occasionally obscure the histological pattern of thyroid neoplasms. Cellular and vascular granulation tissue of organising hematoma or necrosis can mimic sarcoma or angiomatous tumors. Fibrosis, papillary hyperplasia, calcification, cholesterol clefts, vascular thrombosis and capsular distortion simulating invasion are other worrisome histological alterations that occasionally follow needling.[40] Changes are, in general, proportionate to the size of the needle used and the number of needle passes.[41] Post-needling alterations are generally less with the fine needle capillary sampling technique[41] described below. Aggressive and repeated needling and using needles thicker than 22 gauge should be avoided at all times. In cases where needling is to be repeated for inadequate or inconclusive cytology, it is wise to allow an interval of a week to 10 days for any artifacts of initial needling to minimize.[42] Rare cases of tumor implantation along the needle track have been documented[43-45]. Use of fine-caliber needles (24 gauge or less) and gentle needling technique are stressed to avoid complications and to maximize patient comfort.

Technical considerations

After examining the thyroid with the patient sitting upright, the patient should be made to lie supine with a pillow behind the neck for hyperextension, which makes the lesion more obvious. The fine needle capillary sampling technique is eminently more suitable in vascular structures like thyroid as it provides cellular material with minimal dilution by blood. After instructing the patient to refrain from swallowing, the lesion is needled with a fine needle (gauge 25–27), quickly and gently at different angles and points of entry. Needling should be concluded before or as soon as material appears at the hub of the needle, the needle then attached to an air-filled syringe, and material deposited and smeared on to clean glass slides. Half of the smears can be air-dried for May Grünwald Giemsa (MGG) or Diff-Quik stain while the rest should be wet-fixed in ethanol for Papanicolaou (PAP) stain (that brings out nuclear details to advantage). If the aspirate is scanty, air-drying with Diff-Quik or MGG stain is better as it ensures retention of 100% of cells on the slide. Rapid smearing is important in bloody samples, as clotting of blood will entangle diagnostic cells and distort morphology. Slow drying of wet samples causes nuclear shrinkage and loss of cytological characteristics. A hair-dryer can be used for rapid drying but should be avoided in samples that may be infectious, to avoid aerosols. Despite cost and compensation issues, bedside evaluation of a Diff-Quik or ultra-fast PAP-stained smear is advantageous to ascertain adequate cellularity and representative sampling and to select cases for ancillary studies.[42,46,47]

In cystic lesions where fluid appears at the hub of the needle, the needle should be withdrawn and FNA done using a 22-gauge needle attached to a syringe that will enable aspiration and possible evacuation of cyst contents. After evacuation, any palpable lesion remaining should be needled to minimize chances of missing a neoplasm in the cyst wall. Needling sometimes causes the cyst to fill up with blood and US-guided repeat needling can be done after resorption of blood. Surgical excision can be postponed until after repeat needling of cytologically indeterminate lesions (done after 7–10 days), which often gives a definitive diagnosis. US-guided needling improves the diagnostic yield, especially in very small nodules, retrosternal or mediastinal lesions and enlarged parathyroid glands.[48,49] In all US-guided cases, pathologist and radiologist should work together with small-caliber needles, completing the procedure quickly to minimise dilution with blood and reduce chances of the sample clotting within the needle. Rapid bedside evaluation of smears is mandatory to ensure representative sampling. In situations where US-guided FNA yields hemorrhagic material and an on-site pathologist is not available, cell blocks may give better results than direct smears.[50]

Poor smearing technique and issues involving specimen transportation to the laboratory have led to increasing use of liquid-based processing (LBP) at some centers.[8] While LBP has the advantage of enabling ancillary tests such as immunostains and molecular techniques,[51] specific tumor categorization was found to be less frequent as compared to conventional smears.[52] While LBP is a good option in situations where the needling and smearing are performed by a variety of personnel, the importance of training the operator in the technique of optimal smear-making cannot be overemphasized. Increasing use of LBP may also lead to diminishing skills in direct smear reading, which is required for on-site assessment. On-site assessment not only helps determine specimen adequacy but helps triage the specimen to methods that optimize its diagnostic value.[8,46]

Ancillary techniques

In recent years a number of immunocytochemical and molecular markers[53] have been applied to cytological material from thyroid. Ethanol fixed smears, destained smears, LBP preparations or cell blocks can be used for immunocytochemistry.

Thyroglobulin, thyroid transcription factor and calcitonin help to identify cell type in less differentiated thyroid cancers. Cytokeratin 19, HBME-1 and CD44 are helpful in distinguishing PC from other thyroid carcinomas. Galectin 3 has been used to predict PC and oncocytic lesions, combination of galectin 3 and CD44v6 in distinguishing FA from FC[54–56] and thyroperoxidase as a marker of benignity.[57] Telomerase activity[58] and microarray analysis[59] have been tried as predictors of malignancy and BRAF mutation to indicate extrathyroidal extension of PC. Cyclin D1 and D3 have been used to predict malignancy in oncocytic lesions.[60]

Morphometric evaluation has been tried, mainly in the distinction of FA from FC, with varying results.[61,62] Nucleolar measurement, numbers and area of silver-stained nucleolar organiser regions (AgNORs)[63] and DNA ploidy[64] are other prognostic indicators in FN. Electron microscopic studies may be useful in selected cases.

CYTOLOGICAL FEATURES

Unless otherwise stated, the appearances described refer to MGG/Diff-Quik stained smears.

A satisfactory sample

While abundant colloid without altered blood or debris usually indicates a benign lesion, the presence of intact and well-fixed follicular cells is obligatory for a smear to be considered as satisfactory. Relaxing the criteria for a satisfactory sample often leads to higher rates of false-negative diagnoses. Many false-negative diagnoses in thyroid cytology are related to poor-quality specimens being reported as nonmalignant.[65] A cytological sample from a benign thyroid nodule can be considered satisfactory if six clusters of benign cells are seen in at least two slides prepared from two needle passes.[66] This criterion can be softened in situations where the pathologist performs the procedure. Two to three needle passes, performed gently and with small-caliber needles, are usually accepted easily by the patient. Increased numbers of needle passes improve the diagnostic rate but often at the cost of patient discomfort. US-guided procedures can greatly diminish non-diagnostic rates, especially when radiologist and pathologist work together.

Normal structures

Follicular epithelial cells and colloid are regular features in normal thyroids and in colloid goiter. Follicular cells show fragile gray-blue or pale-blue cytoplasm with indistinct or fuzzy cell borders. Coarse blue (paravacuolar) cytoplasmic granules may be seen (Fig. 6.1). Bare nuclei, similar in shape and size to normal lymphocytes, are common. Some cells may show small nucleoli.

In non-bloody specimens, thin colloid stains blue, violet or pink and forms a thin membrane-like coating or film, with folds and cracks due to drying of colloid on the slide (Fig. 6.2A,B). Colloid may wash off from the slide while

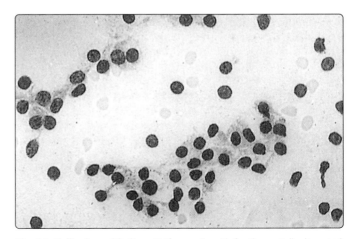

Fig. 6.1 Follicular epithelium Uniform cells with fragile, partially disrupted cytoplasm; bare lymphocyte-like nuclei in a background of thin colloid (MGG, HP).

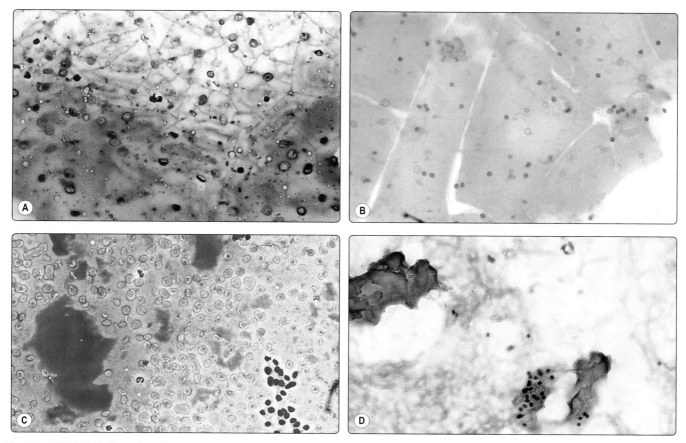

Fig. 6.2 Colloid (**A, B**) Thin colloid forms a varnish-like coat of relatively homogenous material, characteristic 'crazy pavement' and cracking artifacts (**A**, MGG IP; **B**, Pap, IP); (**C, D**) Thick colloid forms irregular dense clumps of material; homogeneous and violet in MGG; variable density and staining in Pap. Compare with Figure 6.3 A and B (**C**, MGG, IP; **D**, Pap, IP).

staining but the parched-earth or crazy-pavement artifact of colloid remains and follicular cells are often seen at the smear margins. Thick colloid appears as round, dense clumps of deep blue, violet or magenta-colored acellular material, or as globular masses with superimposed follicular cells, especially in samples from NG. Colloid can be mistaken for hyalinized collagenous stroma (collagenous spherules) or amyloid. Skeletal muscle fragments appear as straps of dark-blue material with pale ovoid nuclei and cross-striations visible in higher magnification. In PAP-stained smears, thin colloid stains pale green or orange, with cracking artifacts seen. Thick colloid appears as clumps of dark green or orange material (Fig. 6.2C,D). The blue violet color and hyaline texture of colloid appear to advantage in MGG-stained smears and distinction from fibrillary collagen and deep magenta staining amyloid is easier (Fig. 6.3). In bloody smears, colloid resembles other protein-rich fluids, including serum.

C-cells resemble medullary thyroid carcinoma cells and need immunocytochemical stains for identification, except in C-cell hyperplasia, where they are present in large numbers. Accidental puncturing of the trachea or larynx during FNA can be suspected if the patient coughs and air enters the syringe. Smears show mucus, respiratory cells and carbon-laden macrophages. Cartilage may be seen, appearing as brilliant magenta flecks with fibrillary edges.

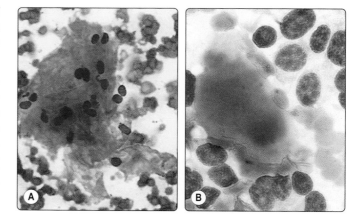

Fig. 6.3 Collagen and amyloid (**A**) Fragment of collagenous stroma; fibrillar texture; red staining; a few nuclei included (MGG, HP); (**B**) Clump of amyloid in medullary carcinoma; structureless but not homogeneously hyaline; magenta color (MGG, HP oil).

Simple colloid goiter

A diffusely enlarged gland with smears showing a normal cytological appearance (or abundant or very thick colloid) indicate a simple colloid goiter which is an early stage in the evolution of NG.

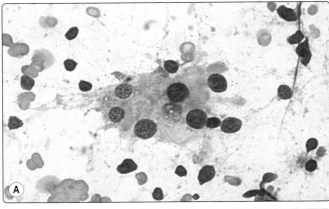

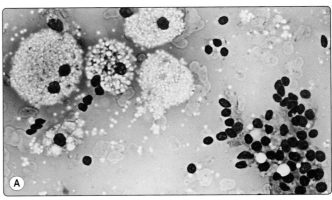

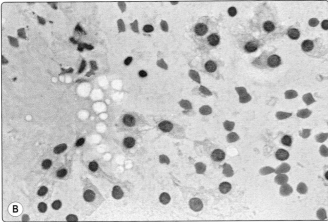

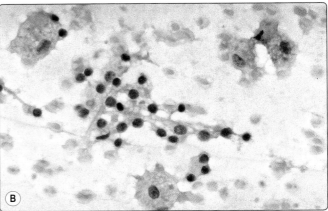

Fig. 6.4 nodular goiter Follicular epithelial cells, some of hyperplastic type with abundant fragile cytoplasm, some of involutional type with small, dark, mainly naked nuclei, background of thin colloid (**A**, MGG, HP; **B**, Pap, HP).

Fig. 6.5 nodular goiter Cystic degeneration: involutional follicular epithelium, foamy macrophages, background of blood and thin colloid (**A**, MGG, HP; **B**, Pap, HP).

Nodular goiter (Figs 6.4–6.7)

DIAGNOSTIC CRITERIA

◆ Abundant thick or thin colloid,
◆ Follicular cells in monolayered sheets, poorly cohesive clusters and single cells,
◆ Hyperplastic, involutional and oxyphilic follicular cells,
◆ Fragile cytoplasm, many bare nuclei,
◆ Pigment laden histiocytes (foam cells),
◆ Degenerative features like old blood and cell debris.

Smears show abundant thick or thin colloid, follicular cells in monolayered sheets, poorly cohesive groups and as single cells, globular colloid masses with superimposed follicular cells, bare nuclei and pigment-laden histiocytes (foam cells) in varying proportions. Involutional follicular cells with small round dark nuclei and fragile, feathery cytoplasm as well as larger, hyperplastic cells with abundant vacuolated cytoplasm or with marginal vacuoles (fire-flares) are seen (see Fig 6.9). The latter may show anisonucleosis. Oxyphilic (Hurthle) cells may be seen.

Macrofollicles disrupted by needling flatten on the slide to form monolayered sheets of epithelial cells. These have a honeycomb structure due to distinct cell membranes (Fig. 6.6A)[3] and frayed edges. Focally, the cytoplasm is indistinct, forming a web-like background to the nuclei. Smaller follicles may be removed intact by the needle. They appear as spherical cell clusters resembling multinucleate giant cells (Fig. 6.6B), that may be enveloped by a basement membrane. Macrofollicles are evidence of benignity and are of diagnostic significance. Hyperplastic papillae containing follicles and intact dilated follicles in cell-block preparations are supportive evidence of a benign nodule. Foam cells, often hemosiderin-laden, suggest degeneration, commonly seen in NG (Fig. 6.5A). Distinction between degenerate epithelial cells and true macrophages is not always possible as transitional forms occur that show epithelioid as well as histiocytoid features and focal atypia. Hyalinized stroma presents as irregular pink/red frayed fragments of vaguely fibrillar material, some with adherent epithelial cells (see Fig. 6.3A).

PROBLEMS AND DIFFERENTIAL DIAGNOSES

◆ Inadequate samples,
◆ Distinction from FN,
◆ Distinction from cystic PC,
◆ Transitional cells (atypical histiocytic versus epithelial cells),
◆ 'Hot' nodules.

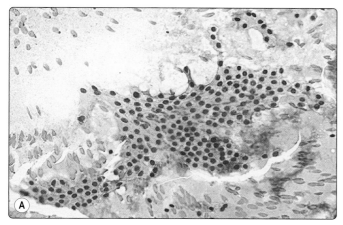

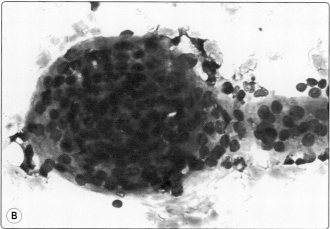

Fig. 6.6 nodular goiter (A) Flat monolayered sheet of epithelial cells representing a flattened macrofollicle; sheet has frayed edges, honeycomb structure (Pap IP); (B) Intermediate-size follicle seen as a three-dimensional ball of cells confined by a basement membrane (MGG, HP).

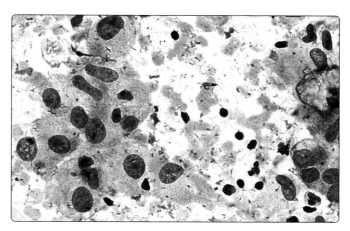

Fig. 6.7 Histiocytes in nodular goiter Histiocytes with abundant cytoplasm and enlarged, irregular nuclei with distinct nucleoli; these could be mistaken for atypical epithelial cells; bare nuclei of degenerate follicular cells in the background (MGG, HP).

Inadequate samples may be obtained from colloid nodules due to low cellularity and degenerative change. If smears contain few or no well-preserved follicular cells, the specimen should be reported as non-diagnostic, unsatisfactory, and repeated.

The cytological appearances of NG can overlap with FN and cytological criteria alone cannot always reliably distinguish between the two. Selective sampling of a microfollicular focus in NG leads to a repetitive pattern of microfollicles or rosettes with no colloid, and distinction from FN may be impossible.[67] However, since this is a focal phenomenon, samples from other areas are likely to show macrofollicles, abundant colloid and degenerative changes recognizable as colloid goiter. In the cytological spectrum of follicular nodules, a large sheet pattern of follicular cells with thin colloid in the background indicates a macrofollicular pattern suggestive of benignity while syncytial clusters with nuclear crowding and overlapping suggest a neoplasm.[68]

Cystic PCs often contain abundant colloid. This can cause diagnostic difficulties if smears are poor in cells, but a close look at the nuclear features should allow a correct diagnosis in most cases, as detailed below. Smears in FV-PC may show well-formed follicles containing colloid.

Groups of large cells with irregular nuclei, not infrequently found in NG, are probably related to degenerative change. Their origin is uncertain; they may be histiocytes or regenerating epithelial cells consistent with repair (Fig. 6.7). Prominent aggregates of histiocytes can in some cases mimic cells of PC due to similar nuclear features.[69]

The value of cytology in hyperfunctioning nodules has been disputed but recent reports suggest that there may be an increased incidence of malignancy in hyperthyroidism and that FNA is a reliable diagnostic method in these cases. It appears reasonable, therefore, to evaluate these lesions cytologically prior to radioactive iodine treatment or surgical intervention.[70]

Cystic nodules

Thyroid cysts are most commonly due to retrogressive changes in NG where they may be small, yielding a few drops of fluid or larger cysts yielding substantial quantities. FNA yields brownish colloid-like fluid with altered blood. Smears show foam cells that may contain hemosiderin and sparse degenerating follicular epithelium (see Fig 6.5).[31,71]

PROBLEMS AND DIFFERENTIAL DIAGNOSES

- ◆ Cystic thyroid neoplasms,
- ◆ Other benign intrathyroid cysts,
- ◆ Parathyroid and thymic cysts.

Cystic change and/or hemorrhage occur in thyroid tumors (25% of PCs, and 20% of FNs in one series).[72] Prevalence of malignancy in resected cystic nodules is 10–15%.[4,31] Partly solid and cystic nodules may also harbor malignancy.

A definitive diagnosis of cystic NG requires adequate sampling of any solid component. Cystic fluid containing only macrophages and no epithelial cells does not rule out a cystic neoplasm. The gross appearance of cyst fluid is not helpful.[31] Presence of atypical cells in a 'cyst fluid only' sample should lead to a 'suspicious' diagnosis (not non-diagnostic).[73] A cystic lesion that can be completely evacuated with no palpable nodule remaining and no epithelial atypia indicates benignity.[71] While 4–40% of cystic lesions can be permanently cured by FNA, others need repeated evacuations. False-negative cytological diagnosis is most common in cystic carcinomas, especially PC, where only up to 60% can be correctly diagnosed.[71,74] Re-biopsy of the cyst bed and of any residual or recurrent swelling, preferably with US-guidance, is advisable. Recurrent cysts, lesions greater than 3–4 cm in diameter and lesions in young males are indications for surgical excision.

Thyroglossal cysts yield clear or mucoid fluid and smears may contain squamous or respiratory epithelium associated with colloid.[75] Foregut cyst of thyroid yields yellowish fluid and smears show detached ciliary tufts and macrophages.[76] Rare epidermoid cysts of thyroid have been described.[77]

Clear fluid aspirated from a lateral cystic lesion suggests a parathyroid cyst and parathormone estimation of the fluid is advised.[78] Thymic cysts yield clear fluid containing lymphocytes.

Acute suppurative thyroiditis

This is an uncommon but potentially life-threatening condition[79] occurring mostly in debilitated or immunosuppressed individuals.[42] Patients present with extremely tender thyroid enlargement, fever and high ESR. Smears show neutrophils, necrotic cells and debris. Intracellular bacteria, (usually Gram-positive cocci), may be present. Less commonly, mycobacteria, viruses, aspergillus, actinomycosis, cryptococcosis and pneumocystis have been observed.[42] Cytologic material can also be sent for culture and sensitivity.

> ### PROBLEMS AND DIFFERENTIAL DIAGNOSES
>
> Smears in AC often show a prominent inflammatory and necrotic component with atypical histiocytoid or fibroblastoid cells. Bacteria (demonstrable by MGG or Gram stain) may be seen in thyroiditis and bizarre giant and spindle cells in AC. Other differential diagnoses of acute thyroiditis are lymphadenitis with abscess, infected thyroid cyst, granulomatous thyroiditis and phlegmonous diffuse neck inflammation that can be resolved by clinical and radiological means.

Autoimmune thyroid disease

The syndromes comprising autoimmune thyroid disease are many intimately related illnesses, the two most common being Graves' disease (GD) (with goiter, hyperthyroidism and, in many patients, associated ophthalmopathy) and Hashimoto's thyroiditis (HT) (with goiter and euthyroidism or hypothyroidism). Immunological mechanisms in these diseases are closely related and the syndromes are connected together by similar thyroid pathology, co-occurrence in family groups, and transition from one clinical picture to another within the same individual over time. Antibodies to thyroid peroxidase (TPO-Ab), produced mainly by intrathyroidal lymphocytes, are the hallmark of autoimmune thyroid disease and are present in most patients with HT and in 75% of patients with Graves' hyperthyroidism.[80]

Graves' disease (primary hyperplasia) (Figs 6.8 and 6.9)[81,82]

> ### DIAGNOSTIC CRITERIA
>
> ◆ Colloid-free bloody background,
> ◆ Moderate to high cellularity,
> ◆ Follicular cells in monolayered sheets, follicular or ring structures,
> ◆ Moderate amounts of pale, cobweb-like, delicately vacuolated cytoplasm,
> ◆ Marginal vacuoles (fire flares).

Cytological study is not usually sought in GD as the clinical and biochemical profile are characteristic in most cases. However, cytology aids distinction from other conditions that present with thyrotoxicity, such as toxic NG, de Quervain's thyroiditis, HT presenting in toxic phase and rarely in thyroid carcinomas.[70]

Smears are bloody with scant colloid. Cellularity is moderate to high with follicular epithelium present as monolayered sheets, rings or follicular structures with suggestion of columnar shape (Fig. 6.8A). Cytoplasm is abundant and cobweb-like and delicately vacuolated, with larger marginal vacuoles giving a characteristic 'fire-flare' appearance.[82] 'Fire-flares' are pale pink/red clumps of material measuring 1–7 μm in diameter, often with a pale center, mainly seen at the rim of the cytoplasm around the edges of aggregates of follicular cells (Fig. 6.9). They may correspond to colloid droplets seen ultrastructurally or to dilated cisternae of endoplasmic reticulum, and are indicative of cellular hyperactivity. They are present in toxic NG, and may be seen in a smaller percentage of cells in HT, diffuse or nodular goiter, and occasionally in neoplasms, including carcinoma.[83,84] In untreated GD, however, up to 100% of cells may show fire-flares. Paravacuolar granules may be seen. There may be moderate to marked nuclear atypia, especially in cases treated with radioactive iodine or neomercazole (Fig 6.8B).[85] Papillary structures may be seen, occasionally resembling PC. Hurthle cells and lymphocytes and rarely multinucleate giant cells or epithelioid cells may be seen.[82]

> ### PROBLEMS AND DIFFERENTIAL DIAGNOSES
>
> Dilution of cells by blood may result in paucicellular, non-diagnostic smears. The bloody, colloid-free, highly cellular cytological appearance in GD with nuclear atypia may be mistaken for a neoplastic lesion, especially in the absence of proper clinical details. The cytoplasm in cells of GD is very delicate and shows a cobwebby, lace-like appearance, unlike the denser cytoplasm and better-defined cell margins seen in neoplastic lesions, especially PC.

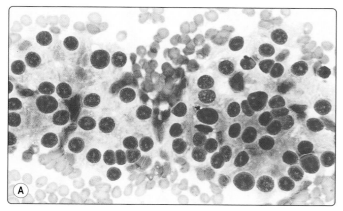

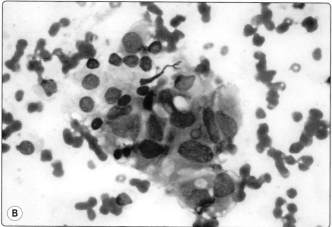

Fig. 6.8 Hyperplasia (A) Clusters of hyperplastic epithelial cells with a follicular arrangement; abundant pale vacuolated cytoplasm and suggestion of columnar shape; (B) Striking anisokaryosis/nuclear atypia in a case of medically treated GD of long duration (MGG, HP).

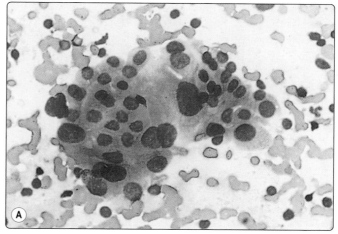

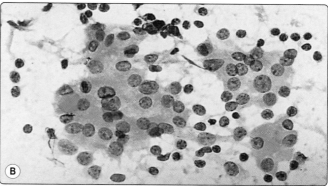

Fig. 6.10 Hashimoto's thyroiditis Aggregates of oxyphil cells; background of blood and lymphocytes; note abundant cytoplasm, anisokaryosis and prominent nucleoli in A, more numerous lymphoid cells in B (A, MGG, HP; B, Pap, HP).

Autoimmune thyroiditis (Hashimoto's thyroiditis/lymphocytic thyroiditis) (Figs 6.10–6.13)[81,86–89]

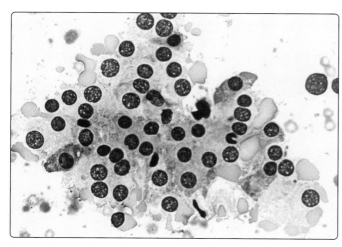

Fig. 6.9 Marginal vacuoles/'fire flares' Loose sheet of hyperplastic follicular cells with abundant cytoplasm and relatively large nuclei; note clumps of homogeneous pale pink material, so-called 'fire flares' around the periphery of the sheet; no clinical evidence of hyperthyreosis in this case (MGG, HP).

DIAGNOSTIC CRITERIA
◆ Lymphoid and plasma cells in the background,
◆ Lymphoid cells impinging on follicular cells,
◆ Lympho-histiocytic collections,
◆ Hurthle cell change (variable),
◆ Multinucleate giant cells and epithelioid cells (variable).

Lymphocytic thyroiditis and HT represent different phases or manifestations of an organ-specific immunologically mediated inflammatory disease. A defect in suppressor T cells makes the gland vulnerable to cytotoxic T cells and stimulates T-helper cells to induce autoantibody production.[90] Patients usually present with diffuse or nodular thyroid enlargement and altered thyroid function caused by gradual immunologically mediated destruction of the gland. Antithyroid antibodies (especially microsomal/TPO-Ab) are significantly elevated in most cases. HT is one of the major manifestations of autoimmune thyroid disease, the other being GD.[91] It is more common in Asians.[92] In multiethnic Malaysia, a study of 88 cases of HT showed it to be more

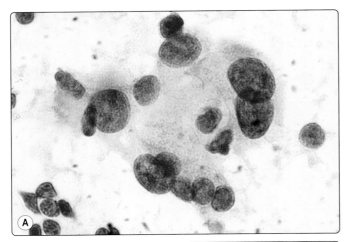

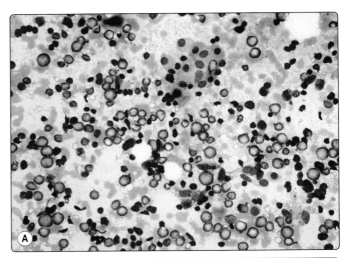

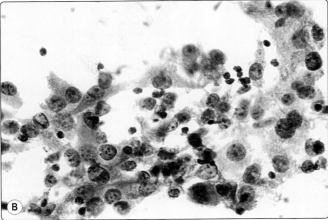

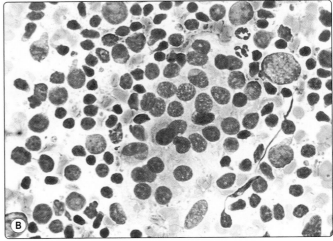

Fig. 6.11 Hashimoto's thyroiditis (A) Syncytial cluster of oxyphil cells; abundant cytoplasm; prominent anisokaryosis; (Pap, HP oil); (B) Poorly cohesive hyperplastic cells showing oxyphil transformation; some resemblance to histiocytes; adherent lymphocytes (Pap, HP).

Fig. 6.12 Florid lymphocytic pattern of HT, 2 cases (A) Polymorphous population of lymphoid cells with high lymphoid:epithelial cell ratio (follicular cells in top center, MGG, IP); (B) Cellular smears, mainly reactive lymphoid cells, cluster of follicular cells in centre (MGG, HP).

common in Indians than Chinese or Malays, and nodular presentation was seen in about one-third of cases.[93]

A bloody background with lymphoid cells, degenerative changes in follicular cells and infiltration of follicular cells by lymphoid cells are characteristic features of HT. Variable features include oxyphilic cells (Hurthle cells), plasma cells, epithelioid cell granulomas and multinucleated giant cells.

The 'lymphocytic' pattern of HT occurs in children and young adults with a shorter history of the disease and absent or low antibody titers.[88] Smears are dominated by a mixed population of lymphoid cells including centroblasts, immunoblasts and dendritic reticulum cells from germinal centers characteristic of a reactive lymphoid proliferation (Fig. 6.12). Germinal center histiocytes have plentiful pale cytoplasm and oval or indented histiocytoid nuclei with granular chromatin. They are often clustered and associated with lymphoid cells, some of which lie within their cytoplasm. Histiocyte-lymphocyte rosettes or lympho-histiocytic clusters may be seen. Lymphoid:follicular cell ratios are often as high as 10:1 with epithelial cells so inconspicuous that smears resemble reactive lymphoid hyperplasia (Fig 6.12 A).

'Classic' or 'florid' HT occurs in older patients (usually women), who are more often hypothyroid and have raised

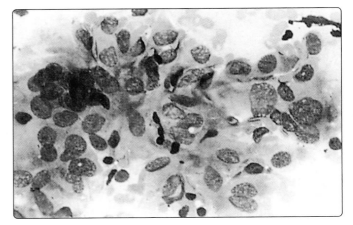

Fig. 6.13 Hashimoto's thyroiditis Plump epithelioid-like oxyphil or histiocytic cells forming a granuloma-like cluster (MGG, HP).

TPO-Ab. The smear background shows lymphocytes with a variable number of plasma cells. There is prominent oxyphilic (Hurthle cell/Askanazy cell) change with single and syncytial aggregates of cells showing abundant, dense, finely granular, gray-blue cytoplasm (MGG), and well-defined cell borders. Nuclei are 2–4 times the size of normal follicular cell nuclei (Figs 6.10 and 6.11) and may show atypia and prominent nucleoli. Normal-appearing follicular cells may be present, showing features of hyperactivity. A characteristic feature is that of lymphocytes (and occasionally plasma cells) seeming to adhere to or infiltrate follicular cells, supporting the theory of direct epithelial damage by lymphocytes. Multinucleated giant cells and epithelioid cells can be seen in up to 40% of cases.[87,93] Neutrophils and eosinophils may be seen adhering to or infiltrating follicular cells in early stages.[42,93]

Seven to thirty-three percent of cases are antibody negative.[87,90,93] In a study of 150 cases of HT, overall Ab positivity was found to be 88.67%.[94] TPO-Ab showed significant correlation with high lymphoid : epithelial ratios but not with cases showing follicular hyperplasia or hashitoxicosis (see below). It appears that antibody positivity may depend on the phase of the disease. Absence of serum antibodies can also be explained on the basis of local antibody production by intrathyroidal lymphocytes.[93]

PROBLEMS AND DIFFERENTIAL DIAGNOSES

◆ Distinguishing bare thyroid nuclei from lymphocytes,
◆ Lymphoid populations in other lesions,
◆ Hyperthyroiditis/hashitoxicosis,
◆ Distinction from lymphoma,
◆ Distinction from follicular and Hurthle cell neoplasms,
◆ Distinction of Hurthle cells from other large nonlymphoid cells,
◆ Granulomatous thyroiditis (GT),
◆ Distinction from fibrosing variant of HT,
◆ Psammoma bodies.

Stripped follicular cell nuclei resemble lymphocyte nuclei in size and shape. However, they have more homogenous chromatin and denser nuclear rim and lack the basophilic rim of cytoplasm seen in lymphocytes. Smears in HT show a polymorphous population of lymphoid cells (including mature and transformed lymphocytes) with lymphoglandular bodies in the backgound.

Lymphoid cells are often seen in smears from PC, especially the diffuse sclerosing and Warthin-like variants.[95,96] Multiple sampling is important to ensure representative sampling so that neoplastic cells are not missed. Histological sections from thyroids resected for NG often show focal collections of lymphoid cells or lymphoid follicles. This does not imply a diagnosis of thyroiditis and review of cytologic smears from such cases rarely show lymphoid cells.[81]

Some cases of HT may present in a hyperthyroid state with increased T3 and T4 levels (hashitoxicosis).[87] In these cases, TPO-Ab are often negative.[94] Smears are highly cellular with hyperplastic follicular cells showing fire-flares. Lymphoid and Hurthle cells may be few or focal, and distinction from GD is often difficult or impossible. Six monthly follow-up of these cases with cytological monitoring and thyroid function tests have shown the patients becoming euthyroid within a few months to 2 years, with concurrently changing smear pattern to reflect the usual features of HT.[42] Awareness of the close kinship between various forms of autoimmune

thyroid disease (GD, HT and postpartum thyroiditis – described later) facilitates diagnosis and management.

While high-grade non-Hodgkin's lymphoma is easily identified on cytological preparations, low-grade and MALT lymphomas are often difficult to distinguish from reactive lymphoid populations seen in thyroiditis. Approximately 75% of lymphomas arise in a background of HT. Focal involvement can cause sampling problems. The smear pattern may be of HT in one part of the gland, that of obvious lymphoma in another (see Fig. 6.65). The 'florid lymphocytic' type of thyroiditis with scant epithelial cells, common in young patients, should be viewed with suspicion if found in elderly individuals, and efforts made to rule out lymphoma. Flow cytometry and molecular assessment of lymphoid infiltrates in fine needle samples are being increasingly used for the distinction of lymphoma from thyroiditis.[97]

Follicular and Hurthle cells in HT may show atypia significant enough to cause concern to the inexperienced observer (Fig. 6.11A). Sometimes, and more often in younger patients with florid lymphocytic thyroiditis, abundant active-looking epithelium may be aspirated, leading to a suspicion of neoplasia. While Hurthle cell atypia in a background of lymphoid cells is recognized as part of the diagnostic spectrum of the disease, selective sampling of lesions of focal nodular hyperplasia constituted by atypical Hurthle or follicular cells (seen in early phase of some cases of HT) with scanty or no lymphoid populations can be easily mistaken for neoplasia.[42,87] In so-called 'burnt-out' HT only oxyphilic cells may be present in smears.[89,98,99] This problem is more pronounced when such a case has a nodular presentation. Multiple sampling offers the best chance of finding evidence of lymphoid infiltration. Disorganized, poorly cohesive masses of oxyphilic cells with prominent nucleoli are more indicative of neoplasia, sheet-like structures infiltrated by lymphocytes of hyperplasia.[100] However, this distinction is not always obvious. Some authors advise against making a diagnosis of follicular/oxyphilic neoplasm in the presence of pleomorphism and abundant lymphoid cells.[82,101,102] The possibility of a neoplasm with surrounding HT should be considered if abundant epithelium and lymphocytes are aspirated.[98,101,103] Coexistence of HT with differentiated thyroid carcinoma (4%) or lymphoma (1%)[42] may have to be considered, especially in cases with nodular presentation, observed in 22–80% cases in various series.[104,105]

Many 'hypertrophic epithelial cells' with abundant cytoplasm are present in early stages of thyroiditis. These lack the dense cytoplasm and well-defined cytoplasmic borders of Hurthle cells. Some may even have 'fire flares' and presumably represent TSH-stimulated cells. Epithelioid-like cells with elongated, spindle-shaped cytoplasm and elongated or bean-shaped nuclei may be seen. These may resemble oxyphilic cells and forms morphologically intermediate between these two types occur (Fig. 6.13). Histiocytes or dendritic reticulum cells from germinal centers could be confused with oxyphilic cells, but lack the characteristic cytoplasmic density.

Cases of HT showing giant cells and/or epithleioid cells[93] may be confused with granulomaotus thyroiditis (GT).[81] The inflammatory infiltrate in GT is not uniformly lymphocytic but is mixed, with evidence of more severe tissue destruction. The smear pattern is dominated by multinucleated giant cells surrounding extruded colloid and epithelioid cell collections. A few cases have showed overlap in cytological features with HT,[106] and thryoid function tests and antibodies are required to clarify the diagnosis.

Fibrosing variant of HT may be confused with Riedel's struma,[42] a rare thyroid manifestation of systemic collagenitis occurring in euthyroid middle-aged women. Smears yield paucicellular material containing collagenous fragments, bland or plump spindle cells and myofibroblasts.[107]

Psammoma bodies have been described in association with HT[108] and in other benign processes. Their presence in smears probably warrants surgical biopsy because of close association with PC. Association of HT per se with PC is also reported.[109]

de Quervain's thyroiditis (subacute thyroiditis; granulomatous thyroiditis) (Figs 6.14–6.17)[42,81,87]

DIAGNOSTIC CRITERIA

◆ Multinucleate giant cells with numerous nuclei, phagocytosed colloid,
◆ Granulomatous aggregates of epithelioid cells,
◆ Degenerating follicular cells, paravacuolar granules,
◆ Dirty smear background with cell debris, colloid, neutrophils, lymphocytes and macrophages.

This is a spontaneously remitting granulomatous inflammation of the thyroid, of possible viral etiology, occurring predominantly in females from the second to the fifth decades. Patients usually present with chills, fever, fatigue and a painful tender goiter that may be unilateral or spread from one lobe to the other.

Smears in GT are dominated by the presence of large multinucleate giant cells with numerous nuclei, granulomatous aggregates of epithelioid cells, degenerating follicular cells, neutrophils, macrophages and lymphocytes in a dirty smear background that shows debris and colloid.

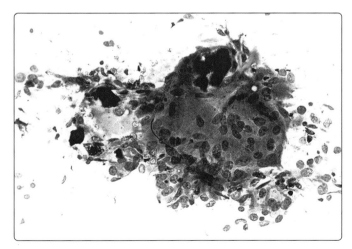

Fig. 6.14 de Quervain's thyroiditis Large multinucleated giant cells; clumps of thick, engulfed colloid (MGG, IP).

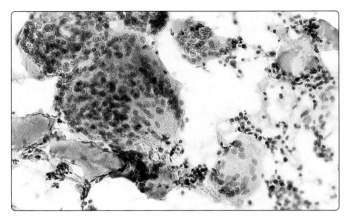

Fig. 6.15 de Quervain's thyroiditis Huge multinucleate histiocytic giant cells, dirty background of clumps of colloid, inflammatory cells and degenerate epithelial cells (Pap, IP).

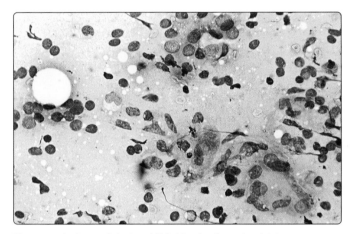

Fig. 6.16 de Quervain's thyroiditis Mixed cell reaction; histiocytes, degenerating epithelial cells and lymphocytes in a 'dirty' background with thin colloid (MGG, HP).

The follicular cells often show degenerative features and contain dark-blue (golden in PAP-stained smears) cytoplasmic 'paravacuolar' granules representing lipofuscin or lysosomal debris. These granules are not a specific feature of this condition and may be seen in involutional follicular cells of NG, in GD and occasionally in PC and FNs.[110] Stripped or crushed nuclei may be present. The giant cells are the hallmark of the disease and are characteristically very large, containing up to 200 nuclei (Figs 6.14 and 6.15), but even without them the diagnosis may be suggested if the other features of the disease are present (Fig. 6.16). Hurthle cells may be seen in some cases.

PROBLEMS AND DIFFERENTIAL DIAGNOSES

◆ Multinucleate and epithelioid cells in other processes,
◆ Hurthle cells,
◆ Pseudogiant cells,
◆ Nodular presentation,
◆ Resolving phase of the disease,
◆ Palpation thyroiditis,
◆ Silent thyrotoxic thyroiditis.

The overlap with cases of HT showing multinucleate giant cells and granulomas has already been discussed. Epithelioid and giant cells may rarely be seen in GD. Giant cells are often seen in PC in association with lymphocytes and therefore PC must be considered in the differential diagnosis.[111] Rarely, the thyroid may be the site of mycobacterial infection, sarcoidosis or other infectious granulomatous processes.[42]

Cases showing Hurthle cells may be confused with HT.[106]

A small follicle withdrawn intact may simulate a multinucleate giant cell. The spherical nature and distinct outline of the structure in contrast with the irregular, flat form of true histiocytic giant cells should prevent confusion (Fig. 6.17A).

Cases with nodular presentation may simulate a lymph node or a neoplasm. Conversely, carcinomatous involvement of thyroid can mimic GT[112,113] or simulate silent thyrotoxic thyroiditis (hyperthyroidism).

Characteristic cytological features of GT may be absent in the resolving phase of the disease.

Vigorous palpation of the gland may cause extrusion of follicular colloid, inciting a giant cell reaction. These granulomas are scanty, minute and clinical and functional profiles of GT are absent.[114]

Silent thyrotoxic thyroiditis (painless thyroiditis, subacute lymphocytic thyroiditis)[88,115,116] usually occurs in women as a sporadic or post-partum condition (post-partum thyroiditis), presenting with a small, diffuse, painless goiter. The disease may go through hyperthyroid, euthyroid, hypothyroid and recovery phases similar to GT. Low titers of TPO Ab are transiently present in two-thirds of cases. Smears show scattered lymphoid cells and giant cells in occasional cases. Unlike GT, there is no pain or any evidence of preceding viral infection and granulomas are uncommon. Rare cases have shown cytologic similarity to HT.[116]

Follicular neoplasms (Figs 6.18–6.24)[23,29,68,117–120]

DIAGNOSTIC CRITERIA

- ◆ Moderate to high cellularity,
- ◆ Bloody, usually colloid-free background,
- ◆ Prominent microfollicular pattern,
- ◆ Rosettes, syncytial groups and equal-sized cell clusters,
- ◆ Nuclear crowding and overlapping,
- ◆ Positive immunostaining for thyroglobulin and TTF-1.

FNs are classified as benign (FA) and malignant (FC). FAs and most FCs are encapsulated tumors, occurring in one of the lobes. Histological diagnosis of a well-differentiated FC requires demonstration of capsular and/or vascular permeation. Most FNs, especially adenomas, have a uniform internal structure that is reflected in the cytological smears. FAs are more common in women and microscopically show a variety of histological patterns such as microfollicular (fetal), normofollicular, macrofollicular, trabecular, solid (embryonal), Hurthle cell and atypical adenomas.[42] Cytologically, follicular lesions include FA, FC, cellular NG and FV-PC.[121]

Smears in FN are cellular in a bloody background that is usually devoid of colloid. Many uniform-sized follicular cell clusters, microfollicles and rosette formations are present. Syncytial aggregates, nuclear crowding and overlapping are also often seen.

The repetitive smear pattern with uniform cell population is in contrast to the variable pattern of different cell types seen in colloid and hyperplastic nodules. Microacinar clusters with a central lumen (that may contain a drop of colloid)

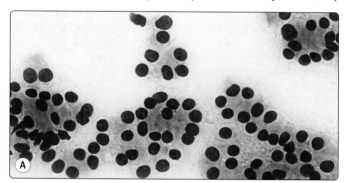

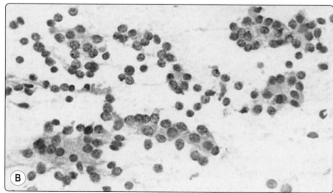

Fig. 6.18 Follicular neoplasm Cellular smears of single cells, microfollicles or rosettes in a repetitive manner; benign adenoma by histology (**A**, MGG, HP; **B**, Pap, HP).

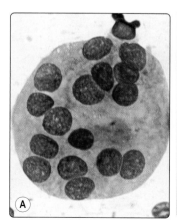
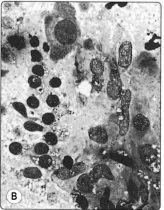

Fig. 6.17 de Quervain's thyroiditis (A) 'Pseudogiant cell'; a small follicle in a smear from NG with a smooth well-defined border and a small amount of colloid in the center; superficial resemblance to a multinucleated giant cell (MGG, HP oil); (**B**) Degenerating epithelial cells with paravacuolar granules (*left*) and epithelioid histiocytes (*right*) in de Quervain's thyroiditis (MGG, HP).

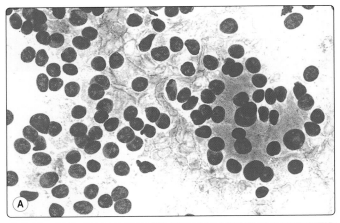

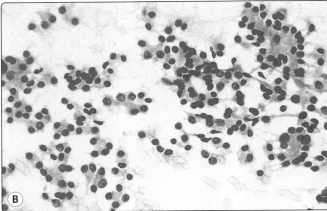

Fig. 6.19 Follicular neoplasm Smears very similar to Figure 6.18; follicular carcinoma with vascular invasion by histology (**A**, MGG, HP; **B**, Pap, HP).

represent microfollicles (Figs 6.18, 6.19 and 6.21B). These are characteristic of FN but may be found focally in NG. Rosette-like groupings without a lumen (Fig. 6.20) suggest a more solid growth pattern. A trabecular pattern is represented by rows and elongated aggregates of epithelial cells that resemble papillary structures when they adhere to strands of vascular stroma (see Fig. 6.33B,C). Small blood vessels with adherent epithelial cells can be found in any type of follicular neoplasm (see Fig. 6.25A).

PROBLEMS AND DIFFERENTIAL DIAGNOSES

◆ Nodular goiter,
◆ Distinction of adenoma from carcinoma,
◆ Atypical adenoma,
◆ FV-PC,
◆ Parathyroid tumors,
◆ Vascularity,
◆ Inspissated colloid mimicking psammoma bodies,
◆ Cystic change.

The distinction between FN and NG is the most common differential diagnostic problem in solitary nodules as cytological appearances overlap (Fig. 6.22). A microfollicular focus in a colloid nodule cytologically resembles a microfollicular neoplasm, while smears from a macrofollicular (colloid) adenoma resemble a dominant nodule

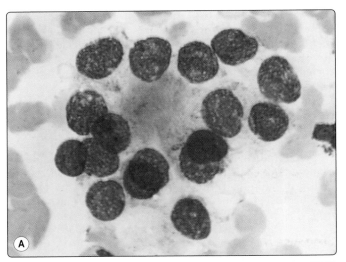

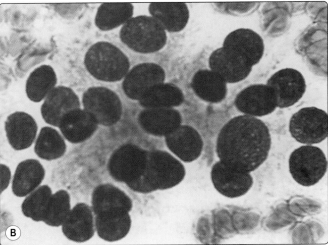

Fig. 6.20 Follicular neoplasm Microfollicular cell clusters/rosettes; some nuclear hyperchromasia and coarseness in both (**A**) follicular adenoma and (**B**) follicular carcinoma (MGG, HP oil).

in multinodular goiter. Jaffar[122] indicated that the presence of hemosiderin within macrophages and follicular cells excludes FN. The false-negative rate of cytology in FN may be 30% or more because of the inability to recognize normofollicular neoplasms.[123] However, these distinctions are of little clinical importance as long as the nodule is recognized as benign and spared from unnecessary surgery.

Most FCs are microfollicular, trabecular or solid, contain little colloid, and will be reported as 'FN' by cytology. Although the failure to recognize FC as neoplastic has been surprisingly high in some series,[7] other studies show high diagnostic sensitivity, with false-negative rates as low as 0–2%.[11,13,28]

Cytological features in FA and FC are similar, with cellular smears composed of syncytial clusters of crowded cells. There is a tendency for uniform nuclear enlargement in FC, whereas FA may show small or large nuclei.[124] These differences are often subtle, with much overlapping (Fig. 6.20).[3,68,125] Cells from a well-differentiated but clinically aggressive FC may not appear obviously atypical or enlarged in smears (Figs 6.23, 6.24B). Anisokaryosis per se is more a feature of non-neoplastic lesions such as NG and thyroiditis.[42]

Most authors are content to use cytology to select cellular FNs for follow-up or surgical excision, and to leave a diagnosis of malignancy to histological assessment of capsular and vascular invasion. Reporting cytological atypia and any suspicion of malignancy, although not diagnostic, may be of

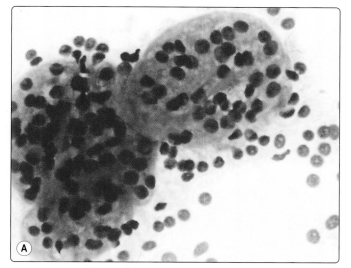

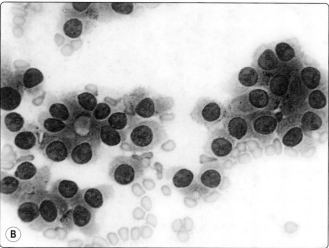

Fig. 6.21 Follicular neoplasm (A) Small intact follicles with basement membrane; small uniform nuclei; follicular adenoma. (B) Microfollicular groups; enlarged nuclei; drop of abnormal colloid in small central lumen; follicular carcinoma (MGG, HP).

some use in making the choice between follow-up and immediate surgical excision. The ultimate prognosis of microfollicular, solid or trabecular adenomas is uncertain and these should probably be excised anyway.

FC has been considered the second most common thyroid cancer, accounting for 10–20% of all thyroid malignancies.[126] The proportion of carcinoma in lesions designated as FN has been reported as ranging from 14% to 44% in previous series.[3,119] In a large series of operated cases from 1994 to 2002 from Bethesda,[127] an 18.2% rate of malignancy was found in cases in which a cytological diagnosis of 'possible FN' was given and 20.9% in cases with a definitive cytological categorization of 'FN'.

Clinicians (and cytopathologists) are conventionally preoccupied with the inability of cytologically distinguishing FA from FC, leading to numerous ancillary investigations to help make this distinction. Computer assisted cell morphometry, ploidy analysis and determination of AgNORs in cytological smears have been tried with variable success.[61,128,129] Results of proton magnetic resonance spectroscopy have been encouraging.[130] However, the most promising technique for the future is probably immunocytochemical demonstration of molecular markers.[131] Positive immunostaining with CD44v6 or galectin 3 (with a score of G2) in combination with FNA[54,55] have been noted to be useful in cases with indeterminate cytology.[56] Telomerase activity[58] and microarray analysis of cytologic samples[59] are other ancillary tests that may aid in distinguishing benign from malignant follicular lesions.

Interestingly, there are studies indicating that FC is gradually becoming a rare entity.[18,22,24,132,133] Prevalence of malignancy in operated cases of FN[118] was 31%, and 9% of these were follicular or Hurthle cell carcinomas. The incidence of FC was only 2% of thyroid cancers in LiVolsi's series[24] and 1% at the University of Chicago Medical Center.[22] Discussing the gradual demise of FC, De May[22] opined that independent of the quality of any diagnostic test employed, statistically speaking, its predictive value would be affected by the prevalence of the disease in question. It stood to reason therefore that, if the prevalence of FC is low, the predictive value of cytology for FC would also tend to be low, although cytology is otherwise an excellent diagnostic modality.

Atypical adenomas show foci of extremely pleomorphic cells that cytologically simulate malignancy (Fig. 6.24A). These are designated as carcinoma only if there is capsular or vascular invasion. Nuclear pleomorphism is not a

Histologic diagnosis	Colloid nodule	FA macrofollicular	FA microfollicular	FC	FV-PC
Cytologic category	Colloid nodule		Follicular neoplasm		
Morphologic features	⟶ Increasing cellularity ⟶ ⟶ Microfollicular structures ⟶ ⟶ Decreasing amounts of colloid ⟶ ⟶ Increasing nuclear size ⟶ Nuclear grooves and inclusions (FV-PC) ⟶				

Fig. 6.22 Follicular neoplasms Rationale for cytological diagnosis.

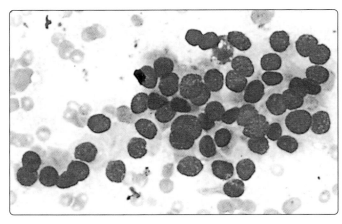

Fig. 6.23 Follicular carcinoma Aspirate of distant lymph node metastasis of disseminated follicular carcinoma; syncytial cluster with some rosetting; bland nuclear chromatin; mild nuclear enlargement and anisokaryosis (MGG, HP).

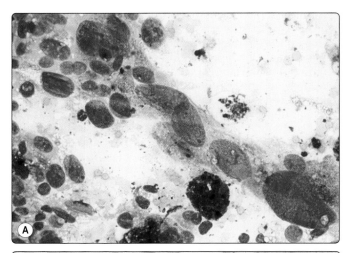

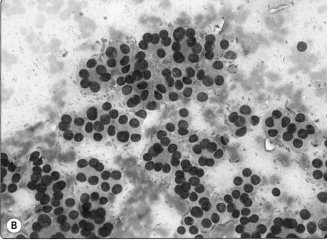

Fig. 6.24 Atypical adenoma and well-differentiated follicular carcinoma (A) Smear from atypical adenoma with bizarre cells; histology showed similar epithelial atypia but no capsular or vascular invasion; uneventful follow-up; (B) Well-differentiated follicular carcinoma metastatic to bone – cellular smear with prominent microfollicular pattern, relatively uniform nuclei and fire-flares (MGG, HP).

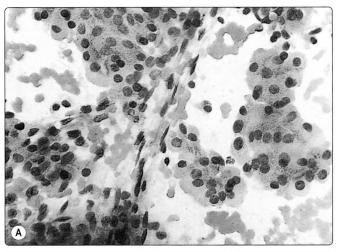

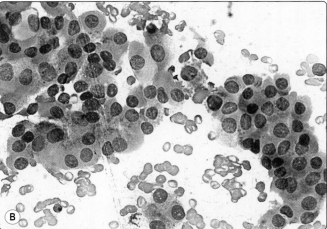

Fig. 6.25 Oxyphil (Hurthle cell) adenoma (A) Sheets of oxyphil cells adherent to capillary blood vessels; histology oxyphil adenoma; (B) Oxyphil cells in a trabecular arrangement; histology oxyphil adenoma (MGG, HP).

common feature of well-differentiated FC and is not considered a cytological criterion of malignancy. On the other hand, it is frequent in dyshormonogenetic goiter, treated GD, and following chemotherapy and radiotherapy.[42,85]

In recent years, FV-PC has attracted much attention. Due to the presence of follicular groupings and colloid in these tumors (see Fig. 6.43), it constitutes a generous proportion of malignancies reported as FN.[21,22,118] However, a proportion of nuclei display typical cytological features of PC (described below in section on PC). In some series, high cytologic accuracy rates for FV-PC[134] with 93–94% sensitivity, specificity, positive and negative predictive values have been demonstrated using ultrafast PAP stain.[135]

No cytological criteria clearly distinguish parathyroid from follicular thyroid neoplasms.[136] Agarwal et al.,[137] performing US-guided FNA of 53 parathyroid adenomas, reported low sensitivity as a major limitation. Smears showed moderate cellularity with monomorphous, round to slightly oval cells predominantly arranged in loose two-dimensional clusters with occasional papillary fragments. The majority of them exhibited stippled nuclear chromatin and bare nuclei were seen in the background. There was no significant pleomorphism, mitotic activity, or prominent nucleoli. Parathyroid adenomas are usually not palpable but radiological examination is capable of locating most non-palpable parathyroid lesions. However, the occasional parathyroid adenoma may be intrathyroidal.[138] Cytohistological overlap in parathyroid and thyroid follicular lesions can be a problem at the time of frozen section evaluation, and intraoperative parathyroid hormone monitoring may be required. In parathyroid carcinomas, clinical, biochemical and radiological findings are usually characteristic. Cytology, combined with clinical, radiological and immunocytochemical findings can enhance diagnostic accuracy.[139] Tseleni-Balafouta[140] felt that due to overlapping morphological features, in order to avoid surgical mismanagement, the possibility of a parathyroid lesion should be stated clearly in cytology reports in all colloid-free cellular follicular lesions. Parathyroid incidentalomas comprise 0.4% of lesions in patients referred for suspected thyroid nodules, and parathyroid hormone analysis in FNA washouts has been found to be a diagnostic aid.[141]

FNs are often highly vascular and aspiration of blood may obscure neoplastic cells. It should be understood that excessively blood-stained smears are not necessarily related to poor technique but may signal the possibility of a neoplasm. Repeat needling using the fine needle capillary sampling technique with a 26 or 27-gauge needle after a gap of a week or two often yields diagnostic material.

Colloid in small follicles is often very dense and may be laminated, but the regular edge is unlike that of a psammoma body.

Variants of follicular neoplasms

- Hurthle (oxyphilic) cell tumors (Figs 6.25 and 6.26),
- Atypical adenoma with bizarre cells (see Fig. 6.24A),
- Neoplasms with clear or signet ring cells.

HCTs, constituting 1.5–10% of thyroid tumors, represent a controversial pathological entity,[142] regarding both their behavior and classification (whether they represent metaplasia in follicular or papillary neoplasms or constitute a distinct entity). Most tumors are encapsulated, and capsular and/or vascular permeation are standard criteria of malignancy. Recent reports suggest that Hurthle cell carcinoma may be a more aggressive tumor, distinct from FC.[143] Rare familial cases of aggressive, metastasising Hurthle cell carcinoma have been reported.[144]

Smears from HCT yield abundant material consisting of large, polygonal Hurthle cells with oval nuclei and abundant, well-defined, granular cytoplasm. Tumor cells appear singly, in acinar arrangement, and in monolayered sheets of variable sizes.[145,146] Nuclei are eccentrically placed. Occasional cells may be ovoid or rounded. Nuclear pleomorphism may be present but is not as common in adenomas as in non-neoplastic lesions like HT. Occasional small syncytial tumor cell clusters and naked nuclei may be seen. Carcinomas show relatively smaller Hurthle cells with monomorphic or pleomorphic nuclei, macronucleoli and ill-defined cytoplasm. Crowded sheets, syncytial tumor cell clusters of variable sizes and naked nuclei may be present.[90] Computerized interactive morphometric analysis of nucleolar features may be helpful in distinguishing benign from malignant lesions.[147] However, due to frequent morphological overlap, a cytological diagnosis of HCT is preferred, with

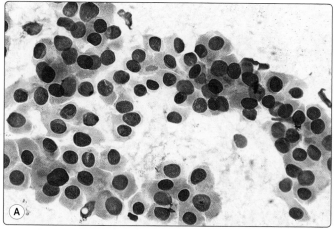

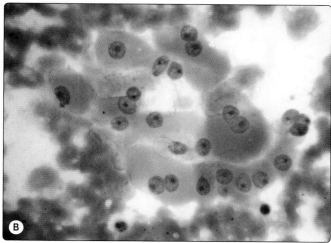

Fig. 6.26 Hurthle cell carcinoma (A) Similar pattern as Figure 6.25B of trabecular groups of oxyphil cells (MGG, HP); (B) Large polygonal cells with well-defined cell margins, basophilic cytoplasm, vesicular nuclei and macronucleoli (MGG, HP).

further categorization deferred for histological study. Galectin 3 immunostain has been shown to stain Hurthle cell adenomas.[55] Combination of galectin 3 and HBME has been demonstrated to show 99% sensitivity and 88% specificity in tumors composed of Hurthle cells (Hurthle cell adenomas, carcinomas and oncocytic variant of PC).[148]

Hurthle cells are seen in a variety of non-neoplastic lesions such as NG, GD, HT and GT. In most of these conditions, they are admixed with other cells that indicate the nature of the lesion, such as lymphoplasmacytic cells in HT, epithelioid cells in GT, etc. A mixture of Hurthle cells and 'normal' follicular epithelial cells is more consistent with a hyperplastic nodule.[99,146] In early stages of HT, needling of proliferating Hurthle cell nodules may lead to a smear pattern dominated by Hurthle cells. The presence of a high percentage of dyshesive Hurthle cells with large nucleoli, with some cells showing significant nuclear enlargement and pleomorphism, are indicative of a neoplastic Hurthle cell lesion.[99,146] Flat sheets of Hurthle cells are more characteristic of thyroiditis, poorly organized and poorly cohesive cell clusters of neoplasia.[100] Neoplastic and non-neoplastic Hurthle cell nodules may develop following irradiation to the head and neck.[149] Smears in such cases often suggest a neoplastic

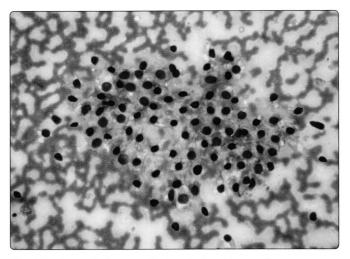

Fig. 6.27 Clear cell change Follicular cells that show a uniform appearance of abundant, delicately vacuolated cytoplasm (MGG, IP).

lesion. These nodules should be excised for careful histological evaluation.

Atypical adenoma with bizarre cells has been discussed above. A rule applicable to all endocrine organs is that nuclear pleomorphism per se cannot be used as a basis for cytological diagnosis of malignancy.

Clear cell change in follicular epithelium may be due to accumulation of glycogen, thyroglobulin, mucin, lipid or varying combinations of these.[90] It may also represent artifacts of formalin fixation or paraffin embedding.[42] While clear cell morphology is well appreciated in tissue sections, cytologic smears show cells with abundant, finely vacuolated, pale but not totally clear cytoplasm (Fig. 6.27). Clear cell change may be a focal or less frequently diffuse phenomenon in FA, FC, HCT[42] and non-neoplastic lesions. Metastatic clear cell carcinoma of renal origin is an important differential diagnosis.[42] Signet ring adenoma containing thyroglobulin as well as mucin, PAS-D and acidic Alcian blue-positive material is a rare finding and could be due to the presence of protein polysaccharide complexes derived from partial degradation of thyroglobulin.[150]

Poorly differentiated thyroid carcinoma

DIAGNOSTIC CRITERIA

- ◆ Hypercellular smears,
- ◆ Single cells, solid, trabecular and insular pattern,
- ◆ Marked cellular crowding and high nuclear : cytoplasmic ratio.

Until recently, thyroid carcinoma with a poorly differentiated insular pattern was considered to be a distinct entity, a thyroglobulin-producing neoplasm, intermediate in aggressiveness between well-differentiated and anaplastic thyroid carcinoma. Reports have appeared documenting cytological features in insular carcinomas such as high cellularity, dispersed and loosely aggregated cells, solid, cohesive trabecular or papilloid structures, intact insulae, fragile, ill-defined, granular cytoplasm, oval, hyperchromatic nuclei, occasional INCIs and/or grooves.[151-155] However, as insular pattern is

often admixed with trabecular and solid growth patterns, the more suitable term 'primordial carcinoma' was suggested for this entity.[156]

The current concept of pure poorly differentiated thyroid carcinoma, as per the Turin proposal[156] is one that shows a histologically mixed solid/trabecular/insular architecture, absence of conventional nuclear features of PC and the presence of one of the following three features: cells with convoluted (raisin-like) nuclei, a mitotic index of ≥3 mitoses/ 10 high-power fields and tumor necrosis. Most tumors are immunohistochemically positive for thyroglobulin and thyroid transcription factor 1, and a subset is also positive for p53.[157] *Ras* mutations are common.

Smears in poorly differentiated thyroid carcinomas are hypercellular with single cells as well as cells in solid, trabecular and insular patterns. There is marked crowding of cells and tumor cells show high nuclear cytoplasmic ratios (Fig. 6.28).[158]

PROBLEMS AND DIFFERENTIAL DIAGNOSES

- ◆ Metastatic carcinoma,
- ◆ Poorly differentiated foci in differentiated thyroid carcinoma.

Distinction from metastatic carcinomas (Fig. 6.29), especially on cytologic smears, requires detailed clinical evaluation, review of sections of previous surgery, prior cytologic smears, if any, and use of ancillary stains (thyroglobulin and TTF-1) where necessary.

Differentiated thyroid carcinomas, especially FC, may show poorly differentiated foci that may be sampled by the needle, missing out the well-differentiated component. MC of small cell type can be distinguished by calcitonin immunostaining.

Papillary carcinoma (Figs 6.30–6.47)[159-162]

DIAGNOSTIC CRITERIA

- ◆ Cellular smears,
- ◆ Cells forming syncytial aggregates and sheets focally with a distinct 'anatomical border' and nuclear crowding and overlapping,
- ◆ Flat sheets, three-dimensional tissue fragments and papillary tissue fragments with or without a fibrovascular core,
- ◆ Enlarged, ovoid, strikingly pale nuclei, finely granular, powdery chromatin (PAP),
- ◆ Intranuclear cytoplasmic inclusions and nuclear grooves,
- ◆ Dense cytoplasm, distinct cell borders,
- ◆ Squamoid or histiocyte-like, 'metaplastic' epithelial cells,
- ◆ Scanty, viscous, stringy (chewing gum) colloid – variable,
- ◆ Psammoma bodies – variable,
- ◆ Macrophages and debris (evidence of cystic degeneration), multinucleate giant cells and lymphocytes – variable,
- ◆ Dual immunostaining for keratin and vimentin; positive immunostaining for CK19, CD44 and HBME.

Papillary carcinoma (PC) is the most common type of thyroid cancer, occurring predominantly in females, in all age groups but most often in the third to fifth decades.[42] It

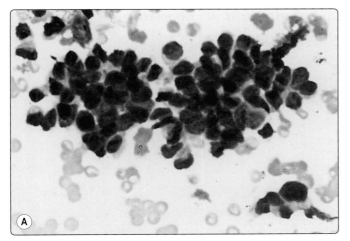

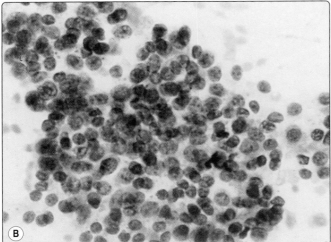

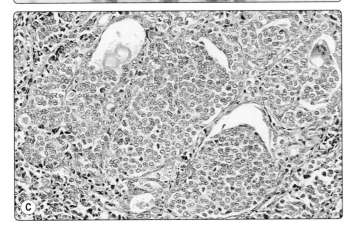

Fig. 6.28 Poorly differentiated carcinoma (**A,B**) Smears showing syncytial clusters of crowded small cells with hyperchromatic nuclei (**A**, MGG, HP; **B**, Pap, HP); (**C**) Tissue section, same case. (H&E, IP).

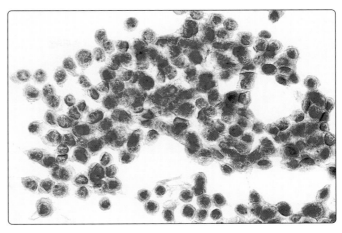

Fig. 6.29 Metastatic carcinoma in thyroid Metastasis to thyroid of breast carcinoma; smear pattern similar to poorly differentiated carcinoma as in Figure 6.28 (Pap, HP).

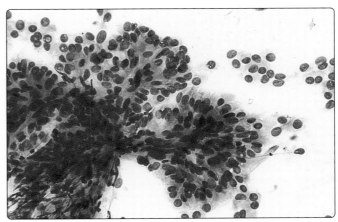

Fig. 6.30 Papillary carcinoma True papillary fragment with a vascular core; columnar cells with oval pale nuclei; intranuclear vacuoles, upper left (MGG, IP).

accounts for 90% of childhood thyroid malignancies. Five to ten percent of cases have had prior head and neck irradiation, usually in the first two decades of life. Most cases show clinically evident metastatic cervical lymphadenopathy at presentation, yet the prognosis is usually good, especially in children and young adults. RET/PTC rearrangements and BRAF mutation are often seen.[159] PC is rarely encapsulated,

infiltrates the thyroid in an irregular manner and is often multifocal with variable degrees of cystic change. Histological hallmarks of the tumor are the branching papillary structures with fibrovascular cores, lined by cuboidal or columnar cells with 'ground-glass' nuclei ('Orphan Annie' eyes). These cells show nuclear grooves and/or INCIs, and psammoma bodies are seen in many cases.

Smears in PC are cellular with numerous three-dimensional and papillary fragments (Fig. 6.30) with or without vascular cores. Often, papillae not removed intact by the needle appear as flat sheets. Sheets of cells show a distinct anatomical border, formed by a row of cuboidal or columnar cells (Fig 6.31A) with focal nuclear crowding and overlapping, features that distinguish sheets of PC from those representing benign macrofollicles (Fig. 6.31B). The tip of a papilla may be seen as a finger-like aggregate of cells with a similar edge (Figs 6.32 and 6.33A). Naked true papillary connective tissue cores are sometimes found and can be diagnostically helpful. Trabecular fragments (Fig. 6.33B) (also present in FN) are represented in smears by cohesive finger-like structures and must not be mistaken for papillae. Seventeen

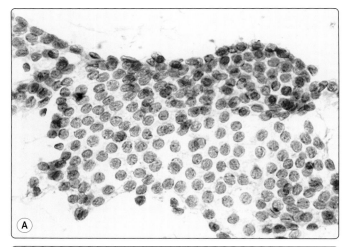

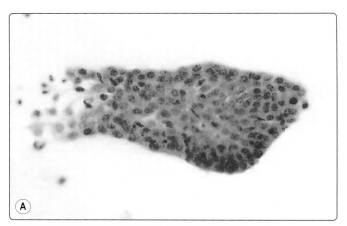

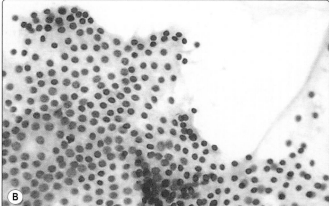

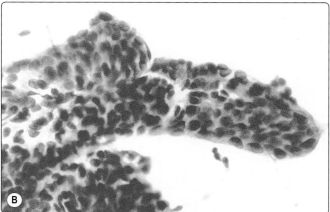

Fig. 6.31 Comparison of sheets of papillary carcinoma and of macrofollicle in nodular goiter (A) Papillary carcinoma. Flat sheet of epithelial cells; partly monolayered, partly with nuclear overlapping; uniformly enlarged, oval nuclei with pale powdery chromatin and small nucleoli; note 'anatomical' edge of a row of cells along upper edge (Pap, HP); (B) Nodular goiter. Flat monolayered sheet of cells from a disrupted macrofollicle; note frayed edges and uniformly small round nuclei (Pap, HP).

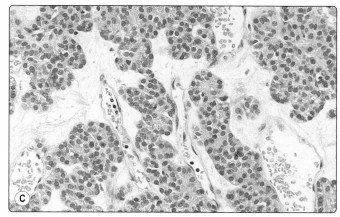

Fig. 6.33 'Papillary' structures (A) Finger-like papilla of papillary carcinoma; distinct lining on three sides by a row of cuboidal/columnar cells (H&E, IP); (B) Finger-like, pseudopapillary fragment from a trabecular thyroid carcinoma (Pap, HP); (C) Tissue section from same case as **B** (H&E, IP).

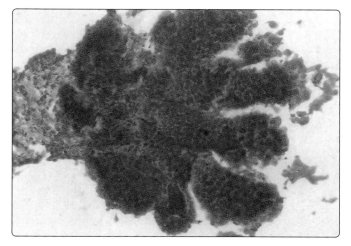

Fig. 6.32 Papillary carcinoma Finger-like papillae with 'anatomical' edges (Pap, IP).

percent of cases show concentrically organized aggregates of tumor cells or 'swirls' (Fig. 6.34), the most peripherally located cells appearing ovoid with nuclei oriented perpendicular to the radius of the swirl.[163] A few cases show only dispersed single cells and syncytial aggregates; diagnosis then relies on identification of nuclear features of PC.

Tumor cells show uniform enlargement with dense cytoplasm and well-defined cell borders. INCIs (Fig. 6.35), characteristic of PC, are seen in up to 90% of cases. They are seen in 5% of the cells (10% if examined under oil

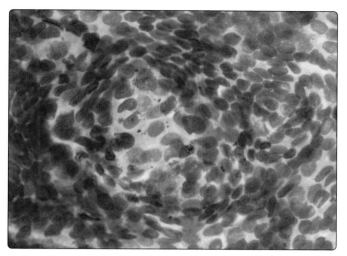

Fig. 6.34 **Papillary carcinoma, swirls** Concentrically arranged tumor cells forming swirls with peripherally located cells appearing perpendicular to radius of the swirl (MGG, HP).

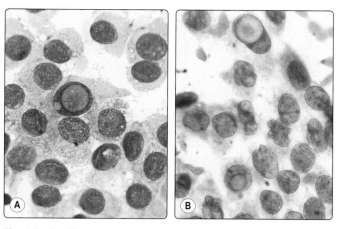

Fig. 6.35 **Papillary carcinoma, intranuclear 'vacuoles'** Large, oval, pale nuclei; several intranuclear cytoplasmic inclusions; pale powdery chromatin most obvious in Pap; note cells with convoluted nuclei in B (A, MGG; B, Pap, HP oil).

immersion under 2–3 planes of focus).[164,165] INCIs, however, are not specific to PC as they can be seen in atypical adenomas,[166] hyalinizing trabecular tumors,[167] MC (see Fig. 6.55),[168] AC (see Fig. 6.59) and rarely in FC,[90] HT[18] and juxta-thyroidal neoplasms (parathyroid adenoma, paraganglioma, etc.).[67,90]

INCIs have sharp, well-defined, membrane-like margins and are not optically clear but resemble the cytoplasmic color and texture. They probably start as trapped cytoplasm in deep nuclear folds (grooves)[169] that eventually invaginate into the nucleus at foci of nuclear membrane weakness. Grooves and inclusions do not usually coexist, possibly due to the pressure of the inclusion unfolding the groove and preventing further groove formation.[170] Artifacts such as superimposed air bubbles or fat droplets can mimic INCIs both in PAP- and MGG-stained material.[27,171] Optically clear vacuoles and poorly defined central areas of pallor (MGG) should not be accepted as inclusions. The clear or ground-glass ('Orphan Annie') nuclei seen in tissue sections are represented in smears by very fine, powdery nuclear chromatin,[164] an important diagnostic criterion and a feature best appreciated in ethanol-fixed, PAP-stained smears (Figs 6.35 and 6.36).

Irregular nuclear shapes, convolutions (Fig. 6.35B) and longitudinal nuclear grooves or creases (Fig. 6.36) are visible in cytologic smears (in 85–100% cases) and in sections.[165,170] Grooves are obvious in alcohol-fixed material but are difficult to discern in MGG preparations. Strict criteria for recognition have been suggested: continuous grooves or creases, clearly defined and running the length of the nucleus.[172] The presence in ≥20% of cells, as counted in selective fields where grooves are frequent, is highly predictive of PC.[173] Grooves, however, may be found in small numbers in 70–80% of non-papillary neoplasms, in 50–60% of non-neoplastic thyroid lesions[172] and in a variety of extrathyroid tumors; hence, metastatic carcinoma and melanoma are included in differential diagnoses.[42]

Tumor cells often show delicate soap-bubble like cytoplasmic vacuolation (septate cytoplasmic vacuoles)[174]or squamoid cytoplasm (metaplastic cells). Dense cytoplasm and

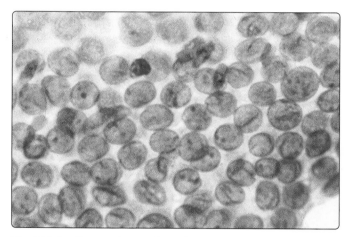

Fig. 6.36 **Papillary carcinoma** Sheet of cells with large, very pale (but not optically clear) crowded nuclei; powdery chromatin; many longitudinal grooves (Pap, HP oil).

well-defined cell margins may simulate Hurthle cells (Fig. 6.37) or squamous cells (Fig. 6.38A). True squamous metaplasia and Hurthle cell change may be present. Cells with abundant vacuolated cytoplasm are seen (Fig. 6.38B) resembling histiocytes (foam cells) but with nuclear features of PC.[162] Such 'foam cell metaplasia' is seen in about 50% of PCs and is best appreciated at the edges of the smear.[42] Foam cell metaplasia may also be seen in cystic NG with papillary hyperplasia[42] and in papillary breast lesions. Macrophages and cell debris may be prominent, especially when cystic change is present. Multinucleate giant cells are frequently seen and, if numerous, have been shown to be associated with larger tumor size and greater likelihood of extrathyroidal extension.[175] Lymphoid cells are present in 30% of cases.[176]

'Chewing gum' colloid presents as strands or chunks of dense, dark-blue (MGG) colloid, rather unlike the colloid found in other thyroid diseases (Fig. 6.39). Concentric, lamellated, calcified (psammoma) bodies are seen in

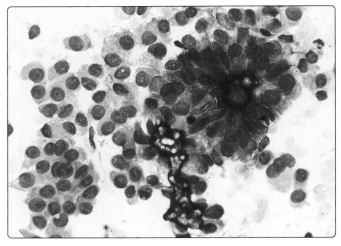

Fig. 6.37 Papillary carcinoma Poorly cohesive cells and a micropapillary cluster; psammoma bodies; abundant dense cytoplasm with distinct cell borders; uniform large nuclei, some nuclear crowding and overlapping (MGG, HP).

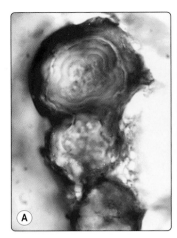 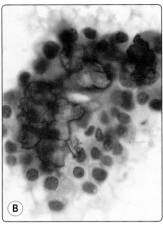

Fig. 6.40 Psammoma bodies (A) Psammoma bodies showing concentric lamellation and variable staining, partly dark blue (MGG, HP oil); (B) Follicular epithelial cells surrounding a central cluster of calcific bodies from a benign colloid nodule with cystic change (Pap, HP).

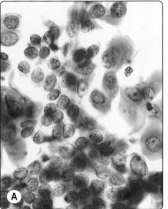 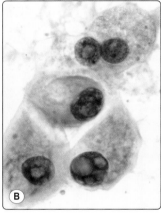

Fig. 6.38 Papillary carcinoma, 'metaplastic' cells (A) Poorly cohesive cells with large, pale, oval nuclei, a few with grooves; some cells with dense 'metaplastic' squamoid cytoplasm (Pap, HP); (B) 'Metaplastic' cells resembling macrophages, but with nuclear features of papillary carcinoma (Pap, HP oil).

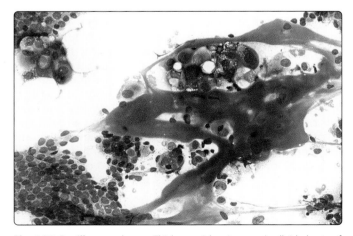

Fig. 6.39 Papillary carcinoma Thick, ropy 'chewing gum' colloid; sheets of cells with enlarged ovoid pale nuclei; some 'metaplastic' cells (MGG, IP).

cytological smears in 0–25% of cases.[177] They look glassy and refractile, measure about 100 μm, stain dark blue with MGG and red with PAP stain, and show concentric lamellations (Fig. 6.40) that distinguish them from non-specific degenerative calcium granules seen in many thyroid lesions. Although not specific to PC, when present in non-neoplastic thyroid tissue or lymph nodes they are an important clue to the presence of occult PC. In smears containing psammoma bodies, laminated hyaline globules, branching hyaline cylinders and irregular hyaline deposits can be seen.[178] Rarely, they show varying numbers of concentric layers of calcium in between the hyaline layers, suggesting an early or precursor form of psammoma bodies (intracellular, targetoid, possible precursor substances were reported in one case).[179]

Multiple criteria must be observed before making a confident cytological diagnosis of PC.[160,162] Logistic regression analysis of the various criteria suggested that a combination of INCIs, papillary structures without adherent blood vessels and dense 'metaplastic' cytoplasm were the three most important variables.[161] The presence of ≥3 of the following features – papillae, psammoma bodies, nuclear grooves, INCIs and fine granular chromatin – has been reported to facilitate cytological diagnosis of PC, with frequent grooves and INCIs being the most dependable.[164] Sensitivity and predictive value of cytological diagnosis in several large series ranged from 60% to over 90%.[30,160,161] Nuclear enlargement, atypia and nucleoli are reported to relate to recurrence.[180] BRAF oncogene mutation, associated with extrathyroidal extension, recurrence and lymph node metastasis, can be identified in cytologic material and can help in optimizing treatment.[181]

As in FC, PC cells show dual immunostaining for cytokeratin and vimentin, a feature of help in identification of distant metastases as of thyroid origin. Immunostaining for cytokeratin 19, CD44, galectin 3 and p63 have been reported to be of value in the diagnosis of PC.[182-184] Nga et al.[185] reported the combination of positive HBME-1 (luminal/membranous) and CK19 (cytoplasmic) staining on smears from PC.

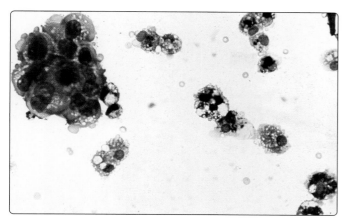

Fig. 6.41 Cystic papillary carcinoma Cystic change in metastatic papillary carcinoma in cervical lymph node; mainly foamy cells with some pigment resembling macrophages; one cluster of degenerate atypical epithelial cells (MGG, HP).

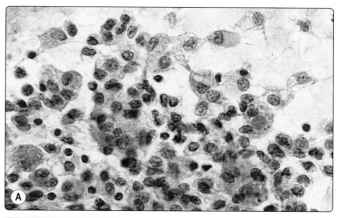

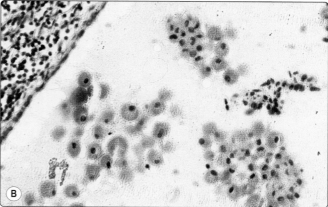

Fig. 6.42 Cystic papillary carcinoma (A) Fluid from cystic papillary carcinoma; numerous macrophages, many with pigment, some clustered; a few nuclei with longitudinal grooves; no well-preserved epithelial cells (Pap, HP); **(B)** Tissue section from a cystic metastatic deposit in lymph node from same case; transition from intact neoplastic epithelium lining the cyst to exfoliated degenerating epithelial cells to 'macrophages' with intracytoplasmic pigment (HE, IP).

PROBLEMS AND DIFFERENTIAL DIAGNOSES

- ◆ Cystic change,
- ◆ Lymphocytes and multinucleated giant cells,
- ◆ Hurthle cell metaplasia,
- ◆ Papillary hyperplasia in other lesions,
- ◆ Hyalinising trabecular tumor,
- ◆ Mimics of PC,
- ◆ FV-PC,
- ◆ Mimics of psammoma bodies.

Fluid aspirated from cystic PC is uncharacteristic, brown or resembles altered blood. The diagnosis can easily be missed if well-preserved epithelial cells are scarce (Fig. 6.41).[30,31,71] Presence of numerous macrophages, with many in cohesive clusters, should raise a suspicion of PC. Some of these cells are probably degenerating tumor cells exfoliated from the cyst lining (Fig. 6.42). They may represent foam cell metaplasia in tumor cells, and careful scrutiny will usually reveal nuclear features of PC. Large cell size, pseudoinclusions, nuclear grooves, and multiple well-defined vacuoles in atypical histiocytoid cells favor a diagnosis of PC.[186]

Tumor cells and tumor fragments in cyst fluid often show attenuation due to pressure of the cyst fluid and may not be recognizable as such in cytological and histological preparations. The sensitivity of FNA diagnosis in cystic neoplasms may be as low as 40%,[31] and all cystic lesions should be managed cautiously. Combining clinical and cytological criteria and using US-guidance while needling minimize false-negative diagnoses.[15] Cervical node metastases of PC are also often cystic and may not yield well-preserved diagnostic epithelial cells; the possibility of metastatic PC should be considered if samples of an abnormal cervical node contain only blood, fluid and histiocytes.

Smears from PC that show lymphocytes and multinucleated giant cells may simulate HT,[42] especially the diffuse sclerosing variant of PC that shows heavy lymphocytic infiltration. Close scrutiny of nuclear features is essential to avoid false-negative diagnosis. Infiltration of follicular and Hurthle cells by lymphoid cells is suggestive of HT, papillary and three-dimensional clusters of cells indicate PC. HT and PC may coexist.[109,187]

Hurthle cell metaplasia of tumor cells may simulate HCT. If all of the tumor cells are of Hurthle cell type, an oxyphilic (Hurthle cell) variant of PC should be considered (described below).

Papillary foci (with rare psammoma bodies) are present in hyperplastic NG and in GD.[188] Such hyperplastic lesions lack nuclear features of PC.

Distinction from hyalinizing trabecular tumor is discussed below.

Many features of PC, such as INCIs, grooves, papillary structures and psammoma bodies, can be seen singly or in various combinations in other neoplasms and non-neoplastic lesions. Calcific debris and inspissated colloid may mimic psammoma bodies, as can also oxalate crystals in benign thyroid lesions, but the latter are birefringent. Intraluminal colloid-associated concretions in clear cell FNs may mimic psammoma bodies. Histiocytic cells in cystic NG can mimic nuclear features of PC; immunostaining for CD68 can be useful in their distinction. Cytological diagnosis of PC should never be made from isolated cytologic characteristics but from the composite cytological picture correlated with the clinical profile. Artifacts occurring during specimen preparation and handling issues such as decalcification, frozen section, and artifacts following FNA are discussed in detail by Baloch and LiVolsi.[189]

Distinction of FV-PC from FN is described in detail in the section on FV-PC. The value of combining CK19 and HBME 1 immunostains has already been described above.[185]

Variants of papillary carcinoma

- Follicular (and macrofollicular encapsulated) variants,
- Oncocytic variant,
- Warthin tumor-like variant,
- Cribriform-morular variant,
- Adenoid cystic variant,
- Variant with fasciitis-like stroma,
- High-grade variants: tall cell, columnar, diffuse sclerosing and solid/trabecular variants.

Follicular variant of PC[134,190–192]

This has attracted great interest in recent years, probably due to difficulties in its cytological distinction from FN. The tumor shows a follicular architecture with a proportion of cells showing nuclear features of PC such as powdery pale chromatin and nuclear grooves. INCIs are less frequent. Pink colloid balls may be present. However, overall cytological features are more akin to FN such as colloid, dispersed cells, acinar and syncytial clusters (Fig. 6.43). Ninety-three to ninety-four percent cytological sensitivity and specificity have been reported in some series,[135] while other studies show that a variable proportion of nodules designated as FN proved to be FV-PC.[18,22,118] The advantage of imprint smears over frozen section was stated earlier. Recent studies indicate that FV-PC may be a heterogeneous disease composed of an infiltrative/diffuse (non-encapsulated) subvariant resembling classic PC in invasiveness and metastatic nodal pattern and an encapsulated form that behaves more like FN.[193]

Macrofollicular encapsulated variant

Characterized histologically by predominance of macrofollicles with nuclear features of PC, this may be diagnosed on cytology as a macrofollicular adenoma or NG.[194,195] Smears show large, cuboidal cells with fine nuclear chromatin, grooves, pseudoinclusions and dense eosinophilic colloid.[195]

Oncocytic variant (Fig. 6.44A,B)

This variant shows papillary and follicular structures populated by oncocytes with abundant, coarsely granular cytoplasm and nuclear features of PC. Smears show papillae and three-dimensional clusters of oncocytes, some with vascular cores.[42,196] INCIs and grooves are present. Maconucleoli are absent, an important distinguishing feature[196] from papillary HCT.[146] Differential diagnosis includes HT that is rarely associated with this variant. As this tumor is often associated with local invasion and can involve cervical lymph nodes, it may require more extensive surgery than classic PC.

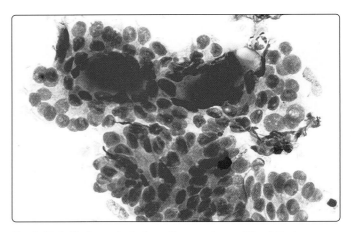

Fig. 6.43 Follicular variant of papillary carcinoma Microfollicular architectural pattern of syncytial clusters and follicles containing colloid, but enlarged, pale nuclei, some with intranuclear vacuoles (right) (MGG, HP).

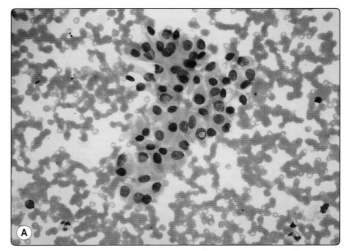

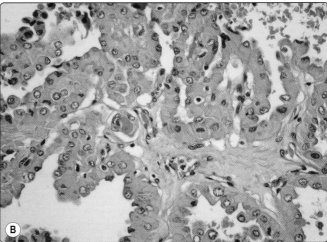

Fig. 6.44 Papillary carcinoma, oncocytic variant (A) Smear showing sheet of oncocytic cells with one cell showing INCI; (B) Tissue section of tumor showing papillae lined by oncocytic cells with nuclear features of PC.

Warthin tumor-like variant

This tumor is characterized by oncocytic tumor cells with nuclear features of PC lining papillary structures, and brisk lymphoplasmacytic infiltrates in the papillary stalks.[197] RET/PTC expression suggests a possible relationship to the oncocytic variant of PC.[198] Cytologically, these lesions appear to be a combination of PC and HT.[42,197] The oncocytes are present as single cells, cohesive and three-dimensional clusters and papillae, show granular eosinophilic cytoplasm, eccentric nuclei, prominent nucleoli and nuclear atypia. Lymphocytes and plasma cells intercalate with the cell clusters, imparting the 'ants at a picnic' appearance of HT.

Cribriform-morular variant[199,200]

This rare subtype is characterized by an admixture of cribriform structures, closely packed follicles, papillae and solid areas with islands of squamoid morules. Some cases show association with familial adenomatous polyposis. Smears show squamoid morules, cribriform structures without colloid, spindle cell whorls and papillae lined by pseudostratified columnar cells. Nuclear chromatin is fine and powdery with occasional grooves and inclusions.

Adenoid cystic variant[201,202]

Smears show papilliform clusters, monolayered sheets, psammoma bodies, many nuclear grooves and INCIs. Follicular formations with colloid are seen, some showing light pink to deep purple hyaline globules giving a laminated appearance and surrounded by neoplastic cells, reminiscent of adenoid cystic carcinoma.[201] Thyroglobulin stained the colloid and follicular cells but not the hyaline globules. Von Kossa stained the psammoma bodies and some of the hyaline globules, suggesting that these globules may be evolving psammoma bodies.

PC with nodular fasciitis-like stroma

Smears show a prominent stromal component with bland spindle cells.[203] Stromal fragments are of irregular shape and size, with extracellular matrix and desmoplasia. Sparse epithelial cell groups show features of PC.

High-grade variants of PC

These variants of PC are clinically more aggressive than the usual type.

Tall cell variant (Fig. 6.45)[134]

This tumor shows solid areas, follicles and papillae lined by oxyphilic cells twice as tall as they are wide with nuclear clearing, grooves and inclusions. Smears show oxyphilic cells with reddish or cyanophilic, granular, septated, or vacuolated cytoplasm, frequent nuclear grooves and inclusions. Lymphocytes are often present. Tadpole-like cells with basal, eccentric nuclei and high MIB-1 labeling have been reported.[204]

Columnar cell variant[205,206]

The least common variant of PC, this tumor has an aggressive course if unencapsulated. It shows a mixed papillary,

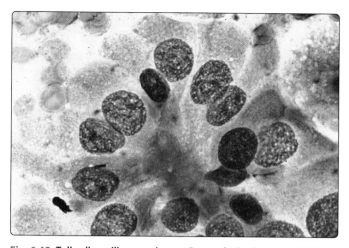

Fig. 6.45 Tall cell papillary carcinoma Group of tall columnar epithelial cells adhering to basement membrane material; abundant cytoplasm, nuclei more atypical than usual papillary carcinoma, nuclear inclusions and grooves were seen in other parts of the smear (MGG, HP oil).

follicular and solid growth pattern with tall columnar, pseudostratified cells lining papilloglandular structures. Smears show papillary and follicular structures lined by tall columnar, pseudostratified cells that resemble respiratory epithelium (Fig. 6.46).[206] Nuclear grooves and inclusions are usually not seen. Dispersed plasmacytoid cells with eccentric nuclei and focal squamous metaplasia may be present.

Diffuse sclerosing variant[95,207]

Histologically, this tumor shows prominent fibrosis, a papillary pattern, squamous metaplasia and many psammoma bodies with moderate lymphoplasmacytic infiltrates. Scattered microcalcifications impart a 'snow-storm' appearance to the US. Clues to cytologic diagnosis are prominence of squamous metaplastic cells, psammoma bodies (Fig. 6.47) and lymphocytes intermingled with tumor cells. INCIs and grooves are present.

Solid/trabecular variant

Comprising 3% of PC, this tumor has an aggressive course in adults but not in children, where it is associated with radiation exposure.[156] Fifty to seventy peercent of the tumor shows a trabecular and/or solid pattern. Nuclear features of PC are seen. Smears show solid masses and anastamotic, 2–10-cell thick trabecular cords, separated by endothelium-lined vascular spaces.[208] Tumor cells show irregular nuclear contours, with some showing grooves and inclusions.

Hyalinizing trabecular tumor
(Fig. 6.48)[167,209,210]

This is a rare thyroid tumor of follicular cell origin with a trabecular pattern of growth and marked intratrabecular hyalinization. It has been mistaken on cytology for MC and paraganglioma with which it shares morphological and architectural similarities. Smears show medium-sized, round,

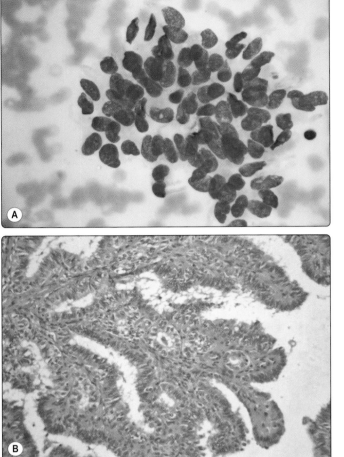

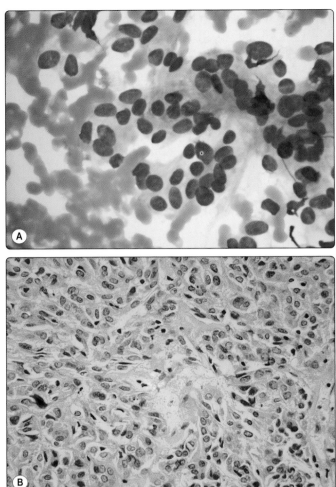

Fig. 6.46 Columnar cell variant of PC (A) Smear showing ovoid to columnar tumor cells with overlapping and pseudostratification; (B) Tissue section showing papillary structures lined by stratified columnar cells.

Fig. 6.48 Hyalinizing trabecular tumor (A) Smear showing tumor cells arranged individually, in small groups and parallel arrays with a few binucleate forms; (B) Tissue section showing tumor with trabecular pattern, intervening areas of hyalinization, and focal binucleate cells.

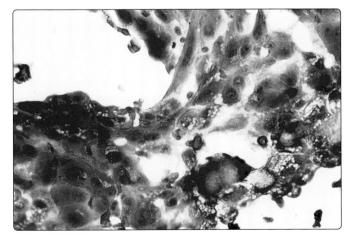

Fig. 6.47 Diffuse sclerosing variant of papillary carcinoma Distorted tissue fragment of mainly 'metaplastic' cells; fibroblasts; many psammoma bodies (*lower right*) (MGG, HP).

oval or polyhedral cells arranged individually, in small groups or parallel arrays. Cells show low nuclear cytoplasmic ratios with moderate to abundant cytoplasm. Nuclei may be eccentrically placed with focal binucleate forms that resemble Hurthle cells or MC. Cohesive aggregates are radially oriented around hyaline material. Nuclear grooves and inclusions, seen in some cases,[167] may simulate PC, while dispersed cell pattern and amorphous amyloid-like or hyaline material in the smears may resemble MC. Intracytoplasmic 'yellow bodies' (giant lysosomes) have been described.[210]

The presence of RET/PTC1 translocations[211] suggests that it may be a variant of PC, but BRAF and *ras* mutations are absent. Strong peripheral cytoplasmic and membranous MIB-1 staining is present.[212] Cases of malignant hyalinizing trabecular tumor have been recorded. However, since most reported cases behaved in a benign fashion, it is considered a benign neoplasm or one of extremely low malignant potential.[211]

Medullary carcinoma (Figs 6.49–6.57)[90,213–222]

Medullary carcinomas (MCs) constitute 5–10% of thyroid cancers[216] and are familial or sporadic with RET proto-oncogene mutations implicated in the former.[217] They are solid, firm, non-encapsulated tumors that show calcitonin-positive, round, polygonal and/or spindle cells in solid, nest-like and organoid patterns in a vascular stroma containing amyloid.[42]

Smears in MC are cellular in a background of blood. The cell pattern is predominantly dissociated with round, oval, polygonal and spindle cells in varying combinations. Plasmacytoid cells or triangular cells with eccentric nuclei are common and they show moderate amounts of cytoplasm

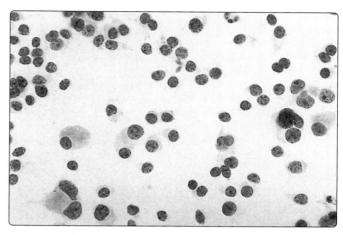

Fig. 6.50 Medullary carcinoma Dispersed cells with a 'plasmacytoid' appearance and several binucleate forms; dark nuclei (Pap, HP).

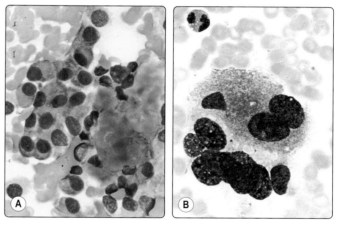

Fig. 6.51 Medullary carcinoma (A) 'Plasmacytoid' cells with abundant well-defined cytoplasm and eccentric nuclei; note clump of magenta-colored amyloid (MGG, HP); (B) Binucleate tumor cell with coarse, red intracytoplasmic granules (MGG, HP oil).

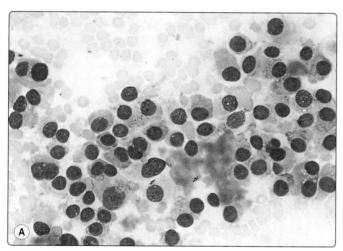

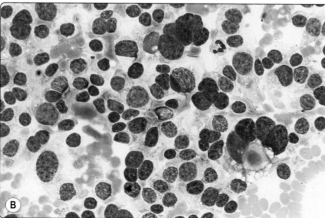

Fig. 6.49 Medullary carcinoma (A) Poorly cohesive cells with a 'plasmacytoid' appearance and moderate anisokaryosis, fragments of magenta-colored amyloid; (B) Cellular smear from another case; dispersed epithelial cells, some lined up in curved rows; anisokaryosis, many cells with two or more nuclei; stippled chromatin; a few tiny specks of amyloid (MGG, HP).

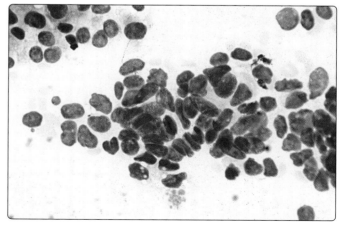

Fig. 6.52 Medullary carcinoma, small-cell pattern Densely clustered cells with ovoid crowded hyperchromatic nuclei; nuclear molding (MGG, HP).

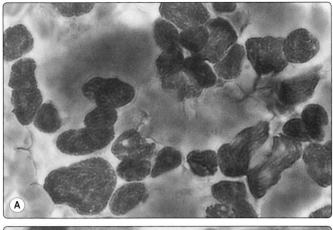

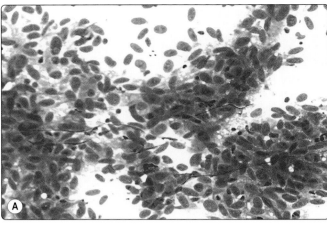

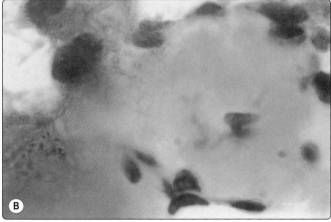

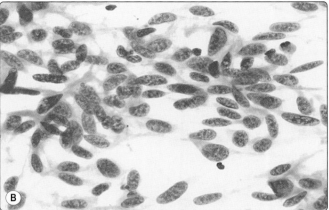

Fig. 6.53 Medullary carcinoma, amyloid (A) Clumps of hyaline material staining a magenta color with MGG; (B) Same in Pap staining pale grayish-green to orange (HP oil).

Fig. 6.54 Medullary carcinoma, spindle cell variant (A) Dispersed and clustered spindle cells with elongated nuclei mimicking a mesenchymal neoplasm (MGG, IP); (B) Spindle cells with speckled nuclear chromatin (Pap, HP).

with well-defined cell margins (Figs 6.49 A, 6.50 and 6.51 A). The small cell type shows scanty cytoplasm, high nuclear cytoplasmic ratio and ovoid nuclei, forming dense clusters, often with nuclear molding (Fig. 6.52). The spindle cell pattern shows cells with elongated, relatively pale nuclei and indistinct attenuated cytoplasm, resembling benign or low-grade spindle cell soft tissue tumors (Fig. 6.54). Nuclear chromatin may be fine and stippled (neuroendocrine-like) or coarsely granular. INCIs have been noted in occasional single cells in up to 55% of cases (Fig. 6.55).[42,90,218]

Anisocytosis is frequent with binucleate, trinucleate and multinucleate forms. Appearances may range from mono-morphic (carcinoid-like) to markedly pleomorphic, mimick-ing AC.[213] Follicular or pseudopapillary patterns may be present.

Some of the cells show coarse reddish cytoplasmic gran-ules (Fig. 6.51B) in Diff-Quik and MGG-stained smears, cor-responding to neurosecretory granules seen on electron microscopy. Calcitonin is prominently present in the granu-lar cells. Amyloid, present in 50–80% of cytological material from MC,[42] appears as dense amorphous clumps, staining variable shades of magenta with MGG and grayish-orange with PAP (Fig. 6.53). Cracking artifacts may be present. Congo-red staining and dichroism confirm the material as amyloid (which may otherwise be confused with hyaline

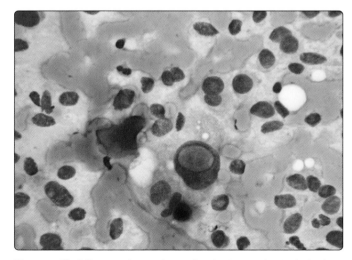

Fig. 6.55 Medullary carcinoma Smear showing intranuclear inclusion in one cell (MGG, HP).

connective tissue, condensed colloid or stroma of hyaliniz-ing trabecular tumor).

Cytologic features suggestive of secretory activity such as cytoplasmic vacuoles, azurophilic granules, marginal vacu-oles, and intracytoplasmic lumina with secretions have been reported.[218] Amyloid-like, intracellular and extracellular material was present that stained with calcitonin, as also the intracytoplasmic lumina. In cytologic smears, calcitonin-positive secretory material appeared to be diffusing out of cells.

Immunocalcitonin staining supports and greatly improves the accuracy of cytological diagnosis in MC.[214,215] The stain works well in air-dried, de-stained and wet-fixed smears and cell block preparations. If calcitonin staining is weak or equivocal, staining for chromogranin and/or carcinoembryonic antigen can be done. Electron microscopic study for demonstration of neurosecretory granules has been largely replaced by immunocytochemistry.

PROBLEMS AND DIFFERENTIAL DIAGNOSES

- Variants of MC,[42,219]
- Mixed medullary and follicular carcinoma,
- Hyalinising trabecular tumor,
- Paraganglioma,
- Amyloid in other conditions.

Papillary, oncocytic, giant cell, small cell, mucinous, squamoid, pigmented and clear cell variants of MC have been described. The small cell variant (Fig. 6.52) is difficult to distinguish from poorly differentiated carcinoma, metastatic small cell carcinoma and malignant lymphoma, the spindle cell variant (Fig. 6.54) from spindle cell mesenchymal lesions and melanoma and the giant cell type (Fig. 6.56) from AC.

Giant cells in MC usually show variation in cell size but not of cell type, as in anaplastic giant cell carcinoma, and bizarre mitoses are uncommon.[213] The oncocytic variant resembles HCT, but cytoplasmic granules in MC are reddish and macronucleoli not as common as in HCT.[42] The papillary variant may show true papillae, INCIs and psammoma bodies. PC cells, however, show dense, non-granular cytoplasm. Definitive diagnosis requires ancillary stains/ techniques. The small cell variant may be calcitonin-negative and positive for keratin and pan-endocrine markers; thus detailed clinical work-up is required to rule out metastatic small cell carcinoma.

Mixed MC and FC (Fig. 6.57)[219A] can be confused with microfollicular pattern in MC, especially if amyloid has been mistaken for colloid. The dual cell population can be highlighted by staining for calcitonin and thyroglobulin (Fig. 6.57B,C) but the possibility of residual follicles being trapped by tumor may be difficult to rule out.

Cytomorphologic overlap and distinction from hyalinising trabecular tumor have been discussed.

Cytological appearance in paraganglioma resembles MC. Clinical and radiological findings may not be of use in rare cases of intrathyroidal paraganglioma.[42] Besides, a paraganglioma-like variant of MC has been described[42] with FNA cytological appearances.[221] Immunoreactivity to a panel of pan-endocrine markers as well as calcitonin and cytokeratin are required to distinguish this from paraganglioma (possible only on cell blocks).

Amyloid may be seen in smears from amyloid goiters as well as in plasmacytoma of thyroid.[42] Attention to the morphology of the accompanying cells facilitates the diagnosis.

C-cell hyperplasia

The finding of calcitonin-positive C-cells in the absence of a discrete nodule raises the possibility of diffuse C-cell

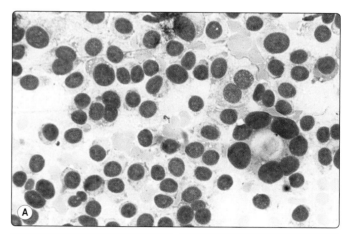

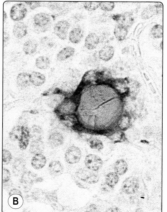
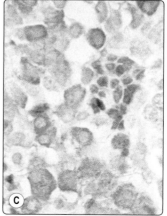

Fig. 6.57 Mixed medullary and follicular carcinoma (A) A cellular smear of dispersed cells consistent with medullary carcinoma but with some distinctly microfollicular structures (*lower right*) (MGG, HP); (B) Microfollicle highlighted by positive thyroglobulin staining; (C) Most cells are calcitonin positive; some groups negative (immunoperoxidase, same case).

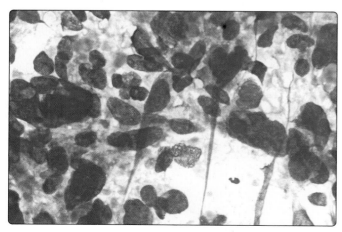

Fig. 6.56 Medullary carcinoma, giant cell variant Large pleomorphic cells resembling anaplastic carcinoma. The cells were strongly positive for calcitonin (MGG, HP).

hyperplasia. This requires further investigation since it may precede development of MC.[222]

Anaplastic carcinoma

(Figs 6.58–6.63)[42,67,213,223–225]

DIAGNOSTIC CRITERIA

◆ Necrotic background with dissociated and/or clustered highly pleomorphic malignant cells,

◆ Multinucleate, bizarre giant cells and/or spindle/squamoid cells showing marked atypia,

◆ Frequent, abnormal mitoses.

The most aggressive of all thyroid cancers, AC presents usually in women above 60 years of age as a rapidly growing, locally infiltrative, hard mass, associated with compression signs. Three major patterns or combinations of these patterns are seen, namely giant cell, spindle cell and squamoid patterns with large intervening areas of necrosis and hemorrhage.

Smears from AC may be cellular or paucicellular, depending on the amount of necrosis and the site of sampling. A malignant background diathesis of necrotic material and neutrophils is often present. Cells are extremely variable in shape and a mixture of spindle and giant cells are seen in about half of the cases. Cells show bizarre nuclei with macro-nucleoli, irregular nuclear membranes and coarsely clumped chromatin. INCIs may be present (Fig 6.59) in a fairly high proportion of cells, as in PC. Mitoses are numerous with abnormal forms. Keratinizing squamous cells may be present and are the dominating population in the squamous variant (Fig 6.60). Osteoclastic giant cells (Fig 6.62), chondroblasto-matous, or osteoblastic differentiation may be seen.[42,226,227] Bizarre cell morphology, the presence of necrosis and mitotic activity and a clinical history of a rapidly enlarging mass clinch the diagnosis. This in turn permits palliative treatment without operative intervention. Smears may show evidence of residual differentiated papillary or follicular cancer.

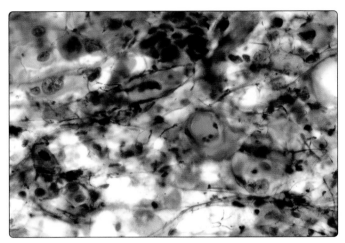

Fig. 6.60 Anaplastic carcinoma, squamous variant Smear showing keratinizing malignant cells in a necrotic background (PAP, HP).

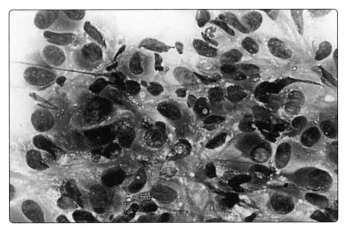

Fig. 6.58 Anaplastic giant cell carcinoma Giant mononuclear and multinucleated tumor cells (MGG, HP).

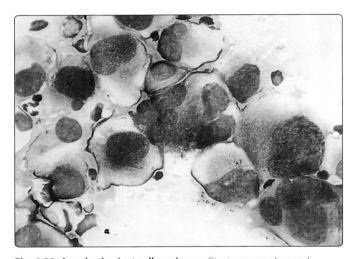

Fig. 6.59 Anaplastic spindle cell carcinoma Cluster of pleomorphic plump spindle cells resembling malignant fibrous histiocytoma; note intranuclear vacuoles (MGG, HP).

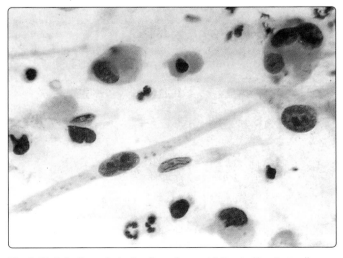

Fig. 6.61 Spindle and giant cell carcinoma Histiocyte-like giant cells; fibroblastoid spindle cells (Pap, HP).

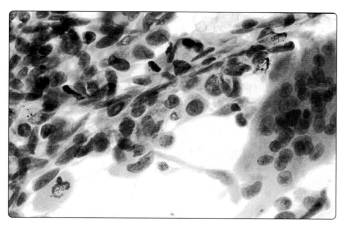

Fig. 6.62 Anaplastic carcinoma with osteoclast-like giant cells Malignant cells of spindle cell type and a multinucleated histiocytic osteoclast-like giant cell (HE, HP).

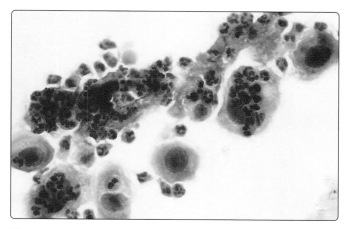

Fig. 6.63 Anaplastic carcinoma, inflammatory type Many clustering polymorphs obscuring scattered single malignant epithelial cells (Pap, HP).

Previous reports of small cell type of AC are in all probability examples of small cell type of MC, lymphoma or poorly differentiated thyroid carcinoma.

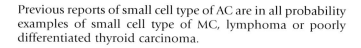

PROBLEMS AND DIFFERENTIAL DIAGNOSES

- Sampling problems leading to false-negative diagnosis,
- Mesenchymal tumors,
- Other thyroid neoplasms,
- Laryngeal carcinoma,
- Metastatic malignancies,
- Reactive changes.

Necrosis, fibrosis and inflammation may dominate the cytological picture, obscuring diagnostic cells (Fig 6.63). Diagnostic reliability in AC is limited mainly by the sampling technique. The false-negative cytologic rate can be as high as 12% and is mainly due to non-representative sampling.[42] In order to ensure adequate sampling, large tumor masses should be subjected to at least 3–4 needle passes at different sites, concentrating on firm areas of the lesion. Paucicellular variants of AC are difficult to diagnose on cytology[225] and may mimic Riedel's thyroiditis.[42]

The spindle cell variant of AC (Fig. 6.59) may be indistinguishable from spindle cell sarcomas. Immunostaining for cytokeratin, if positive, supports a diagnosis of AC. However, cytokeratin positivity is not always present and it may be focal (personal observation). Lack of thyroglobulin immunostaining helps distinguish it from poorly differentiated foci of differentiated thyroid carcinoma.

AC may contain remnants of pre-existing follicular or papillary neoplasms.[42] If the needle has only sampled the differentiated component, the diagnosis of AC can be missed. Presence of INCIs in AC (Fig. 6.59) may cause confusion with high-grade PC. Grossly abnormal nuclear chromatin, tumor necrosis, mitotic activity and loss of expression of thyroglobulin suggest AC. MC of giant cell type may resemble AC cytologically; immunostaining for calcitonin and CEA are required.

Laryngeal carcinoma can occasionally extend and infiltrate the thyroid. If smears show a dominant squamoid pattern,

a laryngoscopic examination is recommended to rule out a primary laryngeal carcinoma.

Giant cell carcinomas of pancreas and lung,[90] sarcomatoid renal cell carcinoma and spindle cell melanomas may metastasize to thyroid and simulate giant cell or spindle cell types of AC, respectively. The value of correlating the cytologic picture with the clinical profile and relevant investigations cannot be overestimated.

Mitotically active, atypical reactive myofibroblasts are occasionally seen in thyroiditis and NG.[90] Follicular cells undergoing repair may show nuclear aytpia with macronucleoli. Radioactive iodine and neomercazole treatment for GD leads to follicular atypia (see Fig. 6.8B). Careful history taking and thorough clinical assessment reduce diagnostic errors in most cases.

Lymphoma (Figs 6.64, 6.65)[90,228,229]

Lymphoma may involve the thyroid secondarily. Primary thyroid lymphoma is rare (1–5% of thyroid malignancies).[230] Most are of B-cell lineage, of MALT type and often occur in a background of HT.[42]

High-grade lymphomas show a dispersed population of predominantly large abnormal lymphoid cells of blastic type (Fig. 6.64). Patients are usually elderly females presenting with rapid thyroid enlargement and pressure symptoms, clinically mimicking AC. Low-grade lymphomas, especially with coexistent HT, present a diagnostic problem, as discussed earlier. A mixed cell population including plasma cells, suggestive of a florid reactive process, may be seen in smears of low-grade lymphoma. Diagnostic difficulties are enhanced by the presence of residual reactive follicles in low-grade MALT lymphoma. Primary thyroid involvement by Hodgkin's disease is rare but has been documented.[42]

PROBLEMS AND DIFFERENTIAL DIAGNOSES

- Low-grade lymphomas,
- Small cell non-lymphoid tumors,
- Langerhans cell histiocytosis.

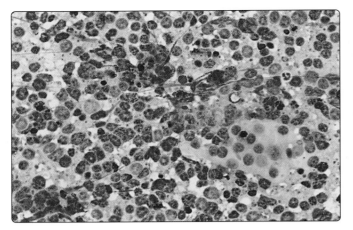

Fig. 6.64 Malignant lymphoma, high grade Highly cellular smear of predominantly large blastic lymphoid cells; note cluster of pale residual follicular epithelial cells (MGG, IP).

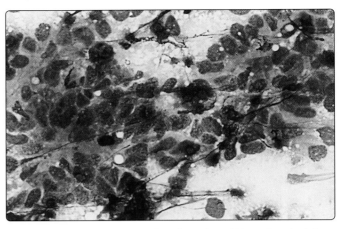

Fig. 6.66 Metastatic carcinoma from large bowel Note microglandular structures, columnar cells and necrotic debris (MGG, HP).

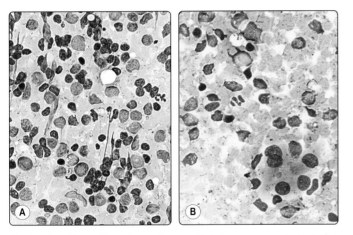

Fig. 6.65 Malignant lymphoma, low grade, in Hashimoto's disease The two figures are from the same case. (**A**) Mixed population of abnormal lymphoid cells, the majority are centrocyte-like; (**B**) Thyroiditis pattern of mixed lymphoid cells and a cluster of oxyphil epithelial cells (MGG, IP).

Distinction of low-grade lymphomas from HT is difficult and requires flow cytometry and immunocytochemical demonstration of monoclonality.[228] Situations where both diseases coexist are further complicated by sampling problems. Selective needling of the recently enlarging nodule often yields diagnostic samples. General principles guiding the distinction of non-Hodgkin's lymphoma from reactive lymphoid infiltrates are covered in Chapter 5.

Apart from the rare small cell variant of MC, true anaplastic small cell carcinoma is extremely rare. Round fragments of pale blue cytoplasm in the background (lymphoglandular bodies) favor lymphoma, while cell clustering, nuclear molding and tear-drop cells favor small cell AC. Metastatic small cell carcinoma should be excluded. Immunostaining is indispensable.

Langerhans cell histiocytosis rarely involves the thyroid as a part of multiorgan disease[231] and may be mistaken cytologically for lymphoma. Admixture with eosinophils and multinucleate giant cells, indentation of nuclei, dendrite-like cytoplasmic processes and positive staining with S-100 protein are clues to the diagnosis.

Uncommon malignancies of thyroid

Mucoepidermoid carcinoma of thyroid can be rarely encountered on FNA where it is usually diagnosed as poorly differentiated carcinoma.[232,233] Brief reports of the cytology of angiosarcoma and Kaposi's sarcoma of thyroid, hemangioendothelioma, osteosarcoma, and metastatic sarcoma are present in the literature.[42,234–236] Teratomas[237,238] occur rarely in the thyroid and are mainly seen in infants or children where they are usually benign.[42] A few teratomas reported in adults were malignant, with the tumor showing a prominent primitive neuroepithelial component. FNA smears in an aggressive and rapidly fatal tumor in a young female[238] showed features suggestive of primitive neuroectodermal tumor with frequent neuroblastoma-like rosettes. Histology of the resected tumor showed neural tubules and neurites, squamous and glandular epithelium with nodal metastasis showing a neuroepithelial pattern.

Metastatic malignancies (Figs 6.29, 6.66 and 6.67)[42]

Metastasis to the thyroid is usually a terminal event in disseminated malignancies, questioning the rationale of conventional treatment. Cytology is very useful in determining whether the lesion in a known case of cancer is a metastasis, a thyroid primary or a non-neoplastic thyroid lesion. Rarely, thyroid metastases may be the presenting feature of an otherwise occult primary (such as renal cell carcinoma).[42] A metastatic tumor can clinically simulate a primary neoplasm or even thyroiditis.[112] Lung, gastrointestinal tract (Fig. 6.66), breast (see Fig. 6.29), kidney, melanoma and lymphoma are the most frequent sites of origin. Breast carcinoma may resemble and be misinterpreted as poorly differentiated follicular carcinoma of thyroid (Fig. 6.67), and the importance of clinical notes cannot be overemphasized. When cytological features are at variance with those seen in primary thyroid cancers, it is a good policy to meticulously go through the clinical notes for any record of other previous primary cancers and to request cytology and histopathology slides of the case for review.

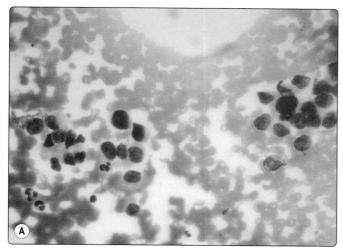

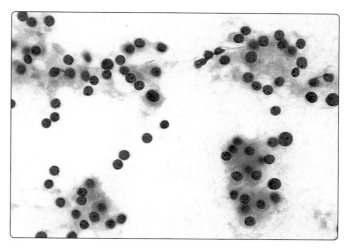

Fig. 6.68 **Parathyroid adenoma** Microfollicular pattern but no colloid; small nuclei, pale fragile cytoplasm, many naked nuclei (Pap, HP).

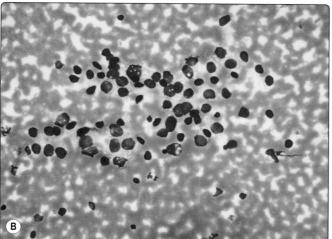

Fig. 6.67 **Metastatic breast and thyroid carcinoma, overlapping cytological features** (A) Smear from breast carcinoma metastatic to thyroid (MGG, HP); (B) Smear from follicular carcinoma metastatic to clavicle (MGG, HP).

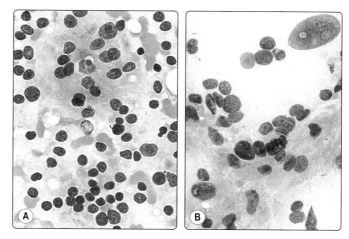

Fig. 6.69 **Parathyroid adenoma** (A) Chief cell type; dispersed cells with small round nuclei, moderate anisokaryosis, most nuclei stripped; (B) Oxyphil parathyroid adenoma; more prominent anisokaryosis, abundant but poorly defined cytoplasm; intranuclear cytoplasmic inclusions (MGG; A, IP; B, HP).

Based on cytomorphologic pattern the following possibilities may be considered and clinical details and relevant ancillary stains used for their distinction:

Clear cell morphology: Metastasis from renal cell carcinoma, salivary gland carcinoma, clear cell melanoma, thyroid and parathyroid tumors showing clear cell change.

Papillary morphology: PC of thyroid, breast carcinoma, rare cases of melanoma.[239]

Oncocytic cells: HCT, oncocytic variants of PC and MC, renal cell carcinoma, salivary gland carcinoma.

Small round cells: Lymphoma, small cell variant of MC, poorly differentiated thyroid carcinoma, metastatic small cell carcinoma, malignant teratoma.

Mucin producing cells: Colonic and lung carcinomas, salivary gland carcinoma, rare mucin-producing variant of MC.

Squamous morphology: AC, laryngeal and lung carcinoma.

Spindle cell morphology: MC, AC, primary and metastatic spindle cell sarcomas, melanoma, sarcomatoid renal, pancreatic and lung carcinomas, atypical reactive myofibroblasts.

Pleomorphic multinucleate giant cells: AC, metastatic pleomorphic sarcomas and giant cell carcinomas of pancreas and lung.

Parathyroid neoplasms (Figs 6.68 and 6.69)[136,240–242]

Parathyroid neoplasms and cysts have been discussed briefly in the earlier section. Cytology is of limited value in the preoperative assessment of patients with hyperparathyroidism. If a parathyroid adenoma cannot be located by surgery, cytology in conjunction with US examination of the neck or mediastinal CT can be tried. High cellularity, aggregates of cohesive cells with small nuclei 6–8 μm in diameter, coarse granular chromatin, some larger nuclei 10–30 μm, numerous bare nuclei, scattered oxyphil cells and absence of colloid or macrophages indicate parathyroid tissue.[240,242,244] Papillae and INCIs (Fig 6.69) have been noted.[243,245] Monolayered sheets and microfollicular structures suggest thyroid origin,[243] but have been seen in parathyroid adenoma (Fig. 6.68); it is agreed that no single cytologic feature can definitely distinguish parathyroid from thyroid follicular nodules.

References

1. Söderstrom N. Puncture of goiters for aspiration biopsy. A preliminary report. Acta Med Scand 1952;144:235–44.

2. Einhorn J, Franzén S. Thin-needle biopsy in the diagnosis of thyroid disease. Acta Radiol 1962;58:321–36.

3. Kini SR. Thyroid. In: Kline TS, editor. Guides to clinical aspiration biopsy, 2nd ed. New York: Igaku-Shoin; 1996.

4. Ashcroft MW, van Herle AJ. Management of thyroid nodules II. Head Neck Surg 1981;3:297–322.

5. Löwhagen T, Granberg PO, Lundell G, et al. Aspiration biopsy cytology (ABC) in nodules of the thyroid gland suspected to be malignant. Surg Clin North Am 1979;59:3–18.

6. Cramer H. Fine-needle aspiration of the thyroid. An appraisal. Cancer (Cancer Cytopathol) 2000;90:325–9.

7. Ashcroft MW, van Herle AJ. Management of thyroid nodules. I. Head, Neck Surg 1981;3:216–30.

8. Layfield LJ, Cibas ES, Gharib H, Mandel SJ. Thyroid aspiration cytology: current status. CA Cancer J Clin 2009;59:99–110.

9. Khalid AN, Hollenbeak CS, Quraishi SA, et al. The cost-effectiveness of iodine 131 scintigraphy, ultrasonography, and fine-needle aspiration biopsy in the initial diagnosis of solitary thyroid nodules. Arch Otolaryngol Head Neck Surg 2006;132:244–50.

10. Yang J, Schnadiq V, Logrono R, Wasseman PG. Fine-needle aspiration of thyroid nodules: a study of 4703 patients with histological and clinical correlations. Cancer 2007;111:306–15.

11. Ravetto C, Colombo L, Dottorini ME. Usefulness of fine-needle aspiration in the diagnosis of thyroid carcinoma. A retrospective study in 37,895 patients. Cancer (Cancer Cytopathol) 2000;90:357–63.

12. Sangalli G, Serio G, Zampatti C, et al. Fine needle aspiration cytology of the thyroid: a comparison of 5469 cytological and final histological diagnoses. Cytopathology 2006;17:245–50.

13. Schmid KW, Ladurner D, Zechmann W, et al. Clinicopathologic management of tumours of the thyroid gland in an endemic goitre area. Combined use of preoperative fine needle aspiration biopsy and intraoperative frozen section. Acta Cytol 1989;33:27–30.

14. Muruganandham K, Sistla SC, Elangovan S. et al. Routine ultrasound-guided aspiration cytology for evaluation of palpable thyroid nodules in an endemic area: is it justified? J Otolaryngol Head Neck Surg 2009;38:222–6.

15. Nabriski D, Ness-Abramof R, Brosh TO, et al. Clinical relevance of non-palpable thyroid nodules as assessed by ultrasound-guided fine needle aspiration biopsy. J Endocrinol Invest 2003;26:3–4.

16. AACE/AME task force on thyroid nodules. American association of clinical endocrinologists and Associazione Medici Endocrinologi medical guidelines for clinical practice for the diagnosis and management of thyroid nodules. Endocr Pract 2006;12:63–102.

17. Cesur M, Corapcioglu D, Bulut S, et al. Comparison of palpation-guided fine needle aspiration biopsy to ultrasound guided fine-nedle aspiration biopsy in the evaluation of thyroid nodules. Thyroid 2006;16:555–61.

18. Dobrinja C, Trevisian G, Ligouri G, et al. Sensitivity evaluation of fine needle aspiration cytology in thyroid lesions. Diagn Cytopathol 2009;37:230–5.

19. Screaton NJ, Berman LH, Grant JW. US-guided core-needle biopsy of the thyroid gland. Radiology 2003;226:827–32.

20. Renshaw AA, Pinnar N. Comparison of thyroid fine-needle aspiration and core needle biopsy. Am J Clin Pathol 2007;128:370–4.

21. Yang GC, Liebeskind D, Messina AV. Should cytopathologists stop reporting follicular neoplasms on fine-needle aspiration of the thyroid? Diagnosis and histologic follow-up of 147 cases. Cancer (Cancer Cytopathol) 2003;99:69–74.

22. De May RM. Follicular lesions of the thyroid. W(h)ither follicular carcinoma? Am J Clin Pathol 2000;114:681–3.

23. Kini SR, Miller JM, Hamburger JI, Smith-Purslowe MJ, et al. Cytopathology of follicular lesions of the thyroid gland. Diagn Cytopathol 1985;1:123–32.

24. LiVolsi VA, Asa SL. The demise of follicular carcinoma of the thyroid gland. Thyroid 1994;4:233–6.

25. Abati A. The National Cancer Institute Thyroid FNA State of the Science Conference: 'Wrapped up'. Diagn Cytopathol 2008;36:388–9.

26. Bibbo M. Thyroid fine needle aspiration. Aca Cytol 2009;53:489–90.

27. Hall TL, Layfield LJ, Philippe A, et al. Sources of diagnostic error in fine needle aspiration of the thyroid. Cancer 1989;63:718–25.

28. Silverman JF, West RL, Larkin EW, et al. The role of fine needle aspiration biopsy in the rapid diagnosis and management of thyroid neoplasm. Cancer 1986;57:1164–70.

29. La Rosa GL, Belfiore A, Giuffrida D, et al. Evaluation of the fine needle aspiration biopsy in the preoperative selection of cold thyroid nodules. Cancer 1991;67:2137–41.

30. Hsu C, Boey J. Diagnostic pitfalls in the fine needle aspiration of thyroid nodules. A study of 555 cases in Chinese patients. Acta Cytol 1987;31:699–704.

31. Sarda AK, Bal S, Dutta Gupta S, et al. Diagnosis and treatment of cystic disease of the thyroid by aspiration. Surgery 1988;103:593–6.

32. Hor T, Lahiri SW. Bilateral thyroid hematomas after fine-needle aspiration causing acute airway obstruction. Thyroid 2008;18:567–9.

33. Park MH, Yoon JH. Anterior neck hematoma causing airway compression following fine needle aspiration cytology of the thyroid nodule; a case report. Acta Cytol 2009;53:86–8.

34. Anastasilakis AD, Polyzos SA, Nikolopoulos P. Subendothelial carotid hematoma after fine-needle aspiration biopsy of a solitary thyroid nodule. J Ultrasound Med 2008;27:1517–20.

35. Alkan S, Kosar AT, Erdurak SC, et al. Transient vocal cord paralysis following ultrasound-guided fine needle aspiratin biopsy for a thyroid nodule. J Otolaryngol Head Neck Surg 2009;38: E14–15.

36. Van den Bruel A, Roelandt P, Drijkoningen M, et al. A thyroid thriller: acute transient and symmetric goiter after fine-neelde aspiration of a solitary thyroid nodule. Thyroid 2008;18:81–4.

37. Nishihara E, Miyauchi A, Matsuzuka F, et al. Acute suppurative thyroiditis after fine-needle aspiration causing thyrotoxicosis. Thyroid 2005;15:1183–7.

38. Musharrefieh UM, Nasrallah MP, et al. Chemical neuritis after fine needle aspiration biopsy of thyroid nodule. J Endocrinol Invest 2006;29:947–8.

39. Das DK, Janardan C, Pathan SK, et al. Infarction in a thyroid nodule after fine needle aspiration. Report of 2 cases with a discussion of the cause of pitfalls in the histopatholgoical diagnosis of papillary thyroid carcinoma. Acta Cytol 2009;53:571–5.

40. Bolat F, Kayaselcuk F, Nursal TZ, et al. Histopathological changes in thyroid tissue after fine needle aspiration biopsy. Pathol Res Pract 2007;203:641–5.

41. Sharma C, Krishnanand G. Histologic analysis and comparison of techniques in fine needle aspiration-induced alterations in thyroid. Acta Cytol 2008;52:56–64.

42. Jayaram G. Atlas and text of thyroid cytology. New Delhi: Arya Publications; 2006.

43. Karwowski JK, Nowels KW, McDougall IR, et al. Needle track seeding of papillary thyroid carcinoma from fine needle aspiration biopsy. A case report. Acta Cytol 2002;46:591–5.

44. Tamiolakis D, Antoniou C, Venizelos J, et al. Papillary thyroid carcinoma metastasis most probably due to fine needle aspiration biopsy. A case report. Acta Dermatovenerol Alp Panonica Adriat 2008;15:169–72.

45. Uchida N, Suda T, Inoue T, et al. Needle track disseminatin of follicular thyroid carcinoma following fine-needle aspiration biopsy: report of a case. Surg Today 2007;37:34–7.

46. Zhu W, Michael CW. How important is on-site adequacy assessment for thyroid FNA? An evaluation of 883 cases. Diagn Cytopathol 2007;35:183–6.

47. Layfield LJ, Bentz JS, Gopez EV. Immediate on-site interpretation of fine-needle aspiration smears. A cost and compensation analysis. Cancer 2001;93:319–22.

48. Baloch ZW, Tam D, Langer J, et al. Ultrasound-guided fine-needle aspiration biopsy of the thyroid: role of on-site assessment and multiple cytological preparations. Diagn Cytopathol 2000;23:425–9.

49. Rosen IB, Azadian A, Walfish PG, et al. Ultrasound-guided fine-needle aspiration biopsy in the management of thyroid disease. Am J Surg 1993;166:346–9.

50. Qiu L, Crapanzano JP, Saqi A, et al. Cell block alone as an ideal preparatory method for hemorrhagic thyroid nodule aspirates procured without onsite cytologists. Acta Cytol 2008;52:139–44.

51. Stamataki M, Anninos D, Brountzos E, et al. The role of liquid-based cytology in the investigation of thyroid lesions. Cytopathology 2008;19:11–18.

52. Ljung BM. Thyroid fine-needle aspiration: smears versus liquid-based preparations. Cancer 2008;114:144–8.

53. Kato MA, Fahey 3rd TJ. Molecular markers in thyroid cancer diagnostics. Surg Clin North Am 2009;89:1139–55.

54. Maruta J, Hashimoto H, Yamashita H, et al. Immunostaining of galectin-3 and CD44v6 using fine-needle aspiration for distinguishing follicular carcinoma from adenoma. Diagn Cytopathol 2004;31:392–6.

55. Penelli G, Mian C, Pelizzo MR, et al. Galectin-3 cytotest in thyroid follicular neoplasia. A prospective, monoinstitutional study. Acta Cytol 2009;53:533–9.

56. Collet JF, Hurbain I, Prengel C, et al. Galectin-3 immunodetection in follicular thyroid neoplasms: a prospective study on fine-needle aspiration samples. Br J Cancer 2005;93:1175–81.

57. Christensen L, Bilchert-Toft M, Brandt M, et al. Thyroperoxidase (TPO) immunostaining of the solitary cold thyroid nodule. Clin Endocrinol 2000;53:161–9.

58. Lerma E, Mora J. Telomerase activity in 'suspicious' thyroid cytology. Cancer 2005;105:492–7.

59. Lubitz CC, Ugras SK, Kazam JJ, et al. Microarray analysis of thyroid nodule fine-needle aspirates accurately classifies benign and malignant lesions. J Mol Diagn 2006;8:490–8.

60. Troncone G, Volante M, Iaccarino A, et al. Cyclin D1 and D3 overexpression predicts malignant behavior in thyroid fine-needle aspirates suspicious for Hurthle cell neoplasms. Cancer Cytopathol 2009;117:522–9.

61. Boon ME, Löwhagen T, Cardozo PL, et al. Computation of preoperative diagnosis probability for follicular adenoma and carcinoma of the thyroid on aspiration smears. Anal Quant Cytol 1982;4:1–5.

62. La Rosa GL, Cavallari V, Giuffrida D, et al. The morphometric analysis of all nuclei from fine needle aspirates of thyroid follicular cells does not improve the diagnostic accuracy of traditional cytological examination. J Endocrinol Invest 1990;13:701–7.

63. Solymosi T, Tóth V, Sápi Z, et al. Diagnostic value of AgNOR method in thyroid cytopathology: correlation with morphometric measurements. Diagn Cytopathol 1996;14:140–4.

64. Bäckdahl M, Wallin G, Lowhagen T, et al. Fine needle biopsy cytology and DNA analysis. Their place in the evaluation and treatment of patients with thyroid neoplasms. Surg Clin North Am 1987;67:197–211.

65. Raab SS, Vrbin CM, Grzybicki DM, et al. Errors in thyroid gland fine needle aspriration. Am J Clin Pathol 2006;125:873–82.

66. Hamburger JI, Husain M, Nishiyama R, et al. Increasing the accuracy of fine needle biopsy for thyroid nodules. Arch Pathol Lab Med 1989;113:1035–41.

67. Droese M. Cytological aspiration biopsy of the thyroid gland, 2nd ed. Stuttgart: Schattauer; 1995.

68. Suen KC. How does one separate cellular follicular lesions of the thyroid by fine needle aspiration biopsy? Diagn Cytopathol 1988;4:78–81.

69. Nassar A, Gupta P, LiVolsi VA, et al. Histiocytic aggregates in benign nodular goitres mimicking cytologic features of papillary thyroid carcinoma (PTC). Diagn Cytopathol 2003;29:243–5.

70. Gul K, Di Ri Doc A, Ki Yak G, et al. Thyroid carcinoma risk in patients with hyperthyroidism and role of preoperative cytology in diagnosis. Minerva Endocrinol 2009;34:281–8.

71. Jayaram G, Kaur A. Cystic thyroid nodules harbouring malignancy. A problem in fine needle aspiration cytodiagnosis. Acta Cytol 1989;33:941–2.

72. Hamburger JI, Hamburger SW. Fine needle biopsy of thyroid nodules: avoiding the pitfalls. NY State J Med 1986;86:241–9.

73. Jaragh M, Carvdis VB, MacMillan C, et al. Predictors of malignancy in thyroid fine-needle aspirates 'cyst fluid only' cases; can potential clues of malignancy be identified? Cancer Cytopathol 2009;117:305–10.

74. Caraway NP, Sneige N, Samaan NA. Diagnostic pitfalls in thyroid fine-needle aspiration: a review of 394 cases. Diagn Cytopathol 1993;9:345–9.

75. Shahin A, Burroughs FH, Kirby JP, et al. Thyroglossal duct cyst: a cytopathologic study of 26 cases. Diagn Cytopathol 2005;33:365–9.

76. Dim DC, Riveros-Angel M, Wong-You-Cheong J, et al. Ultrasound guided fine needle aspiration cytology diagnosis of a foregut cyst in the thyroid. A case report. Acta Cytol 2009.

77. Chen KT. Fine-needle aspiration cytology of epidermoid cyst of the thyroid: report of a case and review of seven cases. Diagn Cytopathol 2007;35:123–4.

78. Lerud KS, Tabbara SO, Del Vecchio DM, et al. Cytomorphology of cystic parathyroid lesions: report of four cases evaluated preoperatively by fine-needle aspiration. Diagn Cytopathol 1996;15:306–11.

79. Paes JE, Burman KD, Cohen J, et al. Acute bacterial suppurative thyroiditis: a clinical review and expert opinion. Thyroid 2010;20:247–55.

80. Trbojevic B, Djurica S. Diagnosis of autoimmune thyroid disease. Srp Arh Celok Lek 2005;133(Suppl. 1):25–33.

81. Persson PS. Cytodiagnosis of thyroiditis. A comparative study of cytological, histological, immunological and clinical findings in thyroiditis. Acta Med Scand 1968;483(Suppl.):7–100.

82. Jayaram G, Singh B, Marwaha RK. Graves' disease. Appearance in cytologic smears from fine needle aspirates of the thyroid gland. Acta Cytol 1989;33:36–40.

83. Volavsek M, Us-Krasovec M, Auersperg M, et al. Marginal vacuoles in fine-needle aspirates of follicular thyroid carcinoma. Diagn Cytopathol 1996;15:93–7.

84. Das DK, Jain S, Tripathi KP, et al. Marginal vacuoles in thyroid aspirates. Acta Cytol 1998;42:1121–8.

85. Sturgis CD. Radioactive iodine-associated cytomorphologic alterations in thyroid follicular epithelium: is recognition possible in fine-needle aspiration specimens? Diagn Cytopathol 1999;21:207–10.

86. Gutteridge DH, Orell SR. Non-toxic goitre: diagnostic role of aspiration cytology, antibodies and serum thyrotrophin. Clin Endocrinol 1978;9:505–14.

87. Jayaram G, Marwaha RK, Gupta RK, et al. Cytomorphologic aspects of thyroiditis. A study of 51 cases with functional, immunologic and ultrasonographic data. Acta Cytol 1987;31:687–93.

88. Poropatich C, Marcus D, Oertel YC. Hashimoto's thyroiditis: fine-needle aspirations of 50 asymptomatic cases. Diagn Cytopathol 1994;11:141–5.

88A. Singh A, Kahlon SK, Chahal KS, et al. Hashimoto's thyroiditis – an unusual presentation as cystic solitary nodule – a diagnostic dilemma. J Cytol 2003; 20(4):193–5.

89. Nguyen G-K, Ginsberg J, Crockford PM, et al. Hashimoto's thyroiditis: cytodiagnostic accuracy and pitfalls. Diagn Cytopathol 1997;16:531–6.

90. De May RM. The art and science of cytopathology-Vol II- aspiration cytology. Chicago: ASCP Press; 1996.

91. Roasai Juan, editor. Rosai and Ackerman's Surgical Pathoogy, 9th ed. St. Louis. MO: Mosby; 2004.

92. Okayasu I, Hatakeyama S, Tanaka Y, et al. Is focal chronic autoimmune thyroiditis an age-related disease? Differences in incidence and severity between Japanese and British. J Pathol 1991;163:257–64.

93. Jayaram G, Iyengar KR, Sthaneshwar P, et al. Hashimoto's thyroiditis; a Malaysian perspective. J Cytology 2007;24:119–24.

94. Singh N, Kumar S, Negi VS, et al. Cytomorphologic study of Hashimoto's thyroiditis and its serologic correlation. A study of 150 cases. Acta Cytol 2009;53:507–16.

95. Kumarasinghe MP. Cytomorphologic features of diffuse sclerosing variant of papillary carcinoma of the thyroid. A report of two cases in children. Acta Cytol 1998;42:983–6.

96. Yousef O, Dichard A, Bocklage T. Aspiration cytology features of the Warthin tumour-like variant of papillary thyroid carcinoma. A report of two cases. Acta Cytol 1997;41:1361–8.

97. Zeppa P, Cossolino I, Peluso AL, et al. Cytologic, flow cytometry and molecular assessment of lymphoid infiltrate in fine-needle cytology samples of Hashimoto thyroiditis. Cancer Cytopathol 2009;117:174–84.

98. Kini SR, Miller JM, Hamburger JI. Cytopathology of Hurthle cell lesions of the thyroid gland by fine needle aspiration. Acta Cytol 1981;25:647–52.

99. Gonzalez JL, Wang HH, Ducatman BS. Fine-needle aspiration of Hurthle cell lesions. A cytomorphologic approach to diagnosis. Am J Clin Pathol 1993;100:231–5.

100. Ravinsky E, Safneck JR. Differentiation of Hashimoto's thyroiditis from thyroid neoplasm in fine needle aspirates. Acta Cytol 1988;32: 854–61.

101. Kollur SM, El Sayed S, El Hag A. Follicular thyroid lesions coexisting with Hashimoto's thyroiditis: incidence and possible sources of diagnostic errors. Diagn Cytopathol 2003;28:35–8.

102. McDonald L, Yadzi HM. Fine needle aspiration biopsy of Hashimoto's thyroiditis. Sources of diagnostic error. Acta Cytol 1999;43:400–6.

103. Carson HJ, Castelli MJ, Gattuso P. Incidence of neoplasia in Hashimoto's thyroiditis. A fine-needle aspiration study. Diagn Cytopathol 1996;14: 38–42.

104. Friedman M, Shimaoka K, Rao U, et al. Diagnosis of chronic lymphocytic thyroiditis (nodular presentation) by needle aspiration. Acta Cytol 1981; 25:513–22.

105. Kini SR, Miller JM, Hamburger JI. Problems in the cytologic diagnosis of the 'cold' thyroid nodule in patients with lymphocytic thyroiditis. Acta Cytol 1981;25:506–12.

106. Bhalotra R, Jayaram G. Overlapping morphology in thyroiditis (Hashimoto's and subacute) and Grave's disease. Cytopathology 1990;1:371–2.

107. Harigopal M, Sahoo S, Recant WM, et al. Fine-needle aspiration of Riedel's disease: report of a case and review of the literature. Diagn Cytopathol 2004;30:193–7.

108. Dugan JM, Atkinson BF, Avitabile A, et al. Psammoma bodies in fine needle aspirate of the thyroid in lymphocytic thyroiditis. Acta Cytol 1987;31:330–4.

109. Cipolla C, Sandonato L, Graceffa G, et al. Hashimoto thyroiditis coexistent with papillary thyroid carcinoma. Am Surg 2005;71:874–8.

110. Sidaway MK, Costa M. The significance of paravacuolar granules of the thyroid. A histologic, cytologic and ultrastructural study. Acta Cytol 1989;33:929–34.

111. Shabb NS, Tawil A, Gergeos F, et al. Multinucleated giant cells in fine-needle aspiration of thyroid nodules: their diagnostic significance. Diagn Cytopathol 1999;21:307–12.

112. Rosen IB, Strawbridge HG, Walfish PG, et al. Malignant pseudothyroiditis: a new clinical entity. Am J Surg 1978; 136:445–9.

113. Prakash R, Jayaram G, Singh RP. Follicular thyroid carcinoma masquerading as subacute thyroiditis diagnosis using ultrasonography and radionuclide thyroid angiography. Australas Radiol 1991;35:174–7.

114. Carney JA, Moore SB, Northcutt RC, et al. Palpation thyroiditis (multifocal granulomatous folliculitis). Am J Clin Pathol 1975;64:639–47.

115. Shigemasa C, Kouchi T, Taniguchi S, et al. Autoimmune thyroiditis with transient thyrotoxicosis: comparison between painful thyroiditis and painless thyroiditis. Horm Res 1991; 36:9–15.

116. Mizukami Y, Michigishi T, Hashimoto T, et al. Silent thyroiditis: A histologic and immunohistochemical study. Hum Pathol 1988;19:423–31.

117. Atkinson B, Ernest CS, Li Volsi V. Cytologic diagnosis of follicular tumours of the thyroid. Diagn Cytopathol 1986;2:1–5.

118. Baloch ZW, Fleisher S, LiVolsi VA, et al. Diagnosis of 'follicular neoplasm': A gray zone in thyroid fine needle aspiration cytology. Diagn Cytopathol 2002;26:41–4.

119. Harach HR. Usefulness of fine needle aspiration of the thyroid in an endemic goitre region. Acta Cytol 1989;33:31–5.

120. Busseniers AE, Oertel YC. Cellular adenomatoid nodules of the thyroid: review of 219 fine-needle aspirates. Diagn Cytopathol 1993;9:581–9.

121. Kapur U, Wojcik EM. Follicular neoplasm of the thyroid-vanishing cytologic diagnosis? Diagn Cytopathol 2007;35:525–8.

122. Jaffar R, Mohanty SK, Khan A, et al. Hemosiderin laden macrophages and hemosiderin within follicular cells distinguish benign follicular lesions from follicular neoplasms. Cytojournal 2009;6:3.

123. Cusick EL, MacIntosh CA, Krukowski ZH, et al. Management of isolated thyroid swellings: a prospective six year study of fine needle aspiration cytology in diagnosis. Br Med J 1990; 301:318–21.

124. Boon ME, Lowhagen T, Willems JS. Planimetric studies on fine needle aspirates from follicular adenomas and follicular carcinomas of the thyroid. Acta Cytol 1980;24:145–8.

125. Nunez C, Mendelsohn G. Fine needle aspiration and needle biopsy of the thyroid gland. Pathol Annu 1989;24(Pt 1):161–98.

126. Kumar VK, Abbas AK, Fausto N. Robbins and Cotran Pathologic basis of disease, 7th ed. Philadelphia, PA: Elsevier Saunders; 2005.

127. Marhefka GD, McDivitt JD, Mohamed Shakir KM, et al. Diagnosis of

follicular neoplasm in thyroid nodules by fine needle aspiration cytology. Does the result, benign vs. suspicious for a malignant process, in these nodules make a difference? Acta Cytol 2009;53:517–23.

128. Frasoldati A, Flora M, Pesenti M, et al. Computer-assisted cell morphometry and ploidy analysis in the assessment of thyroid follicular neoplasms. Thyroid 2001;11:941–6.

129. Camargo RS, Shirata NK, di Loreto C, et al. Significance of AgNOR measurement in thyroid lesions. Anal Quant Cytol Histol 2006;28:188–92.

130. King AD, Yeung DK, Ahuja AT, et al. In vivo IH MR spectroscopy of thyroid carcinoma. Eur J Radiol 2005;54:112–17.

131. Baloch ZW, LiVolsi VA. Fine-needle aspiration of the thyroid: today and tomorrow. Best Pract Res Clin Endocrinol Metab 2008;22:929–39.

132. Clark OH. Predictors of thyroid tumor aggressiveness. West J Med 1996;165:156–7.

133. Mihai R, Parker AJ, Roskell D, et al. One in four patients with follicular thyroid cytology (THY3) has a thyroid carcinoma. Thyroid 2009;19:33–7.

134. Das DK, Mallik MK, Sharma P, et al. Papillary thyroid carcinoma and its variants in fine needle aspiration smears. A cytomorphologic study with special reference to tall cell variant. Acta Cytol 2004;48:325–36.

135. Yang GC, Liebeskind D, Messina AV. Diagnostic accuracy of follicular variant of papillary thyroid carcinoma in fine-needle aspirates processed by ultrafast Papanicolaou stain: histologic follow-up of 125 cases. Cancer 2006;108:174–9.

136. Bondeson L, Bondeson AG, Nissborg A, et al. Cytopathological variables in parathyroid lesions: a study based on 1,600 cases of hyperparathyroidism. Diagn Cytopathol 1997;16:476–82.

137. Agarwal AM, Bentz JS, Hungerford R, et al. Parathyroid fine-needle aspiration cytology in the evaluation of parathyroid adenoma: cytologic findings from 53 patients. Diagn Cytopathol 2009;37:407–10.

138. Odashiro AN, Nguyen GK. Fine-needle aspiration cytology of an intrathyroid parathyroid adenoma. Diagn Cytopathol 2006;34:790–2.

139. Chang TC, Tung CC, Hsiao YL, et al. Immunoperoxidase staining in the differential diagnosis of parathyroid from thyroid origin in fine needle aspirates of suspected parathyroid lesions. Acta Cytol 1998;42:619–24.

140. Tseleni-Balafouta S, Gakiopoulou H, Kavantzas N, et al. Parathyroid proliferations: a source of diagnostic pitfalls in FNA of thyroid. Cancer 2007;111:130–6.

141. Kwak JY, Kim EK, Moon HJ, et al. Parathyroid incidentalomas detected on routine ultrasound-directed fine-needle aspiration biopsy in patients referred for thyroid nodules and the role of parathyroid hormone analysis in the samples. Thyroid 2009;19:743–8.

142. Cannizzaro M, Fiorenza G, Garofalo L, et al. [Hürthle-cell thyroid neoplasms: a clinical enigma. Ann Ital Chir 1999;70:503–8; discussion 508–509.

143. Mills SC, Haq M, Smellie WJ, et al. Hürthle cell carcinoma of the thyroid: Retrospective review of 62 patients treated at the Royal Marsden Hospital between 1946 and 2003. Eur J Surg Oncol 2009;35:230–4.

144. Yaqub A. Familial Hurthle cell carcinoma of the thyroid: case reports and review of the literature. W V Med J 2009;105:23–8.

145. Nguyen GK, Husain M, Akin MR. Cytodiagnosis of benign and malignant Hürthle cell lesions of the thyroid by fine-needle aspiration biopsy. Diagn Cytopathol 1999;20:261–5.

146. Kaur A, Jayaram G. Thyroid tumors: cytomorphology of Hurthle cell tumors, including an uncommon papillary variant. Diagn Cytopathol 1993;9:135–7.

147. Pambuccian SE, Becker Jr RL, Ali SZ, et al. Differential diagnosis of Hurthle cell neoplasms on fine needle aspirates. Can we do any better with morphometry? Acta Cytol 1997;41:197–208.

148. Volante M, Bozzalla-Cassione F, DePompa R, et al. Galectin-3 and HBME-1 expression in oncocytic cell tumors of the thyroid. Virchows Arch 2004;445:183–8.

149. Jayaram G, Kakar A. Hurthle cell nodules of thyroid following irradiation: neoplastic or non-neoplastic? Ind J Radiol Imag 1994;4:67–8.

150. el-Sahrigy D, Zhang XM, Elhosseiny A, et al. Signet-ring follicular adenoma of the thyroid diagnosed by fine needle aspiration. Report of a case with cytologic description. Acta Cytol 2004;48:87–90.

151. Pietribiasi F, Sapino A, Papotti M, et al. Cytologic features of poorly differentiated 'insular' carcinoma of the thyroid, as revealed by fine-needle aspiration biopsy. Am J Clin Pathol 1990;94:687–92.

152. Sironi M, Collini P, Cantaboni A. Fine needle aspiration cytology of insular thyroid carcinoma. A report of four cases. Acta Cytol 1992;36:435–9.

153. Kuhel WI, Kutler DI, Santos-Buch CA. Poorly differentiated insular thyroid carcinoma. A case report with identification of intact insulae with fine needle aspiration biopsy. Acta Cytol 1998;42:991–7.

154. Nguyen GK, Akin MRM. Cytopathology of insular carcinoma of thyroid. Diagn Cytopathol 2001;25:325–30.

155. Layfield LJ, Gopez EV. Insular carcinoma of the thyroid. Report of a case with intact insulae and microfollicular structures. Diagn Cytopathol 2000;23:409–13.

156. Volante M, Collini P, Nikiforov YE, et al. Poorly differentiated thyroid carcinoma: the Turin proposal for the use of uniform diagnostic criteria and an algorithmic diagnostic approach. Am J Surg Pathol 2007;31:1256–64.

157. Bongiovanni M, Sadow PM, Faquin WC. Poorly differentiated thyroid carcinoma: a cytologic-histologic review. Adv Anat Pathol 2009;16:283–9.

158. Bongiovanni M, Bloom L, Krane JF, et al. Cytomorphologic features of poorly differentiated thyroid carcinoma: a multi-institutional analysis of 40 cases. Cancer Cytopathol 2009;117:185–94.

159. Henderson YC, Shellenberger TD, Williams MD, et al. High rate of BRAF and RET/PTC dual mutations associated with recurrent papillary thyroid carcinoma. Clin Cancer Res 2009;15:485–91.

160. Kini SR, Miller JM, Hamburger JI, et al. Cytopathology of papillary carcinoma of the thyroid by fine needle aspiration. Acta Cytol 1980;24:511–21.

161. Miller TR, Bottles K, Holly EA, et al. A step-wise logistic regression analysis of papillary carcinoma of the thyroid. Acta Cytol 1986;30:285–93.

162. Kaur A, Jayaram G. Thyroid tumors: Cytomorphology of papillary carcinoma. Diagn Cytopathol 1991;7:462–8.

163. Szporn AH, Yuan S, Wu M, et al. Cellular swirls in fine needle aspirates of papillary thyroid carcinoma: a new diagnostic criterion. Mod Pathol 2006;19:1470–3.

164. Das DK, Sharma PN. Diagnosis of papillary thyroid carcinoma in fine needle aspiration smears. Factors that affect decision making. Acta Cytol 2009;53:497–506.

165. Das DK, Sharma PN. Intranuclear cytoplasmic inclusions and nuclear grooves in fine needle aspiration smears of papillary thyroid carcinoma and its variants. Advantage of the count under an oil immersion objective over a high power objective. Analyt Quant Cytol Histol 2005;27:83–94.

166. Sato K, Shimode Y, Hirokawa M, et al. Thyroid adenomatous nodule with bizarre nuclei: a case report and mutation analysis of the p53 gene. Pathol Res Pract 2008;204:191–5.

167. Casey MB, Sebo TJ, Carney JA. Hyalinizing trabecular adenoma of the thyroid gland: cytologic features in 29 cases. Am J Surg Pathol 2004;28: 859–67.

168. Ryska A, Cap J, Vaclavikova E, et al. Paraganglioma-like medullary thyroid carcinoma: fine needle aspiration cytology features with histological correlation. Cytopathology 2009;20: 188–94.

169. Deligeorgi-Politi H. Nuclear crease as a cytodiagnostic feature of papillary thyroid carcinoma in fine needle aspiration biopsies. Diagn Cytopathol 1987;3:307–10.

170. Das DK. Intranuclear cytoplasmic inclusions in fine-needle aspiration smears of papillary thyroid carcinoma: a study of its morphological forms, association with nuclear grooves, and mode of formation. Diagn Cytopathol 2005;32:264–8.

171. Christ ML, Haja JH. Intranuclear cytoplasmic inclusions (invaginations) in thyroid aspirations; frequency and specificity. Acta Cytol 1979;23:327–31.

172. Gould E, Watzak L, Chamizo W, et al. Nuclear grooves in cytologic preparations. A study of the utility of this feature in the diagnosis of papillary carcinoma. Acta Cytol 1989; 33:16–20.

173. Alkuwari E, Khetani K, Dendukuri N, et al. Quantitative assessment of nuclear grooves in fine needle aspirates of the thyroid: a retrospective cytohistologic study of 94 cases. Analyt Quant Cytol Histol 2009;31:161–9.

174. Miller JM, Kini SR, Hamburger JI. Needle biopsy of the thyroid: current concepts. New York: Praeger Publishers; 1983.

175. Brooks E, Simmons-Arnold L, Naud S, et al. Multinucleated Giant Cells' Incidence, Immune Markers, and Significance: A Study of 172 Cases of Papillary Thyroid Carcinoma. Head Neck Pathol 2009;3:95–9.

176. Suen KC. Altlas and text of aspiration biopsy cytology. London: Williams and Wilkins; 1990.

177. Leung CS, Hartwick RWJ, Berard YC. Correlation of cytologic and histologic features in variants of papillary carcinoma of the thyroid. Acta Cytol 1993;37:645–50.

178. Das DK, Mallik MK, Haji BE, et al. Psammoma body and its precursors in papillary thyroid carcinoma: a study by fine-needle aspiration cytology. Diagn Cytopathol 2004;31:380–6.

179. Das DK, Sheikh ZA, George SS, et al. Papillary thyroid carcinoma: evidence for intracytoplasmic formation of precursor substance for calcification and its release from well-preserved neoplastic cells. Diagn Cytopathol 2008;36:809–12.

180. Shih SR, Li HY, Hsiao YL, et al. Prognostic significance of cytologic features in fine-needle aspiration cytology samples of papillary thyroid carcinoma: preliminary report. Thyroid 2006;16:775–80.

181. Yip L, Nikiforova MN, Carty SE, et al. Optimizing surgical treatment of papillary thyroid carcinoma associated with BRAF mutation. Surgery 2009;146:1215–23.

182. Khurana KK, Truong LD, LiVolsi VA, et al. Cytokeratin 19 immunolocalization in cell block preparation of thyroid aspirates. An adjunct to fine-needle aspiration diagnosis of papillary thyroid carcinoma. Arch Pathol Lab Med 2003;127:579–83.

183. Bonzanini M, Amadori PL, Sagramoso C, et al. Expression of cytokeratin 19 and protein p63 in fine needle aspiration biopsy of papillary thyroid carcinoma. Acta Cytol 2008;52:541–8.

184. Sanabria A, Caravalho AL, Piana de Andrade V, et al. Is Galectin-3 a good method for the detection of malignancy in patients with thyroid nodules and a cytologic diagnosis of 'follicular neoplasm'? A critical appraisal of the evidence. Head Neck 2007;29:1046–54.

185. Nga ME, Lim GS, Soh CH, et al. HBME-1 and CK19 are highly discriminatory in the cytological diagnosis of papillary thyroid carcinoma. Diagn Cytopathol 2008;36:550–6.

186. Harshan M, Crapanzano JP, Aslan DL, et al. Papillary thyroid carcinoma with atypical histiocytoid cells on fine-needle aspiration. Diagn Cytopathol 2009;37:244–50.

187. Bradly DP, Reddy V, Prinz RA, et al. Incidental papillary carcinoma in patients treated surgically for benign thyroid diseases. Surgery 2009;146:1099–104.

188. Khayyata S, Barroeta JE, LiVolsi VA, et al. Papillary hyperplastic nodule: pitfall in the cytopathologic diagnosis of papillary thyroid carcinoma. Endocr Pract 2008;14:863–8.

189. Baloch ZW, LiVolsi VA. Cytologic and architectural mimics of papillary thyroid carcinoma. Diagnostic challenges in fine-needle aspiration and surgical pathology specimens. Am J Clin Pathol 2006 Jun;125(Suppl.):S135–44.

190. Jain M, Khan A, Patwardhan N, et al. Follicular variant of papillary thyroid carcinoma: a comparative study of histopathologic features and cytology results in 141 patients. Endocr Pract 2001;7:79–84.

191. Aron M, Mallik A, Verma K. Fine needle aspiration cytology of follicular variant of papillary carcinoma of the thyroid: Morphologic pointers to its diagnosis. Acta Cytol 2006;50:663–8.

192. Wu HH, Jones JN, Grzybicki DM, et al. Sensitive cytologic criteria for the identification of follicular variant of papillary thyroid carcinoma in fine-needle aspiration biopsy. Diagn Cytopathol 2003;29:262–6.

193. Liu J, Singh B, Tallini G, et al. Follicular variant of papillary thyroid carcinoma: a clinicopathologic study of a problematic entity. Cancer 2006;107:1255–64.

194. Fadda G, Fiorino MC, Mule A, et al. Macrofollicular variant of papillary thyroid carcinoma as a potential pitfall in histologic and cytologic diagnosis. A report of three cases. Acta Cytol 2002;46:555–9.

195. Lugli A, Terracciano LM, Oberholzer M, et al. Macrofollicular variant of papillary carcinoma of the thyroid: a histologic, cytologic, and immunohistochemical study of 3 cases and review of the literature. Arch Pathol Lab Med 2004;128:54–8.

196. Moreira AL, Waisman J, Cangiarella JF. Aspiration cytology of the oncocytic variant of papillary adenocarcinoma of the thyroid gland. Acta Cytol 2004;48:137–41.

197. Baloch ZW, LiVolsi VA. Fine-Needle Aspiration Cytology of Papillary Hurthle Cell Carcinoma with Lymphocytic Stroma 'Warthin-Like Tumor' of the Thyroid. Endocr Pathol 1998;9:317–23.

198. D'Antonio A, De Chiara A, Santoro M, et al. Warthin-like tumour of the thyroid gland: RET/PTC expression indicates it is a variant of papillary carcinoma. Histopathology 2000;36:493–8.

199. Chuah KL, Hwang JSG, Ng SB, et al. Cytologic features of cribriform-morular variant of papillary carcinoma of the thyroid. A case report. Acta Cytol 2005;49:75–80.

200. Jung CK, Choi YJ, Lee KY, et al. The cytological, clinical, and pathological features of the cribriform-morular variant of papillary thyroid carcinoma and mutation analysis of CTNNB1 and BRAF genes. Thyroid 2009;19:905–13.

201. Haji BE, Ahmed MS, Prasad A, et al. Papillary thyroid carcinoma with an adenoid cystic pattern: report of a case with fine-needle aspiration cytology and immunocytochemistry. Diagn Cytopathol 2004;30:418–21.

202. Ustün H, Atalay FO, Ekinci C. Adenoid cystic variant of papillary thyroid carcinoma: a case report with fine-needle aspiration cytology. Diagn Cytopathol 2008;36:64–6.

203. Leal II, Carneiro FP, Basílio-de-Oliveira CA, et al. Papillary carcinoma with nodular fasciitis-like stroma–a case report in pregnancy. Diagn Cytopathol 2008;36:139–41.

204. Urano M, Kiriyama Y, Takakuwa Y, et al. Tall cell variant of papillary thyroid carcinoma: Its characteristic features demonstrated by fine-needle aspiration

cytology and immunohistochemical study. Diagn Cytopathol 2009;37: 732–7.

205. Ylagan LR, Dehner LP, Huettner PC, et al. Columnar cell variant of papillary thyroid carcinoma. Report of a case with cytologic findings. Acta Cytol 2004;48:73–7.

206. Jayaram G. Cytology of columnar cell variant of papillary thyroid carcinoma. Diagn Cytopathol 2000;22:227–9.

207. Lee JY, Shin JH, Han BK, et al. Diffuse sclerosing variant of papillary carcinoma of the thyroid: imaging and cytologic findings. Thyroid 2007;17: 567–73.

208. Nguyen GK, Lee MW. Solid/trabecular variant papillary carcinoma of the thyroid: Report of three cases with fine-needle aspiration. Diagn Cytopathol 2006;34:712–4.

209. Jayaram G. Trabecular adenoma of the thyroid. Fine needle aspiration cytologic and histologic features in a case. Acta Cytol 1999;43:978–80.

210. Kuma S, Hirokawa M, Miyauchi A, et al. Cytologic features of hyalinizing trabecular adenoma of the thyroid. Acta Cytol 2003;47:399–404.

211. Nosé V, Volante M, Papotti M. Hyalinizing trabecular tumor of the thyroid: an update. Endocr Pathol 2008;19:1–8.

212. Casey MB, Sebo TJ, Carney JA. Hyalinizing trabecular adenoma of the thyroid gland identification through MIB-1 staining of fine-needle aspiration biopsy smears. Am J Clin Pathol 2004;122:506–10.

213. Kaur A, Jayaram G. Thyroid tumors: cytomorphology of medullary, clinically anaplastic, and miscellaneous thyroid neoplasms. Diagn Cytopathol 1990;6:383–9.

214. Forrest CH, Frost FA, de Boer WB, et al. Medullary carcinoma of the thyroid. Accuracy of diagnosis by fine-needle aspiration cytology. Cancer (Cancer Cytopathol) 1998;84:295–302.

215. Papaparaskeva K, Nagel H, Droese M. Cytologic diagnosis of medullary carcinoma of the thyroid gland. Diagn Cytopathol 2000;22:351–8.

216. Moo-Young TA, Traugott AL, Moley JF. Sporadic and familial medullary thyroid carcinoma: state of the art. Surg Clin North Am 2009;89:1193–204.

217. Chang TC, Wu SL, Hsiao YL. Medullary carcinoma. Pitfalls in diagnosis by fine needle aspiration cytology and relationship of cytomorphology to RET proto-oncogene mutations. Aca Cytol 2005;49:477–82.

218. Das DK, Mallik MK, George SS, et al. Secretory activity in medullary thyroid carcinoma: a cytomorphological and immunocytochemical study. Diagn Cytopathol 2007;35:329–37.

219. Rekhi B, Kane SV, D'Cruz A. Cytomorphology of anaplastic giant cell type of medullary thyroid carcinoma – a diagnostic dilemma in an elderly female: a case report. Diagn Cytopathol 2008;36:136–8.

219A. Duskova J, Janotova D, Svobodova E, et al. Fine needle aspiration biopsy of mixed medullary-follicular thyroid carcinoma: a report of two cases. Acta Cytol 2003;47:71–7.

220. Marcus JN, Dise CA, LiVolsi VA. Melanin production in a medullary thyroid carcinoma. Cancer 1982; 49:2518–26.

221. Jayaram G, Hayati JN, Yip CH, et al. Cytologic, histologic and immunocytochemical features in fine needle aspirates of paraganglioma-like variant of medullary carcinoma. Acta Cytol 2008;52:119–21.

222. Aulicino MR, Szporn AH, Dembitzer R, et al. Cytologic findings in the differential diagnosis of C-cell hyperplasia and medullary carcinoma by fine needle aspiration. A case report. Acta Cytol 1998;42:963–7.

223. Luze T, Totsch M, Bangerl I, et al. Fine needle aspiration cytodiagnosis of anaplastic carcinoma and malignant haemangioendothelioma of the thyroid in an endemic goitre area. Cytopathol 1990;6:305–10.

224. Us-Krasovec M, Golouh R, Auersperg M, et al. Anaplastic thyroid carcinoma in fine needle aspirates. Acta Cytol 1996;40:953–8.

225. Deshpande AH, Munshi MM, Bobhate SJ. Cytological diagnosis of paucicellular variant of anaplastic carcinoma of thyroid: report of two cases. Cytopathol 2001;12:203–8.

226. Mehdi G, Ansari HA, Siddiqui SA. Cytology of anaplastic giant cell carcinoma of the thyroid with osteoclast-like giant cells–a case report. Diagn Cytopathol 2007;35:111–12.

227. Cerilli LA, Frable WJ, Spafford MF. Anaplastic carcinoma of the thyroid with chondroblastoma features mimicking papillary carcinoma. A case report. Acta Cytol 2007;51:825–8.

228. Tani E, Skoog L. Fine needle aspiration cytology and immunocytochemistry in the diagnosis of lymphoid lesions of the thyroid gland. Acta Cytol 1989;33:48–52.

229. Sangalli G, Serio G, Zampatti C, et al. Fine needle aspiration cytology of primary lymphoma of the thyroid: a report of 17 cases. Cytopathol 2001; 12:257–63.

230. Gupta N, Nijhawan R, Srinivasan R, et al. Fine needle aspiration cytology of primary thyroid lymphoma: a report of ten cases. Cytojournal 2005;9(2):21.

231. Zhu H, Hu DX. Langerhans cell histiocytosis of the thyroid diagnosed by fine needle aspiration cytology. A case report. Acta Cytol 2004;48: 278–80.

232. Jayaram G, Wong KT, Jalaludin MA. Mucoepidermoid carcinoma of the thyroid: a case report. Malaysian J Pathol 1998;20:45–8.

233. Das S, Kalyani R. Sclerosing mucoepidermoid carcinoma with eosinophilia of the thyroid. Indian J Pathol Microbiol 2008;51:34–6.

234. Isa NM, James DT, Saw TH, et al. Primary angiosarcoma of the thyroid gland with recurrence diagnosed by fine needle aspiration: a case report. Diagn Cytopathol 2009;37:427–32.

235. Poniecka A, Ghorab Z, Arnold D, et al. Kaposi's sarcoma of the thyroid gland in an HIV-negative woman. A case report. Acta Cytol 2007;51:421–3.

236. Tong GX, Hamele-Bena D, Liu JC, et al. Fine-needle aspiration biopsy of primary osteosarcoma of the thyroid: report of a case and review of the literature. Diagn Cytopathol 2008; 36:589–94.

237. Majhi U. Primary malignant teratoma of the thyroid in a child with nodal metastases. Indian J Pathol Microbiol 2009;52:234–6.

238. Jayaram G, Cheah PL, Yip CH. Malignant teratoma of thyroid with predominantly neuroepithelial differentiation-fine needle aspiration cytologic, histologic and immunocytochemical features in a case. Acta Cytol 2000;44:375–9.

239. Baloch ZW, Sack MJ, Yu GH, et al. Papillary formations in metastatic melanoma. Diagn Cytopathol 1999;20:148–51.

240. Abati A, Skarulis MC, Shawker T, et al. Ultrasound-guided fine-needle aspiration of parathyroid lesions: a morphological and immunocytochemical approach. Human Pathol 1995;26:338–43.

241. Layfield LJ. Fine needle aspiration cytology of cystic parathyroid lesions. Acta Cytol 1991;35:447–50.

242. Glenthoj A, Karstrup S. Parathyroid identification by ultrasonically guided aspiration cytology. Is correct cytological identification possible? APMIS 1989;97:497–502.

243. Davey DD, Glant MD, Berger EK. Parathyroid cytopathology. Diagn Cytopathol 1986;2:76–80.

244. Chan SP, Hew FL, Jayaram G, et al. A case report of primary hyperthyroidism with severe bony involvement and nephrolithiasis. Ann Acad Med 2001;30:66–70.

245. Goellner JR, Caudill JL. Intranuclear holes (cytoplasmic pseudoinclusions) in parathyroid neoplasms, or 'holes happen.' Cancer (Cancer Cytopathol) 2000;90:41–6.

CHAPTER 7

Breast

Joan Cangiarella and Aylin Simsir

CLINICAL ASPECTS

Although most countries in Europe continue to perform fine needle aspiration biopsy (FNB) as their first choice in the investigation of breast lesions in both screening and symptomatic populations, the use of core needle biopsy (CNB) is increasing.[1] Centers that continue to use FNB have utilized a multidiscipinary approach to the diagnosis of breast lesions.[2] A significant advantage of FNB is the low cost and the ability to render a diagnosis to the clinician and patient at the time of the procedure thus allowing treatment decisions to be made immediately. The presence of a cytopathologist with expertise in FNB provides superior diagnostic results and low inadequate rates.[3] However, the inability of FNB to definitely diagnose invasion and the preference of pathologists who are not trained in cytopathology to interpret histologic samples rather than cytologic samples have contributed to the increase in the use of core biopsy. The initial investigation of breast lesions by core biopsy started with the 14-gauge spring-loaded cutting core needle guided by ultrasound or by stereotaxis. Now, many institutions use a vacuum-assisted larger-bore (8 to 11-gauge) cutting core needle (VACB), for the investigation of microcalcification, mass lesions and architectural distortion. For a detailed description of the techniques see Wong et al.[4] Recent evidence suggests that the vacuum assisted core biopsy (11 gauge to 8 gauge) has better sensitivity and specificity than the 14-gauge core biopsy or FNB for architectural distortion or microcalcification and that the 14-gauge core biopsy provides better sensitivity and specificity than FNB for other lesions.[5] Besides the ability to give an unequivocal diagnosis of invasion, other advantages of core biopsy include a higher proportion of definitive malignant diagnoses, more type-specific diagnoses, and a more specific diagnosis of benign lesions.[6-10] The technique can be a substitute for open biopsy for the diagnosis of benign lesions and in the preoperative planning of surgery in malignant lesions. In some multidisciplinary assessment centers in Australia, CNB is the only diagnostic method now used, whereas in others FNB is used alone or in combination with CNB. Some countries have developed clear guidelines for the use of FNB and CNB, with core biopsy used in cases with discrepant

cytologic and radiologic findings, inconclusive FNB or in cases of microcalcification.[1]

We consider breast FNB and CNB to be complementary techniques, and both should be available in any modern multidisciplinary clinic. Both are sampling methods and have their advantages, limitations and specific indications.[11]. For example, radiologically low-grade microcalcifications may be better investigated by VACB than by FNB. On the other hand, most high-grade DCIS are malignant by FNB, and CNB is not significantly more reliable than FNB to exclude focal invasion in these lesions. CNB is of great value both in nonpalpable and palpable lesions where initial FNB is suspicious but not diagnostic of malignancy, as is often the case in low-grade cancers, particularly in tubular carcinoma and invasive lobular carcinoma.[12] Some clinical problems, such as opacities occurring postoperatively, are better diagnosed by CNB, as FNB cannot definitely diagnose scar tissue.

Cost factors must also be taken into account, given the large volume of work generated by breast cancer screening.[13] The instrumentation and disposables used for CNB and particularly for VACB are much more expensive than for FNB. This must be weighed against the cost of surgical open biopsy.[8] Approximately two-thirds of screen-detected cancers can be confidently diagnosed by FNB. This means a considerable cost saving compared to CNB if CNB is used for all patients, even if a number of patients may have to undergo both tests. Ultrasound (US)-guided FNB is rapid and usually causes little discomfort to the patient. In the 'assessment center' setting, where the pathologist is on site, FNB smears can be checked immediately for adequacy. An on-the-spot diagnosis can be given to decide on management and to advise the patient without further delay.

The challenge now is to integrate the use of the alternative techniques for the greatest benefit to the patient and for maximal cost effectiveness.

Palpable lesions

A palpable breast lump is a common clinical problem that presents to surgeons, gynecologists and general practitioners. While excisional biopsy was the accepted practice in the past, current practices utilize radiological imaging in combination with needle biopsy, reducing the need for unnecessary surgical excision of benign breast lesions.

A preoperative diagnosis offers several advantages:

1. Immediate diagnosis relieves the patient's anxiety and saves time.
2. A definitive treatment plan can be prepared and discussed with the patient in advance.
3. If cancer is confirmed, additional imaging studies (bone scan, liver scan, etc.) can be done preoperatively to determine stage.
4. With the triple test assessment, many benign conditions can be confidently diagnosed by FNB or CNB and surgery avoided.
5. It has been shown to be cost-effective, allowing one-step definitive surgery including lymph node sampling in malignant cases.
6. The need for frozen section diagnosis is reduced.

The investigation of palpable breast lumps in successful breast programs utilizes a multidisciplinary approach that centers around the 'triple test', analyzing clinical and radiologic findings in conjunction with the pathologic features to diagnose the lesion and determine the best treatment plan for the patient.[1] There has been a dramatic increase in general practitioner (GP) referral of patients with breast lumps for FNB as a first-line investigation in the work-up of these lesions. Given the lower clinical expertise of the GP compared to a surgeon, this places a unique responsibility on the cytopathologist. The cytopathologist must use his or her clinical acumen in addition to the cytological findings in recommending the need for further investigations such as radiological assessment, follow-up, referral to a specialist surgeon, or local excision. While some surgeons may continue to perform CNB of palpable lesions in their office, most lesions today are biopsied under radiologic guidance.

The trend towards more conservative surgery and individualized treatment has increased the importance of close correlation of clinical, radiological, and pathologic findings. Material obtained through preoperative biopsy (through cell block material from FNB or by CNB) is increasingly being used for hormone receptor analysis and for the evaluation of other prognostic parameters by various ancillary techniques. The ctology of palpable nodules in irradiated breast tissue has become a more frequently encountered problem as a result of conservative treatment of cancer by lumpectomy followed by irradiation. FNB is also useful in the evaluation of skin or chest wall lesions in patients post mastectomy.

The place of FNB and CNB in the investigative sequence

While FNB of a palpable breast lump should generally be preceded by mammographic and/or ultrasonographic examination, as the radiological findings help to select the most appropriate area to be biopsied, FNB may be performed as the first-line investigation, especially in symptomatic and screening populations.[14,15]. Caution should be exercised that if FNB is done first, post-biopsy hemorrhage may interfere with the interpretation of the films. The referring doctor normally receives a written report of the cytological findings the following day, with a phone call placed to the referring physician immediately, if necessary. Further steps can then be discussed with the patient and this will relieve anxiety and avoid unnecessary delay. If the decision to perform CNB of a palpable abnormality is made, the majority will be performed with radiographic guidance, either stereotaxically or, more commonly, with ultrasound guidance.

The main purpose of FNB or CNB of breast lumps is to confirm cancer preoperatively and to avoid unnecessary surgery in specific benign conditions.

The role of FNB in the assessment of a breast lump includes:

1. the diagnosis of simple cysts,
2. the investigation of suspected recurrence or metastasis in cases of previously diagnosed cancer,
3. the confirmation of inoperable, locally advanced cancer,
4. the preoperative confirmation of clinically suspected cancer,
5. the investigation of any palpable lump, clinically benign or malignant, as a guide to clinical management,
6. the ability to obtain tumor cells for special analysis and research, e.g. hormone receptor studies, DNA analysis, immunohistochemistry, cell kinetics and molecular studies.

The role of CNB in the assessment of breast lumps is similar to FNB with the exception that it is not routinely used in the diagnosis of simple cysts.

FNB and CNB in the follow-up of breast cancer

The FNB diagnosis of local recurrence of breast cancer is generally straightforward, involving a distinction between cancer and suture granuloma, fat necrosis and scarring.[16–19] However, reactive atypia in reparative granulation tissue, in fat necrosis or in seroma cavities can cause diagnostic problems, and radiation-induced atypia in benign glandular epithelium can be misinterpreted as recurrent malignancy (Fig. 7.1). CNB can also be used; however, fat necrosis may be misinterpreted as invasive carcinoma on core, leading to a false-positive diagnosis of malignancy.[20] Sampling error by core biopsy should always be considered in cases where the suspicion of recurrence is high.

Accuracy of diagnosis in FNB and CNB

As noted above, a significant advantage of CNB is the ability to diagnose invasiveness and thus allow the patient to undergo a single operation including sentinel node biopsy in cases diagnosed as invasive. However, in our experience the presence of malignant cells on FNB in a palpable mass yields invasive carcinoma at excision in approximately 98% and thus the addition of a CNB only adds additional information in a few cases.[21] It must also be recognized that a CNB diagnosis of ductal carcinoma in situ will be upgraded to a diagnosis of invasive carcinoma at surgical excision in approximately 20% of cases.[22] Core biopsy is favored in lesions that appear fibrotic or collagenous and in cases suspected to be invasive lobular carcinoma, as these lesions can be paucicellular on FNB.[23]

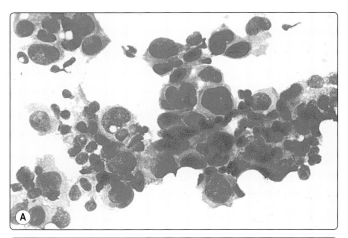

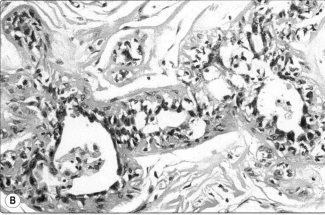

Fig. 7.1 Radiation-induced atypia (A) The epithelial cells in this irregular cluster show considerable nuclear enlargement, pleomorphism and hyperchromasia, but also some degenerative changes such as loss of nuclear structure (MGG, HP); (B) Corresponding tissue section (H&E, IP).

The reported sensitivities, specificities and positive and negative predictive values for FNB vary depending on how insufficient samples are considered (as positive, negative or excluded) and how atypical samples are categorized (positive or negative).[24] When insufficent samples and atypical and benign findings are presumed to be negative, sensitivities range from 43.8% to 95%, specificities from 89.8% to 100%, positive predicitive values from 76.2% to 100% and negative predicitive values from 46.3% to 98.8%. If insufficient samples are excluded, sensitivities and specificities improve to a range of 58.3% to 100% and 55% to 100%, respectively, with a slight change in the negative predictive value to between 46.6% and 98.6%. The variability in reported sensitivities and specificities depends on the expertise and skill of the aspirator and of the interpreter. The aim should be a sensitivity of no less than 95% and this can be achieved with increasing experience. Sensitivity is lower for low-grade carcinomas (invasive and in situ), for lobular carcinoma, and for very small and very large cancers.[25,26] The positive predictive value of a malignant diagnosis is approximately 99%, and, although rare, occasional false-positive diagnoses of malignancy are recorded in most series.[27-30]

The results of studies comparing FNB to CNB are difficult to evaluate due to numerous variables that influence accuracy. Skill and experience are important in performing the biopsy and in the preparation and reading of the smear. Although the technique is simple, training and continuous practice are essential to acquire and to maintain skill. Significant improvement in accuracy occurs with experience. Centers with experienced physicians performing and interpreting FNBs have shown a high diagnostic accuracy. In general, the best results are achieved if the pathologist who reads the smears either performs the biopsies or works directly with the surgeon and radiologist in a multidisciplinary team.[31] The reason for this is that the microscopic examination, immediate or with some delay, provides the pathologist a feedback on the adequacy and quality of the smears causing repeat sampling and the ability to obtain additional diagnostic material, if necessary. For core biopsy, training and skill in the technique and the number and size of the cores will influence accuracy.[32,33] Some studies have shown CNB to be more accurate than FNB in the diagnosis of nonpalpable breast lesions and in the diagnosis of LCIS and infiltrating lobular carcinoma.[34-36] Other studies have shown CNB and FNB to be similar in sensitivity, positive predictive value and inadequate rate, with only statistical differences in specificity.[37] Studies have shown FNB to be more accurate than CNB in distingushing benign from malignant papillary lesions[38] and in diagnosing malignancy in palpable breast cancers.[39] In one study, tumor size influenced accuracy, with tumors less than 2 cm and greater than 5 cm showing similar accuracies by CNB and FNB. However, with tumors between 2 cm and 5 cm in size, CNB showed a higher sensitivity and a lower inadequate rate as compared to FNB.[40] Some studies have shown the inadequate rate to be much higher with FNB as compared to CNB;[23] however, the presence of a cytopathologist at the procedure noticeably lowers inadequacy rates.[3] For core biopsies, specificities range from 99% to 100%, sensitivities from 94% to 99%, negative predictive values from 94% to 99% and positive predictive values from 94% to 100%.[24]

A positive cytological diagnosis is possible in 75–80% of palpable cancers. Definitive treatment can often be based on the cytological diagnosis without the need for histological confirmation in centers with a large volume of cases and specialty trained cytopathologists unless there is disagreement between cytology and clinical and/or mammographic assessment. Approximately 98% of palpable masses with unequivocally malignant FNB cytology are invasive cancers, the remaining few are high-grade DCIS.[21] Studies that compared FNB to CNB for palpable breast carcinoma showed a higher sensitivity (97.5% vs. 90%) for FNB regardless of the size of the tumor, its subtype or its degree of differentiation.[39] In situ carcinoma constitutes a special problem.[41] While high-grade/large cell DCIS (classic comedocarcinoma) is easily recognized as malignant in smears, low-grade DCIS may be impossible to distinguish from atypical but benign epithelial proliferations. Smears from low-grade DCIS are usually reported as atypical or suspicious with a recommendation for CNB or open biopsy. Furthermore, cytological examination on its own can not definitely diagnose invasion. Mammographic and US findings of a tissue density in most cases reflect invasive growth to be confirmed by CNB, while characteristic microcalcifications in the absence of a mass lesion suggests DCIS. However, focal invasion in a predominantly in situ carcinoma can only be assessed by

Table 7.1 Cytology reporting categories

Cytological category	Description/definition
Malignant	Unequivocal diagnosis; can be used for definitive management if consistent with radiological findings and treatment protocols
Suspicious	Suggests malignancy; insufficient evidence for definitive management; histological confirmation needed
Atypical/indeterminate	Diagnosis uncertain; further investigation needed
Benign – specific diagnosis	Cyst; fibroadenoma; intramammary lymph node
Benign – non-specific	Smears of cells of non-neoplastic breast tissue. The number of cells required varies between operators. Not possible to confirm that the smear is representative, the responsibility stays entirely with the radiologist
Unsatisfactory sample	Fat and fibrous tissue only. No cellular material, or bloody samples with poorly preserved cells

histologic examination of the excised lesion. If present, a second-stage extended surgery usually follows. In some cases, additional information about the presence of invasion and the exact tumor type may be required to decide surgical management. This may be provided by CNB or by intraoperative frozen section. The major limitation of core biopsy is sampling error. As noted above, the finding of in situ ductal carcinoma on CNB does not rule out the chance of finding invasive disease at surgical excision. The presence of other benign and high-risk lesions such as radial scars, papillary lesions, atypical ductal hyperplasia, atypical lobular hyperplasia and lobular carcinoma in situ on CNB have been shown to underestimate the presence of carcinoma at surgical excision.

Cytologic categories for the reporting of breast FNB are described in Table 7.1. Indecisive cytology reports such as 'suspicious of malignancy' or 'cytological atypia not diagnostic of malignancy' are neither false-negative nor false-positive diagnoses and should be understood as expressing the need for CNB or open biopsy. A positive report should never be issued if smears are quantitatively or qualitatively unsatisfactory or if there is the slightest doubt of malignancy. Such a policy inevitably results in a number of indecisive reports inversely proportional to experience. Rare false-positive FNB diagnoses occur even in centers of excellence.[29] In our experience, the greatest risk of making a false-positive diagnosis is in cases of fibroadenoma with prominent epithelial atypia, papillary lesions with or without infarction, radial scars,[30] apocrine adenosis[42] tubular adenomas[43] and sclerosing adenosis.[42] False-positive diagnosis by CNB is unusual but can be seen in fat necrosis,[20] complex sclerosing lesions, sclerosing adenosis and adenomyoepitheliomas.[44] The rare occurrence of false-positive diagnosis is an extremely important issue given the risk of overtreatment of a benign condition

with adverse effects to the patient, and medicolegal consequences. A summary of diagnostic pitfalls is presented at the end of this chapter.

The false-negative rate for FNB is generally less than 5%, but significantly higher than the false-positive rate. It is mainly due to sampling error. Most false-negative FNB are due to low-grade carcinomas, such as lobular and tubular carcinomas and carcinomas with abundant sclerosis. Most false negatives can be attributed to a lack of cytologic atypia in well-differentiated lesions rather than misinterpretation.[45] The false-negative rate for CNB is approximately 2%, mainly due to sampling error or missed targeting of a lesion.[46] Ultrasound guidance has been shown to decrease the false-negative rate.[47]

The complete sensitivity of image-guided FNB is about 90%, compared with about 95% for direct FNB of palpable lesions, and the absolute sensitivity is 60–70% compared with 75–80% for direct FNB. The false-negative rate is 5–10%, higher than for palpable lesions.[48–50]

Most high-grade DCIS lesions are diagnosed as malignant at FNB. Most low-grade DCIS lesions on FNB show abnormal cell patterns requiring excision, but relatively few are given an unequivocal diagnosis of malignancy. DCIS lesions associated with dispersed 'powdery' microcalcifications are those most likely to be inadequately sampled. Our experience, and that of others, suggests that this type of lesion (mammographically 3B microcalcifications) is better examined by VACB since representative and diagnostic material is not easily obtained either by FNB or by conventional CNB. In a series of 124 cases of suspicious microcalcifications reported by Dahlstrom et al., no calcification was found in the CNB samples in one-quarter of the cases.[51] The reason for this may be that microcalcifications often occur in soft, mainly fatty tissue offering little substance to the sampling needle, whereas the target is fixed by the vacuum applied by the mammotome. Symmans et al., however, found that stereotaxic FNB of benign microcalcifications had a high negative predictive value, higher than CNB.[48]

Approximately two-thirds of screen-detected cancers are given a definitive cancer diagnosis by FNB as part of triple diagnosis. The other one-third requires further investigation by CNB or open biopsy to give the go-ahead for more extensive definitive surgery. The reason may be discordance with radiological findings, technical difficulties to obtain satisfactory smears, doubts about invasion, or a relatively bland cytology as in low-grade cancers, especially tubular carcinoma and lobular carcinoma of classic type. The rate of atypical or inconclusive cytology is moderately higher from impalpable than from palpable lesions, and the proportion of cancers given an atypical/inconclusive report by image-guided FNB is higher, mainly due to the larger numbers of DCIS and small low-grade lesions.[52] The percentage of cancers in excised lesions with indeterminate cytological diagnoses is lower for image-guided samples than for direct FNB.

It has been found that with experience the accuracy of ultrasound-guided FNB of opacities is comparable to that of stereotactic guidance. The complete sensitivity in the diagnosis of cancer is 90–95%.[49,53] Ultrasound guidance increases accuracy for lesions under 2 cm. Since US guidance is faster and technically less demanding, it has become by far the most commonly used modality for biopsy guidance, except for microcalcifications without a tissue density, for lesions close to the chest wall, and for lesions that are not clearly seen by US. Alkuwari et al. reported a sensitivity of 65% in the ultrasound-guided FNB of metastatic breast carcinoma in nonpalpable axillary lymph nodes in breast cancer patients.

Can a cytology report[54] of a benign breast lesion ever be regarded as diagnostic? If smears are satisfactory and adequate and cytological criteria are met, well-circumscribed lesions such as simple cysts, lipomas, most fibroadenomas, intramammary lymph nodes and fat necrosis can be diagnosed with confidence. Poorly circumscribed lesions – the common hormonal mastopathy-fibrocystic disease-fibroadenosis-mammary dysplasia – cannot be confidently diagnosed by FNB to the exclusion of malignancy. This is particularly true in the presence of epithelial hyperplasia, papillomatosis and adenosis. However, if multiple aspirates with a satisfactory yield of cells are obtained from different parts of the lesion and if the result is consistent with the clinical and mammographic evaluation, conservative management based on clinical follow-up is justified.

For core biopsy, a 1-year follow-up is recommended for definitive benign cases such as fibroadenoma where the imaging and pathologic findings are concordant. For other benign concordant diagnosis, 6-month follow-up is recommended.[55]

While false-negative diagnoses can occur, a missed cancer is rare if the triple test is used as the gold standard. Triple diagnosis, the combination of clinical examination, mammography and pathologic examination, and the multidisciplinary approach increase the quality of FNB and CB and decrease its diagnostic limitations. The use of all three modalities in parallel has led to further improvement in preoperative diagnosis.[56] If all three investigations are in agreement that a lesion is either benign or malignan diagnostic accuracy is over 99%.[57] This is based on the condition that the diagnosis by each modality was reached completely independently of the others. For example, radiological findings must not influence the initial cytological evaluation.

The unsatisfactory sample

When should an FNB sample of a breast lesion be regarded as unsatisfactory? What is the definition of a satisfactory sample? These questions have been discussed in many editorials and articles, and there are no simple answers.[58,59] It depends very much on specific circumstances, for example if samples were taken by an experienced pathologist, or if smears were prepared by clinical staff and submitted to the laboratory. If the lesion sampled is a paucicellular fibrous mastopathy, a sclerosed fibroadenoma, a desmoplastic carcinoma, or hypertrophic adipose tissue, smears are naturally very low in cells. A hypocellular smear must be evaluated on the basis of clinical findings and consideration to the consistency of the tissue felt through the biopsy needle must be given. Poorly prepared smears with crush or drying artifacts or with cells trapped in clotted blood should be rejected as unsatisfactory. Attempts have been made to set quantitative criteria for the minimum cell yield that can be accepted as satisfactory.[28,30] However, rigid criteria are unrealistic for the reasons mentioned above, and monitoring the laboratory's own results on an ongoing basis is the best way of ensuring

accuracy. Skill affects adequacy, and targeted training to sub-optimal aspirators can help improve the quality of their FNB specimens.[60]

For lesions sampled by ultrasound or stereotactic FNB at least three and sometimes up to six passes are used, depending on whether the needle position is satisfactory, and depending on the quality of the smears. If multiple FNB passes from a radiologically indeterminate or suspicious lesion consistently produce a poor yield, CNB is more likely to provide a diagnosis. The significance of a scanty smear in the context of triple diagnosis can only be jointly decided by the assessment team. Overall, about 20% of samples will have scanty cell content. The figure is higher for microcalcifications. However, 'unsatisfactory' samples are mainly seen in benign lesions, and sampling of malignant microcalcifications is much more satisfactory.

Unsatisfactory specimens for CNB most often are due to missed sampling of a lesion but may be caused by fibrotic or sclerotic lesions that are difficult to sample. A CNB specimen obtained for mammographic calcification that does not contain microcalcification on the slide after X-ray of the tissue block should be considered unsatisfactory. Obtaining only skin or fatty tissue (except in suspected lipomas) should also be considered unsatisfactory.

Standardized reporting of FNB and CNB samples and quality assurance

Standard approaches to reporting FNB samples from the breast are recommended. A national conference sponsored by the National Institute of Health in the USA compiled the views of opinion leaders on information required on request forms, technical aspects of sampling, cytologic categories and information to be included in the cytopathology report.[58,61] Five categories of FNB reports are recommended: benign, atypical/indeterminate, suspicious/probably malignant, malignant and unsatisfactory. In each category there should be an attempt to place the findings into a specific pathologic entity such as that used in a surgical pathology diagnosis. A slightly modified version of this system is used in Europe. The benign category is subdivided into 'benign specific' and 'benign NOS'. The rational for this is that if a benign specific diagnosis such as cyst, fibroadenoma, fat necrosis, etc. can be made and if this is in accordance with radiological findings, the sample can be regarded as representative of the lesion. Benign NOS, on the other hand, means simply non-neoplastic breast tissue was obtained and radiologic and clinical follow-up is mandated to consider the sample representative of the lesion. Several surveys have studied the diagnostic criteria used in routine cytological practice or the accuracy achieved in interlaboratory comparisons in non-screening and screening settings.[25,28,62,63] Guidelines for best practices in diagnostic interventional breast procedures and standards have recently been published by the European Society of Breast Imaging.[5] A similar review of prevailing recommendations and contemporary practices in breast FNA has also recently been published.[64] Core biopsies should be reported similarly to surgical excision specimens. Audits of CNB diagnoses and comparison to final surgical excision diagnoses should be performed as part of quality assurance and improvement.

Complications

Complications for both FNB and CNB are uncommon. Major hematomas are unusual. Vasovagal reactions can occur. Pneumothorax is a rare but important complication, occurring more commonly in thin patients when the medial breast or axilla is sampled.[65,66] A tangential approach to needling should be used. Patients may complain of sudden severe pain and a chest X-ray may reveal a pneumothorax. However, some patients do not experience pain until several hours after the procedure. No life-threatening cases have been reported, but there is the potential for medicolegal problems if the patient has not been made aware of the possibility before giving consent. Subpleural hematoma has also been described. Tumor implantation in a fine needle track is a very rare event but a few cases have been recorded in which local recurrence was ascribed to tumor seeding.[67] Hematogeneous dissemination of breast tumor cells after FNB has been noted by RT-PCR.[68] Long-term follow-up of large series of cases has not shown any adverse influence of FNB on tumor spread and prognosis.[69]

FNB does cause some disruption of tissue, even with good technique. A range of changes including hemorrhage, infarction and epithelial implantation resembling invasion have been described.[70] Similar problems occur with CNB where epithelial displacement after core biopsy may imitate stromal or vascular invasion.[71] Epithelial displacement can also lead to the misdiagnosis of DCIS as an invasive carcinoma.[72] The risk of needle track seeding of mucinous carcinoma and perhaps some other malignancies should be kept in mind and the biopsy be planned so that the needle track is included in the subsequent surgical excision. There has been some concern about the risk of cutaneous seeding by CNB, but long-term experience is still insufficient to conclude if the risk is real.[73] Removal of the entire lesion by CNB can be problematic if a post-biopsy clip was not placed. Accurate measurement of tumor size, and thus stage, also becomes difficult if most of a small lesion is removed by the CNB.

In patients with breast prostheses, accidental puncture of a breast prosthesis (silicone) can be avoided by careful positioning of the lesion, ultrasound guidance, and using the nonaspiration technique.[74] Ultrasound-guided sampling with rapid compression of the aspiration site is a better alternative than stereotactic biopsy in patients with bleeding disorders. The venous compression, dependence of the breast and inability to compress the site during stereotactic biopsy encourage bruising.

Contraindications

There are no contraindications to FNB or CNB of breast lumps. Anticoagulation therapy is not a contraindication, but should be noted.

Technical considerations

Aspirates are best obtained with needles of 23–27 gauge. FNB without aspiration is preferable for benign and malignant breast lesions with a high cell content. The difference in tissue consistency between a ductal carcinoma of the usual type, a scirrhous cancer, a medullary carcinoma, a fibroadenoma, adipose tissue and a cyst wall is obvious when the needle is held directly with the fingertips. The feel of the consistency through the needle is a very valuable piece of information, and it helps to secure a representative specimen. We use aspiration only if the sample by the needle alone is too scanty, and in cystic lesions. Cellularity is lower in stereo-guided than in ultrasound-guided samples or in direct samples of palpable lesions, particularly for benign lesions. Several factors are involved. With stereotactic guidance the operator is less able to fix rubbery benign breast tissue and there is a lesser degree of movement of the needle through the lesion. The radiologist may need to withdraw the needle 1 cm above the lesion to allow a 'run-up' – a more vigorous movement through the lesion. There is also a tendency for smears to be more bloodstained, which results in some loss of bare oval nuclei in the background and sometimes in distortion of the cells.

We feel routinely rinsing the needle and syringe used in FNB with fixative, which is then filtered through a Millipore or a Nucleopore filter, is unnecessary if an adequate direct smear can be obtained. ThinPrep processed smears have been shown to be excellent for hormone receptor assessment and other prognostic markers but the use in routine diagnosis should not occur without adequate training.[75] The choice of fixation and staining depends on personal experience. If possible, both alcohol-fixed and air-dried smears should be studied. Cyst fluid is processed in a similar manner to effusions.

Over time, needles used for CNB have increased in size from 18 gauge, now to 8–9-gauge needles. CNB requires local anesthesia and sterile conditions. Although core biopsy carries a higher incidence of local complications as compared to FNB the rate is still quite low. In desmoplastic carcinoma and other fibrous paucicellular lesions it may be impossible to obtain a sufficient number of cells by FNB, and a CNB may be the only alternative to a formal surgical biopsy.

Imprint smears can easily be made from CNBs by stamping or rolling the core on a dry, clean slide, then fixed and stained the same as a FNB smear. This allows an immediate preliminary assessment of the adequacy of the biopsy and may help to reduce the number of samples.[76] Some surgeons find an immediate assessment to be of value when advising the patient.

For assessment of her-2-neu on core biopsy, recommendations for fixation time in formalin has not been fully addressed but is suggested to be at least 1 hour.

FNB for measurement of biological factors for diagnosis or prognostication

Subjective nuclear grading in FNB smears correlates well with nuclear grade in tissue sections and shows some correlation with prognosis.[77–79] Since much of the prognostic information of histologic grading depends on the measurement of mitotic activity, the good correlation between mitotic counts in tissue sections and staining for proliferation markers in smears is promising.[80] Multiple variables, such as nuclear morphometry, ploidy and cell kinetics, can be measured in cell samples or cell blocks, by microspectrophotometry, flow cytometry and video image analysis.[81,82] Tumor-cell proliferation fraction measured by MIB-1 count in tissue samples has been shown to be a useful prognostic parameter in breast cancer.[83] Immunohistochemical quantitation of ER and PR at the cellular level is an important development in breast pathology, and measurement in smears or cell blocks is as accurate as in tissue.[84,85] Newer molecular techniques for detecting p53 gene mutations by PCR, gene alterations by fluorescence in situ hybridization or c-erb B2 oncoprotein by immunocytochemistry or fluorescence in situ hybridization can be applied to FNB material.[82,86]

Emerging molecular techniques such as genomic and proteomic profiling has been successfully used in cytologic material to identify patients at high risk for the development of carcinoma, for prediction of patient outcome and response to treatment and for tumor characterization.[2] Studies have shown the successful use of FNB samples for cDNA microarray[87] and protein microarray analyses.[88]

While prognostic marker studies can be performed on FNB, preference should be to perform ancillary studies on core biopsy or excision specimens.[64] Prognostic and predictive factors that can be reliably assessed on core biopsy include tumor type, tumor grade, tumor size, extent of in situ component, presence of microinvasion, presence of lymphovascular invasion, and the presence of tumor necrosis.[89] Biomarker assessment has included the study of molecular markers that have predictive and prognostic value including her-2, ER and PR. Other markers studied include p53, bcl-2, MIB-1, EGFR, and human milk fat globule membrane.[89] High-throughput gene expression profiling have been performed on core biopsy specimens.[90]

CYTOLOGICAL FINDINGS

Non-neoplastic glandular breast tissue

A comparison between the basic benign pattern (non-neoplastic glandular tissue) and the most common malignant pattern (low-grade carcinoma of no special type) in FNB of breast lesions is given in Table 7.2 (Figs 7.2–7.4).

The basic benign pattern is common to normal glandular breast tissue. Variations occur with the menstrual cycle and with the age of the patient, depending upon the variable proportions between epithelial cells and fibrous stroma. The yield of the needle biopsy is usually scanty and multiple biopsies should always be made to increase the likelihood that the material is representative.

The bimodal pattern of cohesive groups of epithelial cells and scattered single, bare, oval/bipolar nuclei is diagnostic of benign, non-neoplastic breast tissue. Ductular epithelial cells – this term is used here to designate cells from the intralobular epithelial structures of the resting breast, which differ distinctly from the acinar epithelial cells seen in pregnancy and lactation (see below) – are cohesive and are seen as small epithelial groups, which represent terminal ductules. The cohesiveness of non-neoplastic epithelium is in contrast to the dyscohesion of malignant cells unless very well differentiated (Figs 7.3 and 7.5). The nuclei are irregularly distributed within the groups and may appear crowded and overlapping (multilayered). They are uniform, small, round or oval, dark, with a granular chromatin. Nucleoli are indistinct or are very small. Cytoplasm is scanty, visible, but without distinct cell borders; it is pale and may show a blue

Table 7.2 Comparison of the benign pattern and low-grade carcinoma in FNB smears

Non-neoplastic breast tissue (Figs 7.2A, 7.3A and 7.4A)	Low-grade carcinoma NOS (Figs 7.2B, 7.3B and 7.4B)
1. Overall low cell yield	1. Variable but higher cell yield
2. Sheets and aggregates of cohesive, small, uniform cells	2. Irregular clusters of less cohesive, small, mildly irregular cells
3. Small rounded nuclei, bland chromatin, some overlapping	3. Slightly larger and darker nuclei, relatively bland chromatin
4. Myoepithelial cell nuclei among epithelial cells	4. Myoepithelial cell nuclei not seen
5. Variable numbers of single, bare, bipolar nuclei scattered in the background	5. Single cells, most with some cytoplasm, identical to those forming clusters; no bare bipolar nuclei

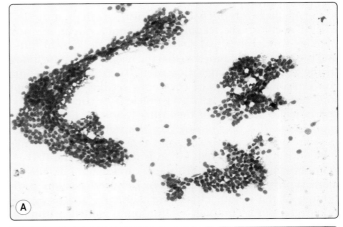

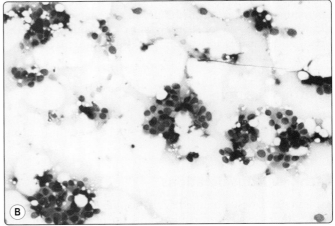

Fig. 7.2 Non-neoplastic glandular breast tissue and low-grade duct carcinoma Low-power view; (A) Bimodal population of epithelial sheets and single bipolar nuclei of non-neoplastic glandular breast tissue; (B) Single population of epithelial cells in low-grade carcinoma (MGG, LP).

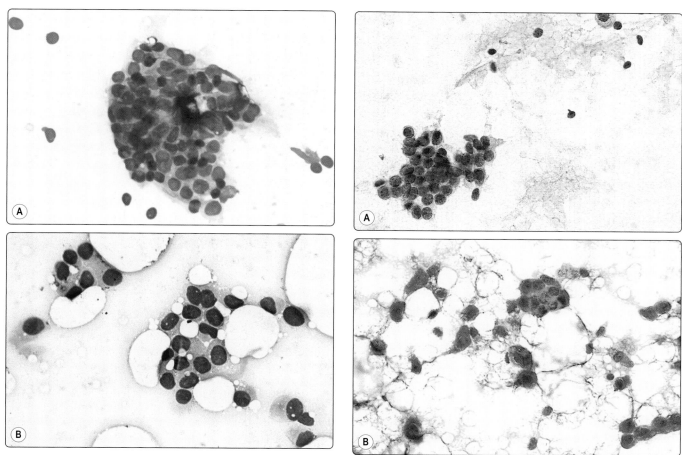

Fig. 7.3 Non-neoplastic glandular breast tissue and low-grade duct carcinoma High-power view, air-dried smears; (**A**) Non-neoplastic glandular breast tissue; (**B**) Low-grade duct carcinoma. Note single bipolar nuclei in **A**, and absence of bipolar nuclei, relatively mild nuclear atypia and some loss of cohesion of malignant cells in **B** (MGG, HP).

Fig. 7.4 Non-neoplastic glandular breast tissue and low-grade duct carcinoma High-power view, Pap-stained smears; (**A**) Bimodal population in smear from non-neoplastic breast; (**B**) Single and clustered cells in low-grade carcinoma; some single cells probably stromal (Pap, HP).

granulation (MGG). Epithelial fragments from larger ducts are sometimes present. They form monolayered sheets of regularly arranged, slightly larger cells with uniform nuclei. The single, bare nuclei scattered in the background are of the same size or a little smaller than those of the epithelial cells. They have a bipolar/oval shape and a very smooth nuclear outline. The chromatin is dense and homogeneous and nucleoli are not seen (Figs 7.3A and 7.4A). The bipolar/oval nuclei sometimes wash off in heavily bloodstained and in wet-fixed smears. Nuclei of similar appearance can also be seen scattered between the cells of the epithelial fragments, distinguishable from these by their smaller size, bipolar shape, and darker staining (Fig. 7.6). They no doubt represent myoepithelial cells, whereas the single nuclei scattered in the background may be either myoepithelial or derived from the specialized, intralobular connective tissue. The number of bipolar/oval nuclei in smears corresponds closely to the cellularity of the lobular stromal component in sections. This is particularly evident in smears from fibroadenoma. However, a recent study of p63 immunoexpression in these cells concluded that the majority was of myoepithelial origin.[91] Small fragments of collagen may be seen, particularly if larger-caliber needles have been used, but are

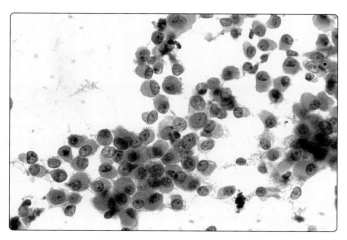

Fig. 7.5 Intermediate-grade duct carcinoma Malignant epithelial cells with intact cytoplasm showing loss of cohesion characteristic of malignancy (Pap, HP).

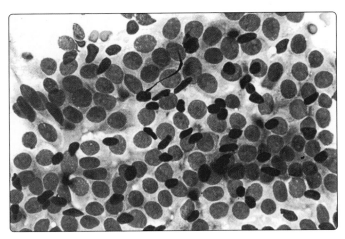

Fig. 7.6 Non-neoplastic glandular breast tissue Sheet of cohesive ductular epithelial cells and scattered small, dark nuclei of myoepithelial cells (MGG, HP).

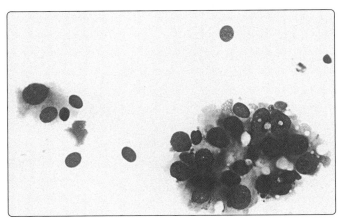

Fig. 7.7 Hormone-induced 'atypia' in non-neoplastic breast Moderate nuclear enlargement and anisokaryosis but bimodal pattern maintained (MGG, HP).

usually inconspicuous, whereas fragments of adipose tissue are frequently present.

Hormone-related changes in non-neoplastic breast tissue

The breast gland is a hormone-responsive organ. Hormonal stimulation causes a hyperplastic response of the epithelial component. This may result in an increased cell content of FNB samples. It may also cause some nuclear enlargement and anisokaryosis, and cell cohesion may be somewhat diminished. The hormone-related 'atypia' that can be seen in pregnancy and in patients on hormone replacement therapy can occasionally cause some concern.[92,93] However, except in late pregnancy and particularly in lactating breast tissue, the biphasic pattern of epithelial fragments and scattered single naked bipolar/oval nuclei characteristic of non-neoplastic breast tissue is maintained (Fig. 7.7).

Breast tissue in pregnancy and lactation (Fig. 7.8)

CRITERIA FOR DIAGNOSIS

- Cellular smears,
- Poorly cohesive, mainly dispersed epithelial cells of acinar type,
- Cells have abundant fragile cytoplasm with secretory vacuoles and frayed borders,
- Rounded vesicular nuclei and central nucleoli,
- Dirty background due to lipid secretion and stripped nuclei with prominent nucleoli,
- Single bipolar nuclei difficult to find.

minimum during pregnancy and lactation. The pattern seen in FNB smears of 'lumps' in a pregnant or lactating breast can be problematic to inexperienced eyes and cause concern for malignancy.[93,94] Smears are usually cellular. The cells

are enlarged and arranged in loose groups or singly. The cells have an abundant fragile cytoplasm, vacuolated and finely granular. Nuclei are round, central, larger than the usual ductular cells, and have distinct small nucleoli (Fig. 7.8B). Some epithelial nuclei are stripped of cytoplasm. Single naked bipolar/oval nuclei are difficult to find. The background of abundant milky secretion with numerous lipid droplets seen as vacuoles is characteristic of actively secreting breast tissue and is the main clue to the diagnosis (Fig. 7.8A).

PROBLEMS AND DIFFERENTIAL DIAGNOSIS

- Breast cancer in pregnancy and lactation.[95]
- The cellularity, the loss of cell cohesion, the lack of a bimodal population and of single bipolar nuclei, and the prominent nucleoli seen in smears of lactating breast tissue could be misinterpreted as carcinoma. The alveolar variant of lobular carcinoma in particular may appear quite similar (see Fig. 7.73A), and the rare secretory variant of breast cancer should also be kept in mind . A false-positive diagnosis is possible in the absence of clinical information. However, the nuclear chromatin is bland, granular and evenly distributed, and the nuclei are uniformly round with a smooth outline. The milky background is the principal key to diagnosis. On the other hand, a malignant lesion could be undercalled due to fears of overdiagnosis of lactational change as cancer. A lump in a lactating breast can thus be a difficult problem for FNB. Clinical correlation and ultrasonography are essential, and CNB or surgical excision may be inevitable in some cases.

Gynecomastia of the male breast[96-98]

Fine needle aspiration biopsy is an extremely valuable tool in the initial evaluation of breast masses in men.[96-98] In one series, gynecomastia was the most common diagnostic entity encountered in men with breast lumps.[96] The cytological pattern of gynecomastia is not specific and the clinical presentation must be known to allow a diagnosis. Smears

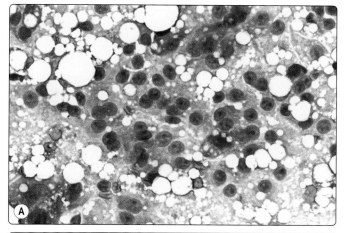

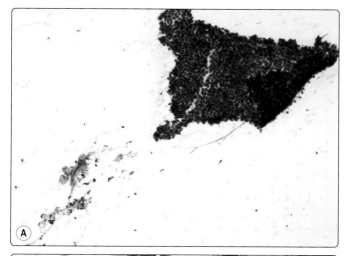

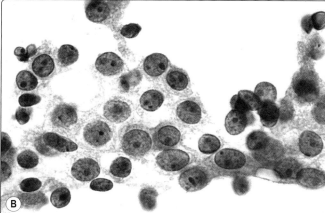

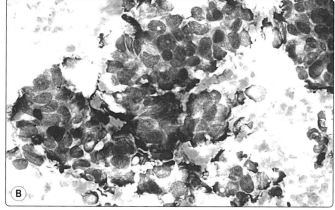

Fig. 7.9 Gynecomastia (A) Usual findings: large epithelial fragments, many single bipolar nuclei, fragments of stroma (MGG, LP); (B) Case showing atypical epithelial cells suspicious of malignancy; histologically benign gynecomastia (MGG, HP).

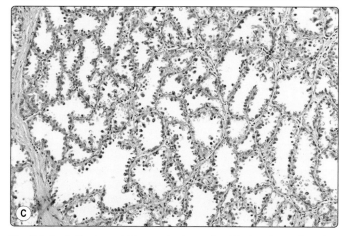

Fig. 7.8 Lactating breast Dispersed acinar cells with abundant pale and fragile cytoplasm, rounded nuclei and prominent central nucleoli; background of lipid secretions (**A**, MGG, HP; **B**, H & E, HP oil); (**C**) Corresponding tissue section (H&E, IP).

are variably cellular, ranging from scanty to markedly cellular. Epithelial fragments are often large as flat/monolayered sheets often with finger-like projections similar to fibroadenoma. Often there is a bimodal pattern of stroma and epithelial cells in addition to single bare bipolar/oval nuclei in the background. Adipose tissue may be present. Moderate nuclear variation and atypia can be allowed in the presence

of a benign bimodal pattern (Fig. 7.9A). In some cases, nuclear atypia and cellularity can be quite prominent and can cause a concern for carcinoma and lead to excision (Fig. 7.9B).[98] In contrast to gynecomastia, carcinoma yields more consistently highly cellular smears with discohesive single malignant cells, more pronounced atypia and lack of bare oval nuclei.

Fibrocystic change

Main features

- Epithelial fragments of usual epithelial cells,
- Scattered single bare bipolar/oval nuclei,
- Background of variable amounts of cyst fluid, macrophages, and apocrine metaplastic cells.

Fibrocystic change may clinically cause an indistinct thickening or 'lump', or an asymmetrical density on the mammogram. Cytologically, it is a variant of the common benign pattern in which 'cyst macrophages', apocrine metaplastic cells and sheets of ductal epithelial cells are found in addition to the usual bimodal cell population of ductular epithelium and single bare oval nuclei. The former components may dominate the smears. Fluid from dilated ducts increases the volume of the aspirate. 'Cyst macrophages' have an abundant, finely vacuolated cytoplasm and may contain pigment, and small round central nuclei. At least some of the 'macrophages' may be degenerating epithelial cells exfoliated from the epithelial lining of dilated ducts, rather than true macrophages. Apocrine metaplastic cells have abundant, dense, finely granular eosinophilic cytoplasm, which stains gray-blue with MGG. The nuclei are round, nuclear size may vary considerably and nucleoli are often prominent. However, the nuclear outline is smooth and the chromatin pattern is uniformly granular (see Fig. 7.13A).

PROBLEMS IN DIAGNOSIS

◆ Representative samples,
◆ Apocrine atypia.

Fibrocystic change' is not a specific cytological diagnosis. These changes are usually poorly circumscribed, and in the same area there may be focal epithelial hyperplasia, atypia or even malignancy. Malignancy can only be ruled out in the tiny area biopsied and the findings in the FNB samples must be evaluated in the context of the clinical and mammographic findings.

The amount of apocrine epithelium aspirated may be large and sometimes the cells show a greater degree of nuclear enlargement. Macronucleoli may also be seen. The atypia can raise a suspicion of carcinoma with apocrine differentiation (see Fig. 7.13B). However, benign apocrine epithelium in fibrocystic breast tissue is cohesive, forming monolayered sheets with few dispersed cells. Even when anisokaryosis is prominent, the N:C ratio is not increased, the nuclei are rounded, the nuclear membrane is smooth and the chromatin rarely shows any obvious abnormality. In contrast, groups of malignant apocrine cells are multilayered and disorganised. Nuclei are markedly pleomorphic and have irregular outlines and abnormal chromatin. If there is a DCIS component, as is often the case, necrotic debris is present in the background.Simple cyst (Figs 7.10–7.14)

CRITERIA FOR DIAGNOSIS

◆ Complete disappearance of the lump after aspiration of the fluid,
◆ Absence of altered blood or necrotic material in the aspirated fluid,
◆ 'Cyst macrophages' and more or less degenerate apocrine epithelial cells,
◆ Inflammatory cells (polymorphs) variable.

Breast cysts are easily diagnosed by US. However, evacuation by FNB may be a more convenient way to immediately relieve patient anxiety. Simple cysts are by far the commonest situation in which a confident benign diagnosis can be rendered by FNB, and a surgical excision avoided.

The aspirated fluid may be thin, clear or turbid, straw colored, brown or green. Smears may be practically cell free (Fig. 7.12A) or contain variable numbers of 'cyst macrophages' and epithelial cells, usually of apocrine metaplastic

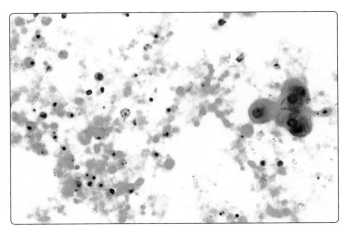

Fig. 7.10 Simple cyst Debris and degenerating 'macrophages'; group of apocrine epithelial cells (Pap, HP).

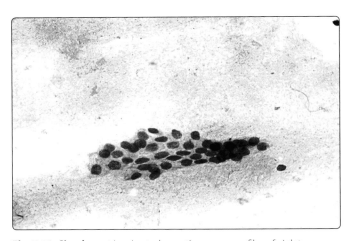

Fig. 7.11 Simple cyst Inspissated secretion seen as a film of violet structureless material; sheet of bland ductal epithelial cells (MGG, IP).

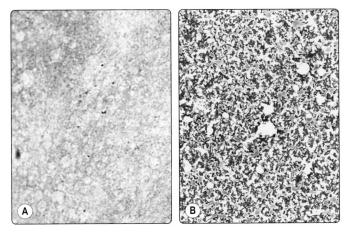

Fig. 7.12 Non-cellular material in breast aspirates (A) Proteinaceous structureless material aspirated from simple cyst; (B) Ultrasound gel contamination (MGG, HP).

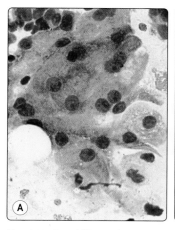
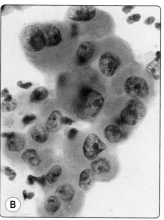

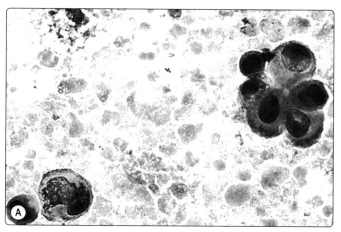

Fig. 7.13 Oxyphil/apocrine cells in cyst fluids (A) Typical sheet of oxyphil cells with abundant cytoplasm and enlarged but bland nuclei (MGG, HP); (B) Sheet of oxyphil epithelium showing prominent nuclear enlargement, anisokaryosis, irregular chromatin and nucleoli, aspirated from simple benign cyst (Pap, HP).

type and more or less degenerate (Fig. 7.13A). Numerous polymorphs are sometimes found in the cyst fluid even in cases with no clinical signs of inflammation.

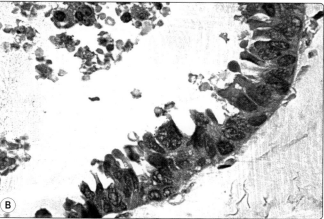

Fig. 7.14 Cystic carcinoma (A) Obviously malignant epithelial cells with a background of debris in aspirated fluid (MGG, HP); (B) Tissue section showing malignant cells lining the cyst wall (H&E, HP).

PROBLEMS AND DIFFERENTIAL DIAGNOSIS

◆ Associated small cancers,
◆ Cystic carcinoma,
◆ Atypical apocrine epithelial cells,
◆ Inspissation/condensation of cyst contents, duct ectasia.

A carcinoma may be present next to a cyst, hidden by a dominant benign cyst. Truly cystic carcinomas are uncommon but do occur, for example intracystic papillary carcinoma.[99] Aspirated cyst fluid may be non-diagnostic. Correlation with radiological findings and re-aspiration of any residual lump after the fluid has been evacuated is essential. Some apparently cystic or partly cystic carcinomas are high-grade tumors with massive central hemorrhage and necrosis. The aspirated fluid is thick, murky and brown due to altered blood. A careful search of the smears may reveal aggregates of cells recognizable as malignant (Fig. 7.14A), or a mass remains after the initial aspiration. Repeat FNB usually yields diagnostic material.

It has been said that malignancy can safely be excluded if no abnormality remains after the cyst has been emptied and if the fluid is not bloody. Microscopic examination of the fluid may then not be necessary.

Apocrine metaplastic cells in cyst fluid often appear atypical, sometimes bizarre and worrying (Fig. 7.13B). They can mimic squamous differentiation and there may be unusual spindle-shaped epithelial cells. However, if all other findings are typical of a simple cyst and in the absence of altered blood or necrotic debris, or of a residual mass after the fluid has been drained, there is no indication for further investigation.

A distinction between inspissated cyst and duct ectasia as defined histologically cannot be made in smears. The

diagnosis is based on the clinical findings. Duct ectasia is usually located close to the nipple, presenting as a subareolar cord-like mass of thickened tissue. It is an unlikely diagnosis in lesions located peripherally in the breast. The presence of chronic inflammatory cells and an occasional sheet of duct epithelium and a total absence of nuclear debris in the condensed secretion of duct ectasia is a clue.

Mastitis (Fig. 7.15)

Common findings.

- A benign bimodal component of non-neoplastic breast tissue,
- Inflammatory cells, chronic and/or acute,
- Regenerative epithelial atypia,
- Histiocytes, epithelioid cells, multinucleated giant cells and plasma cells (granulomatous pattern),
- Microorganisms (infectious mastitis).

There are four types of mastitis recognized; acute, chronic, granulomatous and non-specific.[93] The diagnosis of acute mastitis and abscess presents no problems. Pregnancy is the most common association, but occasionally cysts become infected (often by coagulase-negative staphylococci). The entity of subareolar abscess is recognized separately (Fig.

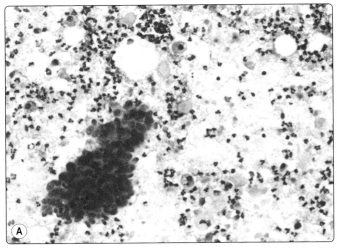

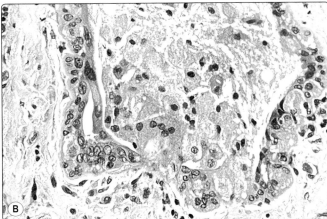

Fig. 7.15 Regenerative epithelial atypia in mastitis (A) Atypical, reactive/regenerating epithelial cells with a background of histiocytes, inflammatory cells and debris (MGG, HP); (B) Corresponding tissue section (H&E, IP).

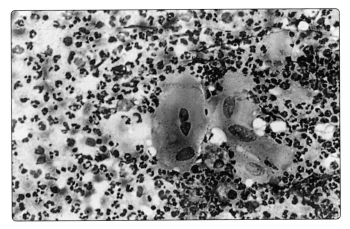

Fig. 7.16 Subareolar abscess Keratinising squamous cells in a background of acute inflammation (MGG, HP).

7.16). Chronic mastitis may be the result of persistence of an acute mastitis, a reaction to retained secretion in fibrocystic disease or duct ectasia, or secondary to previous surgery.

Granulomatous mastitis is an uncommon condition. It may mimic carcinoma radiographically and clinically;

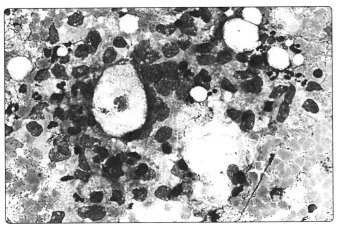

Fig. 7.17 Granulomatous mastitis Atypical epithelial cells, histiocytes and inflammatory cells; no distinctly granulomatous pattern in this example (MGG, HP).

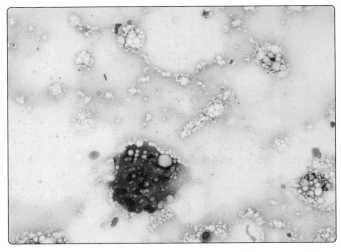

Fig. 7.18 Silicone granuloma A giant cell with some foreign material from palpable nodule adjacent to breast prosthesis (MGG, HP).

etiology is variable, ranging from tuberculosis, fungal, silicone, tumor related, sarcoidosis, fat necrosis, foreign body to non-specific. Aspiration reveals epithelioid histiocytes, multinucleate giant cells. Lymphocytes and plasma cells, may also be seen.

Epithelial atypia can be worrying in some cases of mastitis (Fig. 7.17). Caution is advised in interpreting cytologic findings within the clinical context. However, open biopsy may be necessary for definitive diagnosis in rare cases.

A foreign-body-type granulomatous reaction to silicone can occur adjacent to a breast prosthesis.[100] FNB of a palpable nodule next to the implant may be performed to exclude malignancy. Great care must obviously be taken to avoid accidental puncture of the prosthesis, and US guidance is therefore required. The smear findings are of a foreign body granuloma with multinucleated giant cells, which may contain silicone particles and fibers (Fig. 7.18). If the nodule is a reaction to escaped silicone, the histiocytes and giant cells often contain vacuoles where the lipid-like material has been dissolved in processing.

Regenerative atypia of duct epithelium in an area of mastitis can look worrying and suspicious (Figs 7.15A and 7.17). In addition, the nuclei of reactive histiocytes may appear large and atypical, particularly in air-dried smears. False-positive diagnoses in cases of chronic mastitis and organizing fat necrosis have been reported. However, large numbers of both acute and chronic inflammatory cells are rarely seen in carcinoma. In medullary carcinoma with lymphocytic infiltration and in comedocarcinoma, in which lymphocytes and histiocytes are mixed with the carcinoma cells, the latter dominate and nuclear morphology is obviously malignant. The presence of necrotic cell debris should evoke a suspicion of malignancy.

Recurring subareolar abscess; lactiferous duct fistula (see Fig. 7.16)

CRITERIA FOR DIAGNOSIS:[101]

◆ Purulent inflammation,
◆ Keratin flakes and debris; mature squamous cells.

The prevailing view about the pathogenesis of this condition is keratinizing metaplasia of lactiferous ducts, perhaps as a pre-existing anomaly of the site, associated with recurrent bouts of inflammation, sometimes leading to a sinus track into areolar skin. Some of these episodes may be a chemical mastitis related to duct rupture, but superimposed infection does occur. The patients are often young and nulliparous. Mature or anucleate squamous cells with a background of pus aspirated from an abscess deep to the areola enable this diagnosis to be made. A specific cytologic diagnosis is of clinical significance, since these lesions generally require surgical treatment including excision of the affected duct system.

Problems in diagnosis.

• Contaminant squamous epithelium,
• Reactive changes in inflammatory and epithelial cells,
• Epidermoid cysts.

Keratinous material from the surface of the skin or from dirty slides may be misleading. There must be relatively abundant squamous material intimately mixed with the inflammatory cells to suggest the diagnosis. Reparative changes/atypia occur but the background of acute inflammation should prevent overdiagnosis.

Infected or ruptured epidermoid cysts produce a similar cytological picture, but occur more laterally and superficially.

Fat necrosis (Fig. 7.19)

CRITERIA FOR DIAGNOSIS

◆ A 'dirty' background of granular debris, fat droplets and fragments of adipose tissue,
◆ Foamy macrophages, multinucleated giant cells and adipocytes with bubbly cytoplasm,
◆ Chronic inflammatory cells,
◆ Absence of epithelial cells.

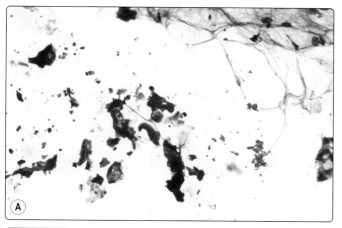

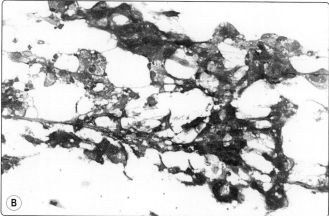

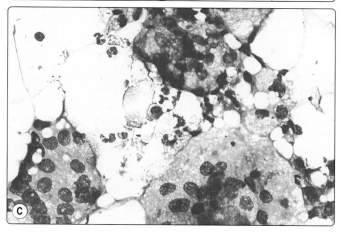

Fig. 7.19 Fat necrosis (A) Postoperative fat necrosis. Necrotic tissue, debris and macrophages; fragment of adipose tissue upper right (MGG IP); (B) Fragments consisting of altered adipocytes, macrophages and fat droplets (MGG, IP); (C) Several multinucleated histiocytes with foamy cytoplasm (MGG, HP).

Postoperative changes in response to prior surgical excision or biopsy give similar findings. Fat necrosis is always in the differential diagnosis of nodules in scars or chest wall after surgery, particularly mastectomy. Vigorous or repeated palpation of breast tissue or previous aspiration of the site can result in the same changes. The aspirate is usually scanty, sometimes of oily fluid, and consists mainly of fat with some foamy macrophages or altered, vacuolated adipocytes and multinucleated histiocytic giant cells. The untidy background of granular debris represents the actual necrosis and is the most specific diagnostic feature (Fig. 7.19A,B).

Problems in diagnosis.

- Lipid cysts,
- Macrophages mistaken for atypical epithelial cells,
- Carcinoma cells with a macrophage-like appearance.

The dissolution of fat leads to a lipid cyst. Lipid cysts can be recognised by radiologists. The liquid is very viscous and may be yellow, clear, or have an unusual appearance of a gray-white color possibly corresponding to saponification. Solidification of the fluid in the test tube occurs after aspiration. The material does not stain with MGG although it may not dissolve completely during staining. A crystalline appearance is sometimes present in unstained slides.

The dispersed presentation of macrophages, particularly if the cytoplasm is dense or nonvacuolated and the nuclei are large with an irregular shape and prominent nucleoli, may mimic a malignant cell pattern, particularly in air-dried MGG smears. Multinucleate forms and foamy cells with similar morphology are helpful in preventing error (Fig. 7.19C).[102] Conversely, some carcinoma cells may resemble macrophages. Immunostaining or excision is sometimes necessary.

'Lipoma' – hypertrophic fat tissue

> **CRITERIA FOR DIAGNOSIS**
>
> - A well-defined, rounded, soft mass,
> - 'Empty' sensation on needling,
> - Fat only in multiple aspirates – fat vacuoles and/or fragments of adipose tissue.

Lesions of this type in the breast are not true lipomas but focal hypertrophy of fat tissue or 'fatty lobules' contained within a fibrous compartment of the breast. Focal fat hypertrophy presents as a discrete, rounded mass, which is often tender. It may be fairly firm to palpation, but at needling, once the thin fibrous capsule has been penetrated, the mass itself has a soft, 'empty' feel. Correlation with mammography is important to ascertain that the biopsy is representative, since the aspirated material is no different from that of normal adipose tissue of the breast or subcutis.

Intramammary and axillary lymph nodes

Lymph nodes are not uncommonly found within the breast, usually in the axillary tail but nodes can occur in any of the quadrants and more centrally.[103] A lymph node may clinically simulate a fibroadenoma or a cyst and can be indeterminate on mammographic examination. Furthermore, malignant lymphoma can present as a breast lump, albeit rarely.[104,105] The differential diagnosis between a reactive lymph node and lymphoma is discussed in Chapter 5, between lymphoid tissue and small cell primary breast carcinoma of neuroendocrine type on page 195.

Axillary or intramammary lymph nodes are usually correctly identified by the radiologist because of the bean shape and the central lucent hilum. Distinction between axillary

node metastasis and primary carcinoma of the upper outer quadrant with a high content of lymphocytes is difficult at times, and node enlargement incidentally noted at mammography could be caused by malignant lymphoma.

US-guided FNA has been successfully utilized for the initial determination of axillary lymph node status in breast carcinoma.[106] Ultrasound is more sensitive than physical examination in determining axillary lymph node status in patients with newly diagnosed breast carcinoma. US-guided FNB provides a more definitive diagnosis in sonographically indeterminate/suspicious lymph nodes compared to information provided by US alone.

Ectopic breast tissue

Breast tissue extending high up in the axilla commonly forms nodules or irregular lumps noted by the patient, especially during pregnancy and lactation, and may be referred for FNB. The ectopic glandular tissue may take part in fibrocystic change, and fibroadenoma or primary carcinoma can occasionally arise from ectopic tissue.[106,107]

Postradiation/chemotherapy effects[17,19,108]

Common findings.

- Anisocytosis; anisonucleosis but preserved N:C ratio,
- Smudged chromatin,
- Cytoplasm abundant, vacuolated, indistinct or basophilic-amphophilic hyaline,
- Preserved spatial arrangement of cells,
- Little dissociation of epithelial cells,
- Presence of myoepithelial cells,
- Clean background.

These features apply to glandular breast tissue undergoing radiation and/or chemotherapy. Post-treatment atypia can be severe and highly suggestive of recurrent carcinoma (see Fig. 7.1A). The key to a correct distinction cytologically between post-treatment atypia and recurrent malignancy is, above all, the awareness of this pitfall and the experience of benign reactive cellular changes from other fields of cytology. High cellularity and dissociation of the abnormal cells, and lack of bare oval nuclei are probably the most reliable criteria of recurrent malignancy in treated tissue. Most smears from benign post-treatment change are relatively low in cellularity. Although pleomorphism can be prominent, the cells are usually in cohesive groups with associated myoepithelial cell nuclei.

Fibroadenoma and phyllodes tumor

Fibroadenoma (Figs 7.20–7.28)

> **CRITERIA FOR DIAGNOSIS**
>
> - Cellular smears with a bimodal pattern containing epithelial and stromal fragments,
> - Large, branching sheets of bland epithelial cells,
> - Numerous single, bare bipolar/oval nuclei,
> - Fragments of fibromyxoid stroma.

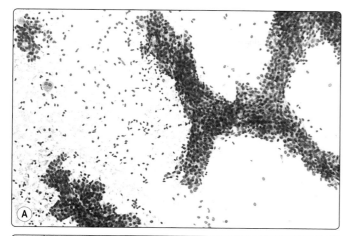

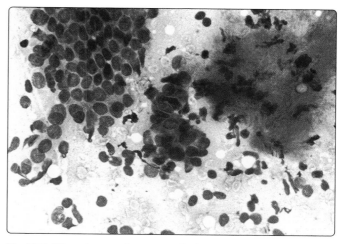

Fig. 7.21 **Fibroadenoma** Aggregates of cohesive epithelial cells, bare bipolar nuclei and a fragment of fibromyxoid stroma (MGG, HP).

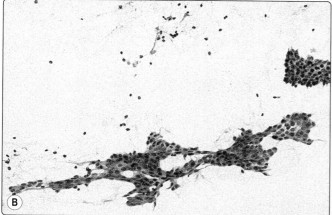

Fig. 7.20 **Fibroadenoma** Cell-rich smear of elongated, branching fragments of ductal epithelium and numerous single bipolar nuclei in the background (**A**, MGG; **B**, Pap; LP).

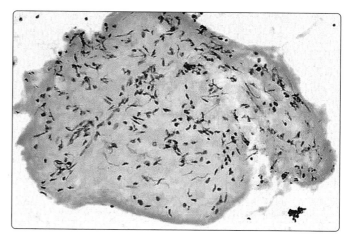

Fig. 7.22 **Fibroadenoma** Fragment of fibromyxoid stroma with many spindle cells (Pap, LP).

Fibroadenoma is one of the most common benign mammary neoplasms sampled by FNB. Aspiration biopsy is a highly reliable diagnostic procedure in the diagnosis of fibroadenoma when combined with clinical and imaging findings with a sensitivity reaching 97% and specificity, positive predictive value and negative predictive value reported to be 94%, 79% and 98%, respectively.[109,110] Fibroadenomas are usually well-circumscribed lesions and have a characteristic rubbery consistency felt through the needle. Smears show a bimodal pattern of non-neoplastic breast tissue but are more cellular (Fig. 7.20). The epithelial fragments of regularly arranged, cohesive cells are large, elongated and branching, stag-horn-like, reflecting the appearance in tissue sections. There is variable nuclear crowding and overlapping. The nuclei are often mildly enlarged but uniform, have a bland granular chromatin pattern and often one or two small, indistinct nucleoli. Single, bare bipolar/oval nuclei are scattered in the background. They are characteristically numerous, much more numerous than in the usual glandular breast tissue, except in fibrotic and sclerosed

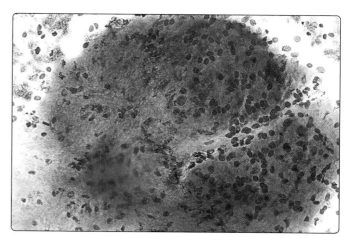

Fig. 7.23 **Fibroadenoma** Fragment of loosely fibromyxoid stroma with many spindle cells in a FNB smear. A cellular stroma per se is not diagnostic of phyllodes tumor (MGG, IP).

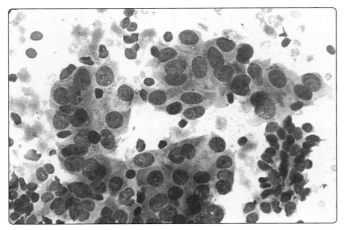

Fig. 7.24 Epithelial atypia in fibroadenoma Aggregates of atypical epithelial cells showing prominent nuclear enlargement and some irregularity; compare the epithelial fragment of bland cells of usual type at lower right; scattered bare bipolar nuclei (MGG, HP).

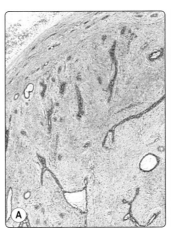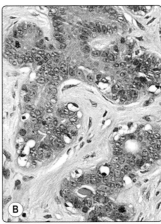

Fig. 7.27 Fibroadenoma Tissue sections from same case as Figure 7.24; (A) Low power: typical appearances of fibroadenoma; (B) High power: ductal structures lined by atypical epithelium with enlarged vesicular nuclei and a few mitoses (H&E).

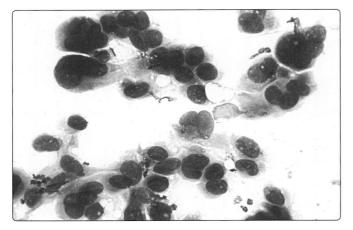

Fig. 7.25 Severe nuclear atypia in fibroadenoma Prominent nuclear enlargement and pleomorphism, hyperchromasia and irregular chromatin. Benign elements typical of fibroadenoma were present in other parts of same smear (MGG, HP).

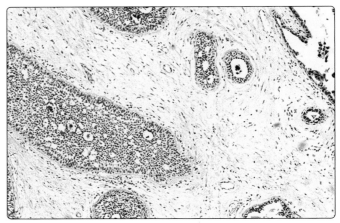

Fig. 7.28 DCIS within a fibroadenoma FNB smears from this lesion showed epithelial atypia, and excision was recommended. Tissue section (H&E, LP).

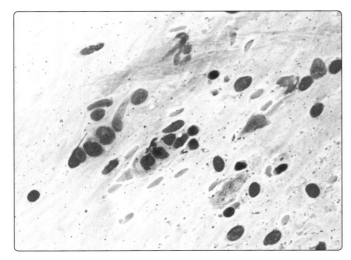

Fig. 7.26 Fibroadenoma Dissociation of ductal cells that can be seen in fibroadenomas (MGG, HP).

fibroadenomas. Myoepithelial cell nuclei are also frequently seen within the epithelial aggregates. Sometimes, epithelial cells with apocrine differentiation may be prominent, and large numbers of foamy macrophages may suggest a cystic component. Fragments of fibromyxoid stroma are obtained from most but not all fibroadenomas. They stain pink to magenta with MGG, pale bluish-green with Pap, have a fibrillary structure and contain spindled fibroblastic nuclei (Figs 7.21–7.23). There may be a film of myxoid ground substance in the background. Smears from fibroadenoma with abundant collagenous stroma and scanty epithelium are less characteristic and may not differ much from the usual non-neoplastic breast tissue or fibrocystic change.

The triad of a cellular smear with a bimodal benign pattern, numerous single bipolar oval nuclei and fragments of stroma is virtually diagnostic of fibroadenoma. In the absence of stroma, numerous single bipolar nuclei are highly suggestive of the diagnosis.

Since a confident diagnosis of fibroadenoma usually means no excision and no further follow-up, diagnostic criteria must be strictly observed. These include the clinical and/or mammographic presentation of a well-defined rounded mass or density. There is some overlap between the smear patterns of proliferative fibrocystic change, or papilloma and fibroadenoma.[109–111] Smears of papilloma may have large, branching epithelial fragments associated with fibrous stroma resembling fibroadenoma, but do not contain numerous single bipolar nuclei and the stroma is not myxoid. Fibrovascular cores and detached columnar cells are usually present. The distinction is more difficult in case of fibroadenoma with a fibrotic stroma. Fragments of myxoid stroma may also be seen in 'fibroadenomatoid hyperplasia'. Fibroadenoma can undergo cystic degeneration, or the ductal structures can become dilated and filled with fluid. Smears from such lesions may contain numerous 'cyst macrophages' and apocrine metaplastic cells and may be interpreted as fibrocystic change.

Prominent nuclear atypia shown by a proportion of the epithelial cells is a common phenomenon in fibroadenoma, particularly in young women and women on hormone replacement therapy. The atypia is in the form of nuclear enlargement, anisokaryosis, some irregularity in shape and nuclear chromatin, prominent nucleoli, sometimes a few mitotic figures, and loss of cohesion (Figs 7.24–7.26). The cohesiveness of the epithelial component and relatively bland apearance of epithelial cells should alert against a diagnosis of carcinoma in such cases. Fibroadenoma is the most common cause of false-suspicious and false-positive diagnoses in breast FNB.[112–115] In the presence of a clearly benign component of single bipolar nuclei, fragments of bland epithelium, and stroma, a malignant diagnosis should not be made regardless of the degree of atypia shown by a proportion of the epithelial cells. The atypia is most likely hormone related, but a consistent correlation with hormone replacement therapy has not been demonstrated. Proliferative fibrocystic changes and apocrine metaplasia are also common sources of atypia. Histologically, fibroadenomas with severe cytological atypia do not differ from the usual type overall, but focally the duct epithelium may show corresponding nuclear atypia when examined with high magnification (Fig. 7.27). Nevertheless, if prominent atypia is found in FNB smears, a recommendation of excision is advised. Carcinoma can rarely arise in a fibroadenoma. We have seen a few cases of DCIS in fibroadenoma (Fig. 7.28), one with focal invasion. In clinical practice, cytologically typical benign fibroadenomas in postmenopausal patients and fibroadenomas which continue to grow in size are often excised, particularly if the lesion is large.

Occasionally, low-grade invasive carcinoma such as tubular carcinoma, lobular carcinoma and intraductal low-grade carcinoma may have a loose fibromyxoid stroma producing a smear pattern that mimics fibroadenoma.[114,115] A false-negative diagnosis of fibroadenoma can be made in such cases. The presence or absence of single bipolar nuclei typical of non-neoplastic breast tissue is of great importance in this context. Fibroadenomas can undergo cystic degeneration, or the ductal structures can become dilated and filled with fluid. Smears from such lesions may contain numerous 'cyst macrophages' and apocrine metaplastic cells and may be interpreted as fibrocystic change. In our experience, some of these cases are difficult to classify even after retrospective review.

In some cases of myxoid fibroadenoma, mucinous (colloid) carcinoma enters the differential diagnosis.[110,116] Myxoid fibroadenoma can be distinguished from mucinous carcinoma by the background containing numerous oval bare nuclei and vascular myxoid stromal fragments, and the absence of dissociated single atypical epithelial cells floating in mucin. Smears of mucinous carcinoma lack oval bare nuclei and usually display free-floating vascular structures instead of stromal fragments. Despite these clues, some myxoid fibroadenomas may ultimately have to be surgically excised for a definitive diagnosis. In addition, in some cases atypia may be of limited value since some fibroadenomas may display more cytologic atypia then colloid carcinoma.

The distinction from phyllodes tumor is discussed below.

Phyllodes tumor (Figs 7.29–7.32)[117–123]

Phyllodes tumor (PT) is a biphasic epithelial/stromal neoplasm of the breast. In contrast to fibroadenoma, PT is a rare tumor comprising less than 0.3% of all breast tumors. It is classified as benign, low grade (borderline) and high grade (malignant) based on histologic features. Stromal cellularity and overgrowth, atypia, mitotic activity, and invasive growth pattern at tumor periphery define whether a PT is benign, low grade or high grade. Benign PTs do not metastasize, but may locally recur if incompletely excised. High-grade PTs behave like sarcomas with higher potential for recurrence and metastasis. Low-grade PTs fall in between.

Aspiration biopsy can accurately diagnose malignant PTs in most cases. On the benign/borderline end of the spectrum, cytologic features of fibroadenoma and PT overlap, making FNA diagnosis difficult (see Fig. 7.23). Precise preoperative distinction is important for optimal patient management. Classic cytologic features in PT are similar to fibroadenoma. However, as opposed to fibroadenoma, stromal fragments are larger, increased in number (stromal overgrowth) and are hypercellular (phyllodes fragments); the single stromal cells in the background are plumper than the typical oval bare nuclei seen in fibroadenoma. These single cells are intact spindled cells with retained cytoplasm (not naked nuclei), and variable degrees of nuclear atypia with nucleoli and pleomorphism. However, some of these features may be entirely lacking in benign and low-grade PTs even after retrospective review of smears, making their differentiation from fibroadenoma virtually impossible. It is not surprising that a

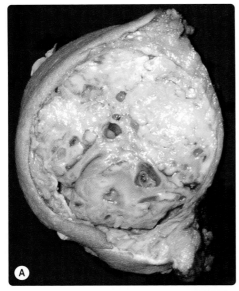

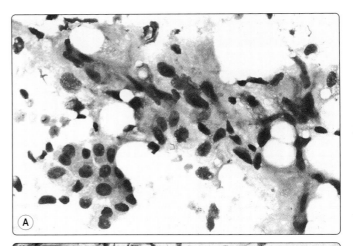

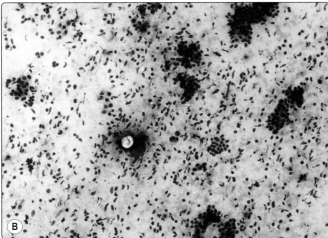

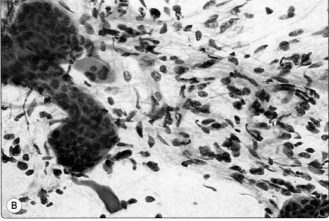

Fig. 7.30 Borderline phyllodes tumor Smears dominated by mildly atypical, both plump and slender spindle cells, single and in loose tissue fragments with fibrous stroma; a few sheets of bland duct epithelium (A, MGG; B, Pap, HP).

Fig. 7.29 Benign phyllodes tumor (A) Huge, slowly growing breast mass in a 40-year-old woman; (B) FNB smears were cellular, dominated by dispersed cells with bare oval or plump spindle nuclei (MGG, HP).

considerable portion of benign and low-grade PTs are initially diagnosed as fibroadenoma on cytology.[117,120,121] This in part reflects sampling problems as hypo- and hypercellular areas tend to alternate within PTs. Another important diagnostic pitfall in PTs is the presence of significant epithelial proliferation including atypical ductal epithelial hyperplasia. If these areas are sampled by aspiration biopsy, this may lead to a false diagnosis of epithelial neoplasm. In our experience, we encountered this problem even with high-grade (malignant) PTs; one such retroareaolar case required core biopsy due to inability of aspiration biopsy to rule out an atypical papillary lesion. In addition, focal malignant transformation may be missed by FNA sampling.

The diagnosis of PT on CNB is equally as challenging (Fig. 7.32). It is especially difficult to differentiate cellular fibroadenoma from benign/low-grade PT. In comparison, in one study, the possibility of PT was raised in 23% on FNB and 65% on core biopsy.[122] In two others, 11 of 44 (25%), and 9 of 23 (39%) of surgically resected PTs were reported as

fibroadenoma or benign on core biopsy.[123,124] Similar to FNB, some PTs are diagnosed as fibroadenoma on core biopsy because of tumor heterogeneity. Marked nuclear pleomorphism and mitotic activity suggest frankly malignant phyllodes tumor (Fig. 7.31A,B).

Other benign entities

Adenomyoepithelioma (Fig. 7.33)

Adenomyoepithelioma, an uncommon biphasic tumor composed of epithelial and myoepithelial cells, usually presents as a single circumscribed nodule.[125] Cytological features include cellular smears with epithelial aggregates, less cohesive myoepithelial cells with pale, fragile cytoplasm, and a variable amount of background stromal tissue (Fig 7.33A).[126–128] Intranuclear cytoplasmic inclusions have been observed.[129] It is important to recognize this entity, as the radiologic and cytologic features can mimic malignancy. However, only rarely can this diagnosis be made definitively on FNA due to overlapping features with other entities such as fibroadenoma, phyllodes tumor, myoepithelioma, and tubular carcinoma. A review of 18 cases collected from the

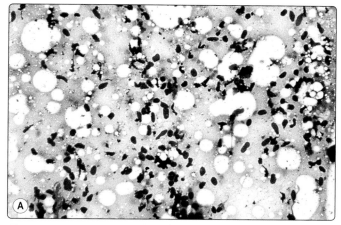

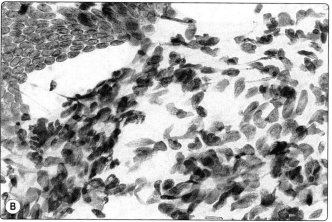

Fig. 7.31 **Malignant phyllodes tumor** (A) Mainly dispersed spindle cells showing moderate nuclear atypia, no epithelial cells. Invasive growth demonstrated in tissue sections; multiple recurrences (MGG, IP); (B) Another case showing numerous spindle cells with more marked atypia and a sheet of bland epithelium (Pap, HP).

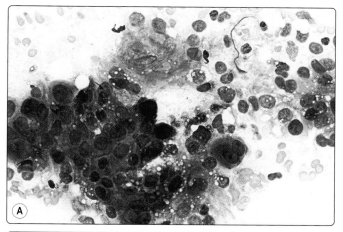

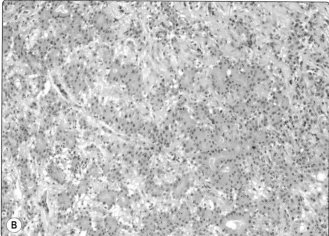

Fig. 7.33 **Adenomyoepithelioma** (A) A biphasic smear pattern of mildly atypical epithelial cells and dispersed myoepithelial cells with abundant pale fragile cytoplasm; scanty fibrous stroma (MGG, HP); (B) Core biopsy showing tubules in a pseudoinfiltrative pattern (H&E, IP).

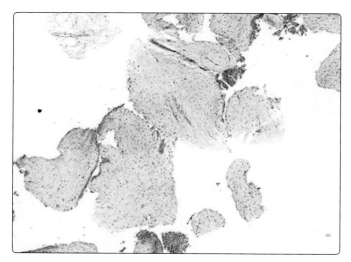

Fig. 7.32 Fibroadenoma mimicking benign phyllodes tumor on core needle biopsy (H&E, IP).

literature showed that the cytological diagnosis of this entity is often difficult and that there is a risk of false-positive reports.[130] False-positive reports of CNBs of adenomyoepithelioma have been reported (Fig. 7.33B).[131] The majority of adenomyoepitheliomas are benign but local recurrences and rarely distant metastases have been described. Rarely, malignant adenomyoepitheliomas can occur. These are usually characterized by cellular pleomorphism, necrosis, high mitotic activity and invasion of the surrounding tissue.

PROBLEMS AND DIFFERENTIAL DIAGNOSIS

◆ Phyllodes tumors: more numerous stromal cells and single spindled stromal cells in PT; single bare nuclei more elongated and abundant in PT,

◆ Myoepithelioma: lacks epithelial component,

◆ Fibroadenoma: can be confused with tubular variant of adenomyoepithelioma; staghorn epithelial groups and fibrillary (rather than dense stroma in adenomyoepithelioma) stroma,

◆ Tubular carcinoma: angular cell clusters and lack of myoepithelial cells,

◆ Adenoid cystic carcinoma: biphasic pattern with three dimensional cribriform epithelial cell clusters and amorphous hyaline globules

Tubular adenoma, adenosis tumor, microglandular adenosis

Specific diagnosis of these entities is usually not possible by FNB. Tubular adenoma usually presents as a palpable mass in young women. Cytologic features include uniform tubules and three-dimensional epithelial balls in a background containing naked nuclei but no stromal fragments.[93] Distinction from fibroadenoma may be difficult. Distinction diagnosis includes tubular carcinoma; in tubular carcinoma, tubules are more angulated and they vary in size and shape; bipolar nuclei are absent. Findings similar to tubular adenoma may be seen in adenosis tumor, which represents localised hyperplasia of lobules/ductules associated with a palpable mass. The cytologic diagnosis of adenosis tumor is difficult due to overlapping features with fibrocystic changes and fibroadenoma. Similarly, a specific cytologic diagnosis of microglandular adenosis is challenging due to overlapping features with other entities described herein. Features are similar to adenosis, with small groups of glycogen filled clear cells showing uniform nuclei and small nucleoli and clusters of fibroblastic cells. The lack of myoepithelial cells may result in an atypical/suspicious diagnosis.

The spectrum of epithelial hyperplasia

The spectrum of epithelial proliferative processes of the breast discussed herein includes usual epithelial hyperplasia, atypical ductal hyperplasia (ADH), papilloma, radial scar and complex sclerosing lesions, and sclerosing adenosis. These entities are histologically relatively well defined but there is a certain overlap that can cause inter-observer disagreement. The overlap is more important in FNB smears, and it is not often possible to seperate a particular case precisely within the spectrum.[132-134] There is also an overlap with nonproliferative lesions that sometimes can give an unusually cell-rich yield.[135] The difficulties are enhanced by the selective nature of FNB sampling. A spectrum of epithelial hyperplasia and atypical epithelial hyperplasia may be present within the same clinically or radiologically defined lesion, and the most abnormal component may not be represented in the sample. In our opinion, it is therefore preferable to report the cytological findings in this category of lesions as consistent with 'proliferative fibrocystic change' with or without atypia. The degree of atypia and any suspicion of malignancy should be specified. The definitive diagnosis is left to histology unless the lesion is considered radiologically and cytologically clearly benign with no indication for core needle or open biopsy.

It is not possible, in our opinion, to list specific cytologic criteria for each one of these processes. We can only describe and compare a number of features as they appear in the main entities – usual epithelial hyperplasia, ADH, and low-grade DCIS. Papilloma, radial scar and complex sclerosing lesions, and sclerosing adenosis will be discussed separately.

Usual epithelial hyperplasia, and ADH

Usual findings with a comparison to low-grade DCIS are listed in Table 7.3 and illustrated in Figs 7.34–7.39.

Table 7.3 Usual epithelial hyperplasia, ADH and low-grade DCIS; cytological findings

Epithelial hyperplasia	ADH	Low-grade DCIS
Cell-rich smears, large sheets of cohesive epithelial cells, few single cells	Cell-rich smears, large sheets of cohesive epithelial cells, few single cells	Cell-rich smears, large and smaller sheets of cohesive epithelial cells, few single cells
Cells often in a 'streaming' pattern; focal crowding and overlapping of nuclei, rarely 'holes'	Focal crowding and overlapping of nuclei; 'holes' suggestive of cribriform pattern in some cases	Focal crowding and overlapping of nuclei; 'holes' suggestive of cribriform pattern common; some papillary cell groups
Nuclear atypia absent or mild	Mild to moderate nuclear atypia	Mild to moderate nuclear atypia
Naked bipolar and myoepithelial nuclei present but may be few; clean background; calcium granules occasionally	Few naked bipolar and myoepithelial nuclei; debris and calcium occasionally present	Naked bipolar and myoepithelial nuclei absent; necrotic debris and calcium often but not invariably present

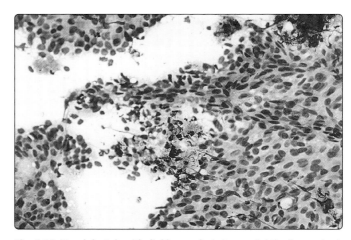

Fig. 7.34 Usual ductal epithelial hyperplasia Large, slightly disorganised sheets of ductal cells; tendency to 'streaming'; a few foamy cells and some bare bipolar nuclei (MGG, IP).

Regarding usual epithelial hyperplasia (Figs 7.34 and 7.37), the correlation between cytological appearances and subsequent histology is imperfect.[134] Criteria such as swirling three-dimensional masses with slit-like irregular lumens are said to be predictive of benign proliferative disease and not seen in DCIS.[136,137] The question is often asked, does cellularity alone constitute a reason for excision, if the pattern is entirely benign? In general, we do not recommend excision on the basis of cellularity alone. Discordant clinical, mammographic or ultrasound findings are usually the main reason for excision. CNB or excision is also recommended if there is cytological atypia such as evidence of papillary

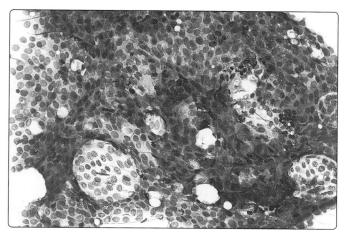

Fig. 7.35 **Atypical ductal hyperplasia (ADH)** Large sheet of mildly atypical cells; 'holes' indicating a cribriform pattern, myoepithelial nuclei not seen (MGG, IP).

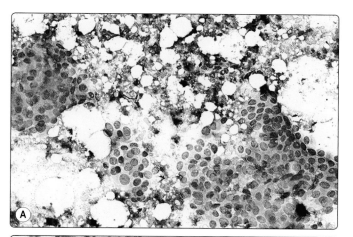

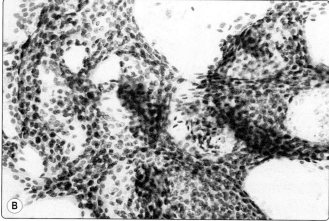

Fig. 7.36 **Low-grade cribriform DCIS** (A) Sheets of mildly atypical ductal epithelial cells; necrotic debris and calcium granules (MGG, IP); (B) Large sheet of ductal epithelium with many 'holes' suggestive of a cribriform pattern; no myoepithelial nuclei (Pap, IP).

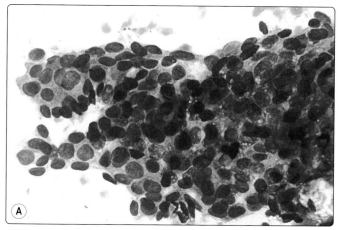

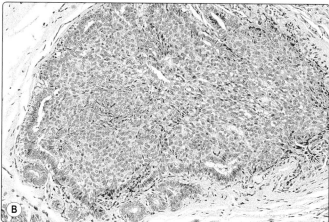

Fig. 7.37 **Usual ductal epithelial hyperplasia** (A) Large aggregate of mildly atypical ductal epithelial cells, nuclear crowding and overlapping; myoepithelial nuclei not obvious (MGG, HP); (B) Corresponding tissue section (H&E, IP).

growth, diminished cell cohesion, nuclear atypia, sparsity of bare bipolar nuclei, and presence of necrosis. Epithelial hyperplasia with or without atypia may be associated with malignancy, particularly in situ carcinoma, and close correlation with clinical and mammographic findings is essential. Malignancy can not be confidently ruled out by FNB alone.

Atypical ductal hyperplasia (ADH) yields similarly cell-rich smears of mainly cohesive sheets and aggregates of epithelial cells (Figs 7.35 and 7.38). Cytological atypia is variable and equals or sometimes even exceeds that of low-grade DCIS. Necrotic debris can sometimes be found. 'Holes' corresponding to the cribriform pattern considered typical of low-grade DCIS may occur also in ADH (Fig. 7.35). Other cases show a lesser degree of cytological atypia and a major component of benign-appearing material. Sneige and Staerkel found both cytological and architectural features of value in identifying atypical or malignant intraductal lesions but there was an overlap with low-grade DCIS and epithelial hyperplasia without atypia.[138] We feel that the overlap is too great to allow a specific diagnosis and that there is no single feature which can confidently separate ADH from low-grade DCIS. The cytologic diagnosis of low-grade DCIS is difficult, and 50% of cases in one study were called atypical on FNB.[41]

Smears from low-grade DCIS are also cell-rich of mainly large cohesive sheets but also smaller aggregates of ductal epithelial cells (Figs 7.36 and 7.39). In a study done by our

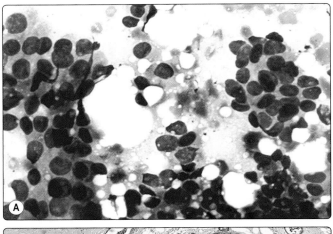

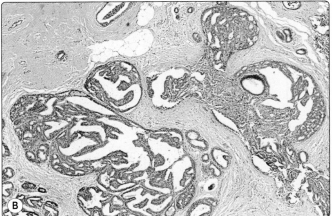

Fig. 7.38 Atypical ductal hyperplasia (ADH) (A) Aggregates of moderately atypical ductal epithelial cells; some loss of cohesion; no myoepithelial nuclei (MGG, HP); (B) Corresponding tissue section (H&E, IP).

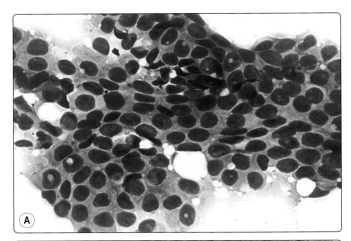

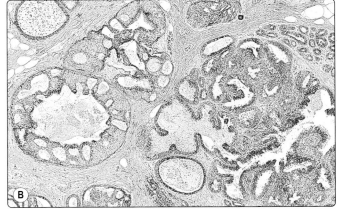

Fig. 7.39 Low-grade cribriform DCIS (A) Sheet of mildly atypical ductal epithelial cells; some crowding of nuclei; no myoepithelial cells; no necrosis or calcium (MGG, HP); (B) Corresponding tissue section; mixed pattern of epithelial hyperplasia and cribriform DCIS (H&E, IP).

group, all low-grade DCIS cases had moderately to highly cellular smears with cohesive, three-dimensional sheets of uniform, small cells with inconspicuous nucleoli arranged around a central lumen, forming cribriform 'punched-out' spaces.[41] Single malignant cells were prominent in only a minority of cases. A study by Sauer et al. demonstrated cribriform architecture in more than 90% of cases and single cells in approximately 30% of cases.[139] As mentioned above, rounded 'holes' in epithelial sheets in smears suggest a cribriform pattern, but are not specific to DCIS. In general, absence of myoepithelial cells and oval bare nuclei favor low-grade DCIS over ADH. However, myoepithelial cells were demonstrated in 51% of the nonhigh-grade DCIS lesions in one study.[139] Cell balls and papillary fragments are features that overlap with those of papillary lesions (see below).

Malignancy in lesions with epithelial hyperplasia is suggested by nuclear atypia, loss of epithelial cell cohesion, necrosis, and absence of myoepithelial cells and single bare bipolar nuclei. However, nuclear atypia in low-grade DCIS is variable and relatively mild. Obvious necrosis in the form of granular debris and calcified granules is highly suggestive of DCIS (Fig.7.36A) but is not diagnostic per se. Similar material can sometimes be found in ADH, and occasionally

in benign proliferative processes. A complete absence of myoepithelial cells and single bipolar nuclei is also in favor of malignancy. In some cases of DCIS, a proportion of the epithelial cells may show more obvious nuclear atypia and chromatin abnormality, increasing the level of suspicion of malignancy.

Correlation with the mammogram is essential and definitive diagnosis is in most cases deferred to histology.

PROBLEMS IN DIAGNOSIS

◆ 'Mild atypia',
◆ Apocrine metaplasia with atypia,
◆ Columnar cell lesions.

The term 'mild atypia' should probably be avoided in reports, because it causes great confusion for clinicians. On the one hand, the pathologist is describing a departure from normal which raises the possibility of malignancy, but, on the other, it is classified as mild and presumably inconsequential. The clinician knows that if there is no further action to investigate the lesion and carcinoma is found later, there may be medicolegal problems. This term is one of the most common reasons for inappropriate open biopsies. The pathologist should generally make a judgment as to whether the degree of atypia is compatible with epithelial hyperplasia (or fibroadenoma, hormonal stimulation, etc.) and report the changes as benign, or whether there is a real possibility of a significant lesion. If the latter decision is made, there should be a recommendation for further investigation. This might be further FNB, CNB or excision, added to mammography and ultrasound examination. The pathologist should not hesitate to recommend CNB or open biopsy if epithelial atypia is more obvious, in view of the overlapping of findings not only in usual hyperplasia, ADH and low-grade DCIS described above, but also in some low-grade invasive carcinomas, notably tubular carcinoma. Overdiagnosis of cancer, on the other hand, is avoided by paying attention to the presence of more than a few clearly benign elements, both ductular epithelium and single bipolar nuclei, in the presence of which great caution should be observed.

A diagnosis of ADH on vacuum-assisted 11-gauge core biopsy warrants excision as 10% to 27% of cases will show carcinoma at surgical excision.[140,141]

An uncommon feature that can cause concern is 'partial' apocrine change, presumably a variant of apocrine metaplasia. Here, the epithelial cells have more cytoplasm than ordinary ductal cells and appear cytologically to be a halfway house to apocrine epithelium. These cells may show loss of cohesion and there may be no bare oval nuclei in the background. The most cellular and worrying cases are usually derived from areas of marked intraductal epithelial hyperplasia. Apocrine metaplasia in areas of adenosis can appear even more worrying.[142] We have noted this phenomenon in association with radial scars and in a ductal adenoma (see Fig. 7.76B).

Columnar cell lesions (CCL) have recently attracted increasing interest in the context of mammographic screening. Histologically, terminal ducts are focally dilated and lined by columnar epithelial cells with cytoplasmic projections (snouts).[143] There may be a variable degree of hyperplasia (columnar cell hyperplasia) with or without atypia. At one end of the spectrum, the atypia equals ADH or low-grade DCIS. Although the premalignant potential is uncertain, awareness of these lesions is important in FNAC since cytological atypia may be considerable with some risk of false-suspicious or positive diagnosis. There are only a few published studies in the cytology literature which describe features of CLLs in aspirates.[144,145] While one study[144] described characteristic features (three-dimensional clusters of enlarged polygonal epithelial cells intermixed with myoepithelial cells and palisading columnar cells peripherally) that allow recognition of this entity in FNA material, the other study[145] concluded that columnar cell lesions cannot be reliably diagnosed on cytology due to cytomorphologic overlap with other lesions, especially with papillary neoplasms and well-differentiated adenocarcinoma. Our own experince agrees with Jensen et al.[145] in that overlapping cytologic findings can also be seen in fibroadenomas and proliferative fibrocystic changes. In Jensen's study, palisading columnar cells were present in only 50% of cases, whereas flat sheets of cells resembling apocrine metaplasia were more prominent. Atypia varied from mild to marked. In summary, it is important to recognize that CLLs

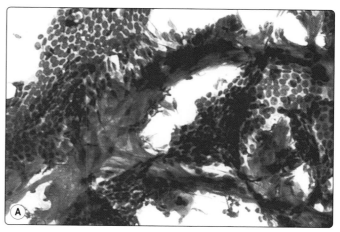

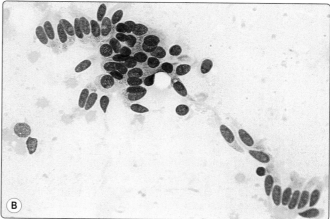

Fig. 7.40 Intraduct papilloma (A) Sheets of bland epithelial cells associated with strands of fibrous or fibrovascular stroma; bipolar nuclei difficult to find (MGG, IP); (B) Clusters of bland epithelial cells, many with an obvious columnar shape and lining up in palisaded rows (MGG, HP).

display a spectrum of cytologic changes that may lead to confusion with other entities including well-differentiated adenocarcinoma.

Papillary lesions (Figs 7.40–7.45)[111,146–148]

CRITERIA FOR DIAGNOSIS

- Cellular smears,
- Complex folded and branching epithelial sheets and finger-like fragments,
- Strands of dense fibrovascular stroma,
- True papillary fragments with stromal cores,
- Dispersed epithelial cells with mild nuclear atypia,
- Rows of palisaded columnar epithelial cells,
- Macrophages and variable amounts of cyst fluid,
- Bare bipolar nuclei (variable, often sparse).

Aspiration of intraductal papilloma often yields a small amount of fluid. Smears may be among the most cellular seen in FNB of the breast, with large aggregates distributed all over the slide as well as many dispersed cells. Intact papillary structures are less often seen. They are most often found

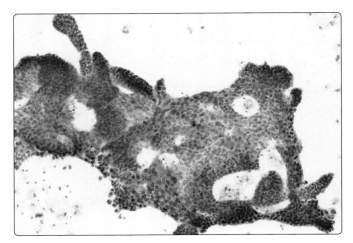

Fig. 7.41 Intracystic papillary carcinoma Complex folded sheet with finger-like extensions/papillaroid edges; background of macrophages (Pap, LP).

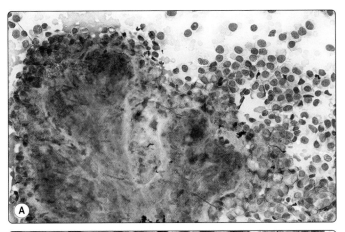

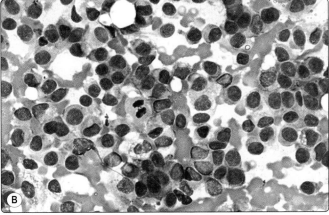

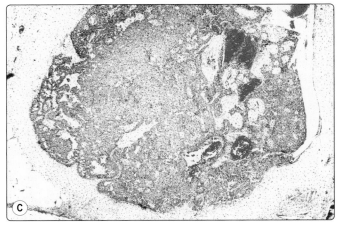

Fig. 7.42 Intracystic papillary carcinoma (A) True papillary tissue fragment with fibrovascular stromal core from thick part of smear (MGG, IP); (B) Dispersed population of atypical epithelial cells with a mitotic figure near center; thin part of same smear as **A**. The presence of true papillary fragments precluded an unequivocal malignant diagnosis (MGG, HP); (C) Corresponding tissue section. There was no evidence of invasive carcinoma (H&E, LP).

in thick bloody parts of the smear, where they have not been disrupted by the smearing pressure. Complex folded sheets associated with collagenous stromal cores are the most characteristic feature (Fig. 7.40A). Frequent rows of palisaded cells with a columnar shape are commonly seen and are a useful indicator of papillary or complex cribriform lesions (Fig. 7.40B). A foamy change of epithelial cells at the margins of aggregates occurs when cells are within a fluid medium. Some of the foamy cells in the smear background may be of epithelial rather than macrophage origin. Hemosiderin pigment and debris may result from minor bleed, which commonly occur in intraductal papilloma. A blood-stained nipple discharge is a common clinical sign. Smears of the discharge show degenerating epithelial cells and hemosiderin-containing macrophages.

The cytological criteria apply to any papillary lesion in the breast and are not specific for papilloma. Cytological diagnosis of papillary lesions shows a significant error rate with overlapping features.[147] Low-grade ductal carcinoma in situ of cribriform or micropapillary type and noninvasive intracystic papillary carcinoma may have all of the above features (Figs 7.41 and 7.42). Cellular atypia and fragments with long and slender papillae with ramifying edges favors papillary carcinoma. Like other forms of epithelial proliferative lesions, peripheral papillomas may be associated with DCIS. Our approach to cytological diagnosis is similar to that of frozen section of such lesions. We report this category as papillary lesions with an assessment of the degree of cytological atypia, if present, and recommend formal excision. Core needle biopsy may allow a more specific diagnosis, but may still not be entirely representative and thus complete excision of any papillary lesion that has not been entirely removed by the initial core biopsy is the optimal management for localized lesions.[148] Most papillary lesions behave indolently, and outcome is usually excellent.

Benign epithelial hyperplasia with papillomatosis may also have some of the above features and may be selected for excision.

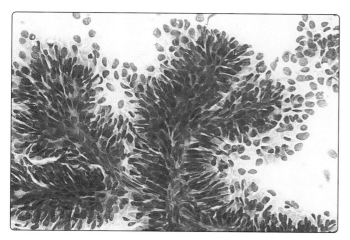

Fig. 7.43 Well-differentiated invasive papillary carcinoma True papillary tissue fragments with fibrovascular stromal cores; crowded and stratified atypical columnar epithelial cells, moderate loss of cohesion (MGG, IP).

PROBLEMS AND DIFFERENTIAL DIAGNOSIS

- ◆ Low-grade papillary carcinoma,
- ◆ Cell dispersal mimicking a malignant smear pattern,
- ◆ Pseudopapillary structures in smears of low-grade invasive duct carcinoma,
- ◆ Overlap with fibroadenoma,
- ◆ Infarcted papilloma.

Cytological atypia is often present to a variable degree in smears from papillary lesions. Although increasing cellularity with nuclear crowding, nuclear enlargement, irregular nuclear shape, and loss of cell cohesion increase the likelihood of malignancy (Figs 7.42 and 7.43), there is no clear distinction cytologically between papilloma with atypia, micropapillary DCIS, noninvasive intracystic papillary carcinoma and low-grade invasive papillary carcinoma. A suspicion of carcinoma can, of course, be expressed in the

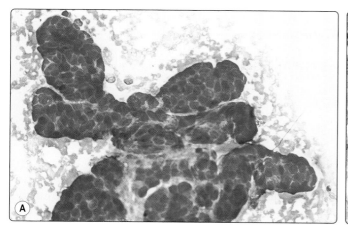

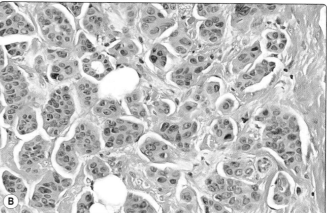

Fig. 7.44 Pseudopapillary pattern in duct carcinoma NOS (A) Many finger-like epithelial fragments with sharp 'anatomical' borders but no columnar or palisading cells and no stromal cores (MGG, HP); (B) Corresponding tissue section. The cords of malignant cells are cohesive and are removed intact by the needle (H&E, IP).

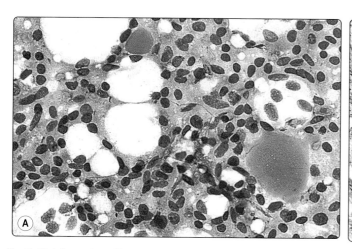

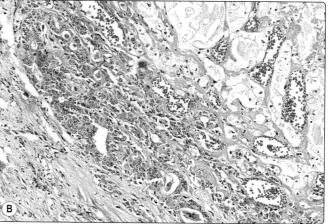

Fig. 7.45 Infarcted papilloma (A) Dispersed atypical cells with oval or spindle nuclei; nuclear hyperchromasia/pyknosis caused by degeneration; globules of hyaline stroma (MGG, HP); (B) Corresponding tissue section; edge of lesion; infarction upper right (H&E, IP).

report if nuclear atypia is worrisome, but the definitive diagnosis is best deferred to histology.

Cells aspirated from an atypical papillomatous lesion are sometimes poorly cohesive and mainly dispersed. Single bare bipolar nuclei may not be obvious. The similarity to the smear pattern of invasive carcinoma is enhanced by numerous single cells with intact cytoplasm, variable nuclear atypia, and sometimes mitotic activity (Fig. 7.42B). An unqualified malignant diagnosis could lead to unnecessary radical surgery of in situ or intracystic papillary carcinoma and should not be made in the presence of a papillary pattern as defined above, but be deferred to histology. Careful examination of the smears is important since papillary structures and/or palisaded columnar cells may be sparsely represented (Fig. 7.42A).

Solid, finger-like epithelial aggregates with a distinct 'anatomical' border of a row of cuboidal cells can be removed intact from a low-grade invasive carcinoma of particularly cohesive cells by FNB. They can be mistaken for fragments of papilloma (Fig. 7.44). However, they do not have a central stromal core, the cells are not columnar in shape and they do not tend to 'ball up' into multilayered fragments. The distinction has clinical importance since the management of a papillary lesion is different from that of invasive carcinoma. A CNB may be necessary to solve the problem.

Papillary-like epithelial fragments and a background of macrophages are sometimes found in fibroadenoma. The finger-like and branching structure of fibroadenoma epithelial aggregates do, however, differ from the more complex of heaped and folded aggregates of papillary lesions, and they do not have stromal cores. The distinction may be difficult in some cases. A background of numerous single bipolar nuclei and fragments of distinctly myxoid stroma strongly favors fibroadenoma.

Infarcting papilloma may produce a combination of findings closely mimicking malignancy.[149] Necrotic or degenerating cells are noncohesive and there may be a completely dispersed population of epithelial cells with a background of debris (Fig. 7.45). Pyknotic change of the nuclei resembles malignant hyperchromasia. Squamous metaplasia may add to an appearance of pleomorphism and there may be other regenerative epithelial changes. The clinical background can be of help in correct assessment. These cases present with a sudden onset of bloodstained discharge and a rapid enlargement or appearance of a breast lump. Dispersed columnar cell forms indicative of a papillary lesion may be found in the smears and even if there are only necrotic columnar shapes, their presence should lead to caution. Papillary stromal cores, which may appear as hyaline rounded bodies, should also alert one to the possibility. Necrosis, infarction or hemorrhage, apart from the confluent masses of granular debris seen in DCIS, is uncommon in small low to intermediate nuclear-grade breast carcinoma and is more common in papilloma and fibroadenoma or associated with pregnancy or lactation. Previous aspiration of papilloma or fibroadenoma may also result in similar changes.

Subareolar duct papillomatosis/ nipple adenoma

In subareolar duct papillomatosis (Fig. 7.46) or nipple adenoma cytologic material can be obtained either by FNB

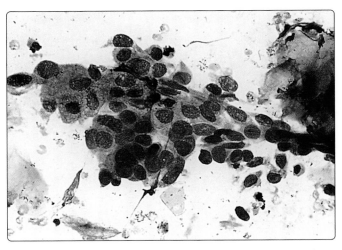

Fig. 7.46 Subareolar duct papillomatosis Nipple scraping. Cohesive but mildly atypical epithelial cells with enlarged nuclei and abundant cytoplasm; background of keratin flakes and some inflammatory cells (MGG, HP).

or by scraping the nipple, depending on the depth of the lesion. In scrape smears, squamous epithelium and some inflammatory cells are mixed with aggregates of mildly atypical epithelial cells of ductal type showing little tendency to dissociate. These are quite different from the single large malignant cells seen in Paget's disease (see Fig. 7.70). Single, bare nuclei of benign type may be inconspicuous.

Complex sclerosing lesions/radial scars (Figs 7.47–7.49)

Common cytologic findings.[93,150–153]

- Aspirates from the central scar poorly cellular (due to fibrosis), more cellular derived from the periphery (due to epithelial hyperplasia).
- Features similar to fibrocystic change (clusters of small bland epithelial cells and bare oval nuclei, foam cells, apocrine cells),
- Epithelial hyperplasia with or without atypia,
- Tubular/angular groups of epithelial cells with mild nuclear atypia,
- Fragments of fibrotic and elastotic stroma.

These lesions are usually discovered by mammography and few are palpable. They are a complex mixture of elastosis, fibrosis and epithelial hyperplasia, often including marked intraductal hyperplasia. The hyperplastic epithelial elements are generally arranged in a radial fashion extending from a central sclerotic scar-like area, which may include some fatty tissue. A number of distorted small tubular epithelial structures are typically present in the central sclerotic area (Fig. 7.47). These are the main cause of difficulties in cytological diagnosis as they closely resemble low-grade tubular carcinoma both cytologically and histologically.

The stellate appearance on mammography resembles that of invasive carcinoma. There are subtle radiological characteristics which allow the diagnosis to be suggested in most cases. The typical image pattern is reflected in the term 'black star'. However, there is an overlap in appearances and about 10% of cases are given an incorrect cancer diagnosis by

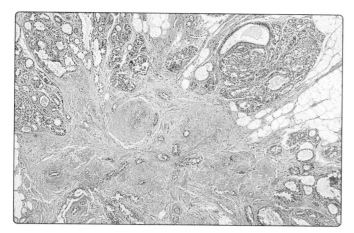

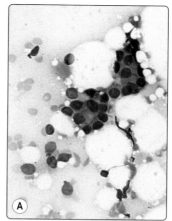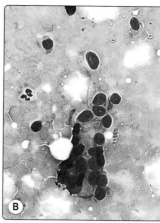

Fig. 7.47 Radial scar/complex sclerosing lesion Tissue section of typical radial scar. Zone of epithelial hyperplasia around periphery; central fibrotic scar with small tubular structures resembling tubular carcinoma (H&E, LP).

Fig. 7.49 Comparison of radial scar and tubular carcinoma (A) Cells from center of radial scar; tubular/angular structure, mild nuclear atypia; occasional single bipolar nuclei; (B) Cells from tubular carcinoma; similar pattern (MGG. HP).

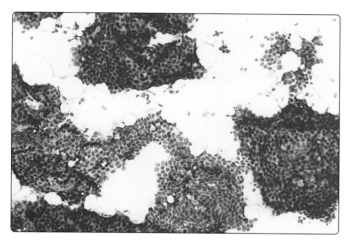

Fig. 7.48 Radial scar/complex sclerosing lesion Cell-rich smear of many large sheets of bland epithelial cells; some single bipolar nuclei. The smear represents usual ductal epithelial hyperplasia at the periphery of the lesion (MGG, LP).

False-positive diagnoses by FNB have occurred in the investigation of radial scars.[152] Although the findings may appear highly suspicious of malignancy, there is usually a coexistent clearly benign component of ductal epithelial fragments and single bipolar nuclei. A definite diagnosis of malignancy should not be made if there is an obvious benign component in the same smears.

Since it is the overall tissue architecture that is diagnostic of radial scar, both FNB and CNB are of limited value. There are only a few series concerning core biopsy in radial scars. One series looking at 43 cases of radial scar on core biopsy showed an incidence of carcinoma at surgical excision of 16%.[153] As mentioned above, lesions thought to be radial scars should be excised regardless of cytological findings. However, FNB or CNB may reveal unequivocal carcinoma, which obviously alters the clinical management.

Sclerosing adenosis

Cytologic features of sclerosing adenosis (Fig. 7.50) may overlap with proliferative fibrocystic change and fibroadenoma.[93] The smears of sclerosing adenosis are moderately to markedly cellular, consisting of small to large groups of benign epithelial cells.[154] Small fragments of dense, hyalinized stroma are found attached to acinar sheets and groups of epithelial cells. Scattered single epithelial cells are present and may cause concern for malignancy. There may be some loss of cell cohesion and mild nuclear atypia, but single bipolar nuclei are usually present. As compared with fibrocystic change, sclerosing adenosis has more abundant cellularity, acinar sheets, single epithelial cells, and hyalinized stroma. Fibroadenomas, in comparison, display more of a branching pattern of epithelial sheets, large sheets and bipolar/oval, naked nuclei and large, hypocellular, fibromyxoid stroma.

Mucocele-like lesions

Epithelial mucin is found in a group of breast lesions. The mucin can dominate the samples obtained by FNB.

mammography. Most radial scars are excised for definitive histological diagnosis because of the difficulty in radiological diagnosis and the not unusual association with ADH and DCIS.

PROBLEMS AND DIFFERENTIAL DIAGNOSIS

◆ Other forms of epithelial hyperplasia,
◆ Tubular carcinoma.

The most common smear pattern is of epithelial hyperplasia with or without atypia representing the zone of hyperplasia around the periphery of the lesion as seen in tissue sections (Figs 7.47 and 7.48). Epithelial atypia should not be ignored since low-grade DCIS is not uncommonly associated with radial scar. If the smear derives mainly from the central sclerotic area, small tubular or angular groups of mildly atypical epithelial cells may be seen associated with stromal elements, including elastotic fragments. This pattern closely resembles that of tubular carcinoma (Fig. 7.49).

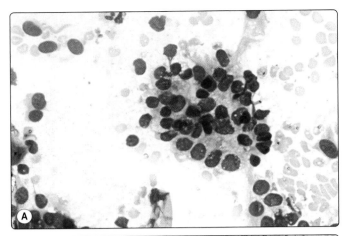

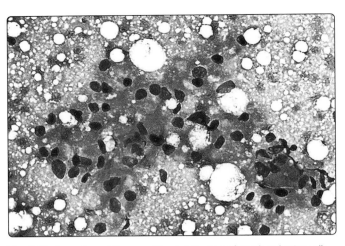

Fig. 7.51 **Granular cell tumor of breast** Clusters of poorly cohesive cells with abundant, dense eosinophilic and granular but fragile cytoplasm with poorly defined cell borders; mildly irregular nuclei. This lesion was mammographically and clinically thought to be carcinoma (MGG, HP).

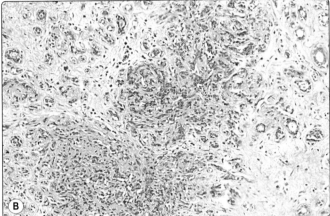

Fig. 7.50 **Adenosis** (A) Cluster of epithelial cells with a microacinar pattern; some single cells and bare bipolar nuclei (MGG, HP); (B) Corresponding tissue section (H&E, LP).

Mucocele-like lesions are a variant of fibrocystic disease, in which ducts are distended by mucin, leading to disruption of some ducts and extravasation of mucin into adjacent tissue. Mucocele-like lesions are most often detected by mammography due to the presence of microcalcifications in the same area. Other examples of mucinous lesions are mucinous fibroadenoma and mucinous DCIS. These lesions are further described in the section on colloid carcinoma, since they constitute an important and sometimes difficult differential diagnosis to colloid carcinoma (see p. 189).

Collagenous spherulosis

This is a stromal reaction most often encountered in areas of fibrocystic disease. It consists of spheres of hyaline basement membrane material closely resembling the hyaline globules of adenoid cystic carcinoma, associated with variable epithelial hyperplasia.[155,156] It may be an incidental finding related to a palpable mass or to a mammographically detected lesion. Overlap with adenoid cystic carcinoma may be problematic (see Fig 7.83).[157] Presence of bare oval nuclei, uniformity of hyaline globules capped by comma-shaped nuclei and benign appearance of epithelial cells favor collagenous spherulosis (see Fig. 7.84).

Benign mesenchymal lesions; rare lesions[158]

Most mesenchymal lesions occurring in the breast are not specific for this site and are described in Chapter 15 (soft tissues). Granular cell tumor can clinically and mammographically mimic breast cancer. The radiological image is of a stellate lesion graded 4 or 5, and the palpation findings are of a hard, irregular lump, not infrequently with skin dimpling. The cytological diagnosis is straightforward if smears are adequate and cells are well preserved, demonstrating the characteristic abundant granular cytoplasm (Fig. 7.51).[159,160] However, the cytoplasm is fragile and may be dispersed in the background, leaving stripped nuclei that may be quite variable in size and shape, some with prominent nucleoli. This pattern could be mistaken for malignancy, particularly if the clinical and radiological diagnosis is of carcinoma. Furthermore, granular macrophage reactions may resemble granular cell tumor, and even immunocytochemistry is not always conclusive.[161] Carcinoma with oxyphil differentiation has a granular cytoplasm and can cause differential diagnostic problems.

A spindle cell lipoma with marked atypia leading to a suspicion of malignancy has been reported.[162] Our approach to unusual spindle lesions of the breast is to recommend local excision for definitive diagnosis. Cases of intramammary schwannoma diagnosed by FNB have been reported.[163]

Fibromatosis/nodular fasciitis can present as a stellate lesion in the breast, clinically and radiologically mimicking primary carcinoma.[158] The yield of FNB can be scanty, but if smears are adequate a correct diagnosis based on the findings of fibrohistiocytic cells, singly and in tissue fragments as in soft tissue lesions of the same type, is possible (Figs 7.52 and 7.53). Reactive reparative processes such as suture granuloma, reparative granulation tissue following previous biopsy, and other scarring processes have similar features.[164]

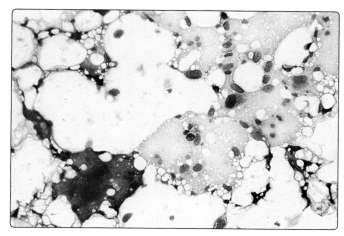

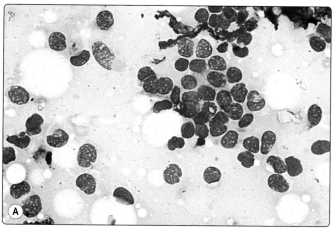

Fig. 7.52 Nodular fasciitis, breast Scanty smear of dispersed spindle cells and a few inflammatory cells; fragments of fibrous stroma (MGG, IP).

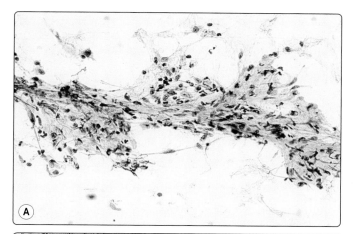

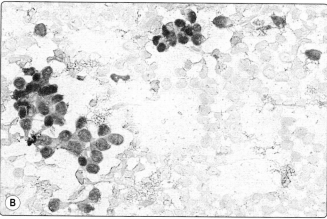

Fig. 7.54 Invasive duct carcinoma NOS, low grade Clustered and single malignant epithelial cells, mild nuclear enlargement and atypia; absence of bipolar nuclei (A, MGG; B, Pap, HP).

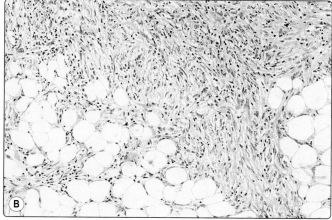

Fig. 7.53 Fibromatosis, breast (A) Disrupted fragment of mesenchymal tissue of spindle cells and intercellular fibrous stroma; some single spindle cells (Pap, IP); (B) Corresponding tissue section (H&E, LP). This lesion was stellate on mammography and suspicious of carcinoma.

Myofibroblastoma is a rare neoplasm mainly occurring in males, characterized by a well-circumscribed mass of spindle cells with eosinophilic cytoplasm in a background of collagenous fibrous tissue. FNB findings are of a benign mesenchymal lesion composed of abundant, randomly arranged single and clustered benign spindle-shaped cells with scant cytoplasm and elongated or oval nuclei displaying a finely granular chromatin pattern and inconspicuous nucleoli.[165]

Primary carcinoma of the breast

Infiltrating ductal carcinoma of no special type
(NOS) (Figs 7.54–7.56 and see Figs 7.2–7.4)

> **CRITERIA FOR DIAGNOSIS**
>
> ◆ Moderately to highly cellular smears,
> ◆ Single population of epithelial cells; no myoepithelial cells, no single bare bipolar nuclei,
> ◆ Variable loss of cell cohesion – irregular clusters and single cells,
> ◆ Single epithelial cells with intact cytoplasm,
> ◆ Moderate to severe nuclear atypia: enlargement, pleomorphism, irregular nuclear membrane and chromatin,
> ◆ Fibroblasts and fragments of collagen (stromal desmoplasia) associated with the atypical cells,
> ◆ Intracytoplasmic neolumina in some cases,
> ◆ Necrosis unusual, more suggestive of DCIS.

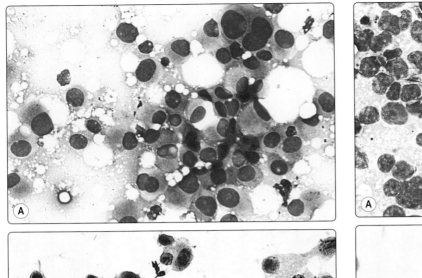

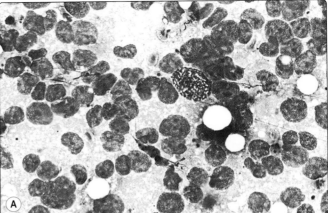

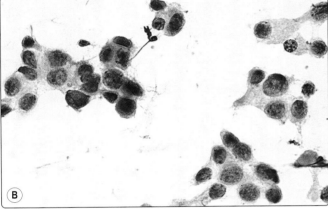

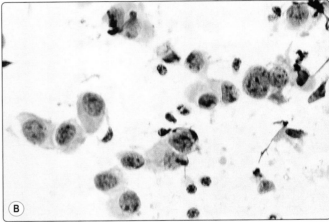

Fig. 7.55 Invasive duct carcinoma NOS, intermediate grade Poorly cohesive malignant cells, single and in clusters; obvious nuclear enlargement and pleomorphism; irregular chromatin (**A**, MGG; **B**, Pap, HP).

Fig. 7.56 Invasive duct carcinoma NOS, high grade Mainly dispersed malignant cells, prominent nuclear enlargement and pleomorphism, coarse chromatin, an occasional mitotic figure; some lymphocytes and fibroblasts in the background but no bipolar nuclei (**A**, MGG; **B**, Pap, HP).

Fine needle aspiration biopsy of most cancers yields a larger number of cells than normal glandular breast tissue. The yield from a scirrhous cancer may be very scanty, but the consistency of such a tumor felt through the needle is so characteristic that this is a suspicious finding on its own. A repeat FNB from the infiltrating edge of the tumor may be more rewarding. Occasionally, a core needle biopsy may prove necessary.

The overall smear pattern (cellularity, presence or absence of a bimodal cell population, cell cohesion, size and shape of cell aggregates, stromal components) is as important to the correct diagnosis as is the cytological detail. A scanty smear does not allow a proper assessment of the overall pattern. A repeat FNB, CNB or open biopsy is therefore mandatory if clinical or radiological findings are suspicious, or if cytological atypia is noted in a scanty smear. Architectural features are studied at low power. Aggregates of malignant cells are irregular, often with an angular or tubular shape. Reduced cell cohesion results in the presence of small clusters of cells, cells in single files, and single cells with intact cytoplasm, whereas single bare bipolar nuclei typical of non-neoplastic breast tissue are absent. Standard cytological criteria of malignancy – nuclear enlargement and pleomorphism, irregular nuclear membranes, irregular distribution of nuclear chromatin, prominent nucleoli, and crowding and overlapping of nuclei within aggregates of cells

– are obvious in high-grade cancers but often subtle in low-grade tumors. Intracytoplasmic neolumina in atypical epithelial cells, sometimes with a 'bull's-eye' inclusion, are an important criterion of malignancy, but are less commonly found in ductal carcinoma (see Fig. 7.74). In poorly differentiated carcinomas, dissociation of cells may be prominent and the smear pattern may resemble that of lymphoma but more often the malignant cells are seen both in aggregates and lying singly. Nuclei are irregularly distributed and overlapping within aggregates of tumor cells and there may be a tendency to microacinar grouping. Single carcinoma cells usually have well-defined cytoplasm but there are exceptions to this rule, particularly infiltrating lobular carcinoma (see below). Fibrous and adipose tissue fragments intimately associated with the cancer cells are suggestive of invasiveness. Stromal material is relatively scanty in most cancers. Nuclei of lymphocytes and fibroblasts derived from the tumor stroma may be present and these must not be mistaken for the bipolar, naked nuclei of benign breast tissue.

The presence of necrosis is strongly suggestive of malignancy. It is particularly characteristic of DCIS, and not often seen in invasive carcinoma. Tumor necrosis must be distinguished from condensed secretion in inspissated cysts and duct ectasia.

Small tumors, tumors obscured by surrounding fibrous tissue, or tumors adjacent to a dominant benign lesion such as a cyst or a lipoma can be missed by the needle. FNB guided by US or stereotaxis has greatly reduced the proportion of nonrepresentative biopsies but has not entirely eliminated this possibility. An overlap between the cytologic findings in fibrocystic disease and low-grade carcinoma can contribute to the problem.[166]

Artifacts (crush artifacts, artifactual disruption of cell aggregates, slow drying of MGG smears, drying artifacts in alcohol-fixed smears) may render interpretation difficult. Nuclear size and texture are altered by poor fixation. Smearing pressure may cause artifactual dissociation of cell aggregates mimicking the loss of cell cohesion in malignancy. Cells mixed with abundant blood or caught in blood clot tend to shrink, and cells dispersed in fat may become distorted and appear to be vacuolated. Aspiration of fat from around a tumor should be avoided, but at the same time cells are more easily obtained from the infiltrating periphery of a cancer.

Smears from low-grade carcinomas with small cells and a desmoplastic stroma (mainly infiltrating lobular but also some ductal carcinomas) may simulate the benign pattern at low magnification.[167] However, the single cells are dispersed malignant cells which may have lost their cytoplasm but still differ from the bare bipolar nuclei of benign breast tissue. The nuclei have an irregular shape and there are usually some remnants of cytoplasm (see Figs 7.2–7.4 and 7.71).

Fibrosclerotic hypocellular lesions may not yield sufficient cells to allow a diagnosis by FNB. This is true of 'scirrhous' carcinoma as well as of sclerosed fibroadenoma. Diagnostic cell material is most likely obtained from the periphery of desmoplastic cancers, as from the peripheral parts of cancers with extensive central necrosis.

Duct carcinoma in situ (DCIS) causes special problems in cytological diagnosis. The cells of large cell DCIS of comedo type are readily recognized as malignant. The overall smear pattern of DCIS is fairly characteristic, but focal invasion can obviously never be ruled out by FNB. Small cell DCIS of papillary or cribriform type are usually reported as epithelial hyperplasia with atypia or as suspicious but not diagnostic of malignancy. Low-grade, tubular invasive carcinoma can also be difficult to recognize as malignant, particularly since naked nuclei of benign type, presumably derived from remnants of the lobular stroma, are often found in the smears.[168]

As described in previous sections, worrying cytological atypia can occur in several benign conditions (fibroadenoma, papilloma and epithelial hyperplasia, gynecomastia,

etc.). Nuclear enlargement and anisokaryosis may be simply related to hormonal stimulation, but nuclei of irregular shape and with irregular contours (buds, indentations, sharp angles, folds, etc.) and chromatin irregularities are indicators of malignancy. To avoid overdiagnosis of malignancy, as a general rule, a definitive malignant diagnosis should not be given if smears include more than a few clearly benign elements in addition to the atypical cells.

If smears from a breast lesion show a malignant pattern not typical of the common forms of primary breast cancer, the alternatives, metastatic carcinoma, sarcoma or lymphoma, must be considered, since mastectomy may not be the appropriate treatment. Further investigation by immunostaining or core needle biopsy may be necessary to solve this problem.

The pitfalls in FNB and CNB of palpable breast lumps are summarized at the end of this chapter.

On CNB, the most significant pitfall in the diagnosis of an invasive carcinoma is confirming invasion in subtle invasive ductal and lobular lesions. Obtaining material from deeper levels can reveal subtle invasive foci, and the use of immunohistochemical stains such as cytokeratin can highlight invasive epithelial cells that have extended outside of the basement membrane.[169] Another pitfall, as mentioned above, is avoiding the misdiagnosis of an invasive component when none exists. This can occur in high-grade DCIS where the stroma is desmoplastic and the ducts appear irregular in shape and mimic invasive foci. Stains for myoepithelial markers should be used to highlight the myoepithelial cells lining these irregularly shaped ducts and confirm the in situ nature of the lesion.

Ductal carcinoma in situ (DCIS) (Figs 7.57, 7.58, and see Figs 7.36, 7.39)[41,138,170–173]

The diagnosis of DCIS in tissue sections and CNB includes an assessment of nuclear grade (high, intermediate and low), growth pattern (solid, cribriform, micropapillary, intracystic papillary) and the presence of necrosis (confluent, comedonecrosis) and calcification. High nuclear grade lesions are

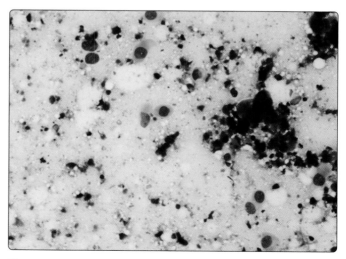

Fig. 7.57 High-grade DCIS (comedocarcinoma) Pleomorphic malignant cells with a background of necrotic debris (MGG, IP).

biologically more aggressive and necrosis appears to impart a worse prognosis in low to intermediate nuclear grade lesions. A specific diagnosis or classification of DCIS cannot be made by FNB. High nuclear grade lesions are cytologically obviously malignant and are reported as high grade, but exclusion of invasion is clearly not possible. The low nuclear grade lesions provide greater difficulty and there is an overlap in appearances with epithelial hyperplasia with atypia. Most cases, however, are recognized as abnormal and recommended for excision.

High nuclear-grade DCIS, solid or comedo growth pattern (Fig. 7.57)

Usual findings.

- Usually cell-rich smears,
- Neoplastic cells in sheets, irregular aggregates and single,
- Large, pleomorphic cells showing obvious malignant nuclear features,
- Necrotic debris, granular calcium, lymphocytes and vacuolated macrophages.

The cells of DCIS of high nuclear grade (large cell, solid, comedo) are large, pleomorphic and show standard cytological criteria of malignancy. The cytoplasm may be abundant and eosinophilic, as in oxyphil cells. The diagnosis of carcinoma is easy. Abundant necrotic debris, often with calcium granules, represents the 'comedo' plugs seen in tissue sections. The absence of a well-defined palpable mass, the mammographic findings of characteristic calcifications without an associated tissue density and the cytologic features, taken together, strongly suggest high-grade DCIS. Invasive growth, if present, is usually suggested by the mammographic appearance, although mass-forming DCIS with periductal fibrosis is a pitfall for all diagnostic methods – radiology, clinical examination and morphology. Certain cytological features listed below are also suggestive of invasion. However, focal invasion can not be reliably excluded by mammography, FNB, or by CNB. Definitive assessment of invasive growth can only be made by excision and histological examination. On CNB, cases of high-grade DCIS can be surrounded by a desmoplastic stroma mimicking invasion. In these cases, the use of immunohistochemical markers for myoepithelial cell markers is useful to demonstrate definitive invasion.

Low-grade DCIS, cribriform, solid or micropapillary, noninvasive intracystic papillary carcinoma (Fig. 7.58, and see Figs 7.36, 7.39)[41,99,138,146,172–174]

Usual findings.

- Epithelial cells mainly cohesive, forming large sheets, often with 'holes' or papillary fragments,
- Bare bipolar nuclei absent,
- Variable, mild to moderate epithelial atypia,
- Necrotic debris, often calcium granules,
- Macrophages.

The findings have been described and the differential diagnosis with other lesions, mainly atypical ductal hyperplasia

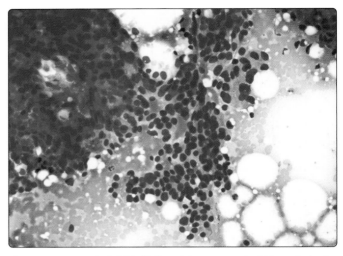

Fig. 7.58 Low-grade DCIS (cribriform) Aggregates of mildly atypical cells in a three-dimensional pattern with 'holes' (*left*) (MGG, IP).

(ADH), has been discussed in the context of epithelial hyperplastic processes on page 175. The pattern also overlaps with that of papillary lesions. It is difficult to distinguish intracystic or intraductal papillary carcinoma from intraductal papilloma or florid papillomatosis. The presence of myoepithelial nuclei suggests benign hyperplasia or papilloma, while nuclear enlargement, nuclear pleomorphism, reduced cell cohesion and the presence of necrosis favor a malignant diagnosis. Correlation with the mammogram is essential and definitive diagnosis must usually be deferred to histology.

Intermediate-grade DCIS is difficult to separate with confidence from high- or low-grade forms, but the malignant nuclear features seen in FNB smears are closer to high-grade than to low-grade DCIS.

Predicting invasion[175–180]

Recent studies have suggested that the finding of tubular or angular epithelial structures, malignant cells adherent to fibrous stroma (Fig. 7.59), the present of intracytoplasmic lumina in malignant cells, fibroblast proliferation and fragments of elastoid stroma were predictive of invasion when associated with a malignant cell pattern. When two features were present the positive predictive value of invasion was 96%. Some workers have found the intimate adherence of malignant cells and fibrous stroma to be the single most useful feature predicting invasion. The presence of epithelial cells in fat tissue has not been confirmed to be a useful sign of invasive growth. Excluding focal invasion is obviously not possible due to the limited sampling. The presence of comedo-like necrosis is a useful sign of the presence of a DCIS component. Cell blocks were found to confirm invasion in 44% of breast FNBs in one study.[180]

The cytological findings described may be of some value in combination with mammographic assessment in deciding management. Clinical presentation is obviously also of significance. Chhieng et al. point out that 97.7% of palpable masses with unequivocally malignant cytology are invasive cancers.[21]

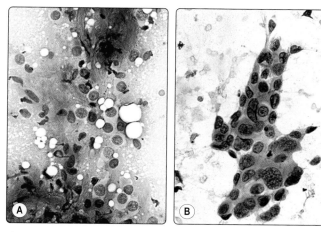

Fig. 7.59 Cytological findings suggestive of invasion (A) Epithelial cells of low-grade carcinoma adherent to or embedded in fibrous stroma (MGG, HP); (B) A fragment of malignant epithelium with a tubular/angular configuration and spiculated edges. Smear from high-grade DCIS with focal invasion (H&E, HP).

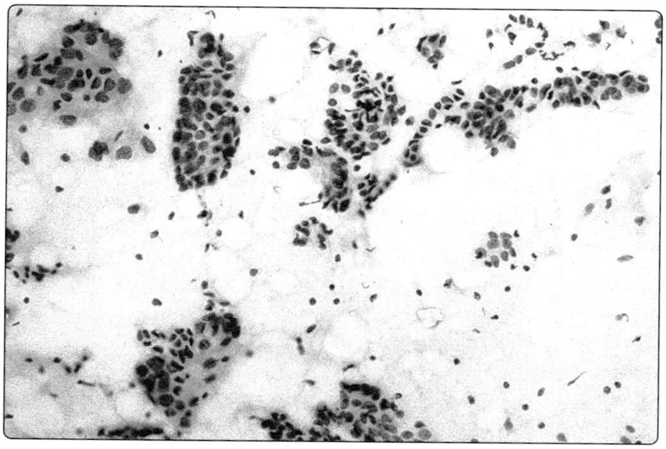

Fig. 7.60 Tubular carcinoma Tubular and angular epithelial fragments of mildly atypical cells; single files of cells; note some single bare nuclei in the background (MGG, LP).

Variants of primary carcinoma

Cytological typing of primary breast carcinoma is of value in correlating the radiological findings with the expected histopathology. For example, medullary and mucinous carcinoma correlate well with a mammographically circumscribed lesion (rounded density), whereas invasive lobular carcinoma correlates with an asymmetrical density. Lobular carcinoma and DCIS tend to be more extensive than indicated by the mammogram. However, in the majority of cases, parameters other than tumor type, such as tumor size and grade, clinical stage, hormone receptor content and other biological factors, will determine the extent of surgery and the need for adjuvant therapy. Nevertheless, familiarity with all the various patterns of breast cancer is necessary to achieve a high level of cytological diagnostic accuracy.[181] The basic diagnostic criteria for infiltrating duct carcinoma (the most common malignant pattern; p. 183) are to some extent applicable to all subtypes.

Tubular carcinoma (Figs 7.60–7.63)[182–187]

Usual findings.

- Moderately cellular smears,
- Cells predominantly in cohesive clusters,
- Epithelial fragments with an angular or tubular shape,
- Relatively uniform, mildly to moderately atypical epithelial cells,
- Absence or paucity of single bipolar nuclei of benign type,
- Fibroblastic cells; fragments of fibromyxoid or elastotic stroma.

This tumor is a cytological challenge, commonly encountered as a small, mammographically detected lesion. The relatively uniform appearance of the nuclei, the preserved cellular cohesion and the presence of bare bipolar nuclei in up to a quarter of cases make a diagnosis of malignancy difficult. Most authors report only half of their cases as

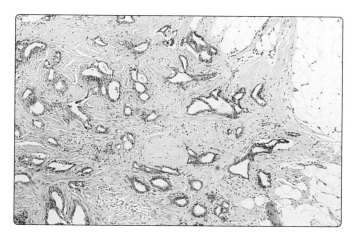

Fig. 7.61 Tubular carcinoma Tissue section of tubular carcinoma showing angulated infiltrating tubules (H&E, IP).

definitely malignant and there is a high false-negative rate. Fortunately, most of these lesions are stellate on mammography and suspicious by ultrasound and are selected for excision. Core biopsy is useful to confirm the diagnosis and to allow definitive treatment without previous excision.

PROBLEMS AND DIFFERENTIAL DIAGNOSIS

- Minor deviation from the benign pattern,
- Mixed tubular and usual ductal carcinoma,
- Complex sclerosing lesion/radial scar, adenosis,
- Fibroadenoma.

Nuclear morphology is usually bland. Nuclear grooves[186] and intracytoplasmic vacuoles are suggestive but not diagnostic features. Large cohesive aggregates of cells may represent a low-grade DCIS component. Many tubular carcinomas have a loose, cellular stroma similar to intralobular connective tissue. Smears may contain single, bare bipolar nuclei,

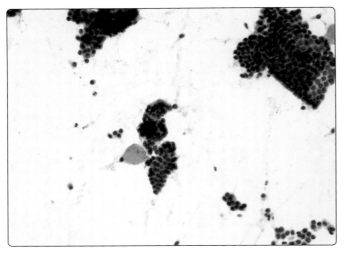

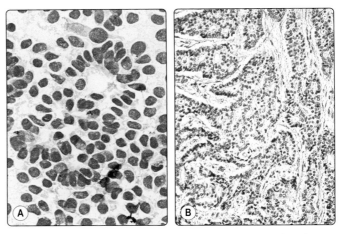

Fig. 7.64 Invasive cribriform carcinoma (A) Cell-rich smear of poorly cohesive small monomorphic cells; some cells are columnar; suggestion of a microacinar/cribriform pattern (MGG, HP); (B) Corresponding tissue section (H&E, IP).

Fig. 7.62 Tubular carcinoma Angulated epithelial cell clusters of angulated epithelial cell clusters; variable nuclear atypia, some cells small bland, some moderately enlarged and atypical, scattered single cells (H&E, IP)

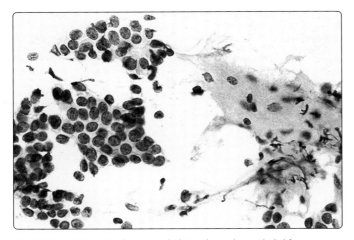

Fig. 7.63 Another case showing tubular and angular epithelial fragments; fibrous stroma, spindle cells and some debris (H & E, HP).

Columnar cell lesions have been associated with tubular carcinomas. On core biopsy, tubular carcinomas should be distinguished from radial sclerosing lesions and sclerosing adenosis. The entrapped ductules in the fibroelastic core of a radial scar may simulate invasive carcinoma, especially tubular carcinomas. The tubules in radial scars are usually elongated and flattened, which contrasts with the angulated tubular glands in tubular carcinoma. Sclerosing adenosis should also be included in the differential. Sclerosing adenosis shows expansion and distortion of lobules secondary to a disordered proliferation of acinar and ductal epithelial cells, myoepithelial cells and intralobular stroma. The lobulocentric nature of the process is helpful in distinguishing this lesion from an invasive carcinoma. The use of myoepithelial markers which are absent in tubular carcinomas can also be of use in distinguishing these lesions.

Mucinous (colloid) carcinoma

(Figs 7.65 and 7.66)[116,188–194]

Usual findings.

- Abundant background mucin (recognizable macroscopically),
- Atypical cells in small solid aggregates and single intact epithelial cells,
- Mild to moderate nuclear atypia,
- Benign epithelial cells and bipolar nuclei absent,
- 'Chicken wire' blood vessels.

Mucinous carcinomas are usually round and well circumscribed, and may be clinically and mammographically mistaken for a benign lesion such as fibroadenoma or cyst. The tumor cells have abundant cytoplasm. Nuclear enlargement and pleomorphism can be relatively mild but the abundance of material, cell dispersal and absence of bare bipolar nuclei generally permit a definite diagnosis of malignancy. The mucin stains bluish violet with MGG. It is less conspicuous and rather pale in smears stained with H&E or Pap. Few mucinous carcinomas demonstrate intracytoplasmic mucin,

as well as spindle cells of fibroblastic type and fragments of fibrous or elastotic stromal material. In the presence of a bimodal cell population, a definitive diagnosis of carcinoma can rarely be made cytologically.

Occasionally, tubular carcinoma may have larger, cohesive, monolayered sheets of epithelial cells which can be mistaken for fibroadenoma, since nuclear enlargement and atypia may occur in both conditions. This resemblance may be heightened by the presence of fragments of loose fibrous stroma. The sparsity of bare bipolar nuclei is against a diagnosis of fibroadenoma and should draw attention to the 'atypical' cell pattern.

Invasive cribriform carcinoma is another variant of low-grade breast cancer related to tubular carcinoma. In keeping with its histological growth pattern, smears from a cribriform carcinoma are usually highly cellular but the neoplastic cells are bland, cuboidal or columnar and show a tendency to an acinar, microglandular or cribriform arrangement (Fig. 7.64).

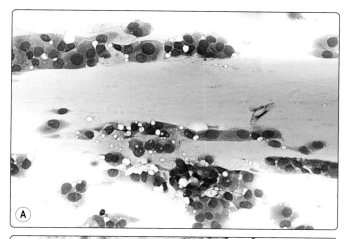

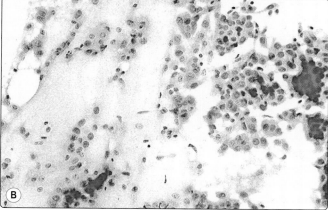

Fig. 7.65 Colloid carcinoma Moderately cohesive epithelial cells with abundant cytoplasm and moderate nuclear enlargement and atypia, suspended in mucus; note single files mainly in **A**. (A, MGG, HP; B, Pap, IP).

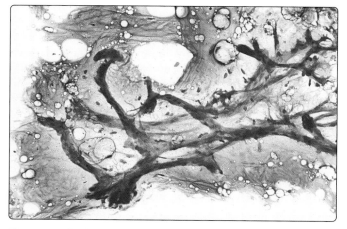

Fig. 7.66 Colloid carcinoma 'Chicken-wire' blood vessels with a background of stringy mucin (MGG, IP).

and signet ring cells are more often seen in other variants, mainly in infiltrating lobular carcinoma.

'Chicken wire' blood vessels are often very prominent in smears of mucinous carcinoma (Fig. 7.66). They are suggestive but not diagnostic of this tumor, and can occur in other lesions, particularly in fibroadenoma.

We usually report a mucinous pattern in FNB samples as a 'component' of mucinous carcinoma since it is often only a focal change in a ductal carcinoma of the usual type.[191] FNB selectively samples the softer mucinous elements.

The differential diagnosis is more complex in impalpable, mammographically detected lesions, as discussed below.

> ### PROBLEMS AND DIFFERENTIAL DIAGNOSIS
>
> ◆ Lack of nuclear pleomorphism,
> ◆ Mucinous DCIS or ADH,
> ◆ Mucocele-like lesions,
> ◆ Mucinous/myxoid fibroadenoma,
> ◆ Myxoid stromal matrix resembling mucin,
> ◆ Metastatic carcinoma,
> ◆ Hemorrhage and necrosis induced by FNB,
> ◆ Ultrasound gel.

The relatively bland nuclear morphology may give a confusingly benign appearance to the smears, but high cellularity, loss of cell cohesion and the absence of single bipolar nuclei are suggestive of malignancy. Mucinous carcinoma must be included in the differential diagnosis of any lesion containing background epithelial mucin.

Mucinous material can be found in smears from several other lesions. In impalpable lesions, mucinous DCIS or ADH are included in the differential diagnosis. These present mammographically as microcalcifications or small opacities. Chicken-wire blood vessels are usually not seen in DCIS and the abnormal cells of DCIS or ADH are usually much more cohesive than in invasive carcinomas, forming large sheets.

Mucocele-like lesions (Figs 7.67 and 7.68) are also most often detected by mammography due to the presence of microcalcifications. They were described initially as benign lesions resembling salivary mucoceles, caused by extravasation of mucin from ruptured ducts with mucinous metaplasia. The lesions occur in the setting of fibrocystic disease. A spectrum of appearances in individual cases has been described, from benign areas to ADH, mucinous DCIS or mucinous carcinoma. Smears from cases of fibrocystic disease with intact ducts distended by mucin are fairly characteristic, showing monolayered sheets of bland, cohesive epithelial cells suspended in a large amount of mucus (Fig. 7.67). Calcium granules are often found. However, diagnostic difficulties can occur in mucocele-like lesions, in which there is rupture and extravasation of mucus into adjacent breast tissue. Smears may then include numerous mucinophages, which can closely resemble the atypical epithelial cells of mucinous carcinoma (Fig. 7.68).[193,194]

Sometimes the myxoid stromal ground substance of fibroadenoma and phyllodes tumor can be mistaken for epithelial mucin. However, the staining properties with MGG differ; epithelial mucin stains bluish violet, whereas myxoid ground substance stains pink/violet. The difference in color is not obvious in smears stained by Pap or H&E. There is a subtle difference in texture; epithelial mucin is homogeneous and structureless; myxoid ground substance is slightly fibrillar and often includes some fibroblastic spindle cells.

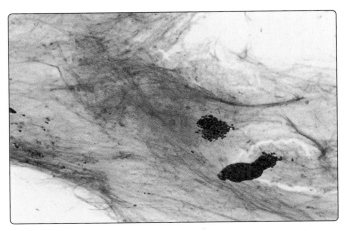

Fig. 7.67 Mucocele-like lesion Background of abundant mucin; cohesive sheets of regular epithelial cells (H&E, LP).

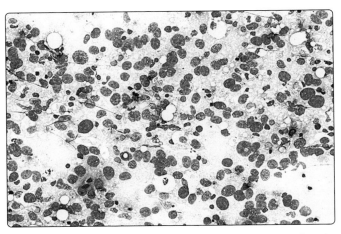

Fig. 7.69 Medullary carcinoma Numerous dispersed malignant cells with large, pleomorphic nuclei; many scattered lymphoid cells (MGG, IP).

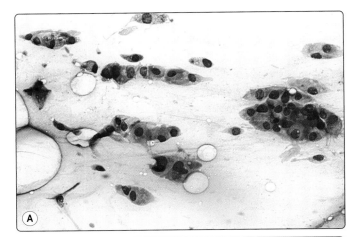

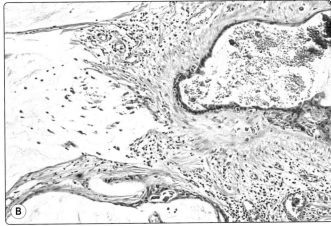

Fig. 7.68 Mucocele-like lesion (A) Many mucinophages forming clusters and runs similar to the atypical epithelial cells of colloid carcinoma; background of mucin (MGG, HP); (B) Corresponding tissue section showing rupture of ducts distended by mucin; extravasation of mucin and a mucinophage reaction in the stroma (H&E, LP).

Metastatic mucinous carcinoma may be difficult to distinguish from a primary mucinous carcinoma.

FNB can cause bleeding into a mucinous carcinoma. We have seen several examples of complete infarction induced by FNB, making frozen section diagnosis difficult.

Distinguishing mucinous lesions by core biopsy may be diagnostically challenging. The diagnosis of mucinous carcinoma on CNB is usually straightforward;[192] however, the presence of extravasated mucin or a mucocele-like lesion on CNB warrants surgical excision to exclude a mucinous carcinoma. Extravasation of mucus and neoplastic cells caused by core needle biopsy has been observed; thus, if a CNB is done the core track should be included in the definitive surgical excision.

Ultrasound gel in smears may resemble mucin and is often accompanied by cellular artifact (see Fig. 7.12B).[195]

Medullary carcinoma (Fig. 7.69)[196]

Usual findings.

- Highly cellular smears,
- Poorly cohesive cells in clusters and singly,
- Large, pleomorphic, obviously malignant nuclei with prominent nucleoli,
- Many lymphocytes and plasma cells.

Like mucinous carcinoma, medullary carcinoma tends to be mammographically rounded and well circumscribed and has a soft feel to the needle. The cytological pattern is not specific but is simply that of a high-grade carcinoma. The presence of numerous lymphocytes in the background may be due to focal lymphocytic infiltration and is not reliable evidence of true medullary carcinoma. Medullary carcinoma is an increasingly rare histological diagnosis, which takes circumscription, tumor cell cytology and lymphocytic infiltration into account. In our cytology reports, we simply comment on the high content of lymphocytes.

PROBLEMS AND DIFFERENTIAL DIAGNOSIS

- High-grade infiltrating ductal carcinoma,
- Metastatic malignancy (melanoma) to axillary nodes,
- Malignant lymphoma,
- High-grade DCIS (comedocarcinoma).

If the lesion is in the upper outer quadrant of the breast, consideration should be given to metastasis of high-grade carcinoma or melanoma in an axillary node. A predominance of lymphoid cells and a mixed population of lymphoid cells including germinal center material and macrophages favor this possibility. Large cell lymphoma also enters the differential diagnosis. Immunohistochemistry and flow cytometry can be useful in distinguishing these lesions.

Cells of both comedocarcinoma and medullary carcinoma have abundant cytoplasm and large, pleomorphic, obviously malignant nuclei. Necrotic debris and foamy macrophages are more typical of comedocarcinoma; loss of cell cohesion is greater in medullary carcinoma. Numerous lymphocytes are not usually seen in smears of high-grade DCIS. As compared to high-grade ductal carcinomas, medullary carcinomas more commonly have syncytial fragments, lack gland formation and have macronucleoli, but there is significant overlap.[196]

Paget's disease of the nipple (Fig. 7.70)[197,198]

CRITERIA FOR DIAGNOSIS

- ◆ Background of keratin, squamous cells, inflammatory cells and debris (scrape smears from nipple).
- ◆ Large malignant cells, singly and in small groups, closely associated with squamous and inflammatory cells.
- ◆ Abundant pale cytoplasm with distinct borders.
- ◆ Obvious nuclear features of malignancy.

Scrape smears from the nipple are an excellent way to diagnose Paget's disease. Any crust or exudate must first be removed carefully. The clean surface is then scraped with a scalpel blade held at a blunt angle. Both alcohol-fixed and air-dried smears are recommended. If there is any palpable mass in the breast, this should also be needled. The tumor cells are of high nuclear grade and usually dispersed or in small groups. Small whorls of cells or cell engulfment are frequently found.

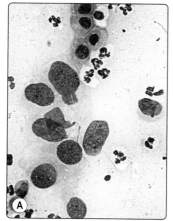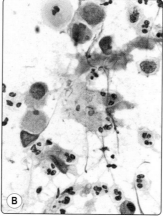

Fig. 7.70 Paget's disease of the nipple Nipple scrapings; mainly single, obviously malignant cells with abundant pale cytoplasm; some squamous cells; many inflammatory cells (**A**, MGG; **B**, Pap, HP).

PROBLEMS AND DIFFERENTIAL DIAGNOSIS

- ◆ Reactive changes secondary to inflammation,
- ◆ Nipple adenoma/subareolar duct papillomatosis,
- ◆ Carcinoma involving nipple from subareolar ducts,
- ◆ In situ squamous carcinoma and melanoma.

Inflammation or ulceration from other causes may produce reactive changes in squamous cells. The reactive cells are usually cohesive and do not show a high degree of nuclear atypia. In nipple adenoma/subareolar duct papillomatosis (see Fig. 7.46), the epithelial cells form cohesive aggregates, they are smaller and more uniform in size and they do not show malignant nuclear characteristics.

A carcinoma arising from a major duct just below the nipple can erupt onto the nipple without infiltrating the epidermis in a pagetoid fashion. In such a case, scrape smears from the nipple contain numerous malignant cells with greater tendency to form syncytial clusters and there is not the intimate mixture of carcinoma cells and squamous epithelial cells typical of Paget's disease.

In situ squamous carcinoma and melanoma are extremely rare in this site. Clinical appearances may be of help, or biopsy and immunohistochemistry for doubtful lesions.

Lobular carcinoma

Infiltrating lobular carcinoma
(Figs 7.71–7.73)[199–208]

Usual findings.

- • A variable, often poor cell yield,
- • Cells single and in small clusters, single files characteristic,
- • Scanty cytoplasm; many naked nuclei; nuclear molding in cell clusters,
- • Small hyperchromatic nuclei of relatively uniform size,
- • Irregularity of nuclear shape with angular, triangular, indented or budding nuclei,
- • Intracytoplasmic lumina/mucin vacuoles/signet ring cells,
- • Few if any naked bipolar nuclei,
- • Thick, eosinophilic background with crushed material interspersed between fatty vacuoles and small fibrous stromal fragments.

The criteria listed apply mainly to infiltrating lobular carcinoma of the classic type. The stroma is abundant, desmoplastic or fibrous, separating small groups and single files of neoplastic epithelial cells. The cells are not easily detached from the desmoplastic stroma and smears therefore tend to be poor in cells. The small cancer cells have a scanty and fragile cytoplasm, nuclear molding is a common finding in cell clusters and single files, and many single nuclei are stripped. In cells with intact cytoplasm, the nuclei tend to be eccentrically placed. The nuclei are only slightly larger than those of benign cells and vary little in size. However, nuclear outline is characteristically irregular, angular rather than rounded, with folds, buds and indentations, and this

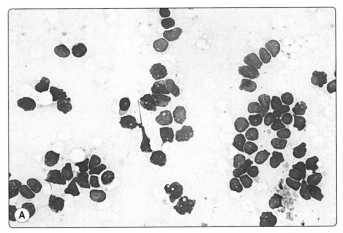

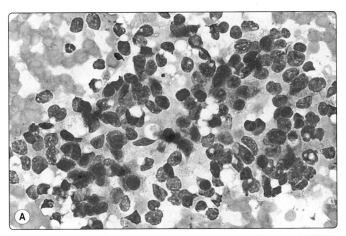

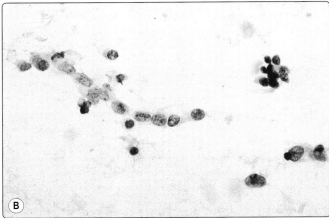

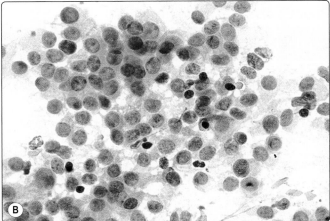

Fig. 7.71 Infiltrating lobular carcinoma, classic type (A) Poorly cohesive cell clusters; single files; uniformly small nuclei with irregular shapes; nuclear molding; indistinct cytoplasm (MGG, HP); (B) Single file of cells with small nuclei of irregular shape (Pap, HP).

Fig. 7.73 Infiltrating lobular carcinoma, alveolar type Cellular smears of poorly cohesive clusters of malignant cells with moderate nuclear atypia; difficult to distinguish from duct carcinoma of similar grade (A, MGG, HP; B, Pap, HP).

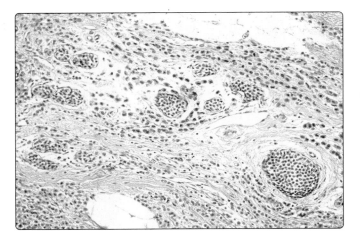

Fig. 7.72 Infiltrating lobular carcinoma, classic type Tissue section corresponding to Figure 7.71 (H&E, LP).

makes it possible to distinguish them from the single bipolar nuclei of benign breast tissue. Fragments of collagen may be seen associated with the tumor cells. The cells are often traumatised, presumably due to the force needed to detach them from the stroma. Non-neoplastic cells are more easily

detached and residual benign ductal elements may be over-represented in the FNB sample.

The cells of some lobular carcinomas have the appearance of signet ring cells with intracytoplasmic neolumina and a central condensed mucin droplet ('bull's-eye' inclusion). This is commonly seen in lobular carcinoma but is not specific and can be found also in duct carcinomas (see Fig. 7.74).

The cytology of the alveolar type of lobular carcinoma can show a rosette-like pattern (Fig. 7.73). Pleomorphic variants cytologically resemble poorly differentiated ductal carcinoma.

PROBLEMS AND DIFFERENTIAL DIAGNOSIS

◆ Sparse cellularity,
◆ Resemblance to non-neoplastic breast tissue on low magnification,
◆ Component of benign epithelium,
◆ Lobular hyperplasia in pregnancy and lactation,
◆ Distinction from low-grade ductal carcinoma,
◆ Intracytoplasmic lumina in other lesions.

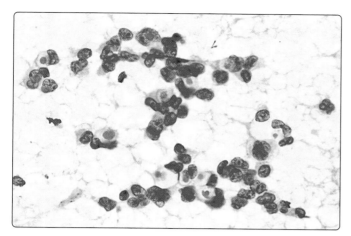

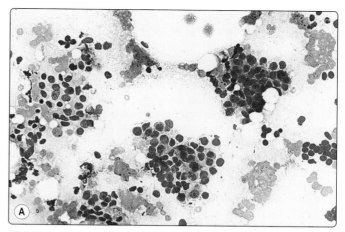

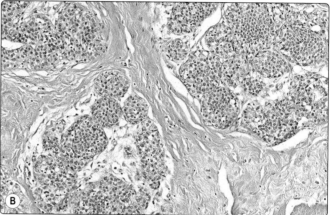

Fig. 7.74 Malignant cells with intracytoplasmic neolumina Malignant cells with intracytoplasmic neolumina are most often seen in lobular carcinoma, but can also occur in invasive duct carcinoma NOS as in this case. Note 'bull's-eye' inclusions (Pap, HP).

Fig. 7.75 Mass-forming lobular carcinoma in situ (LCIS) (A) Loosely cohesive clusters of mildly atypical cells with small round nuclei and pale, fragile cytoplasm (MGG, IP); (B) Corresponding tissue section. There was no evidence of invasion in this case (H&E, IP).

Lobular carcinoma is an important source of false-negative diagnosis in breast FNB. A smear from a lobular carcinoma, overall poor in cells with small clusters of cells and single naked nuclei, can easily be misread as a benign lesion. A scanty sample from a clinically suspicious lesion in an older woman may be due to lobular carcinoma and is always worth a second look, especially since mammography and US are less sensitive in this tumor type. At high-power examination the irregular, abnormal shape of the nuclei, including those of single cells with stripped nuclei, becomes evident. Epithelial cells with irregular, eccentric nuclei and dense cytoplasm and cells with intracytoplasmic lumina or mucin droplets are suggestive of the diagnosis.

Lobular carcinoma is characteristically poorly circumscribed and extends far into the surrounding glandular tissue. This growth pattern tends to leave residual non-neoplastic ducts within the tumor. Residual benign epithelial cells may be preferentially removed by the needle and may dominate a scanty smear to the extent that the malignant cells are overlooked.

Not surprisingly, the cells of low-grade lobular carcinoma of the alveolar type resemble those of hyperplastic acinar cells in pregnancy and lactation (compare Figs 7.8A and 7.73). Cells of both have pale vacuolated cytoplasm and rounded nuclei. Smears of alveolar lobular carcinoma are quite cellular, showing poorly cohesive multilayered clusters of cells, and lack the background of lipid secretion typical of lactating breast tissue.

The distinction between lobular and ductal carcinoma is not always possible. Some low-grade ductal carcinomas have equally small, relatively uniform neoplastic cells. Conversely, cells of lobular carcinoma of higher nuclear grade or of alveolar type are larger and have larger nuclei similar to those of ductal carcinoma NOS (compare Figs 7.5 and 7.73B).[199,207] The distinction has some practical significance in the correlation with mammographic findings, as a lobular carcinoma is often more extensive than suggested by clinical and mammographic findings.

Dispersed atypical cells with intracytoplasmic lumina are a significant observation suggestive but not diagnostic of invasive lobular carcinoma. Aspirates from lobular carcinoma in situ (LCIS) and atypical lobular hyperplasia (ALH) may show these cells. Cells with intracytoplasmic neolumina are not specific for lobular neoplasia and may be found in ductal carcinomas, tubular carcinomas, colloid carcinomas, secretory carcinomas, medullary carcinomas and papillary carcinomas.[208] However, even small numbers of dispersed signet ring cells or cells with intracytoplasmic lumina and a central targetoid ('bull's-eye') mucin droplet are a strong indicator of a significant lesion requiring excision. This does not apply to similar cell changes in cohesive sheets, where vacuoles may be seen in benign hyperplasias, possibly within myoepithelial cells.[204]

Lobular carcinoma in situ/atypical lobular hyperplasia (LCIS, ALH) (Figs 7.74, 7.75)[209–212]

In the past, LCIS was a rare incidental finding in palpable breast lesions subjected to FNB. Few reports of its cytological features can be found in the literature. The cytologic findings in these cases include moderately cellular samples with tight or loosely cohesive clusters of atypical epithelial cells with mild nuclear atypia (Figure 7.74). The cells were small, with prominent nucleoli and occasional cells had intracytoplasmic lumina. In the majority of described cases a definitive diagnosis of LCIS could not be made but the presence of atypical cells warranted excision. In some cases, a diagnosis of infiltrating lobular carcinoma was made on aspiration biopsy[209] as there is overlap in cytologic features between LCIS and infiltrating lobular carcinoma.

Distinction of LCIS from invasive lobular carcinoma may not be possible in some cases even when clinical and radiological findings are correlated with cytology. The existence of mass-forming LCIS needs to be kept in mind when a cytological diagnosis of invasive lobular carcinoma is made, and confirmation by CNB before proceeding to radical surgery may be considered. A definitive diagnosis of LCIS is left to histopathologic examination. A CNB diagnosis of ALH and LCIS warrants surgical excision, as carcinoma is seen in 16% and 25% of the cases, respectively.[212] The main differential on core biopsy of LCIS is the small cell solid type of low-grade DCIS or cancerization of lobules by DCIS. Immunohistochemistry with E-cadherin, a transmembrane glycoprotein, is helpful as it is positive in ductal lesions but lacking in LCIS and invasive lobular carcinomas.

Some uncommon variants of carcinoma[213]

Breast cancer in the male[96–98,214–216]

Most breast cancers in male patients are infiltrating duct carcinoma NOS, identical to the common duct carcinoma in women. DCIS also occurs in the male breast. Metastatic cancer is perhaps as common as primary carcinoma. Smears of gynecomastia can occasionally show worrisome atypia (see Fig. 7.9B) and false-positive diagnoses have been reported. Correlation with clinical and mammographic findings is therefore important, as in female patients.

'Inflammatory' carcinoma[217]

The clinical presentation of 'inflammatory' carcinoma is a diffuse increase in the consistency of the breast without a distinct mass, and thickening and erythema of the skin due to extensive intralymphatic spread of tumor causing lymph stasis and edema. Imaging may detect a mass lesion, making sampling easier. Random sampling from central parts of the breast or intracutaneous sampling with a 25-gauge needle introduced tangentially may produce enough malignant cells to allow a confident diagnosis. The tumor cells occur in small aggregates and show malignant pleomorphism. A diagnosis can often be made on small amounts of material. Inflammatory cells are not seen. CNB, especially with the mammotome device, may prove more useful in the diagnosis of inflammatory breast carcinoma as compared to FNB.[218]

Carcinoma with apocrine (oxyphil) differentiation (Figs 7.76A and 7.77)[219,220]

Invasive carcinoma of purely oxyphil type is rare. DCIS with prominent apocrine metaplasia is more commonly seen, and in MGG preparations cells of high-grade breast carcinoma of no special type may have an apocrine-like appearance. Cancer cells of oxyphil type have large, pleomorphic nuclei, a coarse and irregular nuclear chromatin and

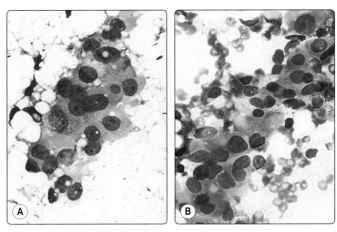

Fig. 7.76 Carcinoma with apocrine differentiation; comparison with atypical apocrine metaplasia (A) Irregular cluster of malignant cells; abundant gray/blue, finely granular cytoplasm; pleomorphic nuclei; prominent nucleoli; (B) Similar atypical oxyphil cells from case of apocrine metaplasia in adenosis; note admixture with usual bland epithelial cells which have smaller nuclei (MGG, HP).

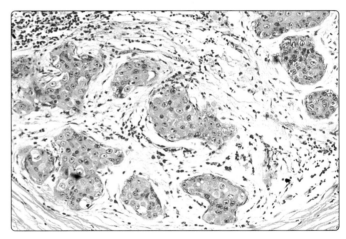

Fig. 7.77 Carcinoma with apocrine differentiation Tissue section corresponding to Figure 7.75A. Case of high-grade DCIS with oxyphil malignant cells and focal invasion (H&E, IP).

macronucleoli. In comparison to the common duct carcinoma cells, apocrine cells have more abundant cytoplasm, which is densely eosinophilic and granular and has more distinct cell borders. Apocrine (oxyphil) metaplasia of epithelial cells in cyst fluids, fibrocystic disease, and lesions with epithelial hyperplasia including fibroadenoma and adenosis often cause concern due to marked atypia and can be the cause of a false-positive diagnosis. Great caution should be observed if atypical apocrine epithelial cells are seen together with benign elements or if they are found in a clinically or mammographically benign lesion, regardless of the degree of cytological atypia. A pure population of severely atypical oxyphil cells with evidence of necrosis and a complete absence of benign epithelium and single bipolar nuclei are features indicating carcinoma. Granular cell tumor and alveolar soft part sarcoma should be included in the differential diagnosis of apocrine carcinoma.

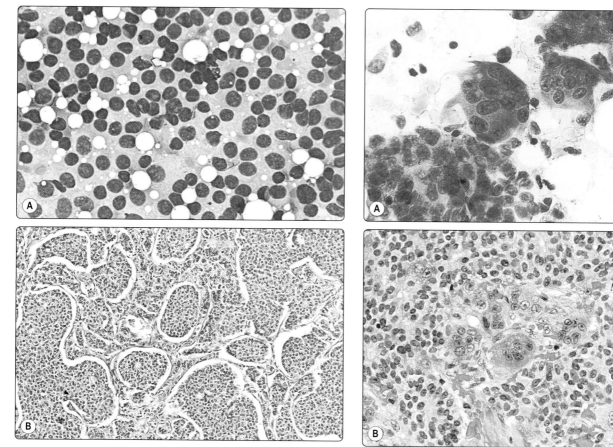

Fig. 7.78 Carcinoma of neuroendocrine type (A) Cellular smear of totally dispersed small cells; relatively uniform nuclei; coarsely granular chromatin (MGG, HP); (B) Corresponding tissue section showing a carcinoid-like pattern; tumor cells were positive for chromogranin (H&E, IP).

Fig. 7.79 Carcinoma with osteoclast-like giant cells (A) Several multinucleated histiocytic giant cells associated with malignant cells similar to intermediate-grade duct carcinoma NOS (MGG, HP); (B) Corresponding tissue section (H&E, IP).

Carcinoma of neuroendocrine type

(Fig. 7.78)[221]

This is an uncommon variant of invasive breast carcinoma. Smears are cellular with mainly dispersed uniform plasmacytoid cells with a coarse granular nuclear chromatin pattern resembling the cells of a carcinoid or other neuroendocrine tumor. The cells may or may not stain positively with neuroendocrine markers such as chromogranin or synaptophysin and contain dense core granules by electron microscopy. The clinical behavior of these tumors does not seem to differ from that of the common duct carcinoma. However, the smear pattern of dispersed, rather uniform cells with scanty cytoplasm could be mistaken for lymphoid tissue, and the possibility of metastatic neuroendocrine carcinoma, for example of bronchogenic origin, has to be considered. Distinction from ductal carcinoma of no special type with dispersed cells and small, relatively uniform nuclei may not be possible without immunohistochemistry but seems to be of no clinical significance as the behavior is similar.

Cytological findings in argyrophilic mucin producing spindle cell carcinoma and in carcinoid tumors in the breast have been reported.[222–224]

Breast carcinoma with osteoclast-like giant cells (Fig. 7.79)[225]

Invasive carcinoma with numerous multinucleated osteoclast-like giant cells is a rare type of breast carcinoma. On aspiration biopsy, the giant cells are intermingled with the malignant epithelial cells. Such tumors tend to be low grade. The giant cells are believed to be derived from fusion of stromal cells, and by electron microscopy are of histiocytic origin. Histiocytic giant cells can occasionally be found also in fibroadenoma and other benign lesions such as granulomatous mastitis.

Invasive micropapillary carcinoma

(Fig. 7.80)[226,227]

Invasive micropapillary carcinoma is another uncommon variant of breast cancer thought to show a more aggressive behavior due to the predilection for lymphatic spread. The findings in smears closely parallel the pattern seen in tissue sections. The smears are of high cellularity with three-dimensional clusters forming rounded balls, morules and micropapillary fragments without a stromal core in addition to malignant discohesive cells. The cells show a moderate

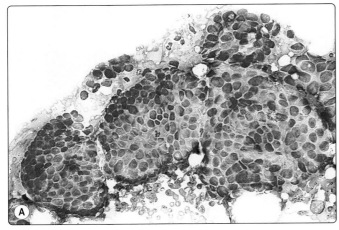

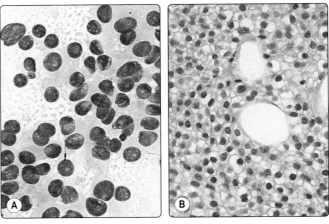

Fig. 7.81 **Glycogen-rich carcinoma** (A) Mainly dissociated malignant cells with abundant pale fragile cytoplasm dispersed in the background (MGG, HP); (B) Corresponding tissue section (H&E, IP.

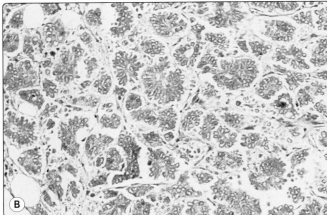

Fig. 7.80 **Invasive micropapillary carcinoma** (A) Many balls and finger-like epithelial fragments with an 'anatomical' border; moderate nuclear atypia, some cuboidal/columnar cells (MGG, HP); (B) Corresponding tissue section (H&E, IP).

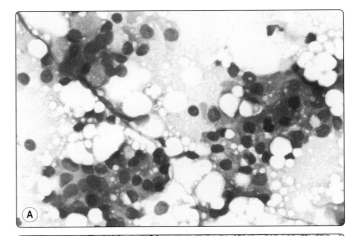

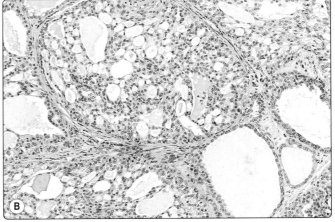

Fig. 7.82 **Secretory carcinoma** (A) Loose clusters of epithelial cells; some single cells; abundant vacuolated cytoplasm; rounded moderately atypical nuclei; some signet ring forms with pink secretory droplets (*upper left*); no bipolar nuclei (MGG, HP); (B) Corresponding tissue section (H&E, IP).

degree of nuclear atypia. Psammoma bodies, malignant apocrine cytology and focal mucin background have also been described.

Clear cell (glycogen-rich) carcinoma
(Fig. 7.81)[228]

Smears are hypercellular with loosely cohesive syncytical groups and single malignant cells. The malignant cells have abundant, pale cytoplasm and moderate to marked nuclear pleomorphism with prominent nucleoli. A tigroid background can be noted. PAS-positive, diastase-sensitive material compatible with glycogen can be seen. The clear cell pattern is much more obvious in paraffin sections due to the high glycogen content. A similar pattern may also be seen in lipid-rich carcinoma.[229]

Secretory carcinoma (Fig. 7.82)[230,231]

Secretory carcinoma is an uncommon variant of ductal carcinoma with a favorable prognosis. Smears are moderately cellular with a background that contains abundant secretion. The cells are arranged in sheets or three-dimensional clusters with small round nuclei and abundant cytoplasm and intracytoplasmic vacuoles. The cells stain positively with a PAS stain.

Case reports describing cystic hypersecretory carcinoma of the breast have been reported in the literature.[232]

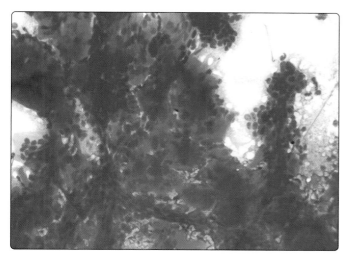

Fig. 7.83 **Adenoid cystic carcinoma** Multilayered aggregates of small cells; relatively uniform hyperchromatic nuclei; some molding; several hyaline globules (MGG, IP).

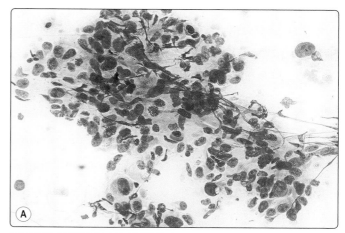

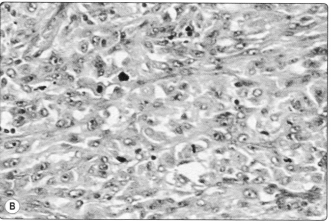

Fig. 7.85 **'Metaplastic' carcinoma** (A) Tissue fragment of poorly cohesive pleomorphic spindle cells suggestive of sarcoma. The cells were positive for cytokeratin and there were more obvious malignant epithelial cells in other parts of the smear (MGG, IP); (B) Corresponding tissue section (H&E, IP).

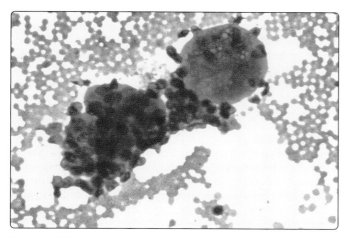

Fig. 7.84 **Collagenous spherulosis** Clusters of small bland epithelial cells attached to a couple of hyaline globules of basement membrane material (MGG, IP).

Adenoid cystic carcinoma (Fig. 7.83)[233,234]

The prognosis for this rare tumor is significantly better than for most other invasive carcinomas. The cytological pattern is identical to that of adenoid cystic carcinoma in other sites, such as salivary glands, lung, etc. Hyaline stromal globules resembling those of adenoid cystic carcinoma can also be associated with collagenous spherulosis, a benign lesion confined to lobular acini or ductules that is seen incidentally with benign proliferative breast lesions (Fig. 7.84). The epithelial cells of collagenous spherulosis are small and uniformly bland whereas the cells of adenoid cystic carcinoma have a high N:C ratio and enlarged, hyperchromatic nuclei with a coarse chromatin and an irregular nuclear membrane. Bipolar nuclei are present in collagenous spherulosis, in contrast to adenoid cystic carcinoma.

Metaplastic carcinoma (Figs 7.85 and 7.86)[235,236]

Some breast carcinomas have a mixed pattern showing metaplasia and variable differentiation. Metaplastic carcinoma is defined as a tumor that has two distinctly different components. There are several variants of 'metaplastic' carcinoma. Spindle cell or sarcomatoid carcinoma closely resembles soft tissue sarcoma (Fig. 7.85). The differential diagnosis between malignant phyllodes tumor and metaplastic spindle cell carcinoma can be particularly difficult both in smears and in core needle biopsy specimens. In malignant phyllodes tumors the stromal overgrowth may be so abundant that it is impossible to distinguish from a pure spindle cell mesenchymal tumor. Sarcomatoid metaplastic carcinoma is confirmed by positive staining of the spindle cells for cytokeratin. Chondroid or osteoid stromal matrix can be found focally in some metaplastic carcinomas (Fig. 7.86).

Squamous differentiation is sometimes seen in poorly differentiated duct carcinoma. Low-grade adenosquamous carcinoma has been described.[237,238] Pure squamous carcinoma has been diagnosed by FNB,[239] including very well-differentiated forms.[240] Cystic change may occur. The alternative of a secondary tumor should be excluded clinically before definitive management is decided.

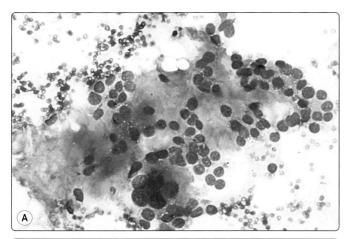

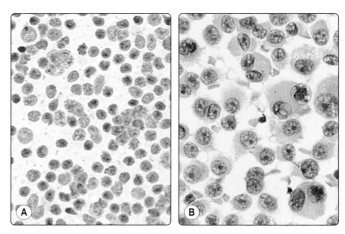

Fig. 7.87 Malignancies of non-breast origin (A) Non-Hodgkin lymphoma, follicular, presenting clinically as a solitary breast lump (MGG, IP); (B) Metastasis of amelanotic melanoma, clinically a solitary breast lump (H&E, HP).

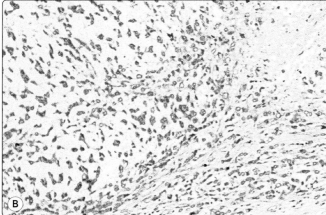

Fig. 7.86 'Metaplastic' carcinoma (A) Carcinoma with chondrosarcomatous areas; note the dense, brightly staining chondroid ground substance (MGG, HP); (B) Corresponding tissue section (H&E, IP). This tumor also contained sarcomatoid spindle cell areas and foci of anaplastic carcinoma.

Other malignant tumors

Metastatic malignancy[241,242]

Metastatic tumor of extramammary origin can occur in the breast, presenting clinically as a solitary lump suggestive of primary breast carcinoma. If the cytological pattern does not fit any of the recognized subtypes of primary breast cancer, the possibility of metastatic malignancy has to be considered. The most common malignant tumors metastasizing to the breast are lymphomas, followed by malignant melanoma and lung carcinoma. Other sites include the ovary, the kidney, the uterine cervix and rarely from sarcomas.

Lymphoma/leukaemia (Fig.7.87A)[243]

Malignant lymphoma rarely presents as a primary breast tumor. The differential diagnosis of malignant lymphoma and reactive lymphoid tissue is described in Chapter 5. Large cell lymphoma may closely resemble poorly differentiated breast carcinoma with a completely dispersed cell population. In large cell lymphoma, many of the cells have a basophilic cytoplasm, an eccentric nucleus with one or multiple nucleolei, and a perinuclear halo. The presence in the background of round basophilic cytoplasmic fragments (lymphoglandular bodies) is a useful indicator of the lymphoid nature of the cells. Breast carcinoma of neuroendocrine type also needs to be considered in the differential diagnosis of lymphoma of small cell type. Leukemia, particularly myeloid, may give rise to mass lesions in the breast.

Sarcoma

Phyllodes tumors have been described on page 171. Malignant phyllodes tumor can be difficult to distinguish from soft tissue sarcoma. Smears contain fragments of highly cellular mesenchymal tissue and dispersed spindle cells showing a variable degree of nuclear atypia and pleomorphism. In some tumors the pattern is obviously malignant, like a spindle cell sarcoma (see Fig. 7.31B); others may have a relatively bland cytology, and the malignant character is suggested by high cellularity and invasive growth (tissue sections). Sheets of epithelial cells may or may not be present, depending on selective sampling. As a rule, the spindle cell component dominates the smears. The epithelial component may appear atypical but does not show malignant criteria. The histological pattern is often variable within the same tumor and a single FNB sample may not be representative, particularly if the tumor is large.

Distinction of primary sarcoma from sarcomatoid carcinoma or malignant phyllodes tumor will generally not be possible by cytomorphology alone and requires immunocytochemical study. An example of primary leiomyosarcoma, which clinically presented as a primary breast cancer, is shown in Figure 7.88. The FNB was reported as a malignant sarcomatous spindle cell tumor. Liposarcoma of the breast diagnosed by FNB has been reported.[244]

In angiosarcoma of the breast, aspiration yields plenty of blood, and tumor cells may be few in numbers and difficult to find.[245,246] This is particularly the case with low-grade tumors, which consist of wide, anastomosing vascular channels lined by atypical endothelial cells showing little

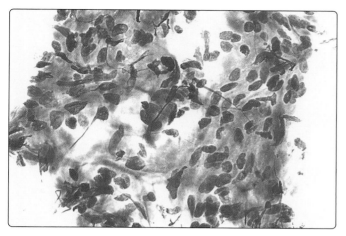

Fig. 7.88 Leiomyosarcoma of breast Tissue fragments of cohesive, moderately atypical spindle cells in a fibrous stroma. FNB of breast mass clinically suggestive of primary breast cancer, reported as low-grade malignant spindle cell tumor inconsistent with primary breast carcinoma. No alternative primary found; leiomyosarcoma confirmed histologically (MGG, HP).

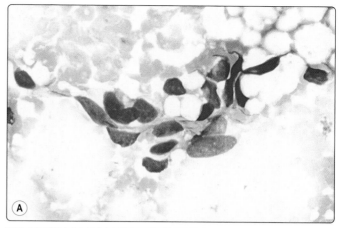

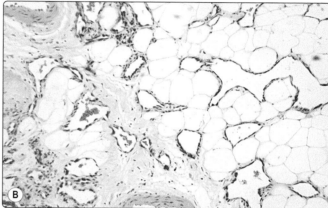

Fig. 7.89 Angiosarcoma (A) Heavily bloodstained smear; few groups of pleomorphic spindle cells of malignant appearance, many fat droplets (MGG, HP); (B) Corresponding tissue section of low-grade angiosarcoma (H&E, LP).

tendency to form solid proliferations. High-grade, more solid tumors are easily recognized as sarcomas. The tumor cells are spindle shaped, they have an attenuated basophilic cytoplasm without distinct borders and dark pleomorphic, elongated or plump spindle nuclei. Most cells occur in syncytial clusters but some are single (Fig. 7.89). There may be a suggestion of vascular structures. The presence of fat tissue fragments in smears is due to the neoplastic vascular channels widely invading adipose tissue. Pitfalls in diagnosis include misinterpreting the spindle cells as derived from benign granulation tissue or other spindle cell lesions, and overlooking a few abnormal cells in a bloodstained, apparently unsatisfactory smear.

Management summaries

Protocols for management are designed to maximize detection of carcinomas while maintaining a low benign to malignant ratio for excised lesions.

- Highly suspicious lesions are excised even if FNB or CNB findings are benign (discordance between radiological and cytological findings). For indeterminate lesions, the FNB findings may determine whether the lesion is excised or whether the patient is followed mammographically. If the smear is cellular, adequate and technically satisfactory, if the findings are consistent with a specific benign diagnosis, and if this is compatible with the radiologic findings, excision is not indicated. If the material is scanty or if any cytological atypia is noted on FNB, further investigation is carried out, with either CNB or excision.
- For lesions of low suspicion radiologically, CNB or excision is recommended if the cytological findings are atypical/equivocal or worse. If the findings are benign non-specific, a multidisciplinary decision needs to be made whether to perform a CNB/excision or to return the patient to normal screening interval. A repeat mammogram at a shorter interval is generally not considered a practical alternative.

FNB or CNB is thus used to:

- establish a definitive benign diagnosis such as cyst or fibroadenoma,
- reinforce a mammographic diagnosis of a benign process,
- shift indeterminate cases into a higher risk group for excision,
- confirm a malignant diagnosis, either as a basis for therapy or to plan further investigations.

Some clinicians suggest that FNB of high-suspicion lesions is of no value because they will be excised whatever the result. However, there is a small but significant number of benign lesions, for example radial scar, nodular fasciitis fibromatosis and granular cell tumor, in this category. Furthermore, preoperative diagnosis gives a much higher likelihood of adequate clearance of cancer at the first operation.[247]

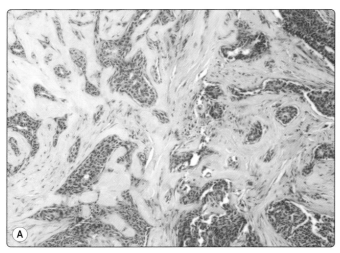
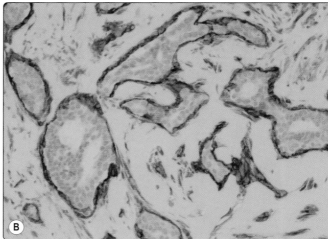

Fig. 7.90 Sclerosed papilloma (A) Infiltration of glands in a sclerotic stroma can mimic infiltrative carcinoma (H&E, IP); (B) Immunohistochemical stain for calponin highlights the myoepithelial layer, confirming a sclerosed papilloma (Calponin, HP).

Summary of main diagnostic pitfalls in breast FNB and CNB[44,169,248]

Conditions in which there is a risk of false-positive diagnosis

1. Papillary lesions

The distinction between intraductal papilloma/florid papillomatosis, intracystic papillary carcinoma/papillary DCIS, and well-differentiated invasive papillary carcinoma is difficult in smears. Infarcted papilloma may closely mimic carcinoma. In general, a definitive cytological diagnosis of malignancy should not be made in papillary lesions but left to histology. Sclerosed papillomas can mimic carcinoma on core biopsy, and immuohistochemical stains for myoepithelial cell markers should be utilised to prevent a false-positive diagnosis (Fig. 7.90).

2. Epithelial hyperplasia with nuclear atypia

Highly cellular smears showing some loss of cell cohesion, and variable nuclear atypia (enlargement and anisokaryosis) can raise a suspicion of malignancy, but the presence of clearly benign elements, in particular of single bare bipolar nuclei, should prevent a cancer diagnosis.

3. Radial scar/complex sclerosing lesion

Groups of atypical epithelial cells derived from the central scar may closely resemble tubular carcinoma, but the presence of benign epithelial cells and single bare bipolar nuclei precludes a malignant diagnosis. Immunohistochemical stains for myoepithelial markers on CNB can help in distinguishing radial scars from tubular carcinomas.

4. Fibroadenoma

Epithelial atypia can be extremely worrisome in some fibroadenomas. Again, the presence of single benign bare bipolar nuclei and sheets of benign epithelium should prevent a false-positive diagnosis. The myxoid stroma characteristic of fibroadenoma is a helpful sign, but similar stroma can occasionally be found in carcinoma of no special type.

5. Regenerative epithelial atypia

In the presence of inflammatory cells, particularly of polymorphs, epithelial atypia should be interpreted with great caution. Regenerative atypia can be prominent in chronic mastitis, granulomatous inflammation and in fat necrosis.

Post-radiation atypia is a special problem which requires experience in the follow-up of postoperative irradiation for breast cancer.

6. Pregnancy and lactation

The smear pattern of dispersed cells resembles cancer at low power but the uniformly round nuclei, the bland nuclear chromatin and, above all, the lipid secretion in the background prevent misdiagnosis.

7. Atypia of ductal epithelium in cysts

Ductal epithelial cells of oxyphil (apocrine) type seen in cyst fluid can look very atypical. If the fluid does not contain altered blood or debris, and if there is no residual lump after evacuation of the fluid, there is practically no likelihood of malignancy.

Conditions in which there is a risk of making a false-negative diagnosis

1. Tumors with central necrosis or sclerosis

Smears from such lesions may be practically acellular. The distinction between scirrhous cancer and sclerosed fibroadenoma, and between necrotic cancer and duct ectasia, may require CNB or excision.

2. A small carcinoma next to a dominant benign lesion

A small cancer situated adjacent to a 'lipoma', a cyst or a lumpy fibroadenosis can easily be missed by FNB or CNB. Radiological guidance (mammography or US) is essential.

3. Complex proliferative lesions

Representative sampling can not be assured in poorly defined complex lesions with epithelial hyperplasia with and without atypia. Such lesions can include foci of in situ or even invasive carcinoma not sampled by FNB or CNB. Close correlation with clinical and mammographic findings is crucial.

4. Low-grade ductal carcinoma

Tubular carcinoma can be a problem, since single, bare, stromal nuclei of benign type are often present in smears from such tumors, and epithelial atypia may be minimal. In most cases, the overall architectural pattern is sufficiently atypical to suggest an open biopsy. Most tubular carcinomas are stellate lesions radiologically, with a high suspicion of carcinoma. Mammography may be more effective than cytology in selecting cases for excision. Another problematic lesion is low-grade DCIS in which fully developed criteria of malignancy are not usually present; however, most cases are diagnosed as 'atypical' or suspicious, with a recommendation of excision.

5. Lobular carcinoma and small cell ductal carcinoma

These lesions are difficult to detect radiologically because they infiltrate diffusely. Cells of infiltrating lobular carcinoma often have uniformly small nuclei and the cell yield is poor due to the highly desmoplastic stroma. The irregular shape of the nuclei, the tendency to form single files or clusters with nuclear molding and the absence of single, bare bipolar nuclei are diagnostic features. Low-grade duct carcinoma NOS may also have uniformly small neoplastic cells. Irregularity of nuclear outline and intracytoplasmic neolumina are helpful clues.

Other issues

1. High-grade DCIS

A combination of large cohesive clusters of malignant cells with a high nuclear grade and a background of necrotic and calcific debris allows a component of high-grade DCIS to be suggested. This finding correlates with pleomorphic or branching calcifications on mammography. FNB cannot reliably exclude invasion. Immunohistochemical stains should be used in cases of high-grade DCIS on CNB to avoid overcalling invasion.

2. Mucinous lesions

A number of lesions may be associated with mucin in smears: invasive mucinous carcinoma, mucinous DCIS or ADH, mucocele-like lesions, and mucinous fibroadenoma. The cell content associated with the mucin is the best guide to the nature of the lesion. Similar problems are seen with CNB.

3. Small sclerotic fibroadenoma

Fine needle aspiration biopsy may not yield enough cell material to be diagnostic in these lesions and CNB is often necessary.

References

1. Kocjan G, Bourgain C, Fassina A, et al. The role of breast FNAC in diagnosis and clinical management: a survey of current practice. Cytopathology 2008;19:271–8.

2. Manfrin E, Mariotto R, Remo A, et al. Is there still a role for fine-needle aspiration cytology in breast cancer screening? Experience with real-time integrated radiopathologic activity (1999–2004). Cancer(Cytopathol) 2008;114:74–82.

3. NIH. The uniform approach to breast fine-needle aspiration biopsy. NIH Consensus Development Conference. Am J Surg 1997;174:371–5.

4. Wong AY, Salisbury E, Bilous M. Recent developments in stereotactic breast biopsy methodologies: an update for the surgical pathologist. Advances in Anatomic Pathology 2000;7:26–35.

5. Wallis M, Tarvidon A, Helbich T, et al. Guidelines from the European Society of Breast Imaging for diagnostic interventional breast procedures. Eur Radiol 2007;17:581–8.

6. Frayne J, Sterrett GF, Harvey J, et al. Stereotactic 14 gauge core-biopsy of the breast: results from 101 patients. Aust NZ J Surg 1996;66:585–91.

7. Britton PD. Fine needle aspiration or core biopsy. The Breast 1999;8:1–4.

8. Liberman L. Percutaneous image-guided core breast biopsy. Radiol Clin N Am 2002;40:483–500.

9. Shannon J, Douglas-Jones AG, Dallimore NS. Conversion to core biopsy in the preoperative diagnosis of breast lesions: is it justified by results? J Clin Pathol 2001;54:762–5.

10. Sun W, Li A, Abreo F, et al. Comparison of fine-needle aspiration cytology and core biopsy for diagnosis of breast cancer. Diagn Cytopathol 2001;24:421–5.

11. Masood S. Fine-needle aspiration biopsy of nonpalpable breast lesions. Challenges and promises. Cancer (Cancer Cytopathology) 1998;84:197–9.

12. Florentine BD, Cobb CJ, Frankel K, et al. Core needle biopsy. A useful adjunct to fine-needle aspiration in select patients with palpable breast lesions. Cancer 1997;81:33–9.

13. Logan-Young W, Dawson AE, Wilbur DC, et al. The cost effectiveness of fine-needle aspiration cytology and 14-gauge core needle biopsy compared with open surgical biopsy in the diagnosis of breast carcinoma. Cancer 1998;82:1867–73.

14. Ahmed I, Nazir R, Chaudhary M Y, Kundi S. Triple assessment of breast lump. J Coll Physicians Surg Pak 2007;17:535–8.

15. NHSBSP. Non-operative diagnosis subgroup of the national coordinating group for breast screening pathology 2001, Publication 50.

16. Gupta RK. Fine-needle aspiration cytodiagnosis of recurrent carcinoma of the breast in operative scars. Diagn Cytopathol 1997;16:14–6.

17. Gupta RK, Gaskell D, Dowle C, et al. Fine needle aspiration cytology of seromas of the breast from irradiated lumpectomy sites. Acta Cytol 2004;48:478–80.

18. Maygarden SJ, Novotny DB, Johnson DE, et al. Fine-needle aspiration cytology of suture granulomas of the breast: a potential pitfall in the cytologic diagnosis of recurrent breast cancer. Diagn Cytopathol 1994;10:175–9.

19. Peterse JL, Thunnissen FB, van Heerde P. Fine needle aspiration cytology of radiation-induced changes in nonneoplastic breast lesions. Possible pitfalls in cytodiagnosis. Acta Cytol 1989;33:176–80.

20. Rakha EA, El-Sayed ME, Reed J, et al. Screen-detected breast lesions with malignant needle core biopsy diagnoses and no malignancy identified in subsequent surgical excision specimens (potential false-positive diagnosis). Eur J Cancer 2009;45:1162–7.

21. Chhieng D, Fernandez G, Cangiarella JF, et al. Invasive carcinoma in clinically suspicious breast masses diagnosed as adenocarcinoma by fine-needle aspiration. Cancer 2000;90:96–101.

22. Rutstein LA, Johnson RR, Poller WR, et al. Predictors of residual invasive disease after core needle biopsy diagnosis of ductal carcinoma in situ. Breast J 2007;13:251–7.

23. Berner A, Davidson B, Sigstad E, et al. Fine needle aspiration cytology vs. core biopsy in the diagnosis of breast lesions. Diagn Cytopathol 2003;29:344–8.

24. Pisano ED, Fajardo LL, Caudry DJ, et al. Fine-needle aspiration biopsy of nonpalpable breast lesions in a multicenter clinical trial: results from the radioloic diagnostic oncology group V. Radiology 2001;219:785–92.

25. Sterrett G, Harvey J, Parsons RW, et al. Breast cancer in Western Australia in 1989: III. Accuracy of FNA cytology in diagnosis. Aust NZ J Surg 1994;64: 745–9.

26. Ciatto S, Bonardi R, Cariaggi MP. Performance of fine-needle aspiration cytology of the breast – multicenter study of 23,063 aspirates in ten Italian laboratories. Tumori 1995;81:13–7.

27. Feichter GE, Haberthür F, Gobat S, et al. Breast cytology. Statistical analysis and cytohistologic correlations. Acta Cytol 1997;41:327–32.

28. Arisio R, Cuccorese C, Accinelli G, et al. Role of fine-needle aspiration biopsy in breast lesions: analysis of a series of 4,110 cases. Diagn Cytopathol 1998;18:462–7.

29. Klijanienko J, Zajdela A, Lussier C, et al. Critical clinicopathologic analysis of 23 cases of fine-needle breast sampling initially recorded as false-positive. The 44-year experience of the Institut Curie. Cancer (Cancer Cytopathol) 2001;93:132–9.

30. Orell SR, Farshid G. False-positive reports in fine needle biopsy of breast lesions. Pathology 2001;33:428–36.

31. Symmans WF, Cangiarella JF, Gottlieb S, et al. What is the role of cytopathologists in stereotaxic needle biopsy diagnosis of nonpalpable mammographic abnormalities. Diagn Cytopathol 2001;24:260–70.

32. Brenner RJ, Fajardo L, Fisher PR, et al. Percutaneous core biopsy of the breast: effect of operator experience and number of samples on diagnostic accuracy. AJR Am J Roentgenol 1996;166:341–6.

33. Helbich TH, Rudas M, Haitel A, et al. Evaluation of needle size for breast biopsy: comparison of 14-, 16- and 18-gauge biopsy needles. AJR Am J Roentgenol 1998;171:59–63.

34. Leifland K, Lagerstedt U, Svane G. Comparison of stereotactic FNB and CNB in 522 non-palpable breast lesions. Acta Radiol 2003;44:387–91.

35. Leifland K, Lundquist H, Lagerstedt U, et al. Comparison of pre-operative simultaneous stereotactic fine needle aspiration biopsy and stereotactic core needle biopsy in ductal carcinoma in situ of the breast. Acta Radiol 2003;44:213–7.

36. Leifland K, Lundquist H, Mare K, et al. Pre-operative simultaneous stereotactic core biopsy and fine-needle aspiration biopsy in the diagnosis of invasive lobular breast carcinoma. Acta Radiol 200;41:57–60.

37. Westenend PJ, Sever AR, Beekman-de Volder HJC, et al. A comparison of aspiration cytology and core needle biopsy in the evaluation of breast lesions. Cancer (Cancer Cytopathol) 2001;93:146–50.

38. Masood S, Loya A, Khalbuss W. Is core needle biopsy superior to fine-needle aspiration biopsy in the diagnosis of papillary breast lesions? Diagn Cytopathol 2003;28:329–34

39. Ballo MS, Sneige N. Can core needle biopsy replace fine needle aspiration cytology in the diagnosis of palpable breast carcinoma. A comparative study of 124 women. Cancer 1996;78:773–7.

40. de Almeida Barra A, Gobbi H, Alencar de L, et al. A comparison of aspiration cytology and core needle biopsy according to tumor size of suspicious breast lesions. Diagn Cytopathol 2008;36:26–31.

41. Cangiarella J, Waisman J, Simsir A. Cytologic findings with histologic correlation in 43 cases of mammary intraductal adenocarcinoma diagnosed by aspiration biopsy. Acta Cytol 2003;47:965–72.

42. Makunura CN, Curling OM, Yeomans P, et al. Apocrine adenosis within a radial scar: A case of false positive breast cytodiagnosis. Cytopathology 1994;5:123–8.

43. Masood S. Core needle biopsy versus fine needle aspiration biopsy: Are there similar sampling and diagnostic issues? Clinics in Lab Med 2005;25:679–88.

44. Hoda SA, Rosen PP. Observations on the pathologic diagnosis of selected unusual lesions in needle core biopsies of breast. The Breast J 2004;10:522–7.

45. Cariaggi MP, Bulgaresi P, Confortini M, et al. Analyses of the cause of false negative cytology reports on breast cancer fine needle aspirates. Cytopathol 1995;6:156–61

46. Lee CH, Philpotts LE, Horvath LJ, et al. Followup of breast lesions diagnosed as benign with stereotactic core needle biopsy: frequency of mammographic change and false negative rate. Radiology 1999;212:189–94.

47. Memarsadeghi M, Pfarl G, Riedl C, et al. Value of 14 gauge ultrasound-guided large-core needle biopsy of breast lesions: own results in comparison with the literature. Rofo 2003;175:374–80

48. Symmans WF, Weg N, Gross J, et al. A prospective comparison of stereotaxic fine-needle aspiration versus stereotaxic core needle biopsy for the diagnosis of mammographic abnormalities. Cancer 1999;85:1119–32.

49. Boerner S, Fornage BD, Singletary E, et al. Ultrasound-guided fine-needle aspiration (FNA) of nonpalpable breast lesions. A review of 1885 FNA cases using the National Cancer Institute-supported recommendations on the uniform approach to breast FNA. Cancer (Cancer Cytopathol) 1999;87:19–24.

50. Mitnick JS, Vazquez MF, Pressman PI, et al. Stereotactic fine-needle aspiration biopsy for the evaluation of nonpalpable breast lesions: report of an experience based on 2,988 cases. Ann Surg Oncol 1996;3:185–91.

51. Dahlstrom JE, Sutton S, Jain S. Histologic-radiologic correlation of mammographically detected microcalcification in stereotactic core biopsies. Am J Surg Pathol 1998;22:246–59.

52. Deb A, Mathews P, Elston CW, et al. An audit of 'equivocal' (C3) and 'suspicious' (C4) categories in fine needle aspiration cytology of the breast. Cytopathol 2001;12:219–26.

53. Sneige N, Fornage BD, Saleh G. Ultrasound-guided fine-needle aspiration of nonpalpable breast lesions. Cytologic and histologic findings. Am J Clin Pathol 1994;102:98–101.

54. Alkuwari E, Auger M. Accuracy of fine-needle aspiration cytology of axillary lymph nodes in breast cancer patients: a study of 115 cases with cytologic-histologic correlation. Cancer 2008;25(114):89–93.

55. Bassett LW, Mahoney MC, Apple SK. Interventional breast imaging: current procedures and assessing for

concordance with pathology. Radiol Clin of N Am 2007;45:881–94.

56. Salami N, Hirschowitz SL, Nieberg RK, et al. Triple test approach to inadequate fine needle aspiration biopsies of palpable breast lesions. Acta Cytol 1999;43:339–43.

57. Kaufman Z, Shpitz B, Shapiro M, et al. Triple approach in the diagnosis of dominant breast masses: combined physical examination, mammography, and fine-needle aspiration. J Surg Oncol 1994;56:254–7.

58. The National Cancer Institute, Bethesda subcommittee. The uniform approach to breast fine-needle aspiration biopsy. Diagn Cytopathol 1997;16:295–311.

59. Abati A. To count or not to count? Diagn Cytopathol 1999;21:142–7.

60. Snead DR, Vryenhoef P, Pinder SE, et al. Routine audit of breast fine needle aspiration (FNA) cytology specimens and aspirator inadequate rates. Cytopathology 1997;8:236–47.

61. The National Cancer Institute, Bethesda conference. The uniform approach to breast fine needle aspiration biopsy. A synopsis. Acta Cytol 1996;40:1120–6.

62. Wells CA. Quality assurance in breast cancer screening cytology: a review of the literature and a report on the U.K. national cytology scheme. Eur J Cancer 1995;2:273–80.

63. Hunt CM, Wilson S, Pinder SE, et al. United Kingdom national audit of breast fine needle aspiration cytology in 1990–91: organization and level of activity. Cytopathology 1996;7:316–25.

64. Abati A, Simsir A. Breast fine needle aspiration biopsy: Prevailing recommendations and contemporary practices. Clin Lab Med 2005:25;631–54.

65. Chen KT, Tschang TP. Pneumothorax: a complication of fine needle aspiration of breast tumors. Acta Cytol 1996;40:844–5.

66. Meyer JE, Smith DN, Lester SC, et al. Large core needle biopsy of nonpalpable breast lesions. JAMA 1999;281:1638–41.

67. Thurfjell MG, Jansson T, Nordgren H, et al. Local breast cancer recurrence caused by mammographically guided punctures. Acta Radiol 2000;48:435–40.

68. Hu XC, Chow LW. Fine needle aspiration may shed breast cells into peripheral blood as determined by RT-PCR. Oncology 2000;59:217–22.

69. Berg JW, Robbins GF. A late look at the safety of aspiration biopsy. Cancer 1962;15:826–7.

70. Lee KC, Chan JK, Ho LC. Histologic changes in the breast after fine-needle aspiration. Am J Surg Pathol 1994;18:1039–47.

71. Youngson BJ, Cranor M, Rosen PP. Epithelial displacement in surgical breast specimens following needling procedures. Am J Surg Pathol 1995;19:1092–4.

72. Diaz LK, Wiley EL, Venta LA. Are malignant cells displaced by large-gauge needle core biopsy of the breast? AJR Am J Roentgenol 1999;173:1303–13.

73. Stolier A, Skinner J, Levine EA. A prospective study of seeding of the skin after core biopsy of the breast. Am J Surg 2000;180:104–7.

74. Fornage BD, Sneige N, Singletary SE. Masses in breasts with implants: diagnosis with US-guide fine needle aspiration biopsy. Radiology 1994:191;339–42.

75. Kontzoglou K, Moulakakis K, Konofaos P, et al. The role of liquid-based cytology in the investigation of breast lesions using fine-needle aspiration: a cytohistopathological evaluation. J Surg Oncol 2005;89:75–8.

76. Sneige N, Tulbah A. Accuracy of cytologic diagnosis made from touch imprints of image-guided needle biopsy specimens of nonpalpable breast abnormalities. Diagn Cytopathol 2000;23:29–34.

77. Robinson IA, McKee G, Kissin MW. Typing and grading breast carcinoma on fine-needle aspiration: is it clinically useful information? Diagn Cytopathol 1995;13:260–5.

78. Zoppi JA, Pellicer EM, Sundblad AS. Cytohistologic correlation of nuclear grade in breast carcinoma. Acta Cytol 1997;41:701–4.

79. Khan MZ, Haleem A, Al Hassani H, et al. Cytopathological grading, as a predictor of histopathological grade, in ductal carcinoma (NOS) of breast, on air-dried Diff-Quik smears. Diagn Cytopathol 2003;29:185–93.

80. Ostrowski ML, Pindur J, Laucirica R, et al. Proliferative activity in invasive breast carcinoma: a comprehensive comparison of MIB-1 immunocytochemical staining in aspiration biopsies to image analytic, flow cytometric and histologic parameters. Acta Cytol 2001;45:965–72.

81. Nizzoli R, Bozzetti C, Naldi N. Comparison of the results of immunocytochemical assays for biologic variables on preoperative fine-needle aspirates and on surgical specimens of primary breast carcinomas. Cancer (Cancer Cytopathol) 2000; 90:61–6.

82. Sneige N. Utility of cytologic specimens in the evaluation of prognostic and predictive factors of breast cancer: current issues and future directions. Diagn Cytopathol 2004;30:158–65.

83. Billgren AM, Tani E, Liedberg A, et al. Prognostic significance of tumor cell proliferation analyzed in fine needle aspirates from primary breast cancer. Breast Cancer Res Treat 2002;71:161–70.

84. Tafjord S, Bohler PJ, Risberg B, et al. Estrogen and progesterone hormone receptor status in breast carcinoma: comparison of immunocytochemistry and immunohistochemistry. Diagn Cytopathol 2002;26:137–41.

85. Löfgren L, Skoog L, von Schoultz E, et al. Hormone receptor status in breast cancer – a comparison between surgical specimens and fine needle aspiration biopsies. Cytopathology 2003;14:136–42.

86. Howes GP, Stephenson J, Humphreys S. Sensitive and reliable PCR and sequencing used to detect p53 point mutations in fine needle aspirates of the breast. J Clin Pathol 1996;49:570–3.

87. Pustazi L, Ayers M, Stec J, et al. Gene expression profiles obtained from fine-needle aspirations of breast cancer reliably identify routine prognostic markers and reveal large-scale molecular differences between estrogen-negative and estrogen-positive tumors. Clin Cancer Res 2003;9:2406–15.

88. Rapkiewicz A, Espina V, Zujewski JA, et al. The needle in the haystack: application of breast fine-needle aspirate samples to quantitative protein microarray technology. Cancer 2007;111:173–84.

89. Rakha EA, Ellis IO. An overview of assessment of prognostic and predictive factors in breast cancer needle core biopsy specimens. J Clin Pathol 2007;60:1300–6.

90. Rody A, Karn T, Gatje R, et al. Gene expression profile of breast cancer obtained from core cut biopsies before neoadjuvant docetaxel, adriamycin, and cyclophosphamide chemotherapy correlate with routine prognostic markers and could be used to identify predictive signatures. Zentralbl Gynakol 2006;128:76–81.

91. Reis-Filho JS, Albergaria A, Milanezi F, et al. Naked nuclei revisited: p63 immunoexpression. Diagn Cytopathol 2002;27:135–8.

92. Carter N, Stephenson TJ, Silcocks PB, et al. Effects of hormone replacement therapy on fine needle aspiration cytology of the breast. Acta Cytol 1995;39:689–92.

93. Levine P, Cangiarella J. Cytomorphology of benign breast disease. Clin Lab Med 2005;25:689–712.

94. Gupta RK, McHutchison AG, Dowle CS, et al. Fine-needle aspiration cytodiagnosis of breast masses in pregnant and lactating women and its impact on management. Diagn Cytopathol 1993;9:156–9.

95. Mitre BK, Kanbour AI, Mauser N. Fine needle aspiration biopsy of breast

carcinoma in pregnancy and lactation. Acta Cytol 1997;41:1121–30.

96. Siddiqui MT, Zakowski MF, Ashfaq R, et al. Breast masses in males: multi-institutional experience on fine-needle aspiration. Diagn Cytopathol 2002;26:87–91.

97. Joshi A, Kapila K, Verma K. Fine needle aspiration cytology in the management of male breast masses; nineteen years of experience. Acta Cytol 1999:43:334–8.

98. MacIntosh RF, Merrimen JL, Barnes PJ. Application of the probabilistic approach to reporting breast fine needle aspiration in males. Acta Cytol 2008;52:530–4.

99. Hummel Levine P, Waisman J, Yang G, et al. Aspiration cytology of cystic carcinoma of the breast. Diagn Cytopathol 2003;28:39–44.

100. Dodd LG, Sneige N, Reece GP, et al. Fine-needle aspiration cytology of silicone granulomas in the augmented breast. Diagn Cytopathol 1993;9:498–502.

101. Silverman JF, Lannin DR, Unverferth M, et al. Fine needle aspiration cytology of subareolar abscess of the breast. Spectrum of cytomorphologic findings and potential diagnostic pitfalls. Acta Cytol 1986;30:413–9.

102. Gottschalk Sabag S, Glick T. The problematic interpretation of foamy cells in breast fine needle aspirates. A report of two cases. Acta Cytol 1997;41:561–4.

103. Schmidt WA, Boudousquie AC, Vetto JT, et al. Lymph nodes in the human female breast: a review of their detection and significance. Hum Pathol 2001;32:178–87.

104. Layfield LJ, Glasgow BJ, Hirschcowitz S, et al. Intramammary lymph nodes: cytologic findings and implications for fine-needle aspiration cytology diagnosis of breast nodules. Diagn Cytopathol 1997;17:223–9.

105. Das DK, Gupta SK, Mathews SV, et al. Fine needle aspiration cytologic diagnosis of axillary accessory breast tissue, including its physiologic changes and pathologic lesions. Acta Cytol 1994;38:130–5.

106. Krishnamurthy S. Current applications and future prospects of fine-needle aspiration biopsy of locoregional lymph nodes in the management of breast cancer. Cancer Cytopathol 2009;25(117):451–62.

107. Vargas J, Nevado M, Rodriguez Peralto JL, et al. Fine needle aspiration diagnosis of carcinoma arising in an ectopic breast. A case report. Acta Cytol 1995;39:941–4.

108. Saad RS, Silverman, JF, Julian T, et al. Atypical squamous metaplasia of seromas in breast needle aspirates from irradiated lumpectomy sites; a potential pitfall for false positive diagnosis of

carcinoma. Diagn Cytopathol 2002;26:104–8.

109. Kollur SM, El Hag IA. FNA of breast fibroadenoma: observer variability and review of cytomorphology with cytohistologic correlation. Cytopathology 2006;17:239–44.

110. López-Ferrer P, Jiménez-Hefferman JA, Vicandi B, et al. Fine needle aspiration cytology of breast fibroadenoma. A cytohistologic correlation study of 405 cases. Acta Cytol 1999;43:579–86.

111. Simsir A, Waisman J, Thorner K, et al. Mammary lesions diagnosed as 'papillary' by aspiration biopsy. 70 cases with follow up. Cancer (Cancer Cytopathol) 2003;99:156–65.

112. Al-Kaisi N. The spectrum of the 'gray zone' in breast cytology. A review of 186 cases of atypical and suspicious cytology. Acta Cytol 1994;38:898–908.

113. Benoit JL, Kara R, McGregor SE, et al. Fibroadenoma of the breast: diagnostic pitfalls of fine-needle aspiration. Diagn Cytopathol 1992;8:643–7.

114. Simsir A, Waisman J, Cangiarella J. Fibroadenomas with atypia: causes of under- and overdiagnosis by aspiration biopsy. Diagn Cytopathol 2001;25:278–84.

115. Rogers LA, Lee KR. Breast carcinoma simulating fibroadenoma or fibrocystic change by fine-needle aspiration. A study of 16 cases. Am J Clin Pathol 1992;98:155–60.

116. Ventura K, Lee I, Cangiarella J, et al. Aspiration biopsy of mammary lesions with abundant extracellular mucinous material: review of 43 cases with surgical followup. Am J Clin Pathol 2003;120:194–202.

117. Bhattari S, Kapila K, Verma K. Phyllodes tumor of the breast. A cytohistologic study of 80 cases. Acta Cytol 2000;44:790–6.

118. Jayaram G, Sthaneshwar P. Fine-needle aspiration cytology of phyllodes tumors. Diagn Cytopathol 2002;26:222–7.

119. Krishnamurthy S, Ashfaq R, Shin HJC, et al. Distinction of phyllodes tumor from fibroadenoma. A reappraisal of an old problem. Cancer (Cancer Cytopathol) 2000;90:342–9.

120. Scolyer RA, McKEnzie PR, Achmed D, et al. Can Phyllodes tumors of the breast be distinguished from fibroadenomas using fine needle aspiration cytology? Pathology 2001;33:437–43.

121. Tse GM, Ma TK, Pang LM, et al. Fine needle aspiration cytologic features of mammary phyllodes tumors. Acta Cytol 2002;46:855–63.

122. Foxcroft LM, Evans EB, Porter AJ. Difficulties in the preoperative diagnosis of phyllodes tumors of the breast: a study of 84 cases. Breast 2007;16(1):27–37.

123. Lee AH, Hodi Z, Ellis IO, et al. Histologic features useful in the distinction of phyllodes tumour and fibroadenoma on needle core biopsy of the breast. Histopathology 2007;51:336–44.

124. Dillon MF, Quinn CM, McDermott EW, et al. Needle core biopsy in the diagnosis of phyllodes neoplasm. Surgery 2006:140:779–84.

125. Hamperl H. The myoepithelia (myoepithelial cells): Normal state; regressive changes; hyperplasia; tumors. Curr Top Pathol 1970;53:161–220.

126. Mercado CL, Toth HK, Axelrod D, et al. Fine-needle aspiration biopsy of benign adenomyoepithelioma of the breast: radiologic and pathologic correlation in four cases. Diagn Cytopathol 2007;35:690–4.

127. Mathur SR, Karak K, Verma K. Adenomyoepithelioma of the breast: a potential diagnostic pitfall on fine needle aspiration cytology. Indian J Pathol Microbiol 2004;47:243–5.

128. Ng W-K. Adenomyoepithelioma of the breast. A review of three cases with reappraisal of the fine needle aspiration biopsy findings. Acta Cytol 2002;46:317–24.

129. Valente PT, Stuckey JH. Fine-needle aspiration cytology of mammary adenomyoepithelioma: report of a case with intranuclear cytoplasmic inclusions. Diagn Cytopathol 1994;10:165–8.

130. Chang A, Bassett L, Bose S. Adenomyoepithelioma of the breast: a cytologic dilemma. Report of a case and review of the literature. Diagn Cytopathol 2002;26:191–6.

131. Doyle AJ, Alder SL, Rohr LR. Myoepithelial lesions of the breast: imaging characteristics and diagnosis with large core needle biopsy in two cases. Radiology 1994;193:787–8

132. Thomas PA, Raab SS, Cohen MB. Is the fine-needle aspiration biopsy diagnosis of proliferative breast lesions possible? Diagn Cytopathol 1994;11:301–6.

133. Sidaway MK, Stoler MH, Frable WJ, et al. Interobserver variability in the classification of proliferative breast lesions by fine-needle aspiration: results of the Papanicolaou Society of Cytopathology study. Diagn Cytopathol 1998;18:150–65.

134. Frost AR, Aksu A, Kurstin R, et al. Can nonproliferative breast disease and proliferative breast disease without atypia be distinguished by fine-needle aspiration cytology? Cancer 1997;81:22–8.

135. Sidaway MK, Tabbara SO, Bryan JA, et al. The spectrum of cytologic features in nonproliferative breast lesions. Cancer (Cancer Cytopathol) 2001;93:140–5.

136. Dawson AE, Mulford DK, Sheils LA. The cytopathology of proliferative breast disease. Comparison with

features of ductal carcinoma in situ. Am J Clin Pathol 1995;103:438–42.

137. Thomas PA, Cangiarella J, Raab SS, et al. Fine needle aspiration biopsy of proliferative breast disease. Mod Pathol 1995;8:130–6.

138. Sneige N, Staerkel GA. Fine-needle aspiration cytology of ductal hyperplasia with and without atypia and ductal carcinoma in situ. Human Pathol 1994;25:485–92.

139. Sauer T, Lomo J, Garred O, et al. Cytologic features of ductal carcinoma in situ in fine-needle aspiration of the breast mirror the histopathologic growth pattern heterogeneity and grading. Cancer 2005;105:21–7.

140. Liberman L, Smolkin JH, Dershaw DD, et al. Calcification retrieval at stereotactic, 11-gauge, directional, vacuum-assisted breast biopsy. Radiology 1998;208:251–60.

141. Plantade R, Hammou JC, Fighiera M, et al. Underestimation of breast carcinoma with 11-gauge stereotactically guided directional vacuum-assisted biopsy. J Radiol 2004;85:391–40.

142. Kaufman D, Sanchez M, Mizrachy B, et al. Cytologic findings of atypical adenosis of the breast. A case report. Acta Cytol 2002;46:369–72.

143. Schnitt SJ, Vincent-Salomon A. Columnar cell lesions of the breast. Adv Anat Pathol 2003;10:113–24.

144. Saqi A, Mazziotta R, Hamela-bena D. Columnar Cell lesions: Fine needle aspiration biopsy features. Diagn Cytopathol 2004;31:370–5.

145. Jensen KC, Kong CS. Cytologic diagnosis of columnar-cell lesions of the breast. Diagn Cytopathol 2007;35:73–9.

146. Michael CW, Buschman B. Can true papillary neoplasms of breast and their mimickers be accurately classified by cytology? Cancer (Cancer Cytopathol) 2002;96:92–100.

147. Tse GM, Ma TK, Lui PC, et al. Fine needle aspiration cytology of papillary lesions of the breast: how accurate is the diagnosis? J Clin Pathol 2008;61:945–9.

148. Ueng SH, Mezzetti T, Tavassoli FA. Papillary neoplasms of the breast: a review. Arch Pathol Lab Med 2009;133:893–907.

149. Greenberg ML, Middleton PD, Bilous AM. Infarcted intraduct papilloma diagnosed by fine-needle biopsy. A cytologic, clinical and mammographic pitfall. Diagn Cytopathol 1994;11:188–94.

150. Greenberg ML, Camaris C, Psarianos T, et al. Is there a role of fine-needle aspiration in radial scar/complex sclerosing lesions of the breast? Diagn Cytopathol 1997;16:537–42

151. Bonzanini M, Gilioli E, Brancato B, et al. Cytopathol features of 22 radial scar/complex sclerosing lesions of the

breast, three of which associated with carcinoma: clinical, mammographic and histologic correlation. Diagn Cytopathol 1997;17:353–62.

152. Orell SR. Radial scar/complex sclerosing lesion – a problem in the diagnostic work-up of screen-detected breast lesions. Cytopathology 1999;10:250–8.

153. Lopez-Medina A, Cintora E, Mugica B, et al. Radial scars diagnosed at stereotactic core-needle biopsy: surgical biopsy findings. Eur Radiol 2006;16:1803–10.

154. Cho EY, Oh YL. Fine needle aspiration cytology of sclerosing adenosis of the breast. Acta Cytol 2001;45:353–9.

155. Highland KE, Finley JL, Neill JS, et al. Collagenous spherulosis. Report of a case with diagnosis by fine needle aspiration biopsy with immunocytochemical and ultrastructural observations. Acta Cytol 1993;37:3–9.

156. Perez JS, Perez-Guillermo M, Bernal AB, et al. Diagnosis of collagenous spherulosis of the breast by fine needle aspiration cytology. A report of two cases. Acta Cytol 1993;37:725–8.

157. Jain S, Gupta S, Kumar N, et al. Extracellular hyaline material in association with other cytologic features in aspirates from collagenous spherulosis and adenoid cystic carcinoma of the breast. Acta Cytol 2003;47(3):381–6

158. Chhieng DC, Cangiarella JF, Waisman J, et al. Fine-needle aspiration cytology of spindle cell lesions of the breast. Cancer (Cancer Cytopathol) 1999;87:359–71.

159. El Aouni N, Laurent I, Terrier P, et al. Granular cell tumor of the breast. Diagn Cytopathol 2007;35:725–7.

160. Pieterse AS, Mahar A, Orell S. Granular cell tumour – a pitfall in FNA cytology of breast lesions. Pathology 2004;36:58–62.

161. Sirgi KE, Sneige N, Fanning TV, et al. Fine-needle aspirates of granular cell lesions of the breast: report of three cases, with emphasis on differential diagnosis and utility of immunostaining for CD68 (KP1). Diagn Cytopathol 1996;15:403–8.

162. Lew WY. Spindle cell lipoma of the breast: a case report and literature review. Diagn Cytopathol 1993;9:434–7.

163. Gupta RK, Naran S, Lallu S, et al. Fine-needle aspiration cytology in neurilemoma (schwannoma) of the breast: report of two cases in a man and a woman. Diagn Cytopathol 2001;24:76–7.

164. Gobbi H, Tse G, Page DL, et al. Reactive spindle cell nodules of the breast after core biopsy or fine-needle aspiration. Am J Clin Pathol 2000;113:288–94.

165. Odashiro AN, Odashiro Miiji LN, Odashiro DN, et al. Mammary

myofibroblastoma: report of two cases with fine-needle aspiration cytology and review of the cytology literature. Diagn Cytopathol 2004;30:406–10.

166. Dey P, Luthra UK. False negative cytologic diagnosis of breast carcinoma. Acta Cytol 1999;43:801–5.

167. Fiorella RM, Kragel PJ, Shariff A, et al. Fine-needle aspiration of well differentiated small-cell duct carcinoma of the breast. Diagn Cytopathol 1997;16:226–9.

168. Bondeson L, Lindholm K. Aspiration cytology of tubular breast carcinoma. Acta Cytol 1990;34:5–20.

169. Hoda S, Rosen PP. Practical considerations in the pathologic diagnosis of needle core biopsies of breast. Am J Clin Pathol 2002;118:101–8.

170. Malamud YR, Ducatman BS, Wang HH. Comparative features of comedo and noncomedo ductal carcinoma in situ of the breast on fine-needle aspiration biopsy. Diagn Cytopathol 1992;8:571–6.

171. Venegas R, Rutgers JL, Cameron BL, et al. Fine needle aspiration cytology of breast ductal carcinoma in situ. Acta Cytol 1994;38:136–43.

172. Theocharous C, Greenberg ML. Cytologic features of ductal carcinoma in situ. Diagn Cytopathol 1996;15:367–73.

173. Bonzanini M, Gilioli E, Brancato A, et al. The cytopathology of ductal carcinoma in situ of the breast. A detailed analysis of fine needle aspiration cytology of 58 cases compared with 101 invasive ductal carcinomas. Cytopathol 2001;12:107–19.

174. Bardales RH, Suhrland MJ, Stanley MW. Papillary neoplasms of the breast: fine-needle aspiration findings in cystic and solid cases. Diagn Cytopathol 1994;10:336–41.

175. Bondeson L, Lindholm K. Prediction of invasiveness by aspiration cytology applied to nonpalpable breast carcinoma and tested in 300 cases. Diagn Cytopathol 1997;17:315–20.

176. Maygarden SJ, Brock MS, Novotny DB. Are epithelial cells in fat or connective tissue a reliable indicator of tumor invasion in fine-needle aspiration of the breast? Diagn Cytopathol 1997;16:137–42.

177. Shin HJC, Sneige N. Is a diagnosis of infiltrating versus in situ ductal carcinoma of the breast possible in fine-needle aspiration specimens? Cancer (Cancer Cytopathol) 1998;84:186–91.

178. McKee GT, Tambouret RH, Finkelstein D. Fine-needle aspiration cytology of the breast: invasive vs. in situ carcinoma. Diagn Cytopathol 2001;25:73–7.

179. Klijanienko J, Katsahian S, Vielh P, et al. Stromal infiltration as a predictor of

tumor invasion in breast fine needle aspiration biopsy. Diagn Cytopathol 2004;30:182–6.

180. Istvanic S, Fischer AH, Banner BF, et al. Cell blocks of breast FNAs frequently allow diagnosis of invasion or histological classification of proliferative changes. Diagn Cytopath 2007;35:263–9.

181. Lamb J, Anderson TJ. Influence of cancer histology on the success of fine needle aspiration of the breast. J Clin Pathol 1989;42:733–5.

182. Dawson AE, Logan-Young W, Mulford DK. Aspiration cytology of tubular carcinoma. Diagnostic features with mammographic correlation. Am J Clin Pathol 1994;101:488–92.

183. Dei Tos AP, Dellaguistina D, De Martin V, et al. Aspiration biopsy cytology of tubular carcinoma of the breast. Diagn Cytopathol 1994;11:146–50.

184. Fischler DF, Sneige N, Ordonez NG, et al. Tubular carcinoma of the breast: cytologic features in fine-needle aspiration and application of monoclonal anti-alpha-smooth muscle actin in diagnosis. Diagn Cytopathol 1994;10:120–5.

185. Cangiarella J, Waisman J, Shapiro RL, et al. Cytologic features of tubular adenocarcinoma of the breast by aspiration biopsy. Diagn Cytopathol 2001;25:311–5.

186. Novak JA, Masood S. Nuclear grooves in fine-needle aspiration biopsies of breast lesions: do they have any significance? Diagn Cytopathol 1998;18:333–7.

187. Javid SH, Smith BL, Mayer E, et al. Tubular carcinoma of the breast: results of a large contemporary series. Am J Surg 2009;197:674–7.

188. Dawson AE, Mulford DK. Fine needle aspiration of mucinous (colloid) breast carcinoma. Nuclear grading and mammographic and cytologic findings. Acta Cytol 1998;42:668–72.

189. Sohn JH, Kim LS, Chae SW, et al. Fine needle aspiration cytologic findings of breast mucinous neoplasms: differential diagnosis between mucocele-like tumour and mucinous carcinoma. Acta Cytol 2001;45:723–9.

190. Jayaram G, Swain M, Chew MT, et al. Cytology of mucinous carcinoma of breast: a report of 28 cases with histological correlation. Malays J Pathol 2000;22:65–71.

191. Stanley MW, Tani EM, Skoog L. Mucinous breast carcinoma and mixed mucinous-infiltrating ductal carcinoma: a comparative cytologic study. Diagn Cytopathol 1989;5:134–8.

192. Wang J, Simsir A, Mercado C, et al. Can core biopsy reliably diagnose mucinous lesions of the breast? Am J Clin Pathol 2007;127:124–7.

193. Yeoh GPS, Cheung PSY, Chan KW. Fine-needle aspiration cytology of mucocelelike tumors of the breast. Am J Surg Pathol 1999;23:552–9.

194. Wong NL, Wan SK. Comparative cytology of mucocele-like lesion and mucinous carcinoma of the breast in fine needle aspiration. Acta Cytol 2000;44:765–70.

195. Molyneux AJ, Coghill SB. Cell lysis due to ultrasound gel in fine needle aspirates; an important new artefact in cytology. Cytopathology 1994;5:41–5.

196. Racz MM, Pommier RF, Troxell ML. Fine-needle aspiration cytology of medulllary breast carcinoma: report of two cases and review of the literature with emphasis on differential diagnosis. Diagn Cytopath 2007;35:313–8.

197. Samarasinghe D, Frost F, Sterrett G, et al. Cytological diagnosis of Paget's disease of the nipple by scrape smears: a report of five cases. Diagn Cytopathol 1993;9:291–5.

198. Gupta RK, Simpson J, Dowle C. The role of cytology in the diagnosis of Paget's disease of the nipple. Pathology 1996;28:248–50.

199. Greeley CF, Frost AR. Cytologic features of ductal and lobular carcinoma in fine needle aspirates of the breast. Acta Cytol 1997;41:333–40.

200. Joshi A, Kumar N, Verma K. Diagnostic challenge of lobular carcinoma on aspiration cytology. Diagn Cytopathol 1998;18:179–83.

201. Jayaram G, Swain M, Chew MT, et al. Cytologic appearances in invasive lobular carcinoma of the breast. A study of 21 cases. Acta Cytol 2000;44:169–74.

202. Menet E, Becette V, Briffod M. Cytologic diagnosis of lobular carcinoma of the breast. Experience with 55 patients in the Rene Huguenin Cancer Center. Cancer (Cancer cytopathol) 2008; 114:111–7.

203. Hwang S, Ioffe O, Lee I, et al. Cytologic diagnosis of invasive lobular carcinoma: factors associated with negative and equivocal diagnoses. Diagn Cytopathol 2004;31:87–93.

204. Sethi S, Cajulis RS, Gokaslan ST, et al. Diagnostic significance of signet ring cells in fine-needle aspirates of the breast. Diagn Cytopathol 1997;16:117–21.

205. Auger M, Huttner I. Fine-needle aspiration cytology of pleomorphic lobular carcinoma of the breast. Comparison with the classic type. Cancer 1997;81:29–32.

206. Abdulla M, Hombal S, Al-Juwaiser A, et al. Cytomorphologic features of classic and variant lobular carcinoma: a comparative study. Diagn Cytopathol 2000;22:370–5.

207. de las Morenas A, Crespo P, Moroz K, et al. Cytologic diagnosis of ductal versus lobular carcinoma of the breast. Acta Cytol 1995;39:865–9.

208. Kelten C, Akbulut M, Zekioglu O, et al. Signet ring cells in fine needle aspiration cytology of breast carcinomas: review of the cytological findings in ten cases identified by histology. Cytopathology 2009;20: 321–7.

209. Üstün M, Berner A, Davidson B, et al. Fine-needle aspiration cytology of lobular carcinoma in situ. Diagn Cytopathol 2002;27:22–6.

210. Salhany KE, Page DL. Fine-needle aspiration of mammary lobular carcinoma in situ and atypical lobular hyperplasia. Am J Clin Pathol 1989;92:22–6.

211. Ayata G, Wang HH. Fine needle aspiration cytology of lobular carcinoma in situ on thinprep. Diagn Cytopathol 2005;32:276–80.

212. Levine P, Simsir A, Cangiarella J. Management issues in breast lesions diagnosed by fine-needle aspiration and percutaneous core breast biopsy. Am J Clin Pathol 2006;125:S124-34.

213. Gorczyka W, Olszewski W, Tuziak T, et al. Fine needle aspiration cytology of rare malignant tumors of the breast. Acta Cytol 1992;36:918–26.

214. Sneige N, Holder PD, Katz RL, et al. Fine-needle aspiration cytology of the male breast in a cancer center. Diagn Cytopathol 1993;9:691–7.

215. Slavin JL, Baird I. Fine needle aspiration cytology in male breast carcinoma. Pathology 1996;28:122–4.

216. Westenend PJ, Jobse C. Evaluation of fine-needle aspiration cytology of breast masses in males. Cancer (Cancer Cytopathol) 2002;96:101–4.

217. Dodd LG, Layfield LJ. Fine-needle aspiration of inflammatory carcinoma of the breast. Diagn Cytopathol 1996;15:363–6.

218. Meloni GB, Dessole S, Becchere MP, et al. Effectiveness of core biopsy by the mammotome device for diagnosis of inflammatory carcinoma. Clin Exp Obstet Gynecol 1999;26;181–2.

219. Johnson TL, Kini SR. The significance of atypical apocrine cells in fine-needle aspirates of the breast. Diagn Cytopathol 1989;5:248–54.

220. Jayaram G, Yaccob RB, Yip CH. Apocrine carcinoma of the breast diagnosed on fine needle aspiration cytology. Acta Cytol 2007;51:664–7.

221. Ng W-K, Poon CSP, Kong JHB. Fine needle aspiration cytology of ductal breast carcinoma with neuroendocrine differentiation. Review of eight cases with histologic correlation. Acta Cytol 2002;46:325–31.

222. Burgan AR, Frierson Jr HF, Fechner RE. Fine-needle aspiration cytology of spindle-cell argyrophilic mucin-producing carcinoma of the breast. Diagn Cytopathol 1996;14:238–42.

223. Wee A, Nilsson B, Chong SM, et al. Bilateral carcinoid tumor of the breast.

Report of a case with diagnosis by fine needle aspiration cytology. Acta Cytol 1992;36:55–9.

224. Ni K, Bibbo M. Fine needle aspiration of mammary carcinoma with features of a carcinoid tumor. A case report with immunohistochemical and ultrastructural studies. Acta Cytol 1994;38:73–8.

225. Cai G, Simsir A, Cangiarella J. Invasive mammary carcinoma with osteoclastic-like giant cells diagnosed by fine-needle aspiration biopsy: review of the cytologic literature and distinction from other mammary lesions containing giant cells. Diagn Cytopathol 2004;30:396–400.

226. Lui PCW, Lau PPL, Tse GMK, et al. Fine needle aspiration cytology of invasive micropapillary carcinoma of the breast. Pathology 2007;39:401–5.

227. Kelten EC, Akbulut M, Duzcan SE. Diagnostic dilemma in cytologic features of micropapillary carcinoma of the breast: a report of 2 cases. Acta Cytol 2009;53:463–6.

228. Akbulut M, Zekioglu O, Kapkac M, et al. Fine needle aspiration cytology of glycogen-rich clear cell carcinoma of the breast: review of 37 cases with histologic correlation. Acta Cytol 2008;52:65–71.

229. Catalina-Fernandez I, Saenz-Santamaria J. Lipid-rich carcinoma of the breast: a case report with fine-needle aspiration cytology. Diagn Cytopathol 2009;37:935–6.

230. Gupta RK, Kenwright D, Naran S, et al. Fine needle aspiration cytodiagnosis of secretory carcinoma of the breast. Cytopathol 2000;11:496–502.

231. Khalbuss WE. Cytomorphology of rare malignant tumors of the breast. Clin Lab Med 2005;25:761–75.

232. Ng WK, Yip WW. Fine needle aspiration cytology findings of cystic hypersecretory ductal carcinoma of the breast: a reappraisal. Acta Cytol 2003;47:513–5.

233. McCluggage WG, McManus DI, Caughley LM. Fine needle aspiration (FNA) cytology of adenoid cystic carcinoma and adenomyoepithelioma of breast: two lesions rich in myoepithelial cells. Cytopathology 1997;8:31–9.

234. Saqi A, Mercado CL, Hamele-Bena D. Adenoid cystic carcinoma of the breast diagnosed by fine-needle aspiration. Diagn Cytopathol 2004;30:271–4.

235. Gupta RK. Cytodiagnostic patterns of metaplastic breast carcinoma in aspiration samples: a study of 14 cases. Diagn Cytopathol 1999;20:10–2.

236. Lui PCW, Tse GM, Tan PH, et al. Fine-needle aspiration cytology of metaplastic carcinoma of the breast. J Clin Pathol 2007;60:529–33.

237. Shizawa S, Sasano H, Suzuki T, et al. Low-grade adenosquamous carcinoma of the breast: a case report with cytologic findings and review of the literature. Pathol Int 1997;47:624–267.

238. Ferrara G, Nappi O, Wick MR. Fine-needle aspiration cytology and immunohistology of low-grade adenosquamous carcinoma of the breast. Diagn Cytopathol 1999;20:13–8.

239. Annam V, Giriyan SS, Kulkarni MH. Diagnosis of pure squamous cell carcinoma of the breast by fine needle aspiration cytology. Acta Cytol 2009;53:722–3.

240. Motoyama T, Watanabe H. Extremely well differentiated squamous cell carcinoma of the breast. Report of a case with a comparative study of an epidermal cyst. Acta Cytol 1996;40:729–33.

241. Shukla R, Pooja B, Radhika S, et al. Fine-needle aspiration cytology of extramammary neoplasms metastatic to the breast. Diagn Cytopathol 2005;32:193–7.

242. David O, Gattuso P, Razan W, et al. Unusual cases of metastases to the breast. A report of 17 cases diagnosed by fine needle aspiration. Acta Cytol 2002;46:377–85.

243. Levine PH, Zamuco R, Yee HT. Role of fine-needle aspiration cytology in breast lymphoma. Diagn Cytopathol 2004;30:332–40.

244. Foust RL, Berry AD, Moinuddin SM. Fine needle aspiration cytology of liposarcoma of the breast. A case report. Acta Cytol 1994;38:957–60.

245. Carson KF, Hirschowitz SL, Nieberg RK, et al. Pitfalls in the cytologic diagnosis of angiosarcoma of the breast by fine-needle aspiration: a case report. Diagn Cytopathol 1994;11:297–9.

246. Pai MR, Upadhyaya K, Naik R, et al. Bilateral angiosarcoma breast diagnosed by fine-needle aspiration cytology Indian J Pathol Microbiol 2008;51:421–3

247. Tartter PI , Kaplan J, Bleiweiss I, et al. Lumpectomy margins, reexecision and local recurrence of breast cancer. Am J Surg 2000;179;81–5.

248. Orell SR, Miliauskas J. Fine needle biopsy cytology of breast lesions. A review of interpretative difficulties. Adv Anat Pathol 2005;12:233–45.

CHAPTER 8

Lung, chest wall and pleura

Amanda Segal, Felicity A Frost and Jan F Silverman

CLINICAL ASPECTS

Lung

Although sporadic reports of the diagnosis of lung carcinoma by fine needle aspiration cytology (FNAC) appeared as early as 1886,[1] the impetus for widespread use of the technique only arose with the development of image intensifiers and television viewing, allowing localization of small parenchymal lesions.[2] Recognition of the high accuracy rate of fine needle biopsy (FNB)[2] and simpler methods to treat pneumothorax combined to bring this diagnostic tool within the reach of most hospital radiologists and pathologists. Infections and some diffuse benign processes may be proven by FNAC, but the main indication remains the diagnosis of localized intrathoracic lesions suspected of being malignant, particularly when less invasive investigations prove to be negative.[3]

The role of FNB has shifted from the diagnosis of malignancy in inoperable patients and the confirmation of metastases, to its use as a first-line diagnostic procedure on which management decisions are based,[4,5] with a shift away from non-invasive methods such as sputum cytology towards FNAC.[6,7] All intrathoracic sites, including mediastinum and deep hilar lung lesions are safely sampled using fine (less than 20 gauge) needles with CT[8] and ultrasound guidance.[9] Lung function and radiological studies can help predict the risk of pneumothorax.[10–12] Transbronchial or transtracheal FNB[13–19] permits sampling of submucosal masses such as carcinoid tumors[20] and mediastinal lesions, enhances the role of FNAC in the staging of lung cancers[13,15,16,21] and may be used for the diagnosis of pulmonary infection[22] and cysts.[23] The more recent addition of ultrasound guided transbronchial and transoesophageal FNB has improved accuracy of targeting perihilar submucosal and mediastinal masses.[24] The presence of the pathologist at the time of the procedure leads to a reduction in the number of needle passes, may decrease the pneumothorax rate,[25] and increase overall sensitivity and accuracy of tumor typing.[15,26] FNAC in immunocompromised individuals has gained greater acceptance, especially for the diagnosis of infectious diseases.[27,28] An important role has also been found in paediatric practice[8] (see Chapter 17). With greater expectations by clinicians regarding tumor typing, demonstration of high rates of cytohistological correlation for the common types of tumors has been achieved.[29–32]

The diagnostic utility of FNB for difficult diagnostic lesions (e.g. neuroendocrine and pleural tumors)[33–44] is now widely accepted, particularly when allied with cell block preparations,[31] and the use of ancillary studies.[45–47] The range of cytological findings in less common tumors such as sarcomas,[48,49] lymphoid lesions[50,51] and metastatic tumors,[52] as well as in second primary tumors,[52,53] along with the most likely mimics of malignancy, have been well described.[54–57] The more recent requirements for molecular assessment of gene mutations relevant to targeted therapy in some lung cancers can be readily achieved by FNB with adequate cell block preparations.[58]

The place of FNAC in the investigative sequence

Fine needle aspiration cytology complements other diagnostic methods.[3] It is often the first choice in lesions which are located in the mediastinum, pulmonary apex, medial upper lobe or peripheral lung. Fiberoptic bronchoscopy (FOB) with brushings and biopsy is usually effective in diagnosing centrally placed pulmonary lesions, while FNB has particular value in those cases in which FOB is non-diagnostic.[3]

Endoscopic bronchial ultrasound (EBUS) localisation with FNB is now playing an increasing role in the sampling of central lesions, staging of lung carcinoma and the diagnosis of sarcoid and lymphoma.[59–63]

There is value in rendering a preoperative diagnosis, as thoracotomy is generally contraindicated for small cell carcinoma, most lymphomas, most metastatic tumors and most infections. A specific diagnosis of benign lesions such as tuberculosis or pulmonary hamartoma helps avoid unnecessary surgical intervention.[64] Additionally, a diagnosis of malignancy in patients at high operative risk allows surgeons to operate without fear that surgery may be unnecessary. FNAC is a cost-effective diagnostic method that can lead to shorter hospitalization, and a reduction in the number of diagnostic thoracotomies.[65]

FNB may be the only way of providing a diagnosis in inoperable patients. An unequivocal diagnosis of carcinoma and distinction between squamous cell carcinoma, small cell carcinoma and adenocarcinoma provides the clinician with sufficient information to select appropriate therapy. Raab et al. reported that FNB coupled with immunohistochemistry is both sensitive and cost effective for subclassifying malignancies in patients with a prior history of extrapulmonary cancers, when compared to bronchoscopy and thoracoscopy.[66] FNB can occasionally be useful intraoperatively in place of frozen section when the use of incisional or large needle biopsy is contraindicated.[67]

Accuracy of diagnosis

The sensitivity of FNB in the diagnosis of malignant pulmonary neoplasms varies according to both the size and the site of the mass,[68] as well as the experience of the radiologist[69] and the pathologist. In experienced hands it now reaches over 90% in both non-academic and academic centers.[70,71] A non-specific negative result on FNB does not exclude malignancy.[3,72] Therefore, repeat aspiration, careful clinical follow-up or additional diagnostic procedures may be necessary for definitive diagnosis. The rate of false-positive diagnoses is usually less than 0.5%.[71] The few false-positive diagnoses of malignancy are often due to reactive bronchiolar epithelial proliferation,[73] squamous metaplasia,[74] reactive mesothelial cell proliferation,[29] or associated with lesions such as tuberculosis, chondroid hamartomas,[75] granulomatous processes,[73] other infections,[76] or pulmonary infarcts. Occasionally, in samples obtained by EBUS, it can be difficult to determine whether the sample is derived from a central lung lesion or nodal deposit, a potential cause of false-positive diagnosis of nodal metastases. Tao advises caution in assuming that a lack of clinical or histological correlation is a result of false-positive cytological diagnosis.[77] He introduced the term 'false false positives' for cases where longer clinical follow-up period or closer histological examination confirms the cytological diagnosis. Well-differentiated adenocarcinomas with minimal cytological atypia and small tumors within larger areas of radiological opacity are prone to this error.

Experienced cytopathologists can reliably identify the histological type in up to 90% of primary lung tumors[29,31,32,70,78,79] and approximately 80% of their predictions of tumor type are correct;[2,30,70] these rates are similar to those achieved with bronchial biopsy.[31,80,81] High levels of cytohistological correlation relate to the combined use of smears and cell blocks, which allow better assessment of tissue architecture.[31] Rapid assessment of aspirated material in the radiology theater enhances accuracy of diagnosis by allowing appropriate triage of material for ancillary techniques. Most cases of small cell carcinoma,[30,35,79,82,83] well-differentiated adenocarcinoma,[84-87] and squamous cell carcinoma[88] are usually identifiable. However, poorly differentiated tumors of glandular or squamous origin and large cell carcinoma are more difficult to separate.[88] More studies of the range of cytological findings in neuroendocrine carcinomas, particularly large cell neuroendocrine tumors, are needed.[36-38] These may be difficult to distinguish from small cell carcinomas or other large cell carcinomas, although in the view of some authorities this distinction may be artificial or arbitrary at times.[89] Pulmonary hamartomas[64,75,90-94] can be accurately diagnosed in the majority of cases. Other benign neoplasms are difficult

to type because their cohesiveness prevents aspiration of adequate diagnostic material. Thin core needle biopsy may add to diagnostic accuracy.[95-97] Radiologists are increasingly prepared to perform core biopsies on intraparenchymal lesions[96,97] and this can be useful in some settings, especially where there are unusual features by FNAC. It is worth noting that a core biopsy will not necessarily provide a diagnosis where FNB has failed, particularly if the FNB sample is extensively necrotic. Cytological evidence of infection including tuberculosis may be gained in up to 80% of cases.[98-103] FNB can be used with a high degree of accuracy to diagnose bacterial, fungal or pneumocystis infection in immunosuppressed patients.[104]

Complications

Fatalities have occurred with 20-gauge or larger needles or in patients who are terminally ill or those with severe underlying pulmonary disease or infection.[105] The most common cause of death is hemorrhage, although there are rare cases of air embolism, tension pneumothorax and cardiac tamponade.[106-110] To our knowledge, no deaths have occurred in our experience of over 5000 cases.

The rate of pneumothorax varies from 6% to 57% and 1.5–20% require intercostal catheterization.[105,111] Emphysema, deeply situated lesions, multiple punctures, older patients and inexperienced operators all contribute to a higher rate of pneumothorax.[10,11,106] Examination of aspirated material in the radiology theater and the use of coaxial needles allows the total number of needle passes to be reduced, thereby reducing the rate of pneumothorax.[25] A small hemorrhage into the surrounding lung occurs in up to 10% of cases without clinical complications. Examples of neoplastic implantation along a thoracic needle track have been reported,[112-115] and one case of skin implantation with fungal organisms.[116] Bacteremia may occasionally be induced.[117]

Contraindications

Patients who do not have a cough reflex, who are unconscious or who cough intractably should not be biopsied. Arteriovenous malformation or aneurysm is usually excluded before attempting FNB, but the risk of bleeding from large hilar vessels is minimal when fine needles are used. There is an increased risk of bleeding in patients with pulmonary hypertension or bleeding disorders and in those undergoing anticoagulant therapy. These patients should be biopsied only in exceptional circumstances, for example in immunosuppressed patients where a positive diagnosis of an infection may lead to curative therapy.[104,118] Most authors do not recommend FNB of suspected hydatid cysts due to the possibility of an anaphylactic reaction to leaking cyst fluid or implantation of germinal epithelium. However, when aspiration of unsuspected cysts occurs, complications are very few.[119,120] Concurrent bilateral biopsies are not recommended.

Technical considerations

Obtaining material

Most radiologists use needles of less than 20 gauge, with a stylet to minimize contamination with tissue from the needle track. Needles of 22–23 gauge provide satisfactory material for cell blocks. Finer needles lessen tissue damage, although their flexibility may reduce the chance of successful puncture in deep lesions. Automated core biopsies are safe for pleural-based or chest wall lesions,[121] and their use in parenchymal lesions is increasing.[96,97]

The puncture site is marked on the skin and local anesthetic introduced down to the pleura. A guide needle makes aiming of the aspiration needles easier, reduces the risk of bending of flexible needles and prevents contamination of the aspirate with chest wall tissues.[122] Non-aspiration techniques often yield adequate material and may be particularly useful in hemorrhagic lesions (e.g. metastatic renal cell carcinoma).[123,124]

CT guidance is generally used although ultrasound may be useful for apical, pleural or chest wall tumors.[125–129] The use of coaxial needles means that repeated re-insertion of the needle is not necessary. Some lesions have distinctive characteristics when aspirated, e.g. pulmonary hamartomas have a rubbery resistance and a tendency to 'move away' from the needle; aspiration of neural tumors may cause intense pain. Adequacy of the aspirated material should be assessed in the radiology theater after rapid staining. The presence of the pathologist at the aspiration optimizes appropriate triage of material. Preliminary assessment in the radiology suite may also identify an unusual lesion where a core sample may be helpful. If the material is heavily bloodstained, collection onto a slide or watch glass (see Chapter 2) enables small clumps of tumor to be recognized as bright translucent fragments against the red background. To reduce blood contamination, these aggregates are selected and smeared onto a separate slide. Carnoys' fixative or acid alcohol are useful for lysing blood. Material is taken for ancillary studies such as flow cytometry, ultrastructural study or submitted for culture depending on the preliminary assessment of the aspirate. Our approach is to generate an adequate fixed smear which is assessed by rapid H&E stain; subsequent material is then triaged according to the appearances of the first aspirate. Other laboratories have found air-dried MGG-stained material to be useful for initial assessment. More smears may need to be assessed if the first pass does not contain diagnostic material or is not consistent with the clinical and radiological findings. However, the days of producing numerous highly cellular smears with no cell block should be over! It should also be remembered that many lung carcinomas will not be resected; the material obtained by FNB may be the only tissue available for subsequent molecular studies, which can determine suitability for a particular treatment, further emphasizing the need to obtain an adequate cell block in all cases.

Use of ancillary techniques[45,46]

We rely heavily on ancillary techniques in FNB of the lung and pleura. Ancillary testing is useful in over 50% of intrathoracic aspirations.[45] O'Reilly et al. used immunocytochemistry in 14.5% of cases, EM in 8%, microbiologic studies in 12%, mucin staining in 21% and cell blocks in 22%. They found the greatest value was in classifying poorly differentiated neoplasms, confirming the diagnosis of well-differentiated adenocarcinoma, identifying neuroendocrine differentiation and establishing primary sites for suspected

metastases.[45] Saleh and Masood found ancillary tests contributed to diagnosis in over 60% of cases.[46] Immunohistochemistry was most often used, but electron microscopy was often helpful. Immunohistochemistry has become the mainstay of cytological diagnosis, especially since the availability of thyroid transcription factor (TTF-1),[130–132] and differential cytokeratin staining.[131,133–135] Currently, EM is seldom used. Flow cytometry has revolutionized the diagnosis of lymphoid lesions.[136–138] PCR-based molecular analysis for gene rearrangements for lymphoma diagnosis and FISH studies for lymphoma (see Chapter 5) and soft tissue tumor diagnosis (see Chapter 15) can be applied to FNB material. PCR studies to identify the presence of gene mutations, e.g. EGFR mutations which are relevant to the selection of particular therapies, can be performed on cell blocks.[58] One can anticipate other techniques such as proteomics and microarray technology being useful.[139,140]

Cell blocks

Architectural features such as gland formation may be more readily appreciated in cell block H&E sections; the main role of cell blocks is to provide material for ancillary studies.

Cytochemistry

Mucin stains (which can be performed on smears or cell block material) aid in subtyping large cell carcinomas and in distinguishing between some primary and metastatic tumors, for example in excluding renal cell or adrenal carcinoma.

Immunocytochemistry

The full range of immunohistochemical markers can be used in cell block preparations. Broad-spectrum antibodies to keratins, S-100 and leukocyte common antigen (CD45) can separate most poorly differentiated carcinomas from melanomas and lymphomas. Calretinin has been the most useful positive marker of mesothelioma in our hands, but also stains some poorly differentiated lung carcinomas and squamous carcinomas; it is most useful in pleural effusion cytology. Neuroendocrine markers such as synaptophysin, chromogranin and CD56 are useful in diagnosing various neuroendocrine tumors. Markers for prostate-specific antigen and thyroglobulin are essential in selected cases. Estrogen receptor (ER) staining helps in identifying metastases of breast carcinoma. Caution is required with particular clones of ER.[141] SP1 clone has a significantly higher rate for positive estrogen receptor expression in pulmonary adenocarcinomas when compared with either 1D5 or 6F11 clones. Caution is required in the use of SP1 antibody alone in distinguishing metastatic breast carcinoma from primary pulmonary adenocarcinoma. Differential cytokeratin staining for CK7 and CK20 can help separate primary adenocarcinomas of the lung (CK7 positive, CK20 negative) from metastatic colonic carcinoma (CK7 negative, CK20 positive).[134,135] CDX2 is an additional positive marker of colonic malignancy. Rarely, primary lung adenocarcinomas of so-called enteric-type are CK20 positive and may also stain for CDX2; they usually retain their CK7 positivity.[142] Squamous cell carcinomas and small cell carcinomas are usually negative for both CK7 and CK20, while squamous cell carcinomas are usually positive for CK5/6 and p63.[143] TTF-1 is relatively specific for lung and thyroid neoplasms[130,131] and is probably the single most useful marker for confirming primary lung adenocarcinoma, although perhaps inevitably there are now reports of cases of various metastatic carcinomas being TTF-1 positive, e.g. ovary, cervix, endometrium, colorectal.[144–146] Antibodies to surfactant protein may also be helpful, but negative results in metastatic tumors have not been validated to the same extent as TTF-1. TTF-1 is said to be positive in 90% of small cell carcinomas,[147] although we have seen several cases of TTF1-negative small cell carcinoma.

Electron microscopy (EM)

The role of EM (see Chapter 2) in the diagnosis of pulmonary neoplasms is declining, but may still be of value in recognizing neuroendocrine tumors, in the diagnosis of occasional cases of melanoma and mesothelioma and some carcinomas, including metastases, when immunocytochemistry has not provided a diagnosis.[45–47,148,149] Demonstration of surfactant granules supports the diagnosis of primary bronchogenic carcinoma. Recent studies have further emphasized the heterogeneity of cell type in lung adenocarcinomas. Tumors may show features of nonciliated bronchiolar cell, alveolar cell, mucus-secreting cells or even mixed features of squamous or neuroendocrine type.[150]

Molecular testing[151–159]

There is a trend toward targeted therapy in oncological practice, usually based on the presence of particular gene mutations. At present, the main molecular testing in lung carcinoma is the assessment of EGFR gene mutations; these mutations are usually found in adenocarcinomas and are limited to exons 18–21, with more than 80% of mutations being short deletions in exon 19 or single point mutations in exon 21.1[51,152] This testing is usually performed only when there is consideration for treatment with small molecule inhibitors of EGFR. In addition, mutations in KRAS are associated with lack of benefit from EGFR inhibitors. Mutations in the EGFR and KRAS genes are almost never seen together in the same tumor.[153] EGFR and KRAS status can be assessed by DNA extraction from cell block samples in which there is adequate tumor representation. PCR and sequencing studies are then performed.[58] When there is insufficient material in a cell block sample, material can be scraped from slides.[154] Bronchioloalveolar carcinoma (BAC), now defined as an in situ adenocarcinoma, is composed of two distinct subgroups – mucinous and non-mucinous. The more frequent non-mucinous BAC which predominates in smokers and often presents as a ground-glass opacity is thought to evolve from the terminal respiratory unit cells and frequently harbors EGFR polysomy/mutations which are considered to be a critical event in the pathogenesis of non-mucinous BAC tumors. The less frequent mucinous BAC, thought to be derived from metaplasia of bronchiolar epithelia, presents more frequently as a pneumonic-type infiltrate, rarely demonstrates EGFR mutations, and more frequently harbors and is driven by a KRAS mutation.[153,155]

There are various other molecular markers, e.g. ERCC1, RRM1, that appear to be of increasing clinical relevance, in particular to predict tumor response to chemotherapeutic agents.[156,157] The recent description of an ALK–ELM translocation which can be detected by FISH and immunohistochemistry, and which is present in a small subset of adenocarcinomas, which will respond dramatically to a particular drug therapy,[158,159] highlights the need to ensure that adequate samples are obtained for cell blocks in order to perform additional studies as required.

Clinical requirements in modern practice[143,160–162]

There are increasing expectations from oncologists to distinguish between adenocarcinoma and squamous cell carcinoma in order to optimize treatment regimens, e.g. bevacizumab is associated with a high risk of bleeding in squamous cell carcinoma and is approved only for adenocarcinoma.[160] This has led to pressure to reduce, if not eliminate, the diagnosis of 'non-small cell carcinoma'. An immunohistochemical panel including CK5/6, p63, CK7 and TTF-1 in poorly differentiated carcinomas, may help to suggest either possible squamous (CK5/6, p63 positive) or glandular (CK7/TTF-1 positive) differentiation.[143] Pardo et al.[161] reduced their diagnosis of large cell carcinoma by 90% in a tissue microarray study, with the use of immunohistochemical panels and Khayyata et al.[143] achieved refinement of diagnosis in 65% of cases of NSCLC to either SCC or adenocarcinoma. While the distinction between adenocarcinoma and squamous cell carcinoma can usually be achieved morphologically in well-differentiated tumors, the addition of immunohistochemical panels may increase diagnostic accuracy in poorly differentiated carcinomas.[162] However, limited sampling, anaplastic tumors, tumor heterogeneity and overlapping immunohistochemical profiles can limit the ability to subclassify some lung carcinomas, and oncologists need to be aware of these issues. It is also worth noting that in some studies there may not have been any 'gold standard' to confirm the immunohistochemical diagnosis. Even in a well-differentiated adenocarcinoma it is still incumbent on the pathologist to ensure that there is adequate cell block material for molecular studies (see above). As new discoveries come to light there may be the need to return to archival material to perform new tests. Once a smear with adequate material has been obtained, further aspirates should be submitted for cell block preparation to ensure sufficient material is available for any additional studies that may be required.

Chest wall and pleura

Chest wall is included here to emphasize that the exact site of origin of lesions in this region may be difficult to ascertain and that it is conceptually useful to consider this site as a 'body compartment'. Lesions arising in rib, chest wall soft tissues, pleura or even breast may extend to underlying lung parenchyma and may be confused with primary lung tumors.[163] Contaminating bone marrow from rib may give rise to diagnostic dilemmas. In some cases, myeloma can be mistaken for an undifferentiated lung carcinoma. There is sometimes difficulty in distinguishing between mesothelioma, anaplastic carcinoma, melanoma, sarcomas of the chest wall and metastases. In our own practice, a chondrosarcoma arising in the rib caused difficulty in diagnosis because the site of origin was not appreciated. A malignant mesothelioma growing along a chest drain site was considered clinically to be a primary breast lesion until FNB was

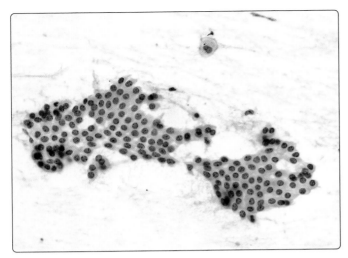

Fig. 8.1 Bronchiolar epithelium Small sheet of regular glandular cells (Pap, HP).

performed. Primary soft tissue lesions of this region are described in Chapter 15.

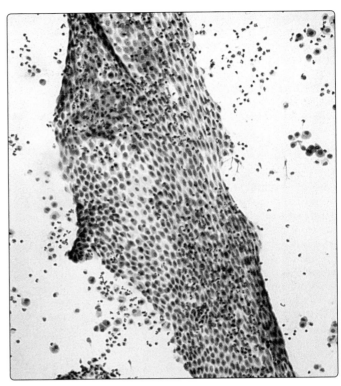

Fig. 8.2 Mesothelial cells Monolayered sheet of cells showing 'spongiotic' separation of individual cells within the sheet (Pap, LP).

CYTOLOGICAL FINDINGS

Lung

The satisfactory smear

A specific benign diagnosis by FNB is generally restricted to the identification of infection, chondroid hamartomas, cysts and a few other disease processes. Non-specific negative findings do not exclude malignancy,[3] and can only be used for patient management in conjunction with clinical and radiological findings. A precise statistical assessment of accuracy rates for a radiology department and a laboratory should be known. In a sense, the only satisfactory sample is one which contains material permitting a specific diagnosis.

Normal structures (Figs 8.1–8.3)

- Bronchial epithelium,
- Bronchiolar epithelium,
- Mesothelium,
- Macrophages,
- Fat/skeletal muscle (chest wall),
- Cartilage/ bone marrow (rib),
- Liver and spleen (right- and left-sided aspirations, respectively).

Bronchial epithelium may be abundant in percutaneous FNB if the needle traverses a medium-sized bronchus or tracks along a bronchial lumen. Transbronchial FNB may also yield abundant bronchial epithelium. Bronchial epithelium appears as small palisaded clusters with a ciliated border. In large aggregates the cells may present as flat sheets with a pavement-like aspect, but ciliated cells can usually be observed at the edges of these sheets.

Bronchiolar epithelium or nonciliated epithelium is seen commonly as sheets of various size (Fig. 8.1). They usually have irregular edges and the component cells display

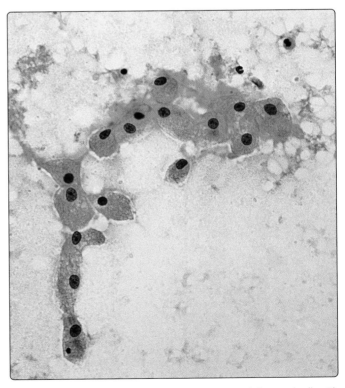

Fig. 8.3 Alveolar macrophages Loose aggregates and dispersed cells with rounded nuclei, small nucleoli, and abundant finely vacuolated cytoplasm (Pap, HP).

variable cell separation. The nuclei are generally small and there is a low nuclear:cytoplasmic (N:C) ratio. Sometimes the nuclear outlines are slightly irregular and small intranuclear cytoplasmic inclusions are observed. Occasionally, atypia of bronchiolar epithelium may be quite pronounced, for example in reactive or inflammatory processes; however, the number of atypical cells is usually small. A diagnosis of malignancy should generally not be made on the basis of small numbers of cells.

Mesothelium can be easily distinguished from bronchiolar epithelium. It is seen as various-sized, flat, monolayered sheets; there is usually more cell separation than in bronchiolar epithelium, which sometimes gives a sponge-like appearance. The cells appear to be joined by intercellular bridges similar to those of squamous epithelium in histological sections. (Fig. 8.2). Reactive mesothelium can appear atypical and be misinterpreted as neoplastic.

Normal lung yields a population of macrophages widely dispersed over the slide (Fig. 8.3); these contain small particles of brown or black particulate matter, some of which is inhaled dust, especially in smokers. Many hemosiderin-laden macrophages usually imply tissue or blood breakdown near the lesion and may add to a suspicion of pulmonary infarction should the clinical background be appropriate.

If stylets are not used, contamination of smears by chest wall tissues such as fat, skeletal muscle, cartilage and bone marrow may occur. Occasionally, intrapulmonary lymph nodes may be aspirated.

Aspirations near the diaphragm can contain liver or splenic tissue and cause concern unless the possibility of inadvertent puncture of abdominal organs is appreciated. Splenic tissue has also been identified in FNB samples from 'thoracic splenosis' following traumatic rupture of the spleen; these are usually pleural based but can occur within the lung.[164,165]

Megakaryocytes are occasionally seen in aspirates of lung[166] or more often from rib marrow.

Inflammatory/non-neoplastic processes[167]

Acute inflammatory material

Common findings

- Several drops of viscous purulent material,
- Many polymorphs,
- Granular and amorphous debris,
- Macrophages, lymphocytes and plasma cells in varying numbers,
- Bacteria.

These findings are not specific unless bacteria are evident, but they can suggest an acute infection. It is worth repeating the aspiration, and sending all the material obtained for aerobic and anaerobic culture. Associated vegetable material may suggest aspiration as a cause.[168]

PROBLEMS AND DIFFERENTIAL DIAGNOSIS

- ◆ Squamous cell carcinoma with necrosis/cavitation/acute inflammation,
- ◆ Caseous necrosis,
- ◆ Fungal infection.

When the center of a necrotic or cavitating carcinoma is aspirated, particularly those of squamous type, acute inflammatory material may result (the so-called carcinomatous lung abscess).[169] Macroscopically, this resembles pus and microscopically only few squamous cells may be present. Small squamous cells with pyknotic nuclei may be difficult to distinguish from degenerate macrophages.

Polymorphonuclear leukocytes are not uncommonly seen in tuberculosis and the background debris may also be rather 'watery', similar to that in some acute inflammatory processes. We stain all inflammatory smears with the Ziehl-Neelsen (ZN) stain and routinely send material for microbiological culture or PCR studies for fungi and mycobacteria, as well as bacteria.

A high polymorph content is usually present in the inflammatory reaction to fungi. A search for a granulomatous component and fungal organisms is mandatory if acute inflammatory material is obtained. With infection by filamentous organisms, e.g. *Nocardia*, the organisms may be identified in the center of distinctive, cohesive neutrophil clusters or rosettes after silver impregnation; this clustering should be a clue to search for such an infection (Fig. 8.4). Similar appearances may also be be seen in streptococcal infection.

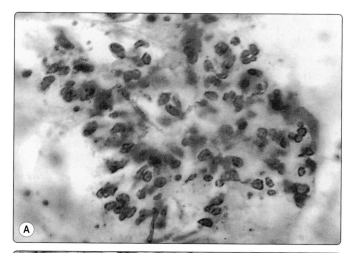

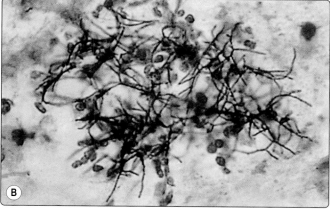

Fig. 8.4 Neutrophil rosette (A) Clump of neutrophils (H&E, HP oil); (B) Fine branching filaments of *Nocardia* (Methemamine silver, HP oil).

Granulomatous inflammation
(Figs 8.5–8.7)[98–103,170–176]

One can make a confident diagnosis of a 'granulomatous process' on aspirated material; however, a more important aspect of the aspiration is to obtain an adequate sample for staining and culture, particularly to distinguish between 'typical' and 'atypical' mycobacteria[101] and for typing fungal organisms. It is best to have a large sample for this purpose and we have not found much value in washings of the needle after a cytology smear has been made. Instead, we advocate sending the whole aspirate for culture. Culture for tuberculosis is more successful in cases with necrotic and inflammatory debris.[99,102] PCR can provide a rapid diagnosis, aids in subtyping and can identify drug resistant strains.[170,171]

Specific diagnosis of most noninfectious granulomatous diseases is not possible, although there are reports of the cytological findings in sarcoidosis,[172–174] Wegener's granulomatosis[175,176] and rheumatoid nodule.[177]

Epithelioid histiocytes are fairly cohesive and form granulomas which are often aspirated intact (Fig. 8.5). Epithelioid cells have an elongated or bean-shaped nucleus and abundant cytoplasm which is rather pale and indistinct both in Pap- and H & E-stained specimens (Fig. 8.5). The cytoplasmic density is higher in MGG-stained material. Multinucleated histiocytes can be seen but are usually sparse. They are mainly free of intracytoplasmic pigment or birefringent material, unlike the multinucleated histiocytes seen in nonspecific reactions in pulmonary tissue. Caseous necrosis has a variable appearance. There may be an amorphous to granular background with little cell outline visible, but sometimes outlines of necrotic cells may be prominent (Fig. 8.6) and often the appearances are merely of nondescript debris, histiocytes and neutrophils. Dahlgren cites granular calcific material as a common accompaniment.[98] Lymphocytes may be plentiful in granulomatous inflammation.

Bailey et al.[99] diagnosed 28 of 34 cases of TB by either auramine rhodamine fluorescence or positive culture; acid-fast bacilli (AFB) were seen in only 38% of cases. In Rajwanshi's[102] and Das's[103] series AFB were identified in approximately half of the cases. Gong et al. found PCR to be about 80% sensitive compared to 40% for ZN staining in FNB material.[171]

Recent advances in mycobacterial genomics and human cellular immunology have resulted in two new blood tests that detect tuberculosis infection by measuring in vitro T-cell interferon-gamma release in response to two unique antigens that are highly specific for *Mycobacterium tuberculosis*, but absent from bacille Calmette-Guérin (BCG) vaccine and most non-tuberculous mycobacteria. These tests appear to be very useful in increasing specificity and sensitivity in the diagnosis of tuberculosis.[178]

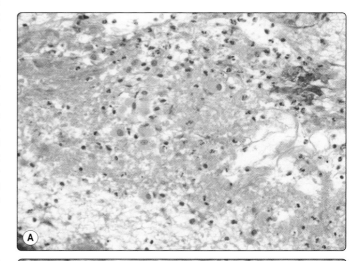

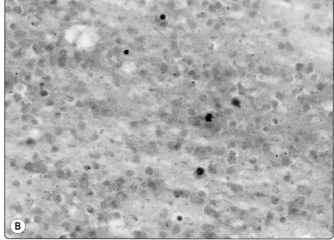

Fig. 8.6 Caseation necrosis (A) Amorphous and granular debris with neutrophils (H&E, MP); (B) Single-cell pattern of necrosis (H & E, HP).

Fig. 8.5 Granulomas Clustered epithelioid histiocytes and lymphocytes (H&E, HP).

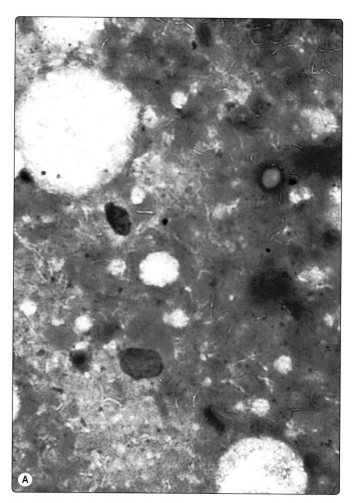

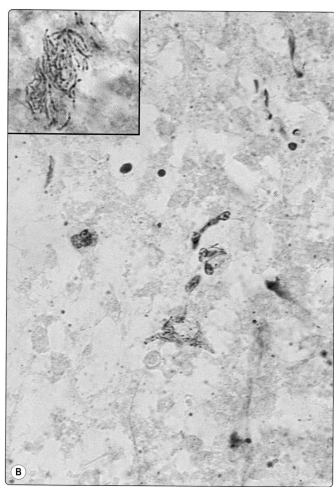

Fig. 8.7 Mycobacterial infection (A) Negative images of bacilli in a background of granular necrotic debris (MGG, HP); (B) Numerous acid-fast bacilli, including clumps of beaded forms (Ziehl-Neelsen, HP; Inset HP oil).

PROBLEMS AND DIFFERENTIAL DIAGNOSIS

◆ Identification of epithelioid histiocytes,
◆ Giant cells in non-specific inflammation,
◆ Giant cell reaction to neoplasm,
◆ Tumor necrosis mimicking caseation and vice versa,
◆ Neutrophil reaction in tuberculosis.

Epithelioid histiocytes may resemble fibroblasts, smooth muscle cells or endothelial cells; they are most characteristically found in clusters and can rarely be identified if they lie singly.

Giant cells which contain pigment are more in keeping with a non-specific reaction than a true granulomatous process.

A granulomatous reaction may develop at the edge of a carcinoma or other neoplasm, particularly squamous cell carcinoma forming keratin; this reaction may be foreign body giant cell in type and yield many multinucleated cells. Histiocytic giant cell reactions also occur in fungal infections, e.g. cryptococcosis[101,179–181] or histoplasmosis,[101] so the

cytoplasm of any giant cells present should be closely examined. It should be remembered that tuberculosis may coexist with carcinoma.

Necrotic tumor may be homogeneous or granular and closely resemble caseous material. Conversely, we have seen cases of tuberculosis where ghost outlines of single cells were distributed across the smear and closely mimicked necrotic tumor (Fig. 8.6).

Acid-fast bacilli are more often seen in cytological material characterized by a mixture of neutrophils, histiocytes, mucoid or necrotic material than in those lesions with a prominent epithelioid cell component,[99,102] though culture is positive in a similar percentage of cases with and without epithelioid cells.[103] Whenever necrotic debris is seen, we restain smears with ZN stains. Maygarden described mycobacteria as negative images in a stained background in MGG material (Fig. 8.7).[182] Silverman reported negative images in both Diff-Quik and Papanicolaou-stained material in a BAL sample from a patient receiving clofazimine treatment for an atypical mycobacterial infection. The reddish, refractile and polarizable drug-derived crystals can impart a pseudo-Gaucher-like appearance to the cells, simulating the negative images of an atypical mycobacterial infection.[183]

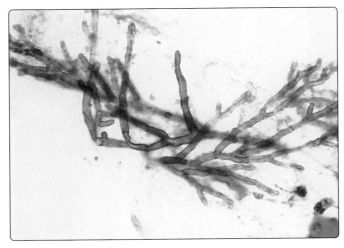

Fig. 8.8 Aspergillus hyphae Acute angled branching, parallel cell walls and septation (Pap, MP).

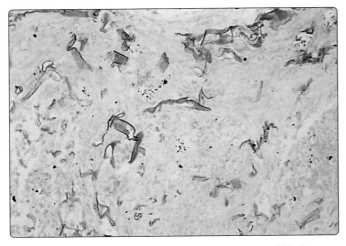

Fig. 8.9 Mucormycosis Broad folded nonseptate hyphae (cell block, H&E, MP).

Other specific infections

In *Aspergillus* (Fig. 8.8) and phycomycete (Fig. 8.9) infections in the lung, fungal hyphae are easily visible in alcohol-fixed material.[184,185] The characteristic appearance of acute-angled branching, parallel cell walls and septa in *Aspergillus* (Fig. 8.8) is shared by several other fungi and culture is necessary for accurate typing.[186] *Pseudoallescheria boydii*, identified as a 'clinically significant mycosis',[187] and *Fusarium* sp. may be morphologically indistinguishable from *Aspergillus*, and even *Candida* resembles this organism on occasion, by forming germ-tube structures with 'septation'.[184] Oxalate crystals are produced by several species of *Aspergillus* and, if identified in cytological material, should lead to a search for organisms.[188,189]

Cryptococci[179–181,190] (Fig. 8.10) have a varied morphology.[181] Later sclerotic foci have a more granulomatous appearance and fewer organisms. In several of our cases of cryptococcosis, organisms were only seen within multinucleated cells. A case of a pulmonary inflammatory myofibroblastic tumor caused by *Cryptococcus* infection, presumed to be the *gattii* species, has been diagnosed by FNAC.[191] Mucicarmine staining of the capsule is a specific and useful criterion for diagnosis and will help distinguish the atypical forms from other yeasts; Fontana-Masson staining of cell

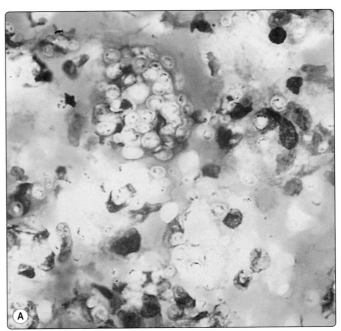

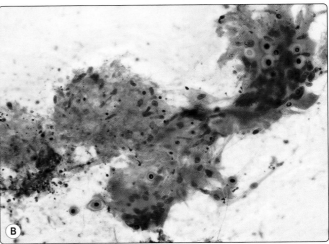

Fig. 8.10 Cryptococcosis (A) Encapsulated yeast organisms (MGG, HP); (B) Necrotizing granulomatous material containing numerous encapsulated organisms. (H&E, MP).

walls will also help distinguish poorly encapsulated forms from *Histoplasma*, *Torulopsis* or *Candida*.[181] Blastomycosis characteristically has more broad-based budding forms.

Histoplasmosis may cause difficulties because the organism is difficult to see in ordinary stains and shows only as small refractile shadows. Methenamine silver preparations are required for diagnosis. *Penicillium marneffei* may mimic *Histoplasma*, as may the small form of *Cryptococcus*.

In some fungal infections, particularly histoplasmosis, organisms are only seen in methenamine silver preparations, although the Pap stain is a superb technique for identifying most other organisms including the filamentous higher bacteria.[192] Destained H&E or Pap-stained smears are as suitable as unstained material for special stains. Culture is necessary for the exact classification of the organism.

Multiple and unusual infections may be encountered in AIDS or post-transplantation.[27,28,193,194] *Pneumocystis* is uncommonly diagnosed by FNB because of the efficacy of

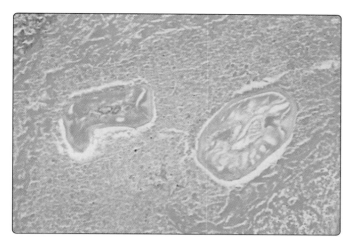

Fig. 8.11 Dirofilariasis Cross-section of parasites in a background of necrosis (cell block, H&E, MP).

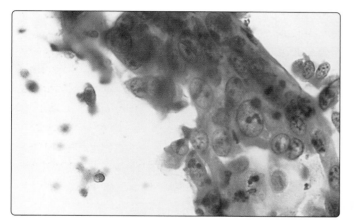

Fig. 8.12 Atypical epithelial repair Cohesive sheet of epithelial cells with enlarged nuclei and prominent nucleoli (Pap, HP).

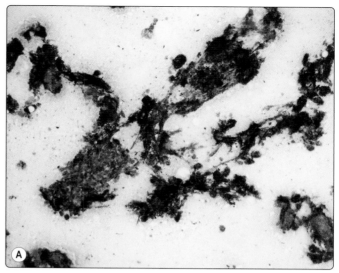

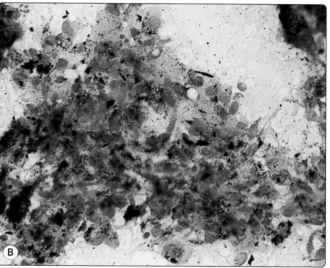

Fig. 8.13 Anthraco-silicosis; progressive massive fibrosis Bilateral upper zone/hilar lung masses in a miner. Dense masses of macrophages and fibrous tissue (**A**, H&E, MP; **B**, H&E, HP).

broncho-alveolar lavage in the diagnosis of diffuse pneumonic disease, but some cases may present with nodular or cavitary lesions in the lung. CMV infection,[195] coccidioidomycosis,[76,196,197] paragonamiasis,[198] amebiasis, hydatid disease[119,120,199] and microfilariasis[200] have all been described in FNB samples.

In coccidioidomycosis,[197] smears show abundant granular eosinophilic debris with a paucity of acute or chronic inflammation; granulomatous inflammation is seldom seen. *Coccidioides immitis* spherules range in size from 20 to 200 μm; fractured or crushed forms are often seen and some are calcified. Endospores are seen only within intact spherules.[196,197] In some cases, the associated reactive cellular changes have been misinterpreted as neoplastic.[76]

According to McCorkell,[120] clear colorless fluid is an indicator of hydatid cyst and should lead to a search for scolices, hooklets or laminated membrane (see Chapter 10). Diagnosis of dirofilariasis[201] requires cell block preparations (Fig. 8.11).

Reparative and reactive change

Squamous metaplasia, epithelial repair reactions, reactive bronchiolar or mesothelial proliferations and reactive histiocytic or fibroblastic cells can all produce significant cellular atypia (Fig. 8.12).[56,73,76] Diagnosis of malignancy in a background of inflammatory change should be made with extreme caution. In FNAC, a malignant diagnosis should also generally be based on highly cellular smears. In this way, the risk of a false-positive diagnosis in reparative or reactive processes can be minimized.[56,167,202]

Pneumoconioses

Birefringent silica and collagenous tissue (Fig. 8.13) or asbestos bodies may help confirm silicosis or exposure to asbestos.[203] However, concomitant malignancy, tuberculosis or other infections may be the cause of the localized opacity in these patients.[204]

Pulmonary infarct

Silverman describes sheets of metaplastic squamous cells showing regenerative changes and histiocytes containing clumped refractile hemosiderin in a clinically

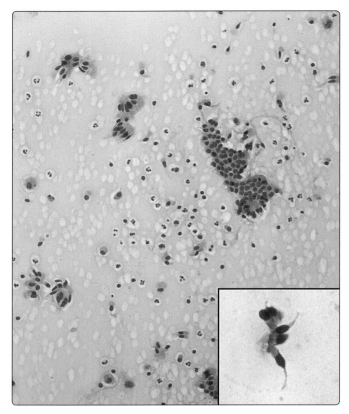

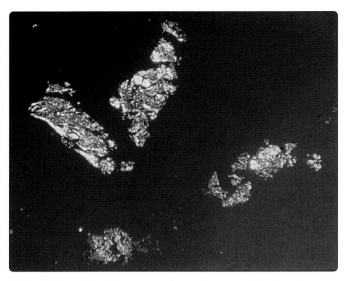

Fig. 8.15 **Amyloidosis** Fragments of amorphous material with apple-green birefringence (Congo red, MP).

Fig. 8.14 **Bronchocele** Rounded mass in mid-lung field. Mucoid material aspirated at FNB. Smears show mucin, scattered macrophages and sheets of bronchial epithelial cells. **Inset**: Ciliated cells. Cytological findings consistent with either bronchogenic cyst or bronchocele. Recent onset of lesion more consistent with bronchcoele (H&E, HP; Inset, Pap, HP oil).

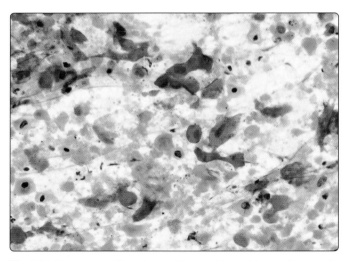

Fig. 8.16 **Squamous cell carcinoma** Dispersed keratinizing malignant cells and necrotic debris (Pap, HP).

unsuspected infarct; FNAC findings led to the diagnosis being suggested. [205]

Other non-neoplastic lesions

Material aspirated from congenital bronchogenic cysts usually consists of mucin and bronchial-type epithelium unless infection supervenes. So-called 'bronchoceles', which represent recent-onset postinflammatory dilated mucin-filled bronchial structures, may yield similar findings, and correlation with clinical and sequential imaging findings is necessary for precise diagnosis. (Fig. 8.14).

Findings in nodular amyloidosis (Fig. 8.15),[206–208] Wegener's granulomatosis,[175,176] extramedullary hemopoiesis[209] and malacoplakia[210] are described. We have seen one case of amyloidosis in consultation, in which amyloid was visible in both smears and cell block preparations. Miller et al. describe FNAC findings of abundant parenchymal material including thickened alveolar walls as being of help in diagnosing 'rolled' or 'rounded' atelectasis in company with consistent CT findings. This entity produces a radiologic appearance of a mass lesion involving pleura and lung, often in the inferior lobes in the posterior basal lateral vertebral area, and is sometimes associated with asbestos-induced pleural disease with underlying lung scarring.[57,211]

Common primary carcinomas

Squamous cell carcinoma (Figs 8.16 and 8.17)

CRITERIA FOR DIAGNOSIS

Keratinizing
- ◆ Predominant single cell presentation,
- ◆ Keratinized malignant cells; cytoplasm refractile and eosinophilic (Pap, H&E); dense, pure blue (MGG),
- ◆ Perinuclear halo,
- ◆ Bizarre cell shapes, spindle and caudate cells,
- ◆ Irregular angular, densely hyperchromatic nuclei,
- ◆ Necrosis.

Non-keratinizing
- ◆ Irregular solid cohesive fragments,
- ◆ Elongated or spindle-shaped nuclei,
- ◆ Variable chromatin density in adjacent cells.

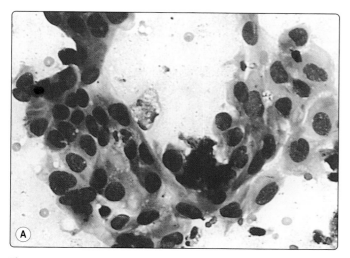
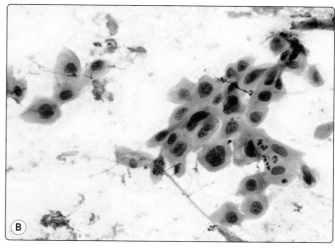

Fig. 8.17 Squamous cell carcinoma Irregular clumps of relatively cohesive nonkeratinizing cells; variation in chromatin density (A, MGG, HP; B, Pap, MP)

Well-differentiated squamous cell carcinoma with keratinizing cells and bizarre cell shapes is not difficult to recognise. The malignant cells are usually dispersed, especially when they are very well differentiated (Fig. 8.16); necrosis is a common accompaniment. Single keratinizing cells are the most reliable indicators of squamous differentiation; when keratinization is not obvious, a perinuclear halo within the cytoplasm and condensation of peripheral cytoplasm are helpful guides to squamous differentiation (Fig. 8.17). Non-keratinizing tumors are usually more cohesive and present as multilayered fragments. Their nuclei are usually spindle shaped or elongated with dense, irregularly distributed chromatin. There is often conspicuous variation in the degree of chromasia of nearby nuclei. Nucleoli vary in size and number, in contrast to adenocarcinoma where nucleolar morphology is more monotonous. Dense cytoplasm and well-defined cell borders are indicators of squamous differentiation, but some adenocarcinomas may have strikingly well-defined borders and very dense cytoplasm.

PROBLEMS AND DIFFERENTIAL DIAGNOSIS

- Necrosis in other carcinomas simulating keratinization,
- Other poorly differentiated carcinomas,
- Inflammation and necrosis, especially in cavitating lesions,
- Giant cell reaction to tumor,
- Very well-differentiated squamous cell carcinoma,
- Teratoma,
- Uncommon carcinomas – mucoepidermoid; basaloid,
- Sarcomatoid tumors/mesothelioma,
- Metastatic squamous cell carcino.

Misinterpreting the cytoplasmic eosinophilia of necrosis for keratinisation is a common source of error (see Fig. 8.30).[30] Necrosis can also impart an angular hyperchromatic appearance to nuclei, similar to squamous carcinomas. This is less of a problem when Pap staining is used because orangiophilia distinguishes between necrosis and keratin better

than H&E or MGG, although cells in heavily bloodstained smears may take on an eosinophilic hue simulating keratinization.

There is an overlap between the appearances of poorly differentiated squamous cell carcinoma, large cell anaplastic carcinoma and poorly differentiated or solid adenocarcinoma in aspirated material. They all present as large, multi-layered fragments corresponding to the solid growth of these carcinomas. Squamous cell carcinoma is overdiagnosed in some series because adenocarcinoma in aspirates may present as pavement-like sheets, mimicking the appearance that squamous cell carcinoma has in sections. The pavement-like appearance of squamous cell carcinoma results only from thin sectioning and does not occur in aspirated material, although it may be seen in sections of cell blocks. Palisading of cells, which may occur at the margins of lobules of nonkeratinizing squamous tumors, may give rise to a false impression of the margin of a gland in smears. There is also a tendency to overestimate the grade of tumor in aspirated material, perhaps because viable rather than maturing or exfoliating new growth is removed. Unusual variants of SCC such as the pseudovascular adenoid form may be easier to recognize as squamous in cytological rather than histological material.[212]

Small-celled forms of poorly differentiated squamous cell carcinoma, and those undergoing degeneration and necrosis, can be confused with small cell carcinoma. Attention to greater cohesion, larger cell size, presence of nucleoli, greater tendency to spindle at the periphery of clusters, denser cytoplasm and occasional keratinized cells should lead to the correct diagnosis. Strong positive p63 and CK 5/6 staining and absence of staining for TTF-1 would favor squamous rather than small cell carcinoma, although rare squamous carcinomas are TTF1 positive.[143,213]

Diagnostic malignant squamous cells may be difficult to find when there is associated acute inflammation and abundant necrosis, especially in cavitating tumors. These aspirates can simulate an abscess, leading to false-negative diagnosis. A comprehensive search for diagnostic malignant keratinized cells is recommended.

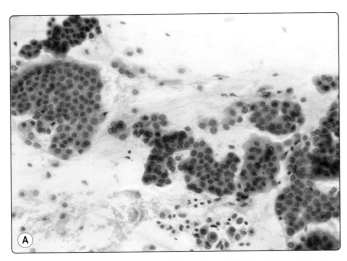 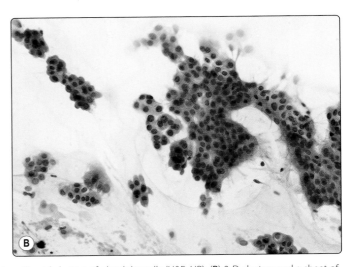

Fig. 8.18 Adenocarcinoma, well differentiated (A) Monolayered sheets and papillaroid clusters of glandular cells (H&E, HP); (B) 3-D clusters and a sheet of glandular cells with a palisaded edge (H&E, HP). Diagnosis of malignancy based on abundance of material and complex architecture.

Keratinizing squamous cell carcinoma, more than other carcinomas, tends to produce a giant cell response in nearby tissues and a false impression of a granulomatous process. A variegated population of many and different types of inflammatory cells, foamy macrophages, mast cells and alveolar cells results from bronchial obstruction associated with the carcinoma. Other types of carcinoma, especially adenocarcinomas, do not usually show this reaction.

Occasionally, only keratinous debris or very well-differentiated squamous cells may be removed from a squamous cell carcinoma and cells with diagnostic malignant nuclei may be absent. Clinical and radiological features may then aid in diagnosis.

Teratoma enters the differential diagnosis, particularly when a lesion has a mediastinal component. In the aspirate from the mature teratomas we have seen, the squamous epithelium was very cohesive, in contradistinction to the dispersed cells of well-differentiated squamous cell carcinoma.

Low-grade mucoepidermoid tumors have been described in FNB samples[214] as well as basaloid squamous carcinoma.[215]

Metastatic squamous carcinoma from head and neck or from anogenital primary sites will often be positive for high-risk HPV DNA, whereas primary lung SCC is rarely HPV positive.[216] PCR studies for HPV DNA on cell block material may be helpful when metastatic disease is being considered.

Adenocarcinoma, including BAC (Figs 8.18–8.24)

CRITERIA FOR DIAGNOSIS

- Medium-sized to large cells with abundant delicate cytoplasm,
- Flat sheets,
- Rosettes, acinar structures or cell clusters/balls,
- Columnar cells,
- Round to oval eccentric nuclei with large solitary nucleoli.

The cellular morphology of adenocarcinoma is similar to that described in brush material. Rosettes, acinar formations or cohesive cell clusters (Figs 8.18 and 8.19) represent anatomical structures removed from the tumor by the needle. The larger the gland formations, the less likely they are to be removed intact and, when only partly removed, deposit on the slide as flat sheets in a monolayer (Fig. 8.18): a useful indicator of glandular differentiation. Artifactual spaces are often seen in large tissue fragments and may be misinterpreted as acinar structures; however, where the spaces have an 'anatomical' rigidity, they may indicate glandular differentiation. Mucin secretion is difficult to identify without the aid of special stains, and vacuolation of the cytoplasm may occur as a result of degeneration or the presence of glycogen. In H&E- or Pap-stained material vacuoles with a central, inspissated, eosinophilic or orangiophilic center are very suggestive of mucin secretion and correspond to the intracellular lumina described ultrastructurally in adenocarcinomas. With MGG staining, mucin may be visible as magenta or purple material within the cytoplasm, either homogeneously or as red granules within a pale vacuole. Well-formed columnar cells or groups of palisaded cells may be a guide to glandular differentiation and terminal plates/bars may also be present. In the 2004 WHO classification,[217] the definition of BAC was limited to a non-invasive process and is now an uncommon diagnosis, requiring full histological assessment; there is currently debate as to whether the term should be used at all, especially since a diagnosis of BAC cannot be rendered on small biopsy samples or cytological samples. However, it is still possible to suggest that a tumor may have a BAC-like component based on cytological features. These include large, cohesive, monolayered sheets which reflect the growth of neoplastic cells in a monolayer along alveolar walls, papillary processes, cell balls and clusters, intranuclear cytoplasmic inclusions and psammoma bodies (Figs 8.18–8.22). The radiogical appearance of a purely ground-glass opacity without a solid component is also suggestive of a BAC.

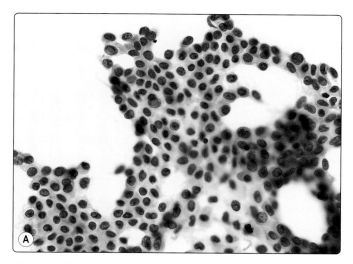

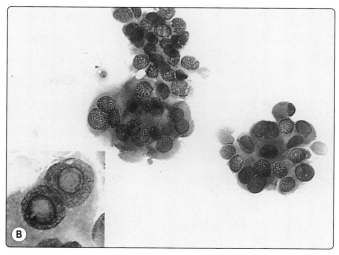

Fig. 8.19 Adenocarcinoma (A) Monolayered sheet of glandular cells showing enlarged hyperchromatic nuclei with irregular outlines and several intranuclear cytoplasmic inclusions (H&E, HP). (B) 3-D clusters of glandular cells (MGG, HP). **Inset**: intranuclear cytoplasmic inclusions (MGG, HP oil).

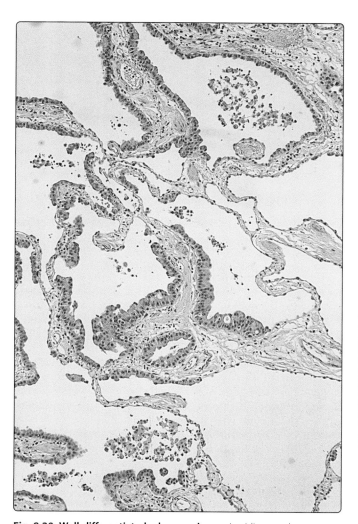

Fig. 8.20 Well-differentiated adenocarcinoma Lepidic growth pattern. Tissue section (H&E, MP).

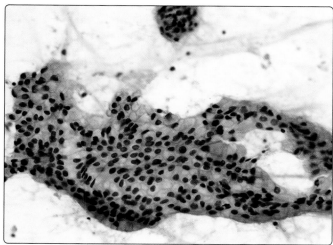

Fig. 8.21 Well-differentiated adenocarcinoma Monolayered sheet of glandular cells with honeycombing and prominent mucin (Pap, HP).

PROBLEMS AND DIFFERENTIAL DIAGNOSIS

◆ Other poorly differentiated large cell carcinomas,
◆ Metastatic adenocarcinoma,
◆ Atypical adenomatous hyperplasia,
◆ Reactive bronchiolar cells,
◆ Other tumors, e.g. neuroendocrine tumors, cystic mucinous neoplasms, mesothelioma.

In adenocarcinomas with meager mucin secretion and little or no glandular formation, the possibility of accurate diagnosis by morphological features is low. The cytoplasmic and nuclear features of large cell carcinoma and of some poorly differentiated squamous cell carcinomas may closely resemble adenocarcinoma; immunostaining for p63, CK5/6 and TTF-1 may be useful.[143,213] If the tumor cells are fairly regular and the nuclei are rounded with large central nucleoli they are more likely to be glandular (Fig. 8.23); this is not, however, a completely reliable criterion.

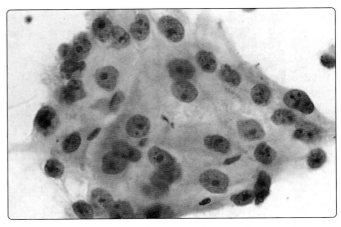

Fig. 8.23 Poorly differentiated adenocarcinoma Delicate cytoplasm, rounded nuclei with single prominent central nucleoli (H&E, HP). Objective criteria of glandular differentiation not present in this aggregate; diagnostic criteria need to be sought elsewhere in smear or cell block.

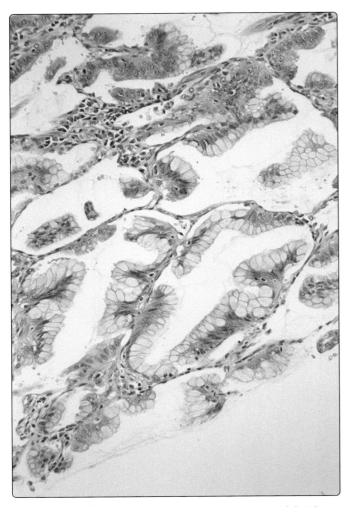

Fig. 8.22 Well-differentiated adenocarcinoma Mucinous with lepidic growth pattern. Tissue section (H&E, MP).

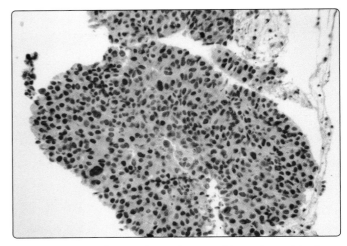

Fig. 8.24 Primary adenocarcinoma Strong positive nuclear staining for TTF-1 (Cell block, IPOX, HP).

There are no absolute cytological criteria for separating primary from secondary adenocarcinomas, although there may be features indicative of a particular organ of origin (see Chapter 5). Immunostaining for TTF-1 provides the best single marker of a primary origin (Fig. 8.24), although it should be recognised that metastic thyroid malignancies and occasionally metastases from other sites may be TTF-1 positive.[144–146]

It is likely that so-called atypical adenomatous hyperplasia (AAH) represents a precursor of peripheral adenocarcinomas of the lung.[218] Foci of AAH are usually small (<5 mm), incidentally found in lung resections and are seldom sampled by FNB. Nevertheless, they potentially represent a source of error in FNAC diagnosis since they can be composed of highly atypical glandular cells, and may produce small opacities.[219] We have encountered one case where the mass lesion seen on CT proved to be an area of non-specific fibrosis at resection and where the small numbers of highly atypical but rather poorly preserved cells seen in FNB samples were derived from adjacent areas of AAH.

It may be difficult to diagnose well-differentiated adenocarcinoma/BAC when there is a low degree of nuclear atypia. The material may mimic benign bronchiolar epithelium, especially when occurring in small sheets. The presence of abundant material should raise the index of suspicion, as should papillae or cell balls. Sometimes there may be only few diagnostic cells so that an overall impression of variation in atypia can be important in reaching a conclusion. Aspirates from non-malignant lesions of the lung frequently contain bronchiolar epithelium, sometimes showing nuclear atypia.[84,167] Reactive sheets are usually small and few in number,[86] and have more irregular borders than malignant sheets. Jarrett and Betsill considered high cellularity, architectural three-dimensionality, intranuclear cytoplasmic inclusions and large nucleolar size to be the most helpful features in distinguishing adenocarcinoma from reactive bronchiolar proliferations.[86] Zaman et al. suggested a predominance of two- and three-dimensional tissue fragments, intranuclear cytoplasmic inclusions and paucity of multinucleated cell forms to be more indicative of malignancy.[202] Silverman found a lack of hyperchromasia, prominence of cell borders, presence of terminal plates, goblet cells and nuclear molding to be more characteristic of benign reactive epithelium.[84]

Confusion with other primary pulmonary neoplasms may occur. Lesions such as carcinoid tumors and rare lesions such as sclerosing hemangioma/pneumocytoma[220–223] yield a uniform cell population similar to that of well differentiated adenocarcinoma. Carcinoid tumors usually consist of regular cells which are smaller and more dispersed than those of adenocarcinoma and their round nuclei have a characteristic stippled 'neuroendocrine' chromatin pattern (see Figs 8.33 and 8.34). We have not seen examples of papillary adenoma in FNB material, but these rare tumors are also likely to provide problems in differential diagnosis. Pulmonary mucinous cystic neoplasms (PMCN) are also rare; distinction from a variety of pulmonary neoplasms, including mucinous BAC, bronchial mucous gland adenoma, mucoepidermoid carcinoma and metastatic mucinous adenocarcinoma, may be difficult.[224] Moran considers that a clear morphological distinction between the benign and malignant forms of PMCN has not been convincingly made and that all lesions should be considered at least potentially malignant.[225] Categorization as a cystic tumor may be important in planning surgery, as circumscribed lesions with minimal invasion are likely to have a good prognosis.

The differential diagnosis between a peripheral well-differentiated adenocarcinoma, including those showing a pseudo-mesotheliomatous growth pattern, and the epithelial form of malignant mesothelioma can usually be resolved by mucin and immunoperoxidase stains; occasionally, ultrastructural studies are required.

Small cell carcinoma (Figs 8.25–8.29)[32,35,36,79,82,83]

CRITERIA FOR DIAGNOSIS

- ◆ Small or medium-sized cells with little or no cytoplasm (larger than in sputum),
- ◆ Dispersed cell presentation; some clusters, including some small tight groups,
- ◆ Nuclear molding and engulfment; irregular nuclei,
- ◆ Uniform finely or coarsely granular nuclear chromatin; small nucleoli,
- ◆ Tear-drop cells, smeared cells and streaks of nuclear material,
- ◆ Engulfment of apoptotic bodies,
- ◆ Numerous mitotic figures.

This group of lung carcinomas is the most aggressive of the common types, having a mean survival of less than 6 months without treatment. Small cell carcinoma is virtually unheard of in non-smokers, while for carcinoid and atypical carcinoid the smoking association is much weaker. It is important to categorize this neoplasm accurately because, in general, chemotherapy rather than surgery will be used in management. In addition, chemotherapy regimens are different from those used for inoperable non-small cell carcinomas. This group is fairly homogeneous in terms of its biology but is more heterogeneous morphologically. Attempts at morphological subclassification have been made; however, the larger 'intermediate' and smaller 'oat cell' subtypes are not reliably separable by expert pathologists and do not have significantly different behavior or response to therapy. The latest WHO classification therefore does not subcategorize small cell carcinoma although it does recognize mixtures with other types of carcinoma.[217]

Cytology is very successful in diagnosing small cell carcinoma in sputum and pleural fluid; in fact, sputum cytology may be more accurate than FNAC in typing this lesion. The criteria for the diagnosis of small cell carcinoma in aspirated material are similar to those in other sample types, but there are some important differences.

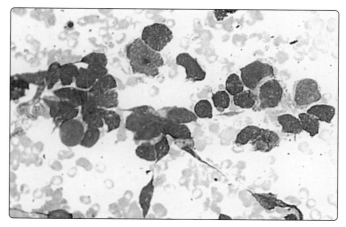

Fig. 8.26 Small cell carcinoma Pleomorphic poorly cohesive cells with little or no cytoplasm; nuclear molding (MGG, HP).

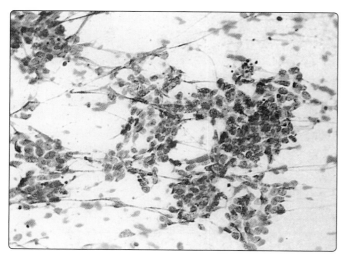

Fig. 8.25 Small cell carcinoma Loose clusters with some dispersal and smearing artifact (Pap, HP).

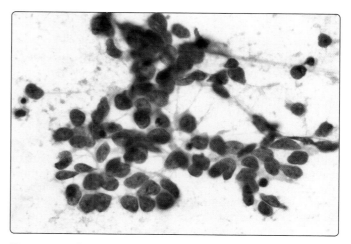

Fig. 8.27 Small cell carcinoma Small loose cluster showing absence of cytoplasm, finely granular chromatin, inconspicuous nucleoli, nuclear molding and teardrop cells (H&E, HP).

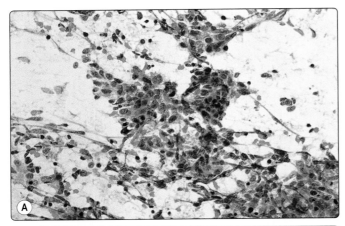

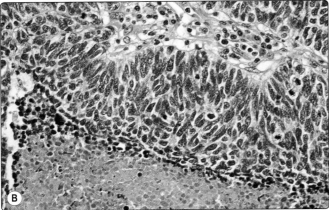

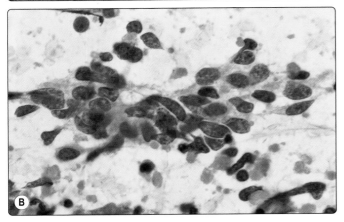

Fig. 8.28 High-grade neuroendocrine carcinoma; small cell carcinoma
(A, B) Smears showing 'intermediate' morphology. Loose aggregates of fragile cells with traumatization artifact and nuclear molding but some background cytoplasm (A, Pap, MP; B, H&E, HP). (C) Tissue section of resected peripheral stage 1 small cell carcinoma (H&E, HP).

Cell pleomorphism is so distinctive that a diagnosis of malignancy is seldom in doubt (Figs 8.25–8.27). The most immediate impression is the absence or sparseness of cytoplasm rather than the small size of the neoplastic cell (Figs. 8.26 and 8.27). In fact, the cell nuclei may appear larger than similar cells in sputum and this may mislead one into making a diagnosis of non-small cell carcinoma. This difference in size between sputum and aspirated material is due to degenerative changes and shrinkage in sputum. It is

sparseness of cytoplasm rather than size which is the most helpful initial clue in differentiating the lesion from other pulmonary carcinomas.

The combination of dispersal with clustering is also important, especially when other small cell neoplasms enter the differential diagnosis (Fig. 8.25). Lymphomas generally do not display such cell cohesion, although large fragments may be dislodged, and in some cases lymphoid cells may form clusters or packets.

Fragility of nuclei is emphasized by tear-drop cells or streaks of smeared nuclear material,[226] and the close nuclear apposition and molding so commonly seen in sputum are also evident (Figs 8.26 and 8.27). Uniform coarsely granular 'salt and pepper' nuclear chromatin is also a well-recognized feature of this cancer in other sites, but one point of difference from sputum is the frequency of small nucleoli in aspirated material; they are less commonly seen in sputum. This may also be related to the better preservation of cells removed directly from tumor; small nucleoli are also often seen in bronchial brush material. Mitotic figures are usually easily found.

Mullins et al. described paranuclear blue inclusions as a common feature of small cell carcinomas;[227] similar inclusions are seen in some non-small cell carcinomas but we have not seen them in lymphoma.

Renshaw et al.,[228] in a review of QA material, found that misclassification of small cell carcinoma as non-small cell carcinoma may reflect a variety of factors, including lack of recognition that some features of non-small cell carcinoma may also be noted in well-preserved cases of small cell carcinoma; there may be increased cytoplasm and cytoplasmic globules (paranuclear blue bodies), or apparent intracytoplasmic lumina. Cases more frequently misclassified as non-small cell carcinoma tended to show better overall cellular and group preservation.

In the largest series the predictive value of a diagnosis of small cell carcinoma by FNB is over 90% and the sensitivity of tumor typing over 80%.[30,82,83] However, there are few series with complete histological follow-up and some series where overall accuracy was lower. Reasonable experience with FNB diagnosis is necessary before the diagnosis can be assumed to be as reliable as by biopsy or sputum cytology.

PROBLEMS AND DIFFERENTIAL DIAGNOSIS

- ◆ 'Intermediate' small cell carcinoma,
- ◆ Large cell neuroendocrine carcinoma,
- ◆ Small celled or basaloid squamous carcinoma,
- ◆ 'Combined' small cell carcinoma,
- ◆ Complement of large cells; mixed small and large cell carcinoma,
- ◆ Low-grade carcinomas, e.g. carcinoid tumor (including spindle cell carcinoid and atypical carcinoid), adenoid cystic carcinoma,
- ◆ Other carcinomas with excessive artifactual smearing,
- ◆ Lymphoma,
- ◆ Metastatic tumors (e.g. melanoma, metastatic neuroendocrine tumors).

Although 'intermediate' small cell carcinoma is no longer recognized as a separate category in international classifica-

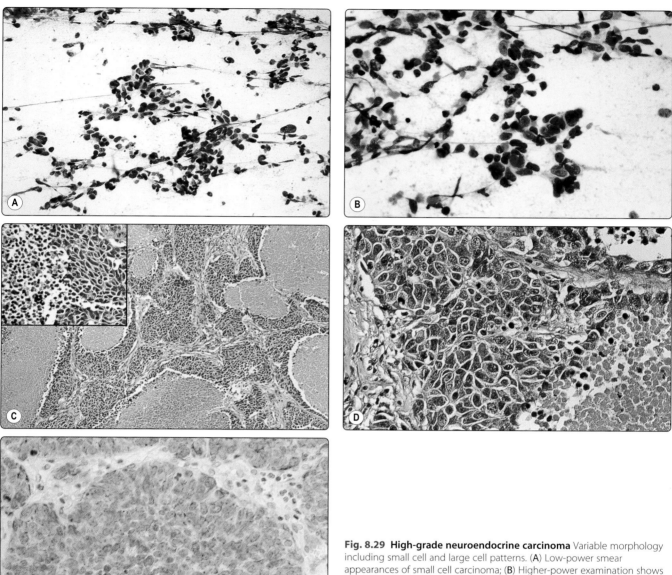

Fig. 8.29 High-grade neuroendocrine carcinoma Variable morphology including small cell and large cell patterns. (**A**) Low-power smear appearances of small cell carcinoma; (**B**) Higher-power examination shows some large cells with prominent nucleoli (**A**, H&E, LP; **B**, H&E, MP). (**C,D**) Tissue sections of resected peripheral stage 1 tumor showing areas of geographic necrosis and a predominance of large cells with prominent nucleoli (**C**, tissue section, H&E, LP, **Inset**, HP; **D**, tissue section, H&E, HP). (**E**) Positive immunostaining for chromogranin in resected specimen (**E**, tissue section, IPOX, HP).

tions, we find it a useful concept to highlight the occasional difficulty in distinguishing between small cell and poorly differentiated non-small cell carcinomas (Figs 8.28 and 8.29). There is overlap in nuclear size between small and large cell carcinomas and a tendency for inexperienced cytologists to include small cell carcinomas with larger than expected nuclei in the non-small cell category. In general, if the nuclear features of a problematical tumor are those of small cell carcinoma – that is, granular chromatin without prominent nucleoli – the neoplasm will usually fall into the small cell carcinoma group histologically, whereas vesicular nuclei with prominent nucleoli would generally be evidence of non-small cell tumor. However, large cell neuroendocrine carcinoma does provide special problems. Our experience is limited but is similar to Yang et al. who described various morphologic patterns in this family of tumors, including small cell-like and mixed small cell/large cell-like FNAC patterns.[37] Cell size is therefore an important criterion and one to be critically evaluated. Tumors with nuclei larger than 2–3 times the diameter of a lymphocyte may be classified as

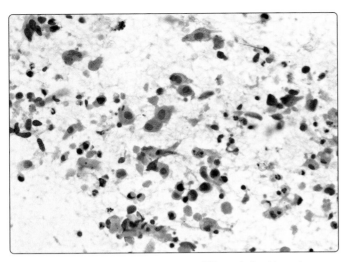

Fig. 8.30 Necrosis simulating squamous differentiation Necrosis, eosinophilia and pyknosis in a metastatic deposit of colonic adenocarcinoma (H&E, HP).

LCNEC histologically, even if nuclear chromatin pattern and other cytological features are similar to those of small cell carcinoma (Fig. 8.29). Our approach is therefore to first come to a diagnosis of 'high-grade neuroendocrine carcinoma' and then to critically examine cell size and morphology to determine the best category – 'small' or 'large'. We do, however, agree with the idea propounded by Marchevsky et al.[89] that the distinction between the two categories may be somewhat artificial in view of the overlap in cell size between the two groups. This is an area which requires close cooperation with oncologists and an acceptance of the limitations of cytological diagnosis. It may be necessary to base management on clinical and staging findings in conjunction with inconclusive cytological tumor typing in some cases.

Cell cohesion is not a feature of small cell cancer and, when present, some caution should be adopted; distinction from small-celled squamous cell carcinoma with minimal cytoplasm may be especially difficult. Basaloid squamous carcinoma, analogous to the tumors described in upper respiratory tract, may rarely occur as a primary lung tumor or more commonly as a metastasis.[229,230] Greater cell cohesion and the presence of even minimal or focal squamous differentiation will be helpful in diagnosis. 'Borderline' tumors exist, where there may be difficulty deciding even histologically between a diagnosis of small cell and non-small cell carcinoma. Combined tumors may occasionally be diagnosed by cytology.[231] Discrepancies between cytological and histological classification can occur because of combined or collision tumors or separate synchronous primaries where cytological sampling may not reveal all tumor elements. Ten percent of predominantly non-small cell tumors have a small cell component histologically.[232] A high percentage of small cell carcinoma cases (28%) are said to show combinations with non-small cell lung cancer, with large cell carcinoma the most common.[233]

A few very large cells are occasionally seen in typical small cell tumors. These usually lie singly and scattered across the smear; however, when clusters of larger cells are present or when these cells are numerous, caution should be exercised.

Combined tumors of mixed small and large cell type are said to have a worse prognosis and to be less sensitive to therapy.[234]

Our approach to problem cases has been to request more biopsy or cytological material for cell block and immunoperoxidase studies. Immunohistochemical demonstration of neuroendocrine differentiation using immunostaining for synaptophysin, chromogranin and CD56 reinforces a diagnosis of small cell carcinoma; however, some studies find up to 25% of small cell carcinomas are negative with all neuroendocrine markers.[235] TTF-1 staining is usually seen in small cell carcinoma (>90% of cases) but is seldom seen in SCC. Strong positive nuclear p63 staining would favor a squamous lesion.[213] A paranuclear CAM 5.2 keratin-positive dot similar to those seen in Merkel cell tumors and some other neuroendocrine tumors is a helpful criterion not seen in other poorly differentiated lung carcinomas. In 'operable' stage I tumors or peripheral tumors, very careful cytological assessment is necessary. Biopsy or lobectomy is advisable when diagnostic difficulty is not resolved by repeated FNB or FOB because some of these tumors will be large cell neuroendocrine carcinomas or atypical carcinoids, best treated by surgery (see Fig. 8.36).[34]

Low-grade carcinomas, e.g. carcinoid or adenoid cystic carcinoma, are also composed of small cells. The regularity and lack of fragility of the former should prevent misdiagnosis. MIB-1 staining also distinguishes low-grade from high-grade neuroendocrine tumors. Lin et al.[236] found that over 50% of nuclei stained in high-grade tumors, compared to less than 25% of nuclei in low-grade tumors. In metastatic adenoid cystic carcinoma in the lung, the appearances are usually easily recognized;[237] however, poorly differentiated adenoid cystic carcinomas can have cytological appearances resembling small cell anaplastic carcinoma. Other lesions such as spindle cell carcinoid, atypical carcinoid and large cell neuroendocrine carcinoma should be considered when the morphology or location of the tumor or clinical features are unusual, for example in small peripheral lesions, polypoid intrabronchial lesions, or in non-smokers.[238]

The cytological distinction of small cell carcinoma from atypical carcinoid is based on prominent nuclear molding and pleomorphism, and abundant mitotic activity and necrosis, including single-cell necrosis, in small cell carcinoma.[35] However, it is safe to heed Frierson's advice that small, peripheral or stage I tumors thought to be small cell carcinoma on cytological or small biopsy histological examination should be further evaluated, because at least some of these would be classified as atypical carcinoids, large cell neuroendocrine carcinomas or 'peripheral small cell carcinoma of lung resembling carcinoid tumor'.[34]

When only small amounts of material are aspirated, artifactual smearing is more common; in these cases the loss of cytoplasm and the disruption of nuclei occurring in other poorly differentiated carcinomas may mimic small cell carcinoma. It is sometimes very difficult to distinguish small cell carcinoma from lymphomas in smears, particularly those of follicular center cell origin with pronounced cell pleomorphism and nuclear irregularity. Cell dispersal together with a rim or a tail of intact cytoplasm in individual cells and a background of round, cytoplasmic fragments staining blue with MGG (lymphoid globules/lymphoglandular bodies) are helpful features in making a diagnosis of lymphoma. Dispersed cells of small cell carcinoma are usually bare nuclei. Some low-grade lymphomas can show pseudomolding due to clustering of the nuclei. Problems can be resolved by immunocytochemistry or flow cytometry.

We have seen one case of metastatic melanoma in which FNB material was virtually indistinguishable from small cell carcinoma. Metastatic neuroendocrine carcinomas from other sites, e.g Merkel cell carcinoma, and high-grade neuroendocrine carcinoma of bladder, cervix, prostate and GIT may also need to be considered.[239]

Large cell carcinoma (Figs 8.31 and 8.32)

Usual findings

- Large, highly pleomorphic cells with abundant cytoplasm,
- Large multilayered fragments of malignant tissue,
- Dispersed cells with a high N:C ratio,
- Tumor giant cells,
- Polymorph ingestion,
- Fragile cytoplasm.

Large cell carcinoma is a diagnosis of exclusion in that cytological features of squamous, glandular or neuroendocrine differentiation are absent in a non-small cell carcinoma.[88] It may be necessary to examine large areas histologically to ensure that differentiation is lacking. This diagnosis can therefore never be established by FNAC alone. Instead, we use the category of poorly differentiated large cell or non-small cell carcinoma to designate non-small cell tumors in which further subtyping is not possible. Many of these prove to be squamous cell carcinoma or adenocarcinoma after histological examination, and the category is virtually eliminated if typing by electron microscopy is used. As previously discussed, attempts should be made to further classify 'non-small cell' carcinoma in cytological specimens using immunohistochemistry. Tumors showing dual differentiation such as adenosquamous carcinoma are uncommonly diagnosed cytologically.[231] Carcinosarcoma (see Fig. 8.54),[240] sarcomatoid/spindle cell carcinoma[241] or blastoma[242] are other considerations in poorly differentiated tumors with a spindle component.

The findings in large cell carcinoma are highly variable; those listed are the common features but have little specific

diagnostic value, and other cytological patterns may occur. For example, in those tumors diagnosed as large cell carcinoma by subsequent histology, there is often a high N:C ratio and cell dispersal may be striking. An appearance resembling melanoma may sometimes be observed. Polymorph ingestion appears to be linked to an abundance of cytoplasm and cell pleomorphism rather than any particular form of differentiation, and virtually any tumor may demonstrate this phenomenon. FNAC findings in lymphoepithelioma-like carcinomas have been described.[243]

Pure giant cell carcinomas have been diagnosed cytologically (Figs. 8.31 and 8.32), although immunostaining is necessary to confirm carcinoma.[244] They are said to be peripheral highly aggressive neoplasms, but occasionally, smaller resectable tumors are encountered.[245]

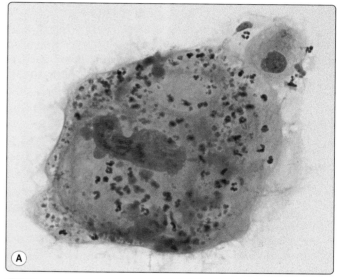

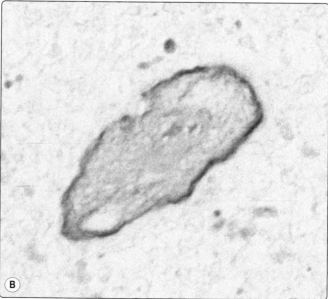

Fig. 8.32 **Giant cell carcinoma** (A) Giant tumor cell with prominent neutrophil ingestion; (B) Positive immunostaining for AE1/AE3 keratins (A, H&E, HP; B, IPOX, HP).

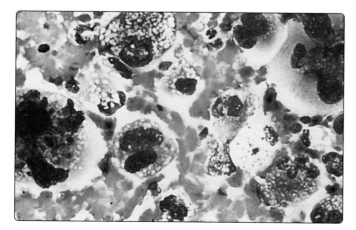

Fig. 8.31 **Giant cell carcinoma** Pure population of multinucleate malignant cells (MGG, HP).

The cytological findings in poorly differentiated squamous cell carcinomas and adenocarcinomas overlap with those of large cell anaplastic carcinoma. In particular, highly eosinophilic cytoplasm simulating squamous differentiation may occur because of necrosis and is a common source of error in classification.

Metastatic neoplasms, especially other anaplastic carcinomas, melanoma, sarcoma and carcinosarcom,a may have similar cytological findings; large cell pulmonary neoplasms may have strikingly similar cytological features to melanoma.

Megakaryocytes, seen in FNB samples of lung either due to contamination from bone marrow, pulmonary capillaries,[166] or extramedullary hematopoiesis,[209] may give rise to suspicion of neoplasia.

Carcinoid tumors (Figs 8.33–8.35)[32–36,238,246,247]

Typical carcinoid[33,35,36,246,247]

Usual findings

- Dispersed cell population with some trabeculae or palisades and small cell clusters,
- A monomorphous population of small neoplastic cells with small amounts of intact cytoplasm,
- Rounded or oval nuclei with stippled/granular nuclear chromatin and small nucleoli,
- Plexiform background of small blood vessels; adherence of cells to vascular cores.

In 'classic' carcinoid tumors, the FNB findings are often distinctive enough to permit diagnosis, with or without ancillary tests such as immunocytochemistry. In contrast, the atypical carcinoids that we have seen were more difficult to classify before resection. Nicholson et al. found similar problems in recognizing a proportion of their neuroendocrine carcinomas, including low- and high-grade tumors, and suggested that 'attention to the presence of loose cell aggregates in a background of singly dispersed cells; feathery patterns created by tumor cells clinging to capillaries; rosette formations; delicate, granular cytoplasm; inconspicuous nucleoli; molding in high-grade tumors; and, most importantly, speckled or dusty chromatin patterns are useful in identifying neuroendocrine differentiation in cytologic specimens'.[36]

In classic carcinoids, the 'neuroendocrine' round or oval nuclei with stippled nuclear chromatin and inconspicuous nucleoli are distinctive; the chromatin pattern may be rather similar to the 'clock face' chromatin of plasma cells (Fig 8.33). Although the cells are not particularly cohesive, small groups and loose clusters are quite common. Dispersed cells usually retain their cytoplasm and the nuclei are rather robust. Even if bare nuclei are prominent, traumatized

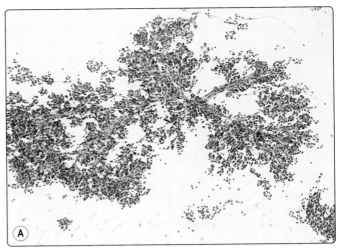

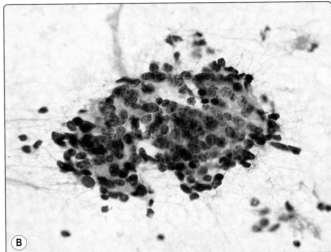

Fig. 8.33 Carcinoid tumor (A) Plexiform aggregate of small blood vessels with adherent tumor cells (Pap, LP); (B) Aggregate of small regular cells with stippled neuroendocrine nuclear chromatin pattern (Pap, HP).

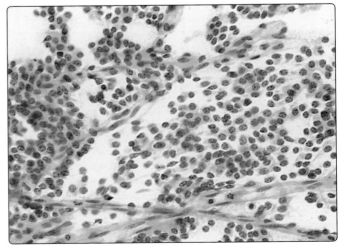

Fig. 8.34 Carcinoid tumor Dispersed regular tumor cells in company with small capillary blood vessels (H&E, HP).

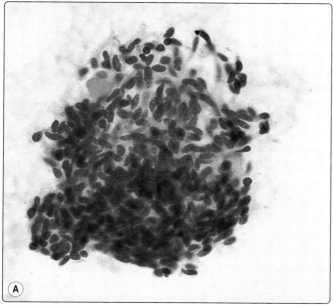

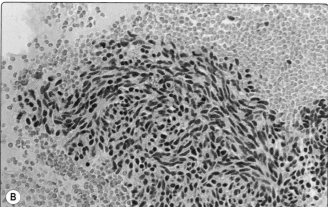

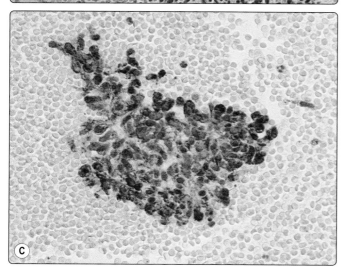

Fig. 8.35 Carcinoid tumor, spindle cell type Tight aggregate of spindle cells with little pleomorphism. Cell block showing no mitotic activity or necrosis. Strong positive immunostaining for synaptophysin (**A**, H&E, HP; **B**, Cell block, H&E, HP; **C**, Cell block, IPOX, HP).

cells, cell debris or streaks of nuclear material are not a feature.

Plexiform leashes of capillaries or venules or vascular cores with adherent tumor cells are a feature of bronchial carcinoids (Fig. 8.33) and are very seldom seen in small cell carcinomas.[246] In Anderson's series, this feature was present in 21 of 23 tumors including spindle and atypical forms.[247] Collins et al. found this feature in only 4 of 19 cases but these were a mixture of pulmonary and metastatic intestinal tumors.[33] In our material, most carcinoids of the classic and atypical type have shown this element when sampled by FNB, in contrast to bronchial brushings where the observation is seldom made.

The amount of cytoplasm varies and we have seen examples with abundant glassy or pale cytoplasm. In a few cases, we observed intracytoplasmic densities corresponding to the intermediate filament 'buttons' seen ultrastructurally and similar to those seen in Merkel cell tumors, salivary small cell carcinomas, some pulmonary small cell carcinomas and mediastinal carcinoids. Intracytoplasmic mucin is present in some cases.

PROBLEMS AND DIFFERENTIAL DIAGNOSIS

- Atypical carcinoid,
- Small cell anaplastic carcinoma,
- Well differentiated adenocarcinoma,
- Pulmonary hamartoma,
- Other small cell tumors; carcinoid variants,
- Metastatic carcinoid,
- Reactive or traumatized bronchiolar epithelium.

Since atypical carcinoid is defined by mitotic activity or necrosis, even when focal, this diagnosis cannot be excluded in cytological material. This may need to be pointed out to clinicians in cytological reports.

Small cell anaplastic carcinoma is usually distinguishable by degree of pleomorphism, absence of cytoplasm, mitotic rate and cell fragility, unless material is minimal or poorly preserved. In small peripheral tumors or apparent stage I small cell tumors, a diagnosis of small cell carcinoma should be given cautiously because some of these tumors may be classified as atypical carcinoids by histopathology.[34] Well-differentiated adenocarcinoma may be composed of very uniform cells; however, the cells are usually much larger, having more abundant cytoplasm and more cohesion than those of carcinoids. Large monolayered sheets are not usually a feature of carcinoids. Some carcinoids of ordinary type can simulate adenocarcinoma and show acinar formations, flat sheets or three-dimensional structures without characteristic neuroendocrine nuclear features.

The epithelial cells of hamartomas may bear some resemblance to carcinoid cells; other small cell lesions such as adenoid cystic carcinoma should also be considered.[247] Bronchiolar cells and plasma cells may resemble neuroendocrine cells.[33,35] Rare tumors such as sclerosing hemangioma resemble carcinoid in smears.[220,223,247,248,249]

Carcinoid variants include those with amyloid stroma, osseous metaplasia, melanin production, psammoma bodies[33] and a papillary structure.

Metastatic carcinoid tumors of, for example, small bowel have similar features to primary tumors of the lung,[33] although, to our knowledge, a plexiform vascular pattern has not yet been detailed in metastases. None of our primary lung tumors has shown the striking red granularity on MGG preparations seen in some small bowel tumors. Immunohistochemistry can aid in the distinction of primary versus metastatic carcinoid; TTF-1 expression is said to be specific for a lung primary in typical and atypical carcinoids and TTF-1-positive carcinoids are predominantly found in a peripheral location.[147,250]

Spindle cell carcinoid[35,238,251]

Peripheral location of a spindle or small cell tumor raises this possibility. We have seen cytological material from several spindle cell carcinoid tumors in which uniformity of nuclear size was a feature which, together with absence of nuclear smearing and background debris, excluded small cell anaplastic carcinoma. Cell clumps were present to a varying degree (Fig. 8.35) and in some smears cell dispersal was more evident. Adherence to proliferative vascular cores led to an appearance much like a vascular tumor in one case. Ultrastructural examination can exclude other spindle cell lesions.[239] One example of a pulmonary tumorlet associated with an opacity on imaging, and providing diagnostic difficulties, has been described.[252] TTF-1 is usually positive in spindle cell carcinoid.[250]

Atypical carcinoid[35,36]

These tumors occupy a position between carcinoid tumors and small cell carcinoma in the spectrum of neuroendocrine carcinomas of lung, in terms of both morphology and biological behavior. In histological material they are defined in the WHO classification as tumors with a carcinoid growth pattern but showing either greater than two mitoses per 2 mm squared, or necrosis.[217,253] They may be associated with pleomorphism/nuclear atypia but this is not a necessary feature for diagnosis. There are examples which are difficult to categorise even when all the tumor is available for histological study, and individual cases may contain mixtures of typical and atypical carcinoid or even foci indistinguishable from small cell carcinoma or large cell neuroendocrine carcinoma. Atypical carcinoid cannot therefore be excluded in FNB samples which suggest carcinoid. We have reviewed cytological material from 15 classic and 11 atypical carcinoids of lung. All the classic tumors were specifically diagnosed; all the atypical cases were recognized as malignant but specific diagnosis was difficult in all. On review, some showed features in common with classic carcinoids such as a combination of cohesive aggregates and dissociation, small to moderate amounts of cytoplasm, neuroendocrine nuclei, trabeculae, palisades and rosettes and plexiform vascularity. Features favoring atypical carcinoid included necrosis and mitotic activity in 5 of 11 cases and more marked pleomorphism in 10 of 11. The absence of widespread molding, smeared fragile nuclei, abundant single-cell necrosis or abundant mitoses and cohesive acinar rosette-like or sheet-like groupings with palisading help exclude small cell carcinoma. Low levels of staining for MIB-1 would also be helpful.[236] Metastatic tumors such as breast carcinoma or prostatic carcinoma may cause differential diagnostic problems.

Adenocarcinoid[35,254,255]

Tumors with prominent glandular differentiation but showing ultrastructural neuroendocrine features are well described and may not be recognizable as being neuroendocrine cytologically.

Large cell neuroendocrine carcinoma
(Fig. 8.36)[36–38,255,256]

Large cell neuroendocrine carcinoma is included as a subtype within the large cell carcinoma category in the WHO classification.[217] This entity is a non-small cell carcinoma without squamous or glandular differentiation, with morphological features suggesting neuroendocrine differentiation, which can be confirmed by immunocytochemistry or EM.[217,255,256] Histologically, cell nesting with peripheral palisading of nuclei, large cells with prominent nucleoli, a high mitotic rate, (>10/10 high-power fields) low nuclear:cytoplasmic ratio, an organoid, trabecular or palisading pattern and large areas of geographic necrosis are features aiding recognition. A 'neuroendocrine' uniformly stippled nuclear chromatin pattern may be present in some tumors. Criteria for recognition by FNB samples have been suggested.[36–38] In our view there is potential for 'misdiagnosis' because of the overlap in appearances between this tumor, small cell carcinoma, atypical carcinoid and basaloid carcinoma. At least some of these carcinomas may have been previously classified as 'intermediate' small cell carcinoma or atypical carcinoids. Yang et al. identified three cytological patterns in a series of 20 cases including small cell-like and mixed small cell and large cell-like tumors. Close attention to nuclear size and prominence of nucleoli are the most important criteria for distinction from small cell carcinoma.[37] In the series of 20 cases reviewed by Wiatrowska, initial diagnoses included a range of non-small cell type tumors. Peripheral palisading of flattened three-dimensional clusters, finely or coarsely granular chromatin and some nuclear molding or crush artifact were features more characteristic of this tumor type than other non-neuroendocrine tumors.[38] TTF-1 positivity has been described in up to 40% of large cell neuroendocrine carcinoma and may be useful in distinguishing this tumor from basaloid squamous carcinoma.[257]

Diffuse idiopathic neuroendocrine cell hyperplasia (DIPNECH)[258,259]

DIPNECH is a putative precursor lesion of carcinoid tumors of the lung.[258,259] As this process may present with multiple nodules radiologically, there is the potential for interpretation as metastatic disease; cytological findings have not yet been reported in the literature.

Primary pulmonary salivary-type neoplasms

Primary pulmonary neoplasms that have similar histological features to those seen in salivary glands are rare. Careful clinical evaluation is necessary to establish the primary pulmonary nature of these tumors and to rule out the possibility of metastasis.[260]

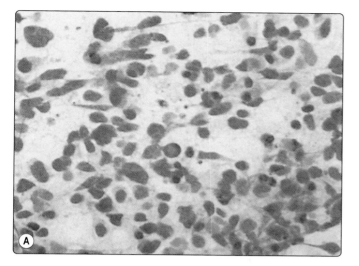

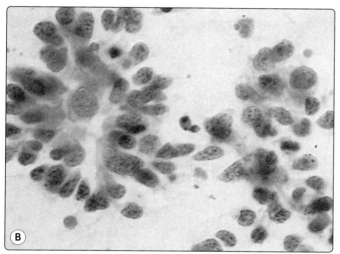

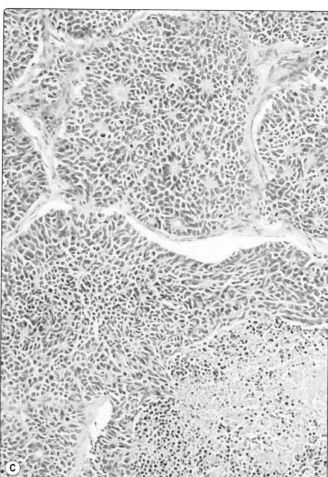

Fig. 8.36 Large cell neuroendocrine carcinoma (A) Cell pattern resembling small cell carcinoma including single-cell necrosis, and pleomorphic fragile cells with minimal cytoplasm (H&E, HP); (B) Cohesive acinar and rosette-like structure (Pap, HP); (C) Sheets, rosette-like structures and foci of confluent necrosis (tissue section; H&E, IP).

Adenoid cystic carcinoma[237,261–264]

Distinction from other small cell malignancies is usually possible if large acellular basement membrane spheres are present (Fig. 8.37). Pitman et al. found diagnosing metastatic tumors to be easily achieved in FNB samples.[237] Ozkara has described FNAC findings of primary pulmonary solid adenoid cystic carcinoma.[261]

Mucoepidermoid carcinoma[214,263,264]

Nguyen[263] describes several low-grade tumors with moderately pleomorphic squamous cells and occasional cytoplasmic mucin vacuoles. Brooks and Baandrup found a mixture of intermediate, squamous and mucin-secreting cells with some spindle cells.[214] Segletes considered the findings to be suggestive in their three cases.[264]

Pleomorphic adenoma[265,266]

This can present as a primary pulmonary lesion or as metastasis from a benign-appearing salivary pleomorphic adenoma; its appearances by FNAC in either setting are identical to those described in the salivary gland.

Bronchial acinic cell carcinoma[267]

Watanabe et al. have described transbronchial FNAC findings in a bronchial acinic cell carcinoma, which were essentially similar to acinic cell carcinomas of the head and neck region.[267]

Other bronchial gland tumors

Cwierczyk et al. described a bronchial oncocytoma.[268] Oncocytomas, carcinoid tumors with oncocytic features and

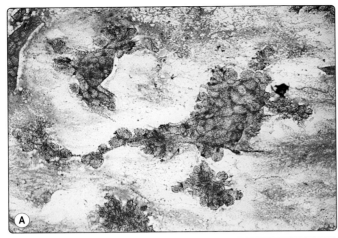

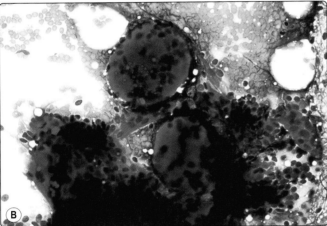

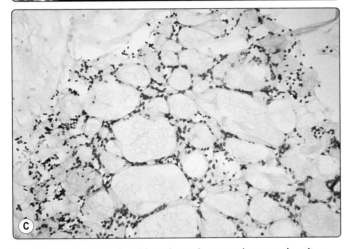

Fig. 8.37 Metastatic adenoid cystic carcinoma; primary oral cavity tumor (A) Large aggregates of tumor cells with a cribriform appearance; (B) Prominent hyaline globules of basement membrane material (A, Pap, LP; B, MGG, HP). (C) Cell block; cribriform pattern around loose basement membrane material (C, Cell block, H&E, IP).

metastatic oncocytic or oxyphilic malignancies may have similar features. An oncocytic carcinoid mimicking granular cell tumor has been described in bronchial brushings.[269] Pulmonary epithelial myoepithelial carcinoma is a rare tumor, usually endobronchial; cytological findings have not yet been described.[270]

Metastatic malignancy[52]

The cytopathologist's approach to the diagnosis of metastases by FNAC is similar to that of the surgical pathologist. Detailed knowledge of the clinical history must be available, together with earlier cytological and histological preparations, for review and comparison with current material. Using these principles, the diagnosis is usually achieved with a high degree of reliability, although some caution is necessary because of the ability of lung carcinoma to mimic other tumors, including sarcomas. Even if the aspirated material cytologically resembles a previous malignancy at another site, a new primary tumor may still be difficult to exclude completely, especially in the case of adenocarcinoma. Perry[57] and Freidman et al.[53] drew attention to the relatively common occurrence of new primary tumors when metastases were suspected clinically. Metastatic carcinoma, particularly from colon and kidney, may show endobronchial growth mimicking primary tumor. Adenocarcinomas from various sites may also show a bronchiolo-alveolar growth pattern along alveolar septa. Specific immunohistochemical stains such as thyroid transcription factor (TTF-1), differential cytokeratins (high and low molecular weight cytokeratins and CK7 versus CK20), CEA, hormone receptors (ER and PR), mammoglobin and gross cystic disease protein (GCDFP-15) may be useful markers in differentiating primary from metastatic carcinoma. Other immunohistochemical stains which are fairly specific for certain malignancies may also be of value, e.g. prostate-specific antigen (PSA), thyroglobulin and S-100, HMB-45 and Melan A for malignant melanoma.

Metastatic colorectal adenocarcinoma

(Figs 8.38–8.40)[271]

Usual findings

- Necrosis,
- Palisading of nuclei; elongated nuclei,
- Large, elongated columnar cells.
- Well-formed gland structures.

Metastatic adenocarcinoma of colorectum usually shows the above features. The 'dirty' necrosis is rather characteristic, with amorphous and granular eosinophilic material and a background of nuclear debris.

We have seen significant necrosis in only one case of well-differentiated, apparently primary carcinoma of the lung and the histological appearances in this case were strikingly similar to those of colonic carcinoma. Palisading of elongated nuclei of columnar cells is often a feature of colonic carcinoma, but not bronchogenic adenocarcinoma. In colonic carcinoma, glandular structures are often evident either within large aggregates (Figs 8.38–8.39) or lying separately; the demonstration of a clear apical space and a brush border in the tumor cells is another characteristic.[271] A CK7/

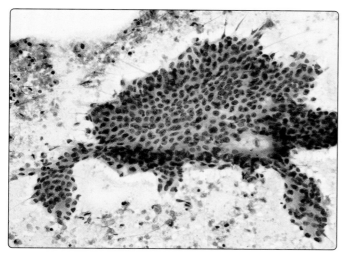

Fig. 8.38 Metastatic colonic carcinoma Well-differentiated tumor with monolayered sheet, gland formation and a background of necrotic tumor (Pap, HP).

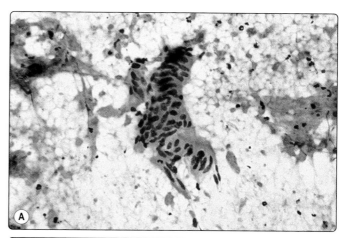

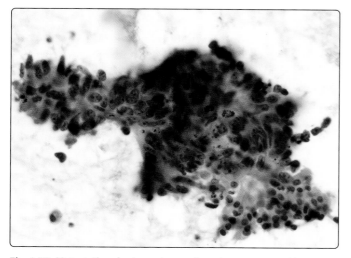

Fig. 8.39 Metastatic colonic carcinoma Complex aggregate with palisading columnar cells, gland openings, mitoses and apoptotic debris (Pap, HP).

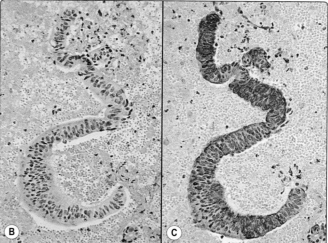

Fig. 8.40 Metastatic colonic carcinoma (A) Strip of tumor tissue with elongated palisaded nuclei, in a background of 'dirty' necrosis; (B) Negative immunostaining for cytokeratin 7 and (C) Strong diffuse cytoplasmic staining for cytokeratin 20 (*right*) in cell-block preparations (A, Pap, MP; B & C, Cell block; IPOX, MP).

TTF-1 negative CK20/ CDX2-positive immunophenotype is generally confirmatory (Fig. 8.40). Some mucinous tumors of the lung may also possess a CK7 negative/CK20 positive phenotype although usually not with such intense or widespread CK20 staining.[272,273] Pulmonary enteric adenocarcinoma can closely resemble colorectal carcinoma but is often CK7 and TTF-1 positive, in addition to being CK20 positive.[142] EM demonstration of junctional complexes and cell surface features of hindgut type in colonic cancer is also helpful.[47]

Other metastatic tumors

Breast carcinoma exhibits variable features including a predominantly dispersed pattern, aggregates, sometimes including cell balls, and linear arrays, the latter mainly in metastatic lobular carcinoma. Positive hormone receptor immunocytochemistry is a valuable criterion (Fig. 8.41). It is worth noting that some clones of estrogen receptor protein can be positive in primary lung adenocarcinoma; SP1 clone has a significantly higher rate of positive estrogen receptor expression in pulmonary adenocarcinomas compared with either 1D5 or 6F11 clones. Caution is required in the use of SP1antibody alone in distinguishing metastatic breast carcinoma from primary pulmonary adenocarcinoma.[141] Recently, cases of primary adenocarcinoma of lung with a TTF-1-negative GCDFP-15-positive phenotype have been described in small samples, further highlighting difficulties in this area.[274]

Renal cell carcinoma presents with aggregates of cells with abundant granular or clear cytoplasm, rounded nuclei and macronucleoli.[275,276] Cytoplasmic clearing may not be evident in smears and is better demonstrated in cell blocks. Immunohistochemistry for RCC antigen and PAX-2 may be

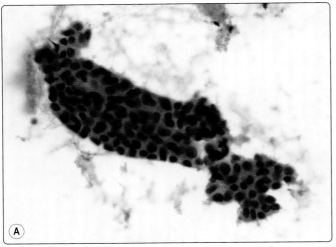

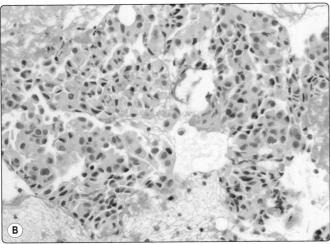

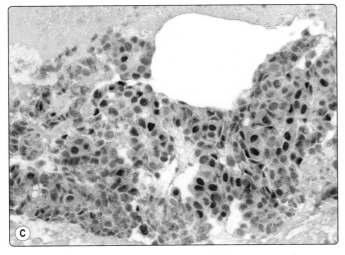

Fig. 8.41 Metastatic breast carcinoma (A) Tubular aggregate of tumor cells (H&E, HP) (B) Cell block; microbiopsy (H&E, HP) (C) Positive nuclear staining for estrogen receptor protein (IPOX, HP).

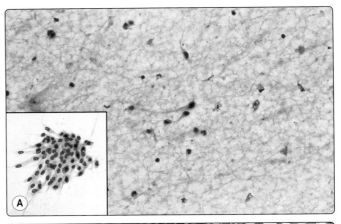

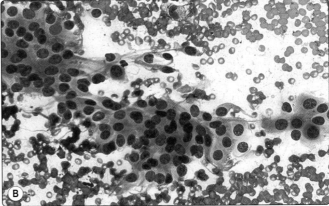

Fig. 8.42 Metastatic urothelial/transitional carcinoma Epithelial cells with strikingly elongated cytoplasmic processes, but without keratinization (**A**, Pap, LP; **Inset**, Pap, HP; **B**, MGG, HP).

of value.[277] Adrenal metastases are essentially similar in appearance to renal cell carcinoma. Benign clear cell ('sugar') tumors may also cause difficulties.[278] Clear cell tumors provide a particular challenge but the site of origin can often be established using cytological features, immunohistochemistry and clinical information.[279] Ancillary studies are valuable in differentiating these and in excluding hepatocellular carcinoma or large cell neuroendocrine carcinoma. Prostatic carcinoma may show rosette-like structures with a central cytoplasmic mass or monolayered sheets similar to BAC; positivity for PSA can be used to confirm the diagnosis. Transitional/urothelial carcinoma (TCC) possesses similar features to primary large cell carcinomas of lung and is difficult to identify specifically, although many cases will be CK7 and CK20 positive, in contrast to large cell carcinomas of lung or adenocarcinomas which are usually CK7 positive and CK20 negative. Johnson and Kini suggest that the most distinctive features were the presence of 'spindled, pyramidal, and/or racquet-shaped malignant cells with eccentric nuclei and cytoplasmic features of both squamous and glandular differentiation including endoplasmic/ectoplasmic interfaces and intracytoplasmic vacuoles', and some glandular features.[280] 'Cercariform' cells, which are non-keratinized cells with a globular body and a cytoplasmic process with a bulbous or fishtail end, have also been suggested as a useful criterion, especially when present in large numbers, and without keratinization (Fig. 8.42).[281,282] Unusual metastases

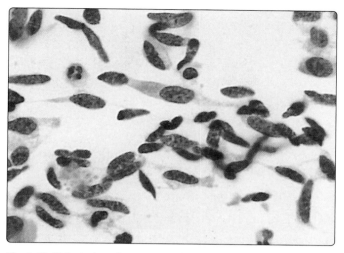

Fig. 8.43 Metastatic melanoma Spindle cell tumor including cells with cytoplasmic tails resembling a mesenchymal neoplasm (H&E, HP).

such as choriocarcinoma,[283] mesothelioma,[284] meningioma,[285] basal cell carcinoma of skin,[286] acinic cell carcinoma of salivary gland,[287] benign giant cell tumor of bone,[288] benign metastasizing leiomyoma,[289] adamantinoma,[290] sacrococcygeal ependymoma[291] and pleomorphic adenoma of salivary gland[265,292] have been diagnosed by FNAC.

Melanoma (Fig. 8.43)[291,292]

An unequivocal diagnosis of metastatic melanoma by FNAC smears alone is difficult without pigment in tumor cells. In Perry's series of 120 cases of melanomas, 60% were amelanotic in FNB samples.[293] Large cell anaplastic carcinomas of lung may exhibit very similar cytological features to melanoma, as may other metastatic carcinomas and sarcomas.

Melanoma cells shed their pigment, which is taken up by surrounding macrophages, often leaving few or no malignant cells containing pigment. Melanin within macrophages cannot be reliably distinguished from lipofuscin or hematoidin using conventional stains. MGG stains all brown pigments blue-black and Fontana-Masson staining is not as reliable in smears. Blaustein reports melanin pigmentation in a metastatic breast carcinoma to the lung.[294] Some carcinoid tumors show intracytoplasmic melanin. S-100, HMB-45 or Melan A staining and negative staining for keratins are prerequisites to FNAC diagnosis of amelanotic melanoma. Spindle cell melanoma should be considered when any spindle cell malignancy is found and especially when there is little or no accompanying connective tissue stroma and when the cells are monotonous or easily dispersed. Some melanomas may closely mimic sarcomas (Fig. 8.43) and possess very fragile, elongated cytoplasmic tails. Other variants include small cell tumors which may resemble lymphoma, small cell carcinoma, or rhabdoid tumors.[295] Metastatic melanoma may have a different immunohistochemical staining profile from the primary melanoma; most commonly, the metastasis will lose Melan A or HMB-45 but occasionally there is loss of S-100 expression.[296] Although rare, it is worth noting that primary melanomas of lung are described and are thought to derive from bronchial melanocytes. FNAC findings are indistinguishable from metastatic melanoma.[297]

Spindle cell lesions of lung
(see Chapter 15)[48,49,298–320]

A wide range of lesions may present as a predominant spindle cell pattern cytologically, including reactive processes, and benign and malignant neoplasms. Benign neural tumors may show alarming nuclear atypia and are a possible source of false-positive diagnoses of malignancy (see also Chapter 15). Although a few false diagnoses were recorded, in the experience of Hummel et al. about 85% of spindle cell lesions may be diagnosed specifically.[298] Nevertheless, in individual cases, definitive diagnosis is often extremely difficult, for example in distinguishing between pleomorphic high-grade sarcoma, melanoma, spindle cell or sarcomatoid carcinoma and mesothelioma. Problems also exist at the low-grade end of the spectrum. Histological material, for example from core biopsies, may be useful; however, we have found immunohistochemistry on small samples, e.g. cell blocks and thin cores, to be unreliable in this setting. Cytogenetics, PCR or FISH studies to detect specific translocations, e.g. t(X;18) of synovial sarcoma, may be diagnostic, however, in the absence of such a specific finding or a known primary elsewhere, resection will usually be required for definitive diagnosis.

Several FNAC series of primary or metastatic sarcomas of lung or pleura have been documented[48,49] and there are reports of metastatic malignant schwannoma,[299,300] malignant fibrous histiocytoma,[301–303] leiomyosarcoma,[304] haemangiopericytoma,[305] dermatofibrosarcoma protruberans,[306] synovial sarcoma,[307] including monophasic forms,[308] metastatic endometrial stromal sarcoma,[309] chondrosarcoma,[310,311] osteosarcoma,[312] epithelioid sarcoma,[313] phyllodes tumor with osteogenesis,[314] and alveolar soft part sarcoma,[315] some presenting for the first time as metastases. Spindle-shaped cells with fragile cytoplasm, which are poorly cohesive and form rather flat cellular aggregates and display many single cells, nuclei with finely granular chromatin and small nucleoli, and bizarre multinucleated cells are all suggested as general indicators of mesenchymal malignancy.[48,49] This contrasts with the three-dimensional cell aggregates and the coarsely granular nuclear chromatin of carcinoma. However, an awareness of the full spectrum of cytological appearances of sarcomas is necessary.

Inflammatory myofibroblastic tumor
(Fig. 8.44)[57,316–320]

Inflammatory pseudotumor is a heterogeneous group of lesions occurring in various organs, and is histologically characterized by fibroblastic and myofibroblastic proliferation, with an inflammatory infiltrate. Inflammatory myofibroblastic tumor is a neoplastic counterpart which often occurs in the lung and which may show aberrant expression of ALK and its gene translocation.[319] ALK positivity by immunohistochemistry has been described in approximately 50% of cases and ALK rearrangement can be detected; however, this has not been documented in FNAC samples. A range of biological behavior is described; most are cured by complete resection; however, recurrences do occur. Up to one-third of patients have fever, weight loss, anemia and elevated ESR. We have seen a few examples of this entity in FNB smears where the smears are often sparsely cellular and contain histiocytes, lymphocytes and plasma cells, sometimes with fibroblastic or ganglion-like cells identified (Fig. 8.44). Hosler et al.[320] found diagnostic accuracy of cytology for IMT to be low (42%). In general, cytological findings are not specific. Histological examination of the whole lesion is necessary for specific diagnosis and to exclude a reaction to other benign or malignant processes.

Other primary lesions of lung

Pulmonary hamartoma (Figs 8.45–8.51)[64,75,90–93,321]

> **CRITERIA FOR DIAGNOSIS**
>
> ◆ Mature cartilage,
> ◆ Myxoid connective tissue/'immature cartilage',
> ◆ Sheets of bronchiolar epithelium,
> ◆ Fat.

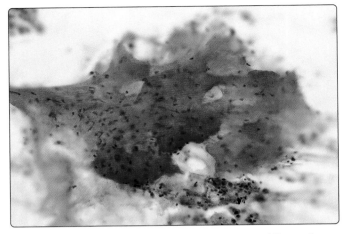

Fig. 8.45 Chondroid hamartoma Fragment of hyaline and fibrocartilage (H&E, MP).

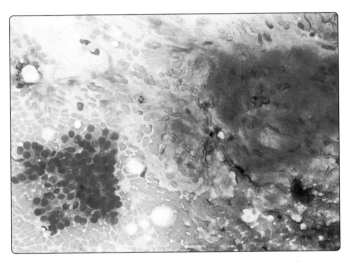

Fig. 8.46 Chondroid hamartoma Magenta chondroid tissue and some bronchiolar epithelial sheets (MGG, HP).

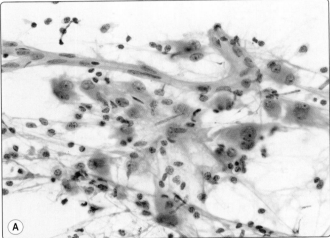

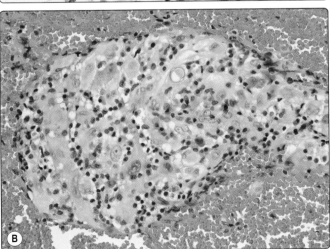

Fig. 8.44 Inflammatory myofibroblastic tumor/pseudotumor (A) Loose collection of large mesenchymal cells with rounded nuclei, binucleation, prominent nucleoli and dense cytoplasm. Background of lymphocytes and plasma cells (Pap, HP). (B) Cell block aggregate of pleomorphic histiocyte-like cells with a background of lymphocytes and plasma cells (H&E, HP).

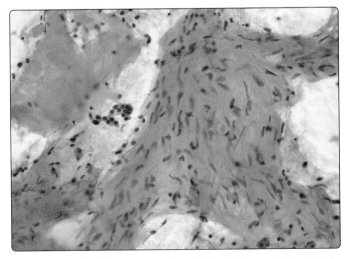

Fig. 8.47 Chondroid hamartoma Chondroid and fibromyxoid tissue and bronchiolar epithelium (H&E, MP).

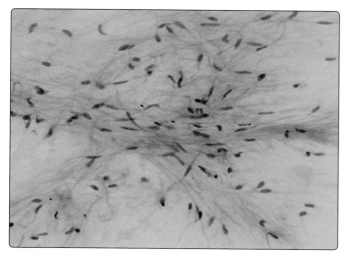

Fig. 8.48 **Chondroid hamartoma** Fibrillar fibromyxoid tissue (Pap, HP).

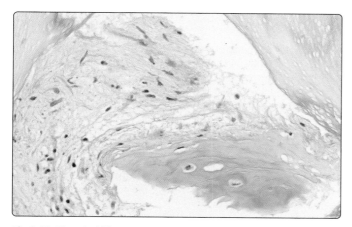

Fig 8.49 **Chondroid hamartoma** Cell block with hyaline cartilage and fibromyxoid tissue (H&E, HP).

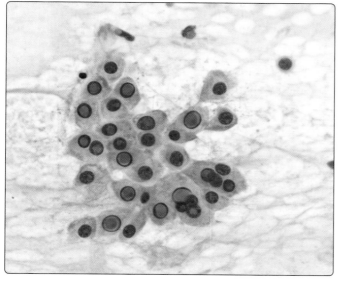

Fig 8.50 **Chondroid hamartoma** Bronchiolar epithelium with prominent intranuclear cytoplasmic inclusions (H&E, HP).

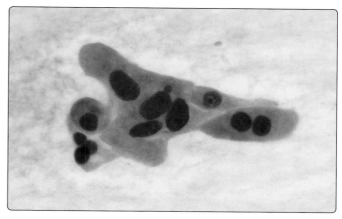

Fig 8.51 **Chondroid hamartoma** Atypical bronchiolar epithelium (H&E, HP).

Pulmonary hamartomas represent approximately 8% of coin lesions[64] and account for 77% of benign lung tumors.[322] Cytogenetic studies support the view that hamartomas are clonal mesenchymal neoplasms.[323] The peripheral location of this lesion and its rounded, well-demarcated border, calcification, or CT densitometric appearances may lead to a strong suspicion of the diagnosis and, if the aspiration needle is deflected by the lesion or bends when inserted into it, this impression is reinforced. Despite its firmness, a good sample of material is often obtained. Aspirated chondroid material may be difficult to express onto the slide. It has an opaque 'glassy' appearance, is firm to gelatinous in consistency and gives a gritty sensation on being smeared. The cytological features correspond to the components of the lesion found in histological sections.

Mature cartilage has a homogeneous waxy, purple-gray appearance in H&E-stained material (Fig. 8.45). It is sparsely cellular; chondrocytes may be seen in lacunae. In contrast, the immature cartilage or myxoid connective tissue has a fibrillar texture (Figs 8.46–8.48). It is pale-staining in H&E, magenta in MGG (Fig. 8.46) and poorly cellular, resembling mucus at first glance. There is, however, a component of spindle cells and the material is usually more cellular than mature cartilage (Fig. 8.49). This material is the most useful diagnostic indicator of hamartoma.[91,93,321] S-100 positivity of the spindle cells has been suggested as an additional criterion.[92,93] The bronchiolar epithelial sheets may show some differences from normal bronchiolar epithelium. There is more abundant pale cytoplasm with less obvious borders; multinucleation may be present. Nuclei are usually rounded, but may be quite large and variable in size (Fig. 8.50). Large intranuclear cytoplasmic inclusions may be evident (Fig. 8.51). Mature fat may or may not be evident. An associated lymphocytic and macrophage component may be present.

In some series, over 90% of hamartomas are recognized by FNAC64,[91,92] and diagnosis by this method is now widely used to justify conservative management,[64] or, in lesions which continue to grow, enucleation rather than lobectomy. Chondromas, which may be seen as part of Carney's triad, are thought to be distinct from pulmonary hamartomas; they consist of well-differentiated cartilage but do not contain fat, spindled cells or entrapped pulmonary epithelium.

PROBLEMS AND DIFFERENTIAL DIAGNOSIS

◆ Tissue from chest wall or bronchus,
◆ Atypia in the epithelial or cartilaginous component,
◆ Difficulty in recognizing myxoid material.

It is possible to aspirate material from the costochondral junctions, especially if a stylet or guide needle is not used and, if found in an aspirate with fat, a diagnosis of hamartoma may be incorrectly assumed.[91]

In one of our cases, the variation in nuclear size and large intranuclear inclusions were sufficient to lead to a false-positive diagnosis of carcinoma; this should not occur if the other components of the lesion are recognized (Figs 8.50 and 8.51), but this is a common source of error in the literature.[75,321]

It may be difficult to discern the myxoid material or cartilage in smears, especially in Pap stains, unless one is familiar with its appearances. The material resembles the myxoid stroma of other entities, for example fibroadenoma of the breast. It is conceivable that other lesions, such as mixed salivary tumors of the bronchial wall, myxoid fibrous neoplasms or amyloidosis,[206] might produce similar cytological pictures but all are extremely rare. The combination of appearances listed above is diagnostic for practical purposes when combined with radiological correlation to support the diagnosis. A 2005 College of American Pathologists Inter-laboratory Comparison Program[321] examining FNB diagnosis of pulmonary hamartoma found the specificity of the interpretation of a benign process was 78%. The false-positive rate was 22%, with the most common false-positive diagnoses being carcinoid tumor, adenocarcinoma, and small cell carcinoma. The overall accuracy for making the correct specific reference diagnosis of pulmonary hamartoma was 26%. The high false-positive rate and the low overall interpretative accuracy was attributed to the failure to recognize the mesenchymal component, which was often subtle on the Papanicolaou-stained slides, and failure to recognize the benign nature of the often very cellular epithelial component. The dominance of the epithelial component was thought to have resulted in incorrectly classifying the lesions as low-grade neoplasms, most often carcinoid tumor and adenocarcinoma.

Sclerosing hemangioma/pneumocytoma[220–223,248,249,324–326]

These lesions are rare benign tumors occurring mainly in middle-aged adults, but are also described in young persons including children. There is a female to male ratio of 5 : 1. They usually present as incidental rounded masses on chest X-ray. The tumors are composed of epithelial elements and stromal-like cells, both of which show positive staining for TTF-1 suggesting a primitive bronchiolar epithelial cell type.[326] The epithelial and stromal cells may or may not show positive staining for keratin and EMA. Sclerosing 'pneumocytoma' is the currently favored terminology.[217] FNAC descriptions include aggregates of epithelial-like cells surrounding a proliferating network of blood vessels or spaces and a stromal-like component,[221,248] and cases with a prominent spindle cell component,[222] or a papillary pattern

in cell block preparations.[221] The epithelial component, when abundant, may lead to an appearance similar to BAC, carcinoid or other tumors. Few cases have been prospectively diagnosed by FNAC. Gal et al.[323] were able to diagnose a case by identifying a two-cell population, both of which were TTF-1 positive. The patient was followed for over 7 years before surgery was necessary due to a growing tumor. Some authors describe frequent progesterone receptor and occasional estrogen receptor positivity in these tumors; however, other studies suggest that hormone receptor positivity is only rarely seen.[325,326]

Figure 8.52 shows our only case. Recognising stromal elements has been suggested as a criterion for avoiding a false-positive diagnosis of BAC. However, we have seen well-differentiated adenocarcinoma with stromal elements resembling those described in sclerosing pneumocytoma. We consider that the clinical and imaging findings, including marked circumscription of the lesion, are likely to provide the best initial clue to a benign diagnosis.

Lymphoid lesions in lung and pleura
(Fig. 8.53)[55,56,302–305]

Non-Hodgkin's lymphomas are uncommon primary lesions and may occur de novo, or in a background of AIDS or pre-existing autoimmune disorders such as Sjögren's syndrome. Primary Hodgkin's lymphoma is rarely seen, but the lung is a common site for relapse. Leukemic infiltration of minor degree is commonly seen in the lung at post-mortem, but clinically significant involvement is rare.

FNAC is valuable in diagnosing focal lung lesions in patients with hematological malignancies. Wong et al., in a series of 67 patients, were able to confirm metastatic lymphoma or leukemia, another lung malignancy or infection, in most samples examined.[327] Confirming spread of lymphoma which has been previously diagnosed may be relatively simple. Recurrent large cell or high-grade lymphomas can usually be diagnosed by FNB, but low-grade lymphomas present more problems. Flow cytometry is an indispensable adjunct (see Chapter 5).[136–138] In Bonfiglio's series, 8 of 10 cases were diagnosed and in two the findings were used as a basis for definitive therapy.[50] In Flint's series of 13 cases of previously diagnosed Hodgkin's disease affecting the lung secondarily, all were diagnosed by FNB.[51] Gattuso et al. found FNAC to be highly specific in diagnosing post-transplant lymphoproliferative disorders.[328] Figure 8.53 shows two examples of NHL seen in our laboratory. The case illustrated in 8.53A was a 17-year-old boy who presented with a 3-month history of viral-like illness, serologically proven EBV infection and multiple hepatic and pulmonary nodules. He also had an orbital lesion with perforation of one eye. The first diagnostic material was from a CT-guided FNB of a lung nodule. The cytological diagnosis was non-Hodgkin's lymphoma of large cell type, excluding infection as a cause. Flow cytometry did not show a clonal population of B cells. A recommendation was made to obtain histological material, and a biopsy of the right eye sclera and orbital tissue gave a diagnosis of EBV-associated angiocentric large B-cell lymphoma. The patient died soon after and autopsy revealed widespread lymphoma involving lung, liver, spleen and bone marrow. The case in Fig. 8.53B was a 55-year-old male with a history of NK/T cell lymphoma involving lung,

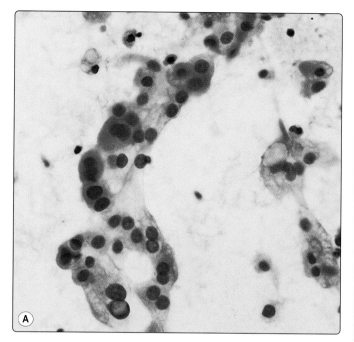

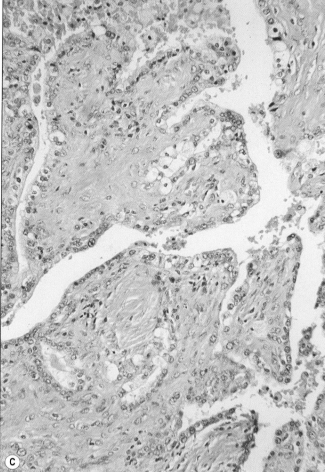

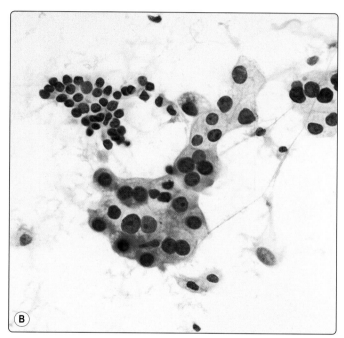

Fig. 8.52 Sclerosing haemangioma/pneumocytoma The patient was a young Asian male with a 10-cm rounded intrapulmonary mass. (**A,B**) Aggregates of moderately pleomorphic glandular epithelial cells including some with prominent intranuclear cytoplasmic inclusions. Note contrast with non-neoplastic bronchiolar cells in **B**; (**C**) Tissue section showing papillary tumor edge with collagenous stromal cores lined by pleomorphic bronchiolar epithelial cells (**A,B**, H&E, HP; **C**, tissue section, MP).

diagnosed on wedge biopsy several years previously. CT-FNA was performed of a recurrent tumor mass in lung. The smears showed a pleomorphic population of dispersed tumor cells consistent with recurrent lymphoma.

PROBLEMS AND DIFFERENTIAL DIAGNOSIS

◆ Dispersed cell pattern of small cell/high-grade neuroendocrine carcinoma,

◆ Pseudomolding and cell aggregation in lymphoma,

◆ Low-grade lymphoproliferative disorders veersus reactive processes.

In small cell carcinoma the neoplastic cells may be dispersed and may resemble a high-grade lymphoma.

Occasional cases of lymphoma demonstrate clustering and even molding of nuclei, resembling small cell carcinoma.

The distinction between lymphoid interstitial pneumonia, reactive lymphoid hyperplasia and low-grade non-Hodgkin's lymphoma may be difficult even in histological sections. Cytological findings are unlikely to be diagnostic because these lesions are all composed of small 'mature' cells. Sending material for flow cytometry or for molecular studies to detect clonal rearrangements of immunoglobulin or T-receptor genes may be helpful.

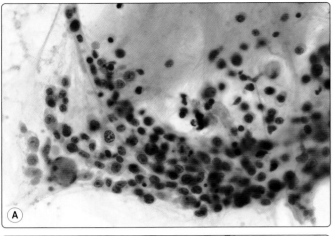

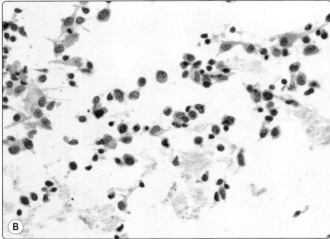

Fig 8.53 High-grade non-Hodgkin's lymphoma (A) Large B-cell lymphoma; (B) NK/T lymphoma (H&E, HP). In general, the diagnosis of even recurrent lymphomas in the lung will require a morphological comparison with the previous tumor and consistent immunophenotyping.

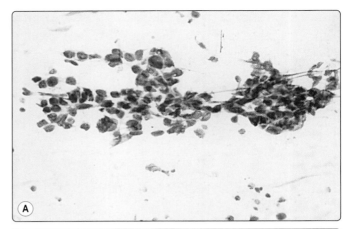

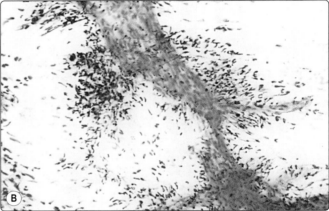

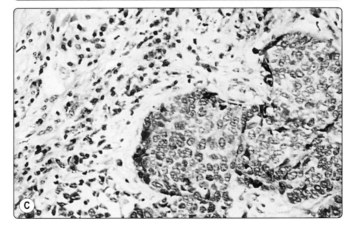

Fig. 8.54 Carcinosarcoma (A) Carcinomatous element (Pap, HP); (B) Mesenchymal elements (Pap, HP); (C) Resection specimen showing biphasic tumor (H&E, MP).

Other rare primary malignancies

Pulmonary blastoma[242,329]

These rare malignant tumors present most commonly in young adult males as peripheral lesions. They resemble fetal lung and show varying mixtures of epithelial tubules with glycogen-rich columnar cells, stromal elements composed of small compact tumor cells and cartilage or smooth or skeletal muscle. FNAC diagnosis is reported, although differentiation from carcinoma or other malignancies is difficult. A related pure epithelial tumor called fetal adenocarcinoma has been described.[330] So-called pleuropulmonary blastoma[331] is a different neoplasm seen in childhood, which lacks an epithelial element, is commonly associated with cystic malformations and has the potential for transformation to multiple sarcomatous types.

Pulmonary carcinosarcoma[240]

These lesions are rare tumors of later decades of life, sometimes presenting as pedunculated lesions of bronchi and

composed of poorly differentiated epithelial and mesenchymal tissue (Fig. 8.54). There is debate over whether they represent sarcomatoid carcinomas or a distinct entity.

Other rare benign tumors[276,332–334]

The literature contains descriptions of benign clear cell tumor,[276] granular cell tumor,[332,333] and primary pulmonary meningioma.[334]

Chest wall and pleura

Malignant mesothelioma (Fig. 8.55)[39–41,43,44,335–338]

Usual findings

- Papillary processes; cell balls or cell clusters (tubulopapillary tumors),
- Flat sheets of epithelial cells with abundant dense cytoplasm and some cell separation (epithelial or biphasic tumors),
- Cytoplasmic vacuolation; intracytoplasmic hyaluronic acid,
- Polygonal cells, dispersed, with binucleation and multinucleation,
- Spindled epithelial cells,
- Spindle cells with a fibroblastic appearance (biphasic or sarcomatous tumors),
- Pleomorphic malignant cells with a multinucleated cell component (anaplastic tumors).

When the clinical findings are consistent and there is a history of asbestos exposure, cytology can offer a clear-cut diagnosis of malignancy and supportive evidence of tumor type. FNAC diagnosis is accepted as a basis for diagnosis and management; material for cell block preparations, immunohistochemistry or ultrastructural studies is necessary for definitive diagnosis.[41,336–338] Membrane-associated EMA staining of epithelial-like cells which also show strong positive nuclear and cytoplasmic staining for calretinin offers strong support of the diagnosis in the correct clinical context. We have now seen FNB material from over 100 cases and the technique is useful for lesions presenting without effusions (approximately 10–15% of pleural cases), in unusual sites such as mediastinum or in metastases.[336] Nevertheless, we try to obtain core biopsy material in all cases where the diagnosis is suspected since this provides a better idea of architecture, and includes spindle cell/mesenchymal elements which are under-represented in smears. In contrast to effusions in which the tumors are mainly epithelial, the full range of growth patterns of malignant mesothelioma is seen in FNAC. The most specific cytological pattern is a combination of sheets of cells, cell groups, dispersed polygonal cells with dense cytoplasm, spindled epithelial cells and spindled fibroblastic cells. Hyaluronic acid vacuoles are commonly seen in FNB specimens; this material has a rather characteristic crumpled membrane-like appearance and stains violet in Pap and magenta in Romanowsky stains.

PROBLEMS AND DIFFERENTIAL DIAGNOSIS

- Well-differentiated adenocarcinoma,
- Other carcinomas/sarcomas,
- Reactive mesothelial proliferation.

A distinction from well-differentiated adenocarcinoma may be difficult, particularly in peripheral lung lesions with a bronchiolo-alveolar growth pattern. Histochemistry and immunohistochemistry are essential for diagnosis. Positive nuclear staining for calretinin and cytoplasmic CK5/6 is a helpful indicator of mesothelioma in the correct context

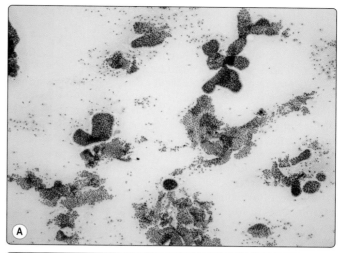
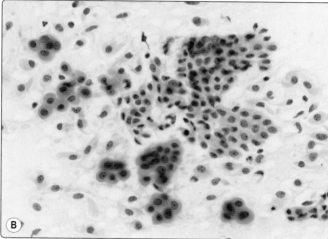
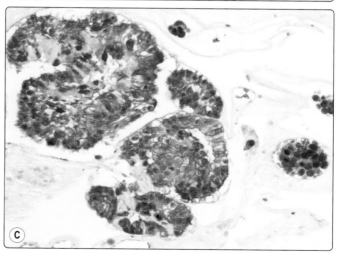

Fig. 8.55 Malignant mesothelioma (A) Highly cellular smear with tubulo-papillary structures, monolayered sheets and some rounded 3-D aggregates (Pap, LP); (B) Sheets and 3-D aggregates with dense cytoplasm (Pap, HP); (C) Cell block; strong nuclear and cytoplasmic staining for calretinin (IPOX, HP).

(Fig. 8.55). The presence of epithelial mucin virtually excludes mesothelioma. Positive staining for glandular markers such as carcinoembryonic antigen (CEA), B72.3, CD15, BerEp4 or TTF-1 also helps to exclude mesothelioma although aberrant staining can be seen in some cases. Vacuoles containing hyaluronic acid display magenta-staining material with MGG, resembling mucin-secreting adenocarcinoma. The prominent finger-like microvilli at the surface of mesothelioma cells, without a glycocalyceal coat, are the most distinctive ultrastructural feature of mesothelioma.

The wide variation in growth patterns and degree of differentiation in mesothelioma is well known and, especially in more poorly differentiated and sarcomatous forms, differentiation from anaplastic epithelial or mesenchymal neoplasms may be impossible with FNAC, even with recourse to electron microscopy and immunostaining. Primary pleural sarcomas are particularly difficult to distinguish from sarcomatous mesothelioma. Similar problems may be encountered in biopsy samples. Correlation with clinical and radiological findings is essential.

Small sheets of reactive mesothelial cells may show some variation in nuclear size and irregularity of nuclear outlines, but differential diagnosis is usually not a problem if one adheres to the rule of making diagnoses of malignancy only when abundant material is present. Strong positive staining for epithelial membrane antigen (EMA) has featured in most malignant mesotheliomas in cell blocks of effusions and pleural biopsy and we have not seen strong widespread mesothelial decoration in reactive conditions. This finding is an extremely useful adjunct in distinguishing between reactive change and malignant mesothelioma.[338,339]

Solitary fibrous tumors (benign; malignant; pleural fibroma) (Fig. 8.56)[340–345]

We have aspirated several solitary fibrous tumors including two histologically malignant metastasizing tumors. Smears were cellular in all cases, including the benign lesions. Many spindle-shaped fibroblastic cells were present; nuclei were moderately pleomorphic and some chromatin clumping was seen, leading to a suspicion of low-grade malignancy in a benign case. Fibers of collagen with adherent spindle cells were included in several cases. Other epithelial-like cells may have been bronchiolar epithelium entrapped within the growing edge of the lesion. In one of the histologically malignant lesions, only material from more benign-appearing areas was aspirated. We recognized only a few of these cases, but believe the combination of a localized, rounded pleural mass yielding dispersed small fibroblastic cells with dark spindled nuclei and background collagen should allow the lesion to be recognized and differentiated from mesothelioma. Cell blocks or core biopsies showing CD34, CD99 and bcl-2 positivity and negative staining for keratins, CEA, EMA and other epithelial markers will also be of value;[344,345] however, resection for histological confirmation is required. Bishop et al.[346] found none of 13 cases of malignant SFT were accurately diagnosed by FNAC, and only six cases were called malignant or suspicious of malignancy. Even in histologically malignant forms, the biological behavior is much less aggressive than malignant tumors of mesothelial origin, and surgical management may be curative; a distinction from mesothelioma or mesenchymal tumors of

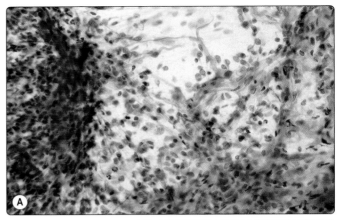
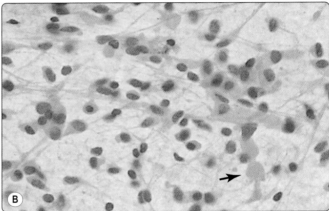
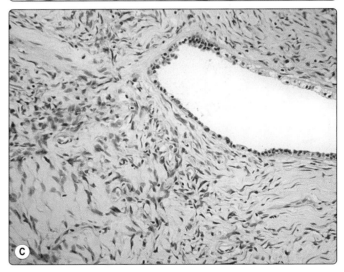

Fig. 8.56 Solitary fibrous tumor of pleura (A) Loose sheets of small oval and elongated spindle fibroblastic cells; (B) Dispersed fibroblastic cells and collagen bundles; (C) Tissue section including a fold lined by mesothelial cells (A, Pap, LP; B, H&E, HP; C, H&E, MP).

other types, such as synovial sarcoma or neural tumors, is important. Occasional intrapulmonary tumors are seen.

Peripheral primitive neuroectodermal tumor/ Ewing's sarcoma (PNET, Askin tumor)[42,347–349]

Peripheral primitive neuroectodermal tumors (PNET) occur mainly in older children and adolescents. They usually involve soft tissue but can extend into pleura and lung. These tumors are further described in Chapters 16 and 17.

Pleural thymoma[350]

Ectopic pleural thymoma can present as solitary or multiple pleural nodules mimicking metastatic disease or mesothelioma; pleural disease may be seen either in association with a thymic mass or in the absence of a thymic mass, where it presumably represents ectopic thymic tissue. The diagnosis can be established by FNB.[350] This is a rare entity but is important to include in the differential diagnosis of an epithelial pleural-based mass, as management and prognosis are very different from mesothelioma or pleural metastasis. We have seen one aspirate from a pleural-based mass which was eventually diagnosed as thymoma by excision; the presence of a mediastinal mass was not appreciated at the time of FNB.

Lesions of rib and soft tissue of chest wall
(see Chapters 15 and 16)[351]

Lesions such as multiple myeloma/plasmacytoma, metastases and occasionally primary sarcomas of bone or soft tissues may present as 'thoracic' tumors and be considered as primary lung lesions clinically. Myeloma can be extremely pleomorphic and mimic epithelial malignancy. Metastases are usually from breast, lung, melanoma or head and neck mucosal tumors.[163] Goel et al. found a very wide range of inflammatory and neoplastic lesions in their series.[351] At least in our experience, granular cell tumor should be kept in mind in the differential diagnosis of this site. We have seen three examples of subcutaneous or deep chest wall lesions, including one malignant tumor with metastases at presentation.

References

1. Menetrier P. Cancer primitif du poumon. Bull Soc Anat 1886;61: 643–7.

2. Dahlgren SE. Aspiration biopsy of intrathoracic tumours. Acta Pathol Microbiol Scand 1967;70:566–76.

3. Levine MS, Weiss JM, Harrell JH, et al. Transthoracic needle aspiration biopsy following negative fiberoptic bronchoscopy in solitary pulmonary nodules. Chest 1988;93:1152–5.

4. Caya JG, Gilles L, Tieu TM, et al. Lung cancer treated on the basis of cytologic findings: an analysis of 112 patients. Diagn Cytopathol 1990;6:313–6.

5. Fraire AE, McLarty JW, Greenberg SD. Changing utilization of cytopathology versus histopathology in the diagnosis of lung cancer. Diagn Cytopathol 1991;7:359–62.

6. Blumenfeld W, Singer M, Glanz S, et al. Fine needle aspiration as the initial modality in malignant lung disease. Diagn Cytopathol 1996;14:268–72.

7. Steffee CH, Segletes LA, Geisinger KR. Changing cytologic and histologic utilisation patterns in the diagnosis of 515 primary lung malignancies. Cancer 1997;81:105–15.

8. Sider L, Davis TM Jr. Hilar masses: evaluation with CT-guided biopsy after negative bronchoscopic examination. Radiology 1987;164:107–9.

9. Knudsen DU, Nielsen SM, Hariri J, et al. Ultrasonographically guided fine needle aspiration biopsy of intrathoracic tumors. Acta Radiol 1996;37:327–31.

10. Fish GD, Stanley JH, Miller KS, et al. Post-biopsy pneumothorax: estimating the risk by chest radiography and pulmonary function tests. Am J Roentgenol 1988;150:71–4.

11. Miller KS, Fish GB, Stanley JH, et al. Prediction of pneumothorax rate in percutaneous needle aspiration of the lung. Chest 1988;93:742–5.

12. Poe RH, Kallay MC. Transthoracic needle biopsy of lung in nonhospitalised patients. Chest 1987;92:676–8.

13. Bhat N, Bhagat P, Pearlman E, et al. Transbronchial needle aspiration biopsy in the diagnosis of pulmonary neoplasms. Diagn Cytopathol 1990;6:14–7.

14. DeCastro FR, Rey A, Caminero J, et al. Transbronchial fine needle aspiration in clinical practice. Cytopathol 1995; 6:22–9.

15. Roche DH, Wilsher ML, Gurley AM. Transtracheal needle aspiration. Diagn Cytopathol 1995;12:106–12.

16. Rodriguez de Castro F, Diaz-Lopez F, Serda GJ, et al. Relevance of training in transbronchial fine needle aspiration technique. Chest 1997;111:103–5.

17. Wang KP, Marsh BR, Summer WR, et al. Transbronchial needle aspiration for diagnosis of lung cancer. Chest 1981;80:48–50.

18. Wang KP. Flexible transbronchial needle aspiration biopsy for histologic specimens. Chest 1985;88:860–3.

19. Xie HB, Cornwell R, Grossman JE, et al. Bronchoscopy-guided transtracheal and transbronchial fine-needle aspiration biopsy: a 5-year institutional review of 111 cases. Diagn Cytopathol 2002;27:276–81.

20. Givens CD Jr, Marini JJ. Transbronchial needle aspiration of a bronchial carcinoid tumour. Chest 1985;88: 152–3.

21. Schenk DA, Bower JH, Bryan CL, et al. Transbronchial needle aspiration

staging of bronchogenic carcinoma. Am Rev Respir Dis 1986;134:146–8.

22. Lorch DG Jr, John JF Jr, Tomlinson JR, et al. Protected transbronchial needle aspiration and protected specimen brush in the diagnosis of pneumonia. Am J Respir Dis 1987;136:565–9.

23. Schwartz AR, Fishman EK, Wang KP. Diagnosis and treatment of bronchogenic cyst using transbronchial needle aspiration. Thorax 1986;41: 326–7.

24. Sun W, Song K, Zervos M, et al. The diagnostic value of endobronchial ultrasound-guided needle biopsy in lung cancer and mediastinal adenopathy. Diagn Cytopathol 2010;38(5):337–42.

25. Johnsrude IS, Silverman JF, Weaver MD, et al. Rapid cytology to decrease pneumothorax incidence after percutaneous biopsy. AJR 1985;144:793–4.

26. Austin JH, Cohen MB. Value of having a cytopathologist present during percutaneous fine needle aspiration biopsy of lung: report of 55 cancer patients and metaanalysis of the literature. Am J Roentgenol 1993;160:175–7.

27. End A, Helbich T, Wisser W, et al. The pulmonary nodule after transplantation. Chest 1995;107: 1317–22.

28. Falguera M, Nogues A, Ruiz-Gonzalez A, et al. Transthoracic needle aspiration in the study of pulmonary infections in patients with HIV. Chest 1994;106: 697–702.

29. Johnston WW. Percutaneous fine needle aspiration biopsy of the lung. A study of 1,015 patients. Acta Cytol 1984;28:218–24.

30. Mitchell ML, King DE, Bonfiglio TA, et al. Pulmonary fine needle aspiration cytopathology. A five year correlation study. Acta Cytol 1984;28:72–6.

31. Pilotti S, Rilke F, Gribaudi G, et al. Transthoracic fine needle aspiration biopsy in pulmonary lesions. Updated results. Acta Cytol 1984;28:225–32.

32. Nguyen GK, Gray JA, Wong EY, et al. Cytodiagnosis of bronchogenic carcinoma and neuroendocrine tumor of the lung by transthoracic fine-needle aspiration. Diagn Cytopathol 2000;23:431–4.

33. Collins BT, Cramer HM. Fine needle aspiration cytology of carcinoid tumors. Acta Cytol 1996;40:695–707.

34. Frierson, HF, Covell JL, Mills SE. Fine needle aspiration cytology of atypical carcinoid of the lung. Acta Cytol 1987;31:471–5.

35. Szyfelbein WM, Ross JS. Carcinoids, atypical carcinoids, and small-cell carcinomas of the lung: differential diagnosis of fine needle aspiration biopsy specimens. Diagn Cytopathol 1988;4:1–8.

36. Nicholson SA, Ryan MR. A review of cytologic findings in neuroendocrine carcinomas including carcinoid tumors with histologic correlation. Cancer 2000;90:148–61.

37. Yang YJ, Steele CT, Ou XL, et al. Diagnosis of high-grade pulmonary neuroendocrine carcinoma by fine-needle aspiration biopsy: nonsmall-cell or small-cell type? Diagn Cytopathol 2001;25:292–300.

38. Wiatrowska BA, Krol J, Zakowski MF. Large-cell neuroendocrine carcinoma of the lung: proposed criteria for cytologic diagnosis. Diagn Cytopathol 2001;24:58–64.

39. Sterrett GF, Whitaker D, Shikin KB, et al. Fine needle aspiration cytology of malignant mesothelioma. Acta Cytol 1987;31:185–93.

40. Kwee W, Utama I. Malignant pleural mesothelioma and thoracic needle biopsy. Chest 1988;93:1115–16.

41. Tao LC. Aspiration biopsy cytology of mesothelioma. Diagn Cytopathol 1989;5:14–21.

42. Kumar PV. Fine needle aspiration cytologic findings in malignant small cell tumor of the thoracopulmonary region (Askin tumor). Acta Cytol 1994;38:702–6.

43. Nguyen GK, Akin MR, Villanueva RR, et al. Cytopathology of malignant mesothelioma of the pleura in fine-needle aspiration biopsy. Diagn Cytopathol 1999;21:253–9.

44. Nguyen GK. Cytopathology of pleural mesotheliomas. Am J Clin Pathol 2000;114(Suppl):S68–81.

45. O'Reilly PE, Brueckner J, Silverman JF. Value of ancillary studies in fine needle aspiration cytology of the lung. Acta Cytol 1994;38:144–50.

46. Saleh H, Masood S. Value of ancillary studies in fine needle aspiration biopsy. Diagn Cytopathol 1995;13:310–15.

47. Davies DC, Russell AJ, Tayar R, et al. Transmission electron microscopy of percutaneous fine needle aspirates from lung: a study of 70 cases. Thorax 1987;42:296–301.

48. Crosby JH, Hoeg K, Hager B. Transthoracic fine needle aspiration of primary and metastatic sarcomas. Diagn Cytopathol 1985;1:221–7.

49. Kim K, Naylor B, Han IH. Fine needle aspiration cytology of sarcomas metastatic to the lung. Acta Cytol 1986;30:688–94.

50. Bonfiglio TA, Dvoretsky PM, Piscioli F, et al. Fine needle aspiration biopsy in the evaluation of lymphoreticular tumors of the thorax. Acta Cytol 1985;29:548–53.

51. Flint A, Kumar NB, Naylor B. Pulmonary Hodgkin's disease. Diagnosis by fine needle aspiration. Acta Cytol 1988;32:221–5.

52. Perry MD, Floyd PB, Johnston WW. Role of fine needle aspiration cytology in medical decision making for metastatic carcinoma of the lungs. Acta Cytol 1984;28:624.

53. Friedman M, Shimaoka K, Fox S, et al. Second malignant tumors detected by needle aspiration cytology. Cancer 1983;52:699–706.

54. Naryshkin S, Young NA. Respiratory cytology: a review of non-neoplastic mimics of malignancy. Diagn Cytopathol 1993;9:89–97.

55. Cagle PT, Kovach M, Ramzy I. Causes of false results in transthoracic fine needle lung aspirates. Acta Cytol 1993;37:16–20.

56. Silverman JF. Inflammatory and neoplastic processes of the lung: differential diagnosis and pitfalls in FNA diagnosis. Diagn Cytopathol 1995;13:448–62.

57. Yi E, Aubry MC. Pulmonary pseudoneoplasms. Arch Pathol Lab Med 2010;134(3):417–26.

58. Shih JY, Gow CH, Yu CJ, et al. Epidermal growth factor receptor mutations in needle biopsy/aspiration samples predict response to gefitinib therapy and survival of patients with advanced nonsmall cell lung cancer. Int J Cancer 2006;118(4):963–9.

59. Sun W, Song K, Zervos M, et al. The diagnostic value of endobronchial ultrasound-guided needle biopsy in lung cancer and mediastinal adenopathy. Diagn Cytopathol 2010;38(5):337–42.

60. Ernst A, Eberhardt R, Krasnik M, et al. Efficacy of endobronchial ultrasound-guided transbronchial needle aspiration of hilar lymph nodes for diagnosing and staging cancer. J Thorac Oncol 2009;4(8):947–50.

61. Ernst A, Anantham D, Eberhardt R, et al. Diagnosis of mediastinal adenopathy-real-time endobronchial ultrasound guided needle aspiration versus mediastinoscopy. J Thorac Oncol 2008;3(6):577–82.

62. Garwood S, Judson MA, Silvestri G, et al. Endobronchial ultrasound for the diagnosis of pulmonary sarcoidosis. Chest 2007;132(4):1298–304.

63. Kennedy MP, Jimenez CA, Bruzzi JF, et al. Endobronchial ultrasound-guided transbronchial needle aspiration in the diagnosis of lymphoma. Thorax 2008;63(4):360–5.

64. de Rooij PD, Meijer S, Calame J, et al. Solitary hamartoma of the lung: is thoracotomy still mandatory? Neth J Surg 1988;40:145–8.

65. Veale D, Gilmartin JJ, Sumerling MD, et al. Prospective evaluation of fine needle aspiration in the diagnosis of lung cancer. Thorax 1988;43:540–4.

66. Raab SS, Slagel DD, Hughes JH, et al. Sensitivity and cost effectiveness of fine needle aspiration with immunocytochemistry. Arch Pathol Lab Med 1997;121:695–700.

67. Capellari JO, Thompson EN, Wallenhaupt SL. Utility of intraoperative fine needle aspiration biopsy in the surgical management of patients with pulmonary masses. Acta Cytol 1994;38:707–10.

68. Layfield LJ, Coogan A, Johnston WW, et al. Transthoracic fine needle aspiration biopsy. Sensitivity in relation to guidance technique and lesion size and location. Acta Cytol 1996;40:687–90.

69. Philips J, Goodman B, Kelly VJ. Percutaneous transthoracic needle biopsy. Pathology 1982;14:211–13.

70. Stanley JH, Fish GD, Andriole JG, et al. Lung lesions; cytologic diagnosis by fine needle biopsy. Radiology 1987;162:389–91.

71. Zarbo J, Fenoglio-Preiser CM. Interinstitutional database for comparison of performance in lung fine needle aspiration cytology. Arch Pathol Lab Med 1992;116:463–70.

72. Afify A, Davila RM. Pulmonary fine needle aspiration biopsy. Assessing the negative diagnosis. Acta Cytol 1999;43:601–4.

73. Mourad WA, Vallieres E, Power RF, et al. Fine needle aspiration cytology of bronchocentric granulomatosis: a potential diagnostic pitfall. Diagn Cytopathol 1996;14: 263–7.

74. Kato H, Konaka C, Kawate N, et al. Percutaneous fine needle cytology for lung cancer diagnosis. Diagn Cytopathol 1986;2:277–83.

75. Curtin CT, Proux J, Davis E. Cartilaginous hamartoma of the lung: a potential pitfall in pulmonary fine

needle aspiration. Acta Cytol 1988;32:764.

76. Chen KTK. Cytodiagnostic pitfalls in pulmonary coccidioidomycosis. Diagn Cytopathol 1995;12:177–80.

77. Tao LC, Weisbrod G, Ritcey EL, et al. False 'false-positive' results in diagnostic cytology. Acta Cytol 1984;28:450–5.

78. Raab SS, Silverman JF. The clinical utility of cytologic typing of lung tumors. Diagn Cytopathol 1994;10:376–82.

79. Delgado PI, Jorda M, Ganjei-Azar P. Small cell carcinoma versus other lung malignancies: diagnosis by fine-needle aspiration cytology. Cancer 2000;90:279–85.

80. Payne CR, Hadfield JW, Stovin PG, et al. Diagnostic accuracy of cytology and biopsy in primary bronchial carcinoma. J Clin Pathol 1981;34:773–8.

81. Bocking A, Klose KC, Kyll HJ, et al. Cytologic versus histologic evaluation of needle biopsy of the lung, hilum and mediastinum. Sensitivity, specificity and tumour typing. Acta Cytol 1995;39:463–71.

82. Sinner WN. Importance and value of a preoperative diagnosis in oat cell carcinoma by radiography and its verification by fine needle biopsy (FNB). Eur J Radiol 1985;5:94–8.

83. Weisbrod L, Cunningham I, Tao LC, et al. Small cell anaplastic carcinoma: cytological-histological correlations from percutaneous fine needle aspiration biopsy. J Can Assoc Radiol 1987;38:204–8.

84. Silverman JF, Finley JL, Park HK, et al. Fine needle aspiration cytology of bronchioloalveolar cell carcinoma of the lung. Acta Cytol 1985;29:887–94.

85. Tao LC, Weisbrod GL, Pearson FG, et al. Cytologic diagnosis of bronchiolo-alveolar carcinoma by fine needle aspiration biopsy. Cancer 1986;57:1565–70.

86. Jarrett DD, Betsill WL. A problem oriented approach regarding the fine needle aspiration cytologic diagnosis of bronchioloalveolar carcinoma of the lung: a comparison of diagnostic criteria with benign lesions mimicking carcinoma. Acta Cytol 1987;31:684.

87. Lozowski W, Hajdu SI. Cytology and immunocytochemistry of bronchiolo-alveolar carcinoma. Acta Cytol 1987;31:717–25.

88. Zusman-Harach SB, Harach HR, Gibbs AR. Cytological features of non-small cell carcinomas of the lung in fine needle aspirates. J Clin Pathol 1991;44:997–1002.

89. Marchevsky AM, Gal AA, Shah S, et al. Morphometry confirms the presence of considerable nuclear size overlap between 'small cells' and 'large cells' in high-grade pulmonary neuroendocrine neoplasms. Am J Clin Pathol 2001;116:466–72.

90. Ramzy I. Pulmonary hamartomas: cytologic appearances of fine needle aspiration biopsy. Acta Cytol 1976;20:15–9.

91. Dunbar F, Leiman G. The aspiration cytology of pulmonary hamartomas. Diagn Cytopathol 1989;5:174–80.

92. Wiatrowska BA, Yazdi HM, Matzinger FR, et al. Fine needle aspiration biopsy of pulmonary hamartomas. Radiologic, cytologic and immunocytochemical study of 15 cases. Acta Cytol 1995;39:1167–74.

93. Wood B, Swarbrick N, Frost F. Diagnosis of pulmonary hamartoma by fine needle biopsy. Acta Cytol 2008;52(4):412–7.

94. Klein JS, Salomon G, Stewart EA. Transthoracic needle biopsy with a coaxially placed 20-gauge cutting needle: results in 122 patients. Radiology 1996;198:715–20.

95. Kim HK, Shin BK, Cho SJ, et al. Transthoracic fine needle aspiration and core biopsy of pulmonary lesions. A study of 296 patients. Acta Cytol 2002;46:1061–8.

96. Tsai IC, Tsai WL, Chen MC, et al. CT-guided core biopsy of lung lesions: a primer. Am J Roentgenol 2009;193(5):1228–35.

97. Yamagami T, Iida S, Kato T, et al. Combining fine-needle aspiration and core biopsy under CT fluoroscopy guidance: a better way to treat patients with lung nodules? Am J Roentgenol 2003;180(3):811–5.

98. Dahlgren SE, Ekstrom P. Aspiration cytology in the diagnosis of pulmonary tuberculosis. Scand J Resp Dis 1972;53:196–201.

99. Bailey TM, Akhtar M, Ashraf Ali M. Fine needle aspiration biopsy in the diagnosis of tuberculosis. Acta Cytol 1985;29:732–6.

100. Robicheaux G, Moinuddin SM, Lee LH. The role of aspiration biopsy cytology in the diagnosis of pulmonary tuberculosis. Am J Clin Pathol 1985;83:719–22.

101. Silverman JF, Marrow HG. Fine needle aspiration cytology of granulomatous diseases of the lung, including nontuberculous mycobacterium infection. Acta Cytol 1985;29:535–41.

102. Rajwanshi A, Bhambbhani S, Das DK. Fine needle aspiration cytology diagnosis of tuberculosis. Diagn Cytopathol 1987;3:13–6.

103. Das DK, Pant CS, Pant JN, et al. Transthoracic (percutaneous) fine needle aspiration cytology diagnosis of pulmonary tuberculosis. Tuber Lung Dis 1995;76:84–9.

104. Batra P, Wallace JM, Ovenfors CO. Efficacy and complications of transthoracic needle biopsy of lung in patients with Pneumocystis carinii pneumonia and AIDS. J Thorac Imaging 1987;2:79–80.

105. Sterrett G, Whitaker D, Glancy J. Fine needle aspiration of lung mediastinum and chest wall. Pathol Annu 1982;17(Part 2):197–228.

106. Sinner WN. Complications of percutaneous transthoracic needle aspiration biopsy. Acta Radiol Diagn (Stockh) 1976;17:813–28.

107. Aberle DR, Gamsu G, Golden JA. Fatal systemic arterial air embolism following lung needle aspiration. Radiology 1987;165:351–3.

108. Cianci P, Posin JP, Shimshak RR, et al. Air embolism complicating percutaneous thin needle biopsy of lung. Chest 1987;92:749–51.

109. Pereira P. A fatal case of cerebral artery gas embolism following fine needle biopsy of the lung. Med J Aust 1993;159:755–71.

110. Kucharczyk W, Weisbrod GI, Cooper JD. Cardiac tamponade as a complication of thin needle aspiration lung biopsy. Chest 1982;82:120–1.

111. Berquist TH, Bailey PB, Cortese DA, et al. Transthoracic needle biopsy. Accuracy and complications in relation to location and type of lesion. Mayo Clin Proc 1980;55:475–81.

112. Sinner WN, Zajicek J. Implantation metastasis after percutaneous transthoracic needle aspiration biopsy. Acta Radiol Diagn (Stockh) 1976;17:473–80.

113. McDonald CF, Baird L. Risk of needle track metastasis after fine needle lung aspiration in lung cancer – a case report. Resp Med 1994;88:631–2.

114. Moloo Z, Finley RJ, Lefcoe MS, et al. Possible spread of bronchogenic carcinoma to the chest wall after a transthoracic fine needle aspiration biopsy. A case report. Acta Cytol 1985;29:167–9.

115. Muller NL, Bergin CJ, Miller RR, et al. Seeding of malignant cells into the needle track after lung and pleural biopsy. J Can Assoc Radiol 1986;37:192–4.

116. Carter RR, Wilson JP, Turner HR, et al. Cutaneous blastomycosis as a complication of transthoracic needle aspiration. Chest 1987;91:917–8.

117. Watts WJ, Green RA. Bacteremia following transbronchial fine needle aspiration. A case report. Chest 1984;85:295.

118. Bhat N, Miller R, Le Riche J, et al. Aspiration biopsy in pulmonary opportunistic infections. Acta Cytol 1977;21:206–9.

119. Das DK, Bhambhani S, Pant CS. Ultrasound guided fine needle aspiration cytology: diagnosis of hydatid disease of the abdomen and thorax. Diagn Cytopathol 1995;12: 173–6.

120. McCorkell SJ. Unintended percutaneous aspiration of pulmonary echinococcal

cysts. Am J Roentgenol 1984;143: 123–6.

121. Arakawa H, Nakajima Y, Kurihawa Y, et al. CT-guided transthoracic needle biopsy: a comparison between automated biopsy gun and fine needle aspiration. Clin Radiol 1996;51:503–6.

122. Mrkve O, Skaarland E, Myking A, et al. Transthoracic fine needle aspiration guided by fluoroscopy: validity and complications with 19 operators. Respiration 1988;53:239–45.

123. Akhtar M, Ashraf Ali M, Huq M, et al. Fine needle biopsy: comparison of cellular yield with and without aspiration. Diagn Cytopathol 1989;5:162–5.

124. Yue X-H, Zheng S-F. Cytologic diagnosis by transthoracic fine needle sampling without aspiration. Acta Cytol 1989;33:805–8.

125. van Sonnenberg E, Casola G, Ho M, et al. Difficult thoracic lesions: CT-guided biopsy experience in 150 cases. Radiology 1988;167:457–61.

126. Knox AM, Fon GT, Orell S. Fine needle aspiration in the chest under CT control. Australas Radiol 1991;35:152–6.

127. Pedersen OM, Aasen TB, Gulsvik A. Fine needle aspiration biopsy of mediastinal and peripheral pulmonary masses guided by real-time sonography. Chest 1986;89:504–8.

128. Pang JA, Tsang V, Hom BL, et al. Ultrasound-guided tissue-core biopsy of thoracic lesions with Trucut and Surecut needles. Chest 1987;91:823–8.

129. Chen CC, Hsu WH, Huang CM, et al. Ultrasound guided fine needle aspiration biopsy of solitary pulmonary nodules. J Clin Ultrasound 1995;23:531–6.

130. Hecht JL, Pinkus JL, Weinstein LJ, et al. The value of thyroid transcription factor-1 in cytologic preparations as a marker for metastatic adenocarcinoma of lung origin. Am J Clin Pathol 2001;116:483–8.

131. Chhieng DC, Cangiarella JF, Zakowski MF, et al. Use of thyroid transcription factor 1, PE-10, and cytokeratins 7 and 20 in discriminating between primary lung carcinomas and metastatic lesions in fine-needle aspiration biopsy specimens. Cancer 2001;93:330–6.

132. Jerome Marson V, Mazieres J, Groussard O, et al. Expression of TTF-1 and cytokeratins in primary and secondary epithelial lung tumours: correlation with histological type and grade. Histopathology 2004;45(2):125–34.

133. Blumenfeld W, Turi GK, Harrison G, et al. Utility of cytokeratin 7 and 20 subset analysis as an aid in the identification of primary site of origin of malignancy in cytologic specimens. Diagn Cytopathol 1999;20:63–6.

134. Johansson L. Histopathologic classification of lung cancer: Relevance of cytokeratin and TTF-1 immunophenotyping. Ann Diagn Pathol 2004;8(5):259–67.

135. Tot T. The value of cytokeratins 20 and 7 in discriminating metastatic adenocarcinomas from pleural mesotheliomas. Cancer 2001;92(10):2727–32.

136. Wakely PE Jr. Aspiration cytopathology of malignant lymphoma: coming of age. Cancer 1999;87:325–45.

137. Young NA, Al-Saleem T. Diagnosis of lymphoma by fine-needle aspiration cytology using the revised European-American classification of lymphoid neoplasms. Cancer 1999;87:325–45.

138. Wakely PE Jr. Fine-needle aspiration cytopathology in diagnosis and classification of malignant lymphoma: accurate and reliable? Diagn Cytopathol 2000;22:120–5.

139. Angeletti C. Application of proteomic technologies to cytologic specimens. A review. Acta Cytol 2003;47:535–44.

140. Rimm DL. Impact of microarray technologies on cytopathology. Overview of technologies and commentary on current and future implications for pathologists and cytopathologists. Acta Cytol 2001;45:111–4.

141. Gomez-Fernandez C, Mejias A, Walker G, et al. Immunohistochemical expression of estrogen receptor in adenocarcinomas of the lung: the antibody factor. Appl Immunohistochem Mol Morphol 2010;18(2):137–41.

142. Inamura K, Satoh Y, Okumura S, et al. Pulmonary adenocarcinomas with enteric differentiation: histologic and immunohistochemical characteristics compared with metastatic colorectal cancers and usual pulmonary adenocarcinomas. Am J Surg Pathol 2005;29(5):660–5.

143. Khayyata S, Yun S, Pasha T, et al. Value of p63 and CK5/6 in distinguishing squamous cell carcinoma from adenocarcinoma in lung fine-needle aspiration specimens. Diagn Cytopathol 2009;37(3):178–83.

144. Kubba LA, McCluggage WG, Liu J, et al. Thyroid transcription factor-1 expression in ovarian epithelial neoplasms. Mod Pathol 2008;21(4):485–90.

145. Siami K, McCluggage WG, Ordonez NG, et al. Thyroid transcription factor-1 expression in endometrial and endocervical adenocarcinomas. Am J Surg Pathol 2007;31(11):1759–63.

146. Xu B, Thong N, Tan D, et al. Expression of thyroid transcription factor-1 in colorectal carcinoma. Appl Immunohistochem Mol Morphol 2010;18(3):244–9.

147. Lin X, Saad RS, Luckasevic TM, et al. Diagnostic value of CDX-2 and TTF-1 expressions in separating metastatic neuroendocrine neoplasms of unknown origin. Appl Immunohistochem Mol Morphol 2007;15(4):407–14.

148. Sehested M, Francis D, Hainau B. Electron microscopy of transthoracic fine needle aspiration biopsies. Acta Pathol Microbiol Immunol Scand (A) 1983;91:457–61.

149. Kurtz SM: Rapid ultrastructural examination of FNAs in the diagnosis of intrathoracic tumours. Diagn Cytopathol 1992;8:289–92.

150. Reyes CV, Jensen JD, Graham G. Adenocarcinoma of the lung: electron microscopy of fine-needle aspiration biopsy specimens – a review of 73 cases. Diagn Cytopathol 1999;20: 257–60.

151. Lynch TJ, Bell DW, Sordella R, et al. Activating mutations in the epidermal growth factor receptor underlying responsiveness of non-small-cell lung cancer to gefitinib. N Engl J Med 2004;350(21):2129–39.

152. Gazdar AF. Activating and resistance mutations of EGFR in non-small-cell lung cancer: role in clinical response to EGFR tyrosine kinase inhibitors. Oncogene 2009;28(Suppl 1): S24–31.

153. Finberg KE, Sequist LV, Joshi VA, et al. Mucinous differentiation correlates with absence of EGFR mutation and presence of KRAS mutation in lung adenocarcinomas with bronchioloalveolar features. J Mol Diagn 2007;9(3):320–6.

154. Smith GD, Chadwick BE, Willmore-Payne C, et al. Detection of epidermal growth factor receptor gene mutations in cytology specimens from patients with non-small cell lung cancer utilising high-resolution melting amplicon analysis. J Clin Pathol 2008;61(4):487–93.

155. Garfield DH, Cadranel J, West HL. Bronchioloalveolar carcinoma: the case for two diseases. Clin Lung Cancer 2008;9(1):24–9.

156. Zheng Z, Chen T, Li X, et al. DNA synthesis and repair genes RRM1 and ERCC1 in lung cancer. N Engl J Med 2007;356(8):800–8.

157. Reynolds C, Obasaju C, Schell MJ, et al. Randomized phase III trial of gemcitabine-based chemotherapy with in situ RRM1 and ERCC1 protein levels for response prediction in non-small-cell lung cancer. J Clin Oncol 2009;27(34):5808–15.

158. Solomon B, Varella-Garcia M, Camidge DR. ALK gene rearrangements: a new therapeutic target in a molecularly defined subset of non-small cell lung cancer. J Thorac Oncol 2009;4(12): 1450–4.

159. Shaw AT, Yeap BY, Mino-Kenudson M, et al. Clinical features and outcome of patients with non-small-cell lung cancer

who harbor EML4-ALK. J Clin Oncol 2009;27(26):4247–53.

160. Johnson DH, Fehrenbacher L, Novotny WF, et al. Randomized phase II trial comparing bevacizumab plus carboplatin and paclitaxel with carboplatin and paclitaxel alone in previously untreated locally advanced or metastatic non-small-cell lung cancer. J Clin Oncol 2004;22(11):2184–91.

161. Pardo J, Martinez-Peñuela AM, Sola JJ, et al. Large cell carcinoma of the lung: an endangered species? Appl Immunohistochem Mol Morphol 2009;17(5):383–92.

162. Idowo MO, Fuller CE, Powers CN. Non-small cell lumg carcinoma; a diagnosis beyond its prime. Pathology Case Reviews 2009;14:199–205.

163. Gattuso P, Castelli M, Reyes AV, et al. Cutaneous and subcutaneous masses of the chest wall: a fine needle-aspiration study. Diagn Cytopathol 1996;15:374–6.

164. Syed S, Zaharopoulos P. Thoracic splenosis diagnosed by fine-needle aspiration cytology: a case report. Diagn Cytopathol 2001;25:321–4.

165. Sarda R, Sproat I, Kurtycz DF, et al. Pulmonary parenchymal splenosis. Diagn Cytopathol 2001;24:352–5.

166. Chen KTK. Megakaryocytes in a fine needle aspirate of the lung. Acta Cytol 1987;31:81–2.

167. Silverman JF. Fine needle aspiration cytology of infectious and inflammatory diseases and other nonneoplastic disorders. In: Kline T, editor. Guides to clinical aspiration biopsy series. New York: Igaku-Shoin; 1991. p. 201.

168. Covell JL, Feldman PS: Fine needle aspiration diagnosis of aspiration pneumonitis (phytopneumonitis). Acta Cytol 1984;38:77–80.

169. Wallace RJ, Cohen A, Awe RJ, et al. Carcinomatous lung abscess. Diagnosis by bronchoscopy and cytopathology. JAMA 1979;242:521–2.

170. Goel MM, Ranjan V, Dhole TN, et al. Polymerase chain reaction vs. conventional diagnosis in fine needle aspirates of tuberculous lymph nodes. Acta Cytol 2001;45:333–40.

171. Gong G, Lee H, Kang GH, et al. Nested PCR for diagnosis of tuberculous lymphadenitis and PCR-SSCP for identification of rifampicin resistance in fine-needle aspirates. Diagn Cytopathol 2002;26:228–31.

172. Pauli G, Pelletier A, Bohner C, et al. Transbronchial needle aspiration in the diagnosis of sarcoidosis. Chest 1984;85:482–4.

173. Vernon SE. Nodular pulmonary sarcoidosis. Diagnosis with fine needle aspiration biopsy. Acta Cytol 1985;29:473–6.

174. Morales CF, Patefield AJ, Strollo PJ, et al. Flexible transbronchial needle aspiration in the diagnosis of sarcoidosis. Chest 1994;106:709.

175. Fekete PS, Campbell WJ Jr, Bernadino ME. Transthoracic needle aspiration biopsy in Wegener's granulomatosis. Morphologic findings in five cases. Acta Cytol 1990;34:155–60.

176. Kaneishi NK, Howell LP, Russell LA, et al. Fine needle aspiration cytology of pulmonary Wegener's granulomatosis with biopsy correlation. A report of three cases. Acta Cytol 1995;39:1094–100.

177. Filho JS, Soares MF, Wal R, et al. Fine-needle aspiration cytology of pulmonary rheumatoid nodule: case report and review of the major cytologic features. Diagn Cytopathol 2002;26:150–3.

178. Lalvani A. Diagnosing tuberculosis infection in the 21st century: new tools to tackle an old enemy. Chest 2007;131(6):1898–906.

179. Whitaker D, Sterrett GF. Cryptococcus neoformans diagnosed by fine needle aspiration cytology of the lung. Acta Cytol 1976;20:105–7.

180. Silverman JF, Johnsrude IS. Fine needle aspiration cytology of granulomatous cryptococcosis of the lung. Acta Cytol 1985;29:157–61.

181. Williamson JD, Silverman JF, Mallak CT, et al. Atypical cytomorphologic appearance of Cryptococcus neoformans. A report of five cases. Acta Cytol 1996;40:363–70.

182. Maygarden SJ, Flanders EL. Mycobacteria can be seen as 'negative images' in cytology smears from patients with acquired immunodeficiency syndrome. Mod Pathol 1989;2:239–43.

183. Silverman JF, Holter JF, Berns LA, et al. Negative images due to clofazimine crystals simulating MAI infection in a bronchoalveolar lavage specimen. Diagn Cytopathol 1993;9:534–9.

184. McCalmont TH, Silverman JF, Geisinger KR. Cytologic diagnosis of aspergillus in cardiac transplantation. Arch Surg 1991;126:394–6.

185. Stanley MW, Deeike M, Knoedler J, et al. Pulmonary mycetomas in immunocompetent patients: diagnosis by fine needle aspiration. Diagn Cytopathol 1992;8:577–9.

186. Fischler DF, Hall GS, Gordon S, et al. Aspergillus in cytology specimens: a review of 45 specimens from 36 patients. Diagn Cytopathol 1997;16:26–30.

187. Walts AE. Pseudallescheria: an underdiagnosed fungus? Diagn Cytopathol 2001;25:153–7.

188. Farley ML, Mabry L, Munoz LA, et al. Crystals occurring in pulmonary cytology specimens. Association with Aspergillus infection. Acta Cytol 1985;29:737–44.

189. Lee SH, Barnes WG, Schaetzel WP. Pulmonary aspergillosis and the importance of oxalate crystal recognition in cytology specimens. Arch Pathol Lab Med 1986;110:1176–9.

190. Hsu C-Y. Cytologic diagnosis of pulmonary cryptococcosis in immunocompromised hosts. Acta Cytol 1993;37:667–72.

191. Kushner YB, Brimo F, Schwartzman K, Auger M. A rare case of pulmonary cryptococcal inflammatory myofibroblastic tumor diagnosed by fine needle aspiration cytology. Diagn Cytopathol 2010;38(6):447–51.

192. Busmanis I, Harney M, Hellyar A. Nocardiosis diagnosed by lung FNA. Acta Cytol 1995;12:56–8.

193. Hajdu SI. Cytology and pathology of acquired immune deficiency syndrome. Acta Cytol 1986;30:599–602.

194. Strigle SM, Gal AA. A review of pulmonary cytopathology in the acquired immunodeficiency syndrome. Diagn Cytopathol 1989;5:44–54.

195. Buchanan AJ, Gupta RK. Cytomegalovirus infection of the lung: cytomorphologic diagnosis by fine needle aspiration cytology. Diagn Cytopathol 1986;2:341–2.

196. Freedman SI, Ang EP, Haley RS. Identification of Coccidioidomycosis of the lung by fine needle aspiration biopsy. Acta Cytol 1986;30:420–4.

197. Raab SS, Silverman JF, Zimmerman KG. Fine needle aspiration biopsy of pulmonary coccidioidomycosis: spectrum of cytology findings in seventy-three patients. Am J Clin Pathol 1993;99:582–7.

198. Rangdaeng S, Alpert LC, Khiyami A, et al. Pulmonary paragonamiasis. Report of a case with diagnosis by fine needle aspiration cytology. Acta Cytol 1992;36:31–6.

199. Kapila K, Verma K. Aspiration cytology diagnosis of echinococcosis. Diagn Cytopathol 1990;6:301–3.

200. Avasthi R, Jain AP, Swaroop K, et al. Bancroftian microfilariasis with pulmonary tuberculosis. Report of a case with diagnosis by fine needle aspiration. Acta Cytol 1991;35:717–8.

201. Hawkins AG, Hsiu JG, Smith RM III, et al. Pulmonary dirofilariasis diagnosed by fine needle aspiration biopsy. A case report. Acta Cytol 1985;29:19–22.

202. Zaman SS, van Hoeven KH, Slott S, et al. Distinction between bronchioloalveolar carcinoma and hyperplastic pulmonary proliferations: a cytologic and morphometric analysis. Diagn Cytopathol 1997;16:396–401.

203. Roggli VL, Johnston WW, Kaminsky DB. Asbestos bodies in fine needle aspirates of the lung. Acta Cytol 1984;28:493–8.

204. Leiman G. Asbestos bodies in pulmonary fine needle aspirates: a more sinister finding than in other

cytologic specimens? Acta Cytol 1986;30:555–6.

205. Silverman JF, Weaver MD, Shaw R, et al. Fine needle aspiration cytology of pulmonary infarct. Acta Cytol 1985;29:162–6.

206. Hsiu JG, Stitik FP, d'Amato NA, et al. Primary amyloidosis presenting as a unilateral hilar mass. Report of a case diagnosed by fine needle aspiration biopsy. Acta Cytol 1986;30:55–8.

207. Dundore PA, Aisner SC, Templeton PA, et al. Nodular pulmonary amyloidosis: diagnosis by fine needle aspiration cytology and a review of the literature. Diagn Cytopathol 1993;9:562–4.

208. Liaw Y-S, Kuo S-H, Yang P-C, et al. Nodular amyloidosis of the lung and the breast mimicking breast carcinoma with pulmonary metastases. Eur Resp J 1995;5:871–3.

209. Walker AN, Feldman PS, Walker GK. Fine needle aspiration of thoracic extramedullary hematopoiesis. Acta Cytol 1983;27:170–2.

210. Lambert C, Gansler T, Mansour KA, et al. Pulmonary malakoplakia diagnosed by fine needle aspiration. A case report. Acta Cytol 1997;41:1833–8.

211. Miller WT Jr, Gupta PK, Grippi MA, et al. Rounded atelectasis: diagnosis by fine-needle aspiration cytology. Diagn Cytopathol 1992;8:617–20.

212. Smith AR, Raab SS, Landreneau RJ, et al. Fine-needle aspiration cytologic features of pseudovascular adenoid squamous-cell carcinoma of the lung. Diagn Cytopathol 1999;21:265–70.

213. Wu M, Wang B, Gil J, et al. p63 and TTF-1 immunostaining. A useful marker panel for distinguishing small cell carcinoma of lung from poorly differentiated squamous cell carcinoma of lung. Am J Clin Pathol 2003;119:696–702.

214. Brooks B, Baandrup U. Peripheral low grade mucoepidermoid carcinoma of the lung – needle aspiration cytodiagnosis and histology. Cytopathol 1992;3:259–65.

215. Mooney EE, Dodd LG, Vollmer RT, et al. Fine needle aspiration biopsy diagnosis of primary bronchial basaloid squamous carcinoma. Diagn Cytopathol 1997;16:187–8.

216. Weichert W, Schewe C, Denkert C, et al. Molecular HPV typing as a diagnostic tool to discriminate primary from metastatic squamous cell carcinoma of the lung. Am J Surg Pathol 2009;33(4):513–20.

217. Travis WD, Brambilla E, Muller-Hemerlink HK, Harris CC, editors. World Health Organization Classification of Tumours. Pathology and Genetics of Tumours of the Lung, Pleura, Thymus and Heart. Lyon: IARC Press: 2004.

218. Ullmann R, Bongiovanni M, Halbwedl I, et al. Is high-grade adenomatous hyperplasia an early bronchioloalveolar adenocarcinoma? J Pathol 2003;201:371–6.

219. Flieder DB. Screen-detected adenocarcinoma of the lung. Practical points for surgical pathologists. Am J Clin Pathol 2003;119(Suppl):S39–57.

220. Wang SE, Nieberg RK. Fine needle aspiration cytology of sclerosing hemangioma of the lung, a mimicker of bronchioloalveolar carcinoma. Acta Cytol 1986;30:51–5.

221. Wojcik EM, Sneige N, Lawrence DD, et al. Fine needle aspiration cytology of sclerosing haemangioma of the lung: case report with immunohistochemical study. Diagn Cytopathol 1993;9:304–9.

222. Kaw YT, Nayak RN. Fine needle biopsy cytology of sclerosing haemangioma of the lung. A case report. Acta Cytol 1993;37:933–7.

223. Gottschalk-Sabag S, Hadas Halpern I, Glick T. Sclerosing hemangioma of lung mimicking carcinoma diagnosed by fine needle aspiration (FNA) cytology. Cytopathol 1995;6:115–20.

224. Gao ZH, Urbanski SJ. The spectrum of pulmonary mucinous cystic neoplasia: a clinicopathologic and immunohistochemical study of ten cases and review of literature. Am J Clin Pathol 2005;124(1):62–70.

225. Moran CA. Mucin-rich tumors of the lung. Adv Anatom Pathol 1995;5:299–305.

226. Davenport RD. Diagnostic value of crush artefact in cytologic specimens. Occurrence in small cell carcinoma of the lung. Acta Cytol 1990;34:502–4.

227. Mullins RK, Thompson SK, Coogan PS, et al. Paranuclear blue inclusions: an aid in the diagnosis of primary and metastatic pulmonary small cell carcinoma. Diagn Cytopathol 1994;10:332–5.

228. Renshaw AA, Voytek TM, Haja J, et al; Cytology Committee, College of American Pathologists. Distinguishing small cell carcinoma from non-small cell carcinoma of the lung: correlating cytologic features and performance in the College of American Pathologists Non-Gynecologic Cytology Program. Arch Pathol Lab Med 2005;129(5):619–23.

229. Dugan JM. Cytologic diagnosis of basal cell (basaloid) carcinoma of the lung. A report of two cases. Acta Cytol 1995;39:539–42.

230. Vesoulis Z. Metastatic laryngeal basaloid squamous cell carcinoma simulating primary small cell carcinoma of the lung on fine needle aspiration lung biopsy. A case report. Acta Cytol 1998;42:783–7.

231. Rollins SD, Genack LJ, Schumann GB. Primary cytodiagnosis of dually differentiated lung cancer by transthoracic fine needle aspiration. Acta Cytol 1988;32:231–4.

232. Roggli VL, Vollmer RT, Greenberg SD, et al. Lung cancer heterogeneity: a blinded and randomized study of 100 consecutive cases. Human Pathol 1985;16:569–79.

233. Nicholson SA, Beasley MB, Brambilla E, et al. Small cell lung carcinoma (SCLC): a clinicopathologic study of 100 cases with surgical specimens. Am J Surg Pathol 2002;26(9):1184–97.

234. Fushimi H, Kukui M, Morino H, et al. Detection of large cell component in small cell carcinoma by combined cytologic and histologic examination and its clinical implication. Cancer 1992;70:599–605.

235. Guinee DG Jr, Fishback NF, Koss MN, et al. The spectrum of immunohistochemical staining of small-cell lung carcinoma in specimens from transbronchial and open-lung biopsies. Am J Clin Pathol 1994;102(4):406–14.

236. Lin O, Olgac S, Green I, et al. Immunohistochemical staining of cytologic smears with MIB-1 helps distinguish low-grade from high-grade neuroendocrine neoplasms. Am J Clin Pathol 2003;120:209–16.

237. Pitman MB, Sherman ME, Black-Schaffer WS. The use of fine-needle aspiration in the diagnosis of metastatic pulmonary adenoid cystic carcinoma. Otolaryngol Head Neck Surg 1991;104:441–7.

238. Craig ID, Finley RJ. Spindle cell carcinoid tumour of lung. Cytologic, histopathologic and ultrastructural features. Acta Cytol 1982;26:495–8.

239. Kaufmann O, Dietel M. Expression of thyroid transcription factor-1 in pulmonary and extrapulmonary small cell carcinomas and other neuroendocrine carcinomas of various primary sites. Histopathology 2000;36(5):415–20.

240. Finley JL, Silverman JF, Dabbs DJ. Fine needle aspiration cytology of pulmonary carcinosarcoma with immunocytochemical and ultrastructural observations. Diagn Cytopathol 1988;14:239–43.

241. Schantz HD, Ramzy I, Tio FO, et al. Metastatic spindle cell carcinoma. Cytologic features and differential diagnosis. Acta Cytol 1985;29:435–41.

242. Cosgrove MM, Chandrasoma PT, Martin SE. Diagnosis of pulmonary blastoma by fine needle aspiration biopsy: cytologic and immunocytochemical findings. Diagn Cytopathol 1991;7:83–7.

243. Chow LT, Chow WH, Tsui WM, et al. Fine-needle aspiration cytologic diagnosis of lymphoepithelioma-like carcinoma of the lung. Report of two

cases with immunohistochemical study. Am J Clin Pathol 1995;103:35–40.

244. Craig ID, Desrosiers P, Lefcoe MS. Giant-cell carcinoma of the lung. A cytologic study. Acta Cytol 1983;27:293–8.

245. Nonomura A, Mizukami Y, Shimizu J, et al. Small giant cell carcinoma of the lung diagnosed preoperatively by transthoracic aspiration cytology. Acta Cytol 1995;39:129–33.

246. Mitchell ML, Parker FP. Capillaries. A cytologic feature of pulmonary carcinoid tumours. Acta Cytol 1991;35:183–5.

247. Anderson C, Ludwig ME, O'Donnell M, et al. Fine needle aspiration cytology of pulmonary carcinoid tumours. Acta Cytol 1990;34:505–10.

248. Chow LT-C, Chan S-K, Chow W-H, et al. Pulmonary sclerosing haemangioma. Report of a case with diagnosis by FNA. Acta Cytol 1992;36:287–92.

249. Krishnamurthy SC, Naresh KN, Soni M, et al. Sclerosing haemangioma of the lung: a potential source of error in fine needle aspiration cytology. Acta Cytol 1994;38:111–12.

250. Du EZ, Goldstraw P, Zacharias J, et al. TTF-1 expression is specific for lung primary in typical and atypical carcinoids: TTF-1-positive carcinoids are predominantly in peripheral location. Hum Pathol 2004 Jul;35(7):825–31.

251. Fekete PS, Cohen C, DeRose PB. Pulmonary spindle cell carcinoid. Needle aspiration biopsy, histologic and immunohistochemical findings. Acta Cytol 1990;34:50–6.

252. Satoh Y, Fujiyama J, Ueno M, et al. High cellular atypia in a pulmonary tumorlet. Report of a case with cytologic findings. Acta Cytol 2000;44:242–6.

253. Travis WD, Rush W, Flieder DB, et al. Survival analysis of 200 pulmonary neuroendocrine tumors with clarification of criteria for atypical carcinoid and its separation from typical carcinoid. Am J Surg Pathol 1998;22(8):934–44.

254. Pilotti S, Rilke F, Lombardi L. Pulmonary carcinoid with glandular features. Report of two cases with positive fine needle aspiration biopsy cytology. Acta Cytol 1983;27:511–4.

255. Nguyen GK, Shnitka TK. Aspiration biopsy cytology of adenocarcinoid tumor of the bronchial tree. Acta Cytol 1986;31:726–30.

256. Travis WD. Lung tumours with neuroendocrine differentiation. Eur J Cancer 2009;45(Suppl 1):251–66.

257. Sturm N, Lantuéjoul S, Laverrière MH, et al. Thyroid transcription factor 1 and cytokeratins 1, 5, 10, 14(34betaE12) expression in basaloid and large-cell neuroendocrine carcinomas of the lung. Hum Pathol 2001;32(9):918–25.

258. Davies SJ, Gosney JR, Hansell DM, et al. Diffuse idiopathic pulmonary neuroendocrine cell hyperplasia: an under-recognised spectrum of disease. Thorax 2007;62(3):248–52.

259. Dacic S. Pulmonary preneoplasia. Arch Pathol Lab Med 2008;132(7):1073–8.

260. Moran CA. Primary salivary gland-type tumors of the lung. Semin Diagn Pathol 1995;12(2):106–22.

261. Ozkara SK, Turan G. Fine needle aspiration cytopathology of primary solid adenoid cystic carcinoma of the lung: a case report. Acta Cytol 2009;53(6):707–10.

262. Smith RC, Amy RW. Adenoid cystic carcinoma metastatic to the lung. Report of a case diagnosed by fine needle aspiration biopsy cytology. Acta Cytol 1985;29:535–6.

263. Nguyen GK. Cytology of bronchial gland carcinoma. Acta Cytol 1988;32:235–9.

264. Segletes LA, Steffee CH, Geisinger KR. Cytology of primary pulmonary mucoepidermoid and adenoid cystic carcinoma. A report of four cases. Acta Cytol 1999;43:1091–7.

265. Zhang Y, Gomez-Fernandez CR, Jorda M, et al. Fine-needle aspiration (FNA) and pleural fluid cytology diagnosis of benign metastasizing pleomorphic adenoma of the parotid gland in the lung: a case report and review of literature. Diagn Cytopathol 2009;37(11):828–31.

266. Ang KL, Dhannapuneni VR, Morgan WE, et al. Primary pulmonary pleomorphic adenoma. An immunohistochemical study and review of the literature. Arch Pathol Lab Med 2003;127(5):621–2.

267. Watanabe K, Ono N, Hoshi T, et al. Fine-needle aspiration cytology of bronchial acinic cell carcinoma: a case report. Diagn Cytopathol 2004;30(5):359–61.

268. Cwierzyk TA, Glasberg SS, Virshup MA, et al. Pulmonary oncocytoma: report of a case with cytologic, histologic and electron microscopic study. Acta Cytol 1985;29:620–3.

269. Ogino S, al-Kaisi N, Abdul-Karim FW. Cytopathology of oncocytic carcinoid tumor of the lung mimicking granular cell tumor. A case report. Acta Cytol 2000;44(2):247–50.

270. Nguyen CV, Suster S, Moran CA. Pulmonary epithelial-myoepithelial carcinoma: a clinicopathologic and immunohistochemical study of 5 cases. Hum Pathol 2009;40(3):366–73.

271. Flint A, Lloyd R. Pulmonary metastases of colonic carcinoma Acta Cytol 1992;36:230–5.

272. Goldstein NS, Thomas M. Mucinous and nonmucinous bronchioloalveolar adenocarcinomas have distinct staining patterns with thyroid transcription factor and cytokeratin 20 antibodies. Am J Clin Pathol 2001;116:319–25.

273. Shah RN, Badve S, Papreddy K, et al. Expression of cytokeratin20 in mucinous bronchioloalveolar carcinoma. Hum Pathol 2002;33(9):915–20.

274. Wang LJ, Greaves WO, Sabo E, et al. GCDFP-15 positive and TTF-1 negative primary lung neoplasms: a tissue microarray study of 381 primary lung tumors. Appl Immunohistochem Mol Morphol 2009;17(6):505–11.

275. Nguyen GK. Fine needle aspiration biopsy cytology of metastatic renal cell carcinoma. Acta Cytol 1988;32:409–14.

276. Saleh H, Masood S, Wynn G, et al. Unsuspected metastatic renal cell carcinoma diagnosed by fine needle aspiration biopsy. A report of four cases with immunocytochemical contributions. Acta Cytol 1994;38:554–61.

277. Gokden N, Gokden M, Phan DC, et al. The utility of PAX-2 in distinguishing metastatic clear cell renal cell carcinoma from its morphologic mimics: an immunohistochemical study with comparison to renal cell carcinoma marker. Am J Surg Pathol 2008;32(10):1462–7.

278. Nguyen GK. Aspiration biopsy cytology of benign clear cell ('sugar') tumour of the lung. Acta Cytol 1989;33:511–5.

279. Hughes JH, Jensen CS, Donnelly AD, et al. The role of fine-needle aspiration cytology in the evaluation of metastatic clear cell tumors. Cancer 1999;87:380–9.

280. Johnson TL, Kini SR. Cytologic features of transitional cell carcinoma. Diagn Cytopathol 1993;9:270–8.

281. Powers CN, Elbadawi A. 'Cercariform' cells: a clue to the cytodiagnosis of transitional cell origin of metastatic neoplasms? Diagn Cytopathol 1995;13:15–21.

282. Hida CA, Gupta PK. Cercariform cells: are they specific for transitional cell carcinoma? Cancer 1999;87:69–74.

283. Craig ID, Shum DT, Desrosiers P, et al. Choriocarcinoma metastatic to the lung: a cytologic study with identification of human choriogonadotropin with an immunoperoxidase technique. Acta Cytol 1983;27:647–50.

284. Ehya H. Cytology of mesothelioma of the tunica vaginalis metastatic to the lung. Acta Cytol 1985;29:79–84.

285. Tao LC. Pulmonary metastases from intracranial meningioma diagnosed by aspiration biopsy cytology. Acta Cytol 1991;35:524–8.

286. Haddad MG, Silverman J. Fine needle aspiration cytology of metastatic basal cell carcinoma of the skin to the lung. Diagn Cytopathol 1994;10:15–9.

287. McCutcheon JM, Mancer K, Dardick I. Acinic cell tumour: a metastasis in the lung diagnosed by electron microscopy

288. van Hoeven KH, Kellogg K, Bavaria JE. Pulmonary metastasis from histologically benign giant cell tumour of bone. Report of a case diagnosed by fine needle aspiration cytology. Acta Cytol 1994;38:412–4.

289. Hafiz MA, Wang K-P, Berkman A. Fine needle aspiration diagnosis of benign metastasising leiomyoma of the lung. A case report. Acta Cytol 1994;38:398–402.

290. Perez-Ordonez B, Bedard YC. Metastatic adamantinoma diagnosed by fine needle aspiration biopsy of the lung. Diagn Cytopathol 1994;10:347–51.

291. Saint Martin GA, Aranha GV, Castelli MJ, et al. Fine needle aspiration diagnosis of metastatic anaplastic sacrococcygeal ependymoma to the lungs. Diagn Cytopathol 1996;15:228–30.

292. Landolt U. Pleomorphic adenoma of the salivary glands metastatic to the lung: diagnosis by FNA cytology. Acta Cytol 1990;34:101–2.

293. Perry MD, Gore M, Seigler HF, et al. Fine needle aspiration biopsy of metastatic melanoma. A morphologic analysis of 174 cases. Acta Cytol 1986;30:385–97.

294. Blaustein RL. Fine needle aspiration of a metastatic breast carcinoma of the lung with melanin pigmentation. Diagn Cytopathol 1990;6:364–5.

295. Slagel DD, Raab SS, Silverman JF. Fine needle aspiration biopsy of metastatic malignant melanoma with 'rhabdoid' features. Frequency, cytologic features, pitfalls and ancillary studies. Acta Cytol 1997;41:1426–30.

296. Zubovits J, Buzney E, Yu L, et al. HMB-45, S-100, NK1/C3, and MART-1 in metastatic melanoma. Hum Pathol 2004;35(2):217–23.

297. Ost D, Joseph C, Sogoloff H, et al. Primary pulmonary melanoma: case report and literature review. Mayo Clin Proc 1999;74(1):62–6.

298. Hummel P, Cangiarella JF, Cohen JM, et al. Transthoracic fine-needle aspiration biopsy of pulmonary spindle cell and mesenchymal lesions: a study of 61 cases. Cancer 2001;93:187–98.

299. Saleh H, Beydoun R, Masood S. Cytology of malignant Schwannoma metastatic to the lung. Report of a case with diagnosis by fine needle aspiration biopsy. Acta Cytol 1993;37:409–12.

300. Silverman J, Weaver MD, Gardner N, et al. Aspiration biopsy cytology of malignant Schwannoma metastatic to the lung. Acta Cytol 1985;29:15–9.

301. Lozowski MS, Mishriki Y, Epstein H. Metastatic malignant fibrous histiocytoma in lung examined by fine needle aspiration: case report and literature review. Acta Cytol 1980;24:350–4.

302. Hsiu JG, Kreuger JK, d'Amato NA, et al. Primary malignant fibrous histiocytoma of the lung. Acta Cytol 1987;31:345–50.

303. Kawahara E, Nakanishi I, Kuroda Y, et al. Fine needle aspiration biopsy of primary malignant fibrous histiocytoma of the lung. Acta Cytol 1988;32:226–30.

304. Krumerman MS. Leiomyosarcoma of the lung: primary cytodiagnosis in two consecutive cases. Acta Cytol 1977;21:103–8.

305. Nickels J, Koivuniemi A. Cytology of malignant haemangiopericytoma. Acta Cytol 1979;23:119–25.

306. Perry MD, Furlong JW, Johnston WW. Fine needle aspiration cytology of metastatic dermatofibrosarcoma protuberans. A case report. Acta Cytol 1986;30:507–12.

307. Kilpatrick SE, Teot LA, Stanley MW, et al. Fine needle aspiration biopsy of synovial sarcoma. A cytomorphologic analysis of primary, recurrent and metastatic tumors. Am J Clin Pathol 1996;106:769–75.

308. Costa I, Lerma E, Esteve E, et al. Aspiration cytology of lung metastasis of monophasic synovial sarcoma. Report of a case. Acta Cytol 1997;41:1289–92.

309. Zaharopoulos P, Wong JY, Lamke CR. Endometrial stromal sarcoma. Cytology of pulmonary metastasis including ultrastructural study. Acta Cytol 1982;26:49–54.

310. Gattuso P, Reddy VB, Castelli MJ. Fine needle aspiration biopsy of paranasal chondrosarcoma metastatic to lung. Acta Cytol 1990;34:102–4.

311. Stanfield B, Powers CN, Desch CE, et al. Fine needle aspiration cytology of an unusual primary lung tumour, chondrosarcoma: a case report. Diagn Cytopathol 1991;7:423–6.

312. Dodd LG, Chai C, McAdams HP, et al. Fine needle aspiration of osteogenic sarcoma metastatic to the lung. A report of four cases. Acta Cytol 1998;42:754–4.

313. Neimann TH, Bottles K. Cytologic diagnosis of metastatic epithelioid sarcoma, a cytologic mimic of squamous cell carcinoma. Am J Clin Pathol 1993;100:171–3.

314. McKenzie CA, Philips J. Malignant phyllodes tumor metastatic to the lung with osteogenic differentiation diagnosed on fine needle aspiration biopsy. A case report. Acta Cytol 2002;46:718–22.

315. Logrono R, Wojtowycz MM, Wunderlich DW, et al. Fine needle aspiration cytology and core biopsy in the diagnosis of alveolar soft part sarcoma presenting with lung metastases. A case report. Acta Cytol 1999;43:464–70.

316. Thunnissen FB, Arends JW, Buchholtz RTF, et al. Fine needle aspiration cytology of inflammatory pseudotumour of the lung (plasma cell granuloma). Report of 4 cases. Acta Cytol 1989;33:917–21.

317. Machicao CN, Sorensen KL, Abdul-Karim FW, et al. Transthoracic fine needle aspiration in inflammatory pseudotumor of the lung. Diagn Cytopathol 1989;5:400–3.

318. Hannah CD, Oliver DH, Liu J. Fine needle aspiration biopsy and immunostaining findings in an aggressive inflammatory myofibroblastic tumor of the lung: a case report. Acta Cytol 2007;51(2):239–43.

319. Gleason BC, Hornick JL. Inflammatory myofibroblastic tumours: where are we now? J Clin Pathol 2008;61(4):428–37.

320. Hosler GA, Steinberg DM, Sheth S, et al. Inflammatory pseudotumor: a diagnostic dilemma in cytopathology. Diagn Cytopathol 2004;31(4):267–70.

321. Hughes JH, Young NA, Wilbur DC, et al.; Cytopathology Resource Committee, College of American Pathologists. Fine-needle aspiration of pulmonary hamartoma: a common source of false-positive diagnoses in the College of American Pathologists Interlaboratory Comparison Program in Nongynecologic Cytology. Arch Pathol Lab Med 2005;129(1):19–22.

322. Arrigoni MG, Woolner LB, Bernatz PE, et al. Benign tumors of the lung. A ten-year surgical experience. J Thorac Cardiovasc Surg 1970;60(4):589–99.

323. Fletcher JA, Longtine J, Wallace K, et al. Cytogenetic and histologic findings in 17 pulmonary chondroid hamartomas: evidence for a pathogenetic relationship with lipomas and leiomyomas. Genes Chromosomes Cancer 1995;12(3):220–3.

324. Gal AA, Nassar VH, Miller JI. Cytopathologic diagnosis of pulmonary sclerosing hemangioma. Diagn Cytopathol 2002;26:163–6.

325. Leong AS, Chan KW, Seneviratne HS. A morphological and immunohistochemical study of 25 cases of so-called sclerosing haemangioma of the lung. Histopathology 1995;27(2):121–8.

326. Devouassoux-Shisheboran M, Hayashi T, Linnoila RI, et al. A clinicopathologic study of 100 cases of pulmonary sclerosing hemangioma with immunohistochemical studies: TTF-1 is expressed in both round and surface cells, suggesting an origin from primitive respiratory epithelium. Am J Surg Pathol 2000;24:906–16.

327. Wong PW, Stefanec T, Brown K, et al. Role of fine-needle aspirates of focal lung lesions in patients with hematologic malignancies. Chest 2002;121:527–32.

328. Gattuso P, Castelli MJ, Peng Y, et al. Post-transplant lymphoproliferative

disorders: a fine needle aspiration study. Diagn Cytopathol 1997;16:392–5.

329. Yokoyama S, Hayashida Y, Nagahama J, et al. Pulmonary blastoma: a case report. Acta Cytol 1992;36:293–7.

330. Lee KG, Cho NH. Fine needle aspiration cytology of a pulmonary adenocarcinoma of fetal type: report of a case with immunohistochemical and ultrastructural studies. Diagn Cytopathol 1991;7:408–14.

331. Gelven PL, Hopkins MA, Green CA, et al. Fine needle aspiration cytology of pleuropulmonary blastoma: case report and review of the literature. Diagn Cytopathol 1997;16:336–40.

332. Husain M, Nguyen GK. Cytopathology of granular-cell tumor of the lung. Diagn Cytopathol 2000;23:294–5.

333. Kintanar EB, Giordano TJ, Thompson NW, et al. Granular-cell tumor of trachea masquerading as Hurthle-cell neoplasm on fine-needle aspirate: a case report. Diagn Cytopathol 2000;22:379–82.

334. Gomez-Aracil V, Mayayo E, Alvira R, et al. Fine needle aspiration cytology of primary pulmonary meningioma associated with minute meningothelial-like nodules. Report of a case with histologic, immunohistochemical and ultrastructural studies. Acta Cytol 2002;46:899–903.

335. Whitaker D, Shilkin KB, Sterrett GF. Cytological appearances of malignant mesothelioma. Malignant mesothelioma. New York: Hemisphere; 1992. pp. 167–82.

336. Whitaker D, Sterrett GF, Shilkin KB. Mesotheliomas. In: Gray W, editor. Diagnostic cytopathology. 2nd ed.

Edinburgh: Churchill Livingstone; 2003.

337. Nguyen GK, Akin MR, Villanueva RR, et al. Cytopathology of malignant mesothelioma of the pleura in fine-needle aspiration biopsy. Diagn Cytopathol 1999;21:253–9.

338. Yu GH, Soma L, Hahn S, et al. Changing clinical course of patients with malignant mesothelioma: implications for FNA cytology and utility of immunocytochemical staining. Diagn Cytopathol 2001;24:322–7.

339. Singh HK, Silverman JF, Berns L, et al. Significance of epithelial membrane antigen in the work-up of problematic serous effusions. Diagn Cytopathol 1995;13:3–7.

340. Dusenbery D, Grimes MM, Frable WJ. Fine needle aspiration cytology of localised fibrous tumor of pleura. Diagn Cytopathol 1992;8:444–50.

341. Caruso RA, LaSpada F, Gaeta M, et al. Report of an intrapulmonary solitary fibrous tumor: fine needle aspiration cytologic findings, clinicopathological and immunocytochemical features. Diagn Cytopathol 1996;14:64–7.

342. Sironi M, Declich P, Di Bella C, et al. Solitary fibrous tumour of the pleura: a cytohistological and immunohistochemical case study. Cytopathol 1996;7:274–8.

343. Ali SZ, Hoon V, Hoda S, et al. Solitary fibrous tumor. A cytologic-histologic study with clinical, radiological and immunohistochemical correlations. Cancer 1997;81:116–21.

344. Apple SK, Nieberg RK, Hirschowitz SL. Fine needle aspiration biopsy of solitary fibrous tumor of the pleura. A report of

two cases with a discussion of diagnostic pitfalls. Acta Cytol 1997;41:1528–33.

345. Clayton AC, Salomao DR, Keeney GL, et al. Solitary fibrous tumor: a study of cytologic features of six cases diagnosed by fine-needle aspiration. Diagn Cytopathol 2001;25:172–6.

346. Bishop JA, Rekhtman N, Chun J, et al. Malignant solitary fibrous tumor: cytopathologic findings and differential diagnosis. Cancer Cytopathol 2010;118(2):83–9.

347. Silverman JF, Berns LA, Holbrook CT, et al. Fine needle aspiration cytology of primitive neuroectodermal tumors. A report of three cases. Acta Cytol 1992;36:543–50.

348. Folpe AL, Hill CE, Parham DM, et al. Immunohistochemical staining of FLI protein expression: A study of 132 round cell tumors with emphasis on CD-99 positive mimics of Ewing's sarcoma / primitive neuroectodermal tumor. Am J Surg Pathol 2000;24:1657.

349. Hummel P, Yang GC, Kumar A, et al. PNET-like features of synovial sarcoma of the lung: a pitfall in the cytologic diagnosis of soft-tissue tumors. Diagn Cytopathol 2001;24:283–8.

350. Kim HS, Lee HJ, Cho SY, et al. Myasthenia gravis in ectopic thymoma presenting as pleural masses. Lung Cancer 2007;57(1):115–7.

351. Goel A, Gupta SK, Dey P, et al. Cytologic spectrum of 227 fine-needle aspiration cases of chest-wall lesions. Diagn Cytopathol 2001;24:384–8.

CHAPTER 9

Mediastinum

Amanda Segal, Felicity A Frost and Kim R Geisinger

CLINICAL ASPECTS

A broad range of mass lesions is found in this site, of which about 40% are malignant. Two major factors in the incidence of different entities are the age of the patient at presentation and the mediastinal compartment in which the mass arose and appears radiographically. Tumors in children are more likely to be neurogenic neoplasms, enterogenous cysts, teratomas, vascular lesions or lymphomas. In adults, the most common mass lesions are metastases and cysts of thymic, pericardial or enteric origin, followed by thymomas, neurogenic tumors, lymphomas and germ cell tumors.[1–3]

Lesions of the anterior/superior mediastinum are more likely to be thymic epithelial neoplasms, thymic cysts, lymphoma, thyroid and parathyroid proliferations and germ cell tumors. Of those in the middle mediastinum, lymphoma and pericardial or bronchogenic cysts predominate. Masses in the posterior mediastinum consist mostly of nerve sheath or neuronal tumors and bronchogenic or enteric cysts.[1–3]

Clinical and laboratory findings may be helpful. For example, such clues include the presence of high levels of circulating human chorionic gonadotrophin (beta-hCG) and alpha-fetoprotein in certain germ cell tumors, myasthenia gravis (although recall that myasthenia is more commonly associated with follicular hyperplasia of the thymus), red cell aplasia, hypogammaglobulinemia in thymoma, and Cushing's syndrome in carcinoids.[1–3]

The mediastinum is a common site for metastases, especially from the lung, and these are far more frequent than primary malignancies. Accordingly, the specific diagnosis of primary thymic carcinoma, neuroendocrine carcinomas and germ cell neoplasms can only be made after exclusion of tumors derived from other sites.

Most lesions are illustrated in other chapters.

The place of FNAC in the investigative sequence

Fine needle aspiration has long been used for the confirmation of metastatic disease and is increasingly accepted as the basis for the management of primary mediastinal malignancies. After imaging, FNB is generally the first-line diagnostic method, although some suggest that core biopsy gives higher rates of specific tumor typing for lymphoma, thymoma and neural tumors (at the cost of lower sensitivity).[4,5] Mediastinoscopy and open thoracotomy and biopsy are still necessary for some primary lesions, particularly Hodgkin lymphoma, rare lesions such as sarcoma where architectural features may be necessary for a fully specific diagnosis or where the initial material is insufficient for immunochemistry, ultrastructure, cytogenetics or molecular analysis, although all of these techniques may be applied to material obtained by FNB. Endoscopic ultrasound (EUS) guided FNB via the transoesophageal or transbronchial routes has become an indispensable method of identifying lymph node metastases in lung cancer diagnosis and staging, and in mediastinal lesions out of the reach of transbronchial or transtracheal sampling.[6–10] Occasionally we have experienced difficulty in verifying the exact site of origin of malignant cells in such specimens as a result of contamination of the sample by malignancy derived from the primary tumor in bronchus or esophagus,[11] despite the use of stilettes. This may limit the use of the technique for staging in some cases. However, one good rule of thumb is that a true metastasis is supported when one microscopically witnesses an intimate admixture of malignant cells and reactive lymphoid elements, especially germinal center fragments.

The selection of cases for EUS-FNB has been the subject of recent study. Eltoum et al. suggest that careful evaluation of pre-test probability of malignancy may help in deciding which patients are likely to benefit from EUS-FNB.[12]

Mediastinal infections are amenable to diagnosis by FNB,[13] as is sarcoidosis.[14]

Accuracy of diagnosis

Most cancers will be diagnosed as malignant, and accurate tumor typing is often possible.[15–37] For example, a diagnosis of a specific germ cell tumor can be achieved with clinical data and conventional cytomorphology supplemented with a small panel of antibodies.[25,36] For example, whereas germinomas yield a highly characteristic cytologic picture, embryonal and endodermal sinus carcinomas are less specific-appearing.

©2012 Elsevier Ltd
DOI: 10.1016/B978-0-7020-3151-9.00009-8

Thymic epithelial neoplasms may prove very challenging, especially when the tumor is lymphocyte rich. The admixture of cytologically bland epithelial cells and reactive lymphoid cells is typical of the mixed thymomas. With pure epithelial tumors, the recognition of relatively benign nuclei in epithelial-appearing cells and the high smear cellularity in the proper clinical context is often sufficient, especially if supported by the results of ancillary testing. Lymphocyte-rich tumors may prove quite challenging, as discussed later. The distinction of benign and invasive thymomas cannot be made on cytomorphology alone. What the radiologist and especially the surgeon have to say is crucial. Thymic carcinomas are rare, have the features of obvious epithelial malignancy, and require accurate clinical data, often aided by the addition of certain ancillary procedures.

It is often difficult to obtain material from sclerotic lesions such as nodular sclerosing Hodgkin lymphoma by fine needle alone, but a combination of cytology and cell blocks or thin core sampling can give diagnostic material.[37] For the non-Hodgkin lymphomas, a specific diagnosis is possible for many lymphomas using a combination of cytomorphology, immunophenotyping by either flow cytometry or immunochemistry on cytospins, cell blocks or thin cores, and at times genetic and cytogenetic tests.[38]

Powers et al.[25] reported a large multi-institutional study of 189 FNA cases with a sensitivity of 87% and a positive predictive value of 97% for a diagnosis of neoplasm. Metastatic small cell carcinoma was the commonest neoplasm, followed by lymphoma and thymoma as the commonest primary tumors. Singh et al.[39] reviewed material from the same institutions, looking specifically at diagnostic pitfalls including 12 cases with discordant cytology and follow-up histology. These included small cell carcinoma resembling lymphoma, Hodgkin lymphoma and large cell lymphoma with prominent spindle cell components suggesting a connective tissue neoplasm, large cell lymphoma diagnosed as Hodgkin lymphoma, thymoma resembling large cell lymphoma, clear cell adenocarcinoma where the possibility of germ cell tumor was raised, thymic carcinoma with insufficient tissue to distinguish from benign thymoma, ectopic thyroid resembling metastatic carcinoma or carcinoid, and a breast carcinoma with a squamous appearance. Sparse cellularity was a contributing factor in most cases and the recommendation for biopsy for definitive typing was often made. Assaad et al. reviewed the results of 157 CT-FNB and were able to make definitive diagnoses in 82% of cases with a high concordance with subsequent histological diagnoses.[40] Geisinger reviewed the range of pitfalls and problems which may be found in cytodiagnosis in this site.[41]

Khan et al. showed 66% sensitivity in the diagnosis of tuberculosis compared with 20% for fibreoptic bronchoscopy.[13]

Complications

The complications of aspiration of this site are no more frequent than in FNA of the lung. Even when superior vena caval obstruction is present, aspiration appears to be very safe, and is the procedure of choice.[16,17,22,24] CT has particular value in this site, as it can localize the needle tip within the lesion far better than fluoroscopy,[16,17] and thus rare complications such as cardiac tamponade can be avoided. Prior CT scanning is used to exclude aneurysm and delineate relationships with adjacent structures, including large vessels. Endoscopic ultrasound (EUS) guided FNA by the transoesophageal and transbronchial routes has further reduced the risk of bleeding or other complications.[7] Nevertheless, as with all deep aspirates, there may be complications. Von Bartheid et al. documented a mediastinal-oesophageal fistula after FNB of TB.[42] Aerts et al. reported a case of mediastinitis after puncture of a necrotic metastatic malignancy in a node.[43] Doi et al. describe needle track tumor implantation in the oesophageal wall after EUS. The clinical background of each case must be considered before embarking on the procedure.[44]

Technical considerations

Obtaining material

Direct FNB is carried out using fluoroscopic, ultrasound[45] or CT guidance, including transthoracic[46] and suprasternal[47] approaches. Transbronchial or transcarinal FNB is especially useful in diagnosing and staging metastatic disease, but may also reveal primary lesions.[7–9,47–50] Endoscopic ultrasound guided FNB has rapidly become an essential tool in the staging of lung carcinomas because of the precision with which needles can be directed into nodal metastases.[7–9] It may be used by transoesophageal or transbronchial routes.[7–9] Mediastinal cystography yields a strong guide to the nature of cysts.[51] Fibrosis and non-specific chronic inflammation sometimes prevent adequate sampling and even mediastinoscopy may not be successful. However, we have found FNA samples to be better than core biopsies on numerous occasions and believe this should be the first-line method, with supplemental material for other tests being based on initial cytological assessment. The thin needle may track into cellular areas better than cores and samples material over a wider area. With the pathologist at the procedure, FNB and core biopsy become complementary. One can evaluate touch preparations of cores at the time of procurement to assess their adequacy, and even assist in diagnosis.

Ancillary testing (Table 9.1)

Our approach to diagnosis is similar to that in other deep sites. The pathologist is present at the aspirate with a microscope to confirm adequacy of material and to prepare for appropriate ancillary studies. We rely particularly on cell-block preparations and immunocytochemistry due to the extraordinary variability of neoplasms of this site; cytological features alone are often not sufficient for the specific diagnosis of some primary tumors. Either repeated aspiration passes or core biopsy using automatic sampling devices is a very useful way of obtaining additional material for ancillary tests and/or for architectural analysis. Neill and Silverman[52] and Taccagni et al.[53] emphasized the value of ultrastructural diagnosis, particularly for thymoma, germ cell tumors, carcinoid tumors and small cell carcinoma. However, today EM is being supplanted by immunophenotyping due to the expense of EM, the greater sampling error with EM, and the

Table 9.1 General outline of ancillary tests in the differential diagnosis of mediastinal tumours[1-3,76]

Tumor	Immunophenotype	Ultrastructure	Comments; other features
Small cell carcinoma	CK+, CEA+, synaptophysin+, chromogranin+, CD57+, CD56+	Sparse dense core neurosecretory granules	SIADH, Eaton-Lambert myasthenic syndrome
Large cell carcinoma	CK+, CD45−, S-100−	Primitive cell junctions; secretory activity or tonofilaments	Note: Some carcinomas have elevated serum markers, but not to the levels in germ cell tumors
Bronchogenic adenocarcinoma	CK7+, CK20−, TTF-1+		
BAC	TTF-1, surfactant protein	Surfactant membrane whorls	
Other metastases	CK7− CK20+ CDX2+ (colon), ER+PgR+GCDFP+ CEA14+ Mammaglobin+(breast), S-100+ HMB-45+ MART-1+ (melanoma), PSA, thyroglobulin	Glycocalyx, terminal rootlets complex junctions, secretory, granules (colon)	
Mesothelioma	CEA−, BER-EP4−, CD15−, B72.3−, EMA+ (membrane) calretinin+,CK5/6+, mesothelin +, HBME1+, thrombomodulin+	Long branching microvilli, absent glycocalyx	
Thymoma (invasive and encapsulated)	CK+ (epithelial cells CD20+; CD57+)	Desmosomal junctions, branching tonofilaments, elongated cell processes and hypogammaglobulinaemia, basal lamina	Myasthenia gravis in 50%; red cell aplasia; autoimmune disease, leukemias
Thymic carcinoma	CK+, CD5+ (some CEA+, B72.3+, CD57+, CD117, CD205, Foxn As above,		Rarely associated with other syndromes. t(15:19)
Thymic carcinoid/ neuroendocrine carcinoma	CK+, synaptophysin+, chromogranin+, ACTH+	Dense core neurosecretory granules	Cushing's syndrome; MEN in some
Large cell non-Hodgkin lymphoma	CD45+, CD20+, CD79a+, light chain restriction (B cell) CD45+, CD3+, CD45RO (UCHL1)+(T cell) CD45+, CD3+/−, CD30+, EMA+, t(2:5) ALK-1+ (Anaplastic T/Null)	Absence of cell junctions; absence of secretory activity or tonofilaments	Compartmentalizing sclerosis common Note: Thymic epithelial cells may be CD20+
Lymphoblastic lymphoma	TdT+, CD1a+/−, CD3+/−, CD4+CD8+ or CD4−CD8− T-receptor gene rearrangements, (T cell); CD79a+, Ig gene rearrangement (B cell)	Absence of cell junctions; high N:C ratio	Note: Similar immunophenotype in immature lymphoid cells in thymomas LBL: 14q/7q abnormality
Hodgkin lymphoma	CD45−, CD15+, CD30+, EBER/LMP1+/− (classical) CD45+, CD15−, CD20+, CD30−, EBER/LMP1− (lymphocyte predominant)		
Germinoma	PLAAP+ (strong, diffuse), CD57+, β-hCG− (focal+), CK− (focal+), CD117+, AFP−, CD45−, S-100−, CEA−, CD15−, CD30−	Giant primitive nucleoli, euchromatin dispersal, absent nuclear membrane chromatin; primitive intercellular junctions	i(12p) cytogenetic abnormality in 80% of GCT Serum β-hCG elevated in some cases, derived from isolated syncytiotrophoblasts
Embryonal carcinoma	PLAAP+, CK+ (strong, diffuse), CD15+, CD57+, CD30+, AFP− (focal+), hCG-(focal+) CD117+	Primitive cell junctions; carcinoma-like features	Elevated serum markers in90% (α-FP, β-HCG), i(12p) cytogenetic abnormality in80% of GCT
Endodermal sinus (Yolk sac) tumor	AFP+, a−1AT+, CK+, PLAP+/−, CEA −/+	Basement membrane material	Elevated serum markers (AFP)+
Choriocarcinoma	βHCG+, CK +/− (50%)	Syncytiotrophoblast/ cytotrophoblast	Elevated serum markers (β-HCG)
Synovial sarcoma	X:18 translocation		

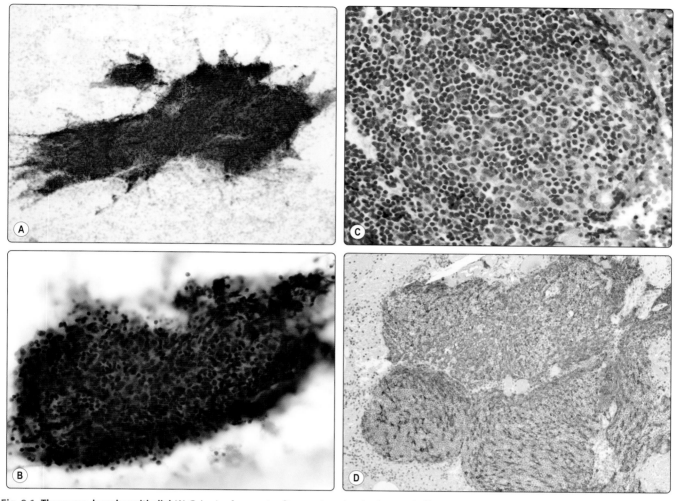

Fig. 9.1 Thymoma, lymphoepithelial (A) Cohesive fragments of tumor tissue in a background of lymphoid cells (Pap, LP); (B) Cohesive cluster. Epithelial cells visible centrally Pap HP; (C) Cell block, indistinct epithelial cells (H&E, HP); (D) Cell block, reticular pattern of epithelial cell staining for AE1+3 keratins (IPOX, LP).

much greater availability of immunochemistry. For example, Akhtar et al.[36,54] and Singh et al.[39] see immunocytochemistry as necessary for confirmation of germ cell tumor type. Immunocytochemistry or flow cytometry are routinely used for diagnosis and typing of non-Hodgkin lymphomas (see Chapter 5). Powers et al. used ancillary tests in 27% of their cases.[25,39] Herman et al. noted lower sensitivity and ability to type tumors accurately in the period before the use of ancillary tests.[23]

It was hoped that molecular analysis may help pinpoint the site of origin in patients with tumors of unknown origin,[55-57] although recent applications of molecular analysis have turned to its use in targeted drug therapy rather than specific tumor typing.

CYTOLOGICAL FINDINGS

Metastatic malignancy

The mediastinum is a common site of metastasis for neoplasms from all sites. In FNA samples, small cell carcinoma of lung is the most frequent metastasis, with lesser numbers of non-small cell tumors of lung, followed by breast carcinoma.[25] Metastatic sarcomas may also be seen, but remember the possibility of origin from a germ cell tumor if a malignant spindle cell neoplasm is encountered. Rare primary sarcomas may also be seen.

Baker et al.[58] suggested that in sampling mediastinal nodes by the transbronchial route, lymphocytes are necessary to confirm specimen adequacy, otherwise bronchial contents may be misinterpreted as originating from mediastinum. As stated above, we agree.

Thymic neoplasms

Thymoma (Figs 9.1–9.6)[18,25-35,59-63]

CRITERIA FOR DIAGNOSIS

- Cohesive tissue fragments with bland polygonal, oval, or spindled 'epithelial' cells (rarely, Hassall's corpuscles),
- Lymphoid cells (mixed thymoma) intermingled with the epithelial component.

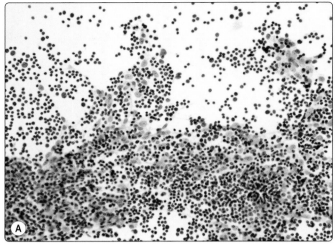

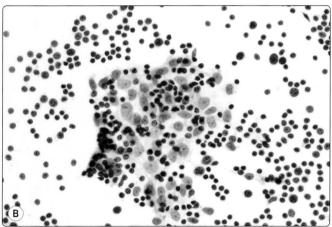

Fig. 9.2 Thymoma, lymphoepithelial (**A**) Less cohesive pattern with loose groups of epithelial cells (Pap, IP); (**B**) Loose group of epithelial cells with pale chromatin and conspicuous nucleoli (Pap, HP).

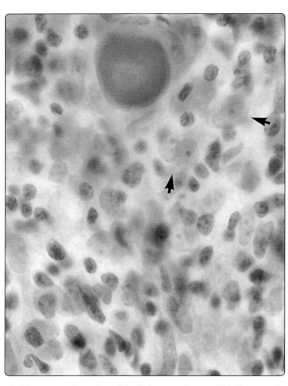

Fig. 9.4 Thymoma, lymphoepithelial; metastatic within lung Biphasic cell population of lymphocytes and epithelial cells with pale nuclei, small nucleoli and indistinct cytoplasm; note the Hassall's corpuscle (Pap, HP oil).

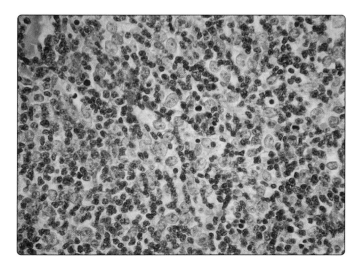

Fig. 9.3 Thymoma, lymphoepithelial Tissue section; biphasic cell population (H&E, HP).

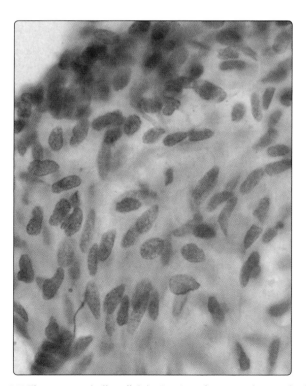

Fig. 9.5 Thymoma, spindle cell Cohesive tissue fragment; elongated pale, regular nuclei; indistinct cell borders (H&E, HP oil).

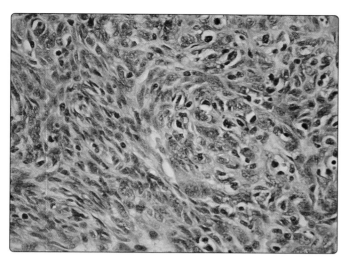

Fig. 9.6 Thymoma, spindle cell Tissue section (H&E, HP).

The histologic classification of thymomas is complex, evolving, and still somewhat controversial. Such subclassification may prove challenging for the histopathologist and this is exaggerated with aspiration cytology. Clearly, there is a wide spectrum in the cytomorphology of thymomas. First, there is a broad range of appearances of benign thymoma cells among and even within some of these neoplasms; this is complicated by the varying proportions of lymphocyes present.

In the benign thymomas, the epithelial cells are usually cohesive (Figs 9.1, 9.5) but may also manifest a reduction in intercellular cohesion (Fig. 9.2). Epithelial cells are not immediately evident in the mixed tumors at low power but are discernible using the higher magnification.[18,29,30] The epithelial cells are polygonal, oval, or spindle shaped with uniform to slightly irregular nuclear outlines possibly with cleaved or folded nuclei. Their nuclear chromatin is homogeneous, finely distributed and pale and, occasionally, small nucleoli are seen. Cell borders are indistinct, but nuclei are separated by moderate amounts of pale cytoplasm (Figs 9.2, 9.5). In one personally examined case of thymoma metastatic to lung, Hassall's corpuscles were evident in the clumps of tumor cells (Fig. 9.4); this is a most unusual manifestation and will not be present in most thymomas. When there is a lymphoid population, the bimodal pattern enables one to make a virtually certain diagnosis.[18,29,30] In pure epithelial or spindle cell forms, definitive diagnosis is more difficult, although in Dahlgren's series[29] most thymomas were diagnosed and in Tao's 37 cases[30] all FNAC diagnoses of thymoma were verified histologically. Ali and Erozan[34] were able to diagnose all of their 14 cases using a combination of cytology, immunocytochemistry and clinical information, and Shin and Katz showed a high accuracy in a range of mediastinal lesions including 14 thymomas.[35] Tao and others describe more variation in the degree of cohesion than we have seen, particularly in pure epithelial/nonspindle cell types.[30] Overall, the most challenging and the most common in our experience are the lymphocyte-rich (type B1) thymomas, as the tumor cells may be obscured by the lymphocytes.

Large cell lymphoma with sclerosis may yield cohesive fragments of tissue, resembling lymphocyte-rich thymomas. Immunophenotyping for lymphoma and ultrastructural or immunoperoxidase demonstration of an epithelial component in thymoma will help resolve the differential diagnosis. The clinical background may be misleading, as in a case of malignant thymoma in an HIV-positive patient.[64] Lymphoma cells compressed within collagen may resemble a spindle cell neoplasm.

Type B1 thymomas contain lymphoid cells of immature thymic type. These may be selectively sampled and give a false impression of lymphoma, especially lymphoblastic lymphoma. Similarly, if material is submitted for flow cytometry, the immature T phenotype may cause confusion. However, a maturing T-cell phenotype is characteristic of thymoma and thus is quite helpful in this situation. The immature cells demonstrate CD1, 2, 4, 5, 7 and 8 positivity and TdT, representing the common or intermediate stage of thymocyte differentiation, a profile similar to that of T-lymphoblastic lymphoma.[65] Some cases also demonstrate apparent 'loss' of various T-cell markers, heightening a suspicion of T-cell lymphoma. In our experience, unless the cytologist reviewing material either in the radiology theatre or in the lab alerts the haematology laboratory to the likelihood of lymphocyte-rich thymoma, there is a very real risk of false-positive diagnosis of lymphoblastic lymphoma by flow cytometry.

Other spindle cell lesions within the mediastinum include benign and malignant connective tissue neoplasms, reactive processes with or without associated neoplasms, granulomas, mesothelioma, melanoma, spindle cell squamous carcinoma and spindle cell carcinoid.[66,67] Connective tissue neoplasms may be cohesive but, especially in neural tumors, have a more abundant and more myxoid stroma than thymomas. Spindle cell squamous carcinoma shows cytological features of malignancy lacking in thymoma; however, primary spindle squamous carcinoma of the thymus (a form of thymic carcinoma) is described. An approach which includes ancillary testing in all cases will help prevent error.

A specific diagnosis of invasive thymoma can only be achieved by histological assessment or in concert with clinical/surgical findings.

Sometimes, non-neoplastic thymic epithelium may be included in an FNB sample and give rise to erroneous tumor typing. Yu et al.[45] described a case of large cell lymphoma in which this occurred and then demonstrated entrapped thymic epithelium in a third of their cases of surgically excised large cell lymphomas. There was reactive proliferation of the epithelium in some cases. Thymic hyperplasia may completely mimic thymoma in smears.[68,69]

The monolayered presentation of mesothelium with intercellular windows allows this to be distinguished from thymic epithelium or neoplastic tissue.

Malignant thymoma (Figs 9.2, 9.7 and 9.8)[1-3,18,25,64,70-74]

Thymic carcinomas are very uncommon cytologically malignant tumors with a wide variety of morphological appearances including keratinizing and nonkeratinizing squamous, sarcomatoid, anaplastic large cell, basaloid, mucoepidermoid, clear cell and small cell types.[1-3] A cytological diagnosis of carcinoma may be made by FNB. Smears are variably cellular and usually dominated by loosely cohesive large malignant cells diagnostic of carcinoma. Most are composed of large tumor cells with solitary clearly malignant nuclei, with or without prominent nucleoli. As expected, their smear appearance resembles the underlying histopathology. Reports of FNB diagnosis of rare subtypes such as basaloid and mucoepidermoid carcinomas area also reported.[73,74]

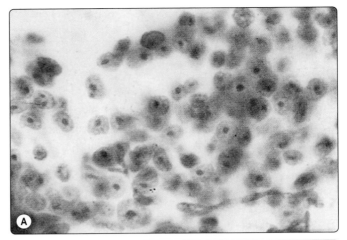

PROBLEMS AND DIFFERENTIAL DIAGNOSIS
◆ Metastatic carcinoma,
◆ Thymic carcinomas of 'borderline' malignancy,
◆ New classifications of thymoma.

Anaplastic carcinoma from other sites is not distinguishable from primary thymic carcinoma on cytomorphology alone. Dorfman et al.[75] found CD5 positivity in tumor cells to be characteristic of primary carcinomas, in contradistinction to benign thymomas and carcinomas from other sites. Newer markers such as Foxn1 and CD205 may also prove useful.[76]

The distinction between thymic carcinoma and invasive thymoma is based on cytological characteristics of malignancy in the former.

A histogenetic classification of thymomas has been accepted by some (see above).[1-3] The older classification (spindle, lymphocytic, epithelial and mixed) and the newer subgrouping (medullary, mixed, predominantly cortical (organoid), cortical and well-differentiated thymic carcinoma) both have prognostic relevance.[2,3,77] The subtypes in these two systems can be related histologically[2,3] although cytological findings alone may not allow accurate prediction of tumor type. Some authors still advocate a simple morphological classification into thymoma, atypical thymoma and thymic carcinoma.[78] All authors acknowledge that staging is a crucial aspect of assessment of biological behavior.[1-3,78] Shimosato et al. trace the conceptual evolution of thymoma and thymic carcinoma classification and staging.[1]

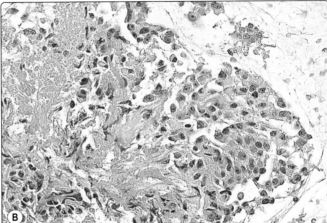

Neuroendocrine neoplasms[66,79-86]

(see also Chapter 8)

Primary neuroendocrine tumors of the mediastinum include carcinomas ranging from low to high grade (carcinoid, atypical carcinoid, large cell carcinoma, and small cell carcinoma).[1-3] Cytomorphologic criteria for diagnosis are quite similar to those in other sites, especially the lung. Although there is a spectrum of biologic behavior correlating with grade, even apparently low-grade neoplasms may show very aggressive clinical behavior in the mediastinum.[83-85] Furthermore, tumors with combined low-grade and high-grade morphologic attributes occur with some relative frequency.[84] The low-grade ones may also produce paraneoplastic syndromes, especially Cushing's syndrome. When combined

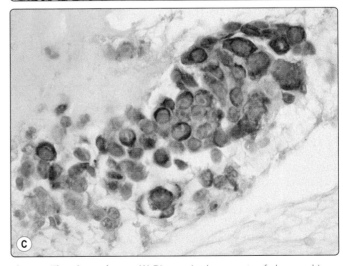

Fig. 9.7 Thymic carcinoma (A) Disorganized aggregate of pleomorphic malignant cells with macronucleoli; (B) Cell block showing poorly differentiated large cell carcinoma; (C) Staining of tumor cells for CD5 (A, Pap, HP; B, Cell block. H&E, HP; C, cell block, IPOX).

with the characteristic radiologic finding of focal calcifications, this may suggest the diagnosis prebiopsy. These tumors are associated with multiple endocrine neoplasm syndromes in about 25% of cases, usually type 1.[87] Gherardi describeed intracytoplasmic paranuclear keratin inclusions similar to those seen in Merkel cell tumors, small cell carcinoma and

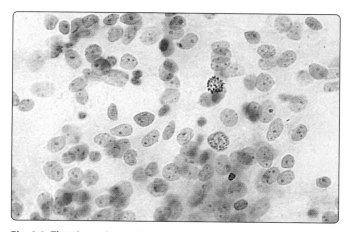

Fig. 9.8 Thymic carcinoma Borderline nuclear criteria of malignancy. Poorly cohesive cells with fragile cytoplasm, rounded or ovoid nuclei, bland chromatin and small but prominent nucleoli; note the mitosis (Pap, HP).

other neuroendocrine neoplasms in three cases sampled by FNB.[79] These structures were best demonstrated in Romanowsky stains as optically clear paranuclear spaces, confirmed by cytokeratin staining in smears, along with Grimelius staining, NSE positivity and Leu-7 or chromogranin staining in several cases. Paranuclear apoptotic material was also observed in some cells and there was discohesion, mitotic activity, single cell necrosis and tingible body macrophages in the background, producing a resemblance to lymphoma. Lymphoglandular bodies were not seen. Wang et al. diagnosed four cases of thymic carcinoid tumor without atypical features.[80] They found Riu's stain or argyrophilia useful for identifying neurosecretory granules in the cytoplasm. One patient had Cushing's syndrome and the tumor cells demonstrated ACTH positivity. In Dusenbury's case, the diagnosis was made by cytology and positive synaptophysin staining.[66] A spindle cell component was described. Smith et al. diagnosed an unusual lipid-rich carcinoid tumor by FNA.[86]

Neural neoplasms (see Chapter 15)

Most mediastinal neural tumors arise in the posterior compartment. *Neurofibromas, schwannomas and ganglioneuromas* occur mainly in adults and are often detected as asymptomatic masses by X-ray, or by pain or other symptoms of local pressure. In the paediatric population, neuroblastoma and ganglioneuroblastoma predominate here. Aspiration may be difficult because of the cohesiveness of tissue, and more vigorous needling and/or core biopsies may be necessary. The cytological findings are described in detail in Chapter 15. In the mediastinum the differential diagnosis includes spindle cell thymoma, carcinoid, other connective tissue neoplasms, lymphoma with associated sclerosis and reactive connective lesions.[67] Cell blocks and immunocytochemistry or electron microscopy are valuable. Diagnosis of malignancy and specific typing of primary malignant nerve sheath tumors is extremely difficult, if not impossible, on aspirated material. Caution should be applied, as some benign lesions are extremely pleomorphic and cellular; mitotic activity and necrosis are more useful criteria in raising the suspicion of malignancy. If a cell block with ample tumor is available, then S-100 protein immunostaining may help. With benign

nerve sheath tumors, staining is diffuse and intense, whereas their malignant counterparts manifest rather weak, focal decoration or are totally negative.

Dahl et al.,[88] Dahlgren and Ovenfors[89] and Zbieranowski and Bedard[90] described series of schwannomas in FNAC. Palombini and Vetrani outlined the FNAC findings in mediastinal *ganglioneuroma and ganglioneuroblastoma.*[91,92] In one case there was a mixture of polyhedral cells including binucleate forms with abundant eosinophilic cytoplasm and smaller oval or spindle cells. The findings suggested ganglioneuroblastoma; elevated VMA levels in serum helped to confirm the diagnosis. In others, a fibrillar background in MGG preparations was a diagnostic clue suggesting neuritic processes.

Pure *neuroblastomas* occur mainly in children and present as small round cell tumors, with a background neuropil.[93,94] Calcifications are common. They are further described in Chapter 17.

Paragangliomas may arise in the mediastinum.[95] Smears are usually highly cellular, but the major tumor cell contour is variable, not only from neoplasm to neeoplasm, but also within a given tumor. Cell shapes include round, plamacytoid and spindled. Nuclei are usually single but bi- and multinucleation may occur, at times frequently. Nuclei tend to be round with disticntly granular chromatin which stains with different intensities; nucleoli are generally inconspicuous. Nuclear diameter may vary tremendously but usually remains smooth and round. Cytoplasm is moderate in volume most often, and, with the MGG stain, is characteristically basophilic with minute red granules.

Lymphoma and lymphoid lesions in the mediastinum (see Chapter 5)

The mediastinum is a characteristic site of presentation of *nodular sclerosing Hodgkin lymphoma* and *sclerosing large cell lymphoma* in young women and *T-lymphoblastic lymphoma in children and adolescent males.* However, all types of non-Hodgkin lymphoma, *angiofollicular lymphoid hyperplasia*[96] and thymoma with a high proportion of lymphocytes enter the differential diagnosis. *Thymic hyperplasia* in children and adults may also provide problems,[97] but can sometimes be suggested on FNB.[76,98] *Small cell anaplastic carcinoma* in the mediastinum may be cytologically difficult to distinguish from lymphoma. Flow cytometry and immunohistochemistry are important adjunctive tests.[99,100] Using a combination of cytomorphology, flow cytometry and molecular/genetic analysis, even rare lymphoma variants may be specifically diagnosed at times.[39,101]

Refer to Chapter 5 for detailed discussion and illustration of lymphoid lesions.

Hodgkin lymphoma[38,39,98,102]

CRITERIA FOR DIAGNOSIS

- Reed-Sternberg cells and mononuclear variants,
- Mixed population of lymphoid cells with a predominance of small mature lymphocytes,
- Consistent immunocytochemical profile (see Table 9.1 and Chapter 5).

In the past, cytological findings alone may have been used as a basis for management in primary mediastinal Hodgkin lymphoma. However, it is now widely accepted that minimum diagnostic criteria include a consistent immunocytochemical profile. Table 9.1 includes a simplified summary of results in Hodgkin and non-Hodgkin lymphomas, with antibodies in routine use in the cytology laboratory. Cell blocks, thin cores or smears and cytocentrifuge preparations may all give good results (see also Chapter 5).

PROBLEMS AND DIFFERENTIAL DIAGNOSIS

- Sampling,
- Large cell non-Hodgkin lymphoma,
- Other anaplastic malignancies,
- Cystic Hodgkin lymphoma.

Fibrotic Hodgkin's disease may provide difficulties in obtaining diagnostic material by FNB.

Large cell non-Hodgkin lymphoma may have very similar cytological and histological findings to Hodgkin's disease, including accompanying fibrosis, an associated reactive lymphoid cell population and multinucleate cells resembling Reed-Sternberg cells. There are also cases with considerable overlap in their immunocytochemical profile and even molecular analysis may not solve the problem. Compared to various small cell lymphomas, large cell forms are often composed of more delicate cells which do not survive flow cytometry as well.

Distinction from anaplastic carcinoma and melanoma can generally be achieved with immunocytochemistry. Reed-Sternberg cells may have less cytoplasm compared to carcinomas and melanomas. The presence of eosinophilic leukocytes in the background may also be a clue to Hodgkin lymphoma.

Hodgkin lymphoma in the mediastinum may be associated with multilocular cystic change in the thymus, with a rim of neoplastic tissue which may not be sampled by the needle, resulting in a false-negative result.[1-3]

Lymphoblastic lymphoma[103-105]

CRITERIA FOR DIAGNOSIS

- High smear cellularity,
- Monotonous population of small to medium-sized lymphoid cells with very high N:C ratios,
- High mitotic rate; tingible body macrophages,
- Delicate nuclear membranes with well-developed irregularities, especially convolutions,
- Finely granular 'dusty' chromatin pattern,
- Minute nucleoli,
- Consistent immunochemical profile.

We find Papanicolaou staining essential to recognize lymphocyte subtypes; MGG staining is also routinely performed, but in our experience does not allow as close a correlation with histological appearances. The variation induced by air-drying sometimes makes it more difficult to appreciate subtle size differences, to compare cells to small lymphocytes and to examine chromatin pattern. Nevertheless, the two stains are complementary.

In the proper clinical setting, the cellular monotony and high mitotic rate may be the first clue to the diagnosis, especially if material is not optimal and nuclear morphology is compromised.

Flow cytometry is technically easier than immunocytochemistry for most laboratories; we select this ancillary method if the diagnosis is suspected at the time of initial examination of smears in radiology. Flow cytometry cannot show monoclonality for T-lymphoblastic tumors, but may show loss of one or more expected T-cell antigens; identification of rearrangements in T-receptor genes will provide this proof. Cytospins are useful for TdT studies, but this can also be assayed by flow cytometry.

PROBLEMS AND DIFFERENTIAL DIAGNOSIS

- Distinction from small lymphocytes,
- Distinction from a follicular hyperplasia pattern,
- Distinction from the immature lymphoid cells in thymoma.

There is a risk of misinterpreting the neoplastic cells as small lymphocytes, especially if preservation is not optimal. In addition, the presence of tingible body macrophages may lure one into considering the changes as reactive hyperplasia. The lymphoid cells in thymomas often have a similar immunophenotype to lymphoblastic lymphoma.[65] As stated above, however, a 'maturing phenotype' is typical of thymoma, whereas there may be deletions of expected T-cell antigens in lymphoblastic lymphoma.

Large cell lymphoma (± sclerosis) (Fig 9.9)[106]

CRITERIA FOR DIAGNOSIS

- Dispersed monomorphic population of large lymphocytes with round or cleaved cells nuclei (centroblasts or immunoblasts),
- Relative absence of small lymphocytes,
- Background of lymphoglandular bodies,[107]
- Consistent immunophenotype.

Figure 9.9 shows material from a 10-cm anterior/superior mass from a 16-year-old male who presented with chest pain. The pathologist examined material in the radiology theater and the initial working diagnosis was large cell lymphoma (Fig. 9.9A). Material was triaged for flow cytometry, smears and cell blocks, and a 20-g core biopsy was also requested and fixed in formalin. The reports on the cytology and histology were prepared in conjunction by the same pathologist. Flow cytometry was non-diagnostic with only 16% of cells identified as lymphoid and no B-cell clonality detected. This situation is quite commonly seen in large cell lymphomas where the neoplastic cells are presumably fragile and disrupted during measurement, and where only robust small lymphoid cells survive the evaluation process. The cell

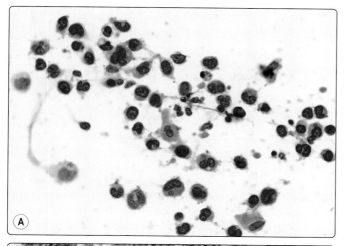

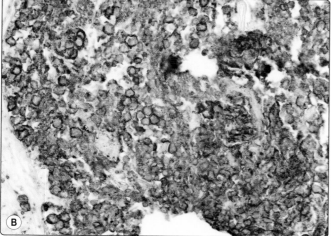

Fig. 9.9 Mediastinal large B-cell lymphoma (A) Dispersed malignant cells with large pleomorphic multilobated nuclei and variable amounts of dense cytoplasm. (H&E, HP); (B) Cell block, intense membrane staining for CD20 (IPOX, HP).

block showed well-preserved tumor cells staining strongly for CD20 (Fig. 9.9B). The thin cores also contained tumor cells infiltrating through fibrous tissue. Immunohistochemistry was performed on cell blocks and cores and there was positive cytoplasmic staining for CD45, and CD30 and nuclear staining for BCL6, but no staining for ALK1, CD10, CD138, cyclin D1, S-100, cytokeratins, PLAAP or CD117. The Ki-67 proliferation index was >60%. FISH analysis on tissue showed no disruption of BCL6-MBR, MYC, IgH, ALK or EWSR1, and no IgH-BCL2 fusion, IgH-MYC fusion or EWSR1-FL11 fusion was detected. The diagnosis was mediastinal diffuse large B-cell lymphoma, most likely of thymic subtype. Management was based on these results.

PROBLEMS AND DIFFERENTIAL DIAGNOSIS

◆ Poor cellularity with distorted spindle cell forms,
◆ Cohesive tissue fragments resembling thymoma,
◆ Hodgkin lymphoma,
◆ Other anaplastic malignancies.

Silverman et al. described specimens where the sample was poorly cellular or composed of microtissue fragments containing distorted spindled lymphoma cells secondary to compression by collagen fibers.[106]

We have seen a case where cohesive fragments were aspirated leading to a misdiagnosis of thymoma based on cytological study alone, emphasizing the value of immunostaining for confirmation of the diagnosis. We are not aware of a similar published example.

Hodgkin lymphoma with a syncytial growth pattern may mimic large cell lymphoma, carcinoma or melanoma.

Other poorly differentiated primary and secondary tumors, including germ cell tumors, must be excluded.

Angiofollicular lymphoid hyperplasia (Castleman disease)[96,108]

This unusual reactive process is probably impossible to diagnose specifically by FNAC. Deschenes et al.[108] found branching capillaries associated with fragments of germinal centers as a constant feature in their cases and in half of the other published case reports, suggesting that these may be useful criteria. However, any lymphoid mass lesion in which a specific diagnosis of lymphoma or thymoma cannot be made should be reaspirated for ancillary testing and/or biopsied or excised for histopathology.

Germ cell neoplasms[36,54,109-117] (see Chapter 13)

Germ cell neoplasms of all types occur in the mediastinum and constitute about 20% of primary mediastinal masses.[1-3] A strong association between germ cell tumors and Klinefelter's syndrome and with hematological neoplasia is recorded.[1-3] The need to confirm metastatic spread of germ cell neoplasms within the thorax will also confront the pathologist. Primary germinomas virtually only occur in young males; other germ cell malignancies also show striking male predominance. On the other hand, cystic teratoma present equally in young women and men. Elevated serum levels of human chorionic gonadotrophin (beta-HCG) and alpha fetoprotein, together with clinical findings, may virtually establish the diagnosis in nonseminomatous tumors. Sampling difficulties may prevent the accurate typing of mixed tumors. Due to the common therapy for all subtypes of nonseminomatous germ cell tumors (this may not be true if there is a choriocarcinomatous component), there is less need for exhaustive histological subtyping in advanced cases with widespread disease; however, specific subcategorization is aimed for in localized forms. All types of germ cell tumors have been diagnosed by a combination of cytology and ancillary testing. Most lesions are discussed and illustrated in Chapter 13.

Teratoma (mature cystic)[110]

Mature cystic teratomas of the mediastinum occur mainly in young women, have similar appearances to the counterpart in the ovary (see Chapter 13) and are benign.

CRITERIA FOR DIAGNOSIS

◆ Keratinous debris, anucleate squamous cells, hair shaft material,
◆ Mature squamous and/or glandular epithelium.
◆ Granulomatous reaction to tumor,
◆ Sampling,
◆ Well-differentiated squamous cell carcinoma.

PROBLEMS AND DIFFERENTIAL DIAGNOSIS

◆ Large cell/anaplastic lymphoma,
◆ Anaplastic carcinoma (thymic or metastatic),
◆ Embryonal carcinoma; yolk sac tumor,
◆ Other metastases, e.g. melanoma,
◆ Cystic change,
◆ Necrosis.

In rare cases, only the granulomatous reaction at the edge of neoplasm may be sampled. If there is only a small amount of cohesive squamous epithelium, the significance may not be appreciated until after resection.

Well-differentiated squamous cell carcinoma usually presents with a dispersed population of keratinized cells, in contrast to the cohesion shown by teratoma. More importantly, the nuclei from a benign teratoma differ greatly form that of keratinizing carcinoma.

Teratoma (immature, malignant)

Immature elements may occur in some tumors. Immature neuroepithelial elements often predominate, resembling neuroblastoma. Other tumors such as carcinosarcoma, blastoma, synovial sarcoma, Wilms' tumor or malignant mesothelioma will enter the differential diagnosis when biphasic lesions are encountered.

Germinoma

CRITERIA FOR DIAGNOSIS

◆ High cellularity and mitotic activity,
◆ Dispersed large cells; small loose groups,
◆ Rounded nuclei, prominent single or multiple nucleoli,
◆ Abundant fragile cytoplasm; vacuolation (glycogen),
◆ 'Tigroid' or streaked cytoplasmic/glycogenic background (MGG),
◆ Lymphocytes; granulomas.

The cytological appearances are identical to seminoma or germinoma elsewhere. The cells are fragile and this results in a so-called 'tigroid' background in Romanowsky stains, described also as frothy, bubbly, lace-like or granular, resulting from disrupted cytoplasm with alternating non-glycogenic and glycogenic areas. This pattern can be seen in other glycogen-rich tumors such as embryonal rhabdomyosarcoma[118] and fetal adenocarcinoma.[119] The pale cytoplasmic crescents and vacuoles seen in MGG-stained intact cells represent glycogen lakes. The nuclei are vesicular with thick membranes and nucleoli. Granulomas and lymphocytic infiltration are variable. This combination can be instantly recognizable, but traumatization of cells or minimal material makes diagnosis a challenge in some instances.

The immunocytochemical profile of germinoma is listed in Table 9.1. Strong diffuse cytoplasmic PLAAP positivity, high glycogen content, absent or minimal focal keratin staining and absent LCA staining are the most useful features.

Large cell/immunoblastic/anaplastic lymphoma may resemble germinoma. The presence of abundant lymphoglandular bodies is strongly suggestive of lymphoma, whereas a tigroid background is not seen in lymphomas. The preservation of true intercellular cohesion and relatively numerous small lymphocytes point to germinoma.

Cell aggregation does occur in germinoma so that it may resemble carcinomas more closely, and when there is moderate pleomorphism, distinction from embryonal carcinoma, yolk sac tumor and anaplastic carcinoma may be difficult. Embryonal carcinoma will often present in three-dimensional aggregates including papillae and lumen formation, which are not expected in germinoma. In addition, N:C ratios tend to be higher. In yolk sac tumor, the neoplastic cells are smaller and usually possess less prominent nucleoli than in germinoma and may be associated with hyaline globules and dense matrix material. Specific diagnosis usually requires ancillary testing.

Germinoma in the mediastinum may be largely cystic with minimal tumor tissue in the wall.[115]

Tumor necrosis may be almost complete; however, the monotonous appearance of the ghost outlines of tumor cells may suggest the diagnosis.[120]

Embryonal carcinoma[109,112–117]

CRITERIA FOR DIAGNOSIS

◆ Cellular smears,
◆ Aggregates and dispersed cells with solitary nuclei and large nucleoli,
◆ Adenocarcinoma-like groups; sheets,
◆ Spindle/mesenchymal cells.

In extragonadal cases, the patients are usually young men and the initial cytological impression is one of an anaplastic epithelial tumor, poorly differentiated adenocarcinoma or even squamous cell carcinoma. In this setting a high index of suspicion for the diagnosis allows serum marker testing and a strongly positive result allows diagnosis without further ancillary testing on tissue. If marker levels are minimally elevated the diagnosis is more problematic, because some carcinomas will secrete beta-HCG and alpha fetoprotein; the clinical background may determine management in these cases.

The immunophenotype of embryonal carcinoma is shown in Table 9.1. Strongly positive diffuse staining for cytokeratins and PLAAP, plus Leu-M1 (CD15) and CD30 positivity will be most helpful. Polyclonal PLAAP cross-reacts with the intestinal alkaline phosphatase in some carcinomas.[113]

Distinction between embryonal carcinoma and the other malignant germ cell neoplasms may be difficult. The cytomorphology may also be very difficult to distinguish from poorly differentiated carcinoma which has spread to the mediastinum, most often from the lung.[101]

Other germ cell tumors

Pure endodermal sinus (yolk sac) tumor is rare in the mediastinum;[54,117] it presents as loosely cohesive epithelial-like cells with mild pleomorphism, rounded nuclei with small nucleoli and vacuolated cytoplasm in a mucoid background. Two forms of vacuolation may be recognized, one due to glycogen (large vacuoles) and the other of uncertain nature. Globular PAS/D-positive intracytoplasmic bodies representing alpha-1 antitrypsin, alpha fetoprotein or laminin may be seen in some cases.[54] They are not, however, specific for this tumor type. A background of extracellular basement membrane-like material may also often be present, and is most easily seen as metachromatic material in MGG preparations; with the Papanicolaou stain it has a pale green hue.[111] This may be the most important clue to the diagnosis in some cases. A fibrillar background may also be observed.[111] The cytological findings may be rather nondescript in some cases, particularly if Papanicolaou stained, but in cell blocks the characteristic reticular or lace-like growth with prominent vessels may be more easily observed. There are numerous histological variants, including a spindle cell form, and these have not been well characterized cytologically.[121] The immunocytochemical profile includes strong alpha fetoprotein and PLAAP positivity and cytokeratin positivity.[54] High serum levels of alpha fetoprotein can be confirmatory.

Choriocarcinoma[109,122] is an extremely rare neoplasm in the mediastinum and distinction from anaplastic carcinoma or other germ cell tumors may be difficult, although serum markers showing very high beta-HCG will be valuable. Sheets of cells representing cytotrophoblast and a giant cell component with multiple obviously malignant nuclei representing syncytiotrophoblast can be seen either lying free or associated with the sheets. Hemorrhage and necrotic debris are characteristic.

Cystic lesions of the mediastinum[21,25,51,123–126]

It is sometimes possible to suggest the nature of a cyst in the mediastinum based on FNB and imaging. In pericardial cysts, the location and injection of radiopaque dye into the lesion which outlines a thin, smooth cyst wall helps make this diagnosis. We found that the cytological findings in cases of presumed pericardial cyst were inconclusive: no mesothelial cells could be identified; macrophages were the main cellular element along with some lymphocytes. Benign neoplasms and some malignant mediastinal lesions may present as largely cystic structures. Developmental or degenerative thymic or parathyroid cysts may be extremely large

and contain lymphocytes and macrophages only. Cystic thymomas may resemble non-neoplastic cysts, until sectioning of their wall reveals small areas of residual neoplasm. Hodgkin lymphoma in young women, germinoma in young men[115] and teratoma may all be largely cystic, the neoplastic element forming only a small part of the cyst or in association with *multilocular squamous-cystic change in the thymus*. This is a non-specific reaction to various disease processes,[124] including AIDS[125] and various neoplasms including low-grade lymphoma. Bronchogenic or gastroenteric cysts are also well described in this site.[123] CT criteria for diagnosing benign cysts include a smooth oval mass with thin walls, homogeneous CT attenuation, near water density, no vascular enhancement or infiltration of nearby mediastinal structures. These, when combined with cytological findings, may allow conservative management in selected cases.[123] Atypical fibroblastic cells in cysts have been reported as mimicking malignancy in this site.[126]

Other lesions

Thyroid lesions

Large retrosternal or ectopic mediastinal *multinodular goiters* may present as superior mediastinal masses. The diagnosis is easily made if colloid and benign thyroid epithelial cells are recognised. This is not as easy without MGG preparations and may be a source of error,[20,25] leading to suspicion of neoplasm. *Ectopic anterior mediastinal thyroid* can also give rise to neoplasms including Hurthle cell tumors.[127,128]

Parathyroid lesions

Parathyroid neoplasms are occasionally sampled by FNB. The cytomorphology consists of a monotous pattern of bland cells with round dark nuclei in loose flat clusters and lying singly. Within aggregates, the cells are uniformly distributed, at times with well-defined cell membranes. Immunohistochemistry on accompanying cell blocks or thin core samples manifest chromogranin and parathormone positivity. In adenomas, one expects a very low proportion of Ki-67 positive nuclei but distinguishing an adenoma from an adenocarcioma may be exceedingly difficult. Vu et al. remind us that aspirate assay for parathormone may be very useful, especially if cell-block parathormone immunocytochemistry is not available.[129] It has been suggested that aspiration may be useful for parathyroid cysts of this site,[130] although there may be some difficulties in interpreting atypical reactive fibroblastic cells in the walls of the cyst.[126]

Other neoplasms

The most common sarcomas of this site include *malignant fibrous histiocytoma* and *liposarcoma*.[131,132] *Synovial sarcoma* is well described.[133] We have seen a single case of monophasic synovial sarcoma of mediastinum diagnosed on transoesophageal EUS FNB by the demonstration of SYT-SSX fusion transcripts by FISH on cell blocks, indicating X:18 translocation (all material shown here is courtesy of Dr. Anita Soma, PathWest QE II AP). (Fig. 9.10) The patient was

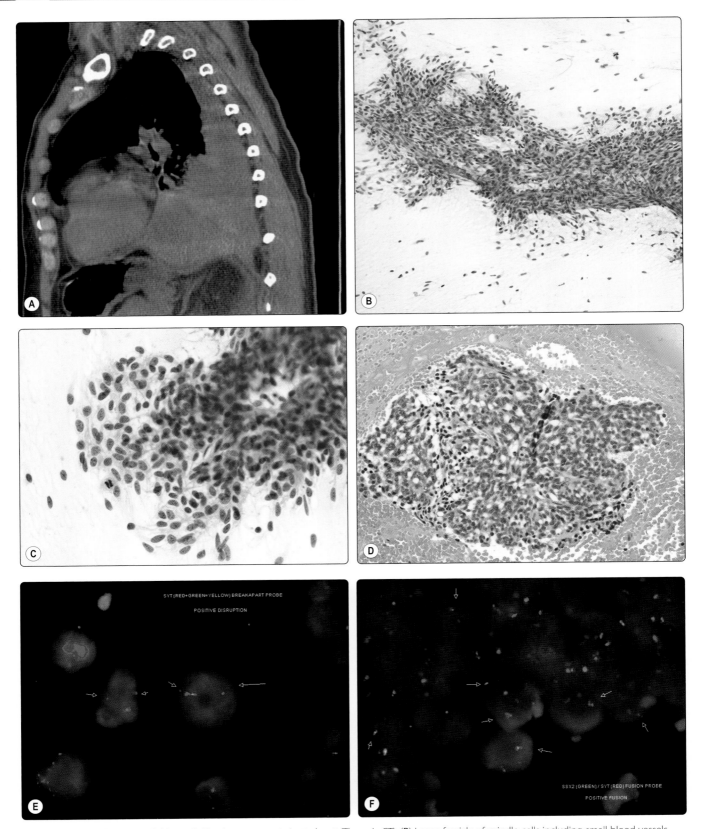

Fig. 9.10 Synovial sarcoma (A) Large infiltrative mass posterior to heart (Thoracic CT); (B) Loose fascicle of spindle cells including small blood vessels. Background of bare tumor nuclei (H&E, LP); (C) Loose cluster of bland spindle cells but with mitotic activity (H&E, HP); (D) Cell block, small spindle tumor cells with non-specific features (H&E, HP);(E) FISH on cell block, breakapart probe for SYT showing positive disruption of red-green-yellow components (FISH, HP); (F) FISH on cell block, fusion probe for SSX2 (green) and SYT (red) probes showing positive fusion of green and red components. (FISH, HP);

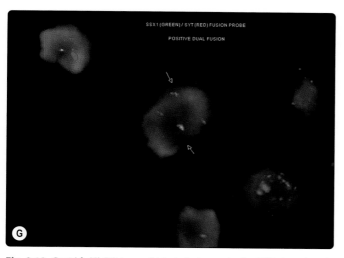

Fig. 9.10 Cont'd (G) FISH on cell block, fusion probe for SSX2 (*green*) and SYT (*red*) probes showing positive fusion of green and red components (FISH, HP).

a 45-year-old male with an 11-cm mass adjacent to the lower oesophagus, displacing the heart. Smears showed a rather bland spindle cell population but with mitotic activity. The cell block immunohistochemistry was negative for cytokeratins, CD117 and smooth muscle markers, making leiomyosarcoma and GIST unlikely. The tumor did show positive staining for CD99, BCL2 and CD34, raising the possibility of solitary fibrous tumor or synovial sarcoma. An SYT-SSX1 fusion transcript was detected by reverse transcriptase PCR, reinforcing the FISH cytogenetics. No other diagnostic procedures were undertaken (Fig 9.10).

Rhabdomyosarcoma should be considered in the differential diagnosis of small round cell tumors, particularly in children.[118] *Thymolipoma* has been diagnosed cytologically.[134]

Extramedullary hematopoiesis (EMH)

Rarely, deposits of *EMH* can present as a mediastinal mass and this entity should be considered when assessing lymphoreticular lesions.[135]

References

1. Shimasato Y, Mukai K, Matsuno Y. Tumours of the mediastinum. AFIP Atlas of Tumor Pathology 4th Series, Fascicle 11, American Registry of Pathology and Armed Forces Institute of Pathology, Washington DC. 2010.

2. Travis WD, Brambilla E, Muller-Hermelink HK, Harris CC, editors. Tumours of the lung, pleura, thymus and heart. Pathology and Genetics. World Health Organisation Histological Classification of Tumours. Lyon: IARC Press; 2004.

3. Rosai J. Mediastinum. In: Rosai J, editor. Akerman's surgical pathology, vol 1. 9th ed. New York: Mosby; 2004.

4. Morrissey B, Adams H, Gibbs AR, Crane MD. Percutaneous needle biopsy of the mediastinum: review of 94 procedures. Thorax 1993;48:632–7.

5. Bocking A, Klose KC, Hauptmann S. Cytologic versus histologic evaluation of needle biopsy of the lung, hilum and mediastinum. Sensitivity, specificity and typing accuracy. Acta Cytol 1995;39:463–71.

6. Medford AR, et al. Mediastinal staging procedures in lung cancer: EBUS, TBNA and mediastinoscopy. Curr Opin Pulm Med 2009;15:334–42.

7. Fritscher-Ravens A, Davidson BL, Hauber HP, et al. Endoscopic ultrasound, positron emission tomography, and computerized tomography for lung cancer. Am J Respir Crit Care Med 2003;168:1293–7.

8. Herth FJ, Becker HD, Ernst A. Ultrasound-guided transbronchial needle aspiration: an experience with 242 patients. Chest 2003;123:604–7.

9. Krasnik M, Vilmann P, Larsen SS, Jacobsen GK. Preliminary experience with a new method of endoscopic transbronchial real time ultrasound guided biopsy for diagnosis of mediastinal and hilar lesions. Thorax 2003;58:1083–6.

10. Kramer H, Sanders J, Post WJ, et al. Analysis of cytological specimens from mediastinal lesions obtained by endoscopic ultrasound-guided fine-needle aspiration. Cancer 2006;108:206–11.

11. Harbaum L, et al. False-positive mediastinal lymph node cytology due to translesional endocopic ultrasound-guided fine-needle aspirtation in a patient with Barrett's early cancer. Endoscopy 2009;41:160–1.

12. Eltoum IA, Chen VK, Chhieng DC, et al. Probabilistic reporting of EUS-FNA cytology: Toward improved communication and better clinical decisions. Cancer 2006;108:93–101.

13. Khan J, Akhtar M, von Sinner WN, et al. CT-guided fine-needle biopsy in the diagnosis of mediastinal tuberculosis. Chest 1994;106:1329–32.

14. Tambouret R, Geisinger KR, Powers CN, et al. The clinical application and cost analysis of fine-needle aspiration biopsy n the diagnosis of mass lesions in sarcoidosis. Chest 2000;117:1004–11.

15. Jereb M, Us-Krasovec M. Transthoracic needle biopsy of mediastinal and hilar lesions. Cancer 1977;40:1354–7

16. Adler O, Rosenberger A. Invasive radiology in the diagnosis of mediastinal masses. Use of fine needle for aspiration biopsy. Radiology 1979;19:169–72.

17. Adler OB, Rosenberger A, Peleg H. Fine needle aspiration biopsy of mediastinal masses: evaluation of 136 experiences. Am J Roentgenol 1983;140:393–6.

18. Sterrett GF, Whitaker D, Shilkin KB, Walters MN-I. Fine needle aspiration cytology of mediastinal lesions. Cancer 1983;51:127–35.

19. Weisbrod GL, Lyons DJ, Tao L-C, Chamberlain DW. Percutaneous fine needle aspiration biopsy of mediastinal lesions. Am J Roentgenol 1984;143:525–9.

20. Bartholdy NJ, Andersen MJ, Thommesen P. Clinical value of percutaneous fine needle aspiration biopsy of mediastinal masses. Analysis of 132 cases. Scand J Thorac Cardiovasc Surg 1984;18:81–3.

21. Linder J, Olsen GA, Johnston WW. Fine needle aspiration biopsy of the mediastinum. Am J Med 1986;81:1005–8.

22. Weisbrod GL. Percutaneous fine needle aspiration biopsy of the mediastinum. Clin Chest Med 1987;8:27–41.

23. Herman SJ, Holub RV, Weisbrod GL, Chamberlain DW. Anterior mediastinal masses: utility of transthoracic needle biopsy. Radiology 1991;180:167–70.

24. Wiersama MJ, Kochman ML, Cramer HM, Wiersama LM. Preoperative staging of non-small cell lung cancer: transesophageal US-guided fine-needle aspiration biopsy of mediastinal lymph nodes. Radiology 1994;190:239–42.

25. Powers CN, Silverman JF, Geisinger KR, Frable J. Fine needle aspiration biopsy of the mediastinum: a multi-institutional analysis. Am J Clin Pathol 1996;105:168–73.

26. Suen K, Quenville N. Fine needle aspiration cytology of uncommon thoracic lesions. Am J Clin Pathol 1981;75:803–9.

27. Pak HY, Yokota SB, Friedberg HA. Thymoma diagnosed by transthoracic fine needle aspiration. Acta Cytol 1982;26:210–6.

28. Sajjid SM, Lukeman JM, Llamas L, Fernandez T. Needle biopsy diagnosis of thymoma. Acta Cytol 1982;26:503–6.

29. Dahlgren S, Sandstedt B, Sunstrom C. Fine needle aspiration cytology of thymic tumors. Acta Cytol 1983;27:1–6.

30. Tao L-C, Griffith Pearson F, Coper JD, et al. Cytopathology of thymoma. Acta Cytol 1984;28:165–70.

31. Miller J, Allen R, Wakefield JSL. Diagnosis of thymoma by fine needle aspiration cytology: light and electron microscopic study of a case. Diagn Cytopathol 1987;3:166–9.

32. Sherman ME, Black-Schaffer S. Diagnosis of thymoma by needle biopsy. Acta Cytol 1990;34:63–8.

33. Pinto MM, Dovgan D, Kaye AD, Chinniah A. Fine needle aspiration for diagnosing a thymoma producing CA-125. A case report. Acta Cytol 1993;37:929–32.

34. Ali SZ, Erozan YS. Thymoma. Cytopathologic features and differential diagnosis on fine needle aspiration. Acta Cytol 1998;42:845–54.

35. Shin HJ, Katz RL. Thymic neoplasia as represented by fine needle aspiration biopsy of anterior mediastinal masses. A practical approach to the differential diagnosis. Acta Cytol 1998;42:855–64.

36. Akhtar M, Al Dayel F. Is it feasible to diagnose germ cell tumours by fine needle aspiration biopsy? Diagn Cytopathol 1997;16:72–7.

37. Moreland WS, Geisinger KR. Utility and outcomes of fine-needle aspiration biopsy in Hodgkin's disease. Diagn Cytopathol 2002;26:278–82.

38. Geisinger KR, Lewis Z. Fine needle aspiration of lymph nodes: pattern recognition. In: Zarka M, editor. Practical Cytopathology. Elsevier Press; in press.

39. Singh HK, Silverman JF, Powers CN, et al. Diagnosis pitfalls in fine-needle aspiration biopsy of the mediastinum. Diagn Cytopathol 1997;17:121–6.

40. Assaad MW, Pantanowitz L, Otis CN. Diagnostic accuracy of image-guided percutaneous fine needle aspiration biopsy of the mediastinum. Diagn Cytopathol 2007;35:705–9.

41. Geisinger KR. Differential diagnostic considerations and potential pitfalls in fine needle aspiration biopsies of the mediastinum. Diagn Cytopathol 1995;13:436–42.

42. von Bartheld MB, van Kralingen KW, et al. Mediastinal-esophageal fistulae after EUS-FNA of tuberculosis of the mediastinum. Gastrointest Endosc 2010;71:210–2.

43. Aerts JG, Kloover J, Los J, et al. EUS-FNA of enlarged necrotic lymph nodes may cause infectious mediastinitis. J Thorac Oncol 2008;3:1191–3.

44. Doi S, Yasuda I, Iwashita T, et al. Needle tract implantation on the esophageal wall after EUS-guided FNA of metastatic mediastinal lymphadenopathy. Gastrointest Endosc 2008;67:988–90.

45. Yu C-J, Yang P-C, Chang D-B, et al. Evaluation of ultrasonically guided biopsies of mediastinal masses. Chest 1991;100:399–405.

46. Van Sonnenberg E, Lin AS, Deutsch AL, Mattrey RF. Percutaneous biopsy of difficult mediastinal, hilar and pulmonary lesions by computed tomographic guidance and modified coaxial technique. Radiology 1983;148:300–2.

47. Belfiore G, Camera L, Moggio G, et al. Middle mediastinal lesions: preliminary experience with CT-guided fine needle aspiration biopsy with a suprasternal approach. Radiol 1997;202:870–3.

48. Schenk DA, Bower JH, Bryan L, et al. Transbronchial needle aspiration staging of bronchogenic carcinoma. Am Rev espir Dis 1986;134:246–8.

49. Roche DH, Wilsher ML, Gurley AM. Transtracheal needle aspiration. Diagn Cytopathol 1995;12:106–12.

50. Pederson BH, Vilmann P, Folke K, et al. Endoscopic ultrasonography and real-time guided fine needle aspiration biopsy of solid lesions of the mediastinum suspected of malignancy. Chest 1996;110:539–44.

51. Nath PH, Sanders C, Holley HC, McElvein RB. Percutaneous fine needle aspiration in the diagnosis and management of mediastinal cysts in adults. South Med J 1988;81:1225–8.

52. Neill JS, Silverman JF. Electron microscopy of fine needle aspiration biopsies of the mediastinum. Diagn Cytopathol 1992;8:272–7.

53. Taccagni G, Cantaboni A, dell'Antonio G, et al. Electron microscopy of fine needle aspiration biopsies of mediastinal and paramediastinal lesions. Acta Cytol 1988;32:868–79.

54. Akhtar M, Ali MA, Sackey K, et al. Fine needle aspiration biopsy diagnosis of endodermal sinus tumor: histologic and ultrastructural correlations. Diagn Cytopathol 1990;6:184–92.

55. Dennis JL, Vass JK, Wit EC, et al. Identification from public data of molecular markers of adenocarcinoma characteristic of the site of origin. Cancer Res 2002;62:5999–6005.

56. Buckhaults P, Zhang Z, Chen YC, et al. Identifying tumor of origin using a gene expression-based classification map. Cancer Res 2003;63:4144–9.

57. Pavlidis N, Briasoulis E, Hainsworth J, Greco FA. Diagnostic and therapeutic management of cancer of an unknown primary. Eur J Cancer 2003;39:1990–2005.

58. Baker JJ, Solanki PH, Schenk DA, et al. Transbronchial fine needle aspiration of the mediastinum. Importance of lymphocytes as an indicator of specimen adequacy. Acta Cytol 1990;34:517–23.

59. Brooks JS. Differential diagnosis of thymic lesions. Acta Cytol 1999;43:527–9.

60. Hajdu SI. The diagnosis of thymomas. Acta Cytol 1998;42:843–4.

61. Chhieng DC, Rose D, Ludwig ME, Zakowski MF. Cytology of thymomas: emphasis on morphology and correlation with histologic subtypes. Cancer 2000;90:24–32.

62. Tao L-C. Lung pleura and mediastinum. In: Kline TS, editor. Guide to clinical aspiration biopsy. New York: Igaku-Skoin; 1988.

63. Wakely Jr PE. Cytopathology of thymic epithelial neoplasms. Semin Diagn Pathol 2005;22:213–22.

64. Fiorella M, Lavin M, Dubey S, Kragel PJ. Malignant thymoma in a patient with HIV positivity: a case report with a review of the differential diagnosis. Diagn Cytopathol 1997;16:267–9.

65. Friedman HD, Hutchison RE, Kohman LJ, Powers CN. Thymoma mimicking lymphoblastic lymphoma: a pitfall in needle aspiration biopsy interpretation. Diagn Cytopathol 1996;14:165–71.

66. Dusenbery D. Spindle-cell thymic carcinoid occurring in multiple endocrine neoplasia I: fine needle aspiration findings in a case. Diagn Cytopathol 1996;15:439–41.

67. Slagel DD, Powers CN, Melaragno MJ, et al. Spindle-cell lesions of the mediastinum: diagnosis by fine-needle aspiration biopsy. Diagn Cytopathol 1997;17:167–76.

68. Geisinger KR, Woodruff RD, Cappellarri JO. True thymic hyperplasia following cytotoxic chemotherapy: A cause of a false positive aspiration biopsy. Pathol Case Rev 2001;6:64–7.

69. Riazmontazer N, Bedayat G. Aspiration cytology of an enlarged thymus presenting as a mediastinal mass. A case report. Acta Cytol 1993;37:427–30.

70. Finley JL, Silverman JF, Strausbauch P, et al. Malignant thymic neoplasms: diagnosis by fine needle aspiration biopsy with histologic, immunocytochemical, and ultrastructural confirmation. Diagn Cytopathol 1986;2:118–25.

71. Kaw YT, Esparza AR. Fine needle aspiration cytology of primary squamous carcinoma of the thymus. A case report. Acta Cytol 1993;37:735–9.

72. Riazmontazer N, Beydat C, Izadi B. Epithelial cytologic atypia in a fine needle aspirate of an invasive thymoma. A case report. Acta Cytol 1992;36:387–90.

73. Posligua L, Ylagan L. Fine-needle aspiration cytology of thymic basaloid carcinoma: case studies and review of the literature. Diagn Cytopathol 2006;34:358–66.

74. Kapila K, Pathan SK, Amir T, et al. Mucoepidermoid thymic carcinoma: a challenging mediastinal aspirate. Diagn Cytopathol 2009 Jun;37(6):433–6.

75. Dorfman DM, Shahsafaei A, Chan JKC. Thymic carcinomas, but not thymomas and carcinomas of other sites, show CD5 immunoreactivity. Am J Surg Pathol 1997;21:936–40.

76. Nonaka D, Henley JD, Chiriboga L, Yee H. Diagnostic utility of thymic epithelial markers CD205 (DEC205) and Foxn1 in thymic epithelial neoplasms. Am J Surg Pathol 2007;31:1038–44.

77. Lewis JE, Wick MR, Scheithauer BW, et al. Thymoma. A clinicopathologic review. Cancer 1987;60:2727–43.

78. Suster S, Moran CA. Thymoma, atypical thymoma, and thymic carcinoma. A novel conceptual approach to the classification of thymic epithelial neoplasms. Am J Clin Pathol 1999;111:826–33.

79. Gherardi G, Marveggio C, Placidi A. Neuroendocrine carcinoma of the thymus: aspiration biopsy, immunocytochemistry and clinical correlates. Diagn Cytopathol 1995;12:158–64.

80. Wang D-Y, Kuo S-H, Chang D-B. Fine needle aspiration cytology of thymic carcinoid tumour. Acta Cytol 1995;39:423–7.

81. Collins BT, Cramer M. Fine needle aspiration cytology of carcinoid tumours. Acta Cytol 1996;40:695–707.

82. Nichols CA, Hopkins MB, Geisinger KR. Thymic carcinoid. Report of a case with diagnosis by fine needle aspiration biopsy. Acta Cytol 1997;41:839–44.

83. Moran CA, Suster S. Neuroendocrine carcinomas (carcinoid tumor) of the thymus. A clinicopathologic analysis of 80 cases. Am J Clin Pathol 2000;114:100–10.

84. Moran CA, Suster S. Thymic neuroendocrine carcinomas with combined features ranging from well-differentiated (carcinoid) to small cell carcinoma. A clinicopathologic and immunohistochemical study of 11 cases. Am J Clin Pathol 2000;113:345–50.

85. Suster S, Moran CA. Neuroendocrine neoplasms of the mediastinum. Am J Clin Pathol 2001;115(Suppl):S17–27.

86. Smith NL, Finley JL. Lipid-rich carcinoid tumor of the thymus gland: diagnosis by fine-needle aspiration biopsy. Diagn Cytopathol 2001;25:130–3.

87. Teh BT, Zedenius J, Kytölä S, et al. Thymic carcinoids in multiple endocrine neoplasia type 1. Ann Surg 1998;228:99–105.

88. Dahl I, Hagmar B, Idvall I. Benign solitary neurilemmoma (Schwannoma). A correlative aspiration cytology and histologic study of 28 cases. Acta Pathol Microbiol Scand (A) 1984;92:91–101.

89. Dahlgren SE, Ovenfors C-O. Aspiration biopsy diagnosis of neurogenous mediastinal tumours. Acta Radiol Diagn (Stockh) 1970;10:408–21.

90. Zbieranowski I, Bedard Y. Fine needle aspiration of Schwannomas. Acta Cytol 1989;33:381–4.

91. Palombini L, Vetrani A, Veccione R, et al. The cytology of ganglioneuroma on fine needle aspiration smear. Acta Cytol 1982;26:259–60.

92. Palombini L, Vetrani A. Cytologic diagnosis of ganglioneuroblastoma. Acta Cytol 1976;20:286–7.

93. Das DK, Pant CS, Rath B, et al. Fine needle aspiration diagnosis of intrathoracic and intra-abdominal lesions: review of experience in the paediatric age group. Diagn Cytopathol 1993;9:383–93.

94. Silverman JF, Dabbs DJ, Ganick J, et al. Fine needle aspiration cytology of neuroblastoma including peripheral neuroectodermal tumor with immunocytochemical and ultrastructural confirmation. Acta Cytol 1988;32:367–76.

95. Varma K, Jain S, Mandal S. Cytomorphologic spectrum of paraganglioma. Acta Cytol 2008;52:549–56.

96. Meyer L, Gibbons D, Ashfaq R, et al. Fine-needle aspiration findings in Castleman's disease. Diagn Cytopathol 1999;21:57–60.

97. Bangerter M, Behnisch W, Griesshammer M. Mediastinal masses diagnosed as thymus hyperplasia by fine needle aspiration cytology. Acta Cytol 2000;44:743–7.

98. Hoerl HD, Wojtowycz M, Gallagher HA, Kurtycz DF. Cytologic diagnosis of true thymic hyperplasia by combined radiologic imaging and aspiration cytology: a case report including flow cytometric analysis. Diagn Cytopathol 2000;23:417–21.

99. Young NA, Al-Saleem T. Diagnosis of lymphoma by fine-needle aspiration cytology using the revised European-American classification of lymphoid neoplasms. Cancer 1999;87:325–45.

100. Wakely Jr PE. Aspiration cytopathology of malignant lymphoma: coming of age. Cancer 1999;87:322–4.

101. Yang GC, Yee HT, Wu CD, et al. TIA-1+ cytotoxic large T-cell lymphoma of the mediastinum: case report. Diagn Cytopathol 2002;26:154–7.

102. Kardos TF, Vinson JH, Behm FG, et al. Hodgkin's disease: diagnosis by fine needle aspiration biopsy: analysis of cytologic criteria from a selected series. Am J Clin Pathol 1986;86:286–91.

103. Jacobs JC, Katz RL, Shabb N, et al. Fine needle aspiration of lymphoblastic lymphoma. A multiparameter approach. Acta Cytol 1992;36:887–93.

104. Kardos TF, Sprague RI, Wakely Jr PE, Frable WJ. Fine needle aspiration biopsy of lymphoblastic lymphoma and leukaemia. A clinical, cytologic and immunologic study. Cancer 1987;60:24–48.

105. Wakely Jr PE, Kornstein MJ. Aspiration cytopathology of lymphoblastic lymphoma and leukemia: the MCV experience. Pediatr Pathol Lab Med 1996;16:243–52.

106. Silverman JF, Raab SS, Park HK. Fine needle aspiration cytology of primary large cell lymphoma of the mediastinum: cytomorphologic findings with potential pitfalls in diagnosis. Diagn Cytopathol 1993;9:209–15

107. Francis IM, Das DK, Al-Rubah NAR, Gupta SK. Lymphoglandular bodies in lymphoid lesions and non-lymphoid round cell tumours: a quantitative assessment. Diagn Cytopathol 1994;11:23–7.

108. Deschênes M, Michel RP, Tabah R, Auger M. Fine-needle aspiration cytology of Castleman disease: case report with review of the literature. Diagn Cytopathol 2008 Dec;36(12):904–8.

109. Sangali G, Livraghi T, Giosano F, et al. Primary mediastinal embryonal carcinoma and choriocarcinoma. A case report. Acta Cytol 1986;30:543–6.

110. Harun MH, Yaacob I. Congenital posterior mediastinal teratoma. A case report. Singapore Med J 1993;34:567–8.

111. Yang GCH. Demonstration of fibrils in the hyaline globules of yolk sac tumor with parietal differentiation in fine needle aspiration smears. Diagn Cytopathol 1994;10:216–20.

112. Collins KA, Geisinger KR, Wakely PE, et al. Extragonadal germ cell tumours: a fine needle aspiration study. Diagn Cytopathol 1995;12:223–9.

113. Motoyama T, Yamamoto O, Iwamoto H, Watanabe H. Fine needle aspiration cytology of primary mediastinal germ cell tumors. Acta Cytol 1995;39: 725–32.

114. Chao TY, Nieh S, Huang SH, Lee WH. Cytology of fine needle aspirates of primary extragonadal germ cell tumors. Acta Cytol 1997;41:497–503.

115. Silverman JF, Olson PR, Dabbs DJ, Landreneau R. Fine-needle aspiration cytology of a mediastinal seminoma associated with multilocular thymic cyst. Diagn Cytopathol 1999;20:224–8.

116. Chhieng DC, Lin O, Moran CA, et al. Fine-needle aspiration biopsy of nonteratomatous germ cell tumors of the mediastinum. Am J Clin Pathol 2002;118:418–24.

117. Yang GC, Hwang SJ, Yee HT. Fine-needle aspiration cytology of unusual germ cell tumors of the mediastinum: atypical seminoma and parietal yolk sac tumor. Diagn Cytopathol 2002;27: 69–74.

118. de Almeida M, Stastny JF, Wakely Jr PE, Frable WJ. Fine-needle aspiration biopsy of childhood rhabdomyosarcoma: reevaluation of the cytologic criteria for diagnosis. Diagn Cytopathol 1994;11:231–6.

119. Geisinger KR, Travis WD, Perkins LA, Zakowski MF. Aspiration cytomorphology of fetal adenocarcinoma of the lung. Am J Clin Pathol in press.

120. Dunsmore N, Sherman ME, Erozan YS. Massive necrosis: a pitfall in the cytopathologic diagnosis of primary mediastinal seminoma. Diagn Cytopathol 1991;7:323–4.

121. Moran CA, Suster S. Yolk sac tumors of the mediastinum with prominent spindle cell features: a clinicopathologic study of three cases. Am J Surg Pathol 1997;21:1173–7.

122. Moran CA, Suster S. Primary mediastinal choriocarcinoma: a clinicopathologic and immunohistochemical study of eight cases. Am J Surg Pathol 1997;21:1007–12.

123. Kuhlman JE, Fishman EK, Wang KP, et al. Mediastinal cysts: diagnosis by CT and needle aspiration. Am J Roentgenol 1988;150:75–8.

124. Suster S, Rosai J. Multilocular thymic cyst. An acquired reactive process. Study of 18 cases. Am J Surg Pathol 1991;15:388–98.

125. Chhieng DC, Demaria S, Yee HT, Yang GC. Multilocular thymic cyst with follicular lymphoid hyperplasia in a male infected with HIV. A case report with fine needle aspiration cytology. Acta Cytol 1999;43:1119–23.

126. Marco V, Carrasco MA, Marco C, Bauza A. Cytomorphology of a mediastinal parathyroid cyst. Report of a case mimicking malignancy. Acta Cytol 1983;27:688–92.

127. Mishriki YY, Lane BP, Lozowski MS, Epstein H. Hurthle-cell tumor arising in the mediastinal ectopic thyroid and diagnosed by fine needle aspiration. Light microscopic and ultrastructural features. Acta Cytol 1983;27:188–92.

128. De Las Casas LE, Williams HJ, Strausbauch PH, Silverman JF. Hurthle cell adenoma of the mediastinum: intraoperative cytology and differential diagnosis with correlative gross, histology, and ancillary studies. Diagn Cytopathol 2000;22:16–20.

129. Vu DH, Erickson RA. Endoscopic ultrasound-guided fine-needle aspiration with aspirate assay to diagnose suspected mediastinal parathyroid adenomas. Endocr Pract 2010;16:437–40.

130. Downey RJ, Cerfolio RJ, Deschamps C, et al. Mediastinal parathyroid cysts. Mayo Clin Proc 1995;70:946–50.

131. Attal H, Jenson J, Reyes CV. Myxoid liposarcoma of the anterior mediastinum. Diagnosis by fine needle aspiration biopsy. Acta Cytol 1995;39:511–3.

132. Munjal K, Pancholi V, Rege J, et al. Fine needle aspiration cytology in mediastinal myxoid liposarcoma: a case report. Acta Cytol 2007;51: 456–8.

133. Suster S, Moran CA. Primary synovial sarcomas of the mediastinum: a clinicopathologic, immunohistochemical, and ultrastructural study of 15 cases. Am J Surg Pathol 2005;29:569–78.

134. Heimann A, Sneige N, Shirkhoda A, DeCaro LF. Fine needle aspiration cytology of thymolipoma. A case report. Acta Cytol 1987;31:335–9.

135. Al-Marzooq YM, Al-Bahrani AT, Chopra R, Al-Momatten MI. Fine-needle aspiration biopsy diagnosis of intrathoracic extramedullary hematopoiesis presenting as a posterior mediastinal tumor in a patient with sickle-cell disease: case report. Diagn Cytopathol 2004;30: 119–21.

Liver and spleen

Bastiaan de Boer*

Liver

The place of FNA in the investigative sequence

Malignancy in the liver, primary or metastatic, is usually inoperable at the time of diagnosis and, as such, portends an ominous prognosis. A diagnostic modality such as FNA, which offers accuracy without significant complications and which requires minimal intervention at low cost, warrants consideration early in the investigative sequence. Portal vein FNA sampling is feasible in patients with hepatocellular carcinoma (HCC) and may be considered as a staging option.[1-3] FNA may become useful after local ablative therapy of liver tumors to determine residual viable tumor.[4,5] In this era of liver transplantation there is some reluctance in performing FNA in patients who are being worked up for a transplant because of the risk of needle track implantation in the setting of immunosuppression, although this is disputed by some.[6-10] Single or multiple focal abnormalities demonstrated by palpation, ultrasonography (US), computed tomography (CT) or nuclear scan constitute the main indications for FNA of the liver. In industrialized countries, metastatic tumor deposits are the most common cause of focal abnormalities. In developing countries, however, hepatocellular carcinoma (HCC) is a major health problem, and is more likely to be encountered in FNA. Approximately 80% of the annual global burden of 560 000 new cases of HCC occurs in Africa and Asia. In these areas, etiology is frequently the hepatitis B virus, with superadded aflatoxin ingestion. HCC in developed countries arises in a background of cirrhosis consequent on chronic alcohol abuse or, more recently, hepatitis C virus.[11]

The differential diagnosis of hepatic mass lesions includes primary liver tumors, benign or malignant, metastatic deposits, congenital and acquired cysts, abscesses and granulomas. Single radiolucencies in the liver are not infrequently found at US scanning of asymptomatic patients. The question raised is that of metastatic cancer versus a primary liver lesion such as hemangioma.

Some workers have advocated the use of FNA in diffuse parenchymal liver disease.[12-14] Most physicians feel that cytological methods lack the precision necessary to be of diagnostic value in processes such as cirrhosis, hepatitis and drug-induced effects.[15,16] The pathologist must nevertheless be familiar with the hepatic changes which may be present as a local reaction adjacent to space-occupying lesions, and with the severe parenchymal abnormality which may represent the cirrhotic background of HCC. The cytological features of normal liver, and various changes associated with diffuse chronic liver disease have been described.[12-14,16-19]

FNA can diagnose certain diffuse processes such as hemosiderosis, amyloidosis and myeloid metaplasia. Metastatic melanoma or carcinoma, particularly of breast and lung, and malignant lymphoma can occasionally cause hepatomegaly by diffuse infiltration, without demonstrable focal abnormalities. These infiltrates may be sampled and can be diagnosed by FNA techniques. FNA has also been used for monitoring liver transplants.[20-25]

Advantages of FNA over conventional core biopsy are: it is less invasive and therefore leads to fewer complications, sampling can be performed over a wide area, either superficial or deep lesions can be targeted, small nodules high in the dome of the right lobe can be sampled, multiple sites including both left and right lobes can be sampled, immediate triage for adequacy can be performed limiting the number of needle passes, and hospitalization is not required. The disadvantages are: the material is limited with less architectural information, and a skilled radiologist and a skilled cytopathologist are required for optimal results. Small focal abnormalities can be missed by either method. Morphologic features must therefore always be correlated with clinical presentation and radiologic findings to determine whether the liver lesion has been fully explained by either modality.

Accuracy of diagnosis

Most studies comparing core needle biopsy and FNA favor the fine needle for focal liver disease,[26-28] although not all,[29] and generally a combination of the two yields the best results.[28,30] Diagnostic sensitivity of FNA in malignancy is usually to around 90% (range 67–100%).[26,28,30-36] Cell typing

*With acknowledgments to Gladwyn Leiman for her work in previous editions

©2012 Elsevier Ltd
DOI: 10.1016/B978-0-7020-3151-9.00010-4

can sometimes be problematic in smears and many centers therefore advocate the additional use of cell blocks for histological assessment and providing multiple sections for immunocytochemistry.[32,37] The use of cell blocks improved reported accuracy of hepatocellular carcinoma typing from around 85%[38,39] to 95%.[40,41] Certain groups report the combined use of aspirates and tissue cores for more definitive diagnosis of focal liver lesions.[30] Recent use of the endoscopic ultrasound guided approach to FNA of the liver appears not only to maintain the high sensitivity and specificity of liver FNA, but also to identify and target lesions too small to be detected by conventional transabdominal ultrasound and CT.[42-44] Whichever modality is used for sampling, we strongly advise the on-site participation of personnel from cytopathology to ensure optimal handling of the sample, rapid interpretation, and triage of the specimen as required.

There are pitfalls which the cytopathologist must be aware of. These include: the clinical history or imaging appearance may be misleading, the sample may be of the liver adjacent to the lesion and therefore non-representative, contamination from structures traversed on the way to the lesion, e.g. stomach, bowel or mesothelium, may predominate.

Complications

No deaths and only one significant complication, an intrahepatic hematoma, occurred in an early report of 2611 cases.[45] A later summary of 7500 FNAs from 11 series recorded no deaths.[46] In an extensive literature review and questionnaire study,[47] Smith collated fatalities following abdominal percutaneous FNA. Of 21 deaths involving liver FNA, he noted that 17 were due to hemorrhage. A needle larger than 0.8 mm (21 gauge) was used in seven. Three of the other 10 followed FNA of vascular tumors (hemangioma 1, angiosarcoma 2). Fatalities due to other causes were rare (sepsis 2, carcinoid crisis 1, uncertain 1). More recently, two deaths due to hemorrhage from among 1750 US guided FNA has been reported.[48]

Allegations of needle track spread of tumor have always dogged FNA, and the liver is no exception in this regard. Of recent concern has been a number of literature reports of subcutaneous seeding of needle tracks from otherwise operable HCCs.[47,49-51] Whereas in some of these reports the procedures comply in every respect with the usual safety precautions advised (0.8-mm/21-gauge needles or smaller, few needle passes, traversal of normal liver parenchyma between abdominal wall and tumor),[52] other reports often included in discussion of this issue have used 18-gauge needles,[53] have traversed one lobe to reach a lesion in the other lobe and have not defined needle size,[54] or are series in which cutting[55] or Trucut[56] needles have been used. Cytopathologists and radiologists performing hepatic FNA should discuss and be very clear about the caliber of needles used.

In those cases in which potentially resectable or transplantable HCC is being investigated, local opinion might preclude preoperative sampling.[9] This is despite studies that show FNA has no significant adverse effect on operability, extrahepatic metastases or long-term survival.[6,8,57] Experience with cases of needle track spread has shown that local treatment by resection has been successful for isolated subcutaneous tumor deposits.[47,49,53-56] In the vast majority of hepatic aspiration procedures, physicians and patients can be assured of very low complication rates (hemorrhage 0.006–0.031%, needle track spread 0.007%).[47]

Contraindications

Hemorrhagic diathesis and anticoagulation are contraindications, and the prothrombin time and the platelet count should be checked before the FNA. The patient should be kept under observation for a few hours after biopsy to monitor pulse, blood pressure and abdominal pain. Hydatid cyst was formerly considered to be a relative contraindication in view of the risk of an anaphylactic reaction.[58] However, no allergic reactions have been observed in two series of 11 hydatid cysts aspirated inadvertently.[59,60] The single documented case of anaphylactic shock, which was reversed, occurred when an 18-gauge needle was used.[58] The risk of hemorrhage by needling of vasoformative tumors exists, but is low if correct techniques are used. This is no longer considered an absolute contraindication.[61-64]

Technical considerations

Whenever possible, the biopsy should be directed rather than blind. If a mass cannot be clearly felt, the biopsy must be guided by radiological imaging. US is the most commonly used modality.[31,32] More recently, clinicians and radiologists have been using endoscopic ultrasound to target some liver lesions, in particular those involving the hilum and left lobe. Great technical expertise is required for good results, and is acquired after significant experience.[43,44,65-67]

Ideally, a cytopathologist or cytologist attends the FNA procedure for rapid review to confirm diagnostic material and to triage the material.[68] Rapid staining (Diff-Quik or H&E) allows immediate screening of samples. The parallel use of MGG and Pap staining is strongly recommended for permanent smears of liver aspirates. Most adjunctive cytochemical or immunocytochemical tests are more easily performed on cell blocks, but some may be useful in smears or in cytocentrifuged and thin-layer preparations. Additionally, demonstration of architectural patterns in sections of tissue fragments increases diagnostic accuracy significantly.[37,40,69-72] If immediate assessment suggests an acute, chronic or granulomatous inflammatory process, material for microbiological assessment should be collected in a sterile container. If a lymphoproliferative disorder is suggested, a separate needle pass should be collected into RPMI or normal saline for flow cytometry. Cytogenetic FISH testing, e.g. for specific translocations, can be performed on cytospin preparations and molecular studies, e.g. for lymphoma clonality, can be conducted on material from cell blocks. Electron microscopy may also contribute to type-specific tumor diagnosis.[70,73] These adjunctive techniques ensure that liver aspirates are highly suited to sophisticated cytohistological interpretation. A core biopsy should occasionally be requested, particularly if architectural assessment is crucial to the diagnosis e.g. hepatic adenoma versus hepatocellular carcinoma. If radiology staff are to prepare the sample they should be trained, appropriate consumables should be supplied and collection of material into fluid for a cell block or cytospin preparations should be encouraged.

CYTOLOGICAL FINDINGS

Liver

Normal structures (Fig. 10.1)

Although the aspirate may appear to consist mainly of blood, it usually contains many liver cells. Cell cohesion is particularly strong, and when the needle content is placed on a slide one can often see small, firm, semitranslucent tissue fragments which are difficult to spread. In comparison, tumor tissue fragments are usually soft, fragile and easily smeared.

In smears, normal hepatocytes form irregular, cohesive sheets and narrow cords 1–2 cells thick (Fig. 10.1A). Single cells are infrequent. The cells are large, round or distinctly polygonal in outline with abundant granular cytoplasm, sometimes vacuolated, staining eosinophilic with H&E, blue with Papanicolaou or gray–blue with MGG (Fig. 10.1B). Nuclei are centrally located, round, with finely granular chromatin which is evenly distributed. Binucleate cells are common. Nucleoli are central and usually small although prominent. The cell membrane is indistinct. Normal hepatocytes may display mild to moderate anisokaryosis due to polyploidy, increasing with the patient's age. Occasional nuclei may be very large in non-neoplastic liver tissue. Coarse, granular intracytoplasmic pigment is commonly present in hepatocytes. It stains green–black with MGG, brown with H&E and is probably lipofuscin rather than bile. Kupffer cells can usually be found and appear as single, bare, comma-shaped nuclei between the hepatocytes. Bile duct epithelial cells form small, regular monolayered sheets. They are palisaded when seen from the side. The cytoplasm is minimal, nuclear chromatin is granular and nucleoli are inconspicuous. These are few in number in samples from normal liver tissue.

Diffuse parenchymal disease (Figs 10.2–10.9)

As already stated, FNA is not primarily suited to diagnosis of non-neoplastic, parenchymal liver disease.[15] However, it is essential that the cytologist recognizes these changes, as they may occur in the region of space-occupying lesions and may themselves mimic neoplasia.

The presence of parenchymal disease is indicated by decreased cohesion of hepatocytes. Smears may be hypercellular and appear quite pleomorphic due to anisocytosis. The hepatocytes are swollen to a variable degree, and the cytoplasm stains less uniformly than usual, paler at the periphery of the cell. Cell membranes which are indistinct in normal

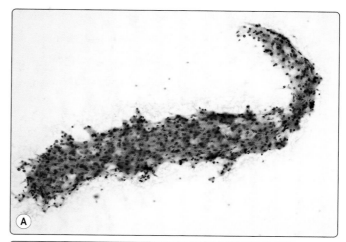

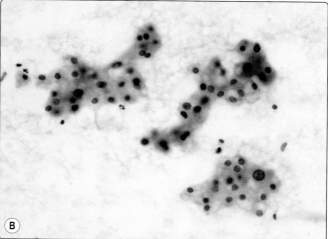

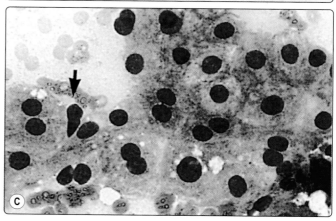

Fig. 10.1 Hepatocytes (A) Irregular cohesive sheet showing a trabecular arrangement (Pap, IP); (B) Cohesive groups of polygonal cells with abundant sometimes vacuolated granular cytoplasm (Pap, HP); (C) Cohesive cells with central round nuclei, granular cytoplasm and indistinct cell borders; note the small wedge-shaped Kupffer cell (*arrow*) (MGG, HP).

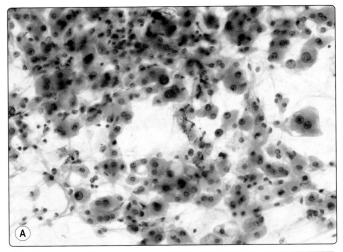

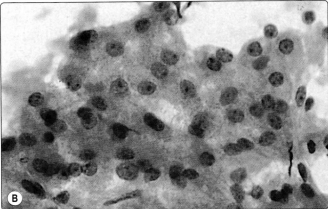

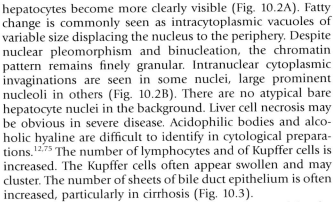

Fig. 10.2 Hepatocyte reactive changes (A) Cells showing decreased cohesion, anisokaryosis and well-defined cell borders; note the scattered Kuppfer cells and lymphocytes (Pap, IP); (B) A sheet of cells showing mild disorganization and prominent nucleoli (H&E, HP).

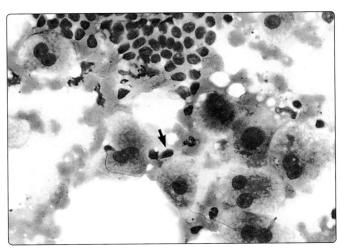

Fig. 10.3 Cirrhosis Poorly cohesive hepatocytes with degenerative/ regenerative features; a sheet of small cohesive bile duct cells; note several Kupffer cells (*arrow*) (MGG, HP).

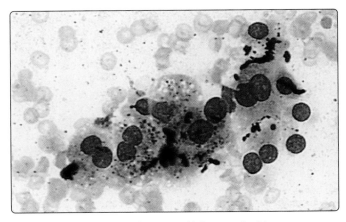

Fig. 10.4 Bile stasis Cords of inspissated bile in canaliculi between hepatocytes (MGG, HP).

hepatocytes become more clearly visible (Fig. 10.2A). Fatty change is commonly seen as intracytoplasmic vacuoles of variable size displacing the nucleus to the periphery. Despite nuclear pleomorphism and binucleation, the chromatin pattern remains finely granular. Intranuclear cytoplasmic invaginations are seen in some nuclei, large prominent nucleoli in others (Fig. 10.2B). There are no atypical bare hepatocyte nuclei in the background. Liver cell necrosis may be obvious in severe disease. Acidophilic bodies and alcoholic hyaline are difficult to identify in cytological preparations.[12,75] The number of lymphocytes and of Kupffer cells is increased. The Kupffer cells often appear swollen and may cluster. The number of sheets of bile duct epithelium is often increased, particularly in cirrhosis (Fig. 10.3).

The degree of parenchymal abnormality varies widely. The reactive change commonly seen adjacent to a neoplasm is an example of mild change, including some dissociation and swelling of hepatocytes and mild to moderate anisokaryosis. In cirrhosis, which may mimic neoplasia radiologically as well as cytologically,[76] there is a marked increase in the number of Kupffer cells and of bile duct epithelial cells, fatty change, and dissociation of hepatocytes. Bile stasis is easily recognized as casts of dense material between hepatocytes,

staining black–green with MGG (Fig. 10.4), yellow–green with Pap or H&E. Nuclear changes and nucleolar enlargement may be quite prominent. In so-called liver cell dysplasia associated with cirrhosis, there is a dominant background of normal hepatocytes among which are scattered atypical cells with considerably enlarged nuclei. The fibrosis of cirrhosis is not often evident on routinely stained smears, but can be demonstrated on smears or on cell block material using a connective tissue stain. Normal liver will demonstrate a fine regular network of reticulin. Cirrhosis is characterized by a disorganized but still intact network (Fig. 10.5). HCC typically shows fragmentation or a complete absence of reticulin framework.[77,78]

Hemosiderosis is recognized by the demonstration of coarse, refractile hemosiderin pigment – golden brown in Papanicolaou, black in Romanowsky stains – in the hepatocytes (Fig. 10.6) and in the Kupffer cells. It is not always easy to distinguish hemosiderin from lipofuscin or even from bile in routinely stained smears; a suitable special stain such as Prussian blue should be used if hemosiderosis is suspected.[14,79] Further, with malignant transformation, iron pigment is lost. Prussian blue negative clusters can be

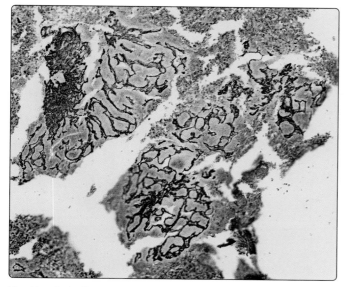

Fig. 10.5 **Reticulin stain** Intact although disorganized sinusoidal network identified in cirrhosis (cell block reticulin, HP).

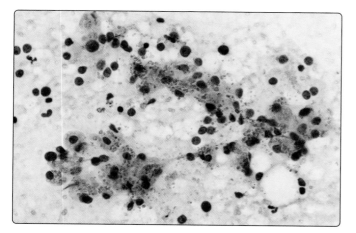

Fig. 10.6 **Hemochromatosis** Hepatocytes showing intracytoplasmic granular brown pigment (Pap, HP).

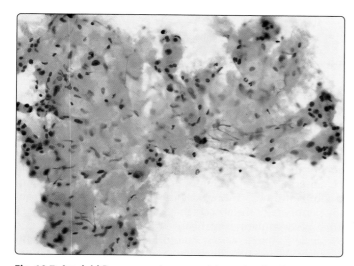

Fig. 10.7 **Amyloid** Dense amorphous material associated with atrophic hepatocytes (H&E, HP).

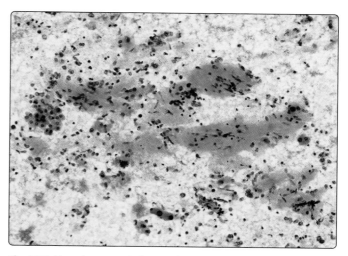

Fig. 10.8 **Granulomatous inflammation** Loose clusters of epithelioid histiocytes and occasional giant cells; note the cluster of hepatocytes mixed in with the inflammation (Pap, IP).

regarded with suspicion in the setting of a mass arising in a background of siderosis.[80] *Amyloidosis* is not common but may cause massive hepatomegaly and is diagnosable cytologically. Amyloid appears in smears as a dense amorphous, waxy material, which stains pink with H&E (Fig. 10.7), magenta with MGG and orangeophilic with Papanicolaou stain. Its presence should be confirmed with special stains such as Congo red. The hepatocytes often appear atrophic.[81–84]

The finding of granulomatous inflammation may either be incidental or represent the lesion being aspirated but does not permit a specific diagnosis.[85] Cytological features include loose aggregates of epithelioid histiocytes which have large elongated plump nuclei, finely granular chromatin, small distinct nucleoli, abundant, pale-staining cytoplasm, Langhans and/or foreign body type giant cells and non-specific inflammation (Fig. 10.8). Caseous necrosis may be seen. The etiology most likely to present as a mass, particularly in the Third World, is infection such as mycobacteria.[86] Material should be collected appropriately for culture and special stains to demonstrate the acid-fast bacilli.[12] Failing this, PCR for mycobacteria can be performed on fresh or fixed material. The list of differential diagnoses for granulomata in the liver is long and their demonstration in FNA smears requires clinical correlation and further investigation to determine their exact etiology.

Non-neoplastic focal lesions

Cysts

Congenital (developmental) cysts

An aspirate from a congenital cyst, in reality a dilatation of a biliary duct, consists of thin, clear fluid but may be bloody or bile stained. A few uniform, cuboidal epithelial cells, single or in monolayered sheets, and some macrophages with vacuolated cytoplasm may be found in the smears (Fig. 10.9A).[87] The columnar cells may balloon if degenerate. The ciliated hepatic foregut cyst can be diagnosed cytologically by observing clusters of ciliated columnar cells in the cyst milieu (Fig. 10.9B).[88,89]

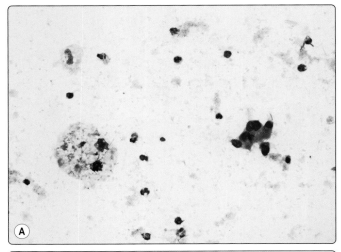

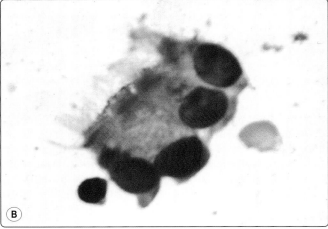

Fig. 10.9 Congenital (developmental) cysts (A) Paucicellular; showing a degenerate macrophage and a cluster of columnar epithelial cells in a background of granular debris (MGG, HP); (B) Ciliated columnar epithelial cells found in fluid aspirated from a hepatic foregut cyst (MGG, HP oil).

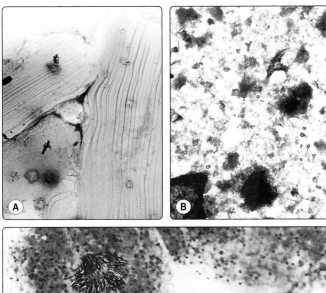

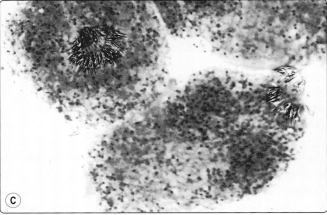

Fig. 10.10 Hydatid cyst (A) Fragments of laminar membrane; (B) Debris and altered blood; note refractile hooklet (*upper right*) (MGG, HP); (C) Full scolices with clearly visible refractile hooklets (MGG, IP).

CRITERIA FOR DIAGNOSIS

◆ Sparsely cellular,
◆ Cuboidal or columnar epithelial cells, usually bland but can be hyperplastic, dysplastic or rarely malignant,
◆ Ciliated cells (in ciliated hepatic foregut cyst) have basal nuclei without prominent nucleoli, abundant apical cytoplasm, terminal plates and fine delicate cilia,
◆ Macrophages and mucin may be present,
◆ Abundant bile pigment in Caroli's disease.

Hydatid cyst

Routine aspiration of a hydatid cyst is not recommended because of the theoretical risk of anaphylaxis should the cyst contents spill into the abdomen.[62,90]

CRITERIA FOR DIAGNOSIS[59,90–92]

◆ The aspirated fluid may be clear or turbid and thick,
◆ Fragments of laminated membrane (stains pink in Papanicolaou smears and magenta with a PAS stain (Fig. 10.10A),
◆ Detached hooklets which are refractile and birefringent (Fig. 10.10B),
◆ Scolices are bulging, rounded, blunt 'heads' with attached suckers and rows of hooklets (Fig. 10.10C) .

Abscess (Fig. 10.11)

Purulent material aspirated from a focal lesion should always be subjected to microbiological investigation. Routine smears should also be prepared and screened for neoplastic cells, as tumor metastases, for example from a primary bowel adenocarcinoma, can undergo central necrosis, simulating an abscess. *Pyogenic abscess* demonstrates a marked neutrophil infiltrate, with necrotic debris.[93] Hepatocytes from the periphery of the abscess may show considerable atypia.[76] The predominant organism in pyogenic abscesses is *Klebsiella*.[93] *Amebic abscess* due to *Entamoeba histolytica*, with contents likened to anchovy paste (thick reddish-brown semi-fluid material), shows abundant necrosis with fewer inflammatory cells. Trophozoites are not found in the central

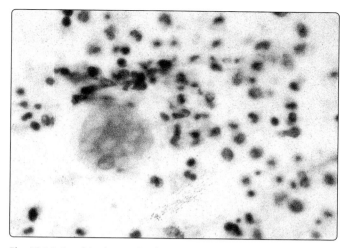

Fig. 10.11 **Amebic abscess** Single trophozoite with a small peripheral nucleus (*upper left*); background of acute inflammatory cells (Pap, HP).

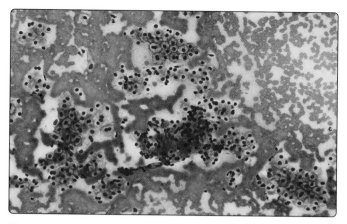

Fig. 10.12 **Focal nodular hyperplasia** Cohesive benign hepatocytes in sheets associated with a fragment of fibrous tissue (MGG, IP).

necrotic area; they should be sought in the viable periphery of the abscess (Fig. 10.11).[93,94] They are globular organisms, with an eccentric spherical nucleus showing a central clear zone with a dot-like karyosome and margination of chromatin. The cytoplasm is vacuolated and contains ingested red blood cells. Amebae stain positive with PAS. They resemble foamy macrophages and may be missed if not suspected. The diagnosis of hepatic *actinomycosis* by FNB has been reported.[95,96] It occurs in a background of systemic actinomycosis, secondary to pulmonary or uterine primary sources of infection.

Focal nodular hyperplasia

(FNH) is a solitary tumor-like lesion of uncertain histogenesis but benign prognosis. It occurs at all ages, predominantly in middle life and in women. Most FNH are detected incidentally in otherwise normal livers. Radiologically and macroscopically, the lesion shows a central radiating scar separating nodules of hepatocytes.

CRITERIA FOR DIAGNOSIS[46,106]

◆ Moderately cellular smears,
◆ Cohesive uniform benign hepatocytes in sheets or clusters (Fig. 10.12),
◆ Trabecular/sinusoidal architecture confirmed on a reticulin stain,
◆ No dispersal or stripped nuclei,
◆ Fragments of fibrous tissue with lymphocytes,
◆ Increased bile ductules.

Distinction from low-grade hepatocellular tumors such as adenoma and well-differentiated hepatocellular carcinoma can be problematic and cell block or core biopsy with a reticulin stain may provide useful architectural information (see section on Hepatocellular carcinoma: Problems and differential diagnoses).

Other non-neoplastic lesions

Focal fatty change in the liver can simulate neoplasia on radiologic imaging, and diagnosis by FNA is of practical importance.[97,98] It is less common than the diffuse form and the etiology is uncertain. The hepatocytes have normal nuclei and the majority contain multiple or single clear vacuoles, bile duct epithelium may be present and the reticulin framework may be distorted by the fat droplets.

Inflammatory pseudotumor is a distinct entity increasingly being identified radiologically and thus entering the ambit of cytodiagnosis. The liver is probably the second most common site after lung for its occurrence.[99] It is a localized lesion of uncertain etiology, representing an atypical immune response or a hypersensitivity reaction to antigen. Histological variants include inflamed granulation tissue, xanthogranuloma, hyaline sclerosing variant and plasma cell granuloma. FNAC can be expected to be equally variable. Hepatocytes and bile duct cells, which can show atypia and plasma cells, lymphocytes, neutrophils ±eosinophils and/or xanthoma cells in a background of fibroblasts, create a mixed picture which should not be overdiagnosed as malignant. Single large abnormal cells with lobulated vesicular nuclei resembling Reed-Sternberg cells have been reported.[100–102]

Nodular extramedullary hemopoiesis occurs typically in the setting of myeloproliferative disease and is recognized by the criteria of the triple cell lines – normoblasts, promyelocytes and megakaryocytes.[103–105] The last mentioned could be mistaken for bizarre malignant cells.

Neoplasms

Primary hepatic tumors of epithelial origin

Hepatobiliary cystadenoma

These solitary multiloculated lesions may reach sizes over 20 cm. They are encountered almost exclusively in females, generally of middle age.[107,108] They are composed of a bland, cuboidal to columnar, nonciliated mucin-secreting epithelium, overlying dense ovarian-like stroma. The cyst contents are mucoid and may show raised CEA and CA 19-9 levels on biochemical testing.[87,107,109]

Tumors have a definite malignant potential and any solid, nodular or polypoid region seen on imaging should be sampled.[110–114]

Liver cell adenoma (Fig. 10.13)

Cytodiagnosis of this entity can hardly be made with confidence by cytology alone and a core biopsy can provide additional architectural information. The cytological pattern must be correlated with clinical presentation and radiological findings.[115] A solitary liver mass found in a young woman with a history of oral contraceptive usage is most likely a hepatocellular adenoma, whereas a mass in an older patient with cirrhosis is more likely either a regenerative nodule or a hepatocellular carcinoma.

The differences in cytological patterns between adenoma and well-differentiated carcinoma can be subtle and will be discussed in the section on hepatocellular carcinoma. The cytoplasm is more abundant, less fragile and better defined with more distinct cell borders in adenoma, the nuclear:cytoplasmic ratio is consistently low, and single, bare neoplastic nuclei are less apparent (Fig. 10.13). Marked anisokaryosis is not a feature. Adenoma and FNH both comprise benign hepatocytes. In the absence of abundant bile duct epithelium, which favors FNH, distinction between them is not possible.[41,106]

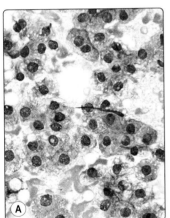
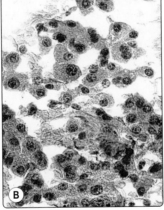
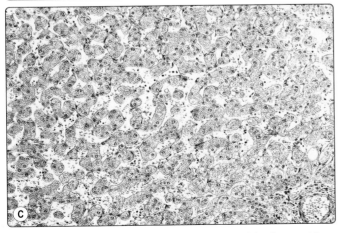

Fig. 10.13 Liver cell adenoma Poorly cohesive epithelial cells resembling hepatocytes, bland nuclei, Kupffer cells but no bile duct epithelium (**A**, H&E, IP; **B**, Pap, HP); (**C**) Corresponding tissue section (H&E, IP).

Hepatocellular carcinoma (Figs 10.14–10.27)

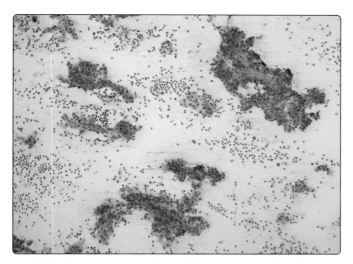

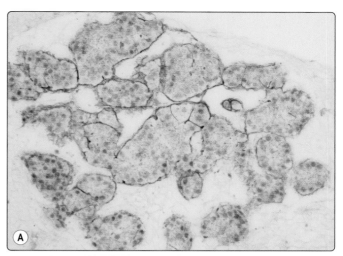

Fig. 10.14 **Hepatocellular carcinoma** Cellular smears with irregular large fragments, clusters and dispersed cells (H&E, LP).

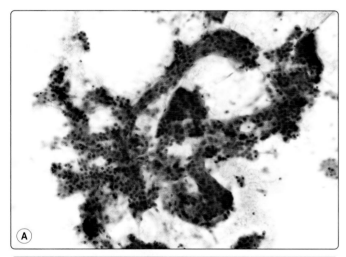

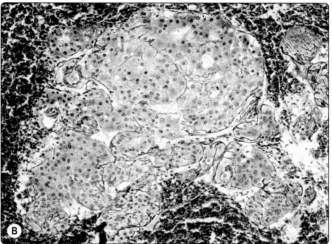

Fig. 10.16 **Hepatocellular carcinoma** A reticulin stain on cell block sections may highlight (**A**) widened trabeculae and/or acinar structures (Reticulin, HP); (**B**) reduced or absent reticulin (cell block reticulin, HP).

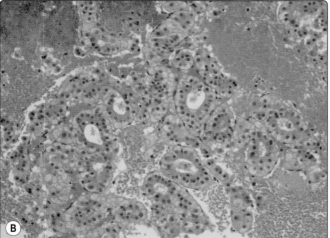

Fig. 10.15 **Hepatocellular carcinoma** (**A**) Cells are typically arranged in widened trabeculae (Pap, IP); (**B**) Less commonly in acinar arrangements (cell block H&E, IP).

The characteristic findings relate to (1) cell groupings, (2) relationship to endothelium and (3) cell morphology.[39,41,72,79,116–132]

The features in any individual FNA sample are extremely variable and largely dictated by tumor differentiation.[116,117,127,132] As the degree of differentiation decreases, the cells become more obviously malignant and their resemblance to hepatocytes decreases.

Smears are typically cellular with large fragments, clusters and dispersed cells (Fig. 10.14). Cell groupings are classically trabecular (Fig. 10.15A), particularly in better-differentiated tumors. Acinar arrangements may be seen in up to 40% of HCC (Fig. 10.15B).[72] With decreasing differentiation, smaller sheets and single-lying cells become more frequent. A reticulin stain on smears or cell block material may highlight the widened trabeculae and/or acinar structures or the reduced or absent reticulin (Fig. 10.16). Endothelial relationships to HCC cell groups are an integral part of the diagnosis. Endothelial cells of sinusoidal capillaries may traverse (Fig. 10.17) or enclose (Fig. 10.18) trabeculae or separate tumor cell groupings.[128] This important diagnostic criterion is diminished and then lost with decreasing differentiation.

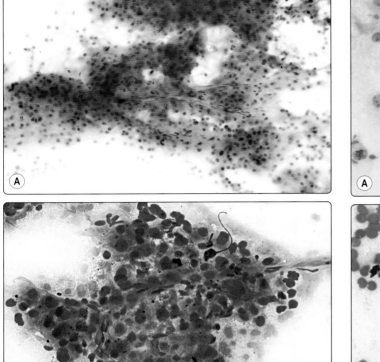

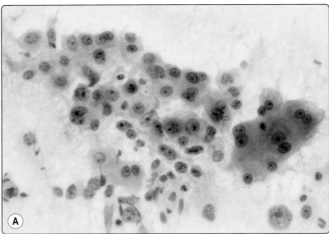

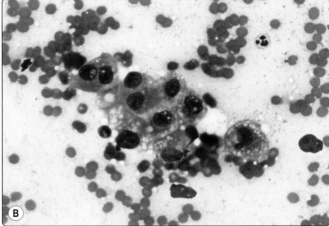

Fig. 10.17 Hepatocellular carcinoma Tissue fragment of malignant cells traversed by spindle endothelial cells representing capillary blood vessels (**A**, Pap, IP; **B**, MGG, HP).

Fig. 10.19 Hepatocellular carcinoma The cells resemble hepatocytes, but are larger with increased nucleocytoplasmic ratios; tumor cells have round nuclei and central large nucleoli; note cluster of benign hepatocytes (*to right in* **A**) (**A**, Pap, HP; **B**, MGG, HP).

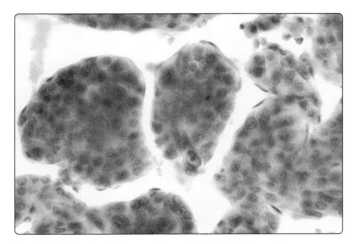

Fig. 10.18 Hepatocellular carcinoma Endothelial cell envelopes seen as thin spindle nuclei surrounding tumor fragments (H&E, HP).

The cells resemble hepatocytes, thus demonstrating polygonal outlines and dense, granular cytoplasm, but with increased nucleocytoplasmic ratios over normal counterparts (Fig. 10.19). Centrally placed nuclei, characterized by granular to coarse chromatin, show cytoplasmic invaginations

(intranuclear inclusions) in up to 70% of cases and large central nucleoli in up to 60% of cases. One of the most outstanding cytological appearances in HCC is the presence of many stripped malignant nuclei with identical characteristics, lying free in the background between cell groups (Fig. 10.20).[126] The presence among malignant cells of occasional tumor giant cells or of bizarre hepatocytes would seem to favor primary liver carcinoma as they are rare in metastatic carcinoma.[72,131] Bile pigment within the cytoplasm and between the cells proves the hepatocellular origin of the tumor, but is demonstrable in only 25% of cases (Fig. 10.21). Fouchet's reagent counterstained with hematoxylin/Sirius red stains bile intensely green (Fig. 2.19). Contaminant benign hepatocytes and bile duct epithelium may be collected from the surrounding non-neoplastic liver, particularly in the setting of cirrhosis. They usually lie apart from the tumor cells.

Cytoplasmic vacuolation is pronounced in clear cell variants of HCC (Fig. 10.22).[133] The clear cytoplasm is due to accumulation of glycogen or fat, and mucin stains are usually negative.[134,135] This is not a defined subtype but rather a morphological pattern usually associated with a component of 'conventional' HCC. Its importance lies in distinguishing it from metastatic clear cell malignancies

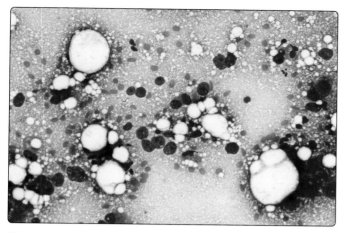

Fig. 10.20 Hepatocellular carcinoma Multiple large round atypical nuclei stripped of their cytoplasm; one or multiple macronucleoli (MGG, HP).

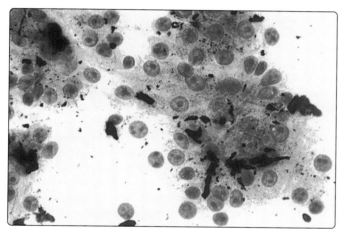

Fig. 10.21 Hepatocellular carcinoma Moderately differentiated tumor with characteristic nuclear morphology; numerous green/black bile thrombi between tumor cells (MGG, HP).

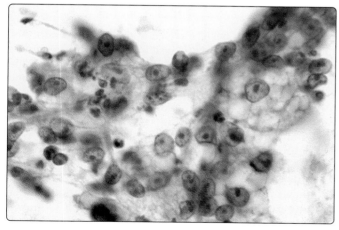

Fig. 10.22 Hepatocellular carcinoma 'Clear cell' variant; large cells with abundant pale vacuolated cytoplasm, large vesicular nuclei, large nucleoli (Pap, HP).

including carcinomas of renal, adrenal, pancreatic and ovarian origin, and sarcomas.[133]

The *fibrolamellar subtype* of HCC occurs as a distinct clinicopathologic variant in the second and third decades of life, without associated parenchymal liver disease and is therefore more often resectable. The neoplastic cells are intermingled with bundles of spindle-shaped fibroblasts and fragments of lamellar collagen (Fig. 10.23A). The tumor cells, readily recognized as of hepatocellular origin, are very large and may be pleomorphic. They have a polygonal shape, abundant, dense, granular cytoplasm, large vesicular nuclei, and large, single, central nucleoli (Fig. 10.23B). Trabeculae and peripheral endothelial wrapping are not observed in this otherwise well-differentiated variant, as the cell population is dispersed or adherent to the fibrous tissue. Intranuclear cytoplasmic inclusions are plentiful and there may be intracytoplasmic hyaline inclusions and pale bodies.[136–138]

PROBLEMS AND DIFFERENTIAL DIAGNOSES

Problems in HCC diagnosis occur at both ends of the differentiation spectrum; well differentiated HCC from benign hepatocellular lesions and poorly differentiated HCC from other primary and secondary malignancies.

The differential diagnosis of HCC depends on the clinical setting. In a patient with known chronic liver disease the major differential diagnosis is macroregenerative nodule (MRN). In a young female patient with a non-cirrhotic liver it is either focal nodular hyperplasia (FNH) or benign hepatocellular adenoma (HA). In an older patient, who may or may not have a past history of a primary malignancy elsewhere, it is metastatic malignancy.

The problem of distinguishing well-differentiated HCC (Fig. 10.24) from a benign regenerative nodule, focal nodular hyperplasia or adenoma has been mentioned. Clinical data such as age and sex, presence or absence of cirrhosis, exposure to steroidal hormones and radiological appearances may help to distinguish between these entities. There is considerable risk of overdiagnosing malignancy in regenerative nodules because nuclear enlargement, anisokaryosis, macronucleoli and dissociation may be prominent. Total absence of bile duct epithelium in a cellular smear favors a neoplasm, benign or malignant. The subtle cytological changes may be insufficient to reach a diagnosis of malignancy, and architectural abnormalities are of great importance. If there are endothelial-lined trabeculae or acini, capillary blood vessels which intersect groups of tumor cells, raised nucleocytoplasmic ratios, macronucleoli, many naked neoplastic nuclei, poorly defined cell borders, overall tumor cell monotony with sporadic tumor giant cells, and mitoses, the lesion is probably HCC.[39–41,72,79,116–132]

Prior to embarking on costly immunotests, a reticulin stain can highlight loss of a normal sinusoidal pattern and shows either widened trabeculae, rounded islands and pseudoglands or just a reduction or total absence of reticulin and distinguish benign from malignant liver lesions (see Figs 10.6 and 10.16).[77–79,120]

CD34 and factor VIII immunostaining have been used in demonstrating the classic endothelial staining pattern of HCC (Fig. 10.25), absent in reactive liver and metastatic

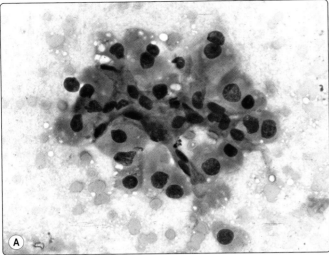

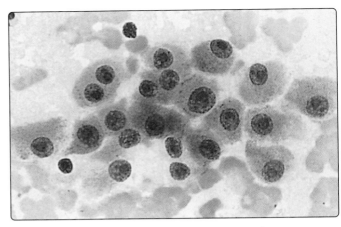

Fig. 10.24 **Hepatocellular carcinoma** Well-differentiated tumor composed of poorly cohesive hepatocytic cells with mild anisokaryosis but large nucleoli; differentiation from adenoma difficult (MGG, HP).

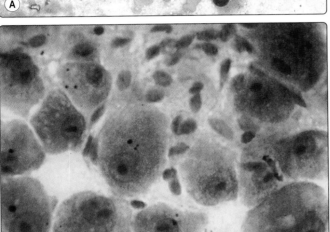

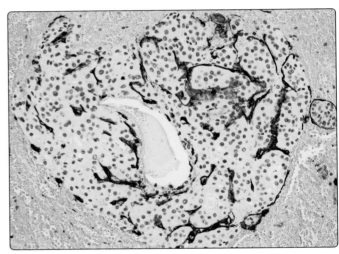

Fig. 10.25 **Hepatocellular carcinoma** CD34 immunostaining demonstrates the classic endothelial staining pattern which is absent in reactive liver cell block (CD34, HP).

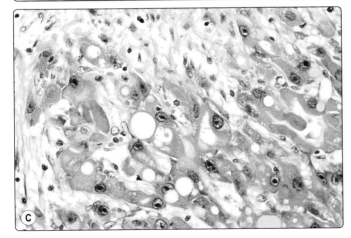

Fig. 10.23 **Hepatocellular carcinoma, fibrolamellar type** (A) Neoplastic cells adherent to fragments of lamellar collagen (MGG, HP); (B) Very large, malignant hepatocytes with prominent nucleoli and abundant granular cytoplasm (MGG, HP oil); (C) Corresponding tissue section (H&E, IP).

differentiation, has been observed in malignant hepatocytes. In several studies on cytological smears, positive staining for Glypican-3 showed a high sensitivity (80–90%) and specificity (>95%) in HCC versus metastatic tumors and benign liver lesions.[142–144]

Image analysis or flow cytometric studies may permit prognostication on the basis of ploidy analysis. Most HCCs are aneuploid, with the remainder euploid (either diploid or polyploid), whereas all benign samples are euploid.[145–147]

Poorly differentiated HCC loses many classic criteria and is difficult to distinguish from metastatic adenocarcinoma, or other undifferentiated malignancies. Most HCC show a spectrum of differentiation and the diagnosis can be reached when the better-differentiated cells show recognisable hepatocellular features. Various cytological features have been identified as useful in discriminating between poorly differentiated HCC and metastatic adenocarcinoma; the presence of trabeculae versus true acinar structures, endothelial

carcinoma,[139] but are limited by partial staining of adenoma and focal nodular hyperplasia. Indeed, they provide little more information than the less expensive reticulin.[131,139–141] Over-expression of Glypican-3, a heparan sulphate proteoglycan that plays an important role in cell growth and

cells lining cell groups or small capillaries transgressing clusters of tumor cells, dissociation and atypical stripped nuclei, polygonal cells with central nuclei rather than columnar or cuboidal cells, round nuclei with one or more large nucleoli or intranuclear cytoplasmic inclusions, eosinophilic granular cytoplasm versus cytoplasmic vacuolation positive staining for glycogen, particularly if metastatic renal cell and adrenocortical carcinoma can be excluded, the presence of cytoplasmic bile, lipid, hyaline globules or Mallory bodies.[72,117,119,148–150]

Along with immunotests, a mucin stain may separate HCC from adenocarcinoma.

Various antibodies have been used to differentiate between hepatocellular carcinoma, cholangiocarcinoma and metastatic malignancies of various types.[151,152] Positive immunoperoxidase staining for alpha fetoprotein favors primary cancer, but is seen in only around 50% of HCCs.[129,153,154] It has good specificity despite also staining some germ cell tumors and occasional hepatoid adenocarcinomas of the gastrointestinal tract.

The demonstration of a characteristic bile canalicular staining pattern in HCC by means of polyclonal carcinoembryonic antigen (pCEA) is useful although it decreases with increasing anaplasia. Whereas metastatic adenocarcinoma displays full cytoplasmic immunostaining, HCC will show staining only along canalicular luminal membrane (Fig. 10.26A).[73,116,129,154–158] Reported sensitivity ranges from 47% to 90%. It is essential that the polyclonal antibody be used; the same results will not be observed with the monoclonal antibody. Staining for CD10 gives the same pattern as CEA but is negative in adenocarcinoma.[159,160]

HepPar-1 is an antibody which recognises mitochondria in both benign and malignant hepatocytes. It has recently proved highly sensitive and specific in the distinction between adenocarcinoma and HCC, producing diffuse granular cytoplasmic staining in the latter (Fig. 10.26B).[156,161,162]

Glypican-3 antigen has also been described as useful in distinguishing HCC from metastatic malignancy. In one study on cytological material, positive staining for Glypican-3 showed a sensitivity of 90% and specificity of 100% for HCC versus metastatic malignancy.[142,144,163]

Cytokeratins 7 and 20 are most often negative in HCC, and may thus be employed as useful adenocarcinoma stains in the liver,[164,165] as may Glut-1 and CA 15-3.[166]

More recently, cytoplasmic staining in HCC for TTF-1 (as opposed to the nuclear staining it produces in pulmonary adenocarcinomas) has been used in the successful discrimination of HCC from metastatic adenocarcinoma.[167,168]

In situ hybridisation for the detection of albumin mRNA has shown positivity in the majority of HCCs.[129,169,170]

Cholangiocarcinoma

Intrahepatic cholangiocarcinoma (CC) is associated with etiological factors such as liver fluke infestation (common in parts of South-east Asia), the primary sclerosing cholangitis/ulcerative colitis complex, congenital conditions such as Caroli's disease and intrahepatic lithiasis. Tumors typically occur at the hilum where they present early with obstructive jaundice. They may be difficult to diagnose although the use of EUS-FNA has reported good results.[66,171]

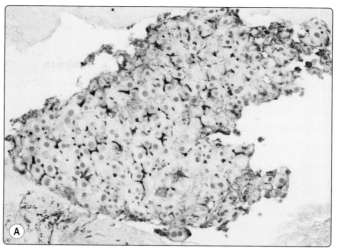

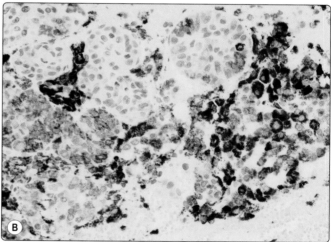

Fig. 10.26 Hepatocellular carcinoma (A) pCEA immunostaining shows cytoplasmic staining along canalicular luminal edges only (pCEA, HP); (B) HepPar-1 produces diffuse granular cytoplasmic staining in distinction to adenocarcinoma, which is negative (HepPar-1, HP).

CRITERIA FOR DIAGNOSIS (Fig. 10.27)[172]

◆ Sheets, clusters and microglandular arrangement showing nuclear crowding and overlapping,
◆ Decreased cell cohesion,
◆ Small to medium cuboidal/columnar cells resembling bile duct epithelium,
◆ Variable nuclear enlargement and pleomorphism,
◆ Prominent nucleoli in the less well-differentiated tumors,
◆ Delicate cytoplasm with fine vacuolization, positive for mucin,
◆ Occasionally fragments of stroma.

Cholangiocarcinomas often have abundant, desmoplastic stroma and may prove difficult to sample by FNA, or CNB for that matter. Although cells from a well-differentiated cholangiocarcinoma may not appear too different from bile duct epithelium, hepatocytes are absent and the number and size of epithelial sheets are larger than are usually obtained from non-neoplastic liver tissue (Fig. 10.27A). The application of P53, bcl-2 and Ki-67 has been reported as useful in discriminating between them.[173] Less well-differentiated carcinomas are indistinguishable from metastatic adenocarcinoma (Fig. 10.27B), particularly those of pancreatic origin. Unfortunately, they are both generally positive for CK7 and CK19 and negative for CK20.[174] Distinction from HCC relies on adenocarcinoma showing positivity for mucin and diffuse cytoplasmic staining for CK7, CK19 and pCEA and HCC staining for alpha fetoprotein and HepPar-1 and others as described earlier in the section on HCC.

Diagnosis depends not only on cytological assessment but on correlation of the clinical and radiological findings, in particularly excluding an extrahepatic malignancy.

The cytology of *combined hepatocellular–cholangiocarcinomas* has been reported.[175,176] They show classic HCC cells, pure glandular cells, and hybrid or intermediate cells with features of both components. A histochemical stain for mucin will confirm intracytoplasmic, brush border or intraluminal mucin. Immunohistochemistry is helpful in confirming the two components. pCEA highlights the canalicular areas of the HCC component and the brush border of the glandular areas.

Hepatoblastoma[177–181]

Hepatoblastoma is a rare, highly malignant tumor of infants and young children, which metastasizes early. It is not associated with chronic liver disease. The alpha fetoprotein level is significantly raised in approximately 90% of cases. Patients can have a good response to surgery and chemotherapy. There is a spectrum of subtypes from anaplastic through embryonal and fetal to macrotrabecular, based on growth pattern and increasing resemblance of component cells from anaplastic towards hepatocyte morphology. A mixed epithelial and mesenchymal pattern includes primitive mesenchyme. The cytological appearance is that of a small round cell childhood tumor, (Fig. 10.28, and also Figs 17.18–17.20), with clusters, ribbons and rosettes of embryonal cells, which are small cells with a high N:C ratio, oval to spindled nuclei, coarse chromatin, prominent, often multiple, nucleoli, and scant to moderate cytoplasm. Fetal epithelial cells, are slightly smaller than hepatocytes with round regular nuclei, fine chromatin, prominent central nucleoli and abundant granular or clear cytoplasm which may contain fat, bile or glycogen. Fragments of mesenchyme may be observed. Foci of extramedullary hemopoiesis are often present. The differential diagnosis is that of other small round cell childhood tumors metastatic to the liver or of HCC, which may occur in older children. HepPar-1 staining of hepatoblastoma can be useful in this regard.[182]

Malignant lymphoma[183,184]

Liver involvement in stage IV malignant lymphoma portends a poor prognosis and has been found in 25% of random FNA biopsies in patients with lymphoma.[185] Primary involvement of the liver is relatively rare. It is often patchy and microscopic and may be missed by either FNA or CNB. The liver tumor may be solitary, multiple or diffuse. Aspirates are usually markedly cellular with dispersed cells and scattered small aggregates without true cohesion, and lymphoglandular bodies are present in the background. Non-Hodgkin lymphoma of diffuse large B cell type (high grade) is the most common type. If on-site rapid evaluation detects a lymphoid lesion, a further needle pass should be performed to obtain

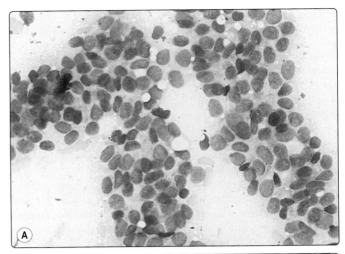

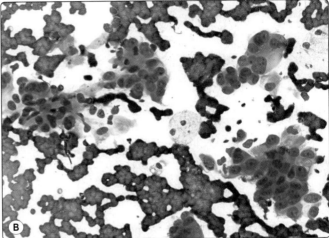

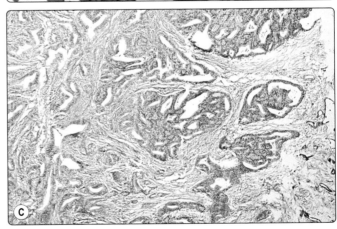

Fig. 10.27 Cholangiocarcinoma (A) Disorganized clusters of irregular but not very pleomorphic tumor cells with pale cytoplasm and relatively small nuclei (MGG, HP); (B) Disorganized cluster of mildly pleomorphic epithelial cells with hyperchromatic nuclei and prominent nucleoli (MGG, HP); (C) Corresponding tissue section (H&E, IP).

cells for phenotyping by immunocytochemistry or flow cytometry, for cytogenetics and for molecular gene rearrangement studies. For detailed cytological criteria for the diagnosis of lymphoma, see Chapter 5. The differential diagnosis of a post-transplant lymphoproliferative disorder (PTLD) should be considered where there is a history of

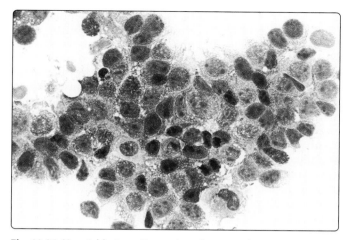

Fig. 10.28 Hepatoblastoma Tumor tissue fragment, showing nuclear crowding and overlapping, increased nucleocytoplasmic ratios, irregular chromatin, minimal cytoplasm (MGG, HP).

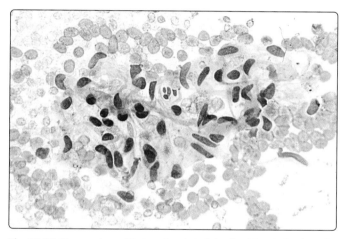

Fig. 10.29 Hemangioma Cluster of endothelial cells with spindle-shaped nuclei in a background of blood (Pap, HP).

organ transplantation. The smears may be either polymorphous with a mixture of lymphocytes, plasma cells and histiocytes, or monomorphous with large atypical lymphocytes. The diagnosis is supported by identifying B-cell monoclonality and the presence of EBV DNA.[183,186,187]

Vascular tumors

Cavernous hemangioma is the most common benign solid lesion in the liver and is not infrequently found by US or by CT in the routine investigation of cancer patients. The diagnosis can often be made by imaging, but in some cases with an atypical appearance a needle biopsy is necessary to confidently exclude metastatic tumor or adenoma.[61,63,64,188,189] In our experience, clusters of benign spindle cells recognizable as endothelial cells are infrequently seen in FNA smears (Fig. 10.29). The diagnosis is based on appropriate clinico-radiological history and aspiration of profuse blood as from a venepuncture, provided the correct positioning of the needle can be ascertained. When diagnostic cells are present, they assume three-dimensional swathes of endothelial cells surrounding cavernous spaces, into which the cell nuclei protrude. Connective tissue fragments may

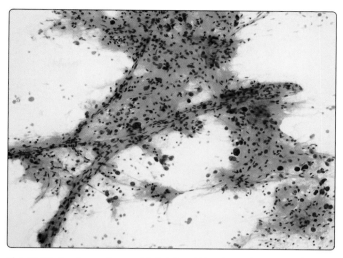

Fig. 10.30 Angiomyolipoma Well-defined blood vessels associated with a mixture of epithelioid and spindle cells showing marked nuclear pleomorphism. Fat cells are not obvious (H&E, IP).

be present. A definitive cytological diagnosis of hemangioma has been made in 27–96% of cases reported in the literature.[61,63,64,188,189]

Epithelioid hemangioendothelioma is a solid vascular-derived tumor with a clinical course intermediate between that of hemangioma and angiosarcoma. Females are more commonly affected than males. The tumor is multifocal and increasingly sclerotic, often pre-empting good FNA yield. The cells are spindled or epithelioid, showing pleomorphism with scattered bizarre tumor giant cells. Intracytoplasmic lumina may be identified.[190] The differential diagnosis includes pleomorphic HCC. Diagnosis is more easily made on cell blocks than on smears and immunohistochemistry for vascular markers is usually positive.[191,192]

Angiosarcoma is a very rare primary hepatic tumor, but reports have appeared in the cytological literature,[191,193,194] in which the FNA findings indicated a malignant spindle-cell neoplasm. Again, diagnosis can be facilitated by the morphology of tissue fragments in cell blocks, which also allow appropriate immunocytochemistry including factor VIII, CD31, CD34 and *Ulex europaeus*.[195] The cytomorphology shows consistently abundant blood, variable cellularity, spindle-shaped tumor cells arranged in anastomosing vessels, papillae or solid groups showing variable pleomorphism, and vasoformative features such as erythrophagocytosis and hemosiderin. As indicated in the preceding section on complications, massive bleeding and death have been reported after FNA of vascular lesions.

Other mesenchymal tumors

Angiomyolipoma of the liver is a rare benign tumor, important not because of its frequency but because of its mimicry of malignancy. As in other sites, it comprises vascular tissue, fat cells, and immature smooth muscle cells with fibrillar cytoplasm, in varying proportions (Fig. 10.30). The muscle cells can be spindled or epithelioid and show pleomorphism with giant cells, but no mitoses or necrosis should be present. Transgressing endothelium may be seen, but no peripheral endothelial wrapping occurs.[196] The diagnosis rests on identifying fat cells as an integral part of the tumor fascicles and

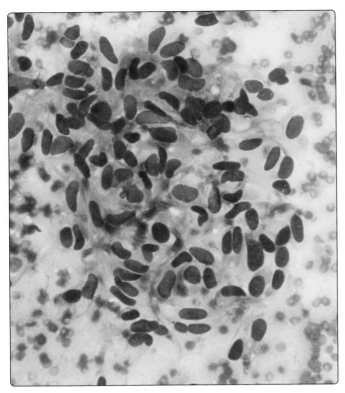

Fig. 10.31 Liver metastasis of gastrointestinal stromal tumor Cohesive cluster of haphazardly arranged spindle cells showing mild anisonucleosis and tapered cytoplasm (MGG, HP).

not regarding them as hepatocytes distended with fat vacuoles. Extramedullary hematopoiesis is a consistent finding. Immunostaining with HMB-45 is confirmatory. Smooth muscle and vascular markers are also positive, as is S-100 in fat cells. In the more pleomorphic forms without fat tissue, absence of keratin staining is an important criterion.[196–198]

Mesenchymal hamartoma is a benign multicystic tumor which may reach very considerable size. It occurs predominantly in male children under the age of 2 years,[199,200] but adult variants have been reported.[201] The mass, which may mimic other paediatric neoplasms clinically and radiologically, yields a biphasic population of small bland rounded epithelial cells of hepatocytic or bile duct origin, admixed with single or aggregated bland spindle cells, often in a myxoid stromal or mucoid background. The spindled component may predominate.[200] Excision is curative. The cytological differential diagnosis includes hepatoblastoma of mixed epithelial and mesenchymal type.

Gastrointestinal stromal tumors (GISTs) are the most frequently encountered sarcoma in the liver (see also Chapter 11). Most are metastatic from the stomach. Diagnosis is accomplished without difficulty if there is an available history, if the morphology is spindled (Fig. 10.31) or if cell blocks are made. Great difficulty arises, however, with the epithelioid variant, which is characterized by small round dissociated cells with clear cytoplasm. The differential diagnosis in these cases is that of metastatic carcinoma. Immunocytochemical positivity for CD117 is diagnostic and CD34 may also be positive.[202–204]

Leiomyosarcoma may arise from the inferior vena cava but is more often a metastatic deposit. It presents as clusters and fascicles of spindle cells with ill-defined bipolar cytoplasm. Pleomorphism, necrosis and mitoses can occur in higher-grade tumors. Immunocytochemistry shows positivity for vimentin, desmin, and smooth muscle actin.[205,206]

Undifferentiated (embryonal) sarcoma is a rare malignant mesenchymal hepatic tumor, occurring predominantly in children under the age of 15 years. Tumor cells occur singly or in clusters. They are polygonal and spindle with large, pleomorphic nuclei, one or several nucleoli and variable poorly defined cytoplasm containing vacuoles and eosinophilic globules which are PAS/D positive. Multinucleated tumor cells are not uncommon and myxoid matrix may be present. Distinction from other paediatric liver tumors is reliant on vimentin, α_1-antichymotrypsin and α_1-antitrypsin positivity.[207–210] Regarding liver tumors in childhood, see also Chapter 17.

Metastatic malignancy (Figs 10.31 and 10.32)

The liver is a common site of metastatic disease because it acts as a filter. Differentiation between primary and secondary tumors on imaging can be problematic. The differential diagnosis between primary hepatocellular carcinoma and metastatic malignancy and the use of immunostaining to discriminate between them has been previously discussed in the section on HCC. Metastatic tumors may be single, multiple or diffusely infiltrating. The metastatic deposit usually shows the morphological characteristics of the primary tumor. Clinical history is very important in making the diagnosis. Review of any previous histology or cytology is recommended.

The clinician needs to know whether liver involvement is present, either from a primary tumor which has already manifested or one which is still occult. The result of FNA will often dictate management such as chemotherapy.[211] Cell typing is thus desirable in most instances. We regard it as particularly important to identify accurately those metastases which are potentially chemosensitive or hormonally manipulable. It is useful to run through a mental checklist to ensure that one is not missing germ cell tumors, neuroendocrine tumors (including small cell undifferentiated carcinomas) or carcinomas of breast, prostatic, endometrium, thyroid or even nasopharyngeal origin.

The macroscopic appearance of the aspirate is usually quite different from that of normal liver tissue. There is frequently less admixture with blood and often a high cell content. The aspirate is easily smeared into a grayish film. Necrosis may be pre-eminent, sometimes to the extent that preserved, diagnostic cancer cells are hard to find. A necrotizing metastatic tumor deposit may present as a cyst.[87] If hepatocytes are found amongst the neoplastic cells, they provide a useful baseline for the evaluation of cell and nuclear size.

The cytologic patterns of metastatic carcinomas and clues to the identification of the primary site of origin are described in Chapter 5 and will not be repeated at length here. Adequate sampling is the key. Colonic adenocarcinoma is probably the most common source of liver metastases. The cytological pattern is characteristic, showing malignant columnar epithelial cells in palisaded rows or microglandular groups with a background of necrotic debris (Fig. 10.32), often with evidence of mucin secretion.[35] Small cell undifferentiated carcinoma of pulmonary or colonic derivation often involves the liver diffusely. Hepatocytes may be numerous and evenly

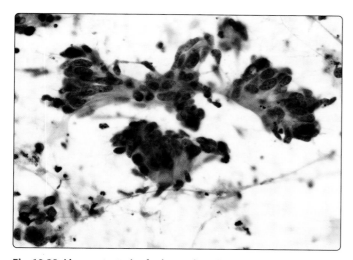

Fig. 10.32 Liver metastasis of colorectal carcinoma Columnar cells arranged in glandular formation on a background of granular debris (Pap, HP).

dispersed between tumor cell groups in smears. Hepatic FNA in these cases has staging value in anticipation of chemotherapy.[212] Carcinoid tumors of bronchogenic, pancreatic or colonic origin are distinguishable from metastatic adenocarcinoma by their endocrine appearance. The nuclei have a rounded shape with 'speckled' granular, hyperchromatic chromatin. Red (MGG) cytoplasmic granularity may be visible. The diagnosis can be confirmed by immunoperoxidase staining for neuroendocrine markers.[213]

Immunohistochemistry can aid in determining the primary site of the metastases.[214,215] Adenocarcinoma of unknown origin remains a diagnostic problem because of lack of specific immunohistochemical markers. It can arise from many different sites, e.g. bronchus, colon, pancreas, breast, stomach, etc. A limited but useful immunoperoxidase panel to determine site of origin of metastatic adenocarcinoma, not otherwise specified in patients in whom clinical history is nondirective, consists of cytokeratins 7 and 20, TTF-1, CDX2 and additional ER/PR in female patients or PSA in male patients.

Spleen

Clinical aspects

The place of FNAC in the investigative sequence

Fine needle biopsy of the spleen is not a commonly performed procedure, although there are increasing reports in the cytological literature, partly due to the advent of endoscopic ultrasound FNA.[216-226] The possible risk of hemorrhagic complications has probably been a discouraging factor and it is uncommon for a patient to present with isolated splenomegaly or a localized splenic lesion which cannot be explained using other diagnostic pathways.

The main purpose of FNA is to diagnose or confirm hematologic or metastatic malignancy.[216,219,226] However, a number of non-neoplastic lesions and disorders involving the spleen can be diagnosed by FNA.[227] Examples are: *cysts*,[228] *abscesses*,[223-229] a variety of infectious and granulomatous processes notably *leishmaniasis, tuberculosis* and *sarcoid*,[224,227,229-233] *myeloid metaplasia*,[234] *inflammatory pseudo-*

tumor,[219,235] *amyloidosis*[236] and, in combination with biochemical investigations, *lipid storage disease*.[237] The cytology is 'normal' in a proportion of cases of isolated splenomegaly and gives no clue to the possible etiology (e.g. in portal hypertension).

Malignant lymphoma most often involves the spleen diffusely, but can occur as solitary or multiple circumscribed deposits.[238] CT scanning or ultrasonography can thus be helpful in selecting the best site for a biopsy. Splenic *metastases* are not uncommon in disseminated carcinoma, but rarely constitute a clinical problem. FNA can replace splenectomy for diagnosis of solitary splenic metastases.[239] Splenic *hamartoma, hemangioma* and *angiosarcoma* are examples of the rare primary tumors of the spleen.[240,241]

Accuracy of diagnosis

Diagnostic sensitivity for neoplasia was 86.4% and specificity 97.5% based on 78 cases with histological correlation in the series by Zeppa et al.[226] Friedlander et al. reported a sensitivity of 94% with a specificity of 84% and a positive predictive value of 79%. They reported four false positives although these included cases they had categorized as 'supicious of malignancy'.[218] In the series from M.D. Anderson Cancer Center there were no false positives and only one false-negative diagnosis in 50 cases, only 10 of whom had subsequent splenectomy. Six biopsies were nondiagnostic.[216] Other series reported accuracy rates of between 80% and 90%.[220,229,242,243]

Diagnostic pitfalls

As FNB of the spleen is not commonly performed there are a number of pitfalls.[218] These include:

- a misleading clinical history directing the cytopathologist in the wrong direction,
- a lack of expert needle placement leading to sampling error,
- a lack of familiarity with the normal appearance of splenic tissue by the cytopathologist, particularly in distinguishing normal from primary vascular lesions of the spleen,
- misleading flow cytometry findings in the diagnosis of splenic lymphoma.

Most of these are not unique to the spleen; however, increased experience with splenic FNA should go some way to minimizing errors related to these pitfalls.

Complications

The risk of a needle biopsy causing rupture and major hemorrhage appears to be small.[218,220] Söderström had no complications in over 1000 FNAs[225] and Selroos et al. had none in 557 cases.[232] However, a few cases of hemorrhagic complications leading to splenectomy have been reported.[224,226,243] Hemorrhagic diathesis and low platelet count are a contraindication. Söderström regarded glandular fever and polycythemia as relative contraindications.[225] Core needle biopsy of the spleen has been advocated by some as it has a greater accuracy, particularly in the diagnosis of of lymphoma,[243-245] but the risk of complications is likely to be greater.[243-247]

Technical considerations

Most FNA samples are obtained using imaging guidance; either percutaneously, or more recently using endoscopic ultrasound FNA.[217,218,242] Direct FNA can be performed into a diffusely enlarged spleen or into a palpable localized mass if no imaging is available. Most splenic aspirates may appear to consist mainly of blood but are, nevertheless, usually quite rich in cells. The material should be smeared thinly, and air-dried MGG-stained smears are essential to allow comparison with blood films and bone marrow aspirates. Immunostaining can be performed on spare slides, cytospins or cell block material, and a cell suspension for flow cytometry should be obtained if lymphoma is considered in the differential diagnosis.

Cytological findings

Non-specific findings in splenomegaly (Fig. 10.33)

> **CYTOLOGIC FEATURES**
>
> ◆ Abundant blood and platelet aggregates,
> ◆ Tissue fragments (lymphoid cells and endothelial cells),
> ◆ Numerous lymphoid cells,
> ◆ Endothelial cells and histiocytes.

It is unlikely that normal spleens are ever subjected to FNA and the normal cytological pattern is therefore not well known. The above features are seen in cases of splenomegaly related to portal hypertension, hemolytic anemia, etc. FNA is performed mainly to exclude hematological malignancy, and does not contribute to a specific diagnosis in these conditions.

Lymphoid cells predominate in FNB samples from the spleen. There is invariably a background of abundant blood and platelet aggregates. The lymphoid cells are more often seen in tissue fragments, trapped in a meshwork of endothelial cells, than as evenly spread, isolated cells. Blast cells constitute a relatively higher proportion of the cell population than in smears from reactive lymph nodes. Diagnostic criteria applied in lymph node cytology should be used with caution when smears from the spleen are examined.

Non-neoplastic processes[225,227]

Myeloid metaplasia (Fig. 10.34)

The findings in myeloid metaplasia include normoblasts, myelocytes and megakaryocytes intermingled with the cells of normal splenic tissue. Normoblasts are easily recognized by their relatively small, round, hyperchromatic nuclei and their homogeneous, dense eosinophilic or amphophilic cytoplasm. Megakaryocytes may be mistaken for malignant neoplastic cells but should be recognizable by the giant, lobulated nucleus and the abundant, granular cytoplasm. Myelocytes have specific cytoplasmic granules. All these features are best seen in MGG-stained smears.[234]

Granulomatous processes

Histiocytes forming granulomatous clusters may be found in several unrelated conditions and do not permit a specific diagnosis when found in splenic aspirates. Well-formed granulomata of epithelioid histiocytes, with or without Langhans giant cells, suggest the main differential diagnoses of *sarcoidosis* and *tuberculosis* (Fig. 10.35).[232,233] Caseous necrosis is characteristic of tuberculosis but is not always seen in smears. The demonstration of AFBs is only possible in some cases of tuberculosis involving the spleen.[231] Material should always be sent for culture where possible. Non-caseating granulomas may also be found in splenic aspirates in cases of *malignant lymphoma*, particularly *Hodgkin's lymphoma*, and the background lymphoid cell population needs to be studied closely.

Others

Conspicuous large histiocytes with foamy cytoplasm indicate lipid storage disease. Histiocytes in *Gaucher's disease* have a characteristic striated cytoplasmic appearance (Fig. 10.36).[237] The foamy histiocytes seen in *Niemann-Pick disease* are less characteristic and the specific diagnosis rests on biochemical analyses. The cytology of *histiocytosis X* is described in Chapter 16 and *amyloidosis*[236] in Chapter 4. Other examples of non-neoplastic lesions in the spleen diagnosed by FNB are splenic *abscess*[223,229,242] and splenic *epidermoid cyst*.[227,248]

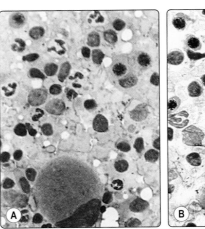

Fig. 10.33 Spleen FNA in non-specific splenomegaly. Mixed population of small and transformed lymphoid cells and a platelet aggregate (MGG, HP).

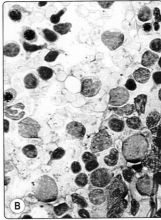

Fig. 10.34 Myeloid metaplasia (A) Megakaryocyte and several erythroblasts adjacent to smeared lymphoid cells (MGG, HP); (B) Erythroblasts, myelocytes, lymphoid cells (MGG, HP).

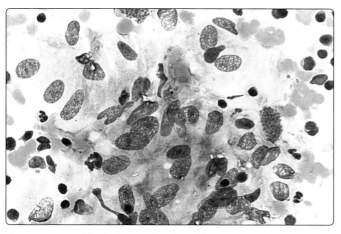

Fig. 10.35 Sarcoidosis Cluster of epithelioid histiocytes with pale elongated (footprint-shaped) nuclei and background of syncytial cytoplasm (MGG, HP).

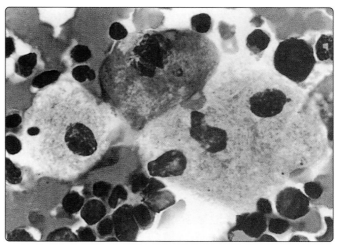

Fig. 10.36 Gaucher's disease Bone marrow smear with large characteristic histiocytes (MGG, HP oil).

Neoplasms

Malignant lymphoma[220,222,226,238]

The findings in malignant lymphoma in splenic aspirates are the same as in other tissues (see Chapter 5). The abnormal lymphoid cells are more dispersed, distributed as single cells, and tissue fragments are less conspicuous than in smears of non-neoplastic splenic tissue. Non-Hodgkin lymphoma of mixed cell type is particularly difficult to diagnose with confidence in splenic aspirates and immune marker studies by flow cytometry or immunohistochemistry are indispensable.[222,249,250] In Hodgkin lymphoma, the diagnosis rests on the demonstration of Reed-Sternberg cells.[251]

Hairy cell leukemia (Fig. 10.37)

CRITERIA FOR DIAGNOSIS

- A monotonous population of abnormal lymphoid cells of B-cell immunophenotype,
- Nuclei ovoid or kidney shaped; larger and paler than those of normal lymphocytes,
- Pale basophilic cytoplasm; fine, hair-like cytoplasmic projections (EM),
- Positive staining for tartrate-resistant acid phosphatase and for acid non-specific esterase,
- Material sent for flow cytometry is useful in confirming the diagnosis.

Splenomegaly is one of the main symptoms in hairy cell leukemia, whereas lymph node involvement appears late in the disease and is less conspicuous. The diagnosis is usually made on examination of a bone marrow aspirate or of peripheral blood but can also be made on a splenic aspirate.[252,253]

Vascular tumors

Very few cases of splenic *hemangioma*,[254] *littoral cell angioma*[255] and of splenic *hamartoma* (*splenoma*)[241,255,256] with FNB have been reported. Splenic hamartoma (Fig. 10.38) is a hamartomatous tumor of the spleen consisting exclusively of red pulp tissue. We have seen one example in which the smears were dominated by numerous spindle cells of endothelial type. The nuclei were elongated and uniform,

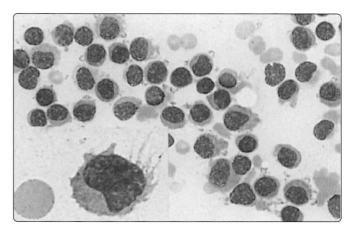

Fig. 10.37 Hairy cell leukemia Uniform lymphoid cells, larger and paler than small lymphocytes and with slightly reniform nuclei (MGG, HP). **Inset:** fine hair-like cytoplasmic processes which may, however, be artifactually produced in other lymphoid cells (MGG, HP oil).

with a bland, finely granular chromatin. FNB was reported as an angiomatous tumor. Distinction between splenic hamartoma and angioma may not be possible in FNA smears.

Angiosarcoma occasionally presents as a primary tumor of the spleen.[240] A case from our files, in which the diagnosis was correctly made by FNA, showed smears which were rich in cells. These were spindly and had elongated, mildly pleomorphic, hyperchromatic nuclei. Most of the cells formed highly cellular tissue fragments which showed a distinctly vasoformative pattern with bunches of radiating spindle cells (Fig. 10.39).

Metastases

Metastases may be solitary or multiple and a history of a primary malignancy elsewhere is not always available. Splenic FNA has value in diagnosis and staging to provide prognostic information and directing further management, e.g. chemotherapy. The more common primary sites include breast, lung, colorectal and ovarian carcinoma and melanoma.[239,257] The cytologic patterns of metastatic malignancies and clues to the identification of the primary site of origin are described in Chapter 5 and will not be repeated here.

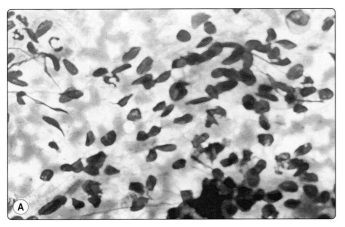
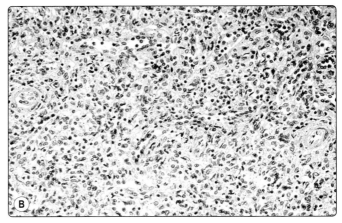

Fig. 10.38 Splenic hamartoma (A) Smear showing many spindle cells of endothelial type with bland nuclei and background of blood (MGG, HP); (B) Corresponding tissue section (H&E, IP).

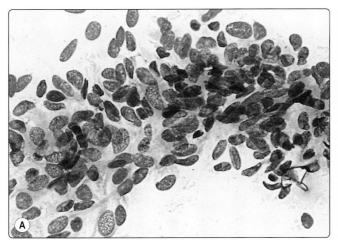
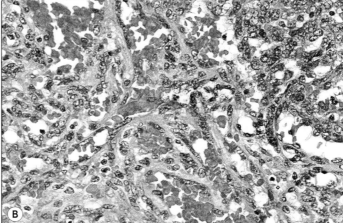

Fig. 10.39 Angiosarcoma of spleen (A) Numerous crowded spindle cells radiating from the center of a loose tissue fragment; variable nuclear size and shape; pale, ill-defined cytoplasm (MGG, HP); (B) Corresponding tissue section (H&E, IP).

References

1. Dusenbery D, Dodd 3rd GD, Carr BI. Percutaneous fine-needle aspiration of portal vein thrombi as a staging technique for hepatocellular carcinoma. Cytologic findings of 46 patients. Cancer 1995 Apr 15;75(8):2057–62.

2. Tarantino L, Francica G, Sordelli I, et al. Diagnosis of benign and malignant portal vein thrombosis in cirrhotic patients with hepatocellular carcinoma: color Doppler US, contrast-enhanced US, and fine-needle biopsy. Abdom Imaging 2006 Sep–Oct;31(5):537–44.

3. Yang L, Lin LW, Lin XY, et al. Ultrasound-guided fine needle aspiration biopsy in differential diagnosis of portal vein tumor thrombosis. Hepatobiliary Pancreat Dis Int 2005 May;4(2):234–8.

4. Lin SM, Kuo SH, Lin DY, et al. Cytologic changes in hepatocellular carcinoma after percutaneous acetic acid injection. Correlation with helical computed tomography findings. Acta Cytol 2000 Jan–Feb;44(1):1–6.

5. Moreland WS, Zagoria RJ, Geisinger KR. Use of fine needle aspiration biopsy in radiofrequency ablation. Acta Cytol 2002 Sep–Oct;46(5):819–22.

6. Bialecki ES, Ezenekwe AM, Brunt EM, et al. Comparison of liver biopsy and noninvasive methods for diagnosis of hepatocellular carcinoma. Clin Gastroenterol Hepatol 2006 Mar;4(3):361–8.

7. Forner A, Vilana R, Ayuso C, et al. Diagnosis of hepatic nodules 20 mm or smaller in cirrhosis: Prospective validation of the noninvasive diagnostic criteria for hepatocellular carcinoma. Hepatology 2008 Jan;47(1):97–104.

8. Ng KK, Poon RT, Lo CML, et al. Impact of preoperative fine-needle aspiration cytologic examination on clinical outcome in patients with hepatocellular carcinoma in a tertiary referral center. Arch Surg 2004 Feb;139(2):193–200.

9. Ohlsson B, Nilsson J, Stenram U, et al. Percutaneous fine-needle aspiration cytology in the diagnosis and

management of liver tumours. Br J Surg 2002 Jun;89(6):757–62.

10. Torzilli G, Olivari N, Del Fabbro D, et al. Indication and contraindication for hepatic resection for liver tumors without fine-needle biopsy: validation and extension of an Eastern approach in a Western community hospital. Liver Transpl 2004 Feb;10(2 Suppl 1):S30–3.

11. Stewart BW, Kleihues P. World cancer report. Lyon: IARC Press; 2003.

12. Brits CJ. Liver aspiration cytology. S Afr Med J 1974 Nov 2;48(53):2207–14.

13. Linsk JA, Franzen S. Clinical aspiration cytology. 2nd ed. Philadelphia: Lippincott; 1989.

14. Perry MD, Johnston WW. Needle biopsy of the liver for the diagnosis of nonneoplastic liver diseases. Acta Cytol 1985 May–Jun;29(3):385–90.

15. Brunetti E, Silini E, Pistorio A, et al. Coarse vs. fine needle aspiration biopsy for the assessment of diffuse liver disease from hepatitis C virus-related

chronic hepatitis. J Hepatol 2004 Mar; 40(3):501–6.

16. Wasastjerna C. Liver. In: Zajicek J, editor. Aspiration biopsy cytology Part 2 Cytology of infradiaphragmatic organs. Basel: Karger; 1979. p. 167–93.

17. Dominis M, Cerlek S, Solter D. Cytology of diffuse liver disorders. Acta Cytol 1973 May–Jun;17(3):205–8.

18. Henriques UV, Hasselstrom K. Evaluation of jaundice: fine-needle aspiration liver cytology as a discriminating tool. Dan Med Bull 1977 Jun;24(3):104–8.

19. Wasastjerna C, Reissell P, Karjalainen J, Ekelund P. Fatty liver in diabetes. A cytological study. Acta Med Scand 1972 Mar;191(3):225–8.

20. Carbonnel F, Samuel D, Reynes M, et al. Fine-needle aspiration biopsy of human liver allografts. Correlation with liver histology for the diagnosis of acute rejection. Transplantation 1990 Oct;50(4):704–7.

21. Hockerstedt K, Lautenschlager I, Ahonen J, et al. Diagnosis of acute rejection in liver transplantation. J Hepatol 1988 Apr;6(2):217–21.

22. Kirby RM, Young JA, Hubscher SG, et al. The accuracy of aspiration cytology in the diagnosis of rejection following orthotopic liver transplantation. Transpl Int 1988 Oct;1(3):119–26.

23. Kubota K, Ericzon BG, Reinholt FP. Comparison of fine-needle aspiration biopsy and histology in human liver transplants. Transplantation 1991 May;51(5):1010–3.

24. Lautenschlager I, Hockerstedt K, Hayry P. Fine-needle aspiration biopsy in the monitoring of liver allografts. Transpl Int 1991 Apr;4(1):54–61.

25. Their M, Lautenschlager I, von Willebrand E, et al. The use of fine-needle aspiration biopsy in detection of acute rejection in children after liver transplantation. Transpl Int 2002 May;15(5):240–7.

26. Babb RR, Jackman RJ. Needle biopsy of the liver. A critique of four currently available methods. West J Med 1989 Jan;150(1):39–42.

27. Jacobsen GK, Gammelgaard J, Fuglo M. Coarse needle biopsy versus fine needle aspiration biopsy in the diagnosis of focal lesions of the liver. Ultrasonically guided needle biopsy in suspected hepatic malignancy. Acta Cytol 1983 Mar–Apr;27(2):152–6.

28. Stewart CJ, Coldewey J, Stewart IS. Comparison of fine needle aspiration cytology and needle core biopsy in the diagnosis of radiologically detected abdominal lesions. J Clin Pathol 2002 Feb;55(2):93–7.

29. O'Connell AM, Keeling F, Given M, et al. Fine-needle trucut biopsy versus fine-needle aspiration cytology with ultrasound guidance in the abdomen. J Med Imaging Radiat Oncol 2008 Jun;52(3):231–6.

30. Franca AV, Valerio HM, Trevisan M, et al. Fine needle aspiration biopsy for improving the diagnostic accuracy of cut needle biopsy of focal liver lesions. Acta Cytol 2003 May–Jun;47(3):332–6.

31. Fornari F, Civardi G, Cavanna L, et al. Ultrasonically guided fine-needle aspiration biopsy: a highly diagnostic procedure for hepatic tumors. Am J Gastroenterol 1990 Aug;85(8):1009–13.

32. Guo Z, Kurtycz DF, Salem R, et al. Radiologically guided percutaneous fine-needle aspiration biopsy of the liver: retrospective study of 119 cases evaluating diagnostic effectiveness and clinical complications. Diagn Cytopathol 2002 May;26(5):283–9.

33. Leiman G, Leibowitz CB, Dunbar F. Fine-needle aspiration of the liver: out of the ivory tower and into the community. Diagn Cytopathol 1989;5(1):35–9.

34. Nazir RT, Sharif MA, Iqbal M, Amin MS. Diagnostic accuracy of fine needle aspiration cytology in hepatic tumours. J Coll Physicians Surg Pak Jun;20(6):373–6.

35. Samaratunga H, Wright G. Value of fine needle aspiration biopsy cytology in the diagnosis of discrete hepatic lesions suspicious for malignancy. Aust N Z J Surg 1992 Jul;62(7):540–4.

36. Wang P, Liu LM, Meng ZQ, et al. [Evaluation of the results of fine-needle aspiration liver biopsies and the complications in 2528 cases.]. Zhonghua Gan Zang Bing Za Zhi 2007 Oct;15(10):758–62.

37. Bell DA, Carr CP, Szyfelbein WM. Fine needle aspiration cytology of focal liver lesions. Results obtained with examination of both cytologic and histologic preparations. Acta Cytol 1986 Jul–Aug;30(4):397–402.

38. Bret PM, Labadie M, Bretagnolle M, et al. Hepatocellular carcinoma: diagnosis by percutaneous fine needle biopsy. Gastrointest Radiol 1988 Jul;13(3):253–5.

39. Sole M, Calvet X, Cuberes T, et al. Value and limitations of cytologic criteria for the diagnosis of hepatocellular carcinoma by fine needle aspiration biopsy. Acta Cytol 1993 May–Jun;37(3):309–16.

40. Sangalli G, Livraghi T, Giordano F. Fine needle biopsy of hepatocellular carcinoma: improvement in diagnosis by microhistology. Gastroenterology 1989 Feb;96(2 Pt 1):524–6.

41. Zainol H, Sumithran E. Combined cytological and histological diagnosis of hepatocellular carcinoma in ultrasonically guided fine needle biopsy specimens. Histopathology 1993 Jun;22(6):581–6.

42. Awad SS, Fagan S, Abudayyeh S, et al. Preoperative evaluation of hepatic lesions for the staging of hepatocellular and metastatic liver carcinoma using endoscopic ultrasonography. Am J Surg 2002 Dec;184(6):601–4; discussion 4–5.

43. Nguyen P, Feng JC, Chang KJ. Endoscopic ultrasound (EUS) and EUS-guided fine-needle aspiration (FNA) of liver lesions. Gastrointest Endosc 1999 Sep;50(3):357–61.

44. tenBerge J, Hoffman BJ, Hawes RH, et al. EUS-guided fine needle aspiration of the liver: indications, yield, and safety based on an international survey of 167 cases. Gastrointest Endosc 2002 Jun;55(7):859–62.

45. Lundquist A. Liver biopsy with a needle of 0.7 MM outer diameter. Safety and quantitative yield. Acta Med Scand 1970 Dec;188(6):471–4.

46. Nguyen GK. Fine-needle aspiration biopsy cytology of hepatic tumors in adults. Pathol Annu 1986;21(Pt 1):321–49.

47. Smith EH. Complications of percutaneous abdominal fine-needle biopsy. Review. Radiology 1991 Jan;178(1):253–8.

48. Drinkovic I, Brkljacic B. Two cases of lethal complications following ultrasound-guided percutaneous fine-needle biopsy of the liver. Cardiovasc Intervent Radiol 1996 Sep–Oct;19(5):360–3.

49. Lundstedt C, Stridbeck H, Andersson R, et al. Tumor seeding occurring after fine-needle biopsy of abdominal malignancies. Acta Radiol 1991 Nov;32(6):518–20.

50. Saborido BP, Diaz JC, de Los Galanes SJ, et al. Does preoperative fine needle aspiration-biopsy produce tumor recurrence in patients following liver transplantation for hepatocellular carcinoma? Transplant Proc 2005 Nov;37(9):3874–7.

51. Tung WC, Huang YJ, Leung SW, et al. Incidence of needle tract seeding and responses of soft tissue metastasis by hepatocellular carcinoma postradiotherapy. Liver Int 2007 Mar;27(2):192–200.

52. Roussel F, Dalion J, Benozio M. The risk of tumoral seeding in needle biopsies. Acta Cytol 1989 Nov–Dec;33(6):936–9.

53. Navarro F, Taourel P, Michel J, et al. Diaphragmatic and subcutaneous seeding of hepatocellular carcinoma following fine-needle aspiration biopsy. Liver 1998 Aug;18(4):251–4.

54. Jourdan JL, Stubbs RS. Percutaneous biopsy of operable liver lesions: is it necessary or advisable? N Z Med J 1996 Dec 13;109(1035):469–70.

55. Huang CJ, Pitt HA, Lipsett PA, et al. Pyogenic hepatic abscess. Changing trends over 42 years. Ann Surg 1996 May;223(5):600–7; discussion 7–9.

56. John TG, Garden OJ. Needle track seeding of primary and secondary liver carcinoma after percutaneous liver biopsy. HPB Surg 1993;6(3):199–203; discussion 4.

57. Regimbeau JM, Fargas O, Vilgrain V, et al. What is the local risk of

recurrence after percutaneous biopsy of hepatocellular carcinoma? Hepato-Gastroenterol 1995;42:601–6.

58. Agarwal PK, Husain N, Singh BN. Cytologic findings in aspirated hydatid fluid. Acta Cytol 1989 Sep–Oct;33(5):652–4.

59. Das DK, Bhambhani S, Pant CS. Ultrasound guided fine-needle aspiration cytology: diagnosis of hydatid disease of the abdomen and thorax. Diagn Cytopathol 1995 Mar;12(2):173–6.

60. Pogacnik A, Pohar-Marinsek Z, Us-Krasovec M. Fine needle aspiration biopsy in the diagnosis of liver echinococcosis. Acta Cytol 1990 Sep–Oct;34(5):765–6.

61. Caturelli E, Rapaccini GL, Sabelli C, et al. Ultrasound-guided fine-needle aspiration biopsy in the diagnosis of hepatic hemangioma. Liver 1986 Dec;6(6):326–30.

62. Langlois SL. Fine-needle biopsy of hepatic hydatids and haemangiomas: an overstated hazard. Australas Radiol 1989 May;33(2):144–9.

63. Nakaizumi A, Iishi H, Yamamoto R, et al. Diagnosis of hepatic cavernous hemangioma by fine needle aspiration biopsy under ultrasonic guidance. Gastrointest Radiol 1990 Winter;15(1):39–42.

64. Solbiati L, Livraghi T, De Pra L, et al. Fine-needle biopsy of hepatic hemangioma with sonographic guidance. AJR Am J Roentgenol 1985 Mar;144(3):471–4.

65. Crowe DR, Eloubeidi MA, Chhieng DC, et al. Fine-needle aspiration biopsy of hepatic lesions: computerized tomographic-guided versus endoscopic ultrasound-guided FNA. Cancer 2006 Jun 25;108(3):180–5.

66. Fritscher-Ravens A, Broering DC, Sriram PV, et al. EUS-guided fine-needle aspiration cytodiagnosis of hilar cholangiocarcinoma: a case series. Gastrointest Endosc 2000 Oct;52(4):534–40.

67. Singh P, Erickson RA, Mukhopadhyay P, et al. EUS for detection of the hepatocellular carcinoma: results of a prospective study. Gastrointest Endosc 2007 Aug;66(2):265–73.

68. Miller DA, Carrasco CH, Katz RL, et al. Fine needle aspiration biopsy: the role of immediate cytologic assessment. AJR Am J Roentgenol 1986 Jul;147(1):155–8.

69. Hall-Craggs MA, Lees WR. Fine needle biopsy: cytology, histology or both? Gut 1987 Mar;28(3):233–6.

70. Pinto MM, Avila NA, Heller CI, Criscuolo EM. Fine needle aspiration of the liver. Acta Cytol 1988 Jan–Feb;32(1):15–21.

71. Tatsuta M, Yamamoto R, Kasugai H, et al. Cytohistologic diagnosis of neoplasms of the liver by ultrasonically guided fine-needle aspiration biopsy. Cancer 1984 Oct 15;54(8):1682–6.

72. Wee A, Nilsson B, Tan LK, Yap I. Fine needle aspiration biopsy of hepatocellular carcinoma. Diagnostic dilemma at the ends of the spectrum. Acta Cytol 1994 May–Jun;38(3):347–54.

73. Silverman JF, Geisinger KR. Ancillary studies in FNA of liver and pancreas. Diagn Cytopathol 1995 Dec;13(5):396–410.

74. Lundquist A, Akerman M. Fine-needle aspiration biopsy in acute hepatitis and liver cirrhosis. Ann Clin Res 1970 Sep;2(3):197–203.

75. Tao LC. Liver and pancreas. In: Bibbo M, editor. Comprehensive Cytopathology. Philadelphia: Saunders; 1991. p. 822–59.

76. Servoll E, Viste A, Skaarland E, et al. Fine-needle aspiration cytology of focal liver lesions. Advantages and limitations. Acta Chir Scand 1988 Jan;154(1):61–3.

77. Bergman S, Graeme-Cook F, Pitman MB. The usefulness of the reticulin stain in the differential diagnosis of liver nodules on fine-needle aspiration biopsy cell block preparations. Mod Pathol 1997 Dec;10(12):1258–64.

78. Gagliano EF. Reticulin stain in the fine needle aspiration differential diagnosis of liver nodules. Acta Cytol 1995 May–Jun;39(3):596–8.

79. Bottles K, Cohen MB. An approach to fine-needle aspiration biopsy diagnosis of hepatic masses. Diagn Cytopathol 1991;7(2):204–10.

80. Terada T, Nakanuma Y. Iron-negative foci in siderotic macroregenerative nodules in human cirrhotic liver. A marker of incipient neoplastic lesions. Arch Pathol Lab Med 1989 Aug;113(8):916–20.

81. Bose S, Kapila K, Verma K. Amyloidosis of the liver diagnosed by fine needle aspiration cytology. Acta Cytol 1989 Nov–Dec;33(6):935–6.

82. Gangane N, Anshu, Shivkumar VB, Sharta S. Cytodiagnosis of hepatic amyloidosis by fine needle aspiration cytology: a case report. Acta Cytol 2006 Sep-Oct;50(5):574–6.

83. Michael CW, Naylor B. Amyloid in cytologic specimens. Differential diagnosis and diagnostic pitfalls. Acta Cytol 1999 Sep–Oct;43(5):746–55.

84. Srinivasan R, Nijhawan R, Gautam U, Bambery P. Potassium permanganate resistant amyloid in fine-needle aspirate of the liver. Diagn Cytopathol 1994;10(4):383–4.

85. Stormby N, Akerman M. Aspiration cytology in the diagnosis of granulomatous liver lesions. Acta Cytol 1973 May–Jun;17(3):200–4.

86. Wee A, Nilsson B, Wang TL, et al. Tuberculous pseudotumor causing biliary obstruction. Report of a case with diagnosis by fine needle aspiration biopsy and bile cytology. Acta Cytol 1995 May–Jun;39(3):559–62.

87. Pinto MM, Kaye AD. Fine needle aspiration of cystic liver lesions. Cytologic examination and carcinoembryonic antigen assay of cyst contents. Acta Cytol 1989 Nov–Dec;33(6):852–6.

88. De J, Rossman L, Kott MM, Deavers MT. Cytologic diagnosis of ciliated hepatic foregut cyst. Diagn Cytopathol 2006 Dec;34(12):846–9.

89. Hornstein A, Batts KP, Linz LJ, et al. Fine needle aspiration diagnosis of ciliated hepatic foregut cysts: a report of three cases. Acta Cytol 1996 May–Jun;40(3):576–80.

90. von Sinner WN, Nyman R, Linjawi T, Ali AM. Fine needle aspiration biopsy of hydatid cysts. Acta Radiol 1995 Mar;36(2):168–72.

91. Singh A, Singh Y, Sharma VK, et al. Diagnosis of hydatid disease of abdomen and thorax by ultrasound guided fine needle aspiration cytology. Indian J Pathol Microbiol 1999 Apr;42(2):155–6.

92. Vercelli-Retta J, Manana G, Reissenweber NJ. The cytologic diagnosis of hydatid disease. Acta Cytol 1982 Mar–Apr;26(2):159–68.

93. Wee A, Nilsson B, Yap I, Chong SM. Aspiration cytology of liver abscesses. With an emphasis on diagnostic pitfalls. Acta Cytol 1995 May–Jun;39(3):453–62.

94. Bhambhani S, Kashyap V. Amoebiasis: diagnosis by aspiration and exfoliative cytology. Cytopathology 2001 Oct;12(5):329–33.

95. Granger JK, Houn HY. Diagnosis of hepatic actinomycosis by fine-needle aspiration. Diagn Cytopathol 1991;7(1):95–7.

96. Shurbaji MS, Gupta PK, Newman MM. Hepatic actinomycosis diagnosed by fine needle aspiration. A case report. Acta Cytol 1987 Nov–Dec;31(6):751–5.

97. Caturelli E, Rapaccini GL, Sabelli C, et al. Ultrasonography and echo-guided fine-needle biopsy in the diagnosis of focal fatty liver change. Hepatogastroenterology 1987 Aug;34(4):137–40.

98. Layfield LJ. Focal fatty change of the liver: cytologic findings in a radiographic mimic of metastases. Diagn Cytopathol 1994 Dec;11(4):385–7.

99. Anthony PP, Telesinghe PU. Inflammatory pseudotumour of the liver. J Clin Pathol 1986 Jul;39(7):761–8.

100. Isobe H, Nishi Y, Fukutomi T, et al. Inflammatory pseudotumor of the liver associated with acute myelomonocytic leukemia. Am J Gastroenterol 1991 Feb;86(2):238–40.

101. Lupovitch A, Chen R, Mishra S. Inflammatory pseudotumor of the liver.

Report of the fine needle aspiration cytologic findings in a case initially misdiagnosed as malignant. Acta Cytol 1989 Mar–Apr;33(2):259–62.

102. Malhotra V, Gondal R, Tatke M, Sarin SK. Fine needle aspiration cytologic appearance of inflammatory pseudotumor of the liver. A case report. Acta Cytol 1997 Jul–Aug;41(4 Suppl): 1325–8.

103. Dardi LE, Marzano M, Froula E. Fine needle aspiration cytologic diagnosis of focal intrahepatic extramedullary hematopoiesis. Acta Cytol 1990 Jul–Aug;34(4):567–9.

104. Lemos LB, Baliga M, Benghuzzi HA, Cason Z. Nodular hematopoiesis of the liver diagnosed by fine-needle aspiration cytology. Diagn Cytopathol 1997 Jan;16(1):51–4.

105. Raab SS, Silverman JF, McLeod DL, Geisinger KR. Fine-needle aspiration cytology of extramedullary hematopoiesis (myeloid metaplasia). Diagn Cytopathol 1993 Oct;9(5):522–6.

106. Ruschenburg I, Droese M. Fine needle aspiration cytology of focal nodular hyperplasia of the liver. Acta Cytol 1989 Nov–Dec;33(6):857–60.

107. Adam YG, Nonas CJ. Hepatobiliary cystadenoma. South Med J 1995 Nov;88(11):1140–3.

108. Logrono R, Rampy BA, Adegboyega PA. Fine needle aspiration cytology of hepatobiliary cystadenoma with mesenchymal stroma. Cancer 2002 Feb 25;96(1):37–42.

109. Filippi de la Palavesa MM, Vasilescu C, et al. Biliary cystadenocarcinoma: sonographic and cytologic findings. J Clin Ultrasound 1999 May;27(4):210–2.

110. Del Poggio P, Jamoletti C, Forloni B, et al. Malignant transformation of biliary cystadenoma: a difficult diagnosis. Dig Liver Dis 2000 Nov;32(8):733–6.

111. Iemoto Y, Kondo Y, Nakano T, et al. Biliary cystadenocarcinoma diagnosed by liver biopsy performed under ultrasonographic guidance. Gastroenterology 1983 Feb;84(2): 399–403.

112. Ishak KG, Willis GW, Cummins SD, Bullock AA. Biliary cystadenoma and cystadenocarcinoma: report of 14 cases and review of the literature. Cancer 1977 Jan;39(1):322–38.

113. Wee A, Nilsson B, Kang JY, et al. Biliary cystadenocarcinoma arising in a cystadenoma. Report of a case diagnosed by fine needle aspiration cytology. Acta Cytol 1993 Nov–Dec;37(6):966–70.

114. Woods GL. Biliary cystadenocarcinoma: Case report of hepatic malignancy originating in benign cystadenoma. Cancer 1981 Jun 15;47(12):2936–40.

115. Tao LC. Are oral contraceptive-associated liver cell adenomas premalignant? Acta Cytol 1992 May–Jun;36(3):338–44.

116. Ali MA, Akhtar M, Mattingly RC. Morphologic spectrum of hepatocellular carcinoma in fine needle aspiration biopsies. Acta Cytol 1986 May–Jun;30(3):294–302.

117. Bottles K, Cohen MB, Holly EA, et al. A step-wise logistic regression analysis of hepatocellular carcinoma. An aspiration biopsy study. Cancer 1988 Aug 1;62(3):558–63.

118. Cohen MB, Haber MM, Holly EA, et al. Cytologic criteria to distinguish hepatocellular carcinoma from nonneoplastic liver. Am J Clin Pathol 1991 Feb;95(2):125–30.

119. Das DK. Cytodiagnosis of hepatocellular carcinoma in fine-needle aspirates of the liver: its differentiation from reactive hepatocytes and metastatic adenocarcinoma. Diagn Cytopathol 1999 Dec;21(6):370–7.

120. de Boer WB, Segal A, Frost FA, Sterrett GF. Cytodiagnosis of well differentiated hepatocellular carcinoma: can indeterminate diagnoses be reduced? Cancer 1999 Oct 25;87(5):270–7.

121. Granados R, Aramburu JA, Murillo N, et al. Fine-needle aspiration biopsy of liver masses: diagnostic value and reproducibility of cytological criteria. Diagn Cytopathol 2001 Dec;25(6): 365–75.

122. Greene CL, Fehrman I, Nery D, et al. Liver transplant aspiration cytology (TAC) at three weeks and one year in healthy recipients with grafts free of histologic abnormality. Transplant Proc 1989 Feb;21(1 Pt 2):2211–2.

123. Kung IT, Chan SK, Fung KH. Fine-needle aspiration in hepatocellular carcinoma. Combined cytologic and histologic approach. Cancer 1991 Feb 1;67(3):673–80.

124. Longchampt E, Patriarche C, Fabre M. Accuracy of cytology vs. microbiopsy for the diagnosis of well-differentiated hepatocellular carcinoma and macroregenerative nodule. Definition of standardized criteria from a study of 100 cases. Acta Cytol 2000 Jul–Aug;44(4):515–23.

125. Noguchi S, Yamamoto R, Tatsuta M, et al. Cell features and patterns in fine-needle aspirates of hepatocellular carcinoma. Cancer 1986 Jul 15;58(2):321–8.

126. Pedio G, Landolt U, Zobeli L, Gut D. Fine needle aspiration of the liver. Significance of hepatocytic naked nuclei in the diagnosis of hepatocellular carcinoma. Acta Cytol 1988 Jul–Aug;32(4):437–42.

127. Pisharodi LR, Lavoie R, Bedrossian CW. Differential diagnostic dilemmas in malignant fine-needle aspirates of liver: a practical approach to final diagnosis. Diagn Cytopathol 1995 Jun;12(4):364–70; discussion 70–1.

128. Pitman MB, Szyfelbein WM. Significance of endothelium in the fine-needle aspiration biopsy diagnosis of hepatocellular carcinoma. Diagn Cytopathol 1995 May;12(3):208–14.

129. Salomao DR, Lloyd RV, Goellner JR. Hepatocellular carcinoma: needle biopsy findings in 74 cases. Diagn Cytopathol 1997 Jan;16(1):8–13.

130. Takenaka A, Kaji I, Kasugai H, et al. Usefulness of diagnostic criteria for aspiration cytology of hepatocellular carcinoma. Acta Cytol 1999 Jul–Aug;43(4):610–6.

131. Wee A, Nilsson B. Highly well differentiated hepatocellular carcinoma and benign hepatocellular lesions. Can they be distinguished on fine needle aspiration biopsy? Acta Cytol 2003 Jan–Feb;47(1):16–26.

132. Wee A, Nilsson B, Chan-Wilde C, et al. Cytological diagnosis from fine needle aspiration biopsy of the liver. Ann Acad Med Singapore 1991 Mar;20(2):208–14.

133. Singh HK, Silverman JF, Geisinger KR. Fine-needle aspiration cytomorphology of clear-cell hepatocellular carcinoma. Diagn Cytopathol 1997 Oct;17(4): 306–10.

134. Buchanan Jr TF, Huvos AG. Clear-cell carcinoma of the liver. A clinicopathologic study of 13 patients. Am J Clin Pathol 1974 Apr;61(4): 529–39.

135. Mathew T, Affandi MZ. Fine needle aspiration biopsy of a hepatic mass. An example of a near error. Acta Cytol 1989 Nov–Dec;33(6):861–4.

136. Davenport RD. Cytologic diagnosis of fibrolamellar carcinoma of the liver by fine-needle aspiration. Diagn Cytopathol 1990;6(4):275–9.

137. Perez Gil MA, Ruiz Recuento J, Relanzon Molinero S, et al. [Focal liver lesions in multiple myeloma: ecography, computed tomography, and magnetic resonance findings. A case report]. Radiologia 2006 Jul–Aug;48(4):251–4.

138. Suen KC, Magee JF, Halparin LS, et al. Fine needle aspiration cytology of fibrolamellar hepatocellular carcinoma. Acta Cytol 1985 Sep–Oct;29(5):867–72.

139. Gottschalk-Sabag S, Ron N, Glick T. Use of CD34 and factor VIII to diagnose hepatocellular carcinoma on fine needle aspirates. Acta Cytol 1998 May–Jun;42(3):691–6.

140. de Boer WB, Segal A, Frost FA, Sterrett GF. Can CD34 discriminate between benign and malignant hepatocytic lesions in fine-needle aspirates and thin core biopsies? Cancer 2000 Oct 25;90(5):273–8.

141. Kong CS, Appenzeller M, Ferrell LD. Utility of CD34 reactivity in evaluating focal nodular hepatocellular lesions sampled by fine needle aspiration biopsy. Acta Cytol 2000 Mar–Apr;44(2):218–22.

142. Kandil D, Leiman G, Allegretta M, et al. Glypican-3 immunocytochemistry in

liver fine-needle aspirates : a novel stain to assist in the differentiation of benign and malignant liver lesions. Cancer 2007 Oct 25;111(5):316–22.

143. Ligato S, Mandich D, Cartun RW. Utility of glypican-3 in differentiating hepatocellular carcinoma from other primary and metastatic lesions in FNA of the liver: an immunocytochemical study. Mod Pathol 2008 Feb 8.

144. Nassar A, Cohen C, Siddiqui MT. Utility of glypican-3 and survivin in differentiating hepatocellular carcinoma from benign and preneoplastic hepatic lesions and metastatic carcinomas in liver fine-needle aspiration biopsies. Diagn Cytopathol 2009 Sep;37(9): 629–35.

145. Cottier M, Jouffre C, Maubon I, et al. Prospective flow cytometric DNA analysis of hepatocellular carcinoma specimens collected by ultrasound-guided fine needle aspiration. Cancer 1994 Jul 15;74(2):599–605.

146. Ng IO, Lai EC, Ho JC, et al. Flow cytometric analysis of DNA ploidy in hepatocellular carcinoma. Am J Clin Pathol 1994 Jul;102(1):80–6.

147. Russo A, Bazan V, Plaja S, et al. Flow cytometric DNA analysis of hepatic tumours on ultrasound-guided fine-needle aspirates. J Surg Oncol 1992 Sep;51(1):26–32.

148. Pitman MB. Fine needle aspiration biopsy of the liver. Principal diagnostic challenges. Clin Lab Med 1998 Sep;18(3):483–506.

149. Renshaw AA, Haja J, Wilbur DC, Miller TR. Fine-needle aspirates of adenocarcinoma/metastatic carcinoma that resemble hepatocellular carcinoma: correlating cytologic features and performance in the College of American Pathologists Nongynecologic Cytology Program. Arch Pathol Lab Med 2005 Oct;129(10):1217–21.

150. Renshaw AA, Haja J, Wilbur DC, Miller TR. Fine-needle aspirates of hepatocellular carcinoma that are misclassified as adenocarcinoma: correlating cytologic features and performance in the College of American Pathologists Nongynecologic Cytology Program. Arch Pathol Lab Med 2006 Jan;130(1):19–22.

151. Kakar S, Gown AM, Goodman ZD, Ferrell LD. Best practices in diagnostic immunohistochemistry: hepatocellular carcinoma versus metastatic neoplasms. Arch Pathol Lab Med 2007 Nov;131(11):1648–54.

152. Saleh HA, Aulicino M, Zaidi SY, et al. Discriminating hepatocellular carcinoma from metastatic carcinoma on fine-needle aspiration biopsy of the liver: the utility of immunocytochemical panel. Diagn Cytopathol 2009 Mar;37(3):184–90.

153. Guindi M, Yazdi HM, Gilliatt MA. Fine needle aspiration biopsy of hepatocellular carcinoma. Value of immunocytochemical and ultrastructural studies. Acta Cytol 1994 May–Jun;38(3):385–91.

154. Johnson DE, Powers CN, Rupp G, Frable WJ. Immunocytochemical staining of fine-needle aspiration biopsies of the liver as a diagnostic tool for hepatocellular carcinoma. Mod Pathol 1992 Mar;5(2):117–23.

155. Rishi M, Kovatich A, Ehya H. Utility of polyclonal and monoclonal antibodies against carcinoembryonic antigen in hepatic fine-needle aspirates. Diagn Cytopathol 1994 Dec;11(4):358–61; discussion 61–2.

156. Wang L, Vuolo M, Suhrland MJ, Schlesinger K. HepPar1, MOC-31, pCEA, mCEA and CD10 for distinguishing hepatocellular carcinoma vs. metastatic adenocarcinoma in liver fine needle aspirates. Acta Cytol 2006 May–Jun;50(3):257–62.

157. Wee A, Nilsson B. pCEA canalicular immunostaining in fine needle aspiration biopsy diagnosis of hepatocellular carcinoma. Acta Cytol 1997 Jul–Aug;41(4):1147–55.

158. Wolber RA, Greene CA, Dupuis BA. Polyclonal carcinoembryonic antigen staining in the cytologic differential diagnosis of primary and metastatic hepatic malignancies. Acta Cytol 1991 Mar–Apr;35(2):215–20.

159. Ahuja A, Gupta N, Kalra N, et al. Role of CD10 immunochemistry in differentiating hepatocellular carcinoma from metastatic carcinoma of the liver. Cytopathology 2008 Aug;19(4):229–35.

160. Lin F, Abdallah H, Meschter S. Diagnostic utility of CD10 in differentiating hepatocellular carcinoma from metastatic carcinoma in fine-needle aspiration biopsy (FNAB) of the liver. Diagn Cytopathol 2004 Feb;30(2): 92–7.

161. Siddiqui MT, Saboorian MH, Gokaslan ST, Ashfaq R. Diagnostic utility of the HepPar1 antibody to differentiate hepatocellular carcinoma from metastatic carcinoma in fine-needle aspiration samples. Cancer 2002 Feb 25;96(1):49–52.

162. Zimmerman RL, Burke MA, Young NA, et al. Diagnostic value of hepatocyte paraffin 1 antibody to discriminate hepatocellular carcinoma from metastatic carcinoma in fine-needle aspiration biopsies of the liver. Cancer 2001 Aug 25;93(4):288–91.

163. Kandil DH, Cooper K. Glypican-3: a novel diagnostic marker for hepatocellular carcinoma and more. Adv Anat Pathol 2009 Mar;16(2):125–9.

164. Centeno BA. Pathology of liver metastases. Cancer Control 2006 Jan;13(1):13–26.

165. Maeda T, Kajiyama K, Adachi E, et al. The expression of cytokeratins 7, 19, and 20 in primary and metastatic carcinomas of the liver. Mod Pathol 1996 Sep;9(9):901–9.

166. Zimmerman RL, Burke M, Young NA, et al. Diagnostic utility of Glut-1 and CA 15-3 in discriminating adenocarcinoma from hepatocellular carcinoma in liver tumors biopsied by fine-needle aspiration. Cancer 2002 Feb 25;96(1):53–7.

167. Lei JY, Bourne PA, diSant'Agnese PA, Huang J. Cytoplasmic staining of TTF-1 in the differential diagnosis of hepatocellular carcinoma vs cholangiocarcinoma and metastatic carcinoma of the liver. Am J Clin Pathol 2006 Apr;125(4):519–25.

168. Wieczorek TJ, Pinkus JL, Glickman JN, Pinkus GS. Comparison of thyroid transcription factor-1 and hepatocyte antigen immunohistochemical analysis in the differential diagnosis of hepatocellular carcinoma, metastatic adenocarcinoma, renal cell carcinoma, and adrenal cortical carcinoma. Am J Clin Pathol 2002 Dec;118(6):911–21.

169. Papotti M, Pacchioni D, Negro F, et al. Albumin gene expression in liver tumors: diagnostic interest in fine needle aspiration biopsies. Mod Pathol 1994 Apr;7(3):271–5.

170. Stephen MR, Oien K, Ferrier RK, Burnett RA. Effusion cytology of hepatocellular carcinoma with in situ hybridisation for human albumin. J Clin Pathol 1997 May;50(5):442–4.

171. Eloubeidi MA, Chen VK, Jhala NC, et al. Endoscopic ultrasound-guided fine needle aspiration biopsy of suspected cholangiocarcinoma. Clin Gastroenterol Hepatol 2004 Mar;2(3):209–13.

172. Jain M, Ahluwalia C, Agarwal K, Pathania OP. Cytological diagnosis of cholangiocarcinoma with rib metastasis in a young female–a case report. Indian J Pathol Microbiol 2004 Jul;47(3):417–20.

173. Tan G, Yilmaz A, De Young BR, et al. Immunohistochemical analysis of biliary tract lesions. Appl Immunohistochem Mol Morphol 2004 Sep;12(3):193–7.

174. Chaudhary HB, Bhanot P, Logrono R. Phenotypic diversity of intrahepatic and extrahepatic cholangiocarcinoma on aspiration cytology and core needle biopsy: case series and review of the literature. Cancer 2005 Aug 25;105(4):220–8.

175. Gibbons D, de las Morenas A. Fine needle aspiration diagnosis of combined hepatocellular carcinoma and cholangiocarcinoma. A case report. Acta Cytol 1997 Jul–Aug;41(4 Suppl):1269–72.

176. Wee A, Nilsson B. Combined hepatocellular-cholangiocarcinoma. Diagnostic challenge in hepatic fine needle aspiration biopsy. Acta Cytol 1999 Mar–Apr;43(2):131–8.

177. Dekmezian R, Sneige N, Popok S, Ordonez NG. Fine-needle aspiration cytology of paediatric patients with primary hepatic tumors: a comparative study of two hepatoblastomas and a

liver-cell carcinoma. Diagn Cytopathol 1988;4(2):162–8.

178. Iyer VK, Kapila K, Agarwala S, Verma K. Fine needle aspiration cytology of hepatoblastoma. Recognition of subtypes on cytomorphology. Acta Cytol 2005 Jul–Aug;49(4):355–64.

179. Parikh B, Jojo A, Shah B, et al. Fine needle aspiration cytology of hepatoblastoma: a study of 20 cases. Indian J Pathol Microbiol 2005 Jul;48(3):331–6.

180. Sola Perez J, Perez-Guillermo M, Bas Bernal AB, Mercader JM. Hepatoblastoma. An attempt to apply histologic classification to aspirates obtained by fine needle aspiration cytology. Acta Cytol 1994 Mar–Apr;38(2):175–82.

181. Wakely Jr PE, Silverman JF, Geisinger KR, Frable WJ. Fine needle aspiration biopsy cytology of hepatoblastoma. Mod Pathol 1990 Nov;3(6):688–93.

182. Fasano M, Theise ND, Nalesnik M, et al. Immunohistochemical evaluation of hepatoblastomas with use of the hepatocyte-specific marker, hepatocyte paraffin 1, and the polyclonal anti-carcinoembryonic antigen. Mod Pathol 1998 Oct;11(10):934–8.

183. Collins KA, Geisinger KR, Raab SS, Silverman JF. Fine needle aspiration biopsy of hepatic lymphomas: cytomorphology and ancillary studies. Acta Cytol 1996 Mar–Apr;40(2):257–62.

184. Rappaport KM, DiGiuseppe JA, Busseniers AE. Primary hepatic lymphoma: report of two cases diagnosed by fine-needle aspiration. Diagn Cytopathol 1995 Aug;13(2):142–5.

185. Jansson SE, Bondestam S, Heinonen E, et al. Value of liver and spleen aspiration biopsy in malignant diseases when these organs show no signs of involvement in sonography. Acta Med Scand 1983;213(4):279–81.

186. Gattuso P, Castelli MJ, Peng Y, Reddy VB. Posttransplant lymphoproliferative disorders: a fine-needle aspiration biopsy study. Diagn Cytopathol 1997 May;16(5):392–5.

187. Raymond E, Tricottet V, Samuel D, et al. Epstein-Barr virus-related localized hepatic lymphoproliferative disorders after liver transplantation. Cancer 1995 Oct 15;76(8):1344–51.

188. Layfield LJ, Mooney EE, Dodd LG. Not by blood alone: diagnosis of hemangiomas by fine-needle aspiration. Diagn Cytopathol 1998 Oct;19(4):250–4.

189. Taavitsainen M, Airaksinen T, Kreula J, Paivansalo M. Fine-needle aspiration biopsy of liver hemangioma. Acta Radiol 1990 Jan;31(1):69–71.

190. Manucha V, Sun CC. Cytologic findings and differential diagnosis in hepatic Epithelioid hemangioendothelioma: a case report. Acta Cytol 2008 Nov–Dec;52(6):713–7.

191. Cho NH, Lee KG, Jeong MG. Cytologic evaluation of primary malignant vascular tumors of the liver. One case each of angiosarcoma and epithelioid hemangioendothelioma. Acta Cytol 1997 Sep–Oct;41(5):1468–76.

192. Soslow RA, Yin P, Steinberg CR, Yang GC. Cytopathologic features of hepatic epithelioid hemangioendothelioma. Diagn Cytopathol 1997 Jul;17(1):50–3.

193. Boucher LD, Swanson PE, Stanley MW, et al. Cytology of angiosarcoma. Findings in fourteen fine-needle aspiration biopsy specimens and one pleural fluid specimen. Am J Clin Pathol 2000 Aug;114(2):210–9.

194. Liu K, Layfield LJ. Cytomorphologic features of angiosarcoma on fine needle aspiration biopsy. Acta Cytol 1999 May–Jun;43(3):407–15.

195. Wong JW, Bedard YC. Fine-needle aspiration biopsy of hepatic angiosarcoma: report of a case with immunocytochemical findings. Diagn Cytopathol 1992;8(4):380–3.

196. Cha I, Cartwright D, Guis M, et al. Angiomyolipoma of the liver in fine-needle aspiration biopsies: its distinction from hepatocellular carcinoma. Cancer 1999 Feb 25;87(1):25–30.

197. Ma TK, Tse MK, Tsui WM, Yuen KT. Fine needle aspiration diagnosis of angiomyolipoma of the liver using a cell block with immunohistochemical study. A case report. Acta Cytol 1994 Mar–Apr;38(2):257–60.

198. Sawai H, Manabe T, Yamanaka Y, et al. Angiomyolipoma of the liver: case report and collective review of cases diagnosed from fine needle aspiration biopsy specimens. J Hepatobiliary Pancreat Surg 1998;5(3):333–8.

199. al-Rikabi AC, Buckai A, al-Sumayer S, et al. Fine needle aspiration cytology of mesenchymal hamartoma of the liver. A case report. Acta Cytol 2000 May–Jun;44(3):449–53.

200. Jimenez-Heffernan JA, Vicandi B, Lopez-Ferrer P, et al. Fine-needle aspiration cytology of mesenchymal hamartoma of the liver. Diagn Cytopathol 2000 Apr;22(4):250–3.

201. Drachenberg CB, Papadimitriou JC, Rivero MA, Wood C. Distinctive case. Adult mesenchymal hamartoma of the liver: report of a case with light microscopic, FNA cytology, immunohistochemistry, and ultrastructural studies and review of the literature. Mod Pathol 1991 May;4(3):392–5.

202. Cheuk W, Lee KC, Chan JK. c-kit immunocytochemical staining in the cytologic diagnosis of metastatic gastrointestinal stromal tumor. A report of two cases. Acta Cytol 2000 Jul–Aug;44(4):679–85.

203. Padilla C, Saez A, Vidal A, et al. Fine-needle aspiration cytology diagnosis of metastatic gastrointestinal stromal tumor in the liver: a report of three cases. Diagn Cytopathol 2002 Nov;27(5):298–302.

204. Wieczorek TJ, Faquin WC, Rubin BP, Cibas ES. Cytologic diagnosis of gastrointestinal stromal tumor with emphasis on the differential diagnosis with leiomyosarcoma. Cancer 2001 Aug 25;93(4):276–87.

205. Smith MB, Silverman JF, Raab SS, et al. Fine-needle aspiration cytology of hepatic leiomyosarcoma. Diagn Cytopathol 1994 Dec;11(4):321–7.

206. Wee A, Nilsson B. Fine needle aspiration biopsy of hepatic leiomyosarcoma. An unusual epithelioid variant posing a potential diagnostic pitfall in a hepatocellular carcinoma-prevalent population. Acta Cytol 1997 May–Jun;41(3):737–43.

207. Garcia-Bonafe M, Allende H, Fantova MJ, Tarragona J. Fine needle aspiration cytology of undifferentiated (embryonal) sarcoma of the liver. A case report. Acta Cytol 1997 Jul–Aug;41(4 Suppl):1273–8.

208. Gupta C, Iyer VK, Kaushal S, et al. Fine needle aspiration cytology of undifferentiated embryonal sarcoma of the liver. Cytopathology Jan 22.

209. Kaur J, Dey P, Das A. Fine needle aspiration cytology of undifferentiated (embryonal) sarcoma of liver in an adult male. Diagn Cytopathol Jul;38(7):547–8.

210. Sola-Perez J, Perez-Guillermo M, Gimenez-Bascunana A, Garre-Sanchez C. Cytopathology of undifferentiated (embryonal) sarcoma of the liver. Diagn Cytopathol 1995 Jul;13(1):44–51.

211. Khalbuss WE, Grigorian S, Bui MM, Elhosseiny A. Small-cell tumors of the liver: a cytological study of 91 cases and a review of the literature. Diagn Cytopathol 2005 Jul;33(1):8–14.

212. Miralles TG, Gosabez F, de Lera J, et al. Percutaneous fine needle aspiration biopsy cytology of the liver for staging small cell lung carcinoma. Comparison with other methods. Acta Cytol 1993 Jul-Aug;37(4):499–502.

213. Prosser JM, Dusenbery D. Histocytologic diagnosis of neuroendocrine tumors in the liver: a retrospective study of 23 cases. Diagn Cytopathol 1997 May;16(5):383–91.

214. Bocking A, Pomjansky N, Buckstegge B, Onofre A. [Immunocytochemical identification of carcinomas of unknown primaries on fine-needle-aspiration-biopsies]. Pathologe 2009 Dec;30(Suppl 2):158–60.

215. Onofre AS, Pomjanski N, Buckstegge B, Bocking A. Immunocytochemical diagnosis of hepatocellular carcinoma and identification of carcinomas of unknown primary metastatic to the liver on fine-needle aspiration cytologies. Cancer 2007 Aug 25;111(4):259–68.

216. Caraway NP, Fanning CV. Use of fine-needle aspiration biopsy in the evaluation of splenic lesions in a cancer center. Diagn Cytopathol 1997 Apr;16(4):312–6.

217. Eloubeidi MA, Varadarajulu S, Eltoum I, et al. Transgastric endoscopic ultrasound-guided fine-needle aspiration biopsy and flow cytometry of suspected lymphoma of the spleen. Endoscopy 2006 Jun;38(6):617–20.

218. Friedlander MA, Wei XJ, Iyengar P, Moreira AL. Diagnostic pitfalls in fine needle aspiration biopsy of the spleen. Diagn Cytopathol 2008 Feb;36(2):69–75.

219. Iwashita T, Yasuda I, Tsurumi H, et al. Endoscopic ultrasound-guided fine needle aspiration biopsy for splenic tumor: a case series. Endoscopy 2009 Feb;41(2):179–82.

220. Lal A, Ariga R, Gattuso P, et al. Splenic fine needle aspiration and core biopsy. A review of 49 cases. Acta Cytol 2003 Nov–Dec;47(6):951–9.

221. Lishner M, Lang R, Hamlet Y, et al. Fine needle aspiration biopsy in patients with diffusely enlarged spleens. Acta Cytol 1996 Mar–Apr;40(2):196–8.

222. Ramdall RB, Cai G, Alasio TM, Levine P. Fine-needle aspiration biopsy for the primary diagnosis of lymphoproliferative disorders involving the spleen: one institution's experience and review of the literature. Diagn Cytopathol 2006 Dec;34(12):812–7.

223. Schwerk WB, Maroske D, Roth S, Arnold R. [Ultrasound-guided fine-needle puncture in the diagnosis and therapy of liver and spleen abscesses]. Dtsch Med Wochenschr 1986 May 30;111(22):847–53.

224. Silverman JF, Geisinger KR, Raab SS, Stanley MW. Fine needle aspiration biopsy of the spleen in the evaluation of neoplastic disorders. Acta Cytol 1993 Mar–Apr;37(2):158–62.

225. Soderstrom N. How to use cytodiagnostic spleen puncture. Acta Med Scand 1976;199(1–2):1–5.

226. Zeppa P, Vetrani A, Luciano L, et al. Fine needle aspiration biopsy of the spleen. A useful procedure in the diagnosis of splenomegaly. Acta Cytol 1994 May–Jun;38(3):299–309.

227. Kumar PV, Monabati A, Raseki AR, et al. Splenic lesions: FNA findings in 48 cases. Cytopathology 2007 Jun;18(3):151–6.

228. Nerlich A, Permanetter W. Fine needle aspiration cytodiagnosis of epidermoid cysts of the spleen. Report of two cases. Acta Cytol 1991 Sep–Oct;35(5):567–9.

229. Kang M, Kalra N, Gulati M, et al. Image guided percutaneous splenic interventions. Eur J Radiol 2007 Oct;64(1):140–6.

230. Haque I, Haque MZ, Krishnani N, et al. Fine needle aspiration cytology of the spleen in visceral leishmaniasis. Acta Cytol 1993 Jan–Feb;37(1):73–6.

231. Rajwanshi A, Gupta D, Kapoor S, et al. Fine needle aspiration biopsy of the spleen in pyrexia of unknown origin. Cytopathology 1999 Jun;10(3):195–200.

232. Selroos O, Koivunen E. Usefulness of fine-needle aspiration biopsy of spleen in diagnosis of sarcoidosis. Chest 1983 Feb;83(2):193–5.

233. Taavitsainen M, Koivuniemi A, Helminen J, et al. Aspiration biopsy of the spleen in patients with sarcoidosis. Acta Radiol 1987 Nov–Dec;28(6):723–5.

234. Sen R, Bhadani PP, Singh H, et al. Myeloid metaplasia in aspirates from enlarged spleens: a clue in the absence of peripheral blood findings characteristic of myelofibrosis. Acta Cytol 2006 Jul–Aug;50(4):379–83.

235. Colovic R, Micev M, Grubor N, et al. [Inflammatory pseudotumours of spleen]. Srp Arh Celok Lek 2009 Mar–Apr;137(3–4):189–93.

236. Pasternack A. Fine-needle aspiration biopsy of spleen in diagnosis of generalized amyloidosis. Br Med J 1974 Apr 6;2(5909):20–2.

237. Domanski H, Dejmek A, Ljung R. Gaucher's disease in an infant diagnosed by fine needle aspiration of the liver and spleen. A case report. Acta Cytol 1992 May–Jun;36(3):410–2.

238. Moriarty AT, Schwenk Jr GR, Chua G. Splenic fine needle aspiration biopsy in the diagnosis of lymphoreticular diseases. A report of four cases. Acta Cytol 1993 Mar–Apr;37(2):191–6.

239. Comperat E, Bardier-Dupas A, Camparo P, et al. Splenic metastases: clinicopathologic presentation, differential diagnosis, and pathogenesis. Arch Pathol Lab Med 2007 Jun;131(6):965–9.

240. Delacruz V, Jorda M, Gomez-Fernandez C, et al. Fine-needle aspiration diagnosis of angiosarcoma of the spleen: a case report and review of the literature. Arch Pathol Lab Med 2005 Aug;129(8):1054–6.

241. Lee SH. Fine-needle aspiration cytology of splenic hamartoma. Diagn Cytopathol 2003 Feb;28(2):82–5.

242. Fritscher-Ravens A, Mylonaki M, Pantes A, et al. Endoscopic ultrasound-guided biopsy for the diagnosis of focal lesions of the spleen. Am J Gastroenterol 2003 May;98(5):1022–7.

243. Gomez-Rubio M, Lopez-Cano A, Rendon P, et al. Safety and diagnostic accuracy of percutaneous ultrasound-guided biopsy of the spleen: a multicenter study. J Clin Ultrasound 2009 Oct;37(8):445–50.

244. Cavanna L, Artioli F, Vallisa D, et al. Primary lymphoma of the spleen. Report of a case with diagnosis by fine-needle guided biopsy. Haematologica 1995 May–Jun;80(3):241–3.

245. Civardi G, Vallisa D, Berte R, et al. Ultrasound-guided fine needle biopsy of the spleen: high clinical efficacy and low risk in a multicenter Italian study. Am J Hematol 2001 Jun;67(2):93–9.

246. Lindgren PG, Hagberg H, Eriksson B, et al. Excision biopsy of the spleen by ultrasonic guidance. Br J Radiol 1985 Sep;58(693):853–7.

247. Lopez JI, Del Cura JL, De Larrinoa AF, et al. Role of ultrasound-guided core biopsy in the evaluation of spleen pathology. APMIS 2006 Jul–Aug;114(7–8):492–9.

248. Goldfinger M, Cohen MM, Steinhardt MI, et al. Sonography and percutaneous aspiration of splenic epidermoid cyst. J Clin Ultrasound 1986 Feb;14(2):147–9.

249. Bonifacio A, Goldberg RE, Patterson BJ, Haider M. Flow-cytometry-enhanced fine-needle aspiration biopsy of the spleen. Can Assoc Radiol J 2000 Jun;51(3):158–62.

250. Zeppa P, Picardi M, Marino G, Troncone G, et al. Fine-needle aspiration biopsy and flow cytometry immunophenotyping of lymphoid and myeloproliferative disorders of the spleen. Cancer 2003 Apr 25;99(2):118–27.

251. Gupta R, Jain P, Bakshi S, Sharma MC. Primary Hodgkin's disease of spleen – a case report. Indian J Pathol Microbiol 2006 Jul;49(3):435–7.

252. Meara RS, Reddy V, Arnoletti JP, et al. Hairy cell leukemia: a diagnosis by endoscopic ultrasound guided fine needle aspiration. Cytojournal 2006;3:1.

253. Pinto RG, Rocha PD, Vernekar JA. Fine needle aspiration of the spleen in hairy cell leukemia. A case report. Acta Cytol 1995 Jul–Aug;39(4):777–80.

254. Barbazza R, De Martini A, Mognol M, et al. Fine needle aspiration biopsy of a splenic hemangioma. A case report with review of the literature. Haematologica 1990 May–Jun;75(3):278–81.

255. Ramdall RB, Alasio TM, Cai G, Yang GC. Primary vascular neoplasms unique to the spleen: littoral cell angioma and splenic hamartoma diagnosis by fine-needle aspiration biopsy. Diagn Cytopathol 2007 Mar;35(3):137–42.

256. Conlon PJ, Procop GW, Fowler V, et al. Predictors of prognosis and risk of acute renal failure in patients with Rocky Mountain spotted fever. Am J Med 1996 Dec;101(6):621–6.

257. Cavanna L, Lazzaro A, Vallisa D, et al. Role of image-guided fine-needle aspiration biopsy in the management of patients with splenic metastasis. World J Surg Oncol 2007;5:13.

CHAPTER 11

Pancreas, biliary tract and intra-abdominal organs

Bastiaan de Boer*

CLINICAL ASPECTS

In the developed world, the incidence of pancreatic cancer has risen threefold since the 1920s. Prognosis is very poor, this tumor accounting for almost a quarter million deaths annually worldwide. In the USA, cancer of the pancreas is now the fourth leading cause of cancer deaths in male and females. The majority of patients have irresectable disease or metastases at the time of diagnosis. Therapeutic options are limited.[1] A diagnostic test such as fine needle biopsy (FNB), which combines accuracy with minimal intervention, is of unchallenged value in these patients.

Ultrasonography (US) and computed tomography (CT) made mass lesions of the pancreas, biliary tree and elsewhere in the abdomen readily accessible to FNB. Teams in Sweden and Denmark were the first to use FNB, guided by angiography or US, to investigate pancreatic masses.[2,3] Endoscopic evaluation of pancreatic and biliary disease has long been part of the work-up of patients with obstructive symptoms or mass lesions, with additional retrograde imaging studies and/or the collection of pancreatobiliary fluid or brushing specimens. However, the recent addition of a fine needle biopsy channel and linear ultrasonographic functions to the endoscope, have made this the method of choice in the early assessment of patients with pancreaticobiliary symptomatology. There are several good reviews,[4–6] and many recent series attest to the value, efficacy and low complication rate of endoscopically performed, ultrasonographically directed (EUS) procedures.[7–14] An alternative method of obtaining a tissue diagnosis is by transduodenal FNB at laparotomy, performed with curative intent, or for surgical bypass of obstructive jaundice.

As confidence in cytological diagnosis has become well established, there is an onus on the cytologist to provide specific information on tumor type as a basis for therapeutic decisions. This has led to use of supplementary techniques such as cell blocks, EM, immunocytochemistry, and analysis of pancreatic cyst fluid.[4–6,15,16] Core needle and wedge biopsies are generally discouraged in the pancreas owing to the propensity for fistula formation, spill of lytic enzymes, fat necrosis of peripancreatic tissues, and tumor track spread (see Complications below).

The place of FNAC in the investigative sequence

Fine needle biopsy of a pancreatic mass is performed after imaging has defined site, dimensions, anatomic relationships, depth and solid or cystic nature. This information is important not only for the biopsy procedure and its safety but also for the subsequent interpretation of the smears. The biopsy should be performed by the radiologist and the pathologist in close cooperation. EUS procedures are done by the endoscopist, usually a gastroenterologist. Again, the presence of a cytologist in the endoscopy suite to effect rapid evaluation is highly advisable. Cytological examination may unexpectedly reveal a benign neoplasm, an islet cell tumor, a metastatic malignancy or a lymphoma instead of the presumed pancreatic adenocarcinoma, with its inherently poorer prognosis. If pancreatic cancer is diagnosed microscopically, staging will determine further management. Unresectable or metastatic lesions may require stent insertion for relief of obstructive jaundice. Stent placement may be performed after FNB, at the same endoscopic procedure. If deemed operable, cancer cases can undergo subsequent surgery with the diagnosis and staging already accomplished.[17]

FNB does not contribute significantly to early diagnosis of pancreatic cancer. Neither is it suited, generally speaking, to the diagnosis of pancreatitis. Inflammatory pancreatic masses, conversely, constitute the chief clinical differential diagnosis of pancreatic neoplasia and must be recognisable to the cytopathologist.[18,19] In pancreatic pseudocyst, FNB can be both diagnostic and therapeutic.[15,20,21] Decompression of an acutely developed cyst may relieve symptoms and facilitate surgical treatment. Some patients are subjected to laparotomy without prior FNB in anticipation of resectability or for biliary bypass palliation to alleviate symptomatic jaundice. Under these circumstances, the FNB can be undertaken easily and with high precision intraoperatively.[22–24A] FNB at operation is done through the wall of the opened duodenum for pancreatic head masses. It has the advantage over the traditional wedge biopsy for frozen section of being

*With acknowledgments to Gladwyn Leiman for her work on previous editions.

©2012 Elsevier Ltd
DOI: 10.1016/B978-0-7020-3151-9.00011-6

virtually free of complications such as hemorrhage and fistula formation. It can be repeated to sample many different parts of a large mass, thereby increasing the probability of obtaining representative material. A thin needle can pass through the stomach or duodenum without risk. Rapid on-site staining and interpretation of intraoperative smears is quicker than cutting and staining frozen sections. With experience, interpretation of technically satisfactory smears is often easier than that of frozen section because of better preservation of cell detail.

Mass lesions of the gastrointestinal tract are, as a rule, investigated by radiological imaging and by endoscopy. FNB can be done percutaneously or endoscopically, an approach well-suited to submucosal neoplasms, and to lymph nodes adjacent to the bowel.[6,25,26] Endoscopically visible lesions in the upper or lower gastrointestinal tract are better sampled by exfoliative means, such as brushing, or by tissue biopsy. The cytopathology of exfoliative gastrointestinal and pancreatobiliary brushings is beyond the scope of this book.

Accuracy of diagnosis

Diagnostic accuracy is related primarily to the adequacy and representativeness of the biopsy, which in turn depends on the site, size and nature of the lesion, and on the expertise of the operator. The relative merits of available radiological techniques in guiding the biopsy are discussed in Chapter 3. The requirement for technical expertise is greatest for EUS-FNA, the success of which is almost entirely operator dependent. Although technical progress continues to improve the quality of radiological tumor imaging, there is still a minimum size of approximately 1.0 cm below which a lesion cannot be clearly demonstrated by traditional US or by CT, and precise needling is not possible. EUS appears to have the capability of detecting lesions of 0.3–1.0 cm. Intraoperatively, under the control of direct palpation, lesions measuring only a few millimeters in diameter can be biopsied successfully. Very large tumors present the difficulty of identifying viable areas from which to obtain well-preserved cells, in a background of extensive necrosis or hemorrhage.

Diagnostic specificity for malignant pancreatic lesions is 100% in nearly all published series. However, occasional false-positive diagnoses have been reported in cases of chronic pancreatitis or in the presence of pancreatic intraepithelial neoplasia (PanIN).[19,27] Diagnostic sensitivity is more variable, particularly in series of US- or CT-directed percutaneous biopsies with reported sensitivity of between 50% and 90%.[19,28–33] Intraoperative FNB achieves sensitivities in excess of 90%.[22–24,34] Recent series of pancreatic EUS-FNA report sensitivies of between 90% and 100%.[9,11,12,14,35–39] Factors influencing the sensitivity include pre-analytical issues such as: the size of the lesion, whether the lesion is solid or cystic, the experience of the operator, the number of needle passes, and the availability of on-site assessment by a cytologist or cytopathologist,[4] as well as analytical issues. It has been reported that repeat EUS-FNA in indeterminate cases further improves the sensitivity.[39,40]

Many of the cited studies focus on solid lesions of the pancreas and it is acknowledged that the sensitivity and specificity in diagnosis of cystic lesions is lower.[4] Biochemical analysis of fluid from cystic lesions improves the sensitivity and specificity of these lesions over cytologic assessment alone (see Intraductal papillary – mucinous and mucinous cystic neoplasms below).[15,41–44]

Complications

Significant complications are rare if thin needles of 0.08 mm (21 gauge) or less are used. Such needles pass through stomach or bowel without causing peritonitis, although caution is recommended in cases of bowel obstruction or distension. In a comprehensive review of the literature, and a questionnaire study, Smith documented six deaths after pancreatic FNB.[45] Of these, five were due to pancreatitis and one followed sepsis post aspiration of a pancreatic pseudocyst. In an earlier review of 184 procedures, Mueller and colleagues reported a 3% incidence of (nonfatal) severe pancreatitis.[46] All of the cases developing pancreatitis in either series had inflammatory mass lesions mimicking carcinoma. Hence, FNB is not recommended for the investigation of classic clinical pancreatitis but should be reserved for cases with a radiologically localized lesion. Major hemorrhage is very rare. The coagulation status should be noted but a full investigation is unnecessary unless the spleen or the liver is involved. A recent study of 1034 pancreatic EUS-FNA identified 10 hemorrhages (0.96%), none of which was fatal, two cases of acute severe pancreatitis (0.19%) and one duodenal perforation (0.09%) which lead to a post-surgical death.[47] Two cases of pancreatic ascites due to fistula formation have received literature attention.[48,49] Both fistulas closed with regression of the ascites.

Tumor seeding in the needle track has been reported in a small number of cases following FNB of pancreatic carcinoma. In a literature review by Smith, the risk of needle track seeding was 4.45 per 100 000 transabdominal FNB procedures in four questionnaire studies of 156 652 patients.[45] Five of 11 instances of needle track spread after FNB of the pancreas used a needle greater than 21 gauge. It is thus apparent that cutaneous needle track seeding is an extremely rare event. More frequently than is clinically realized, however, may be the tracking of cells to the peritoneal surfaces as a result of FNB. Some authors have reported a significant increase in incidence of exfoliated malignant cells within operative peritoneal washings after FNB,[50] while others have failed to confirm this.[51] More recently, it has been shown that EUS-FNA results in positive peritoneal cytology significantly less often than percutaneous FNB.[52] The significance of this positive peritoneal cytology remains uncertain, with some authors finding that it was an indicator of unresectability, advanced disease, early metastasis and short survival,[51] others identified a trend to decreased survival,[53] while others did not show any survival disadvantage.[54] The latter group concluded that cell spillage into the peritoneum at FNB did not render the procedure unsafe, particularly if neoadjuvant chemo-radiation was part of the management protocol. Clinicians wishing to minimise this potential hazard may prefer the transduodenal route of FNB offered by EUS, or by intraoperative sampling.

Technical considerations

Transperitoneal deep FNB is done as a hospital procedure and performed in the radiology or endoscopy departments where all the facilities for tumor imaging are available. The

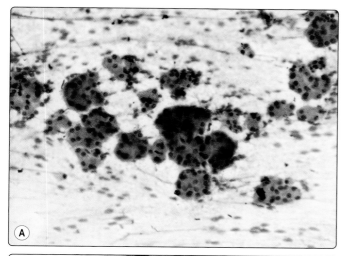

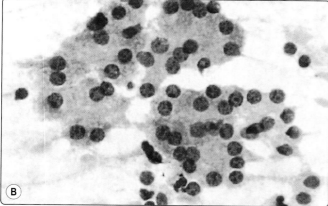

Fig. 11.1 Pancreatic acinar cells (A) Cohesive clusters of exocrine epithelial cells forming rounded acini (Pap, IP); (B) Acinar cells showing granular cytoplasm and eccentric small round uniform nuclei (H&E, HP).

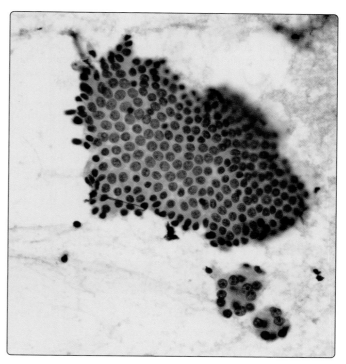

Fig. 11.2 Pancreatic ductal cells Monolayered sheet of uniform ductal epithelial cells; note the adjacent clusters of benign acinar cells (Pap, HP).

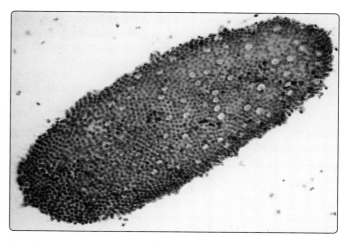

Fig. 11.3 Duodenal surface epithelium Monolayered sheet of duodenal epithelial cells with interspersed goblet cells (Pap, LP).

presence of a cytologist or cytopathologist in the endoscopy suite to effect rapid evaluation is highly advisable. Smears should be prepared and stained immediately so that the adequacy of the specimen can be checked and the aspiration repeated if necessary. A cell block should be made whenever possible to allow histochemical and immunocytochemical staining if necessary. These ancillary tests can also be performed on smears, either air-dried or wet-fixed, or liquid based preparations. If a lymphoid lesion is suspected, collection of a cellular specimen into RPMI or saline for flow cytometry is mandatory. Culture is rarely required in pancreatic FNB. Collection of fluid from cystic lesions for biochemical analysis should always be considered.

CYTOLOGICAL FINDINGS

The pancreas and biliary tract

Normal structures (Figs 11.1–11.3)

- Exocrine epithelial cells in rounded acinar clusters,
- Ductal epithelial cells in monolayered sheets,
- Naked single nuclei resembling nuclei of small lymphocytes.

Fine needle biopsy smears from normal pancreatic tissue can occasionally be surprisingly cellular. Most of the cells are acinar unless the needle traverses a major duct. Acinar cells have indistinct cell borders; their acinar arrangement suggests an individual triangular shape to the cells, the nuclei being disposed in a circle at the periphery of small, round clusters (Fig. 11.1). Larger fragments are composed of multiple acini held together by sparse fibrovascular stroma, often surrounding an intact duct. The nuclei are uniformly small, round and of similar size and shape to those of small lymphocytes. Many cells are represented by single, naked nuclei.

The nuclear chromatin is densely granular and evenly distributed. There may be a single, prominent nucleolus or multiple small nucleoli. The cytoplasm is dense and granular. The ductal epithelial cells form monolayered sheets (Fig. 11.2). Cell borders are usually visible, the cytoplasm is pale and the nuclei are regularly spaced within the sheets. The nuclei are larger than those of the acinar epithelial cells and are more ovoid. They are paler and have finely granular chromatin and small, usually single, nucleoli. Palisading may be seen along the edge of sheets. Ductal epithelial cells from major bile ducts look similar and cannot be clearly distinguished from those of major pancreatic ducts in smears. Columnar cells of duodenal origin, however, although also in monolayers, are distinguished by the presence of goblet cells within the sheets (Fig. 11.3).

Pancreatitis (Fig. 11.4)

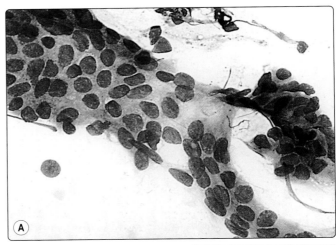

CRITERIA FOR DIAGNOSIS

◆ Normal, degenerate or regenerating admixed acinar and ductal epithelial cells,

◆ Variable acute and chronic inflammatory cells,

◆ Foamy macrophages, some multinucleated,

◆ Abundant mucous or serous exudate and debris.

Acute diffuse hemorrhagic pancreatitis is unlikely to be subjected to FNB. Percutaneous FNB is not a suitable method to confirm clinically suspected chronic pancreatitis, partly because the inflammatory cells found in smears are often too sparse to be diagnostic, partly because of the risk of the biopsy causing exacerbation of pre-existing pancreatitis.[18,19] However, it may be utilized if fibrosis with resultant nodularity leads to a radiological presentation which is suspicious of a neoplastic mass, and, if on surgical exploration, the gland is felt to be increased in size and/or consistency, whether focally or diffusely. Since duct obstruction, edema and inflammation peripheral to a carcinoma can simulate true pancreatitis, multiple biopsies should be taken both proximal to the mass and from different parts of the abnormal area to exclude malignancy. This can be done endoscopically or intraoperatively without significantly increasing the risk of local complications.

In severe chronic pancreatitis much of the exocrine parenchyma may be destroyed and be replaced by fibrous tissue. In such cases, remaining ductal, acinar and endocrine epithelium can show prominent reactive/regenerative atypia which can be difficult to distinguish from well-differentiated adenocarcinoma (Fig. 11.4). There may be crowding of nuclei and microglandular arrangement of cells with nuclear enlargement and variation in nuclear size and shape. The atypia is usually variable in degree between cells.

Infectious pancreatitis is uncommon in immunocompetent hosts, and occurs more frequently in circumstances of immune suppression. It may be caused by a variety of pathogens, including viruses, parasites, bacteria and fungi.[55] Organisms gain access to the pancreas either by the hematogenous route in systemic infections, or from the intestinal tract through the pancreaticobiliary system.

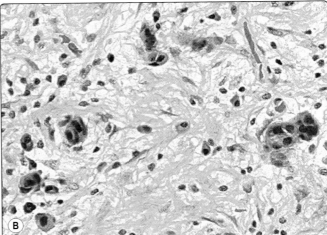

Fig. 11.4 Chronic pancreatitis, epithelial atypia (A) Aggregate of glandular cells showing acinar pattern and prominent nuclear atypia (MGG, HP); (B) Corresponding tissue section; fibrous tissue with small islands of residual epithelium showing prominent atypia (H&E, HP).

PROBLEMS IN DIAGNOSIS

◆ Paucity of inflammatory cells,

◆ Regenerative epithelial atypia which may simulate well-differentiated carcinoma.

Cysts

Cysts in the pancreas can be congenital or post-pancreatitic pseudocysts. Some tumors are inherently and primarily cystic; in addition, any neoplasm, benign or malignant, may undergo cystic degeneration. Evaluation of cysts by radiologic or endoscopic features alone can sometimes be problematic.[56] Cytologic evaluation of aspirated cyst fluid is widely used and often fully diagnostic of the nature of the cyst, although sampling and interpretative errors are acknowledged.[57,58] Sensitivity of cytodiagnosis of pancreatic cystic lesions was considerably lower than that of solid lesions (64% vs 98%) in one study.[57] Biochemical analysis of fluid from cystic lesions improves the sensitivity and specificity over cytologic assessment alone (see Intraductal papillary mucinous and mucinous cystic neoplasms below).

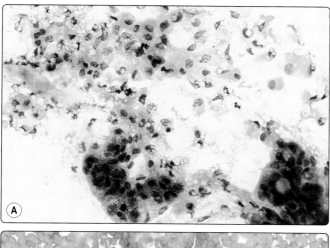

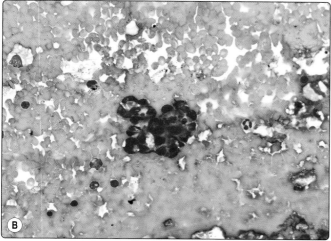

Fig. 11.5 Pancreatic pseudocyst (A) Mainly debris, inflammatory cells and macrophages; a few clusters of degenerating epithelial cells (Pap, IP); (B) These degenerating epithelial cells may be interpreted as atypical and are a pitfall leading to false-positive diagnoses (MGG, HP).

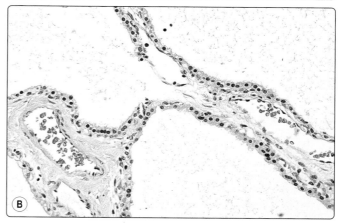

Fig. 11.6 Serous cystadenoma (A) Watery aspirate with a few monolayered sheets of epithelial cells with small round uniform nuclei and moderate pale cytoplasm; see inset (Pap, HP); (B) Corresponding tissue section (H&E, IP).

Pseudocyst (Fig. 11.5)

These non-neoplastic cysts are the most commonly encountered pancreatic cysts. Being fluid collections occurring in post-pancreatitic states, they are not true cysts and as such are lined by granulation tissue, not by epithelium. Aspiration yields copious turbid watery fluid which contains debris, occasional inflammatory cells including histiocytes, possible fibroblasts and bile, and perhaps rare fragments of epithelial tissue from the surrounding gland. Raised enzyme levels, e.g. amylase and lipase, and low or absent tumor marker levels are found in the aspirated cyst fluid. The fluid is nonmucinous, but may demonstrate background fibrinous strands. Should the aspirate appear purulent, it should be submitted for culture to confirm secondary infection.

Serous cystadenoma (microcystic/glycogen-rich adenoma) (Fig. 11.6)

These are uncommon benign lesions, often incidental findings in older individuals. Their presentation must be familiar to cytopathologists, as failure to identify the constituent bland monolayered sheets might result in an erroneous 'nonrepresentative' report. Histopathologically, these tumors demonstrate classic microcysts, lined by bland, uniform glycogen-rich mucin-negative cells (Fig. 11.6).[59] Several reports have appeared in the literature on FNB cytodiagnosis.[58,60,61] The aspirate is clear and watery, some are acellular, while others contain a sparse exfoliate of monomorphic round cells with finely vacuolated, glycogen-positive, mucin-negative cytoplasm, and centrally disposed nuclei containing fine chromatin. Occasionally, larger monolayered sheets may be obtained (Fig. 11.6). The cell groups may resemble mesothelial cells or bland acinar cells. Cell features are thus non-specific, but are assessed in conjunction with the watery nature of the aspirate and the very characteristic radiological picture of small microcysts within a well-demarcated round mass lesion arising anywhere in the pancreas. A PAS stain will highlight the glycogen-rich cytoplasm.

Biochemical analysis of cyst fluid generally shows a low viscosity and low CEA and amylase levels.[62] A recent study which combined imaging, biochemical and cytological data in reaching a diagnosis concluded that the preoperative diagnosis of serous cystadenomas remains a challenge.[63]

Solid-psedopapillary neoplasm (Figs 11.7 and 11.8)

This relatively uncommon low malignant potential pancreatic neoplasm, with its many pseudonyms, occurs almost exclusively in young women under the age of 20 years.[64] They usually behave in a benign manner but 10–15% of cases show spread or metastases. Still considered to be of uncertain histogenesis, this tumor is thought to be hormonally dependent. Occurring anywhere along the length of the pancreas, the mass is usually sizeable at presentation, averaging 8 cm. Grossly, as well as on imaging studies, it is characterized by good circumscription, multiloculation and solid and cystic areas. The histopathologic features, which are specific and diagnostic, are mirrored exactly by the cytologic pattern in FNB smears. Initial tumor growth is solid, but degeneration results in clefts, eventually enlarging to cysts, between vascularized cell fragments, which then appear 'pseudopapillary'.

Fifty isolated case reports or limited series attesting to the ability of FNB to confidently identify this unusual but widely reported neoplasm were summarized in 2002 by Pettinato and colleagues in a definitive paper.[64] Richly cellular smears demonstrate characteristic pseudopapillae and pseudorosettes, composed of small tumor cells adherent to delicate metachromatic fibrovascular stalks. Recognition of this stromal component is essential in distinguishing this tumor of relatively good prognosis from similar small-celled pancreatic neoplasms. The outline of both the pseudopapillae and the pseudorosettes appears irregular, due to exuberant exfoliation of single cells into the smear background. These vascular-based aggregates vary from large grape-like branching structures to single capillaries with leaf-like single-cell linings (Fig. 11.7). These cells are small, round to oval, plasmacytoid or cuboidal and extremely monotonous. Cytoplasm is variably preserved, vesicular to faintly granular, containing characteristic eosinophilic, hyaline intracytoplasmic globules, which are PAS positive.

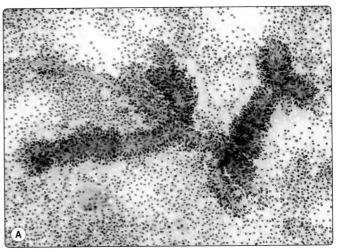

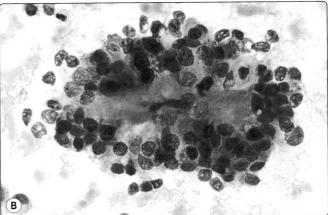

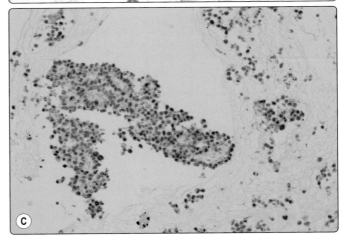

Fig. 11.7 Solid-pseudopapillary neoplasm (A) Vessel associated pseudopapillary fragment (Pap, LP); (B) Pseudopapillary fragment. Note small tumor cells and irregular outer border with detached tumor cells (MGG, IP); (C) Cell block section showing positive staining for progesterone receptors (PR, IP).

Nuclei are round and even, with grooves but no major irregularities or significant pleomorphism. Chromatin is described as finely granular, without clumping or clearing. Small nucleoli may be appreciated and are occasionally multiple. In the background, foam cells, multinucleated giant cells, debris and laminated psammoma bodies reflect the cystic and papillary nature of the parent tumor. Mucus

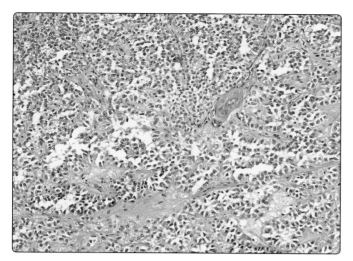

Fig. 11.8 Solid and cystic papillary neoplasm Corresponding tissue section from Figure 11.7 (H&E, IP).

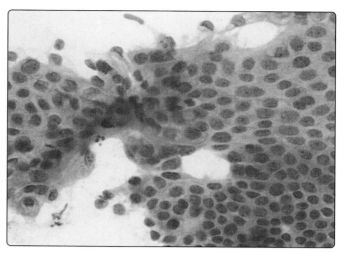

Fig. 11.9 Adenocarcinoma (pancreas) Very well-differentiated adenocarcinoma presenting as cohesive, monolayered epithelial sheets; note nuclear crowding, overlapping and nuclear atypia present focally (H&E, HP).

is absent. Diagnostic accuracy of EUS-FNA has been reported as 75% in a series of 28 cases.[65]

Immunocytochemistry is extremely variable but most neoplasms studied stain positively for vimentin, α_1-antitrypsin, α_1-antichymotrypsin and progesterone receptor (Fig. 11.7C). Unlike PET, they are typically negative for chromogranin, cytokeratin, EMA and specific pancreatic hormones. Both tumors may express CD10, synaptophysin and CD56.[64,66-69] More recently, nuclear expression of beta-catenin together with loss of normal membrane localization of E-cadherin have been proposed as useful in separating the two entities.[66,67,69]

Morphologic recognition is critical to extract these slow-growing, operable and potentially curable tumors of young women from the very much larger pool of usual pancreatic cancers with their abysmal prognosis.

PROBLEMS AND DIFFERENTIAL DIAGNOSIS

◆ Islet cell tumors,
◆ Papillary variant of usual pancreatic ductal carcinoma,
◆ Other cystic neoplasms.

Adenocarcinoma (Figs 11.9–11.11)

CRITERIA FOR DIAGNOSIS[33,70-73]

◆ Disordered monolayer sheets, microglandular patterns, nuclear crowding; loss of cell cohesion,
◆ Nuclear criteria of malignancy with contour irregularity and fairly distinctive margination of chromatin,
◆ Moderate amount of cytoplasm, often mucin vacuoles, indistinct cell borders,
◆ Evidence of necrosis, mitoses, macronucleoli and hyperchromasia in poorly differentiated forms.

Almost all adenocarcinomas arising in the pancreas are of ductal origin, without unique features permitting absolute distinction from carcinomas arising in the biliary tree. The characteristic FNB pattern is of crowded 'drunken'

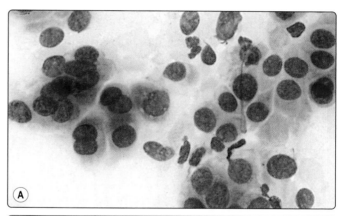

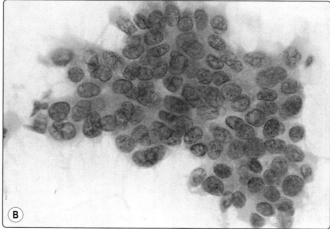

Fig. 11.10 Adenocarcinoma (pancreas) Well-differentiated adenocarcinoma; relatively mild nuclear atypia, but nuclear crowding and some dissociation, and in **B** a tendency to microacinar arrangement (A, MGG, HP; B, H&E, HP).

monolayered sheets, with moderately tall columnar palisading cells at luminal edges. Smaller aggregates commonly show rounded glandular structures with feathered edges, or three-dimensionality. Cytoplasmic borders may be very well demarcated in better-differentiated forms; in other cases, the

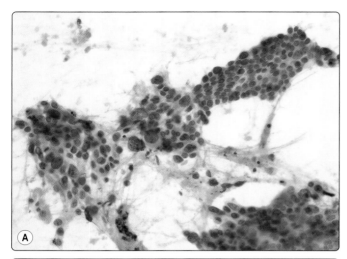

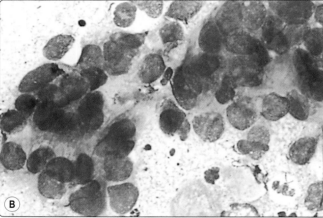

Fig. 11.11 Adenocarcinoma (pancreas) moderately differentiated
(A) Sheets showing disorganization and nuclear pleomorphism; background of necrotic debris (H&E, IP); (B) Disorganized clusters with some acinar arrangements (MGG, HP).

monolayer sheets appear syncytial. The diagnosis of malignancy ultimately depends on nuclear features, which range from very subtle alterations to overly malignant criteria with decreasing differentiation (Figs 11.9–11.11). In an assessment of individual criteria by regression analysis, Cohen and colleagues extracted as most important: anisocytosis (4:1), nuclear enlargement and molding, with combined sensitivity of 98% using all three criteria to distinguish malignant from benign.[70] In a similar study, Robins, Katz and Evans ascribed major status to nuclear crowding, contour and chromatin irregularity, minor status to single cells, mitoses and enlarged nuclei,[33] requiring two major, or one major and two minor criteria for the definitive diagnosis of malignancy. Focusing specifically on the most challenging area, the recognition of well-differentiated carcinoma, Lin and Staerkel listed the following features: nuclear enlargement >2 rbc (99%), anisonucleosis 4:1 (97%), nuclear membrane irregularity (97%), and crowding/overlapping/three-dimensionality (92%).[73]

The use of ancillary studies has been advocated to improve sensitivity. The mucin profile of MUC1+/MUC2−/MUC5AC+ has been reported as discriminating between a benign and malignant glandular epithelial cells.[74,75]

Immunohistochemistry for mesothelin and prostate stem cell antigen (PSCA) was also found to be useful,[76] as was a combination of P53, DPC4 (MAD4) and Kras mutation.[77] Some authors have also reported molecular analysis for K-ras mutation improves the sensitivity of FNB cytology.[78,79]

PROBLEMS AND DIFFERENTIAL DIAGNOSIS

◆ Well-differentiated adenocarcinoma,
◆ Regenerative atypia,
◆ Islet cell tumors,
◆ High-grade tumors – pleomorphic carcinoma and metastases.

Carcinoma variants comprise as many as 10–15% of ductal carcinomas. Of these, *adenosquamous carcinoma* is the most common, accounting for up to 5% of pancreatic neoplasms. The percentage of cells showing glandular and squamous differentiation is highly variable, particularly in FNB specimens. The glandular component is usually moderately or poorly differentiated; the squamous component may be keratinizing or not. The prognosis of this variant is as poor as that of usual ductal cancer.[80–82]

Mucinous tumors of the pancreas

These tumors are best categorized into four subgroups,[83] each of which has implications for cytodiagnosis:

• intraductal papillary-mucinous neoplasm (IPMN),
• mucinous cystic neoplasm (MCN),
• ductal adenocarcinoma of mucinous type, noncystic (colloid),
• ductal adenocarcinoma of signet ring type.

Of these, the last two mentioned require little further expansion, both being rare variants of ductal adenocarcinoma. *Mucinous adenocarcinoma/colloid carcinoma* is a solid ductal carcinoma in which greater than 50% of the tumor is of mucinous type, revealing tall columnar morphology and demonstrable intracytoplasmic and extracellular mucus. The radiologic appearance of a solid neoplasm separates it from both IPMN and MCN. Mucinous or colloid carcinomas occur mainly in the pancreatic head and have identical gender, age and prognostic implications as the usual adenocarcinoma. *Signet ring carcinoma* is exceptionally rare, and often difficult to distinguish histologically from chronic pancreatitis because of its diffuse infiltrative characteristics. It is cytologically recognizable by the presence of classic single-lying signet ring cells, bloated with mucin, seen in pools of mucin. This subtype, too, carries no prognostic advantage.

Intraductal papillary mucinous and mucinous cystic neoplasms (Figs 11.12–11.14)

CRITERIA FOR DIAGNOSIS

◆ Abundant background mucin,
◆ Cohesive sheets and papillary aggregates,
◆ Cuboidal to columnar, mucin-filled cells,
◆ Spectrum of nuclear changes

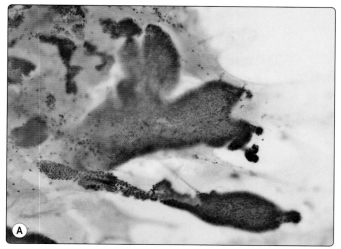

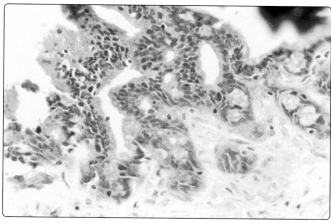

Fig. 11.13 Intraductal papillary-mucinous neoplasm (IPMN) Tissue section corresponding to Figure 11.12 (H&E, IP).

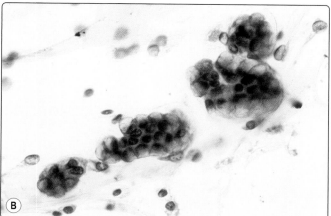

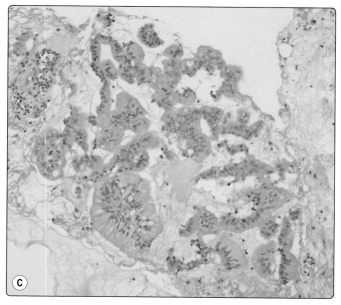

Fig. 11.12 Intraductal papillary-mucinous neoplasm (IPMN) (A) Large multilayered papillary structures; note the smooth borders (H&E, IP); (B) Small papillary clusters of cuboidal epithelial cells with mucin vacuoles; the pale mucin in the background is not easily seen (Pap, HP); (C) Cell block showing strips and papillary formations of atypical columnar epithelium (H&E, IP).

Distinction between IPMN and MCN on cytologic grounds is problematic and requires correlation with clinical, imaging and endoscopic findings as the clinico-radiologic characteristics are very different.

Intraductal papillary-mucinous neoplasms (IPMN) were first described as a distinct entity in the 1980s.[83] They are now well characterized as tumors of better prognosis as they have a long intraductal course but eventually will invade into periductal pancreatic parenchyma, and then go on to nodal and distant metastases.[84] Both sexes can be affected, but elderly males predominate. IPMN usually involves the main duct in the head of the pancreas but can arise in side branches. As the name implies, the lining epithelium is both papillary and mucinous. The duct system is filled with viscous mucus, leading to a very characteristic endoscopic appearance, where the ampulla of Vater is often seen to be patulous, and draining mucin. The cytology is distinctive (but not entirely specific), showing abundant background mucin, in which sheets and papillary aggregates of cuboidal to columnar, mucin-filled cells are seen (Figs 11.12 and 11.13). Several reports attest to the ability of cytology to diagnose these good-prognosis tumors preoperatively, in conjunction with radiologic and endoscopic features.[84–86] In a series of 19 patients, a sensitivity of 82% and specificity of 100% was reported.[87]

The classic *mucinous cystic neoplasm (MCN)* is an indolent tumor of middle-aged females, the majority occurring in the tail of the pancreas. These tumors show a spectrum of grade and behavior including benign cystadenomas, borderline forms, and malignant cystadenocarcinomas. The latter obviously has a poorer prognosis if invasion has occurred. Radiologic studies identify a usually discrete and obviously cystic mass in the pancreatic tail. As there is no communication with the pancreatic ductal system, endoscopy does not demonstrate mucinous discharge from a patulous ampulla. As with IPMN, cytology shows a background of copious extracellular mucin, in which cohesive monolayered sheets of mucinous columnar cells are found (Fig. 11.14). These demonstrate regular to irregular honeycombing, with a spectrum of nuclear changes depending on the stage of tumor progression. Epithelial cell cytoplasm is distended with mucin vacuoles.[88–91]

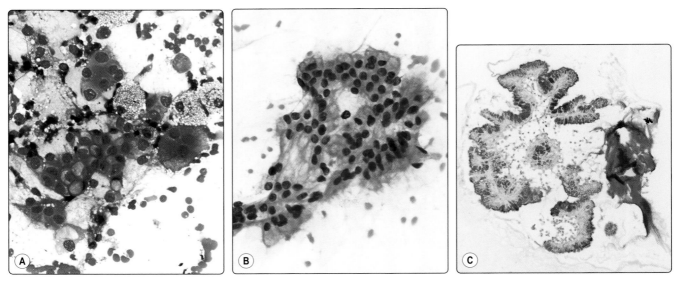

Fig. 11.14 Mucinous cystic neoplasm (MCN) (A, B) Clusters and sheets of relatively monotonous malignant glandular cells showing intracytoplasmic mucin vacuoles (A, MGG, HP; B, H&E, HP); (C) PAS diastase stain on cell block material highlights the intra- and extracellular mucin (PAS/D, IP).

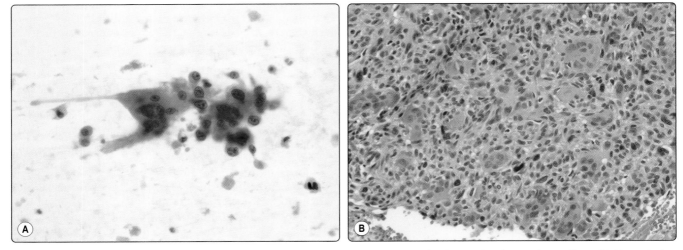

Fig. 11.15 Osteoclastic adenocarcinoma (pancreas) (A) Two osteoclastic type giant cells mixed with a poorly cohesive cluster of large, highly atypical epithelial cells (H&E, HP); (B) Cell block section corresponding to A (H&E, IP).

Biochemical analysis of fluid from cystic lesions improves the sensitivity and specificity over cytologic assessment alone. Various parameters have been measured including the presence of mucin, viscosity, CEA, CA 19-9, amylase, lipase.[21,44] Amylase levels are a normal.[16] CEA appears to be the most helpful for diagnosing IPMN and MCN[15,42,43,92] and some authors state that cytologic analysis adds little to biochemical analysis of the cyst fluid.[92,93] A very high levels of CEA (>6000 ng/mL) can predict malignancy.[42,94]

Analysis of the mucin expression profile (MUC1, MUC2 and MUC5AC) has been reported as useful in discriminating between mucinous versus non-mucinous lesions as well as between benign versus malignant mucinous neoplasms.[31,75,86] More recently, there have been studies suggesting various molecular analyses on cyst fluid such as k-*ras* mutation and loss of heterozygosity, may be similarly useful.[95–98]

Other variants of pancreatic cancer

Pure *osteoclastic giant cell tumors* of the pancreas also require cytologic recognition as their behavior pattern may be more indolent than that of usual ductal carcinoma.[99] Osteoclastic cells, with clustered bland nuclei disposed in dense cytoplasm, are interspersed with mononuclear cells displaying identical, uniform nuclei (Fig. 11.15).[99,100] It is mandatory to distinguish this from another carcinoma variant, *pleomorphic giant cell tumor* (sometimes called anaplastic carcinoma) of the pancreas, which, as its name implies, also contains giant cells but with anisokaryotic daughter nuclei and macronucleoli (Fig. 11.16). Phagocytosis of inflammatory cells by tumor cells is common, and residual recognizable adenocarcinoma may be seen. This is the most lethal of all the pancreatic malignancies.[101,102] Interestingly, mixed forms, containing

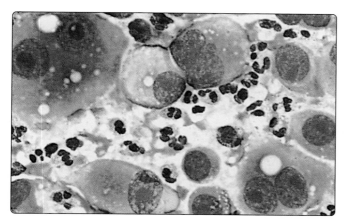

Fig. 11.16 Anaplastic pancreatic carcinoma Highly pleomorphic mainly dispersed mononuclear and multinucleated tumor cells with macronucleoli (MGG, HP).

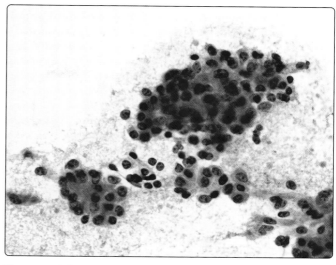

Fig. 11.17 Acinar cell adenocarcinoma Loosely cohesive sheet of large, mildly pleomorphic cells with poorly defined granular cytoplasm, large nuclei with smooth nuclear membranes and prominent nucleoli (H&E, HP).

both osteoclastic and pleomorphic giant cells, occur.[103,104] Most reports indicate the prognosis to be extremely poor, approximating that of the pleomorphic variant.

Deposits of metastatic cancer within the pancreas or adjacent lymph nodes occur from a wide variety of primary sites, predominantly lung, kidney and breast. The possibility of a non-pancreatic primary should be considered whenever the cytological pattern deviates from that of typical adenocarcinoma. A pancreatic adenocarcinoma of ductal type is cytologically indistinguishable from extrahepatic bile duct carcinoma. Diagnosis is facilitated when the patient has had a history of a previous primary tumor; conversely, the pancreas may be the presenting site of a tumor originating elsewhere.[105,106] Comparison of current cytomorphology with previous aspirates or tissue sections will solve many cases of suspected metastasis. Alternately, immunocytochemistry may be utilized to distinguish metastases from various sites. Differential cytokeratin 7 and 20 staining, together with TTF-1 (for lung), ER and PR (for breast), CD10 (for kidney) and melanoma markers, form a useful panel.

Pancreatic *lymphoma* is rare, but nodal lymphomas in the peripancreatic region are not. These may cause space-occupying lesions and biliary obstruction, mimicking pancreatic neoplasia. Rapid on-site evaluation will detect a lymphoid lesion, and will prompt collection of a separate needle pass into an appropriate medium (RPMI) for flow cytometry, or cell block material for lymphoma immunophenotyping. The majority of pancreatic lymphomas are reported to be diffuse large-cell non-Hodgkin's lymphomas; a few cases have been small non-cleaved cell lymphomas of B lineage.[105]

Rarest of all exocrine tumors of the pancreas is the highly aggressive *acinar cell adenocarcinoma*.[107-112] The few cytologic case reports describe and illustrate highly cellular smears, with the cells in loosely cohesive aggregates, sometimes showing acinar formations. The cells having poorly defined granular cytoplasm, large smooth central nuclei, irregularly clumped chromatin, prominent chromatin clearing and large cherry-red nucleoli (Fig. 11.17).[107,110,111] Distinction from islet cell tumor, which can be a problem, is generally made using immunocytochemical staining for exocrine enzymes and neuroendocrine markers, respectively.[113] Zymogen granules are demonstrable, as are microvilli on ultrastructural examination.[107,110,112]

Islet cell tumours (Figs 11.18–11.20)

CRITERIA FOR DIAGNOSIS

◆ Many single and loosely grouped cells, pseudorosettes,
◆ Rounded monotonous nuclei, mild to moderate anisokaryosis,
◆ Speckled chromatin and 1–3 small nucleoli,
◆ Poorly defined, finely granular cytoplasm, often dispersed in the background,
◆ Nuclei eccentric if cytoplasm intact.

These functional or nonfunctioning tumors of adults are situated mainly in the body and tail of the pancreas. The tumors are well within the scope of EUS cytodiagnosis.[114,115] The neoplastic cells are mainly dissociated, but often form loose acinar or follicular clusters and curved or circular rows (Fig. 11.18). In the majority of cases, nuclei are characteristically round to oval and uniformly small. Occasionally, nuclear anisokaryosis may be prominent, but the nuclear chromatin pattern varies little between cells. The chromatin is evenly distributed, coarsely granular or 'speckled'. The small nucleoli are not easily seen in Giemsa-stained smears. Due to its fragility, the cytoplasm is often dispersed in the background. When it is preserved, nuclei are eccentrically situated within defined cell borders. A very fine, red granularity is often discernible in MGG smears with high magnification. Clumps of amyloid may occasionally be seen, but necrosis is not observed.[113,116-119] The cytological pattern of most islet cell tumors is sufficiently characteristic to be easily distinguished from that of pancreatic adenocarcinoma. Production and secretion of specific hormone products cannot

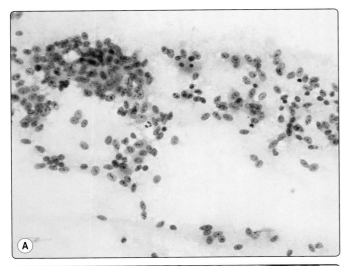

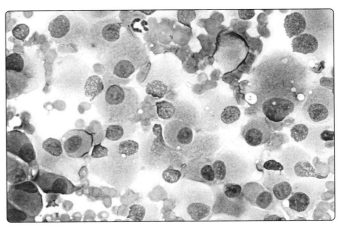

Fig. 11.20 Malignant islet cell tumor Poorly cohesive cells of endocrine appearance; no obvious cytologic features to suggest malignancy. This tumor metastasized to the liver (MGG, HP).

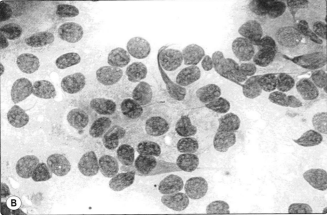

Fig. 11.18 Islet cell tumor (A) Poorly cohesive sheets and dispersal; cells with oval nuclei, stippled chromatin and small nucleoli (Pap, IP); (B) Mainly dispersed cells with uniformly round nuclei, speckled chromatin, moderate anisokaryosis; delicate cytoplasm; a suggestion of pseudorosettes (MGG, HP).

be distinguished on the basis of routine cytological smears alone. If the secretory products of the neoplastic cells can be identified by immunocytochemical methods, a more specific diagnosis can be made with confidence. General neuroendocrine markers will usually be positive, such as neuron-specific enolase, synaptophysin, chromogranin-A, PGP9.5 and CD56. Specific secretory products, e.g. insulin can be marked by appropriate antibodies but this does not necessarily correlate with raised serum levels. Electron microscopy will demonstrate dense-core neurosecretory granules. A decision on whether a tumor is benign or malignant is problematic. Even histopathology is poorly predictive of aggressive behavior. In general, nuclear atypia and pleomorphism cannot be relied on as cytological criteria of malignancy (Fig. 11.20). More aggressive behavior correlates with a raised proliferation index assessed using Ki-67 immunohistochemistry (>2%).[120] This is a parameter in the WHO 2004 histology based-grading system.[121,122] Only documentation of metastasis finally provides proof of malignancy.[123,124]

PROBLEMS AND DIFFERENTIAL DIAGNOSIS

◆ Normal pancreatic acini mimic islet tumor architecture,
◆ Solid and cystic papillary neoplasm may have acinar configuration,
◆ Acinar cell adenocarcinoma.

Pancreatoblastoma

These unusual, large pancreatic primary tumors are encountered in children and adolescents. They demonstrate solid and acinar architecture with interspersed squamous corpuscles and osseous and/or chondroid metaplasia. Cytologic reports are scant, but mention cellular smears, detached small cells, primitive 'blastemal' epithelial cells with even chromatin and delicate cytoplasm, rare squamous

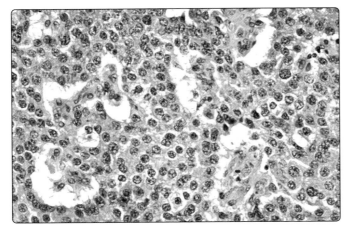

Fig. 11.19 Islet cell tumor Tissue section corresponding to Figure 11.18 showing a trabecular and solid pattern (H&E, IP).

corpuscles and mesenchymal fragments. The most obvious differential diagnosis, particularly if mesenchyma is present and squamous differentiation absent, is the solid-cystic papillary tumor encountered in young women (see also Chapter 17).[125-127]

Intra-abdominal tumors

Endoscopic ultrasonograph guided FNB is increasingly being used as a modality of choice in sampling of lymph nodes, extraluminal masses in the region of the bowel and gastrointestinal wall lesions.[128] Mucosal lesions encountered at endoscopy in the upper gastrointestinal tract may be sampled by endoscopically obtained brushings. Further, depending on adjunctive clinical and radiologic studies, brush devices may be passed through the ampulla of Vater into the biliary tree at endoscopy, offering an innovative and low intervention mechanism of collection of cytologic material for diagnosis of lesions involving the extrahepatic and pancreatic ductal systems.[1,129-131] However, exfoliative techniques, results and morphologic features are not in the scope of this book. Should endoscopic techniques not be available, or not be successful, access to intra-abdominal mass lesions may be gained by transabdominal FNB, with US or CT guidance.

Adenocarcinoma of the gastrointestinal tract may be well or poorly differentiated and glandular, signet ring, or mucinous in type. The origin of the tumor is usually revealed by clinical and radiological findings but may be suggested by cytological features. For example, a poorly differentiated signet ring adenocarcinoma with intracytoplasmic mucin vacuoles is most likely of gastric origin; a well-differentiated adenocarcinoma of columnar cells showing a palisaded arrangement and with tumor necrosis is probably of colonic origin. An example of anal carcinoma of cloacogenic type is illustrated in Figure 11.21. However, distinction between adenocarcinoma of the pancreas, the biliary tract or the female genital tract may not be possible on the basis of routine smears. Differential cytokeratin immunostaining may be helpful.

The cytological characteristics of *carcinoid tumors* are described in Chapter 8. The pattern is similar to that of pancreatic islet cell tumors and immunostaining for neuroendocrine markers, particularly synaptophysin and chromogranin, is positive.[118]

Gastrointestinal stromal tumors (GISTs), formerly classified as smooth muscle tumors, have now been extracted as a distinct entity. They are mesenchymal tumors, arising in the wall of the gastrointestinal tract, showing a spectrum of benign, borderline and malignant behavior. They are typically spindled but there is also an epithelioid variant showing the same antigen profile. Cytodiagnosis of the spindle-celled variant is relatively simple, showing fascicles of spindled cells with elongated, cigar- or comma-shaped nuclei, often set in a wispy filamentous background (Fig. 11.22A and B). The epithelioid variant presents greater difficulty, resembling epithelial tumors. The cells are round, cytoplasm distinct with a perinuclear halo, and nuclei vesicular (Fig. 11.22C).

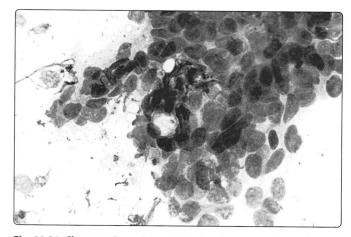

Fig. 11.21 Cloacogenic carcinoma FNB of anal tumor; multilayered tumor fragment of malignant basaloid cells with high N:C ratio, no microarchitectural pattern (MGG, HP).

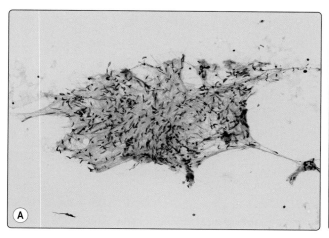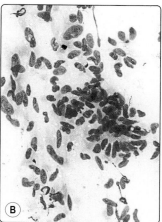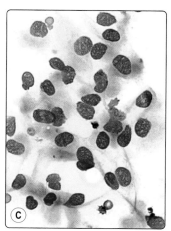

Fig. 11.22 Gastrointestinal stromal tumor (GIST) (A, B) Spindle cell variant; typical pattern (A, Pap, LP; B, MGG, IP); (C) Epithelioid variant (MGG, HP).

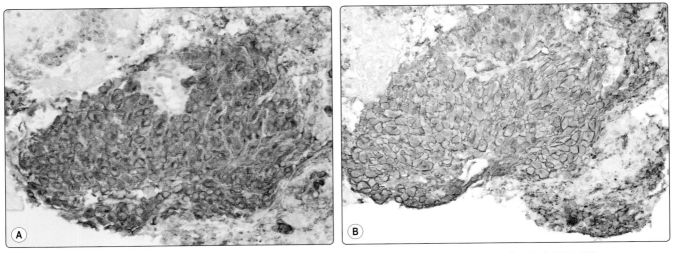

Fig. 11.23 Gastrointestinal stromal tumor (GIST) (A, B) Cell block sections stained for C-kit (CD117) and CD34 (A, C-kit, HP; B, CD34, HP).

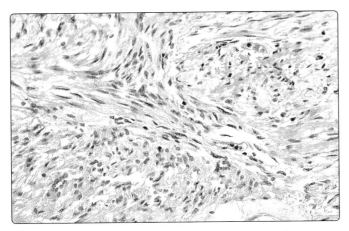

Fig. 11.24 Gastrointestinal stromal tumor (GIST) Tissue section corresponding to Figure 11.22B (H&E, IP).

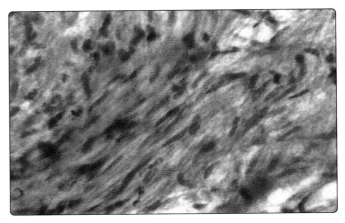

Fig. 11.25 Gastrointestinal autonomic nerve tumor Cohesive tissue fragment of bland-looking spindle cells resembling schwannoma. Result of immunohistochemistry; see text (Pap, HP).

The tumors express CD117 (C-kit) and CD34 (Figs 11.23 and 11.24), but are negative for desmin, S-100 and keratin. Cytopathologists must be 'GIST-conscious' owing to the responsiveness of these tumors to Gleevec, which can induce tumor regression and long-term response, even in metastases.[132–136]

An example of a very uncommon tumor arising from small bowel wall, a *gastrointestinal autonomic nerve tumor* (GANT), is shown in Figures 11.25 and 11.26. This is a spindle cell tumor of neural origin. It is a biologically aggressive neoplasm with metastatic potential. Neurosecretory granules are frequent, and staining with antibodies to synaptophysin, S-100, NSE and vimentin is observed, staining for desmin is negative. Intra-abdominal *desmoplastic small cell round tumor*, a relatively new entity, is a rare, highly aggressive malignant neoplasm of the serosa of the abdominal cavity, seen mainly in young male patients. The findings in FNB smears have been reported.[137–140] A description is given in Chapter 17, and a case is illustrated in Figure 11.27.

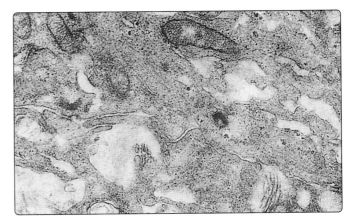

Fig. 11.26 Gastrointestinal autonomic nerve tumor Several interleaving tumor cell processes showing numerous microtubules and irregularly arranged cytoplasmic filaments. EM of fine needle aspirate × 34 100 (Courtesy of Dr. D. V. Spagnolo).

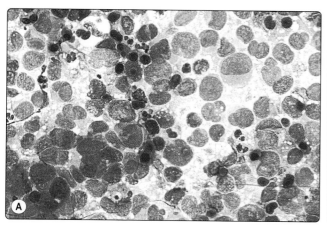
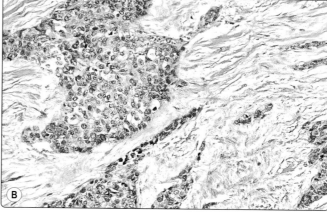

Fig. 11.27 Desmoplastic small round cell tumor (A) FNB of disseminated intra-abdominal tumor in a young male; highly cellular smear of a small round cell malignant tumor; some necrotic debris (MGG, HP); (B) Corresponding tissue section (H&E, IP).

References

1. Stewart CJ, Mills PR, Carter R, et al. Brush cytology in the assessment of pancreatico-biliary strictures: a review of 406 cases. J Clin Pathol 2001 Jun; 54(6):449–55.

2. Hancke S, Holm HH, Koch F. Ultrasonically guided percutaneous fine needle biopsy of the pancreas. Surg Gynecol Obstet 1975 Mar;140(3):361–4.

3. Oscarson J, Stormby N, Sundgren R. Selective angiography in fine-needle aspiration cytodiagnosis of gastric and pancreatic tumours. Acta Radiol Diagn (Stockh) 1972 Nov;12(6):737–50.

4. Bellizzi AM, Stelow EB. Pancreatic cytopathology: a practical approach and review. Arch Pathol Lab Med 2009 Mar;133(3):388–404.

5. Jhala NC, Jhala DN, Chhieng DC, et al. Endoscopic ultrasound-guided fine-needle aspiration. A cytopathologist's perspective. Am J Clin Pathol 2003 Sep;120(3):351–67.

6. Stelow EB, Bardales RH, Stanley MW. Pitfalls in endoscopic ultrasound-guided fine-needle aspiration and how to avoid them. Adv Anat Pathol 2005 Mar;12(2):62–73.

7. Brandwein SL, Farrell JJ, Centeno BA, et al. Detection and tumor staging of malignancy in cystic, intraductal, and solid tumors of the pancreas by EUS. Gastrointest Endosc 2001 Jun;53(7):722–7.

8. Faigel DO, Ginsberg GG, Bentz JS, et al. Endoscopic ultrasound-guided real-time fine-needle aspiration biopsy of the pancreas in cancer patients with pancreatic lesions. J Clin Oncol 1997 Apr;15(4):1439–43.

9. Fritscher-Ravens A, Izbicki JR, Sriram PV, et al. Endosonography-guided, fine-needle aspiration cytology extending the indication for organ-preserving pancreatic surgery.

Am J Gastroenterol 2000 Sep;95(9):2255–60.

10. O'Toole D, Palazzo L, Arotcarena R, et al. Assessment of complications of EUS-guided fine-needle aspiration. Gastrointest Endosc 2001 Apr;53(4):470–4.

11. Raut CP, Grau AM, Staerkel GA, et al. Diagnostic accuracy of endoscopic ultrasound-guided fine-needle aspiration in patients with presumed pancreatic cancer. J Gastrointest Surg 2003 Jan;7(1):118–26; discussion 27–8.

12. Shin HJ, Lahoti S, Sneige N. Endoscopic ultrasound-guided fine-needle aspiration in 179 cases: the M. D. Anderson Cancer Center experience. Cancer 2002 Jun 25;96(3):174–80.

13. Ylagan LR, Edmundowicz S, Kasal K, et al. Endoscopic ultrasound guided fine-needle aspiration cytology of pancreatic carcinoma: a 3-year experience and review of the literature. Cancer 2002 Dec 25;96(6):362–9.

14. Zamboni GA, D'Onofrio M, Idili A, et al. Ultrasound-guided percutaneous fine-needle aspiration of 545 focal pancreatic lesions. AJR Am J Roentgenol 2009 Dec;193(6):1691–5.

15. Pinto MM, Meriano FV. Diagnosis of cystic pancreatic lesions by cytologic examination and carcinoembryonic antigen and amylase assays of cyst contents. Acta Cytol 1991 Jul–Aug;35(4):456–63.

16. Silverman JF, Geisinger KR. Ancillary studies in FNA of liver and pancreas. Diagn Cytopathol 1995 Dec;13(5):396–410.

17. Gress FG, Hawes RH, Savides TJ, et al. Role of EUS in the preoperative staging of pancreatic cancer: a large single-center experience. Gastrointest Endosc 1999 Dec;50(6):786–91.

18. Hollerbach S, Klamann A, Topalidis T, et al. Endoscopic ultrasonography (EUS) and fine-needle aspiration (FNA) cytology for diagnosis of chronic pancreatitis. Endoscopy 2001 Oct;33(10):824–31.

19. Jorda M, Essenfeld H, Garcia E, et al. The value of fine-needle aspiration cytology in the diagnosis of inflammatory pancreatic masses. Diagn Cytopathol 1992;8(1):65–7.

20. Centeno BA. Fine needle aspiration biopsy of the pancreas. Clin Lab Med 1998 Sep;18(3):401–27, v–vi.

21. Hammel P, Levy P, Voitot H, et al. Preoperative cyst fluid analysis is useful for the differential diagnosis of cystic lesions of the pancreas. Gastroenterology 1995 Apr;108(4):1230–5.

22. Blandamura S, Costantin G, Nitti D, et al. Intraoperative cytology of pancreatic masses. A 10-year experience. Acta Cytol 1995 Jan–Feb;39(1):23–7.

23. Hyoty MK, Mattila JJ, Salo K, et al. Intraoperative fine needle aspiration cytologic examination of pancreatic lesions. Surg Gynecol Obstet 1991 Sep;173(3):193–7.

24. Saez A, Catala I, Brossa R, et al. Intraoperative fine needle aspiration cytology of pancreatic lesions. A study of 90 cases. Acta Cytol 1995 May–Jun;39(3):485–8.

24A. Forsgren L, Orell SR. Aspiration cytology in carcinoma of the pancreas. Surgery 1973;73:38–42.

25. Vilmann P, Hancke S, Henriksen FW, et al. Endosonographically-guided fine needle aspiration biopsy of malignant lesions in the upper gastrointestinal tract. Endoscopy 1993 Oct;25(8):523–7.

26. Wiersema MJ, Wiersema LM, Khusro Q, et al. Combined endosonography and fine-needle aspiration cytology in the

evaluation of gastrointestinal lesions. Gastrointest Endosc 1994 Mar–Apr; 40(2 Pt 1):199–206.

27. Jarboe EA, Layfield LJ. Cytologic features of pancreatic intraepithelial neoplasia and pancreatitis: Potential pitfalls in the diagnosis of pancreatic ductal carcinoma. Diagn Cytopathol Aug 20.

28. Brandt KR, Charboneau JW, Stephens DH, et al. CT- and US-guided biopsy of the pancreas. Radiology 1993 Apr; 187(1):99–104.

29. Di Stasi M, Lencioni R, Solmi L, et al. Ultrasound-guided fine needle biopsy of pancreatic masses: results of a multicenter study. Am J Gastroenterol 1998 Aug;93(8):1329–33.

30. Gupta RK. Value of image guided fine-needle aspiration cytology in the diagnosis of pancreatic malignancies. Diagn Cytopathol 1995 Aug;13(2): 120–3.

31. Paksoy N, Lilleng R, Hagmar B, et al. Diagnostic accuracy of fine needle aspiration cytology in pancreatic lesions. A review of 77 cases. Acta Cytol 1993 Nov–Dec;37(6):889–93.

32. Pinto MM, Avila NA, Criscuolo EM. Fine needle aspiration of the pancreas. A five-year experience. Acta Cytol 1988 Jan–Feb;32(1):39–42.

33. Robins DB, Katz RL, Evans DB, et al. Fine needle aspiration of the pancreas. In quest of accuracy. Acta Cytol 1995 Jan–Feb;39(1):1–10.

34. Parsons Jr L, Palmer CH. How accurate is fine-needle biopsy in malignant neoplasia of the pancreas? Arch Surg 1989 Jun;124(6):681–3.

35. Afify AM, al-Khafaji BM, Kim B, et al. Endoscopic ultrasound-guided fine needle aspiration of the pancreas. Diagnostic utility and accuracy. Acta Cytol 2003 May–Jun;47(3):341–8.

36. Eloubeidi MA, Jhala D, Chhieng DC, et al. Yield of endoscopic ultrasound-guided fine-needle aspiration biopsy in patients with suspected pancreatic carcinoma. Cancer 2003 Oct 25;99(5): 285–92.

37. Fisher L, Segarajasingam DS, Stewart C, et al. Endoscopic ultrasound guided fine needle aspiration of solid pancreatic lesions: Performance and outcomes. J Gastroenterol Hepatol 2009 Jan;24(1):90–6.

38. Mitsuhashi T, Ghafari S, Chang CY, et al. Endoscopic ultrasound-guided fine needle aspiration of the pancreas: cytomorphological evaluation with emphasis on adequacy assessment, diagnostic criteria and contamination from the gastrointestinal tract. Cytopathology 2006 Feb;17(1):34–41.

39. Tadic M, Kujundzic M, Stoos-Veic T, et al. Role of repeated endoscopic ultrasound-guided fine needle aspiration in small solid pancreatic masses with previous indeterminate

and negative cytological findings. Dig Dis 2008;26(4):377–82.

40. Payne M, Staerkel G, Gong Y. Indeterminate diagnosis in fine-needle aspiration of the pancreas: reasons and clinical implications. Diagn Cytopathol 2009 Jan;37(1):21–9.

41. Brugge WR. Pancreatic fine needle aspiration: to do or not to do? JOP 2004 Jul;5(4):282–8.

42. Linder JD, Geenen JE, Catalano MF. Cyst fluid analysis obtained by EUS-guided FNA in the evaluation of discrete cystic neoplasms of the pancreas: a prospective single-center experience. Gastrointest Endosc 2006 Nov;64(5):697–702.

43. Ryu JK, Woo SM, Hwang JH, et al. Cyst fluid analysis for the differential diagnosis of pancreatic cysts. Diagn Cytopathol 2004 Aug;31(2):100–5.

44. Shami VM, Sundaram V, Stelow EB, et al. The level of carcinoembryonic antigen and the presence of mucin as predictors of cystic pancreatic mucinous neoplasia. Pancreas 2007 May;34(4): 466–9.

45. Smith EH. Complications of percutaneous abdominal fine-needle biopsy. Review. Radiology 1991 Jan; 178(1):253–8.

46. Mueller PR, Miketic LM, Simeone JF, et al. Severe acute pancreatitis after percutaneous biopsy of the pancreas. AJR Am J Roentgenol 1988 Sep;151(3): 493–4.

47. Carrara S, Arcidiacono PG, Mezzi G, et al. Pancreatic endoscopic ultrasound-guided fine needle aspiration: complication rate and clinical course in a single centre. Dig Liver Dis Jul;42(7): 520–3.

48. Rosenbaum DA, Frost DB. Fine-needle aspiration biopsy of the pancreas complicated by pancreatic ascites. Cancer 1990 Jun 1;65(11):2537–8.

49. Sims J, Carroll D, Turner JR, et al. Cardiac and metabolic activity in mild hypertensive and normotensive subjects. Psychophysiology 1988 Mar; 25(2):172–8.

50. Warshaw AL. Implications of peritoneal cytology for staging of early pancreatic cancer. Am J Surg 1991 Jan;161(1): 26–9; discussion 9–30.

51. Leach SD, Rose JA, Lowy AM, et al. Significance of peritoneal cytology in patients with potentially resectable adenocarcinoma of the pancreatic head. Surgery 1995 Sep;118(3):472–8.

52. Micames C, Jowell PS, White R, et al. Lower frequency of peritoneal carcinomatosis in patients with pancreatic cancer diagnosed by EUS-guided FNA vs. percutaneous FNA. Gastrointest Endosc 2003 Nov;58(5): 690–5.

53. Meszoely IM, Lee JS, Watson JC, et al. Peritoneal cytology in patients with potentially resectable adenocarcinoma

of the pancreas. Am Surg 2004 Mar;70(3):208–13; discussion 13–4.

54. Johnson DE, Pendurthi TK, Balshem AM, et al. Implications of fine-needle aspiration in patients with resectable pancreatic cancer. Am Surg 1997 Aug;63(8):675–9; discussion 9–80.

55. Dassopoulos T, Ehrenpreis ED. Acute pancreatitis in human immunodeficiency virus-infected patients: a review. Am J Med 1999 Jul;107(1):78–84.

56. Ahmad NA, Kochman ML, Lewis JD, et al. Can EUS alone differentiate between malignant and benign cystic lesions of the pancreas? Am J Gastroenterol 2001 Dec;96(12): 3295–300.

57. Brugge WR. Role of endoscopic ultrasound in the diagnosis of cystic lesions of the pancreas. Pancreatology 2001;1(6):637–40.

58. Centeno BA, Lewandrowski KB, Warshaw AL, et al. Cyst fluid cytologic analysis in the differential diagnosis of pancreatic cystic lesions. Am J Clin Pathol 1994 Apr;101(4):483–7.

59. Alpert LC, Truong LD, Bossart MI, et al. Microcystic adenoma (serous cystadenoma) of the pancreas. A study of 14 cases with immunohistochemical and electron-microscopic correlation. Am J Surg Pathol 1988 Apr;12(4): 251–63.

60. Laucirica R, Schwartz MR, Ramzy I. Fine needle aspiration of pancreatic cystic epithelial neoplasms. Acta Cytol 1992 Nov–Dec;36(6):881–6.

61. Nguyen GK, Suen KC, Villanueva RR. Needle aspiration cytology of pancreatic cystic lesions. Diagn Cytopathol 1997 Sep;17(3):177–82.

62. van der Waaij LA, van Dullemen HM, Porte RJ. Cyst fluid analysis in the differential diagnosis of pancreatic cystic lesions: a pooled analysis. Gastrointest Endosc 2005 Sep;62(3):383–9.

63. Belsley NA, Pitman MB, Lauwers GY, et al. Serous cystadenoma of the pancreas: limitations and pitfalls of endoscopic ultrasound-guided fine-needle aspiration biopsy. Cancer 2008 Apr 25;114(2):102–10.

64. Pettinato G, Di Vizio D, Manivel JC, et al. Solid-pseudopapillary tumor of the pancreas: a neoplasm with distinct and highly characteristic cytological features. Diagn Cytopathol 2002 Dec;27(6):325–34.

65. Jani N, Dewitt J, Eloubeidi M, et al. Endoscopic ultrasound-guided fine-needle aspiration for diagnosis of solid pseudopapillary tumors of the pancreas: a multicenter experience. Endoscopy 2008 Mar;40(3):200–3.

66. Burford H, Baloch Z, Liu X, et al. E-cadherin/beta-catenin and CD10: a limited immunohistochemical panel to distinguish pancreatic endocrine

neoplasm from solid pseudopapillary neoplasm of the pancreas on endoscopic ultrasound-guided fine-needle aspirates of the pancreas. Am J Clin Pathol 2009 Dec;132(6): 831–9.

67. Kim MJ, Jang SJ, Yu E. Loss of E-cadherin and cytoplasmic-nuclear expression of beta-catenin are the most useful immunoprofiles in the diagnosis of solid-pseudopapillary neoplasm of the pancreas. Hum Pathol 2008 Feb;39(2):251–8.

68. Pelosi G, Iannucci A, Zamboni G, et al. Solid and cystic papillary neoplasm of the pancreas: a clinico-cytopathologic and immunocytochemical study of five new cases diagnosed by fine-needle aspiration cytology and a review of the literature. Diagn Cytopathol 1995 Oct; 13(3):233–46.

69. Serra S, Salahshor S, Fagih M, et al. Nuclear expression of E-cadherin in solid pseudopapillary tumors of the pancreas. JOP 2007;8(3):296–303.

70. Cohen MB, Egerter DP, Holly EA, et al. Pancreatic adenocarcinoma: regression analysis to identify improved cytologic criteria. Diagn Cytopathol 1991; 7(4):341–5.

71. Francillon YJ, Bagby J, Abreo F, et al. Criteria for predicting malignancy in fine needle aspiration biopsies (FNAB) of the pancreas and biliary tree. Acta Cytol 1996;40:1084.

72. Hejka AG, Baernacki EG. Cytopathology of well-differentiated columnar adenocarcinoma of the pancreas diagnosed by fine needle aspiration. Acta Cytol 1990;34:716.

73. Lin F, Staerkel G. Cytologic criteria for well differentiated adenocarcinoma of the pancreas in fine-needle aspiration biopsy specimens. Cancer 2003 Feb 25;99(1):44–50.

74. Giorgadze TA, Peterman H, Baloch ZW, et al. Diagnostic utility of mucin profile in fine-needle aspiration specimens of the pancreas: an immunohistochemical study with surgical pathology correlation. Cancer 2006 Jun 25;108(3): 186–97.

75. Wang Y, Gao J, Li Z, et al. Diagnostic value of mucins (MUC1, MUC2 and MUC5AC) expression profile in endoscopic ultrasound-guided fine-needle aspiration specimens of the pancreas. Int J Cancer 2007 Dec 15; 121(12):2716–22.

76. McCarthy DM, Maitra A, Argani P, et al. Novel markers of pancreatic adenocarcinoma in fine-needle aspiration: mesothelin and prostate stem cell antigen labeling increases accuracy in cytologically borderline cases. Appl Immunohistochem Mol Morphol 2003 Sep;11(3):238–43.

77. van Heek T, Rader AE, Offerhaus GJ, et al. K-ras, p53, and DPC4 (MAD4) alterations in fine-needle aspirates of

the pancreas: a molecular panel correlates with and supplements cytologic diagnosis. Am J Clin Pathol 2002 May;117(5):755–65.

78. Bournet B, Souque A, Senesse P, et al. Endoscopic ultrasound-guided fine-needle aspiration biopsy coupled with KRAS mutation assay to distinguish pancreatic cancer from pseudotumoral chronic pancreatitis. Endoscopy 2009 Jun;41(6):552–7.

79. Maluf-Filho F, Kumar A, Gerhardt R, et al. Kras mutation analysis of fine needle aspirate under EUS guidance facilitates risk stratification of patients with pancreatic mass. J Clin Gastroenterol 2007 Nov–Dec;41(10):906–10.

80. Leiman G, Markowitz S, Svensson LG. Intraoperative cytodiagnosis of pancreatic adenosquamous carcinoma: a case report. Diagn Cytopathol 1986 Jan–Mar;2(1):72–5.

81. Rahemtullah A, Misdraji J, Pitman MB. Adenosquamous carcinoma of the pancreas: cytologic features in 14 cases. Cancer 2003 Dec 25;99(6):372–8.

82. Wilczynski SP, Valente PT, Atkinson BF. Cytodiagnosis of adenosquamous carcinoma of the pancreas. Use of intraoperative fine needle aspiration. Acta Cytol 1984 Nov–Dec;28(6): 733–6.

83. Fukushima N, Mukai K. Pancreatic neoplasms with abundant mucus production: emphasis on intraductal papillary-mucinous tumors and mucinous cystic tumors. Adv Anat Pathol 1999 Mar;6(2):65–77.

84. Adsay NV, Conlon KC, Zee SY, et al. Intraductal papillary-mucinous neoplasms of the pancreas: an analysis of in situ and invasive carcinomas in 28 patients. Cancer 2002 Jan 1;94(1): 62–77.

85. Emerson RE, Randolph ML, Cramer HM. Endoscopic ultrasound-guided fine-needle aspiration cytology diagnosis of intraductal papillary mucinous neoplasm of the pancreas is highly predictive of pancreatic neoplasia. Diagn Cytopathol 2006 Jul;34(7):457–62.

86. Stelow EB, Stanley MW, Bardales RH, et al. Intraductal papillary-mucinous neoplasm of the pancreas. The findings and limitations of cytologic samples obtained by endoscopic ultrasound-guided fine-needle aspiration. Am J Clin Pathol 2003 Sep;120(3):398–404.

87. Fernandez-Esparrach G, Pellise M, Sole M, et al. EUS FNA in intraductal papillary mucinous tumors of the pancreas. Hepatogastroenterology 2007 Jan–Feb;54(73):260–4.

88. Compagno J, Oertel JE. Mucinous cystic neoplasms of the pancreas with overt and latent malignancy (cystadenocarcinoma and cystadenoma). A clinicopathologic

study of 41 cases. Am J Clin Pathol 1978 Jun;69(6):573–80.

89. Dodd LG, Farrell TA, Layfield LJ. Mucinous cystic tumor of the pancreas: an analysis of FNA characteristics with an emphasis on the spectrum of malignancy associated features. Diagn Cytopathol 1995 Mar;12(2):113–9.

90. Gupta RK, Scally J, Stewart RJ. Mucinous cystadenocarcinoma of the pancreas: diagnosis by fine-needle aspiration cytology. Diagn Cytopathol 1989;5(4):408–11.

91. Vellet D, Leiman G, Mair S, et al. Fine needle aspiration cytology of mucinous cystadenocarcinoma of the pancreas. Further observations. Acta Cytol 1988 Jan–Feb;32(1):43–8.

92. Brugge WR, Lewandrowski K, Lee-Lewandrowski E, et al. Diagnosis of pancreatic cystic neoplasms: a report of the cooperative pancreatic cyst study. Gastroenterology 2004 May;126(5):1330–6.

93. Lim SJ, Alasadi R, Wayne JD, et al. Preoperative evaluation of pancreatic cystic lesions: cost-benefit analysis and proposed management algorithm. Surgery 2005 Oct;138(4):672–9; discussion 9–80.

94. Maire F, Voitot H, Aubert A, et al. Intraductal papillary mucinous neoplasms of the pancreas: performance of pancreatic fluid analysis for positive diagnosis and the prediction of malignancy. Am J Gastroenterol 2008 Nov;103(11): 2871–7.

95. Khalid A, Nodit L, Zahid M, et al. Endoscopic ultrasound fine needle aspirate DNA analysis to differentiate malignant and benign pancreatic masses. Am J Gastroenterol 2006 Nov;101(11):2493–500.

96. Khalid A, Zahid M, Finkelstein SD, et al. Pancreatic cyst fluid DNA analysis in evaluating pancreatic cysts: a report of the PANDA study. Gastrointest Endosc 2009 May;69(6):1095–102.

97. Sawhney MS, Devarajan S, O'Farrel P, et al. Comparison of carcinoembryonic antigen and molecular analysis in pancreatic cyst fluid. Gastrointest Endosc 2009 May;69(6):1106–10.

98. Schoedel KE, Finkelstein SD, Ohori NP. K-Ras and microsatellite marker analysis of fine-needle aspirates from intraductal papillary mucinous neoplasms of the pancreas. Diagn Cytopathol 2006 Sep; 34(9):605–8.

99. Manci EA, Gardner LL, Pollock WJ, et al. Osteoclastic giant cell tumor of the pancreas. Aspiration cytology, light microscopy, and ultrastructure with review of the literature. Diagn Cytopathol 1985 Apr–Jun;1(2):105–10.

100. Chopra S, Wu ML, Imagawa DK, et al. Endoscopic ultrasound-guided fine-needle aspiration of undifferentiated carcinoma with

osteoclast-like giant cells of the pancreas: a report of 2 cases with literature review. Diagn Cytopathol 2007 Sep;35(9):601–6.

101. Moore JC, Hilden K, Bentz JS, et al. Osteoclastic and pleomorphic giant cell tumors of the pancreas diagnosed via EUS-guided FNA: unique clinical, endoscopic, and pathologic findings in a series of 5 patients. Gastrointest Endosc 2009 Jan;69(1):162–6.

102. Silverman JF, Finley JL, Berns L, et al. Significance of giant cells in fine-needle aspiration biopsies of benign and malignant lesions of the pancreas. Diagn Cytopathol 1989;5(4):388–91.

103. Combs SG, Hidvegi DF, Ma Y, et al. Pleomorphic carcinoma of the pancreas with osteoclast-like giant cells expressing an epithelial-associated antigen detected by monoclonal antibody 44-3A6. Diagn Cytopathol 1988;4(4):316–22.

104. Layfield LJ, Bentz J. Giant-cell containing neoplasms of the pancreas: an aspiration cytology study. Diagn Cytopathol 2008 Apr;36(4):238–44.

105. Benning TL, Silverman JF, Berns LA, et al. Fine needle aspiration of metastatic and hematologic malignancies clinically mimicking pancreatic carcinoma. Acta Cytol 1992 Jul–Aug;36(4):471–6.

106. Carson HJ, Green LK, Castelli MJ, et al. Utilization of fine-needle aspiration biopsy in the diagnosis of metastatic tumors to the pancreas. Diagn Cytopathol 1995 Feb;12(1):8–13.

107. Geisinger KR, Silverman JF. Fine-needle aspiration cytology of uncommon primary pancreatic neoplasms: a personal experience and review of the literature. In: Schmidt WA, Miller TR, Katz RL, editors. Cytopathology Annual. Baltimore: Williams & Wilkins; 1992. p. 23–38.

108. Ishihara A, Sanda T, Takanari H, et al. Elastase-1-secreting acinar cell carcinoma of the pancreas. A cytologic, electron microscopic and histochemical study. Acta Cytol 1989 Mar–Apr;33(2):157–63.

109. Klimstra DS, Heffess CS, Oertel JE, et al. Acinar cell carcinoma of the pancreas. A clinicopathologic study of 28 cases. Am J Surg Pathol 1992 Sep;16(9):815–37.

110. Samuel LH, Frierson Jr HF. Fine needle aspiration cytology of acinar cell carcinoma of the pancreas: a report of two cases. Acta Cytol 1996 May–Jun;40(3):585–91.

111. Stelow EB, Bardales RH, Shami VM, et al. Cytology of pancreatic acinar cell carcinoma. Diagn Cytopathol 2006 May;34(5):367–72.

112. Villanueva RR, Nguyen-Ho P, Nguyen GK. Needle aspiration cytology of acinar-cell carcinoma of the pancreas: report of a case with diagnostic pitfalls

and unusual ultrastructural findings. Diagn Cytopathol 1994;10(4):362–4.

113. Labate AM, Klimstra DL, Zakowski MF. Comparative cytologic features of pancreatic acinar cell carcinoma and islet cell tumor. Diagn Cytopathol 1997 Feb;16(2):112–6.

114. Gines A, Vazquez-Sequeiros E, Soria MT, et al. Usefulness of EUS-guided fine needle aspiration (EUS-FNA) in the diagnosis of functioning neuroendocrine tumors. Gastrointest Endosc 2002 Aug;56(2):291–6.

115. Jhala D, Eloubeidi M, Chhieng DC, et al. Fine needle aspiration biopsy of the islet cell tumor of pancreas: a comparison between computerized axial tomography and endoscopic ultrasound-guided fine needle aspiration biopsy. Ann Diagn Pathol 2002 Apr;6(2):106–12.

116. Chang F, Vu C, Chandra A, et al. Endoscopic ultrasound-guided fine needle aspiration cytology of pancreatic neuroendocrine tumours: cytomorphological and immunocytochemical evaluation. Cytopathology 2006 Feb;17(1):10–7.

117. Chatzipantelis P, Salla C, Konstantinou P, et al. Endoscopic ultrasound-guided fine-needle aspiration cytology of pancreatic neuroendocrine tumors: a study of 48 cases. Cancer 2008 Aug 25;114(4):255–62.

118. Collins BT, Cramer HM. Fine-needle aspiration cytology of islet cell tumors. Diagn Cytopathol 1996 Jul;15(1):37–45.

119. Figueiredo FA, Giovannini M, Monges G, et al. Pancreatic endocrine tumors: a large single-center experience. Pancreas 2009 Nov;38(8):936–40.

120. Chatzipantelis P, Konstantinou P, Kaklamanos M, et al. The role of cytomorphology and proliferative activity in predicting biologic behavior of pancreatic neuroendocrine tumors: a study by endoscopic ultrasound-guided fine-needle aspiration cytology. Cancer Cytopathol 2009 Jun 25;117(3):211–6.

121. Capella C, Heitz PU, Hofler H, et al. Revised classification of neuroendocrine tumours of the lung, pancreas and gut. Virchows Arch 1995;425(6):547–60.

122. Heitz PU, Komminoth P, Perren A, et al. Tumours of the endocrine pancreas. In: DeLellis RA, Lloyd RV, Heitz PU, Eng C, editors. World Health Organization Classification of Tumours: Pathology and Genetics of Tumours of Endocrine Organs. Lyon, France: IARC Press; 2004.

123. al-Kaisi N, Weaver MG, Abdul-Karim FW, et al. Fine needle aspiration cytology of neuroendocrine tumors of the pancreas. A cytologic, immunocytochemical and electron microscopic study. Acta Cytol 1992 Sep–Oct;36(5):655–60.

124. Shaw JA, Vance RP, Geisinger KR, et al. Islet cell neoplasms. A fine-needle

aspiration cytology study with immunocytochemical correlations. Am J Clin Pathol 1990 Aug;94(2):142–9.

125. Hasegawa Y, Ishida Y, Kato K, et al. Pancreatoblastoma. A case report with special emphasis on squamoid corpuscles with optically clear nuclei rich in biotin. Acta Cytol 2003 Jul–Aug;47(4):679–84.

126. Henke AC, Kelley CM, Jensen CS, et al. Fine-needle aspiration cytology of pancreatoblastoma. Diagn Cytopathol 2001 Aug;25(2):118–21.

127. Silverman JF, Holbrook CT, Pories WJ, et al. Fine needle aspiration cytology of pancreatoblastoma with immunocytochemical and ultrastructural studies. Acta Cytol 1990 Sep–Oct;34(5):632–40.

128. Wiersema MJ, Vilmann P, Giovannini M, et al. Endosonography-guided fine-needle aspiration biopsy: diagnostic accuracy and complication assessment. Gastroenterology 1997 Apr;112(4):1087–95.

129. Govil H, Reddy V, Kluskens L, et al. Brush cytology of the biliary tract: retrospective study of 278 cases with histopathologic correlation. Diagn Cytopathol 2002 May;26(5):273–7.

130. Vadmal MS, Byrne-Semmelmeier S, Smilari TF, et al. Biliary tract brush cytology. Acta Cytol 2000 Jul–Aug;44(4):533–8.

131. Ylagan LR, Liu LH, Maluf HM. Endoscopic bile duct brushing of malignant pancreatic biliary strictures: retrospective study with comparison of conventional smear and ThinPrep techniques. Diagn Cytopathol 2003 Apr;28(4):196–204.

132. Dong Q, McKee G, Pitman M, et al. Epithelioid variant of gastrointestinal stromal tumor: Diagnosis by fine-needle aspiration. Diagn Cytopathol 2003 Aug;29(2):55–60.

133. Gu M, Ghafari S, Nguyen PT, Lin F. Cytologic diagnosis of gastrointestinal stromal tumors of the stomach by endoscopic ultrasound-guided fine-needle aspiration biopsy: cytomorphologic and immunohistochemical study of 12 cases. Diagn Cytopathol 2001 Dec;25(6):343–50.

134. Li SQ, O'Leary TJ, Buchner SB, et al. Fine needle aspiration of gastrointestinal stromal tumors. Acta Cytol 2001 Jan–Feb;45(1):9–17.

135. Rader AE, Avery A, Wait CL, et al. Fine-needle aspiration biopsy diagnosis of gastrointestinal stromal tumors using morphology, immunocytochemistry, and mutational analysis of c-kit. Cancer 2001 Aug 25;93(4):269–75.

136. Wieczorek TJ, Faquin WC, Rubin BP, et al. Cytologic diagnosis of gastrointestinal stromal tumor with emphasis on the differential diagnosis

with leiomyosarcoma. Cancer 2001 Aug 25;93(4):276–87.

137. Akhtar M, Iqbal MA, Mourad W, et al. Fine-needle aspiration biopsy diagnosis of small round cell tumors of childhood: A comprehensive approach. Diagn Cytopathol 1999 Aug;21(2): 81–91.

138. Caraway NP, Fanning CV, Amato RJ, et al. Fine-needle aspiration of intra-abdominal desmoplastic small cell tumor. Diagn Cytopathol 1993 Aug;9(4):465–70.

139. Ferlicot S, Coue O, Gilbert E, et al. Intraabdominal desmoplastic small round cell tumor: report of a case with fine needle aspiration, cytologic diagnosis and molecular confirmation. Acta Cytol 2001 Jul–Aug;45(4):617–21.

140. Insabato L, Di Vizio D, Lambertini M, et al. Fine needle aspiration cytology of desmoplastic small round cell tumor. A case report. Acta Cytol 1999 Jul–Aug; 43(4):641–6.

CHAPTER 12

Kidney, adrenal and retroperitoneum proper

Svante R. Orell and Jerzy Klijanienko

CLINICAL ASPECTS

The place of FNAC in the investigative sequence

By the 1960s, Scandinavian workers had already demonstrated the value of FNAC in the diagnosis of *solid renal masses*.[1-3] Since then, several series of kidney tumors investigated by FNAC have been published, reporting good results.[4-8] Two recent developments have had an important influence on the practice of FNAC in this area. Advances in radiological imaging technique, particularly computed tomography (CT), have considerably increased diagnostic accuracy, reducing the need for a preoperative tissue diagnosis by needle biopsy. On the other hand, the revised classification of renal tumors and the definition of new subtypes with different behavior and prognosis have produced a greater need for specific preoperative tumor typing to allow more conservative surgical treatment in selected cases.[9] Immunophenotyping and cytogenetics play an increasing role in this context, and FNB is an ideal, minimally invasive way of providing cell material for such studies. The most rational approach to diagnosis seems to be the combination of radiological imaging and FNB in the same session.[10]

Generally accepted indications for FNB of solid renal masses are:

- Cases in which the radiological findings are atypical or doubtful,
- If preoperative embolization or irradiation is considered,
- When nephrectomy is contraindicated or the tumor is advanced and considered inoperable,[11]
- A suspicion of secondary tumor or lymphoma,[12]
- Lesions likely to be benign or low grade, in which surgery may be avoided or conservative,[13] for example angiomyolipoma and some variants of renal cell tumors with a favorable prognosis,
- To guide the management of small size (< 4 cm) tumors;[14] small size favors benign or low grade but does not exclude high-grade malignancy.

Puncture and aspiration through a thin needle has been the standard procedure to confirm simple *renal cysts*. Today, the diagnostic accuracy of ultrasound (US) examination has rendered cytological confirmation of simple cysts unnecessary, whereas FNB still has a place in the investigation of complex cysts such as multicystic nephroma and cystic renal cell carcinoma. Material from a renal abscess for microbiological investigation can be obtained by FNB.

For a review of the indications and usefulness of FNAC of lesions in the kidney based on current experience, see Puttaswamy et al.[15]

With regard to the *adrenal*, FNAC has mainly been used to investigate lesions detected by abdominal CT in the preoperative work-up of potentially resectable lung tumors. Mass lesions found incidentally by upper abdominal CT examination, so-called 'incidentalomas', may be primary adrenal tumors, metastatic malignancies or non-neoplastic lesions, with an approximately equal probability of neoplasms being metastatic or primary.[16,17] The efficacy of image-guided FNB in the diagnosis of adrenal lesions has been demonstrated in several studies.[18-21] Appropriate radiological and biochemical investigations may reduce the need for biopsy.[13]

For tumors of the *retroperitoneum proper*, percutaneous image-guided FNB is a valuable supplement to preoperative radiological investigations. For example, the distinction between tumor recurrence and retroperitoneal fibrosis as the cause of ureteric obstruction in patients treated for cancer of this region is of great clinical importance.[22,23] In advanced inoperable disease, a cytological diagnosis may be a sufficient basis for palliative radiotherapy or chemotherapy without the need for a formal surgical biopsy. Cytological diagnosis of primary soft tissue tumors of the retroperitoneum is difficult and a type-specific diagnosis may not be possible, but the exclusion of metastatic malignancy or lymphoma is of clinical value. If smears prove to be nondiagnostic on immediate checking, a core needle biopsy can be performed in the same session.

Abdominal and retroperitoneal lymphadenopathy are a common targets for image-guided FNB, to distinguish metastatic malignancy, malignant lymphoma and reactive lymphadenopathy.[24,25] In metastatic malignancy the cytology often suggests the site and type of the primary tumor. FNB is a valuable supplement to lymphangiography or CT in the preoperative staging of urogenital cancer.[26,27]

©2012 Elsevier Ltd
DOI: 10.1016/B978-0-7020-3151-9.00012-8

FNAC in the investigation of renal, adrenal and retroperitoneal lesions in the paediatric age group is presented in Chapter 17.

Accuracy of diagnosis

As in other sites, diagnostic accuracy is highly dependent on representative and adequate samples and on expertly prepared smears. Diagnostic criteria are well established for the commonly occurring tumors, less so for unusual entities. If a type-specific diagnosis is not possible, a categorization of disease with a differential diagnosis as a guide to further investigation and management is still of clinical value. Histochemical, immunohistochemical, ultrastructural and cytogenetic examination of FNB samples can provide more precise information of the histogenesis and phenotype of the tumor cells. However, expensive supplementary techniques should be used selectively in order to avoid nonproductive increase in costs.

In a literature review of 1585 cystic and solid *renal and adrenal masses*, the false-positive rate was 2.3% if cases reported as suspicious of malignancy were included. The diagnostic sensitivity was 86% for 603 malignant tumors, specificity was 98% and the predictive value of a positive result was 96%.[4] More recent series recorded similar levels of accuracy.[5–10,28] The commonest causes of false-negative diagnosis are insufficient diagnostic cells in cystic tumors, small tumors, or large tumors with extensive necrosis and hemorrhage. False-positive diagnoses have been recorded in angiomyolipoma, in inflammatory processes such as pyelonephritis with regenerative epithelial atypia, and in infarcts.[29,30]

Large series of FNB of *adrenal lesions* have been reported, but histologic correlation is often lacking. Only two incorrect diagnoses were made in 81 primary adrenal lesions reported from M. D. Anderson Cancer Center.[17] Others have reported similar results and a 100% specificity for the diagnosis of malignancy.[18–20,31] Tumor size is an important parameter in the diagnosis of adrenal tumors, underlining the importance of clinical and radiological correlation.[32]

The accuracy of image-guided FNB of abnormal *retroperitoneal lymph nodes* has been analyzed in the context of staging urogenital cancer.[23,33] FNB may reveal metastatic involvement of nodes that appear radiologically normal.

Complications and contraindications

The complications of puncture of renal cysts were analyzed in a large number of cases accumulated from several institutions in the USA by Lang in 1977.[34] Hemorrhage, infection and pneumothorax did occur after puncture, but the rate was low and was reduced by experience and technical modifications. Complications have been recorded in about 0.4% of FNB of solid renal masses.[4,27] A few cases of tumor seeding in the needle track following FNB of renal cell carcinoma have been reported.[28,35] The risk is considered higher for transitional cell carcinoma.[28,36] Needle size is not always specified in the reports and some involved core needle biopsy.[37] This serious complication is extremely rare but should not be ignored.[38] Infarction of renal cell carcinoma following FNA has been reported.[39]

There is a documented risk of causing a hypertensive crisis by needling adrenal pheochromocytoma.[40,41] The expertise and facilities to deal with such an event must therefore be immediately available at the procedure, which should only be performed in major hospitals.[42]

Aortic or other arterial aneurysm must obviously be excluded before an abdominal/retroperitoneal mass is subjected to FNB. An aneurysm may be occluded by organizing thrombus, may not pulsate and may appear solid on US examination.

Technical considerations

The biopsy technique is described in detail in Chapters 2 and 3. Image guidance is the routine, even in palpable masses, to ensure representative samples avoiding necrosis, cystic change, hemorrhage and major vessels. The parallel use of air-dried, MGG/Diff-Quik-stained and wet-fixed Pap-stained smears is recommended. Cell blocks are often of great value and are better suited for immunohistochemical studies than smears. The pros and cons of FNB and core needle biopsy (CNB) in renal tumors have been discussed in a review by Volpe et al.,[28] concluding that the methods are complementary. We feel that FNB, correctly carried out, is less traumatic and less costly than CNB and should be the first line of investigation. Immediate checking of samples during the procedure allows the selective use of CNB.

CYTOLOGICAL FINDINGS

The kidney

Normal structures; cortical pseudotumor
(Figs 12.1 and 12.2)[3]

- Tubular epithelial cells from different levels of the nephron,
- Whole glomeruli or fragments of glomeruli,
- Absence of necrosis or hemorrhage.

Non-neoplastic epithelial cells and other components of renal cortical tissue may be sampled by FNB in three different

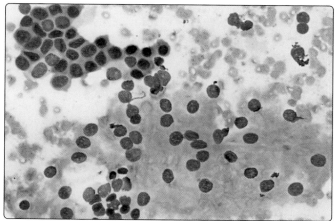

Fig. 12.1 Kidney, normal cortical tissue Sheet of large cells with abundant granular cytoplasm, invisible cell borders and small dark nuclei, representing proximal convoluted tubule, and sheet of smaller epithelial cells with dense cytoplasm from distal tubule (*upper left*) (MGG, HP).

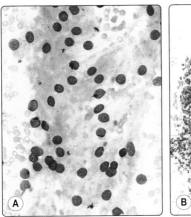
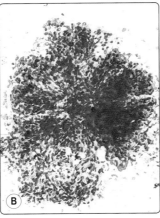

Fig. 12.2 Kidney, normal cortical tissue (A) Monolayered sheet of cells from proximal convoluted tubule (MGG, HP); (B) Glomerulus with some separation of lobules (MGG, LP).

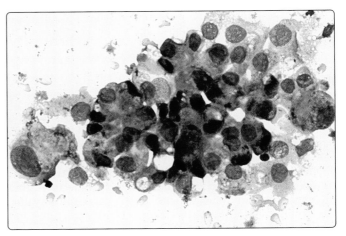

Fig. 12.3 Renal cyst macrophages Clustered atypical-looking macrophages in fluid aspirated from a simple renal cyst (MGG, HP).

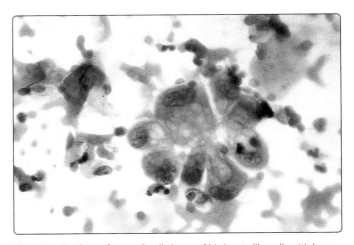

Fig. 12.4 Cystic nephroma Small cluster of histiocyte-like cells with large, eccentric, pleomorphic nuclei representing the 'hob-nail' epithelial cells lining cystic spaces (Pap, HP) *(Courtesy of Dr. B. H. Coombes, Southport, Queensland).*

ways: (1) The needle may inadvertently sample normal tissue adjacent to the target; (2) focal hyperplasia of renal cortical tissue, either as a mass at the convexity (cortical pseudotumor) or as a rounded expansion of a medullary pyramid (inversion of renal lobule or lobular dysmorphism), may mimic an avascular solid tumor radiologically; (3) an ectopic kidney may be radiologically mistaken for a neoplasm.[43] Smears from non-neoplastic renal tissue may be surprisingly cellular, suggestive of a low-grade renal cell tumor, a possible pitfall for the inexperienced observer. The hallmark of non-neoplastic renal cortical tissue is the coexistence in smears of tubular epithelial cells from different parts of the nephron looking distinctly different. Glomeruli are not always found.

Large epithelial cells from the proximal convoluted tubules usually dominate the smears. The cytoplasm is abundant, pale eosinophilic (gray–violet in MGG), finely granular with indistinct cell borders. Nuclei are round, central, relatively small and uniform, with small indistinct nucleoli. Cytoplasmic vacuolation is not a feature of normal tubular epithelial cells. Single cells and stripped nuclei may be seen but most of the cells form monolayered sheets. The nuclei are often arranged in rows. Cells of intermediate size, from the distal convoluted tubules, also lack distinct cell borders. The smaller tubular epithelial cells from the loop of Henle and from the collecting tubules have scanty, dense cytoplasm and distinct cell borders and form monolayered sheets or short tubular segments (Fig. 12.1). Some of the cells contain coarse, dark, cytoplasmic granules, probably lipofuscin. Aggregates of tubular epithelial cells may include strands of pink (MGG) hyaline material, contributing to the resemblance to renal cell tumors. Glomeruli are seen as rounded tissue fragments of tightly cohesive, small, spindly endothelial cells with indistinct cytoplasm and strands of stroma. They have a lobulated shape similar to glomeruli in tissue sections, but more or less distorted by smearing (Fig. 12.2).[44]

Benign and inflammatory conditions

Renal cysts (Fig. 12.3)

The diagnosis of simple renal cyst is usually made by US examination alone and cytological confirmation is not often necessary, but the aspirated fluid is often routinely submitted for cytological examination. The fluid is typically thin, clear, containing small numbers of degenerate epithelial cells and macrophages, but the number of cells can occasionally be surprisingly large. Macrophages in air-dried smears may appear atypical with moderately enlarged irregular nuclei, and may be clustered (Fig. 12.3).[45] This could raise a suspicion of a cystic tumor, but if the radiological features are typical of a cyst and if the aspirated fluid is clear, there is no cause for concern. On the other hand, if the aspirate contains old blood and/or necrotic debris, a cystic neoplasm has to be excluded by further investigations, even if no tumor cells are found in the smears. Carcinoma within the wall of an apparently solitary simple cyst is a rare but well-recognized event in which the malignant component can be missed by needle biopsy.[46,47] Accurate radiological guidance is essential.

Cystic nephroma (multilocular renal cyst) (Figs.12.4, 12.5)

Cystic nephroma is most common in children and is related to Wilms' tumor, but also occurs in adults. In adults, tumors

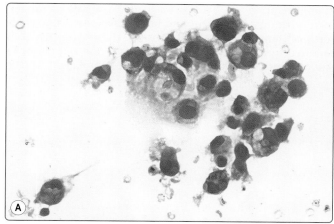

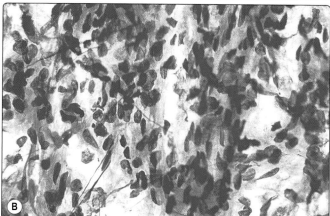

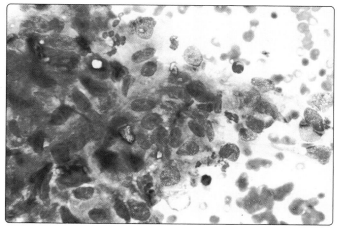

Fig. 12.6 Xanthogranulomatous inflammation Cluster of reactive macrophages; nuclear crowding, atypia and pleomorphism; (MGG, HP).

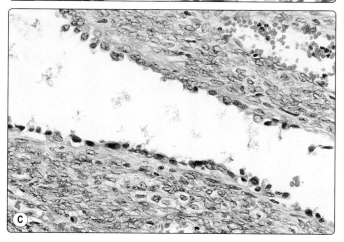

Fig. 12.5 Cystic nephroma (A) Loose cluster of cells, which could be either macrophages or atypical, degenerate epithelial cells; cyst fluid; (B) Cellular tissue fragment of spindle cells with bland nuclei; smear from a solid part of the same lesion (MGG, HP); (C) Corresponding tissue section; spaces lined by 'hob-nail' epithelial cells and septae of cellular mesenchymal tissue (H&E, IP).

of this type are now often reclassified as other entities unrelated to nephroblastoma. It is included here as a cystic lesion of the kidney. Cytological findings have been reported in a number of single cases.[48–51] Aspiration yields mainly cyst fluid. The cell content of the fluid is fairly low, but the cells often appear atypical and may be mistaken for cystic renal cell carcinoma. The atypical cells, which are both clustered

and single, represent the hobnail type of epithelial cells lining the cystic spaces (Fig. 12.4). In one reported paediatric case, the cytology showed features mimicking a malignant small round cell tumor.[52] The cystic spaces are separated by septa of solid connective tissue, which is usually densely fibrous with no blastema and which does not contribute cells to the smears.

In one of our adult cases, smears contained highly cellular tissue fragments of spindle cells in addition to epithelial cells of hobnail type (Fig. 12.5B). The histological counterpart was multifocal thickening of cyst walls and septa by cellular stroma of spindle cells reminiscent of ovarian cortex. The possibility of a *mixed epithelial and stromal tumor of the kidney*,[53] a recently defined entity that was previously regarded as adult mesoblastic nephroma or as a variant of cystic nephroma with cellular stroma, was therefore considered. However, this lesion should also contain an epithelial component of immature tubules, which was not present in our case. Morgan and Greenberg reported a similar case with spindle cells of smooth muscle type, incorrectly diagnosed as angiomyolipoma.[50]

Abscess

The aspirate is purulent and smears show mainly degenerating polymorphs and macrophages. A few normal or degenerating tubular epithelial cells may be present. Part of the aspirate should be submitted for culture.

Xanthogranulomatous pyelonephritis[3,54]

Macrophages in FNB smears from xanthogranulomatous pyelonephritis can be numerous and look quite atypical, and can be mistaken for malignancy. They have a vacuolated cytoplasm and the nuclei appear enlarged and irregular, particularly in air-dried smears. Chronic inflammatory processes involving adipose tissue in other sites in the retroperitoneum can show a similar cytological pattern (Fig. 12.6). The clinical and radiological findings, the generally inflammatory character of the smear, and the recognition of the 'atypical' cells as histiocytes (easier in alcohol-fixed smears) point to the correct diagnosis.

Angiomyolipoma of kidney (Figs 12.7–12.11)[55–58]

CRITERIA FOR DIAGNOSIS

◆ Spindle cells with features of smooth muscle cells,
◆ Cohesive syncytial tissue fragments and some single cells,
◆ A background of blood, prominent fat droplets and often adipocytes,
◆ Segments of small blood vessels (variable),
◆ Positive immunostaining for smooth muscle actin and HMB-45, EMA negative.

Conservative surgical intervention may be required to control hematuria in angiomyolipoma, but nephrectomy is generally not indicated. A definitive diagnosis by FNB may therefore be important.

The cytological findings are fairly characteristic. Aspirates tend to be bloody but contain a variable number of tissue fragments, syncytial cell clusters and single cells. The cells have elongated or spindle-shaped nuclei, some with truncated ends. Their size and shape are moderately variable. Nuclear chromatin is bland and mitoses are rare. The abundant fragile eosinophilic cytoplasm appears as a background to the nuclei, and cell borders are generally not visible (Fig. 12.8). Large fat vacuoles and some adipocytes are intimately associated with the spindle cells. Strands of endothelial cells and short segments of small vessels are often, but not always present in smears (Fig. 12.7). Tallada et al. found vascular structures in only one of four cases.[56]

PROBLEMS AND DIFFERENTIAL DIAGNOSIS

◆ A round cell pattern resembling an epithelial tumor,
◆ Nuclear atypia and pleomorphism suspicious of malignancy,
◆ Heavy admixture with blood common.

Some angiomyolipomas include highly cellular areas composed predominantly of epithelioid cells of leiomyoblastic type with rounded nuclei (Figs 12.10 and 12.11).[59] Nuclear enlargement, anisokaryosis and hyperchromasia of moderate degree may be present and be mistaken for a low-grade renal cell tumor. Several false-positive diagnoses have been reported in the literature.[4,5,30,55] However, the cytoplasm of smooth muscle cells is not granular or vacuolated but pale

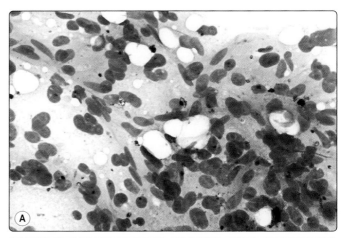

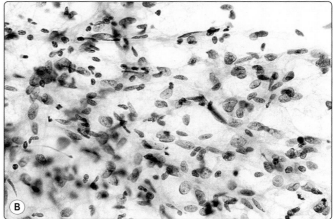

Fig. 12.8 Angiomyolipoma (A) Loosely clustered spindle cells with abundant cytoplasm and indistinct cell borders; plump spindled or rounded nuclei; some anisokaryosis but bland chromatin; many fat droplets (MGG, HP); (B) Similar appearances in Pap-stained smear (HP).

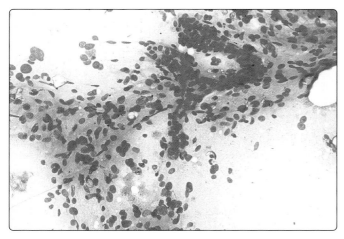

Fig. 12.7 Angiomyolipoma Tissue fragment of spindle cells with abundant cytoplasm and indistinct cell borders; a small branching blood vessel; fat droplets (MGG, IP).

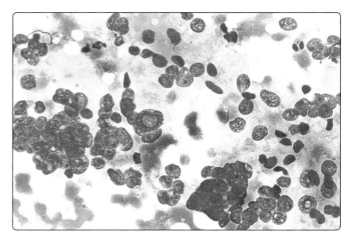

Fig. 12.9 Angiomyolipoma (atypical) Cellular smear of clustered cells with mainly round, moderately enlarged and pleomorphic nuclei; some intranuclear inclusions; a small number of usual bland spindle cells (MGG, HP). Conservative surgical resection confirmed benign angiomyolipoma.

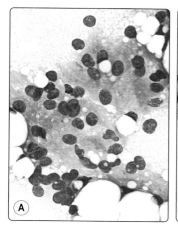
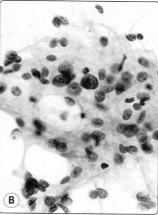
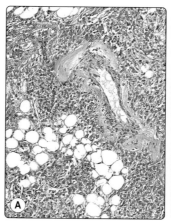
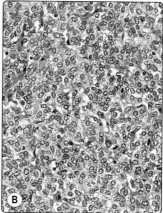

Fig. 12.10 Angiomyolipoma (round-cell epithelioid pattern) The round nuclei and the abundant cytoplasm with many vacuoles convey a resemblance to renal cell carcinoma, but the cytoplasm is syncytial, eosinophilic, non-granular, there are many large lipid droplets, nuclei are bland and some are spindle-shaped (**A**, MGG; **B**, H&E, HP).

Fig. 12.11 Angiomyolipoma Tissue sections; same case as Fig. 12.10. (**A**) Typical pattern (H&E, IP); (**B**) Round cell pattern (H&E, HP).

eosinophilic, and the nuclear chromatin is bland. Some typical spindle-shaped nuclei can usually be found also in predominantly round cell areas. A background of fat droplets and adipocytes is usually seen in angiomyolipoma, whereas strands of basement membrane material with adhering tumor cells are characteristic of renal cell tumors. Prominent nuclear atypia and pleomorphism can occur also in angiomyolipoma of the usual spindle cell type raising a suspicion of malignancy (Fig. 12.9). Correlation with clinical and radiological findings and immunostaining (EMA, SMA, HMB-45) is helpful in atypical cases.[55]

Heavy admixture with blood is common and can make a cytological diagnosis difficult. In such cases, a cell block preparation may contain diagnostic tissue fragments including a vascular component.[60] CNB has been successfully used in some cases to confirm the diagnosis.

Oncocytoma and metanephric adenoma

See pages 323 and 325.

Renal cell tumors[4,5,9,18,61,62]

The current classification of renal cell tumors (WHO 2004) includes the following entities:

- Clear cell renal cell carcinoma, including a multilocular cystic subtype,
- Papillary renal cell carcinoma, types 1 and 2,
- Chromophobe renal cell carcinoma,
- Collecting duct carcinoma,
- Renal medullary carcinoma,
- Renal carcinoma associated with Xp11.2 translocations,
- Mucinous tubular and spindle cell carcinoma,
- Renal oncocytoma,
- Renal cell carcinoma unclassified.

Sarcomatoid change can occur in any of the types and is not classified as a separate entity. The granular type is included with the clear cell tumors.

Clear cell renal cell carcinoma (Figs. 12.12–12.16)

> **CRITERIA FOR DIAGNOSIS**
>
> ◆ Variable cellularity, background of fresh and altered blood and necrotic debris,
> ◆ Cells mainly in loosely cohesive tissue fragments; some single cells,
> ◆ Abundant fragile pale eosinophilic cytoplasm, vacuolated or granular but not truly clear; visible cell borders,
> ◆ Rounded nuclei, variable anisokaryosis; pleomorphic in high-grade tumors,
> ◆ Nuclear size, chromatin and nucleoli vary with tumor grade,
> ◆ Intranuclear cytoplasmic inclusions common,
> ◆ Tumor cells adhering to endothelial cells and strands of stromal (basement membrane) material,
> ◆ Co-expression of vimentin and L.M.W. cytokeratin; EMA, RCC antigen and CD10 positive.

About three-quarters of renal cell tumors (RCC) are histologically of the classic *clear cell type*. Although the clear cell appearance is not well reproduced in cytological preparations, the findings in low- and intermediate-grade tumors are fairly characteristic. Cells have abundant, pale eosinophilic, granular and vacuolated cytoplasm, and cell borders are generally distinct. The cells are relatively cohesive, forming sheets and solid, trabecular or pseudopapillary aggregates. There are variable numbers of single cells and stripped nuclei due to cytoplasmic fragility. Cell cohesion is reduced and single cells are more common in less well-differentiated tumors. The cells are polygonal and have a low nuclear:cytoplasmic ratio. Nuclei are rounded, relatively small and uniform in low-grade tumors (Fig. 12.12), and are enlarged and of variable size, shape and chromatin pattern in intermediate and high-grade tumors (Fig. 12.13). Nucleoli are hardly visible in low-grade tumors, and are large to very large in high-grade tumors. The pattern is less characteristic at the poorly differentiated end of the spectrum, but some cells with abundant pale vacuolated cytoplasm can usually be found (Fig. 12.14). A characteristic feature in smears is tumor cells adhering to strands of stromal material staining pink with MGG, probably derived from the wall of sinusoidal blood vessels (Fig. 12.13). This pseudopapillary pattern must not be mistaken for true papillae. Intranuclear

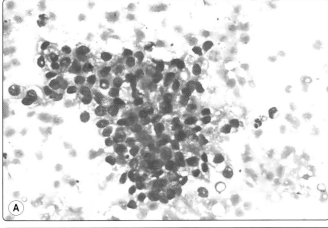

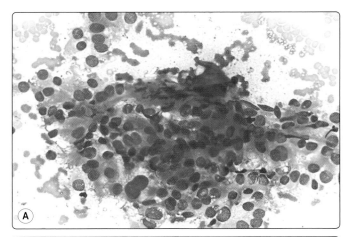

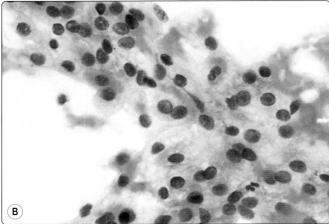

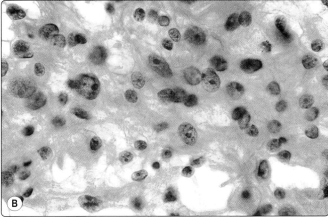

Fig. 12.12 Low-grade renal cell carcinoma, clear cell type Loosely cohesive cell clusters; abundant fragile, vacuolated cytoplasm, relatively uniform small nuclei; inconspicuous nucleoli; stromal material not obvious in this example but there are a few endothelial cells (**A**, DQ, HP; **B**, Pap, HP).

Fig. 12.13 Intermediate-grade renal cell carcinoma, clear cell type Poorly cohesive cells with abundant fragile vacuolated and granular cytoplasm; indistinct cell borders; strands of stroma and some endothelial cells; moderate nuclear enlargement and anisokaryosis. Nucleolar prominence best seen in H&E (**A**, DQ; **B**, H&E, HP).

cytoplasmic inclusions can be found in about one-third of RCCs. Intracytoplasmic hyaline eosinophilic globules have been observed but can be found also in large cell carcinomas of other sites.[63] Finally, fresh and altered blood, necrotic material and foamy or hemosiderin-containing macrophages are commonly present in the background.

The cytology of RCC, at least of low or intermediate grade, is usually characteristic enough to be recognized also in FNB samples from metastatic sites (Fig. 12.15).[64,65] Co-expression of cytokeratin and vimentin by the tumor cells, and positive staining for RCC antigen and CD10, although not specific, can be helpful in the identification of unsuspected metastatic RCC.[66,67] Higher specificity has been claimed for two new markers, PAX-2 and H2AX.[68]

Malignant cells of *granular cell type* are most commonly seen focally in clear cell carcinoma but occur also in other types of RCC. A separate granular cell variant is no longer recognized. Cells of this type usually have high-grade nuclear morphology. The cytoplasm is abundant, but eosinophilic and finely granular rather than vacuolated (Fig. 12.16).[69]

Multilocular cystic renal cell carcinoma is a rare subtype of clear cell carcinoma with a generally very good prognosis.[70] Conservative, nephron-sparing surgery may be suitable for this tumor, but to our knowledge the potential of preoperative diagnosis by needle biopsy has not yet been documented.

Papillary renal cell carcinoma

CRITERIA FOR DIAGNOSIS

◆ Cell-rich smears,

◆ Cells forming papillary fragments/clusters with fibrovascular cores, and dispersed single cells,

◆ Small epithelial cells, mainly basophilic, with low-grade uniformly small nuclei, some grooved (type 1), or larger, acidophilic cells with larger nuclei of intermediate grade (type 2),

◆ Abundant foamy macrophages and hemosiderin pigment (type 1); background of blood and necrotic debris,

◆ Psammoma bodies commonly present,

◆ Immunoprofile similar to clear cell carcinoma, but vimentin is variable.

Ten to fifteen percent of RCCs are of the *papillary type* (Figs 12.17 and 12.18).[71,72] The cells of the type 1 variant are small with a small amount of dense cytoplasm showing no obvious vacuolation or granularity. Nuclei are small, uniform and bland-looking, and nucleoli are inconspicuous. Intranuclear vacuoles occur. True papillary fragments are often

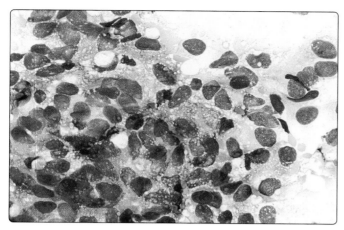

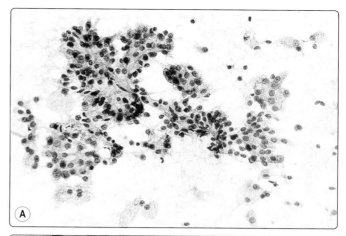

Fig. 12.14 High-grade renal cell carcinoma, clear cell type Tissue fragment of pleomorphic malignant cells; variable N:C ratio; some cells with abundant finely vacuolated cytoplasm (MGG, HP).

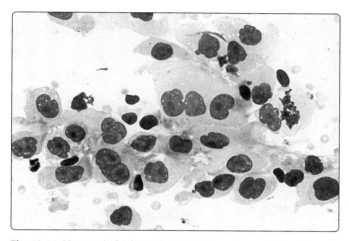

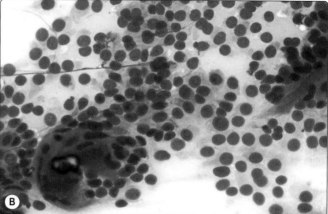

Fig. 12.17 Renal cell carcinoma, papillary type (A) Cell clusters and papillary fragments; small uniform nuclei; moderate amount of pale cytoplasm; some of the single cells are foamy macrophages (Pap, IP); (B) Poorly cohesive small cells with round uniform nuclei; stromal fragments from disrupted papillae; psammoma body lower left (DQ, HP).

Fig. 12.15 Metastatic, high-grade renal cell carcinoma Cluster of poorly cohesive large cells; abundant pale cytoplasm with some vacuoles; relatively distinct cell borders; large pleomorphic nuclei; prominent nucleoli; mitotic figure (MGG, HP).

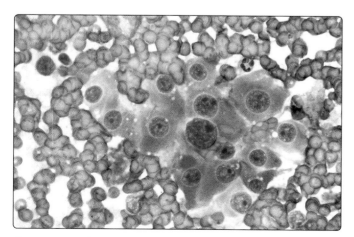

prominent in smears. Psammoma bodies are commonly found. Numerous vacuolated macrophages are a characteristic component when present and intracytoplasmic hemosiderin is often seen.[73,74] Distinction of type 1 from renal cortical adenoma is mainly based on size. Metastases have been observed from tumors as small as 1 cm[75] and tumors larger than 5 mm are now classified as RCC. A conservative approach and radiological follow-up may be an option in very small, incidentally discovered tumors, but if FNB findings are of a clear cell pattern or high nuclear grade the tumor should probably be regarded as RCC regardless of size. Metanephric adenoma also enters the differential diagnosis (see below).

Papillary RCC type 2 can be mistaken for clear cell carcinoma due to higher nuclear grade and more abundant eosinophilic cytoplasm. It is CK7+ in only a small proportion of cases whereas most type 1 tumors are strongly positive. EMA is usually negative in type 2, positive in type 1 and in clear cell RCC. Prognosis is generally less favorable than for type 1 but varies with tumor size and nuclear grade.

Fig. 12.16 Renal cell carcinoma, granular cell pattern Cluster of epithelial cells with abundant, dense, finely granular cytoplasm, malignant nuclear features (MGG, HP).

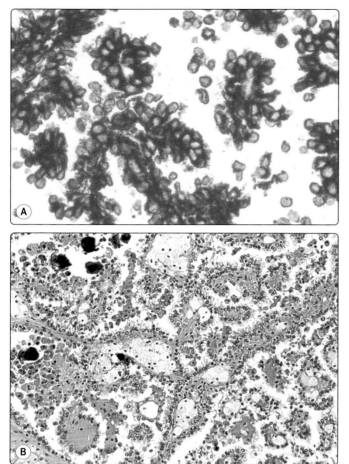

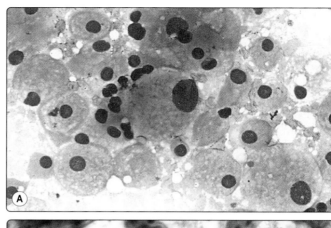

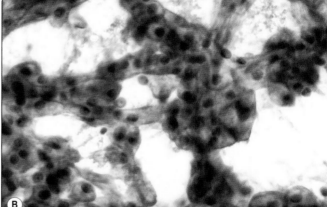

Fig. 12.18 Renal cell carcinoma, papillary type (A) Tumor cells strongly positive for CK7; same case as Fig. 12.17 (immunostaining, HP); (B) Tissue section from same case. Papillary pattern; interstitial foam cells; psammoma bodies (H&E, LP).

Fig. 12.19 Renal cell carcinoma, chromophobe type Clustered cells, majority with abundant granular and vacuolated cytoplasm, some much smaller cells; moderate anisokaryosis, some cells with small nucleoli. Cytoplasm condensed peripherally, perinuclear pale area, best seen in Pap (**A**, MGG; **B**, Pap, HP).

Chromophobe renal cell carcinoma

CRITERIA FOR DIAGNOSIS

- Moderately to highly cellular smears,
- Small, loosely cohesive monolayered sheets and single cells with intact cytoplasm,
- Mixture of large cells with abundant, pale, flocculent cytoplasm and smaller cells with dense cytoplasm, flocculent,
- Thick cell membrane, cytoplasm dense peripherally, pale centrally (halo),
- Nuclear grade usually 2, anisokaryosis, binucleation common, small nucleoli,
- No stromal material, no necrosis,
- CK7+, vimentin−, RCC antigen variable, CD10−, CD117+.

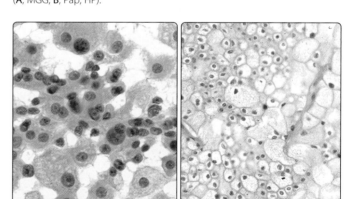

Fig. 12.20 Renal cell carcinoma, chromophobe type (A) A dual population of large and smaller cells more obvious in this example (H&E, HP); (B) Corresponding tissue section (H&E, IP).

Five percent of RCCs are of the *chromophobe type* (Figs 12.19 and 12.20). Smears of chromophobe RCC are cellular, showing both single cells and small sheets. There is a conspicuous variation in the size of the cells. Most cells are large with abundant, vacuolated cytoplasm of a flocculent texture. The cytoplasmic density varies; it is dense at the periphery and pale in the center, like a perinuclear halo. Cell membranes are thick. There are also groups of smaller cells with dense cytoplasm, giving an impression of a dual population. There is moderate anisokaryosis, but the nuclear:cytoplasmic ratio is consistently low. Nuclei are moderately hyperchromatic and nucleoli are small. Nuclear grade is mainly 2. The nuclear membranes have been described as irregular and 'raisinoid'. Binucleation is a common feature, and small nuclear inclusions occur.[76-78]

Renal oncocytoma is the main differential diagnosis in FNB smears. Cells of oncocytoma have dense granular eosinophilic cytoplasm and small bland nuclei of uniform size.[79] Immune markers are helpful in this distinction.[80,81]

Uncommon variants of renal cell carcinoma

Sarcomatoid renal cell carcinoma is no longer distinguished as a subtype since this pattern can occur focally in any type of RCC. The tumor tissue is poorly differentiated of highly pleomorphic, anaplastic and often with spindle-shaped cells (see Fig. 12.21). This pattern, which resembles a pleomorphic sarcoma, is seen focally in 1.5% of RCC and suggests a poor prognosis.[82,83]

The *collecting duct type* of renal carcinoma is rare. Smears show small groups and single cells of glandular or intermediate type with malignant nuclear features. A tubular or papillary arrangement may be present. Fragments of fibrous stroma may reflect desmoplasia seen in tissue sections (Fig. 12.22). Metastatic carcinoma, papillary RCC and TCC should be included in the differential diagnosis.[84-86]

A few cases of FNB of the rare *medullary carcinoma* of the kidney have been reported. Distinction from other types of high-grade carcinoma including RCC, TCC and collecting duct carcinoma is difficult by cytology and clinical correlation is important.[87] The tumor occurs almost exclusively in patients with sickle cell hemoglobinopathy (trait).

Another entity, *Xp11.2 translocation carcinoma*, has recently been separated from clear cell RCC on the basis of cytogenetic findings. It is most common in children but also occurs in adult patients and has a very aggressive behavior.[88] The histological features are a mixed pattern of clear cell and papillary components, prominent vascularity and in some cases hyaline globules and psammoma bodies. Positive nuclear staining for TFE3 has been reported. These features may be reflected in FNB smears as shown by a few single case reports.[89]

Mucinous tubular and spindle cell carcinoma is also a recently defined variant of RCC but of low grade. A preoperative diagnosis may be important in view of the good prognosis. Only single case reports of the cytology are available and criteria have yet to be defined.[90,91]

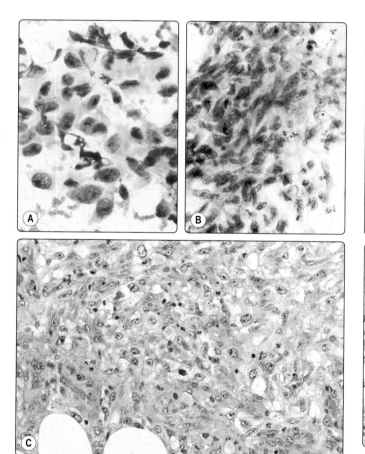

Fig. 12.21 Renal cell carcinoma, sarcomatoid type Moderately cohesive, pleomorphic spindle cells with malignant nuclear features (**A**, MGG; **B**, H&E; HP); (**C**) Corresponding tissue section (H&E, IP).

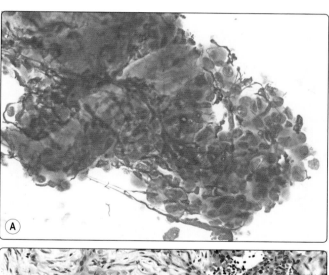

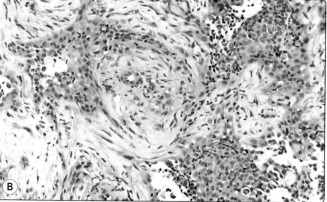

Fig. 12.22 Collecting duct RCC (A) Tissue fragment of obviously malignant epithelial cells resembling TCC; note stromal fragments representing desmoplasia (DQ, HP); (B) Corresponding tissue section (CNB, H&E, IP).

Grading of renal cell carcinoma

Histological grading of all variants of RCC based on nuclear and nucleolar size, nuclear irregularity, chromatin pattern and mitotic activity has been found to be a useful indicator of prognosis.[92] Cytological nuclear grading on similar principles correlates well with histological grade as demonstrated in several reported series.[1,62,93,94] There may be a tendency for the cytological grade to be lower than the histological, probably because of limited sampling.

Renal oncocytoma (Fig. 12.23)

CRITERIA FOR DIAGNOSIS

◆ Moderately cellular smears of loosely cohesive sheets and single cells,
◆ Cells uniformly large with abundant eosinophilic granular cytoplasm and visible cell borders,
◆ Nuclei uniformly small, round, with small nucleoli,
◆ Clinical and radiological correlation important.

Renal oncocytoma should be separated from low-grade RCC because of its favorable prognosis.[95] The main differential diagnosis is low-grade clear cell carcinoma and chromo-phobe carcinoma. The cells of oncocytoma are uniformly of oncocytic type and have abundant dense, finely granular, eosinophilic cytoplasm and small bland nuclei with inconspicuous nucleoli. Cell borders are distinct.[96,97] An oncocytic pattern may occur focally in RCC, and selective sampling of a heterogenous tumor may result in an erroneous diagnosis. A confident diagnosis of renal oncocytoma should therefore probably not be based on cytology alone, but should take clinical and radiological features such as a well-circumscribed lesion, a central scar and low vascularity into account. Immunocytochemistry is helpful,[80,81,98] although reported results are somewhat inconsistent. Vimentin, RCC antigen and CK7 are negative in most cases, CD117 is positive. Hemorrhage, necrosis, mitotic figures and obvious nuclear atypia are not seen in oncocytoma and, if present, favor renal cell carcinoma.

PROBLEMS AND DIFFERENTIAL DIAGNOSIS IN RENAL CELL TUMORS

◆ Representative sampling,
◆ Xanthogranulomatous pyelonephritis and other inflammatory processes,
◆ Angiomyolipoma, renal oncocytoma and other benign renal tumors,
◆ Adrenal cortical tumors,
◆ Tumors metastatic to the kidney.

Diagnostic cell material can be difficult to obtain in cystic tumors and in large tumors with extensive necrosis or hemorrhage. Necrotic material aspirated from a renal mass should raise a suspicion of carcinoma even in the absence of intact neoplastic cells. Small tumors can be missed, and cells aspirated from adjacent non-neoplastic cortical tissue can be confusing (see p. 316).

Histiocytes in xanthogranulomatous pyelonephritis and other chronic inflammatory conditions can appear disturbingly atypical, particularly in air-dried MGG smears (see p. 317). Foamy histiocytes may be prominent in smears from some tumors, particularly papillary RCC. Silverman et al.[29] have drawn attention to the regenerative epithelial atypia that may be seen in aspirates from renal infarcts.

The distinction from cellular angiomyolipoma with a predominance of round epithelioid cells can be difficult. The differential diagnosis is briefly discussed in the section on angiomyolipoma. The cytological pattern of renal oncocytoma has been described above. Metanephric adenoma is mentioned on page 325. The distinction of these benign tumors from low-grade RCC is obviously essential in view of the differences in prognosis and clinical management.

The cytological features of RCC may in some cases resemble endocrine tumors: poorly cohesive cells with abundant fragile cytoplasm and uniformly round nuclei, cells arranged in curved rows or loose follicles, prominent vascularity (Fig. 12.24). Adrenal cortical neoplasms are the main problem in view of the anatomical proximity to the kidney, but other tumors such as paraganglioma may also be considered. Immune marker studies (Inhibin, Melan A, RCC antigen, CD10, etc.) are helpful in this situation.

Metastatic tumors to the kidney are discussed below.

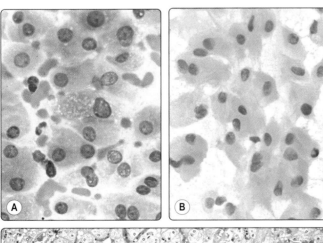

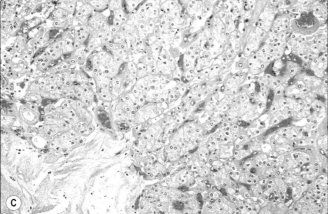

Fig. 12.23 Renal oncocytoma Uniform population of epithelial cells with bland nuclei and abundant, eosinophilic, finely granular cytoplasm; distinct cell borders (**A**, MGG; **B**, H&E, HP); (**C**) Corresponding tissue section. Note central scar lower left (H&E, IP).

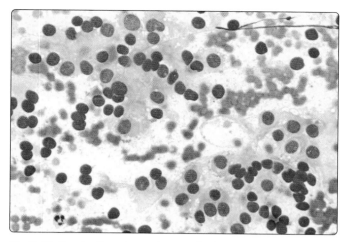

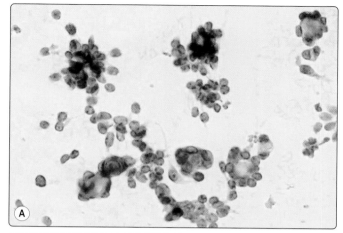

Fig.12.24 Renal cell carcinoma, low-grade The pattern of poorly cohesive cells forming curved rows shows some resemblance to a neuroendocrine neoplasm. Abundant fragile cytoplasm; mild anisokaryosis; bland chromatin (DQ, HP).

Other tumors of the kidney

Metanephric adenoma[99–102]

Metanephric (embryonal) adenoma is a rare benign renal tumor arising from metanephric blastema, most often seen in middle-aged women. A few cases with cytology have been reported. Smears are relatively cellular of monomorphous cells with small oval overlapping nuclei, bland chromatin and scanty cytoplasm. The cells are arranged in micropapillary or trabecular clusters and rosette-like, small tubular or micro-follicular groups. The cell groups are associated with scanty stromal, basement membrane-like material sometimes forming a thin central core in small rounded clusters (Fig. 12.25). Figure 12.26 is of similar FNB findings from a solitary, well-circumscribed renal lesion in a 70-year-old woman, radiologically thought to be a cyst. It had been present for 15 years, showing no change. The cytology in conjunction with the clinical/radiological findings was consistent with metanephric adenoma, and surgery was not performed.

The main differential diagnoses are well-differentiated Wilms' tumor and papillary RCC. Patel et al.[100] propose a battery of immune markers (WT1, CD57, CD56, AMACR, CK7) to help in this distinction.

Wilms' tumor (Figs 12.27 and 12.28)[103–105]

CRITERIA FOR DIAGNOSIS

- Numerous undifferentiated small cells, single and in tight clusters (blastema),
- Small, round or ovoid, hyperchromatic nuclei; multiple small nucleoli,
- Scanty cytoplasm,
- Epithelial differentiation: rosettes, tubular structures or cords (commonly present),
- Mesenchymal differentiation: spindle cells (sometimes present).

Wilms' tumor (nephroblastoma) is predominantly a tumor of childhood and is dealt with in more detail in Chapter 17. However, it can also occur in adults. Smears are usually

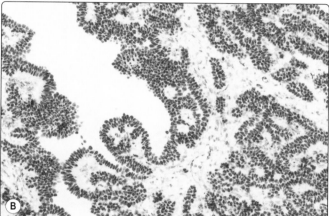

Fig.12.25 Metanephric adenoma (A) Single and clustered cells forming small trabecular and follicular groups, some with hyaline stromal material in the center (Pap; HP); (B) Tissue section, immunostaining for WT1 (IP) *(Courtesy Dr. L. Francis, Brisbane).*

dominated by small, undifferentiated malignant cells representing blastema. A specific diagnosis requires in addition evidence of epithelial and mesenchymal differentiation, but this may only be obvious in the better-differentiated tumors. Individual cells generally appear undifferentiated. Epithelial differentiation is suggested by microarchitectural patterns such as rosettes, tubules or cords (Fig. 12.27), which are not always present in smears. Correlation with clinical and radiological findings is important. The diagnosis may be supported by ancillary studies. The results of immunostaining are variable, depending on differentiation. Useful markers are vimentin, LMWCK, EMA and WT1. Heterogeneous cytogenetic abnormalities can be demonstrated in a proportion of tumors.

The differential diagnosis with other malignant small round cell tumors of the abdominal organs, primary and metastatic, is also discussed in detail in Chapter 17. Ancillary techniques are usually necessary since distinguishing features in routine smears may be subtle. Nuclear molding is prominent in classic small cell anaplastic carcinoma, cytoplasm is minimal and nucleoli are absent. Tight cell clusters are not a common feature in lymphoma, lymphoid globules (round cytoplasmic fragments) are present in the background, and cells with more abundant pale-blue cytoplasm and a perinuclear pale zone are usually found. Rhabdomy-

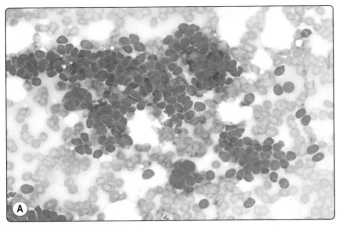

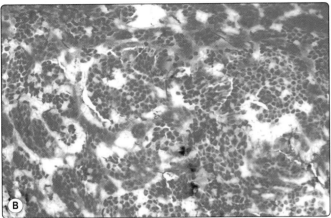

Fig.12.26 **Metanephric adenoma** (A) Cellular smear of clusters of small cells with uniform oval bland nuclei and scanty cytoplasm, some cells forming small round tubular groups; (B) The same smear contained tissue fragments almost like a cell block, showing microarchitectural features of trabecular or tubular groups separated by stroma (A, DQ, HP; B, IP).

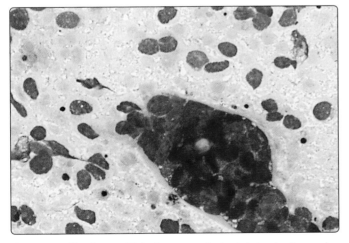

Fig. 12.27 **Wilms' tumor** Biphasic tumor; cohesive tubular structure and undifferentiated mesenchymal cells (MGG, HP).

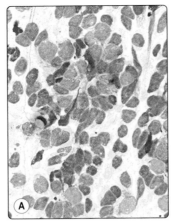
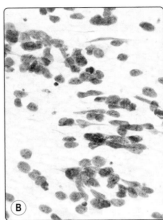

Fig. 12.28 **Wilms' tumor** Small round cell tumor pattern of undifferentiated blastema (**A**, MGG; **B**, Pap, HP).

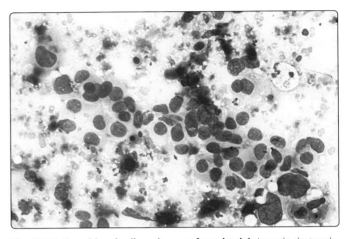

Fig. 12.29 **Transitional cell carcinoma of renal pelvis** Loosely clustered malignant epithelial cells; pleomorphic hyperchromatic nuclei; moderate amount of dense cytoplasm; necrotic debris (MGG, HP).

chemistry and cytogenetics to reach a confident, type-specific diagnosis.

Transitional cell carcinoma (Figs 12.29–12.31)[106,107]

CRITERIA FOR DIAGNOSIS

◆ High cellularity; cells single and in syncytial clusters; rarely papillary structures,

◆ Large pleomorphic nuclei; variable hyperchromasia; coarse chromatin,

◆ Eccentric nuclei within a dense cytoplasm,

◆ Prominent nucleoli,

◆ Cercariform cells often present,

◆ Most tumors are CK7+ and CK20+.

---

oblasts with eccentric nuclei and a 'tail' of dense eosinophilic cytoplasm are indicative of rhabdomyosarcoma. Tumor cell rosettes with finely fibrillar material in the center (neuropil) suggest neuroblastoma. Ultrastructural characteristics are particularly helpful in this group of tumors and FNB samples can and should be used for EM examination, immunocyto-

Transitional cell carcinoma (TCC) developing from the epithelial lining of the renal pelvis involves the parenchyma by invasion and the malignant cells may therefore be intimately mixed with non-neoplastic tubular epithelial cells in FNB smears (Fig. 12.29). Most of the tumors subjected to FNB are solid and high grade, and true papillary structures

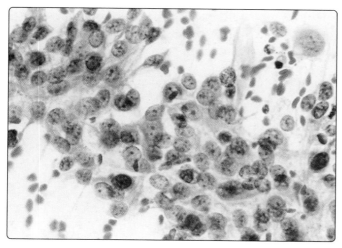

Fig. 12.30 Transitional cell carcinoma of renal pelvis Poorly cohesive malignant cells with relatively high N:C ratio; pale cytoplasm; vesicular nuclei; prominent nucleoli (Pap, HP).

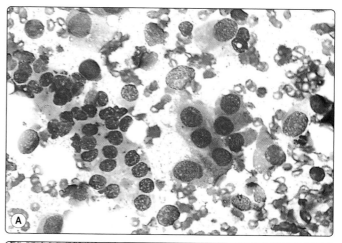

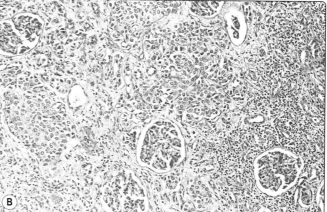

Fig. 12.31 Transitional cell carcinoma (A) Mixed population of non-neoplastic tubular epithelium and malignant cells with dense cytoplasm and eccentric nuclei (MGG, HP); (B) Corresponding tissue section; carcinoma cells infiltrating between normal renal structures (H&E, IP).

are not often found. A tendency to squamous differentiation is not uncommon, some tumors have a spindle cell pattern and some are highly anaplastic and cannot easily be identified as of transitional cell origin. So-called 'cercariform' cells, which have long unipolar cytoplasmic processes with a thickening at the tail, are regarded as a clue to the recognition of TCC in smears.[108,109]

The distinction between RCC and TCC is not always easy. TCC sometimes has a clear cell appearance in tissue sections and correspondingly a pale vacuolated cytoplasm in smears. This is usually a focal phenomenon; the nuclear:cytoplasmic ratio is still relatively high and the nuclei are hyperchromatic with a coarse, irregular chromatin. Tumor cells are positive for CK7, usually also for CK20, high molecular weight cytokeratin and thrombomodulin, negative for RCC antigen and CD10.

Some uncommon primary renal tumors

Carcinoid tumors and *small cell carcinoma* of neuroendocrine type primary in the kidney are a rare occurrence, which has been associated with horseshoe kidney in several cases.[110,111] A single case with FNB cytology has been reported.[112] *Juxtaglomerular cell tumors* are diagnosed by clinical (hypertension) and radiological findings. A variety of mesenchymal tumors can also arise in the kidney or renal pelvis. The cytological findings in *leiomyosarcoma* of the kidney have been reported.[113,114]

Metastatic carcinoma and malignant lymphoma

Metastatic carcinoma is not uncommon in the kidney and may be solitary mimicking a primary tumor. This possibility should be kept in mind if there is a past history of extrarenal malignancy and must be considered if the cytological findings are not typical of a primary renal tumor. In the series reported by Gattuso et al. 21% of malignant renal tumors were metastatic.[115] Giashuddin et al.[116] reported eleven cases, all accurately diagnosed by FNB as metastatic to the kidney. A correct diagnosis is essential in view of the different management. Clinical and radiological data are usually helpful.

In the reverse situation, a patient presenting with metastatic deposits form an unknown primary, RCC is usually not difficult to recognize in FNB samples.[64–67] This may be of clinical importance since metastatic RCC is often a solitary lesion that may be considered for surgical excision. Tumors of the thyroid, salivary glands and breast showing a clear cell or oncocytic pattern can cause differential diagnostic problems. Large pleomorphic nuclei with macronucleoli in cells with relatively abundant cytoplasm are seen in both high-grade RCC and in adrenal cortical carcinoma, hepatocellular carcinoma and large cell anaplastic carcinoma of lung or pancreas. Immunocytochemistry is helpful in this situation.[68]

Malignant lymphoma may involve the kidneys and may cause bilateral diffuse enlargement. It is rarely the first manifestation of systemic lymphoma but can occasionally be an unexpected finding in the investigation of a mass in the kidney by FNB.[117]

The adrenal

Non-neoplastic lesions

Adrenal hemorrhage is not always symptomatic and an *old hematoma* is sometimes discovered incidentally as a mass on abdominal CT scan. An adrenal hematoma can be either spontaneous or secondary to a neoplasm. This distinction may not be possible by FNB. Macrophages in a background of altered blood and debris can be difficult to distinguish from single degenerate neoplastic cells.

Fluid aspirated from adrenal *cysts*, most of which lack an epithelial lining, is usually acellular or contains only a few macrophages.[118] *Tuberculosis* is a possible cause of adrenal enlargement. Epithelioid histiocytes, giant cells and granular necrotic material in smears suggest this diagnosis, to be confirmed by the demonstration of acid-fast bacilli.

Smears from *myelolipoma*, adrenal and extra-adrenal, show a characteristic mixture of fat droplets, adipocytes and hematopoietic cells. The combination of these features in this site is diagnostic.[119] Single megakaryocytes can be mistaken for pleomorphic malignant cells but are the hallmark of hematopoietic tissue in any site.

Metastatic carcinoma

The confirmation or exclusion of metastatic carcinoma is the main indication for FNB of the adrenal (see p. 314). In this context, the primary is usually known and is most commonly in the lung. The cytological findings in metastatic tumors and clues to their origin are described elsewhere.

Primary adrenal cortical tumors[17–19,120,121]

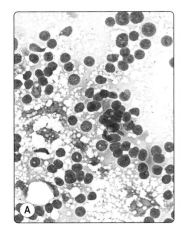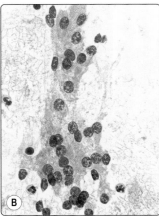

Fig. 12.32 Adrenal cortical adenoma Sheets and single cells; small, round uniform nuclei; numerous small cytoplasmic lipid vacuoles (A, MGG; B, H&E, HP).

CRITERIA FOR DIAGNOSIS

◆ Moderately to highly cellular smears,
◆ Microarchitecture varies from tissue fragments with prominently vascular stroma to loose clusters or sheets of cells, to single cells, in variable proportions,
◆ Abundant granular, sometimes vacuolated, cytoplasm; indistinct cell borders; many stripped nuclei; small lipid droplets,
◆ Nuclei generally eccentric, rounded, variably enlarged; anisokaryosis, pleomorphism and atypia variable,
◆ High cellularity, necrosis, nuclear pleomorphism, abnormal chromatin, mitoses, prominent nucleoli and large tumor size are indicative of malignancy,[121]
◆ Melan A (A103) and inhibin usually positive, cytokeratin (AE1/AE3) often negative.[122,123]

Most *cortical adenomas* subjected to FNB are asymptomatic lesions detected by abdominal CT in the preoperative investigation of patients with potentially resectable lung tumors, or incidentally by abdominal CT for other reasons ('incidentaloma'). The main purpose of FNB is to exclude metastatic cancer. Smears are moderately cellular. The cells are poorly cohesive and appear single, in groups and in loose monolayered sheets without a distinctive architectural pattern. There are numerous stripped nuclei with a background of lipid droplets, but some cells have an abundant granular and vacuolated cytoplasm (Fig. 12.32). Lipofuscin pigment may be seen. The nuclei are generally small and uniformly round and have one or several small nucleoli, but anisokaryosis can be prominent in some tumors. Nuclear chromatin is granular and evenly distributed. Saboorian et al.[17] emphasize the importance of precise positioning of the needle at biopsy

since cells of an adenoma are not easily distinguished from those of normal adrenal cortex.

As in other endocrine tumors, the cytological pattern is not a good predictor of biological behavior and features overlap between adenoma and *adrenal cortical carcinoma*. Tumor size is an important parameter. In general, adenomas are less than 3–4 cm in diameter, carcinomas over 5 cm.[21,121] Cells of well-differentiated adrenal cortical carcinoma to a variable degree resemble those of cortical adenoma, whereas cells of poorly differentiated carcinomas display severe nuclear pleomorphism, abnormal nuclear chromatin and very large nucleoli (Figs 12.34 and 12.35). Ren et al.,[121] in an analysis of 20 cases, found high cellularity, necrosis, nuclear pleomorphism, mitoses and prominent nucleoli to be the most useful indicators of malignancy. Clinical, radiological and immunocytochemical findings must be correlated with the cytology.

FNB findings in *oncocytic variants of both adrenal cortical adenoma and adrenocortical carcinoma* have been described.[124,125] We have seen one example of oncocytic adrenal cortical adenoma, a large tumor of uncertain malignant potential, which was originally diagnosed by FNB as a renal cell tumor with a predominantly granular cell pattern (Fig. 12.33).

PROBLEMS AND DIFFERENTIAL DIAGNOSIS

◆ Renal cell tumors,
◆ Metastatic carcinoma,
◆ Pheochromocytoma and low-grade neuroendocrine tumors.

Distinction between adrenal cortical adenoma or low-grade carcinoma and low-grade renal cell tumor can be a problem.[126] Both are composed of cells with abundant, vacuolated cytoplasm, a low nuclear:cytoplasmic ratio and small, round, bland nuclei. Vascular structures are prominent in both, but are of sinusoidal type in RCC, more like a network of capillaries with adherent tumor cells in adrenal tumors.

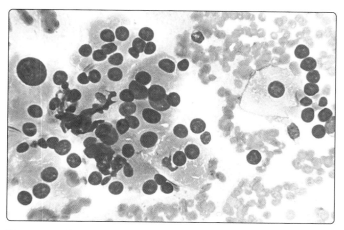

Fig. 12.33 Adrenal oncocytic adenoma Loose clusters of epithelial cells with a suggestion of acinar groupings and rows of cells; prominent anisokaryosis; bland chromatin; abundant relatively dense oxyphil cytoplasm. Smears are from a large tumor of uncertain malignant potential. FNB initially reported as low-grade renal cell tumor (MGG, HP).

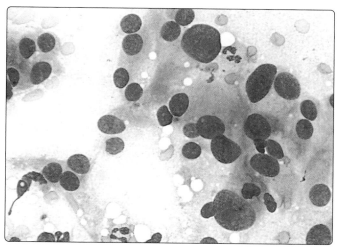

Fig. 12.36 Phaeochromocytoma Loosely clustered cells with prominent anisokaryosis; nuclear chromatin uniformly granular; some large nucleoli; fragile, finely granular cytoplasm (MGG, HP).

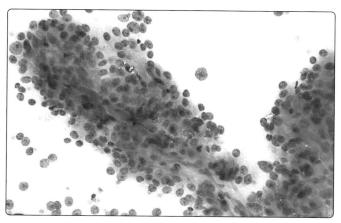

Fig. 12.34 Adrenal cortical carcinoma Well-differentiated tumor; trabecular tissue fragment with prominent fibrovascular stromal cores; crowded nuclei; moderate anisokaryosis, some nucleolar prominence (DQ, IP).

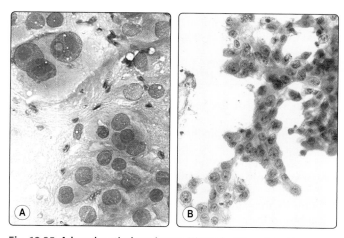

Fig. 12.35 Adrenal cortical carcinoma (A) Poorly differentiated tumor. Obviously malignant cells with large pleomorphic nuclei and large nucleoli; resemblance to high-grade renal cell carcinoma or hepatocellular carcinoma (DQ, HP); (B) Moderately differentiated tumor; trabecular aggregates; moderate anisokaryosis, some nucleolar prominence (Pap, IP).

Dispersal of cells, predominance of naked nuclei and discrete small lipid vacuoles favor cortical adenoma. Positive staining for Melan A (A103) is a good marker for adrenal cortical cells, both normal and neoplastic, and staining for inhibin and CD10 may also be helpful.[122,123,127] Investigation of the vascular supply of the tumor by angiography, and histochemical and ultrastructural examination of the aspirate may be helpful in establishing a correct diagnosis.

Anaplastic carcinomas, both primary and metastatic, display severe nuclear pleomorphism, abnormal nuclear chromatin and very large nucleoli. Malignancy is obvious, but the origin of the tumor can be difficult to decide. Pheochromocytoma, metastatic melanoma, hepatocellular carcinoma and, of course, renal cell carcinoma need to be considered in the differential diagnosis. Some tumors have a spindle cell pattern that could be suggestive of a mesenchymal tumor.[128]

Distinction from pheochromocytoma and other neuroendocrine tumors is discussed below.

Pheochromocytoma (Figs 12.36, 12.37)[128–131]

CRITERIA FOR DIAGNOSIS

◆ Bloody smears, variable cellularity, poor cell cohesion, often vascular components,
◆ Abundant, pale syncytial cytoplasm with anastomosing strands and indistinct cell borders form a web-like background to nuclei; fine red granulation in some of the cells,
◆ Loosely formed acinar or trabecular patterns; linear or curved rows of nuclei,
◆ Striking anisokaryosis of neuroendocrine type: single very large, often spindle or bizarre nuclei or binucleate cells scattered in a relatively uniform population,
◆ Relatively uniform nuclear chromatin; may be coarse, 'speckled',
◆ Nucleoli inconspicuous to prominent,
◆ Neuroendocrine markers (NSE, chromogranin A, synaptophysin, CD56) positive; S-100 highlights the sustentacular cells; cytokeratin usually negative.

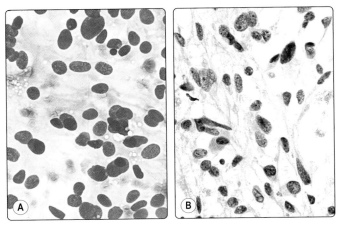
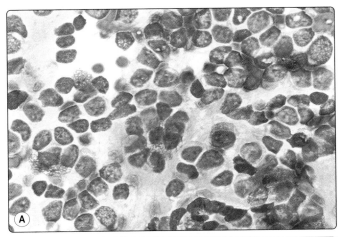

Fig. 12.37 Phaeochromocytoma Mainly dispersed cells, rounded or spindled; anisokaryosis; bland chromatin, abundant fragile cytoplasm with anastomosing strands (**A**, MGG; **B**, Pap, IP).

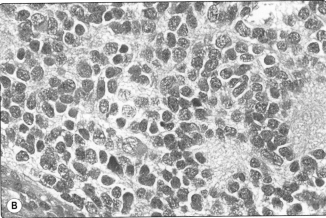

Fig. 12.38 Neuroblastoma (**A**) Cell-rich smear; small round cell pattern with a suggestion of rosettes and a small amount of fibrillar intercellular material; irregular hyperchromatic nuclei (MGG, HP); (**B**) Corresponding tissue section showing some rosettes with neuropil (H&E, HP).

Needle biopsy of suspected pheochromocytoma is generally discouraged in view of the risk of precipitating a hypertensive crisis, but is not an absolute contraindication if necessary precautions are taken. In any case, since pheochromocytoma may be an unexpected finding and may occur in extra-adrenal sites, the cytopathologist must be familiar with its cytological pattern.

Smears are usually bloody but relatively cellular. Cells are poorly cohesive but may be arranged in a loosely acinar or trabecular pattern, or in semicircular rows, and associated with vascular elements. The cytoplasm is abundant and fragile, syncytial, without distinct cell borders, often with anastomosing strands creating a web-like background. There is a fine, red cytoplasmic granulation (MGG) in a proportion of cells. Nuclei vary in size and shape, round, oval or often spindled, sometimes bizarre. Anisokaryosis is typically prominent, seen as scattered very large nuclei in an otherwise relatively uniform population. Bi- or multinucleated cells are common. Nuclear chromatin is granular, evenly distributed and relatively uniform. Nucleoli are inconspicuous to prominent, single or multiple. Intranuclear inclusions are not uncommon, and intracytoplasmic hyaline globules (H&E) are found in some cases.

The pattern closely resembles that of medullary carcinoma of the thyroid, non-chromaffin paraganglioma and other neuroendocrine tumors. A case cytologically mimicking small cell anaplastic carcinoma has been reported.[130] Immunostaining for neuroendocrine markers is helpful. A bloody aspirate can successfully be processed as a cell block to be used for this purpose.

Neuroblastoma (see Chapter 17)

The cytology of *neuroblastoma, ganglioneuroblastoma and ganglioneuroma* seen in FNB smears is described in Chapter 17, where several references are also given. The pattern is basically of a malignant small round cell tumor common to a range of neoplasms including small cell anaplastic carcinoma, Wilms' tumor, embryonal rhabdomyosarcoma, etc. Characteristic rosettes of tumor cells, in the center of which there is finely fibrillar, pink staining (MGG) material (neuropil), are often found but are not specific (Fig. 12.38). As with other malignant small round cell tumors, a type-specific diagnosis should be supported by immunocytochemical, ultrastructural or other ancillary studies, which can be carried out on FNB samples (see p. 428).

Retroperitoneum proper

The soft tissues of the retroperitoneum can give rise to a great variety of neoplasms, both benign and malignant. Liposarcoma, malignant fibrous histiocytoma and leiomyosarcoma are the most frequent malignant soft tissue tumors encountered in the retroperitoneum. Rhabdomyosarcoma is mainly seen in children and is most often of the embryonal type. Fibrosarcoma and neurogenic sarcoma are rare in this site. Among benign soft tissue tumors are the fibromatoses, xanthogranuloma, lipoma (much less common than liposarcoma), leiomyoma (rare), neurinoma, neurofibroma and angiomatous tumors. The cytological findings in soft tissue tumors are described and illustrated in Chapter 15. However, a few entities, which we have

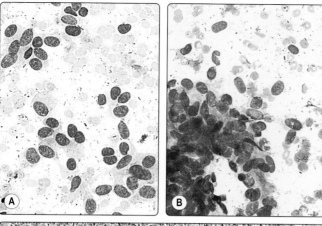

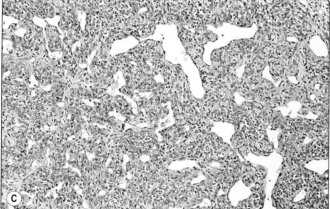

Fig. 12.39 Malignant haemangiopericytoma (A) Dispersed plump spindle cells; uniform bland nuclei and indistinct cytoplasm; (B) Cohesive tissue fragment of spindle cells fanning out from a stromal core (MGG, IP); (C) Corresponding tissue section; classic pattern (H&E, LP).

A 62-year-old man had some months' history of increasing pelvic pain on defecation. A firm mass was felt between the sacrum and the posterior rectal wall. Transrectal FNB yielded abundant blood and numerous neoplastic cells, some single but mainly clusters and small tissue fragments (Fig. 12.39). The cells were elongated or spindle shaped with a moderate amount of pale fragile cytoplasm. Some were attached to strands of basement membrane-like material. The nuclei were relatively uniform, ovoid or elongated and measured on average 10 × 30 μm. Nucleoli were inconspicuous. Even though the nuclear morphology appeared bland and no mitoses were found, the high cellularity was considered suspicious of low-grade malignancy. Histologically, the tumor was reported as a hemangiopericytoma, probably malignant on the basis of its large size, the presence of necrosis (not seen in the FNB samples) and its focally infiltrating borders. Some months after surgery, a solitary lung metastasis appeared.

Predominantly solid variants of hemangiopericytoma may not show any suggestion of a vasoformative pattern, and are more likely to be reported as spindle cell sarcoma. Variants with larger cells may be mistaken for epithelial papillary tumors. EM and/or immunostaining of FNB samples can render a type-specific diagnosis possible.[132]

Extra-adrenal paraganglioma (Fig. 12.40)[133,134]

Extra-adrenal paraganglioma of the sympathetic system of the retroperitoneum down to the pelvic floor is a rare tumor. It is often functional and often malignant. Paragangliomas of the parasympathetic system of the head and neck with a similar cytomorphology are described in Chapter 4. A case of malignant metastasizing paraganglioma of the retroperitoneum is illustrated in Figure 12.40. Intranuclear inclusions are sometimes a feature of this tumor.[133]

encountered mainly in the retroperitoneum, are included in this section.

Aneurysm

Needle biopsy is obviously contraindicated in case of arterial aneurysm. However, an aneurysm occluded by organizing old thrombus can be mistaken for a solid tumor clinically and radiologically and subjected to FNB. Smears of the semisolid aspirated material show altered blood, amorphous debris and a few macrophages with intracytoplasmic lipid droplets and blood pigment, similar to material aspirated from an old hematoma in any site. Degenerate cells and nuclei of uncertain nature may raise a suspicion of necrotic tumor. Further noninvasive investigations should be recommended.

Hemangiopericytoma (see also Chapter 15)

The cytology of hemangiopericytoma (most adult hemangiopericytomas may now be reclassified as solitary fibrous tumor) seen in FNB smears has been described. One example is illustrated in Figure 12.39 from a case presenting with a retroperitoneal mass.

A 40-year-old man presented with a large palpable retroperitoneal mass. CT-guided FNB was done as one of the initial investigations and smears showed moderate numbers of cells, single and in loose acinar/follicular clusters resembling thyroid follicular epithelial cells. Nuclei were uniformly round and relatively small and showed moderate anisokaryosis. The nuclear chromatin was granular and evenly distributed; nucleoli were indistinct. The cytoplasm was pale, without distinct cell borders. Many cells showed a fine red cytoplasmic granularity (MGG). The overall pattern suggested a neuroendocrine tumor (Fig. 12.40A). The differential diagnosis included paraganglioma as well as other neuroendocrine tumors such as carcinoid and pheochromocytoma, but also metastasis of follicular thyroid carcinoma and of low-grade renal cell carcinoma. Surgical biopsy confirmed the diagnosis of paraganglioma. Serum catecholamines were not significantly raised, but abundant neurosecretory granules were demonstrated by EM. There were widespread metastases, and the patient died 4 months later.

The striking similarity between the cytology of thyroid carcinoma and that of paraganglioma is illustrated by an FNB smear of a para-aortic lymph node metastasis in a case of follicular carcinoma of the thyroid (Fig. 12.40B). The distinction between paraganglioma and medullary or

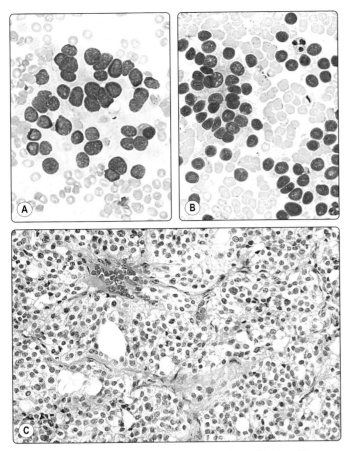

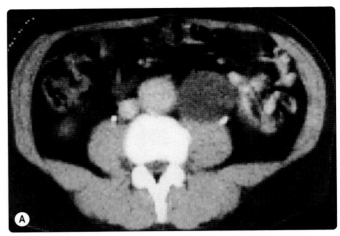

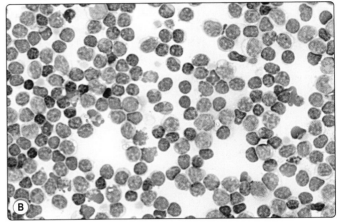

Fig. 12.40 Paraganglioma; malignant, comparison with thyroid carcinoma (A) Paraganglioma; loose cluster of cells with microfollicular groupings; small round dark relatively uniform nuclei; indistinct cytoplasm; fine cytoplasmic granulation not evident on photograph; (B) Metastasis of thyroid follicular carcinoma to retroperitoneal lymph node (MGG, HP); (C) Tissue section from the same case as in (A) (H&E, IP).

Fig. 12.41 Cystic lymphangioma, retroperitoneum (A) Abdominal CT scan; low-density round lesion left of aorta; (B) Smear of cyst fluid; numerous mainly small lymphocytes (MGG, HP).

follicular carcinoma of the thyroid, whether in a primary site in the neck or metastatic to other sites, requires immune marker studies.

Cystic lymphangioma[135]

Smears of fluid aspirated from a cystic lymphangioma contain only lymphoid cells, mainly small lymphocytes, in variable numbers. A case from our files is illustrated in Figure 12.41.

A 66-year-old man was investigated for suspected abdominal aortic aneurysm. A CT scan demonstrated a round mass below the left kidney between the aorta and the psoas muscle which was clearly separated from the aorta (Fig. 12.41A). The mass appeared to be cystic on ultrasonography. FNB yielded milky fluid and the mass decreased considerably in size. Smears of the fluid showed numerous normal lymphocytes. A diagnosis of cystic lymphangioma was made, there was no surgical intervention and follow-up was uneventful.

Idiopathic retroperitoneal fibrosis[136,137]

Fine needle biopsy may be called upon to urgently investigate the cause of ureteric obstruction, whether it is due to tumor recurrence or postradiation fibrosis.[22,23] This problem occurs mainly in patients with a history of surgery and/or radiotherapy for urogenital cancer. Idiopathic fibrosis or metastases from other sites or lymphoma may also enter the differential diagnosis. Smears from idiopathic or postradiation fibrosis are likely to be hypocellular and only a positive finding of neoplastic cells is diagnostic.

Retroperitoneal lymph nodes

Cancers of the urogenital tract, large bowel and pancreas are the main sources of metastases to retroperitoneal nodes. The cytological findings in metastatic carcinoma in lymph nodes from different sources and of malignant lymphoma are described in Chapter 5.

The possibility of a *germ cell tumor*, primary or metastatic, should be considered in cases without a known primary.[138] A primary in the testis may be small and clinically undetected, but may be revealed by radiological imaging. Germ cell tumors have a fairly characteristic cytological pattern and the diagnosis can be supported by immunostaining (see Chapter 13). The most common germ cell tumors in the paediatric age group are teratoma, embryonal carcinoma and yolk sac tumor; in the adult, all types can occur in this site.

The tendency to fibrosis shown by some malignant lymphomas of retroperitoneal nodes can make it difficult to obtain sufficient numbers of cells by FNB, or can mimic a chronic inflammatory process. Core needle biopsy may be necessary to obtain diagnostic material and tissue for immune marker studies.

References

1. Von Schreeb T, Franzén S, Ljungqvist A. Renal adenocarcinoma. Evaluation of malignancy on a cytologic basis: a comparative cytologic and histologic study. Scand J Urol Nephrol 1967;1: 265–9.

2. Kristensen JK, Holm HH, Rasmussen SN, et al. Ultrasonically guided percutaneous puncture of renal masses. Scand J Urol Nephrol 1972;6(Suppl 15):49–56.

3. Zajicek J. Aspiration biopsy cytology. Part 2. Cytology of infradiaphragmatic organs. Basel: Karger; 1979.

4. Orell SR. The diagnosis of solid renal and adrenal masses by aspiration cytology. In: Luciani L, Piscioli F, editors. Aspiration cytology in the staging of urological cancer. Berlin: Springer; 1988. p. 215–23.

5. Leiman G. Audit of fine needle aspiration cytology of 120 renal lesions. Cytopathology 1990;1:65–72.

6. Kelley CM, Cohen MB, Raab SS. Utility of fine-needle aspiration biopsy in solid renal masses. Diagn Cytopathol 1996; 14:60–3.

7. Renshaw AA, Granter SR, Cibas ES. Fine-needle aspiration of the adult kidney. Cancer (Cancer Cytopathol) 1997;81:71–88.

8. Truong LD, Todd TD, Dhurandhar B, et al. Fine-needle aspiration of renal masses in adults. Analysis of results and diagnostic problems in 108 cases. Diagn Cytopathol 1999;20:339–49.

9. Renshaw AA, Lee KR, Madge R, et al. Accuracy of fine needle aspiration in distinguishing subtypes of renal cell carcinoma. Acta Cytol 1997;41: 987–94.

10. Garcia-Solano J, Acosta-Ortega J, Perez-Guillermo M, et al. Solid renal masses in adults: Image-guided fine-needle aspiration cytology and imaaging techniques – 'Two heads better than one?' Diagn Cytopathol 2008;36:8–12.

11. Niceforo JR, Coughlin BF. Diagnosis of renal cell carcinoma: value of fine-needle aspiration cytology in patients with metastases or contraindications to nephrectomy. AJR 1993;161: 1303–5.

12. Rybicki FJ, Shu KM, Cibas ES, et al. Percutaneous biopsy of renal masses: sensitivity and negative predictive value stratified by clinical setting and size of masses. A J R 2003;180:1281–7.

13. Wood BJ, Khan MA, McGovern F, et al. Imaging guided biopsy of renal masses: indications, accuracy and impact on clinical management. J Urol 1999;161: 1470–4.

14. DeRoche T, Walker E, Magi-Galluzzi C, et al. Pathologic characteristics of solitary small renal masses. Can they be predicted by preoperative clinical parameters? Am J Clin pathol 2008; 130:560–4.

15. Puttaswamy S, Bagby J, Turbat-Herrera EA. Pathology Case Reviews 2006;11:161–8.

16. Gross MD, Shapiro B. Clinically silent adrenal masses. J Clin Endocrinol Metab 1993;77:885–8.

17. Saboorian MH, Katz RL, Chamsangavej C. Fine needle aspiration cytology of primary and metastatic lesions of the adrenal gland. A series of 188 biopsies with radiologic correlation. Acta Cytol 1995;39:843–51.

18. Nguyen GK. Percutaneous fine-needle aspiration biopsy cytology of the kidney and adrenal. Pathol Annu 1987;22(pt 1):163–91.

19. Wadih GE, Nance KV, Silverman JF. Fine needle aspiration cytology of the adrenal gland. Fifty biopsies in 48 patients. Arch Pathol Lab Med 1992; 116:841–6.

20. De Agustin P, López-Ríos F, Alberti N, et al. Fine-needle aspiration biopsy of the adrenal glands: a ten-year experience. Diagn Cytopathol 1999;21:92–7.

21. Lumachi F, Borsato S, Brandes AA, et al. Fine-needle aspiration cytology of adrenal masses in noncancer patients. Clinicoradiologic and histologic correlations in functioning and nonfunctioning tumors. Cancer (Cancer Cytopathol) 2001;93:323–9.

22. Freiman DB, Ring EJ, Oleaga JA, et al. Thin needle biopsy in the diagnosis of ureteral obstruction with malignancy. Cancer 1978;42:714–6.

23. Barbaric ZL, MacIntosh PK. Periureteral thin-needle aspiration biopsy. Urol Radiol 1981;2:181–5.

24. Al-Mofleh IA. Ultrasound-guided fine needle aspiration of retroperitoneal, abdominal and pelvic lymph nodes. Diagnostic reliability. Acta Cytol 1992;36:413–5.

25. Memel DS, Dodd GD, Esola CC. Efficacy of sonography as a guidance technique for biopsy of abdominal,

pelvic and retroperitoneal lymph nodes. AJR 1996;167:957–62.

26. Luciani L, Piscioli F. Aspiration cytology in the staging of urological cancer. Berlin: Springer; 1988.

27. Chagnon S, Cochand-Priollet B, Gzaeil M, et al. Pelvic cancers: staging of 139 cases with lymphography and fine-needle aspiration biopsy. Radiology 1989;173:103–6.

28. Volpe A, Kachura JR, Geddie WR, et al. Techniques, safety and accuracy of sampling of renal tumors by fine needle aspiration and core biopsy. J Urol 2007;178:379–86.

29. Silverman JF, Gurley M, Harris JP, et al. Fine needle aspiration cytology of renal infarcts: cytomorphologic findings and potential diagnostic pitfalls in two cases. Acta Cytol 1991;35:736–41.

30. Zardawi IM. Renal fine needle aspiration cytology. Acta Cytol 1999;43: 184–90.

31. Fassina S, Borsato S, Fedeli U. Fine needle aspiration cytology (FNAC) of adrenal masses. Cytopathol 2000;11:302–11.

32. Candel AG, Gattuso P, Reyes CV, et al. Fine-needle aspiration biopsy of adrenal masses in patients with extraadrenal malignancy. Surgery 1993; 114:1132–6.

33. Wajsman Z, Gamarra M, Park JJ, et al. Transabdominal fine needle aspiration of retroperitoneal lymph nodes in staging of genito-urinary tract cancer. J Urol 1982;128:1238–40.

34. Lang EK. Renal cyst puncture and aspiration: a survey of complications. AJR 1977;128:723–7.

35. Von Schreeb T, Arner O, Skovsted G, et al. Renal adenocarcinoma. Is there a risk of spreading tumour cells in diagnostic puncture? Scand J Urol Nephrol 1967;1:270–6.

36. Slywotzky C, Maya M. Needle tract seeding of transitional cell carcinoma following fine needle aspiration of a renal mass. Abdom Imaging 1994;19:174–6.

37. Lee IS, Nguyen S, Shanberg AM. Needle tract seeding after percutaneous biopsy of Wilms tumor. J Urol 1995;153: 1074–6.

38. Powers CN. Complications of fine needle aspiration biopsy: the reality behind the myths. In: Schmidt WA,

editor. Cytopathology. Chicago: ASCP Press; 1996. p. 69–91.

39. Malatskey A, Fields S, Shapiro A. Complete hemorrhagic necrosis of renal adenocarcinoma following percutaneous biopsy. Urology 1989;33:125–6.

40. Heaston DK, Handel DB, Ashton PR, et al. Narrow gauge needle aspiration of solid adrenal masses. AJR 1982;138: 1143–8.

41. Cassola G, Nicolet V, van Sonnenberg E, et al. Unsuspected pheochromocytoma: risk of blood pressure alterations during percutaneous adrenal biopsy. Radiology 1986;159:733–5.

42. Bernardino ME, Walther MM, Phillips VM, et al. CT guided adrenal biopsy; accuracy, safety and indications. AJR 1985;144:67–9.

43. Goreagonkar R, Viswanathan S, Merchant NH, et al. Diagnostic dilemmas in fine needle aspiration cytology of an ectopic kidney. A case report. Acta Cytol 2009;53:83–5.

44. Pasternack A, Helin H, Törnroth T, et al. Aspiration biopsy of the kidney with a new fine needle: a way to obtain glomeruli for morphologic study. Clin Nephrol 1978;10:79–84.

45. Horwitz CA, Manivel JC, Inampudi S, et al. Diagnostic difficulties in the interpretation of needle aspiration material from large renal cysts. Diagn Cytopathol 1994;11:380–4.

46. Khorsand D. Carcinoma within solitary renal cysts. J Urol 1965;93:440–4.

47. Todd TD, Dhurandhar B, Mody DM, et al. Fine-needle aspiration of cystic lesions of the kidney. Morphologic spectrum and diagnostic problems in 41 cases. Am J Clin Pathol 1999;111:317–28.

48. Clark SP, Kung IT, Tang SK. Fine-needle aspiration of cystic nephroma (multilocular cyst of the kidney). Diagn Cytopathol 1992;8:349–51.

49. Drut R. Cystic nephroma: cytologic findings in fine-needle aspiration cytology. Diagn Cytopathol 1992;8:593–5.

50. Morgan C, Greenberg ML. Multilocular renal cyst: a diagnostic pitfall on fine-needle aspiration cytology: case report. Diagn Cytopathol 1995;13: 66–70.

51. Hughes JH, Niemann TH, Thomas PA. Multicystic nephroma: report of a case with fine-needle aspiration findings. Diagn Cytopathol 1996;14:60–3.

52. Gupta R, Dhingra K, Singh S, et al. Multicystic nephroma. A case report. Acta Cytol 2007;51:651–3.

53. Adsay NV, Eble JN, Strigley JR, et al. Mixed epithelial and stromal tumor of kidney. Am J Surg Pathol 2000;24: 958–70.

54. Sease WC, Elyanderani MK, Belis JA. Ultrasonography and needle aspiration

in diagnosis of xanthogranulomatous pyelonephritis. Urology 1987;29:231–5.

55. Bonzanini M, Pea M, Marignoni G, et al. Preoperative diagnosis of renal angiomyolipoma: fine needle aspiration cytology and immunocytochemical characterization. Pathology 1994;26:170–5.

56. Tallada N, Martinez S, Raventos A. Cytologic study of renal angiomyolipoma by fine-needle aspiration biopsy: report of four cases. Diagn Cytopathol 1994;10:37–40.

57. Wadih GE, Raab SS, Silverman JF. Fine needle aspiration cytology of renal and retroperitoneal angiomyolipoma. Report of two cases with cytologic findings and clinicopathologic pitfalls in diagnosis. Acta Cytol 1995;39: 945–50.

58. Crapanzano JP. Fine-needle aspiration of renal angiomyolipoma: Cytological findings and diagnostic pitfalls in a series of five cases. Diagn Cytopathol 2005;32:53–7.

59. Mojica WD, Jovanoska S, Bernacki EG. Epithelioid angiomyolipoma: appearance on fine-needle aspiration – report of a case. Diagn Cytopathol 2000;23:192–5.

60. Handa U, Nanda A, Mohan H. Fine-needle aspiration of renal angiomyolipoma: a report of four cases. Cytopathol 2007;18:250–4.

61. Franzén S, Brehmer-Andersson E. Cytologic diagnosis of renal cell carcinoma. Prog Clin Biol Res 1982;100:425–32.

62. Cajulis RS, Katz RL, Dekmezian R, et al. Fine needle aspiration biopsy of renal cell carcinoma. Cytologic parameters and their concordance with histology and flow cytometric data. Acta Cytol 1993;37:367–72.

63. Unger P, Hague K, Klein G, et al. Fine needle aspiration of a renal cell carcinoma with eosinophilic globules. Acta Cytol 1993;39:201–4.

64. Linsk JA, Franzén S. Aspiration cytology of metastatic hypernephroma. Acta Cytol 1984;28:250–60.

65. Nguyen GK. Fine needle aspiration biopsy cytology of metastatic renal cell carcinoma. Acta Cytol 1988;32: 409–14.

66. Saleh H, Masood S, Wynn G, et al. Unsuspected metastatic renal cell carcinoma diagnosed by fine needle aspiration biopsy. A report of four cases with immunocytochemical contributions. Acta Cytol 1994;38: 554–61.

67. Hughes JH, Jensen CS, Donnelly AD, et al. The role of fine-needle aspiration cytology in the evaluation of metastatic clear cell tumors. Cancer (Cancer Cytopathol) 1999;87:380–9.

68. Wasco MJ, Pu RT. Comparison of PAX-2, RCC antigen and

antiphosphorylated H2AX antibody in diagnosing metastatic renal cell carcinoma by fine needle aspiration. Diagn Cytopathol 2008;36:568–73.

69. Tickoo SK, Amin MB, Linden DM, et al. Antimitochondrial antibody (113–1) in the differential diagnosis of granular renal cell tumors. Am J Surg Pathol 1997;21:929–30.

70. Suzigan S, Lopez-Beltran A, Montironi R, et al. Multilocular cystic renal cell carcinoma: a report of 45 cases of a kidney tumor of low malignant potential. Am J Clin Pathol 2006;125: 217–22.

71. Flint A, Cookingham C. Cytologic diagnosis of the papillary variant of renal-cell carcinoma. Acta Cytol 1987; 31:325–9.

72. Dekmezian R, Sneige N, Shabb N. Papillary renal-cell carcinoma: fine-needle aspiration of 15 cases. Diagn Cytopathol 1991;7:198–203.

73. Granter SR, Perez-Atayde AR, Renshaw AA. Cytologic analysis of papillary renal cell carcinoma. Cancer (Cancer Cytopathol) 1998;84:303–8.

74. Wang S, Filipowicz EA, Schnadig VJ. Abundant intracytoplasmic hemosiderin in both histiocytes and neoplastic cells: a diagnostic pitfall in fine-needle aspiration of cystic papillary renal-cell carcinoma. Diagn Cytopathol 2001;24:82–5.

75. Ligato S, Ro JY, Tamboli P, et al. Benign tumors and tumor-like lesions of the adult kidney. Part I: benign renal epithelial neoplasms. Advances in Anatomic Pathology 1999;6:1–11.

76. Granter SR, Renshaw AA. Fine-needle aspiration of chromophobe renal cell carcinoma. Analysis of six cases. Cancer (Cancer Cytopathol) 1997;81: 122–8.

77. Salamanca J, Alberti N, Lopez-Rios F, et al. Fine needle aspiration of chromophobe renal cell carcinoma. Acta Cytol 2007;51:9–15.

78. Tejerina E, Gonzalez-Peramato P, Jimenez-Heffernan JA. Cytological features of chromophobe renal cell carcinoma, classic type. A report of nine cases. Cytopathol 2009;20:44–9.

79. Wiatrowska BA, Zakowski MF. Fine-needle aspiration biopsy of chromophobe renal cell carcinoma and oncocytoma. Comparison of cytomorphologic features. Cancer (Cancer Cytopathol) 1999;87:161–7.

80. Garcia E, Li M. Caveolin-1 immunohistochemical analysis in differentiating chromophobe renal cell carcinoma from renal oncocytoma. Am J Clin Pathol 2006;125:392–8.

81. Memeo L, Jhang J, Assaad AM, et al. Immunohistochemical analysis for cytokeratin 7, KIT, and PAX2. Value in the differential diagnosis of chromophobe cell carcinoma. Am J Clin Pathol 2007;127:225–9.

82. Delahunt B. Sarcomatoid renal cell carcinoma: the final common dedifferentiation pathway of renal epithelial malignancies. Pathology 1999;31:185–90.

83. Auger M, Katz RL, Sella A, et al. Fine-needle aspiration cytology of sarcomatoid renal cell carcinoma; a morphologic and immunocytochemical study of 15 cases. Diagn Cytopathol 1993;9:46–51.

84. Layfield LJ. Fine-needle aspiration biopsy of renal collecting duct carcinoma. Diagn Cytopathol 1994;11:74–8.

85. Caraway NP, Wojcik EM, Katz RL, et al. Cytologic findings of collecting duct carcinoma of the kidney. Diagn Cytopathol 1995;13:304–9.

86. Bejar J, Szvalb S, Maly B, et al. Collecting duct carcinoma of kidney: a cytologic study and case report. Diagn Cytopathol 1996;15:136–8.

87. Assad L, Resetkova E, Oliveira VL, et al. Cytologic features of renal medullary carcinoma. Cancer (Cancer Cytopathol) 2005;105:28–34.

88. Meyer PN, Clark JI, Flanigan RC, et al. Xp11.2 translocation renal cell carcinoma with very aggressive course in five adults. Am J Clin Pathol 2007;128:70–9.

89. Schinstine M, Filie AC, Torres-Cabala C, et al. Fine-needle aspiration of a Xp11.2 translocation/TFE3 fusion renal cell carcinoma metastatic to the lung: report of a case and review of the literature. Diagn Cytopathol 2006;34:751–6.

90. Otani M, Shimizu T, Serizawa H, et al. Mucinous tubular and spindle cell carcinoma of the kidney. Report of a case with imprint cytology features. Acta Cytol 2006;50:680–2.

91. Owens CL, Argani P, Ali SZ. Mucinous tubular and spindle cell carcinoma of the kidney. Cytopathologic findings. Diagn Cytopathol 2007;35:593–6.

92. Fuhrman S, Lasky L, Lims C. Prognostic significance of morphologic parameters in renal cell carcinoma. Am J Surg Pathol 1982;6:655–63.

93. Kelley CM, Cohen MB, Raab SS. Utility of fine-needle aspiration biopsy in solid renal masses. Diagn Cytopathol 1996;14:14–9.

94. Al Nazer M, Mourad WA. Successful grading of renal-cell carcinoma in fine-needle aspirates. Diagn Cytopathol 2000;22:223–6.

95. Hartwick RWJ, El-Naggar AK, Ro JY, et al. Renal oncocytoma and granular renal cell carcinoma. A comparative clinicopathologic and DNA flow cytometric study. Am J Clin Pathol 1992;98:587–93.

96. Nguyen GK, Amy RW, Tsang S. Fine needle aspiration biopsy cytology of renal oncocytoma. Acta Cytol 1985;29:33–6.

97. Caputo V, Repetti ML, Bordoni V, et al. Preoperative diagnosis of renal oncocytoma by fine needle aspiration. Cytopathology 1996;7:366–71.

98. Liu J, Fanning CV. Can renal oncocytomas be distinguished from renal cell carcinoma on fine-needle aspiration specimens? A study of conventional smears in conjunction with ancillary studies. Cancer (Cancer Cytopathol) 2001;93:390–7.

99. Zafar N, Spencer D, Berry AD. Embryonal adenoma of the kidney: a report of two cases. Diagn Cytopathol 1997;16:42–6.

100. Khayyata S, Grignon DJ, Aulicino MR, et al. Metanephric adenoma vs. Wilms' tumor. A report of 2 cases with diagnosis by fine needle aspiration and cytologic comparisons. Acta Cytol 2007;51:464–7.

101. Francis LP, James DT. Pitfalls in the cytological diagnosis of metanephric adenoma. Cytopathol 2008;19 (suppl 1):abstract 135.

102. Patel NP, Geisinger KR, Zagoria RJ, et al. Fine needle aspiration biopsy of metanephric adenoma. A case report. Acta Cytol 2009;53:327–31.

103. Hazarika D, Narasimhamurthy KN, Rao CR, et al. Fine needle aspiration cytology of Wilms' tumor. A study of 17 cases. Acta Cytol 1994;38:355–60.

104. Ellison DA, Silverman JF, Strausbauch PH, et al. Role of immunocytochemistry, electron microscopy and DNA analysis in fine-needle aspiration biopsy diagnosis of Wilms' tumor. Diagn Cytopathol 1996;14:101–7.

105. Li P, Perle MA, Scholes JV, et al. Wilm's tumor in adults: aspiration cytology and cytogenetics. Diagn Cytopathol 2002;26:99–103.

106. Nguyen G-K, Schumann GB. Needle aspiration cytology of low-grade transitional cell carcinoma of the renal pelvis. Diagn Cytopathol 1997;16:437–41.

107. Ho CC, Nguyen G-K, Schumann GB. Needle aspiration cytology of metastatic high-grade transitional-cell carcinomas of the urinary tract. Diagn Cytopathol 1998;18:409–15.

108. Powers CN, Elbadawi A. 'Cercariform' cells: a clue to the cytodiagnosis of transitional cell origin of metastatic neoplasms. Diagn Cytopathol 1995;13:15–21.

109. Dey P, Amir T, Jogai S, et al. Fine-needle aspiration cytology of metastatic transitional cell carcinoma. Diagn Cytopathol 2005;32:226–8.

110. Têtu B, Ro JY, Ayala AG, et al. Small cell carcinoma of the kidney. A clinicopathologic, immunohistochemical and ultrastructural study. Cancer 1987;60:1809–14.

111. Quinchon JF, Aubert S, Biserte J, et al. Primary atypical carcinoid of the kidney: a classification is needed. Pathology 2003;35:353–5.

112. Bhalla R, Popp A, Nassar A. Case report: metastatic renal carcinoid to the thyroid diagnosed by fine needle aspiration biopsy. Diagn Cytopathol 2007;35:597–600.

113. Tsun-Cheung Chow L, Chan S-K, Chow W-H. Fine needle aspiration cytodiagnosis of leiomyosarcoma of the renal pelvis. A case report with immunohistochemical study. Acta Cytol 1994;38:759–63.

114. Villaneuva RR, Nguyen-Ho P, Nguyen G-K. Leiomyosarcoma of the kidney. Report of a case diagnosed by fine needle aspiration and electron microscopy. Acta Cytol 1994;38:568–72.

115. Gattuso P, Ramzy I, Truong LD, et al. Utilization of fine-needle aspiration in the diagnois of metastatic tumors to the kidney. Diagn Cytopathol 1999;21:35–8.

116. Giashuddin S, Cangiarella J, Elgert P, et al. Metastases to the kidney: eleven cases diagnosed by aspiration biopsy with histological correlation. Diagn Cytopathol 2005;32:325–9.

117. Truong LD, Caraway N, Ngo T, et al. Renal lymphoma. The diagnostic and therapeutic roles of fine-needle aspiration. Am J Clin Pathol 2001;115:18–31.

118. Scheible W, Coel M, Siemers PT, et al. Percutaneous aspiration of adrenal cysts. AJR 1977;128:1013–6.

119. Dunphy CH. Computed tomography-guided fine needle aspiration biopsy of adrenal myelolipoma. Case report and review of the literature. Acta Cytol 1991;35:353–6.

120. Her-Juing H, Cramer HM, Kho J, et al. Fine needle aspiration cytology of benign adrenal cortical nodules. A comparison of cytologic findings with those of primary and metastatic adrenal malignancies. Acta Cytol 1998;42:1352–8.

121. Ren R, Guo M, Sneige N, et al. Fine-needle aspiration of adrenal cortical carcinoma. Cytologic spectrum and diagnostic challenges. Am J Clin Pathol 2006;126:389–98.

122. Fetsch PA, Powers CN, Zakowski MF, et al. Anti-alpha-Inhibin. Marker of choice for the consistent distinction between adrenocortical carcinoma and renal cell carcinoma in fine-needle aspiration. Cancer (Cancer Cytopathol) 1999;87:168–72.

123. Shin SJ, Hoda RS, Ying L, et al. Diagnostic utility of the monoclonal antibody A103 in fine-needle aspiration biopsies of the adrenal. Am J Clin Pathol 2000;113:295–302.

124. Wragg T, Nguyen G-K. Cytopathology of adrenal cortical oncocytoma. Diagn Cytopathol 2001;24:222–3.

125. Krishnamurthy S, Ordonez NG, Shelton TO, et al. Fine-needle aspiration cytology of a case of oncocytic adrenocortical carcinoma. Diagn Cytopathol 2000;22:299–303.

126. Sharma S, Singh R, Verma K. Cytomorphology of adrenocortical carcinoma and comparison with renal cell carcinoma. Acta Cytol 1997;41:385–92.

127. Yang B, Ali SZ, Rosenthal DL. CD10 facilitates the diagnosis of metastatic renal cell carcinoma from primary adrenal cortical neoplasm in adrenal fine-needle aspiration. Diagn Cytopathol 2002;27:149–52.

128. Nance KV, McLeod DL, Silverman JF. Fine-needle aspiration biopsy of spindle cell neoplasms of the adrenal gland. Diagn Cytopathol 1992;8:235–41.

129. Nguyen GK. Cytopathologic aspects of adrenal pheochromocytoma in a fine needle aspiration biopsy. A case report. Acta Cytol 1982;26:354–8.

130. Deodhare S, Chalvardjian A, Lata A, et al. Adrenal pheochromocytoma mimicking small cell carcinoma on fine needle aspiration biopsy. A case report. Acta Cytol 1996;40:1003–6.

131. Shidham VB, Galindo LM. Pheochromocytoma. Cytologic findings on intraoperative scrape smears in five cases. Acta Cytol 1999;43:207–13.

132. Geisinger KR, Silverman JF, Cappellari JO, et al. Fine-needle aspiration cytology of malignant hemangiopericytomas with ultrastructural and flow cytometric analyses. Arch Pathol Lab Med 1990;114:705–10.

133. Vera-Alvarez J, Marigil-Gómez M, Abascal-Agorreta M, et al. Malignant retroperitoneal paraganglioma with intranuclear vacuoles in a fine needle aspirate. Acta Cytol 1993;37:229–33.

134. Jimenez-Hefferman JA, Vicandi B, Lopez-Ferrer P, et al. Cytologic features of Pheochromocytoma and retroperitoneal paraganglioma. A morphologic and immunohistochemical study of 13 cases. Acta Cytol 2006;50:372–8.

135. Sarno RC, Carter BL, Bankoff MS. Cystic lymphangiomas: CT diagnosis and thin needle aspiration. Br J Radiol 1984;57:424–6.

136. Stein AL, Bardawil RG, Silverman SG, et al. Fine needle aspiration biopsy of idiopathic retroperitoneal fibrosis. Acta Cytol 1997;41:461–6.

137. Dash RC, Liu K, Sheafor DH, et al. Fine-needle aspiration findings in idiopathic retroperitoneal fibrosis. Diagn Cytopathol 1999;21:22–6.

138. Collins KA, Geisinger KR, Wakely PE, et al. Extragonadal germ cell tumours: A fine-needle aspiration biopsy study. Diagn Cytopathol 1995;12:223–9.

CHAPTER 13

Male and female genital tract

Miguel Perez-Guillermo and Svante R. Orell

Male genital tract, prostate and testis

Miguel Perez-Guillermo

Introduction

Transrectal fine needle aspiration (tFNA) of the prostate was introduced in 1960.[1] In Europe, tFNA was the technique of choice for investigating palpable abnormalities of the prostate for more than two decades. It became popular in the United States only later, in the 1980s.[2-4] Despite the initial success, tFNA has been gradually superseded by the biopsy-gun technique and pathologists who trained after 1990 generally have had little experience with tFNA of the prostate.[5] Thin-needle core biopsy (TNCB) yields thin 15–20 mm-long tissue cylinders, which provide Gleason scores for prostate cancer based on histopathology, as required by urologists. However, the predictive value of TNCB in selecting patients for radical prostatectomy (RP) has been brought into question.[6] In one study, only 55% of patients who met the criteria for RP had tumors that were organ confined.[7] The utility of tFNA of palpable lesions of the prostate,[5,8,9] and its continuing role into the twenty-first century have been discussed elsewhere.[10] A promising future for tFNA has been foretold.[11]

Testicular germ cell tumors (TGCT) usually present as a nodule or painless swelling of one testicle. A dull ache or heaviness in the scrotum or lower abdomen, and a swelling mistaken for epididymitis may be the presenting symptoms.[12] Incisional biopsy is contraindicated because of the risk of spread, locally and to regional lymph nodes. Ultrasonography (US) is the primary imaging modality for investigating scrotal pathology.[12,13] Serum tumor markers (STM) may be helpful.[12] However, scrotal content pathology still poses diagnostic problems for urologists. US and STM are not readily accessible in some countries. The impact of delay, by patients or healthcare providers, in the diagnosis of testicular cancer has been addressed by several authors.[14-16] Diagnostic delay is highly correlated with stage and survival in non-seminomatous TGCT.[16]

In experienced hands, the information provided by FNA is more useful than that provided by US and STM. FNA can avoid the 'shuttle syndrome' and the 'wait and see' approach. We and others believe that FNA has an important place in the diagnosis of intrascrotal pathology and in the evaluation of male fertility.[17-25]

The same technique as for tFNA of the prostate can be used to biopsy lesions of the female genital tract via the vagina or rectum. A detailed account of clinical applications and limitations of transvaginal and tFNA in gynecology can be found elsewhere.[26]

Prostate

Clinical aspects

The place of FNA in the investigative sequence

The utility and practice of tFNA of the prostate and the reasons for its success in our hospital have been reported previously.[8-10] Provided the pathologist is able to pinpoint nodules and indurations of the prostate by palpation with the index finger, and has dexterity in performing tFNA, the results of FNA match those obtained by TNCB.[10]

The three-tiered cytological classification for grading prostate cancer proposed by Esposti[27] has been shown to have prognostic value. An estimation of Gleason score can also be made on tFNA samples.[10] As recently as 2007, Maksen et al.[5] stated that gland size roughly determines Gleason pattern in liquid-fixed FNA samples. Prostatic intraepithelial neoplasia (PIN) should not be diagnosed by FNA alone. However, a highly cellular smear with pronounced atypia seems to rule out PIN.[28] Immunostaining has proven useful in FNA of the prostate.[5,29]

tFNA is likely to continue to be used in view of economic considerations and recent health budget restraints because it is a simple and comparatively much cheaper technique than TCNB. We acknowledge that nowadays tFNA has been relegated in most Western countries, but it may still play a key role in developing countries.

DOI: 10.1016/B978-0-7020-3151-9.00013-X

Indications

- Palpable nodules,
- Focal or diffuse stony indurations,
- Patients older than 75 years with PSA >30 ng/mL, or with PSA >20 ng/mL and suspicious digital rectal examination,[30]
- Pathological fracture even if the prostate has been deemed benign on palpation,
- Control of the effect of hormonal treatment,[27,31]
- To establish prostate origin in metastatic carcinomas of unknown primary,
- Guidelines for the use of digitally guided tFNA and US-guided TNCB have been proposed.[32,33]

Accuracy of diagnosis

Transrectal fine needle aspiration and US-guided TNCB using automated biopsy devices have a high and essentially equal accuracy in diagnosing prostate cancer.[4,5] A recent review of the literature[10] produced a list of references commenting on the correlation between cytological grading and Gleason score and the accuracy of digitally guided tFNA compared with thick and US-guided TNCB. Prerequisites for acquisition of an acceptable level of competence in performing tFNA and interpreting the smears have been defined.[34]

Tannenbaum et al.[4] and Maksen et al.[5] have described the features of benign prostatic cytology, the sources of atypical cells, the cytology of carcinoma, and the causes of false-negative and false-positive cytological diagnoses in liquid-fixed FNA collections, and Willems et al.[34] in conventional smears. The most common cause of a false-negative FNA is an inadequate sample. Dexterous pathologists rarely make a false-positive diagnosis. We have previously commented on the diagnostic challenges posed by atypical cells in smears of granulomatous prostatitis[8] and on pitfalls and infrequent findings in FNA of the prostate.[9] Basic rules to avoid pitfalls in FNA in different contexts have been put forward.[35] See also Chapter 5 in the seminal monograph by Zajicek[36] and Chapter 11 in the book by Linsk and Franzén.[37]

Complications

The rare complications of tFNA were analyzed in a review of 14 000 patients with follow-up.[38] Transient hematuria is not uncommon. Fever may develop within 24 hours. Patients should be instructed to report promptly in both situations. In our experience of more than 10 000 tFNAs (using 23-gauge needles), no tumor seeding in the needle track has been observed after 5 to 10 years' follow-up.

Contraindications

The only contraindication is symptomatic febrile prostatitis.[36] We have performed tFNAs in patients with inadvertent acute prostatitis without complications. tFNA can be performed in patients with hemorrhagic diathesis and in patients on anticoagulation therapy.

Technical considerations

Patients should be verbally informed of the whole procedure by the examining pathologist and a written informed consent requested. No special preparations for biopsy and no sedation are necessary. tFNA is carried out as an outpatient procedure. A urological lubricant helps to introduce the palpating finger. The most comfortable position for both patient and examining pathologist is the lithotomy position on a gynecological examination couch (Fig. 13.1A,B). A rapid feedback to urologists is essential to achieve success.

Appropriate training should ensure that the operator properly masters the technique of tFNA using the Franzén guide and a 20-cm long 23-gauge needle fitted to a disposable syringe and a Cameco holder (Cameco AB, Box 5519, Täby, S-183 05 Sweden, Pat no. 3819091). This is essential to minimise the proportion of unsatisfactory specimens and to increase the accuracy of the procedure. The examining pathologist must be proficient in digital examination of the prostate. Details about the biopsy technique can be found elsewhere.[34,37]

We perform one or two tFNAs from each abnormal palpable zone; additional aspirates are taken from the opposite lobe even if apparently normal on palpation. This approach enables us to suggest at least a T2C stage if cancer cells are found in aspirates from both lobes. We use Diff-Quik (DQ)™ and Pap stain in parallel.

The gross aspect of the yield may predict the diagnosis even before microscopic examination: abundant, granular

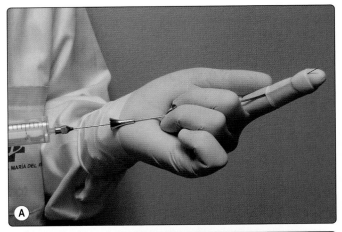

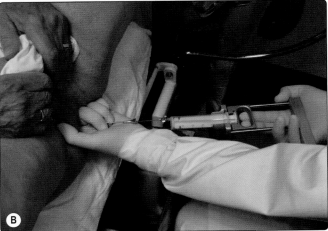

Fig. 13.1 t-FNA of the prostate (A) The Franzén guide fitted to the left index finger covered with a finger cot; (B) Performing a tFNA of the prostate.

yield suggests carcinoma; a drop of blood-tinged fluid with particulate material suggests hyperplasia; hemorrhagic yield indicates that the needle is out of the prostate; a 'non-representative' smear obtained by a dexterous operator suggests stromal hyperplasia; abundant fluid suggests either urine or a cyst.

The importance of proficient training in smearing and distributing the yield onto several slides cannot be overemphasised (see Chapter 2). The three-step smearing technique is recommended for fluid yields in order to concentrate solid fragments into two bands. The yield is suitable for molecular studies.

Cytological findings

Benign prostatic hyperplasia (BPH)
(Fig. 13.2)[4,5,34,36,37,39]

> **CRITERIA FOR DIAGNOSIS**
>
> ◆ A watery aspirate with particulate material,
> ◆ Monolayered sheets of glandular epithelial cells,
> ◆ Distinct cell membranes; low N:C ratio,
> ◆ Evenly distributed, uniform, rounded nuclei; bland granular chromatin,
> ◆ Tiny nucleoli/chromocenters,
> ◆ Coarse intracytoplasmic granules (variable).

Cohesive monolayered sheets of glandular epithelial cells can be quite large with distinct boundaries; most cells are seen on end and appear polygonal with centrally placed nuclei. The abundant pale cytoplasm and the distinct cell membranes give the sheet a honeycomb appearance (Fig. 13.2A,B). Only at the periphery are some cells seen in profile as columnar.

The main criteria of benignity are the uniform distribution of nuclei within monolayered sheets, distinct cell membranes, low N:C ratio and intracytoplasmic secretory granules (Fig. 13.2A). The granules stain dark magenta with DQ but are less conspicuous in alcohol-fixed Pap-stained smears.

Although granules are not present in all benign epithelial cells, they are rarely present in carcinoma cells and absent in epithelial cells from rectal mucosa.

Other common findings in smears of BPH are: inflammatory cells, macrophages, metaplastic squamous epithelial cells, clumps of condensed secretion, fragments of calculi and corpora amylacea. Tiny fragments of stromal smooth muscle tissue are sometimes seen. Cytologic features of the central zone have been described in scrape smears of surgical specimens.[40]

Prostatitis (Figs 13.3 and 13.4)[4,36,37,39]

> **CRITERIA FOR DIAGNOSIS**
>
> ◆ Many inflammatory cells: polymorphs, lymphocytes and macrophages,
> ◆ Mild epithelial atypia.

Mild epithelial atypia is acceptable in the presence of significant inflammation (Fig. 13.3). The distribution of cells in epithelial sheets may be less regular than normal and the cell membranes less distinct. Nuclei may be mildly enlarged

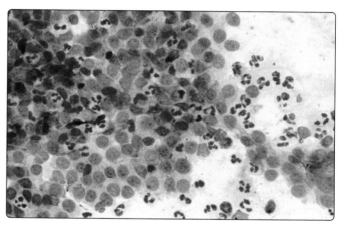

Fig. 13.3 Prostatitis (acute) Irregular epithelial sheet with mildly enlarged nuclei; background of neutrophils (DQ, HP).

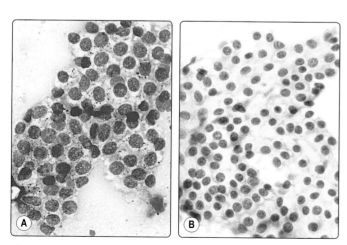

Fig. 13.2 Prostate, benign hyperplasia Honeycomb-like sheets of uniform glandular epithelial cells; note visible cell borders and coarse cytoplasmic granules in **A** (**A**, DQ; **B**, Pap, HP).

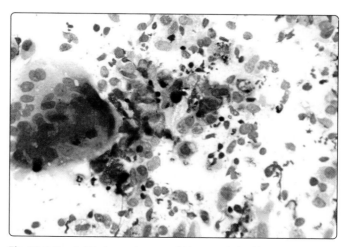

Fig. 13.4 Prostatitis (granulomatous) Many epithelioid histiocytes, multinucleated giant cell with phagocytosed secretion; many neutrophils (DQ, IP).

and varying in size. Cytoplasmic granules are often absent, while degenerative changes such as cytoplasmic vacuolation are often seen. However, prominent nuclear enlargement and pleomorphism, nucleolar enlargement and chromatin abnormalities do not occur. There is little tendency to dissociation of epithelial sheets, and microacini are not seen. As inflammation may coexist with carcinoma, epithelial atypia must be carefully evaluated. We require the presence of epithelial sheets encrusted with polymorphonuclears to arrive at the diagnosis of acute prostatitis.

Granulomatous prostatitis (Fig. 13.4)[36,37,39] remains a diagnostic dilemma since both clinical and cytological findings may mimic carcinoma. The cytological diagnosis of non-specific granulomatous prostatitis or tuberculous prostatitis, respectively, is based on the presence of epithelioid granulomas or obvious caseous necrosis. Nuclear overlapping, anisonucleosis, occasionally striking atypia, naked nuclei and some acinar formation may result in a false-positive diagnosis. Epithelial atypical cells in granulomatous prostatitis show a typical basophilia in DQ-stained smears; this basophilia is not seen in prostate carcinoma cells.

The diagnostic challenges posed by epithelioid aggregates and reactive changes in both duct/acinar and metaplastic cells have been discussed elsewhere.[8]

The cytological findings in *malacoplakia* of the prostate by FNA have been described.[41]

Adenocarcinoma of prostate
(Figs 13.5–13.8)[4,5,27,34,36,37,39]

CRITERIA FOR DIAGNOSIS

- ◆ Cell-rich smears (if derived from a solid carcinoma nodule),
- ◆ Decreased cell cohesion, variable numbers of single cells,
- ◆ Three-dimensional clusters, microacini,
- ◆ Interconnected large mono- or bilayered sheets with honeycomb pattern (well-differentiated carcinoma),
- ◆ Indistinct cell membranes; high N:C ratio,
- ◆ Nuclear and nucleolar enlargement; variable pleomorphism,
- ◆ Intracytoplasmic granules only rarely present,
- ◆ Positive staining for PSA and/or PSAP, absence of cytokeratin-positive basal cells.

In smears of prostatic carcinoma, sheets of benign glandular epithelial cells are commonly seen side-by-side with aggregates of malignant cells (Fig. 13.6), reflecting the diffusely infiltrative growth of the tumor. Benign and malignant cells can be directly compared (very helpful clue) and differences in cytoarchitectural features are easily appreciated. Nuclear enlargement is one of the most important criteria of malignancy. Nucleolar enlargement is better demonstrated in Pap-stained smears.

Absence of visible cell membranes, nuclear crowding and overlapping and dissociation of cells are other important criteria. The presence of coarse intracytoplasmic secretory granules makes malignancy unlikely, but they can occasionally be found in cells from well-differentiated adenocarcinoma. Cytoplasmic vacuolation may be seen in both benign and malignant cells. Nuclear pleomorphism and chromatin abnormalities are obvious in less well-differentiated cancers but may be subtle in well-differentiated carcinomas, render-

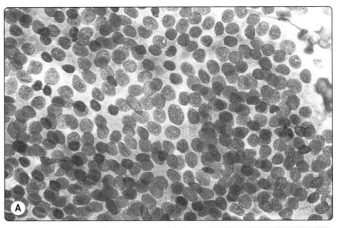

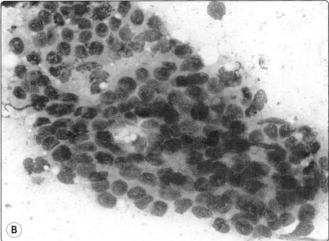

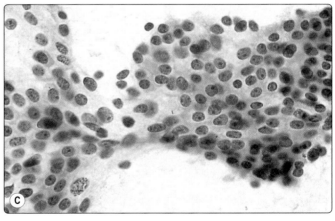

Fig. 13.5 Well-differentiated adenocarcinoma Cohesive sheets of atypical glandular epithelium; mild nuclear enlargement and anisokaryosis; crowding of nuclei; absence of cytoplasmic granules. Note microacinar pattern in **B** and prominent nucleoli and a mitotic figure in **C** (A and B, DQ; C, Pap, HP).

ing a definitive malignant diagnosis difficult (Fig. 13.5). Demonstration of basal epithelial cells by immunocytochemistry may be of help in the distinction between well-differentiated adenocarcinoma and adenosis or basal cell hyperplasia,[5] but interpretation is more difficult than in histologic sections. Immunostaining is a useful tool for the diagnosis of prostate cancer at metastatic sites.[42] Results may

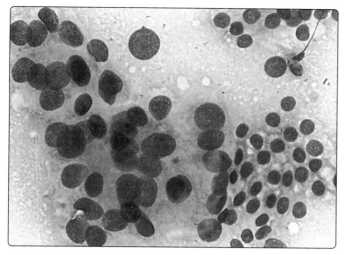

Fig. 13.6 Moderately-differentiated adenocarcinoma Aggregate of malignant cells; marked nuclear enlargement and nuclear pleomorphism; nuclear crowding; microacinar pattern: indistinct cell borders. Note contrasting honeycomb sheet of benign epithelium (DQ, HP).

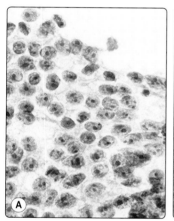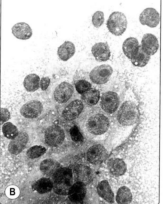

Fig. 13.7 Moderately-differentiated adenocarcinoma Cellular smears of less cohesive malignant glandular epithelial cells; vesicular nuclei; prominent nucleoli. Note fragile vacuolated cytoplasm suggestive of a clear cell pattern in **B** (**A**, Pap; **B**, DQ, HP).

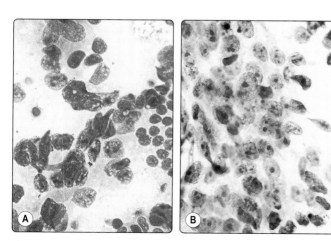

Fig. 13.8 Poorly-differentiated adenocarcinoma Poorly cohesive malignant cells with large vesicular malignant nuclei and large nucleoli. Note small sheet of benign epithelium on right in **A** (**A**, DQ; **B**, Pap, HP).

be conflicting in metastases of poorly differentiated carcinomas.

If only a small number of atypical cells are found in a predominantly benign cell population, great caution should be observed in making a definitive diagnosis of malignancy. Sources of atypical cells have been referred to elsewhere.[4,5,8,9] In case of doubt, the patient should be submitted to systematic TNCB taken according to a standardized protocol.

Regarding cytological grading of prostatic adenocarcinoma, see below and Figures 13.5 to 13.8.

PROBLEMS AND DIFFERENTIAL DIAGNOSIS

◆ Suboptimal aspirates (few diagnostic cells, poor smearing and/or staining),
◆ Basal cell hyperplasia,
◆ Well-differentiated carcinoma and high-grade prostatic intraepithelial neoplasia (PIN),
◆ Contamination by rectal mucosa,
◆ Seminal vesicular epithelium,
◆ Transitional cell carcinoma invading the prostate,
◆ Prostatic duct adenocarcinoma,
◆ Ganglion cells,
◆ Tight clusters of atrophic epithelium.

Not infrequently, smears from BPH contain a few cohesive aggregates of cells with frank atypia that may represent PIN, basal cell or atypical hyperplasia, and can be mistaken for malignancy (Figs 13.9 and 13.10). However, they fall short of clear-cut criteria of malignancy; cell cohesion is maintained and microacini are rarely seen. The atypical cells usually constitute only a minor proportion of the cell population. The presence of nucleolar enlargement in some cells should not lead to the diagnosis of carcinoma since they may correspond to focal atypical hyperplasia.

PIN should not be diagnosed by tFNA alone.[28] We use the term 'atypical cells' when the atypia and cellularity are below the requirements needed to reach a confident diagnosis of malignancy, and submit the patient for systematic TNCB. Histology of these cases almost always reveals either high-

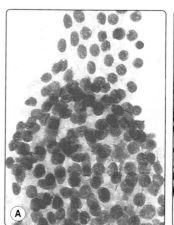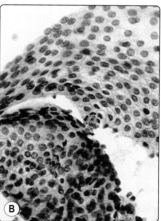

Fig. 13.9 Basal cell (atypical) hyperplasia Sheets of glandular epithelial cells showing mild nuclear enlargement and nuclear crowding contrasting with normal epithelium (**A**, DQ; **B**, Pap, HP).

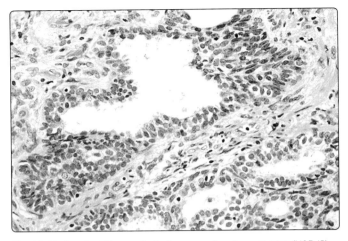

Fig. 13.10 Basal cell hyperplasia Corresponding tissue section (H&E, IP).

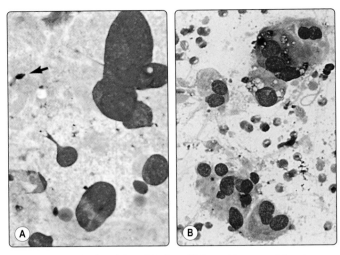

Fig. 13.12 Seminal vesicle epithelium (A) Large bizarre nuclei; note occasional spermatozoa in the background (*arrow*) (DQ, HP); (B) Single epithelial cells with large pleomorphic nuclei; note coarse intracytoplasmic pigment (DQ, HP).

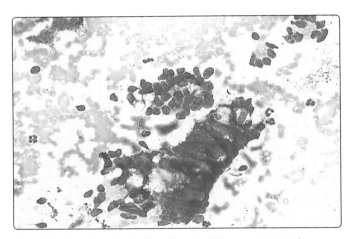

Fig. 13.11 Rectal contamination Microglandular aggregates and palisading columnar epithelial cells; some mucin (DQ, IP).

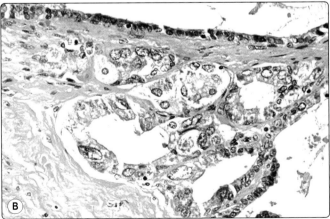

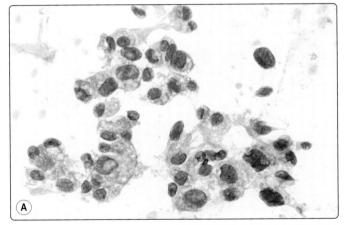

Fig. 13.13 Seminal vesicle epithelium (A) Vaguely glandular aggregates of epithelial cells with pleomorphic and hyperchromatic nuclei; abundant cytoplasm with vacuoles and brown pigment granules (Pap, HP); (B) Corresponding tissue section (H&E, HP).

grade PIN or low-grade carcinoma. Pathologists should refrain from making a definitive diagnosis of malignancy when the smears contain only a small proportion of cells with malignant features.

Contamination of samples by epithelial cells from the *rectal mucosa* is common when tFNA is performed by an inexperienced operator.[36,37] Isolated tall cylindrical cells, palisaded rows, glandular structures and goblet cells intermingled with mucin and rectal content indicate rectal mucosal origin. Rectal cells lack intracytoplasmic granules (Fig. 13.11).

Inadvertent aspiration of the *seminal vesicle* may yield large atypical cells that may mislead the unwary into an erroneous diagnosis of poorly differentiated carcinoma. Large hyperchromatic, often multilobated, pleomorphic, even bizarre, nuclei are seen.[9,36,37] Coarse intracytoplasmic granules of lipofuscin, which stain dark green–blue with DQ, brown with Pap or H&E, quite different from the secretory granules of prostate epithelium (Figs 13.12 and 13.13), dense aggregates of basophilic amorphous material and spermatozoa in the background indicate origin from seminal vesicle.

Ganglion cells may mimic malignant cells (Fig. 13.14).[9]

The differential diagnosis between prostatic adenocarcinoma and transitional cell carcinoma is discussed below.

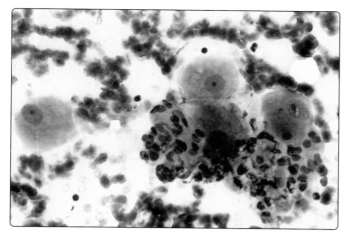

Fig. 13.14 Ganglion cells Three large ganglion cells with prominent nucleoli next to a cluster of malignant cells. Notice a malignant acinus at the bottom-right corner. (DQ IP).

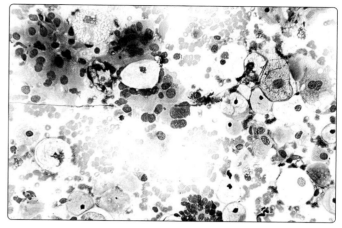

Fig. 13.15 Prostate, hormonal effect Metaplastic squamous cells; large glycogenized cells and clusters of epithelial cells, some with enlarged nuclei. Hormonal response in confirmed prostatic adenocarcinoma (DQ, IP).

Pitfalls and infrequent findings in prostate aspirates, a list of benign conditions mimicking carcinoma and clues to diagnosis have been published elsewhere.[9]

Grading of adenocarcinoma[4,5,27,34,36,37,39]

The cytologic presentation is related to the tumor grade. Three grades are recognized.[27] Differentiation may vary within the same tumor. Grading is decided by the most malignant pattern seen in available smears, which may not be representative of the whole tumor. Although the correlation between cytological grade and survival has been shown to be very good in a large series of cases,[27] most urologists require Gleason grading based on systematic TNCB taken according to a standardized protocol if RP is considered.

Well-differentiated carcinoma may go unnoticed if normal epithelial cells are not present for comparison. The number of cells aspirated tends to be much greater than in samples of BPH, and the amount of background secretion is less. High cellularity on its own may raise a suspicion of malignancy and suggests further investigation by systematic TNCB and serum PSA.

Well-differentiated carcinoma (Fig. 13.5)

- Malignant microacini: abundant ill-defined cytoplasm occupying the central zone encircled by a crown of nuclei. Microacini vary noticeably in size and shape. The high frequency of microacini is one of the most important diagnostic criteria,[36]
- Mono- and bilayered large interconnected strands of epithelium,
- Few single cells,
- Mild anisonucleosis,
- Mild hyperchromasia,
- Mild or even absent nuclear atypia,
- Inconspicuous nucleoli (Pap enhances nucleoli).

Moderately-differentiated carcinoma (Figs 13.6, 13.7)

- Microacini showing frank nuclear atypia,
- Frequent obviously malignant irregular three-dimensional clusters,
- Nuclear hyperchromasia,
- Conspicuous nucleoli,

- Some dissociated well-preserved malignant cells,
- The smear may be overrun by malignant irregular three-dimensional clusters.

Poorly-differentiated carcinoma (Fig. 13.8)

- Malignant irregular three-dimensional clusters and numerous dissociated cells,
- Obvious increase of N:C ratio,
- Large nuclei and nucleoli,
- Intense hyperchromasia,
- Rare or absent microacini with frank atypia,
- Dispersed cells or naked nuclei may dominate the smear. Nuclei may be smudged. Caveat: do not mistake for high-grade lymphoma.

Effects of hormonal treatment and radiotherapy (Fig. 13.15)[9,27,31,36,37,39]

CRITERIA FOR DIAGNOSIS

- ◆ Squamous metaplasia,
- ◆ Large cells with abundant transparent cytoplasm resembling a fried egg ('glycogen cells'),
- ◆ Nuclear pyknosis,
- ◆ Loss of nucleoli,
- ◆ Nuclear shrinkage,
- ◆ Well-preserved malignant cells may persist associated with squamous metaplasia or 'glycogen cells'.

Transitional cell carcinoma (Figs 13.16 and 13.17)[9,37]

CRITERIA FOR DIAGNOSIS

- ◆ Cells single and in clusters with no distinct microarchitectural pattern.
- ◆ Moderate amount of dense cytoplasm with well-defined borders; eccentric nuclei.
- ◆ Pleomorphic, hyperchromatic nuclei; nucleoli variable.
- ◆ Nuclear chromatin coarse and irregular, varies from cell to cell.
- ◆ Negative immunostaining for PSA and PSAP.

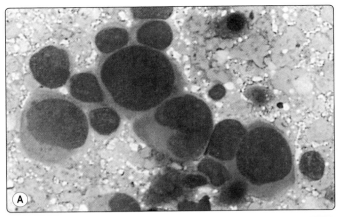

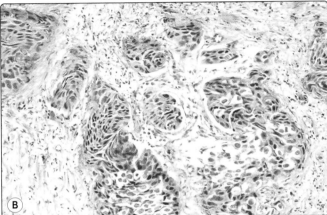

Fig. 13.16 Transitional cell carcinoma (A) Pleomorphic malignant cells; hyperchromatic eccentric nuclei; dense cytoplasm (tFNA of prostate; DQ, HP); (B) Corresponding tissue section of transitional cell carcinoma invading the prostate (H&E, IP).

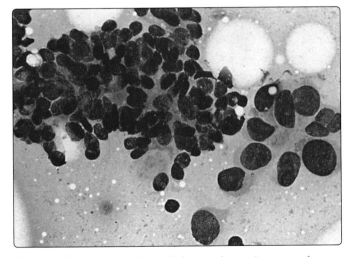

Fig. 13.17 Combined transitional/adenocarcinoma Aggregate of well-differentiated adenocarcinoma with nuclear crowding and microacinar pattern; adjacent group of larger, more pleomorphic malignant transitional cells (DQ, HP).

Transitional cell carcinoma may invade the prostate from the urinary bladder or it may arise from periurethral ducts within the prostate itself. Coexistence of transitional cell carcinoma and adenocarcinoma of the prostate is not rare (Fig. 13.17). It is important to distinguish transitional cell carcinoma

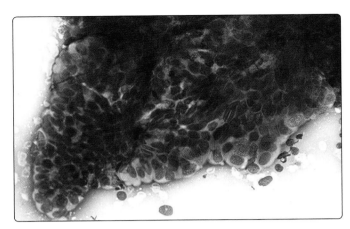

Fig. 13.18 Ductal cell adenocarcinoma A papillary cluster. Notice nuclear palisading and monomorphism (DQ, HP).

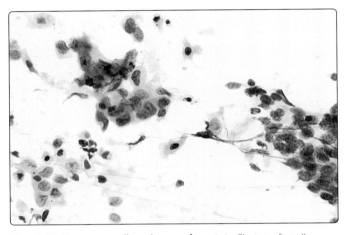

Fig. 13.19 Squamous cell carcinoma of prostate Clusters of small malignant cells, some showing squamous differentiation including a few orangeophilic cells (*center and upper left*) (Pap, IP).

from adenocarcinoma, since the former does not respond to hormonal treatment.

Transitional cell carcinomas involving the prostate are usually deeply invasive, high-grade tumors (see also Figs 12.29–12.31). Squamous differentiation is seen in some tumors, whereas papillary structures are rare.

PROBLEMS AND DIFFERENTIAL DIAGNOSIS

The distinction from prostatic adenocarcinoma is essential. Cells from a prostatic adenocarcinoma of comparable differentiation show a lesser degree of nuclear pleomorphism, the nuclei are paler, vesicular, and the cytoplasm is indistinct and fragile. The nuclei are also fragile and some are smudged. Microacini can nearly always be found in adenocarcinoma except in truly anaplastic tumors. Palisading at the periphery of cell aggregates from a transitional cell carcinoma should not be mistaken for glandular differentiation. Immunostaining for PSA, PSAP, 34βE12, Uroplakin III and p63 is helpful in difficult cases although interpretation may be troublesome.

Rare tumors of the prostate[9]

Cytologic descriptions and differential diagnoses of 'foamy cell carcinoma', prostatic ductal adenocarcinoma (papillary or endometrioid) (Fig. 13.18), mucinous (colloid), small cell carcinoma, squamous cell carcinoma (Fig. 13.19),

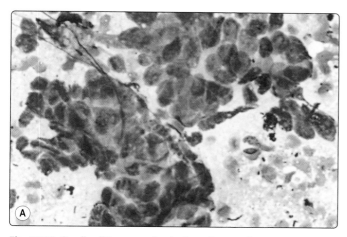

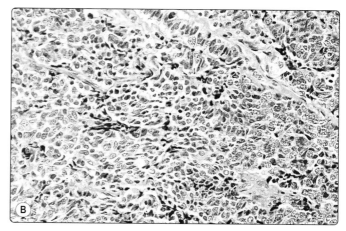

Fig. 13.20 Small cell (neuroendocrine) carcinoma of prostate (A) Clusters of malignant cells with a high N:C ratio and some nuclear molding (DQ, HP); (B) Tissue section, same case (H&E, IP). Immunostaining for chromogranin was positive.

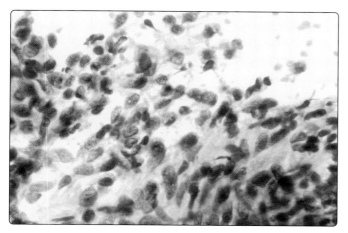

Fig. 13.21 Leiomyosarcoma of prostate Tissue fragment of moderately pleomorphic spindle cells with eosinophilic cytoplasm; some loss of cell cohesion (H&E, HP).

metastatic solid tumors within the prostate, and mesenchymal tumors have been described elsewhere.[9] The differential diagnosis between ductal cell carcinoma, prostatic adenocarcinoma and transitional cell carcinoma has been discussed. Nuclear grooves are a helpful clue for diagnosis of ductal cell carcinoma.[43]

A morphologic and immunohistochemical study of small cell carcinomas of the prostate has been published.[44] The cytological pattern is similar to small cell tumors in other sites (Fig. 13.20). A review of *adenoid cystic/basal cell carcinoma* of the prostate has been reported.[45] We are not aware of any report of cytological findings of this tumor.

Rarely, *lymphomas* may involve the prostate and cause enlargement and clinical symptoms. This could be mistaken for small-cell or anaplastic carcinoma in smears. The diagnosis can be confirmed by immunostaining.

Sarcomas of the prostate are rare. These are mainly rhabdomyosarcomas in children, leiomyosarcomas (Fig. 13.21) or fibrosarcomas in adults (see Chapter 15).[9,46]

Testis

Clinical aspects

The place of FNA in the investigative sequence

Pathologists attempting cytological diagnosis of testicular masses must be fully conversant with the WHO classification of tumors of the testis[12] and with the bewildering patterns shown by these tumors.[12,47–49] This is also essential in the proficient identification of extragonadal germ cell tumors, primary and metastatic, in FNA samples.[50–56] FNA sampling and subsequent microscopy should ideally be performed by the same pathologist to enable cytological interpretation in the light of clinical findings.[14,18]

In our hospital, after clinical examination by the urologist, the patient is referred to the clinical cytology unit. The pathologist explains the procedure and obtains a written consent from the patient. A provisional diagnosis of benign or malignant, and if malignant of seminoma versus nonseminoma, is provided to the urologist on site. The whole procedure takes less than 30 minutes. In case of malignancy, orchidectomy follows 3–7 days after diagnosis. Rapid feedback to the urologist is essential.

FNA does not replace histological diagnosis. The aim is mainly to provide a triage of cases of testicular swelling into those who do not require surgery as the first-choice treatment and those who do.[14] Seminoma represents about 50% of TGCT and 40–45% of all testicular neoplasms.[48] This means that familiarity with the cytologic patterns of seminoma enables the pathologist to identify about 50% of TGCT in FNA samples.

Accuracy of diagnosis

The experience of cytologic features of germ cell tumors (GCT), primary and metastatic, accrued over two decades, permits not only a confident diagnosis of malignancy but also correct tumor typing in most cases.[14,50–66] The proper use of FNA of testicular masses reduces the need for surgery considerably.[21,58–61] Gupta et al.[20] underlined the role of FNA in the differential diagnosis of epididymal nodules, avoiding surgical biopsy and other investigations. See also Chapter 12 in the monograph by Linsk and Franzén,[65] and Chapter 4 in that by Zajicek.[66]

Limitations of FNA of testicular tumors are:[14]

- Samples may be inadequate (insufficient diagnostic cells),
- Samples may not be fully representative particularly in large mixed TGCT,
- Cytologic training and experience in this area may be inadequate.

A few additional specific problems should be emphasized:

- The pleomorphism seen in smears of normal testis could be mistaken for TGCT or lymphoma.
- A careful search for concealed diagnostic cells in the presence of necrosis and hemorrhage is mandatory.
- Intrascrotal fluid may conceal a tumor. The testicle must be re-examined after evacuation of fluid from a hydrocele or hematocele.[14]

Complications

Fine needle aspiration may be painful in benign conditions and in fertility studies. The pain usually irradiates to the homolateral inguinal zone. It subsides in an hour and can be relieved by painkillers. FNA of malignant conditions and acute scrotum syndrome is almost painless. We have seen microscopic hemorrhage and necrosis in the subsequent surgical specimen, possibly caused by the needle, but this has never prevented histological diagnosis.

The only contraindication to testicular FNA mentioned in the literature is acute orchitis accompanied by cellulitis of the scrotum.[65]

Tumor seeding in the needle track has not been recorded in a number of studies.[58,65–67] Tumor stage (TNM) was not modified following FNA in a series of malignant testicular tumors.[61] In our experience of more than 120 TGCT with 5–10 years' follow-up, there has been no evidence of dissemination caused by FNA. The benefit of a rapid and reliable diagnosis of malignancy outweighs the unproven risk of dissemination.

Technical considerations

We do not use local anesthesia for testicular FNA. Infiltration of the spermatic cord has been advocated in sequential aspirations for the evaluation of male infertility and for sperm retrieval.[68] We use 25-gauge needles, only exceptionally 23 gauge, and only one or two biopsies with one or two passes each time. US guidance may be helpful in partly cystic tumors, in non palpable US-detected lesions, in cases of retroperitoneal GCT (burnt-out TCGT), and in the follow-up of patients with lymphoma or leukemia.

Adequate training and experience in performing FNA and handling of samples is of paramount importance (see Chapter 2). Some points are of particular importance in testicular tumors. It is essential that the needle remains within the target during aspiration and that the negative pressure is released before withdrawing the needle. Smear pressure must be carefully balanced to avoid crush artifacts, particularly in seminoma. Bloody samples must be smeared quickly and are most often suboptimal.

Gross examination of the samples at smearing often gives valuable hints to the nature of the target lesion (author's unpublished results). We strongly recommend the parallel use of DQ and Pap staining, but DQ takes preference over Pap stain. We do not use immunocytochemistry routinely in FNA of suspected testicular tumors. We believe that its use exceeds the basic aim of FNA in this field: a triage separating benign from malignant lesions. However, immunostaining for OCT 3/4, EMA, AE1/AE3, S-100, and appropriate lymphoid markers is useful to establish germ cell origin for a metastatic poorly differentiated neoplasm in a young man because of the potential for specific curative chemotherapy.[69] Immunostaining for PLAP has been used in an attempt to detect noninvasive testicular cancer in cryptorchid men.[70]

Cytological findings

The non-neoplastic testis (Figs 13.22 and 13.23)

Smears from normal testicular tissue contain cells which represent all stages of spermiogenesis, from spermatogonia to spermatozoa, in varying proportions. Spermatozoa and late spermatids are easily recognized by the nuclear size,

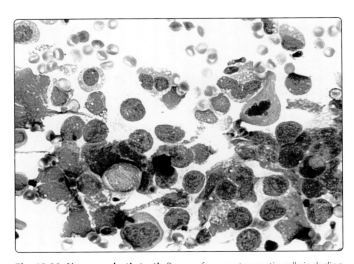

Fig. 13.22 Non-neoplastic testis Range of spermatogenetic cells including a few mature sperms; note resemblance to lymphoid cells (DQ HP).

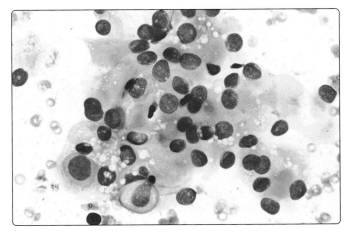

Fig. 13.23 Sertoli cells Clustered cells with abundant cytoplasm, some vacuolation, and indistinct cell borders (DQ, HP).

shape and hyperchromasia, whereas the less mature forms resemble lymphoid cells of blastic type, particularly in air-dried DQ-stained smears (Fig. 13.22). Dark and pale spermatogonia can be recognized by their chromatin density, primary spermatocytes in pachytene; the latter are larger and have easily discernible thick, long chromatin threads frequently parallel to each other. Normal spermiogenesis must not be mistaken for lymphoma or TCGT. The presence of normal spermiogenesis excludes neoplasia, unless the target has been missed.

Sertoli cells, single or in groups, are easily identified, particularly in smears from atrophic testicular tissue. Sertoli cells have pale, round nuclei, prominent nucleoli and abundant, relatively dense, vacuolated cytoplasm with indistinct borders. They often appear as naked nuclei (Fig. 13.23). Sertoli cells predominate in infancy, cryptorchidism, cirrhosis, infections and following hormonal blockage for prostate cancer. In 'Sertoli cell only syndrome' there is a complete absence of the germinal line; this condition cannot be distinguished from diffuse severe atrophy.

Leydig cells are difficult to recognize in FNA smears of normal testis regardless of the staining method. Nuclei are perfectly round and characteristically have one or two eccentric nucleoli. The chromatin pattern is denser than that of Sertoli cells, and the cytoplasm is better defined, dense eosinophilic and granular. Reinke's crystals are difficult to spot except in Leydig cell tumors.[71] Leydig cells predominate in aspirates from patients with Klinefelter's syndrome. In the appropriate clinical setting, this diagnosis is suggested if smears show abundant Leydig cells and connective tissue strands and absence of cells of germ lineage.

Detailed accounts of the cytology of spermatogenesis as seen in FNA smears were published more than two decades ago.[72,73] FNA has achieved great popularity in India and Middle Eastern countries for the study of male infertility.[21–23,74–77] It has been used to locate areas of sperm production to guide sperm extraction procedures in men with non-obstructive azoospermia.[68,78] An interesting scheme for reporting FNA testicular biopsies has been proposed by Dajani.[75] See also Linsk & Franzen[65] and Zajicek.[66]

In *acute orchitis*.[60,65,66] the testicle is swollen and hard, and FNA is painful. Aspirates usually have abundant entangled fibrin threads, leukocytes, histiocytes, debris and fragments of necrotic seminiferous tubules. Chromatin threads may be found (Fig. 13.24).

Embryonal carcinoma, mixed TGCT and seminoma must be ruled out before making a diagnosis of acute orchitis.

Chronic orchitis[66] is a rare condition. Aspirates are scanty due to fibrosis. Lymphocytes, plasma cells, histiocytes and sparse polymorphs may be present.

Granulomatous orchitis[60,65,66] (Fig. 13.25) is usually cryptogenic but may be tuberculous or due to other infections. Aspirates resemble chronic orchitis but also include aggregates of epithelioid histiocytes and multinucleated giant cells. Caseous necrosis is frequently seen in tuberculous orchitis.

Tuberculous orchitis is almost always associated with tuberculous epididymitis, but isolated tuberculous epididymitis does occur. Increased consistency of a mobile epididymis does not suggest tumor, but an enlarged epididymis fixed to the testis as occurs in tuberculous epididymitis can mimic a tumor. Tuberculous orchitis can also mimic

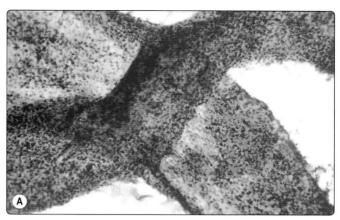

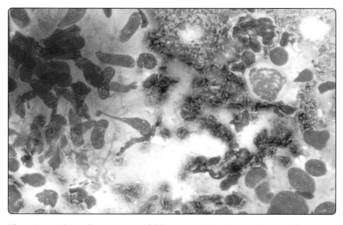

Fig. 13.24 Acute orchitis (**A**) Two intersected seminiferous tubules filled with necrotic and inflammatory cells; (**B**) Dirty background, naked nuclei of Sertoli cells, degenerate germinal cells (upper-right corner), tailless spermatozoa and debris (**A** Pap, LP; **B** DQ, HP).

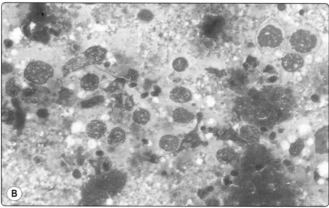

Fig. 13.25 Granulomatous orchitis An epithelioid granuloma (*left*). Notice a primary spermatocyte in the upper-right corner and reactive atypical nuclei at the lower-right corner. (DQ, HP)

testicular malignancy.[79] The correct diagnosis of tuberculous epididymitis and epididymo-orchitis may prevent unnecessary orchidectomy.[17,25,80]

Chronic and granulomatous orchitis must be distinguished from seminoma. Eighty per cent of seminomas contain lymphocytic infiltrates and 50% contain epithelioid granulomas.[66] Seminoma may present with a clinical history suggestive of chronic orchitis.[66] Seminoma must be ruled out

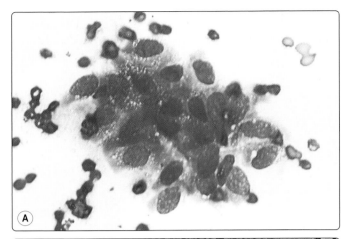

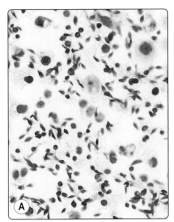

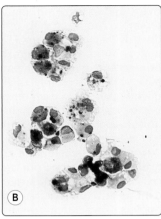

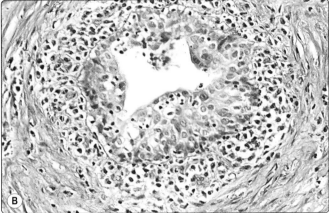

Fig. 13.27 Testicular/epididymal cysts (A) Spermatocele. Numerous sperms, some nucleated cells, probably sperm precursor cells (Pap, IP). (B) Hydrocele. Clusters of vacuolated and pigmented macrophages (MGG, IP);

Fig. 13.26 Chronic epididymitis (A) Cluster of atypical, somewhat degenerate epithelial cells and inflammatory cells (MGG, HP); (B) Corresponding tissue section (H&E, IP).

whenever smears contain abundant lymphocytes or epithelioid cells. In our experience, the differential diagnosis between granulomatous orchitis, seminoma and non-Hodgkin lymphoma is easier cytologically than in tissue sections. Spermatic granuloma also enters the differential diagnosis in granulomatous lesions.[81]

Epididymitis[60,66] FNA smears from acute and chronic epididymitis are dominated by inflammatory cells intermingled with sparse epididymal cells, single or forming monolayered sheets. Quite atypical-looking cells may be found, probably representing regenerative atypia (Fig. 13.26). Surgical exploration may be inevitable if the lesion cannot be clearly separated from the testis clinically or radiologically. Tuberculosis should always be considered in epididymal lesions with or without testicular enlargement (see above). FNA provides adequate material for both cytologic and microbiologic examination and avoids orchidectomy.[25] We amplify by PCR the highly conserved IS6110 genomic sequence for the identification of *Mycobacterium tuberculosis* species.

The role of FNA in the diagnosis of epididymal nodules has been discussed by Gupta et al.[20]

Miscellaneous

Hydrocele[60,65] usually presents as a concentric swelling. The aspirate is pale or dark amber. A pale aspirate is sparsely cellular of just a few mesothelial cells and lymphocytes. A dark amber sample contains numerous cells including polymorphs, typical and reactive mesothelial cells singly or forming three-dimensional balls, histiocytes and debris (Fig. 13.27B) representing a hydrocele of long evolution. If numerous three-dimensional balls with spherical or scalloped borders are seen, a mesothelioma of the tunica vaginalis should be considered. Japko et al. gave the first description of the cytology of malignant mesothelioma of the tunica vaginalis in hydrocele fluid.[82]

Hematocele[60,65] aspirates are hemorrhagic and bright or dark red in color. A bright aspirate contains preserved erythrocytes, a dark aspirate lysed erythrocytes and hemosiderophages. Hematoceles are generally secondary to problems of venous drainage, coagulation disorders, or to trauma. The possibility of underlying neoplasia must always be considered and the testis reexamined after evacuation of the fluid with repeat FNA in case of doubt.[66]

Spermatocele is usually peripheral and may mimic a tumor. The aspirate is typically milky and the presence of numerous immobile spermatozoids, balls of spermatozoids, histiocytes, spermiophages and some monolayered sheets of epididymal cells allows a confident diagnosis (Fig. 13.27A). A spermatocele can often be completely evacuated by FNA, leaving no residual lesion. FNA is both diagnostic and therapeutic in hydroceles, hematoceles and spermatoceles.[60]

Scrotal hernia presents as a scrotal tumor with negative transillumination. Aspirates contain clusters of typical or reactive mesothelial cells and fibroadipose tissue. Mucosecretory epithelium is usually not seen since the needle generally only penetrates as far as the pre-hernial lipoma. The possibility of teratoma must be considered if mucous and intestinal epithelium is aspirated.[60]

Spontaneous spermatic cord torsion and testicular trauma[60] account for an increasing number of consultations. Cytological findings are very similar. FNA is completely painless and aspirates consist of blood in variable quantity and state of preservation, cell debris and ghost germinal cells. Fragments of necrotic seminiferous tubules may be seen (Fig. 13.28A,B).

Spermatic granuloma smears show inflammatory cells and tailless spermatozoids, epithelioid granulomas and

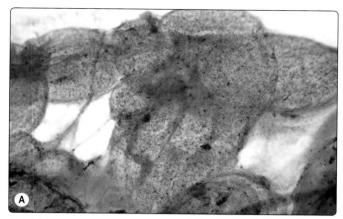

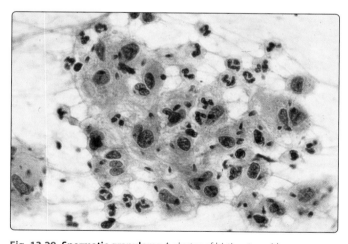

Fig. 13.28 **Acute torsion** (A) A twisted seminiferous tubule filled with debris. (Pap, LP); (B) A cast of a seminiferous tubule with ghost cells (DQ, IP).

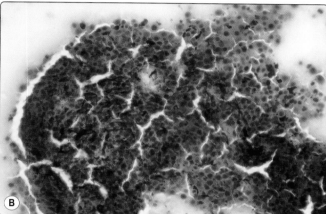

Fig. 13.29 **Spermatic granuloma** A cluster of histiocytes with phagocytosed spermatozoa (Pap, HP).

macrophages engulfing spermatozoids. Caseous necrosis is not seen. Neoplasia or benign tumor may be suspected clinically. The differential diagnosis has been discussed above (Fig. 13.29).[81]

Scrotal epidermal cysts are common, easily recognized on clinical examination. Smears show keratinized or non-keratinized squames, multinucleated foreign body giant cells, polymorphs and histiocytes.

Neoplasms[14,58–61,63,65,66]

The great majority of malignant testicular tumors are GCT. The cytologic features of TGCT described here are based on our personal experience on FNA of primary testicular tumors.

Since TGCT can include more than one component not all necessarily sampled by FNA, a definitive type-specific diagnosis is generally deferred to histological examination. Familiarity with the cytology of TGCT permits the recognition of extragonadal GCT, mainly in the mediastinum and retroperitoneum. The diagnosis is of great clinical importance since treatment and prognosis are different from that of other malignancies occurring in these sites. The diagnosis may be supported by immunostaining.[51,69] Note that spermiogenesis is not seen in satisfactory FNA samples of TGCT.

Detailed accounts of the utility and limitations of FNA at extragonadal sites and of cytologic features of extragonadal GCT have been published.[51,52]

Seminoma (Figs 13.30 and 13.31)[14,50,57–63,65,66]

CRITERIA FOR DIAGNOSIS

◆ Cell-rich smears,

◆ Dispersed cells, little tendency to clustering,

◆ Highly fragile cytoplasm and nuclei ('tigroid background' (TB) and nuclear trailing),

◆ Large rounded vesicular nuclei; distinct nucleoli, smaller than in embryonal carcinoma,

◆ Irregular chromatin with some clearing,

◆ Abundant fragile, pale/clear cytoplasm; some marginal vacuoles (punched-out vacuoles),

◆ Lymphocytes, plasma cells,

◆ Tangled chromatin threads (seminoma cells and lymphocytes),

◆ Some epithelioid histiocytes, epithelioid granulomas (variable),

◆ Striking contrast in size between seminoma cells and the background of lymphocytes and plasma cells.

◆ Immunocytochemistry: cells positive for PLAP, c-kit (CD117) and OCT 3/4, and negative for CD30, AE1/AE3, and CK7, CK8, CK18 and CK19, although focal pancytokeratin-positive cells may be seen.

Seminoma is a highly cellular neoplasm of poorly cohesive cells and little stroma. The presence of a lace-like tigroid background (TB), and the high cellularity including lymphocytes account for the intense navy-blue color of the smears. This may suggest the diagnosis even before microscopic study. Comments about the origin of TB and the distinction from 'lymphoglandular bodies' have been made elsewhere.[60] TB may go unnoticed in Pap-stained smears, but is more conspicuous in DQ smears (Fig. 13.30). A diagnosis of seminoma should not be based solely on the presence of TB or TB-like material. We have observed TB-like material also in aspirates of embryonal carcinoma. The contrary is also true: seminoma should not be ruled out simply because the pathologist is unable to identify TB.[14] Large seminomas may show prominent necrosis. Necrosis is a major cause of false negatives in testicular FNA.[59] Tumor giant cells or syncytiotrophoblastic cells may be seen in aspirates of seminoma, but can also be found in embryonal carcinoma, mixed TGCT and in trophoblastic tumors.

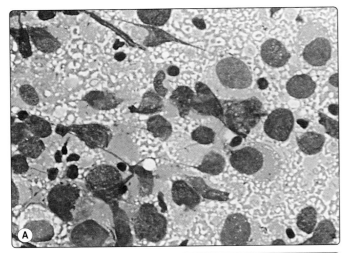

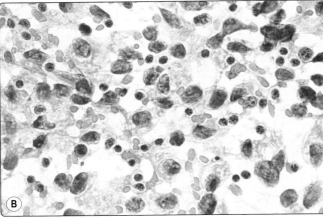

Fig. 13.30 Seminoma (A) Dispersed cells with large pale nuclei and poorly defined cytoplasm; note 'tigroid' background, smudged nuclei and small lymphocytes (MGG, HP); (B) Dispersed cells; moderately pleomorphic vesicular nuclei; single or multiple prominent nucleoli; many scattered lymphocytes (Pap, HP).

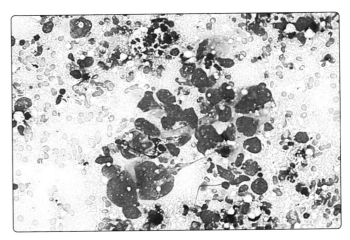

Fig. 13.31 Mediastinal seminoma Smear from large mediastinal mass clinically thought to be thymic carcinoma. Cluster of poorly cohesive, obviously malignant cells and some necrotic debris. Cytoplasmic vacuolation and nuclear fragility suggest malignant germ cell tumor; some lymphocytes present but specific typing not possible. Histology confirmed seminoma (MGG, HP).

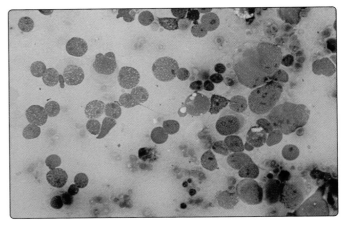

Fig. 13.32 Spermatocytic seminoma Note evident nuclear size variation, spireme chromatin (*half left side*) and absence of tigroid substance (DQ, HP).

The plasmatic membrane is well-defined in seminoma, but it is difficult to see in embryonal carcinoma. When lymphocytes, plasma cells, histiocytes and epithelioid granulomas are abundant and seminoma cells scarce, a diagnosis of granulomatous orchitis may be entertained: the absence of spermatozoids and of the germinal line suggest a seminoma.[60]

Chromatin trailing may be prominent, particularly if the sample was smeared vigorously. This artifact has no diagnostic value in itself, since it may occur also in embryonal carcinoma, yolk sac tumors, lymphomas and acute orchitis. When the smear is dominated by this artifact, and there are no acute inflammatory cells and no spermatogenesis, the pathologist must search carefully for preserved diagnostic cells. In this situation, a tentative diagnosis of seminoma may be made.[14]

Lymphocytes, plasma cells and even 'lymphoglandular bodies' may be prominent in smears of seminoma and may lead to an erroneous diagnosis of lymphoma. Lymphoblasts may also be mistaken for seminoma cells.

Familiarity with the cytology of testicular seminoma helps in the recognition of extragonadal seminoma and metastatic seminomas (Fig. 13.31). Immunostaining may be of help in doubtful cases.[69]

Seminomas with a greater degree of cellular pleomorphism, higher mitotic rate and scarce stromal lymphocytes have been called anaplastic seminoma or atypical seminoma.[12] These seminomas may be mistaken for embryonal carcinoma.[65]

Spermatocytic seminoma (Fig. 13.32)[14,64]

CRITERIA FOR DIAGNOSIS

◆ Cell-rich smears,
◆ Occasionally edematous background,
◆ PAS-negative tumor cells,
◆ Round cells showing noticeable pleomorphism: lymphocyte-like, intermediate-sized cells, and mono- or rarely multinucleated large cells,
◆ Some tumor cells display a filamentous or spireme chromatin pattern resembling spermatocytes,
◆ Frequent mitoses,
◆ Not seen: tigroid background, 'lymphoglandular bodies', epithelioid granulomas and necrosis.

Saran et al.[64] have listed the cytomorphological features that distinguish spermatocytic seminoma from classical seminoma. The markers useful in other TGCT are generally negative.[12]

Embryonal carcinoma
(Figs 13.33 and 13.34)[14,58–61,63,65,66]

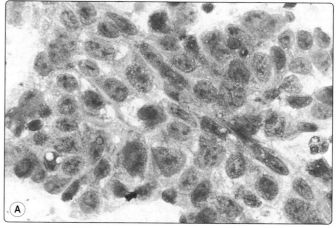

CRITERIA FOR DIAGNOSIS

◆ Cell-rich smears,
◆ Frequent three-dimensional clusters,
◆ Occasional tendency to acinar and microglandular grouping,
◆ Large vesicular, obviously malignant nuclei, large nucleoli,
◆ Indistinct cell borders,
◆ Basophilic to amphophilic, sometimes pale, vacuolated cytoplasm,
◆ Immunocytochemistry: cells positive for PLAP, OCT 3/4, CD30, AE1/AE3 and CK7.

The vesicular nuclei of embryonal carcinoma are larger and more pleomorphic than those of seminoma, the chromatin is coarse and irregular and nucleoli are large, occasionally huge, and eosinophilic. The cytoplasm is pale and distinctly vacuolated, but not 'bubbly'. It is not highly fragile and a TB as in seminoma is not seen. Cytoplasmic boundaries are poorly defined (Fig. 13.33). Hemorrhage and tumor necrosis may be prominent and may hamper the identification of diagnostic cells. It is usually not seen in smears of seminoma. Chromatin threads and reticulated material resembling TB can occur. Large syncytiotrophoblastic cells may be found. Prominent lymphoid/plasma cell infiltrates or mucus are not seen. The presence of cellular mesenchyme on its own does not warrant a designation of teratoma (Figs. 13.33B and 13.34).[49]

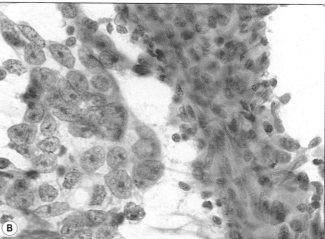

Fig. 13.33 Embryonal carcinoma (A) Adenocarcinoma-like tissue fragment of large malignant cells with large vesicular nuclei, coarse chromatin, prominent nucleoli; prominent cytoplasmic vacuolation (MGG, HP); (B) Fragment of undifferentiated mesenchymal tissue right; cluster of malignant epithelial cells with large vesicular nuclei and prominent large nucleoli (H&E, HP) left.

Tumors of more than one histologic type
(mixed forms) (Figs 13.35 and 13.36)[14,60,63,65]

While the basic GCT types are infrequent in pure forms they are very frequent in mixed forms. Embryonal carcinoma and teratoma are each present in 47% of cases, and yolk sac tumors in 41%; 40% of TGCT contain varying numbers of syncytiotrophoblastic cells.[12]

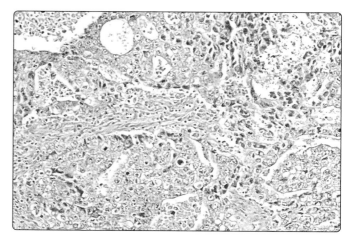

Fig.13.34 Embryonal carcinoma Tissue section corresponding to Fig. 13.33B (H&E, IP).

CRITERIA FOR DIAGNOSIS

◆ Cellular aspirates; necrosis and hemorrhage frequent,
◆ Three-dimensional clusters of epithelial malignant cells as described above
◆ Coexisting teratomatous structures represented by mature or immature tissues originating from one or more blastodermal leaf: fusiform naked nuclei embedded in a myxoid background resembling embryonal mesenchyme; islets of cartilage; sheets of epithelial cells, which may be squamous, ciliated or intestinal (with goblet cells); bundles of fusiform cells with blunt ends reminiscent of leiomyoma; tight clusters of deeply stained bare nuclei may correspond to primitive neuroectodermal tissue.

The diagnosis of mixed forms is simple when malignant elements of an epithelial nature coexist with clear-cut teratomatous structures. Necrosis may obscure the neoplastic cells and the teratomatous component may be only minor or even absent. This can be explained by its greater cohesion causing under-representation in FNA samples. As a result, the differential diagnosis between mixed TGCT and embryonal carcinoma is sometimes difficult or impossible.[14,59–61,65,66] The presence of multinucleated syncytial cells is not diagnostic of choriocarcinoma.

Yolk sac tumor (Figs 13.37 and 13.38)[14,53–56,59–61,63]

Most cytologic reports are based on FNA performed on metastatic sites. A detailed account of the morphologic spectrum of endodermal sinus tumor has been reported by Akhtar et al.[53]

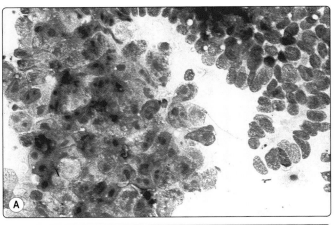

Fig. 13.35 Tumor of more than one histological type (mixed form) Large bisected tumor occupying most of the enlarged testicle in a male 19 years of age. Note hyalinized, degenerate and cystic areas.

CRITERIA FOR DIAGNOSIS

- ◆ Mucoid background,
- ◆ Glomeruloid structures,
- ◆ Schiller-Duval bodies (characteristic finding when present),
- ◆ Very immature cells, prominent nucleolus, basophilic cytoplasm,
- ◆ Small naked nuclei,
- ◆ Intra- or extracellular PAS-positive hyaline globules (AFP positive),
- ◆ Prominent cytoplasmic vacuoles and distinct cell boundaries confer a clear-cell appearance,
- ◆ Immunocytochemistry: focal staining for AFP, AE1/AE3 and PLAP; negative for OCT ¾.

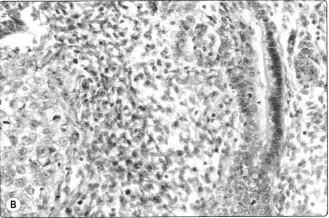

Fig. 13.36 Tumor of more than one histological type (mixed form) (A) Well-differentiated glandular epithelium (*right*), large malignant cells similar to embryonal carcinoma (*left*) (MGG, HP); (B) Corresponding tissue section (A, H&E, IP; B, PAP, IP).

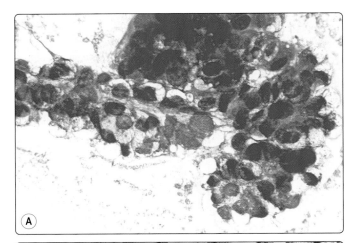

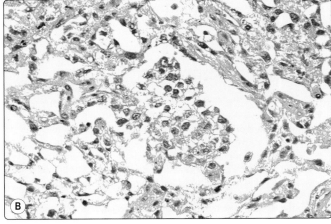

Fig. 13.37 Endodermal sinus tumor (A) Polypoid epithelial fragment of large malignant cells with pale, almost clear, vacuolated cytoplasm (MGG, HP); (B) Corresponding tissue section (H&E, IP).

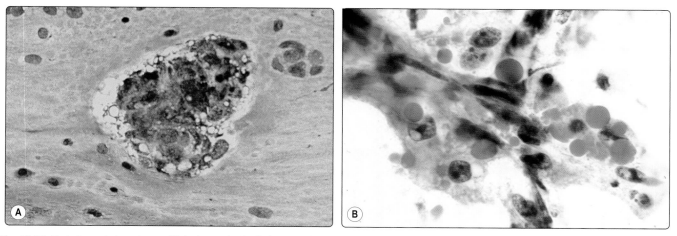

Fig. 13.38 Endodermal sinus tumor (A) A glomeruloid cell cluster with vacuolated cytoplasm on a mucoid background (DQ, IP); (B) Cell cluster with a vascular stalk and several hyaline globules.

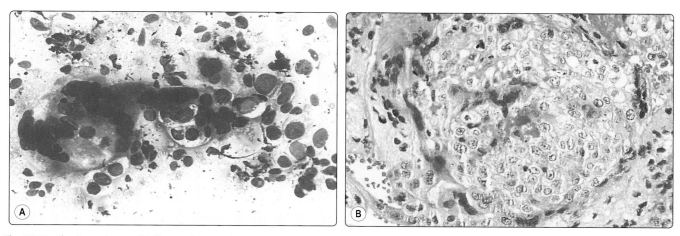

Fig. 13.39 Choriocarcinoma (A) Cluster of cytotrophoblastic and syncytiotrophoblastic cells (MGG, HP); (B) Corresponding tissue section (H&E, IP).

Pure yolk sac tumors are almost always encountered in infants and young children but rare in the first 6 months of life.[49] In adults, this pattern is seen in approximately 40% of nonseminomatous GCT;[12] however, it can easily be mistaken for embryonal carcinoma in FNA smears. This is why most reported cases are of metastatic tumors. Hyaline globules and eosinophilic membrane-like material are hints to the diagnosis of this tumor type (Fig. 13.38B). In infants and young children, the aforementioned cytological criteria permit a confident diagnosis by FNA.

Choriocarcinoma (Fig. 13.39)[59,63,66]

These tumors most commonly present with symptoms referable to metastases[12] and most FNA reports are of extratesticular metastases. Immunostaining for βHCG is helpful to identify syncytiotrophoblastic cells. Large syncytiotrophoblastic cells may also be aspirated from classical seminomas, embryonal carcinomas and mixed TGCT.

Teratoma (Fig. 13.40)[14,59,63,66]

CRITERIA FOR DIAGNOSIS

- ◆ Cells representing a variety of epithelial and mesenchymal tissues, which may be mature or immature,
- ◆ Mature components: epithelial sheets (keratinizing and non-keratinizing squamous, ciliated, intestinal), cartilage, leiomyomatous bundles (Fig. 13.40A),
- ◆ Immature components (fetal-like tissues): primitive mesenchymal tissue of tightly packed spindle cells with an eosinophilic stroma, fusiform naked nuclei in a myxoid background and syncytial clusters of round to oval naked nuclei resembling primitive neuroectoderm (Fig. 13.40B,C).

It is difficult to specify diagnostic criteria for this entity because of the variability of histologic patterns.[14,58] In our experience, the main problem is that small foci of embryonal carcinoma may be missed. Organising testicular infarction

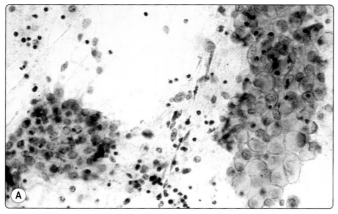

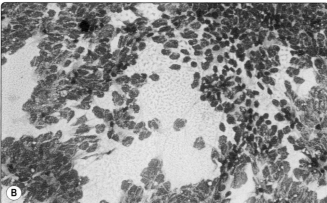

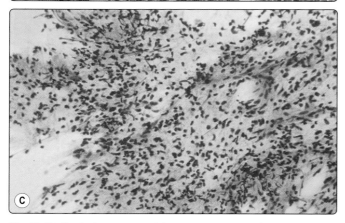

Fig. 13.40 Testicular teratoma (A) Mature components (squamous and mucus secretory) (Pap, IP); (B) Primitive neuroectoderm; (C) Immature mesenchyma (fetal-like tissue) (B,C; DQ, IP).

may lead the unwary to an erroneous diagnosis of teratoma.[14] If the needle samples a cystic component of a teratoma, acellular fluid may be obtained, resulting in a false-negative diagnosis. In such cases, the pathologist must reexamine the testis, and any persistent testicular mass must be rebiopsied.

The finding of palisading cylindrical cells and mucus should raise the possibility of a scrotal hernia and this diagnosis should be ruled out before making a diagnosis of mature teratoma. Readers are referred to the monograph by Zajicek[66] for descriptions of pure teratoma We reported the cytologic features in a case of epidermoid cyst.[83]

Sex cord-gonadal stromal tumors

Leydig cell tumor (Fig. 13.41)[60,61,66,71]

Numerous Leydig cells may also be obtained from testicles of patients with Klinefelter's syndrome and from the so-called testicular tumor of the adrenal genital syndrome, but the clinical setting is different.

The finding of intracytoplasmic lipofuscin pigment and several intracytoplasmic as well as intranuclear Reinke's crystals serve to clinch the diagnosis on FNA.[71] Cytologic features do not permit the separation of benign from malignant Leydig cell tumors.

Other sex cord-gonadal stromal tumors

The cytologic features of *Sertoli cell tumor*[61,66] and *juvenile granulosa cell tumor*[84] have been described.

Hematopoietic tumors

The clinicopathological features of *primary testicular and paratesticular lymphomas* have been described by Al-Abbadi et al.[85]

A malignant lymphoid infiltrate found in FNA of the testis raises three possibilities with different clinical implications: a terminal testicular leukemic or lymphomatous infiltration, the initial manifestation of a previously undiagnosed lymphoma, and a primary testicular lymphoma.

The distinction between testicular lymphoma, seminoma, embryonal carcinoma and granulomatous orchitis is easier in cytologic specimens than in tissue sections. Misinterpretation can occur, especially in cases presenting at an age similar to that for TGCT. Appropriate immunostaining may be of help.

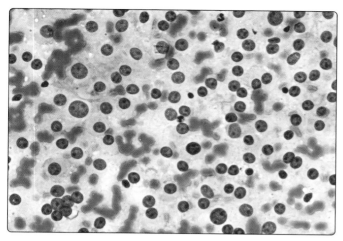

Fig. 13.41 **Leydig cell tumor of testis** Isolated naked nuclei with a prominent nucleolus, mild anisokaryosis. (DQ, HP).

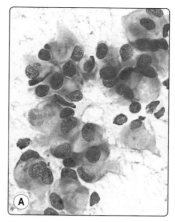
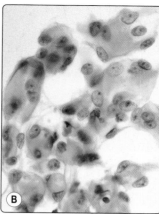

Fig. 13.42 **Adenomatoid tumor** Clusters of plump spindle cells resembling mesothelial cells; abundant well-defined cytoplasm; a few vacuoles; mild nuclear atypia (**A**, DQ; **B**, Pap, HP).

FNA has been used for early detection of *testicular involvement and relapse of acute lymphoblastic leukemia* in children.[86,87] Granulocytic sarcoma may involve the testis; only rarely has this entity been diagnosed by FNA.[88]

Secondary tumors of the testis

Rarely, *metastatic carcinoma* may simulate a primary testicular tumor. The origin of the cancer is most often in the lung or the prostate. We have seen a gastric signet ring cell carcinoma metastatic to the testis. A clinicopathological analysis of 26 cases has been recently published.[89]

Tumors of paratesticular structures

Adenomatoid tumor (Fig. 13.42)[90]

CRITERIA FOR DIAGNOSIS

- ◆ Pink, finely granular, or amorphous proteinaceous background,
- ◆ Moderate to abundant cellularity,
- ◆ Monolayered sheets, naked nuclei, well-defined multilayered clusters of small monotonous cells; vaguely glandular pattern occasionally,
- ◆ Abundant, poorly defined cytoplasm,
- ◆ Pink–clear paranuclear vacuoles,
- ◆ Intercellular windows visible but not prominent,
- ◆ Round to oval, eccentric nuclei; one small nucleolus; finely reticular, evenly distributed chromatin,
- ◆ Scanty stromal fragments.

The clinicocytologic presentation of adenomatoid tumors is unique and easily recognized by FNA cytology, which permits its differentiation from primary testicular neoplasms.[90] However, the diagnosis of adenomatoid tumor can be problematic in an atypical location as it may be mistaken for seminoma.[24]

Mesothelioma (Fig. 13.43)

We have studied two cases displaying cytological features similar to those found in pleural effusions. The main

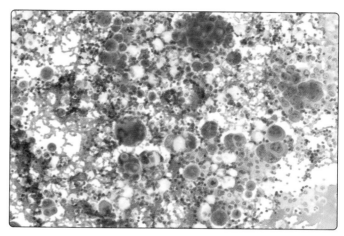

Fig. 13.43 **Mesothelioma** Numerous malignant morules. Notice only one malignant cell population on a background of erythrocytes and inflammatory cells (Pap, IP).

differential diagnoses are longstanding hydrocele with reactive mesothelial cells forming numerous three-dimensional balls, and metastatic carcinoma. FNA findings in intrascrotal mesothelioma have been described in a few cases, some with a well-documented history of asbestos exposure.[82,91,92] The immunohistochemical profile of malignant mesotheliomas of the tunica vaginalis has been reported.[93]

Other tumors

Liposarcoma and leiomyosarcoma are the most common sarcomas of the scrotum in adults, *paratesticular rhabdomyosarcoma* in children.[12] A few case reports with FNA have been published.[19,67,94,95] The cytology of a *congenital malignant rhabdoid tumor* has been described.[96] Paratesticular sarcomas may mimic a primary testicular tumor clinically and ultrasonographically. FNA is helpful to rule out a TGCT.[19,67,94,96]

The cytologic findings of a testicular *papillary serous cystadenoma* have recently been described.[97]

A case of primary *melanoma* of scrotum in 55-yr-old man diagnosed by FNA has been reported.[98]

Penis

Primary squamous cell carcinoma of the penis can be diagnosed by scrape smears directly from the surface of the lesion. Secondary carcinoma involving the deeper tissues of the shaft of the penis from primary tumors in the prostate or bladder can be diagnosed by FNA using a 25–27-gauge needle. This is well tolerated by patients without significant complications. A series of FNA of penile lesions have been reported by Skoog et al.[99]

Female genital tract

Svante R. Orell

CLINICAL ASPECTS

The place of FNAC in the investigative sequence

The main use of FNAC in gynecological practice is in the investigation of suspected pelvic recurrence or metastasis in patients treated for gynecological cancer. A palpable mass in the vaginal vault or in the pelvic tissues detected during routine follow-up and clinically suspicious of recurrent tumor may simply be due to local edema, inflammation or repair. FNAC is the simplest and least invasive method of biopsy confirmation in these circumstances.[100–103]

The role of FNAC in the preoperative investigation of ovarian tumors and of ovarian cysts at laparoscopy remains controversial mainly due to the proven risk of intraperitoneal seeding.[104–108] It is also argued that preoperative biopsy is unnecessary since surgical exploration is mandatory anyway. On the other hand, cytological assessment may allow selective treatment in some cases, for example preoperative irradiation of anaplastic carcinoma.[5] Aspirated material can be used for ancillary studies. FNB of the contralateral ovary during laparotomy for ovarian tumor can be of value when preservation of ovarian function is important.[6,7] FNB may be considered in patients who are poor surgical risks, have disseminated cancer at presentation or have suspected recurrence of previously diagnosed tumor.

Most ovarian cysts detected at laparoscopy are functional cysts but a few may be neoplastic. Hormonal assay of aspirated cyst fluid helps to distinguish between functional and neoplastic cysts.[109–111] Laparoscopic cyst aspiration in conjunction with US findings (size, multiloculation, solid areas) and with hormonal assay can reduce the need for surgery in selected cases.[10,112] However, peritoneal dissemination following laparoscopic FNB of cystic carcinoma has been observed.[113]

Accuracy of diagnosis

Cytological diagnosis of recurrent or metastatic cancer is usually not difficult if samples are adequate, of good quality and contain unequivocally malignant cells, and if the histology of the primary is known. However, postradiation atypia of epithelial or stromal cells can cause problems and full knowledge of any given treatment is essential.[114]

The diagnostic accuracy of preoperative FNB of ovarian tumors has been reported as 90–95%.[5–7] A type-specific diagnosis may not be possible, particularly in ovarian stromal and other uncommon tumors. Accuracy is lower in cystic tumors but can be improved by supplementing cytological examination with biochemical assay. One study showed a high proportion of unsatisfactory samples and a low diagnostic sensitivity for FNB of ovarian cystic lesions, but specificity was high.[13]

Complications

Septicemia has been recorded following transrectal FNB of cystic ovarian tumors, and a transvaginal approach is therefore favored. As mentioned above, peritoneal seeding of tumor cells can occur following transabdominal FNB of cystadenocarcinoma.[14] The true incidence of this serious complication is uncertain, but the risk is real and an extraperitoneal approach should be chosen if malignancy is suspected.[5]

Technical considerations

The technique described for FNB of the prostate is applicable to any palpable pelvic mass. FNB can be performed as an office procedure, or coordinated with other procedures requiring general anesthesia, such as bimanual palpation, diagnostic curettage or cystoscopy.

Transvaginal puncture is more likely to sample a solid portion of a cystic ovarian tumor than a transabdominal approach.[5] The possibility that the aspirate is of peritoneal fluid rather than fluid from a cystic lesion should be considered since the exact position of the needle at biopsy can be difficult to decide. Parallel use of MGG/Diff-Quik and Papanicolaou staining is recommended. Spare smears, cell blocks or liquid-based preparations for special stains and immunostaining may be needed in selected cases.

CYTOLOGICAL FINDINGS

Lower female genital tract

Most palpable lesions in the lower female genital tract are accessible to FNB.[115] Malignant tumors subjected to FNB are mainly recurrent or metastatic squamous cell carcinomas or adenocarcinomas.[1–3] Examples of recurrent carcinoma in the pelvis, retroperitoneum and vaginal vault confirmed by transvaginal FNB are illustrated in Figures 13.44 to 13.46. Malignant melanoma should be remembered in the differential diagnosis of poorly differentiated malignancies.

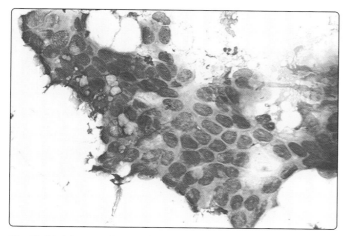

Fig. 13.44 Adenocarcinoma of uterine cervix FNA smear of pelvic recurrence. Sheet of atypical glandular epithelial cells; nuclear crowding and overlapping, moderate pleomorphism (MGG; HP).

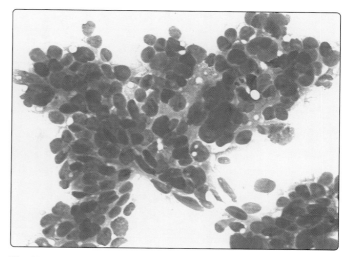

Fig. 13.45 Retroperitoneal metastasis of adenocarcinoma of fallopian tube Pattern of moderately differentiated adenocarcinoma without specific features (DQ; HP).

Postoperative inflammation and repair may be clinically suspicious of recurrent cancer. Smears from such lesions can be highly cellular, and reactive histiocytes can appear atypical, particularly in air-dried smears. Postradiation atypia of non-neoplastic cells causes diagnostic difficulties in some cases.

Cytological findings in *malacoplakia* of the vagina have been described.[116] Smears show many histiocytes with intracytoplasmic PAS-positive Michaelis-Gutmann bodies. Benign and malignant vulval tumors are easily accessible to FNB.[3] The cytological patterns of *papillary hidradenoma*[117] and of *adenoid cystic carcinoma* of Bartholin's gland[118] have been reported.

Pelvic endometriosis (Fig. 13.47)

CRITERIA FOR DIAGNOSIS

◆ Coexistence in smears of both glandular cells and stromal spindle cells,
◆ Background of altered blood, debris and hemosiderin-containing macrophages.

Endometriosis is a relatively common lesion in the pelvic peritoneum, abdominal wall and genital tract. A history of cyclic symptoms in a premenopausal woman suggests the diagnosis, but it may present as a mass lesion suspicious of neoplasia. The diagnosis is based on the identification of both glandular epithelial cells and spindle stromal cells in the smears. The epithelial component may appear atypical (see Fig. 13.48B), but this should not cause concern in the appropriate setting.[119,120]

Uterus

Uterine leiomyoma (Fig. 13.48)

Uterine leiomyomas are not often subjected to FNB. The consistency of the tissue felt through the needle is characteristically hard and tough. Smears are scanty, containing tissue

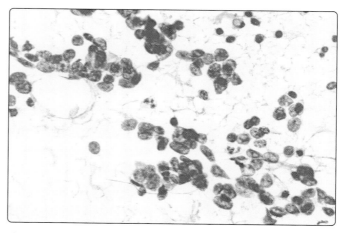

Fig. 13.46 Small-cell neuroendocrine carcinoma vagina FNA smear of recurrent tumor of the vaginal vault. Irregular clusters of small cells with hyperchromatic nuclei; some nuclear molding (Pap; HP).

fragments of spindle cells and intercellular collagen, and few single cells. The cells have syncytial eosinophilic cytoplasm and bland nuclei. There are no mitoses and no evidence of necrosis.

The distinction between highly cellular leiomyoma and low-grade leiomyosarcoma may not be possible, since mitotic counts are not reliable in FNB samples.[121]

Malignant tumors

The primary diagnosis of *endometrial adenocarcinoma* is made by other means, but FNB may be used to confirm tumor recurrence or metastasis (Fig. 13.49).[122]

The cytological findings in uterine *leiomyosarcoma* are of a spindle cell sarcoma. Smooth muscle differentiation is suggested by a dense, eosinophilic cytoplasm and truncated nuclei, but a type-specific diagnosis should be supported by immunostaining (see Chapter 15). High cellularity, reduced cell cohesion, nuclear pleomorphism, chromatin abnormalities and the presence of necrosis suggest malignancy. Mitotic

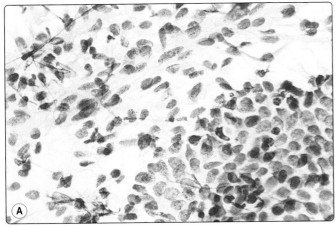

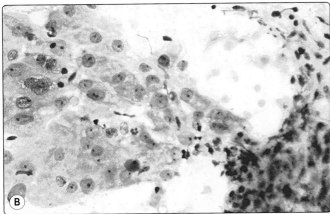

Fig. 13.47 Endometriosis Fragments of spindle cell stroma and sheets of glandular epithelium; mild nuclear atypia in (B); (A, Pap; B, MGG; HP).

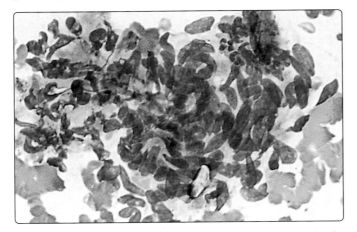

Fig. 13.48 Cellular leiomyoma Cohesive cluster of spindle cells; high cell yield gave rise to suspicion of malignancy; the tumor was considered histologically to be of borderline malignancy (MGG, HP).

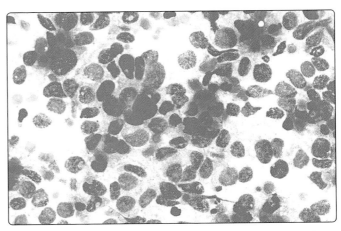

Fig. 13.49 Intermediate-grade endometrial adenocarcinoma Poorly cohesive malignant epithelial cells; some microglandular groups (MGG, HP). *(Courtesy Dr. J. Klijanienko, Curie Institute, France.)*

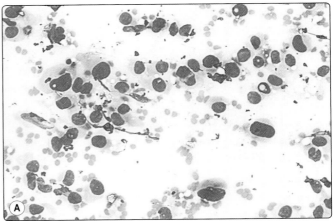

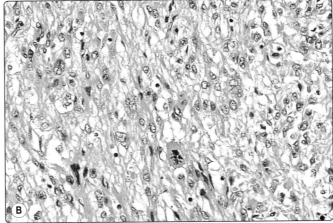

Fig. 13.50 Uterine leiomyosarcoma (A) Epithelioid pattern; dispersed, pleomorphic malignant cells of predominantly rounded shape, pale fragile cytoplasm (MGG, HP); (B) Corresponding tissue section; note abnormal mitotic figure (H&E, IP).

counts are unreliable in FNB samples.[22] Leiomyosarcoma with a round cell epithelioid pattern can be mistaken for carcinoma unless immune marker studies are added (Fig. 13.50).

FNA smears of *endometrial stromal sarcoma* are highly cellular.[123,124] The cells are plump spindled, eosinophilic with anastomosing cytoplasmic processes. In low-grade tumors (endolymphatic stromal myosis), the cells are relatively small and uniform with bland nuclei, and form cohesive clusters. In high-grade tumors, cells are mainly dispersed and there is no architectural pattern. Nuclei are oval, vesicular, enlarged and moderately pleomorphic, with granular chromatin and small nucleoli. Mitotic figures are frequently observed (Fig. 13.51). Positive staining for CD10 is helpful in the distinction from other spindle cell lesions.

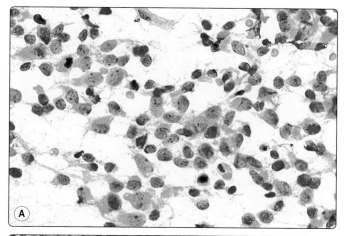

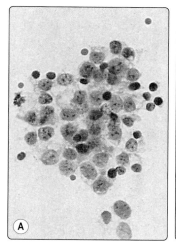

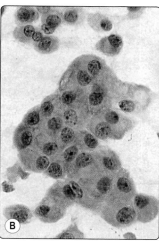

Fig. 13.52 Functional ovarian cysts (A) Follicular cyst. Loose aggregate of small cells with pale nuclei, indistinct cytoplasm; many apoptotic cells; note mitosis (*left*) (H&E, HP); (B) Cystic corpus luteum. Papillary-like clusters of cohesive luteinized cells with abundant well-defined cytoplasm (Pap, HP).

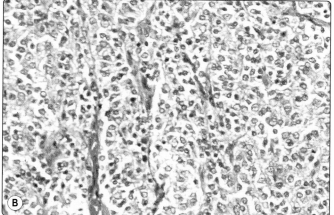

Fig. 13.51 Endometrial stromal sarcoma (A) Poorly cohesive plump spindle cells with pale ovoid nuclei and small nucleoli; note anastomosing strands of eosinophilic cytoplasm and a few mitoses (H&E, IP); (B) Corresponding tissue section (H&E, IP).

Coexistence of malignant glandular epithelial cells and malignant mesenchymal cells in smears from a uterine or ovarian tumor suggests a *malignant mixed Mullerian tumor* or *carcinosarcoma*. A few cases diagnosed by FNB have been reported.[125,126] Mesenchymal elements are not often demonstrated in metastatic deposits of this tumor.[27]

Ovary

Non-neoplastic ovarian cysts

Simple cysts including surface epithelial inclusion cysts, parovarian and fimbrial cysts, regressing follicular cysts and simple serous cysts, fall into this category. The cysts are lined by a single layer of columnar, cuboidal or flat, sometimes ciliated cells. Aspirated fluid contains mainly 'cyst macrophages'. These have small central nuclei and abundant well-defined pale, vacuolated cytoplasm often containing hemosiderin pigment. Distinction from degenerate epithelial cells may be difficult. Hormone assay of the cyst fluid can identify functional cysts.[8,127]

Functional cysts (Fig. 13.52). Kovacic et al.[128] have described the cytology of follicular cysts, corpus luteum and theca lutein cysts separately and in detail.

The cytological findings are distinctive. The fluid is often cell-rich. Cells are single and in loose clusters. Single cells resemble macrophages. Anisokaryosis may be prominent and nuclear diameter varies from 10 to over 20 microns. Granulosa cell nuclei are rounded, showing only minor irregularities. The chromatin is granular, resembling nuclei of neuroendocrine cells. There are many single apoptotic cells with pyknotic nuclei. Mitotic figures are frequently found (Fig. 13.52A).

Luteinized granulosa cells have a larger amount of dense, granular and vacuolated cytoplasm with better-defined cell borders (Fig. 13.52B). Cells from a corpus luteum are more cohesive, forming solid cords, which can mimic papillary fragments but lack stromal cores. Blood and fibrin are often prominent in the background.

Fluid aspirated from follicular cysts has a high estradiol content.[12,28] Intracellular estrogen may also be demonstrated in smears by immunostaining.

Endometriotic cysts. The aspirate usually consists of dark brown fluid or creamy material. Smears show mainly numerous hemosiderin-containing macrophages with a background of altered blood. A specific diagnosis of endometriosis is only possible if epithelial cells and spindle stromal cells are both present in smears (see Fig. 13.47). This is often the case in extraovarian endometriosis but rarely in aspirates from endometriotic cysts. Cell block preparations are useful in this setting, but overall diagnostic specificity of FNA for

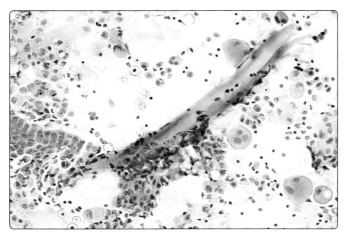

Fig. 13.53 Benign cystic teratoma Anucleate squamous cells and a small sheet of benign glandular epithelial cells (*lower left*); hair shafts, macrophages, debris (Pap, IP).

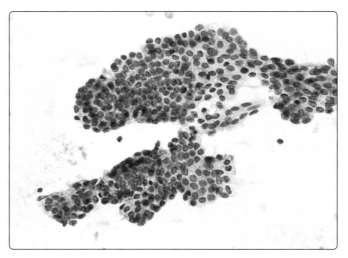

Fig. 13.54 Benign serous ovarian cystadenoma Intraoperative cyst fluid aspiration. Sheets and papillary clusters of small, round epithelial cells and small relatively uniform nuclei (Pap, HP).

ovarian endometriosis is low.[28] Old blood and hemosiderin-containing macrophages are non-diagnostic, present also in functional cysts, extra-uterine pregnancy and some tumors.

Benign neoplasms

Smears of *ovarian fibroma and thecoma* are paucicellular, showing a few spindle cells similar to those of uterine leiomyoma. Thecoma cells have plumper and more irregular nuclei and a larger amount of indistinct, fragile cytoplasm. Intracytoplasmic fat droplets are demonstrated by oil-red-O staining of air-dried smears.

We have no personal experience of the cytology of *Brenner tumors*. The cytological pattern has been described as sheets of epithelial cells of benign appearance with ovoid, grooved ('coffee bean') nuclei.[6] Extracellular, large, hyaline, eosinophilic globules are characteristic in smears of this tumor. The cytology of a malignant Brenner tumor in a metastatic site has also been reported.[129]

Smears from *benign cystic teratoma* (dermoid cyst) show mainly amorphous non-cellular material and some anucleate squames. The presence of fragments of hair shafts and, occasionally, of benign cells from other differentiated tissues supports the diagnosis (Fig. 13.53).[130]

CRITERIA FOR DIAGNOSIS

- Thick, greasy, yellowish aspirate,
- Background of thick amorphous material,
- Anucleate keratinized squames,
- Some inflammatory cells, macrophages and foreign body giant cells,
- Fragments of hair shafts,
- Cells from other differentiated tissues.

The finding of keratinous debris or mature squamous cells in FNB samples is equivocal. This may represent contaminant squamous cells from laboratory staff handling, or from the vaginal mucosa in transvaginal FNB.

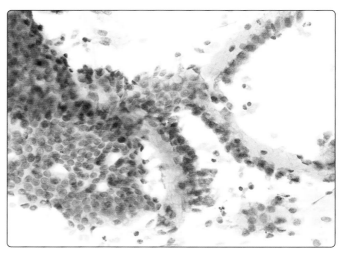

Fig. 13.55 Benign mucinous ovarian cystadenoma Sheets and strips of columnar epithelial cells with abundant pale vacuolated cytoplasm and uniform bland nuclei. Background mucus seen in other parts of smear (Pap, HP).

Cystadenoma, serous and mucinous[104,105]

Cyst fluid from *benign serous cystadenoma* of ovary is usually poor in cells, and any cells present are often degenerate or show shrinkage artifacts making a type-specific diagnosis difficult. Cell blocks are often helpful. Well-preserved cells form papillary aggregates, have small, dark, bland nuclei and may have vacuolated cytoplasm (Fig. 13.54). However, papillary tufts of mesothelial cells from the broad ligament closely resemble those of a serous cystadenoma, and may appear atypical if reactive. This possibility must be kept in mind when examining ovarian aspirates. Tall columnar cells with basal nuclei and empty-looking cytoplasm, and viscous mucus in the background suggest *mucinous cystadenoma* (Fig. 13.55).

Malignant neoplasms[5,6,31]

Cell-rich smears of serous or mucinous epithelial cells showing nuclear atypia of moderate degree raise a suspicion

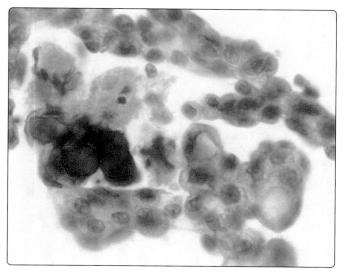

Fig. 13.56 Serous cystadenoma, 'borderline' Clusters of atypical cells showing moderate nuclear enlargement and pleomorphism; some prominent nucleoli; some cytoplasmic vacuoles; psammoma bodies in center left. Histologically borderline serous tumor (Pap, HP).

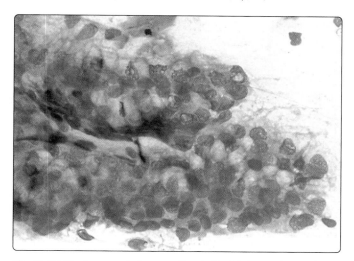

Fig. 13.57 Mucinous cystadenoma, 'borderline' Cohesive sheets of atypical mucin-secreting columnar cells; multilayering and nuclear crowding. Histologically borderline mucinous tumor (MGG, HP).

of malignancy. This is a difficult problem and it is probably not possible to distinguish cytologically between ovarian tumors of *'borderline' malignancy* and well-differentiated cystadenocarcinoma (Figs 13.56 and 13.57).[131] Psammoma bodies are more often a feature of borderline or malignant than of benign serous tumors. Nuclear folds are said to be common in both benign and borderline tumors.[132]

Serous cystadenocarcinoma (Fig. 13.58)

CRITERIA FOR DIAGNOSIS

- ◆ Mucoid, turbid fluid of variable viscosity,
- ◆ Single cells and papillary, glandular and/or syncytial aggregates,
- ◆ Columnar cells, relatively high N:C ratio,
- ◆ Nuclear criteria of malignancy,
- ◆ Psammoma bodies (some tumors),

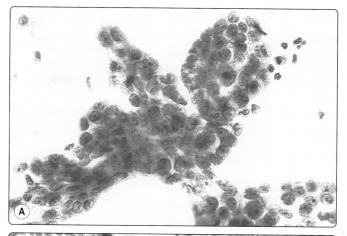

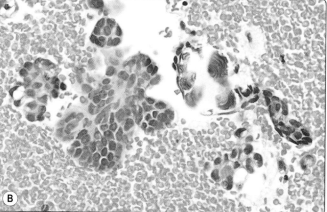

Fig. 13.58 Serous cystadenocarcinoma (A) Papillary tissue fragment of crowded atypical glandular cells; large overlapping nuclei; prominent nucleoli; scanty pale cytoplasm (Pap, HP); (B) Cell block. Papillary tumor fragments, psammoma bodies(*upper right*) (H & E, HP).

The tumor cells generally have a moderate amount of cyanophilic (Pap) cytoplasm, which may be vacuolated but stains negative for mucin. A papillary microarchitectural pattern is not always obvious. Finger-like aggregates of cells with a well-defined border on three sides are more commonly seen than true papillary structures with stromal cores. The microarchitectural pattern is best shown in cell blocks (Fig. 13.58B). Psammoma bodies showing concentric lamellation are a helpful sign when present.

Mucinous cystadenocarcinoma (Fig. 13.59)

CRITERIA FOR DIAGNOSIS

- ◆ Mucinous, highly viscous, sticky fluid,
- ◆ Smear background of stringy mucin,
- ◆ Mainly cohesive sheets and aggregates of cells (well differentiated),
- ◆ Columnar, mucin-secreting cells,
- ◆ Nuclear criteria of malignancy.

Smears are usually cell rich. However, the sample may consist only of mucinous secretion with few cells, mainly mucinophages or bland-looking, spindly epithelial cells similar to those of pseudomyxoma peritonei. The cells resemble

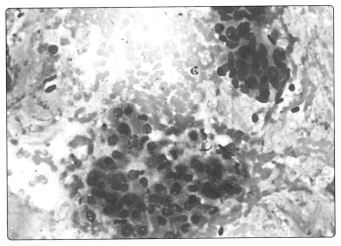

Fig. 13.59 **Mucinous cystadenocarcinoma** Clusters of pleomorphic malignant glandular cells with a background of mucus (DQ, HP).

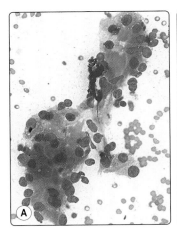
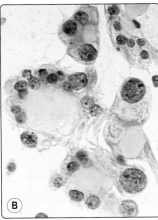

Fig. 13.61 **Clear cell carcinoma** Papillary clusters of cells with abundant, pale, finely vacuolated cytoplasm. Globular cores of hyaline stromal material (A, MGG, IP; B, H&E, HP) *(Courtesy Dr. J. Philips, Sydney, NSW.)*

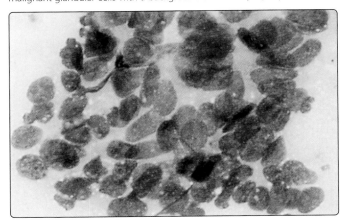

Fig. 13.60 **Endometrioid carcinoma** Loose cluster of malignant glandular cells with an acinar pattern and some nuclear palisading (MGG, HP).

those of mucinous cystadenoma but show a variable degree of nuclear enlargement and crowding, an increased N:C ratio and nuclear criteria of malignancy, more obvious in less well-differentiated cancers. The background is of thick, stringy mucus, which stains bluish-violet with MGG. Distinction from metastatic adenocarcinoma may be difficult.

Endometrioid adenocarcinoma (Fig. 13.60)

The cytological features of endometrioid carcinoma are not very specific.[23] The cells have an eosinophilic granular cytoplasm and the microarchitectural pattern is glandular, cribriform and partly solid. Mucin is absent or sparse. It may be difficult to distinguish from serous adenocarcinoma, but the main differential diagnosis is metastatic adenocarcinoma, particularly of colonic origin.

Immunocytochemistry is helpful in the differential diagnosis between primary ovarian carcinoma and metastatic adenocarcinoma. Primary ovarian carcinoma is usually CK7+, CK20– and CDX2–, whereas colonic cancer is CK7–, CK20+ and CDX2+.

Clear cell carcinoma (Fig. 13.61)

Clear cell carcinoma is an adenocarcinoma in which the cells have abundant, pale, finely granular and vacuolated cytoplasm containing glycogen. The cells form papillary clusters with globoid stromal cores of hyaline, basement membrane-like material (Fig. 13.61B).[133] These structures have been called 'raspberry bodies' and are of diagnostic significance in ascitic fluid. 'Hobnail' cells, as seen in histological sections, may be recognizable also in smears. Nuclear pleomorphism can be relatively mild. The smear background appears 'tigroid' and intracytoplasmic glycogen can be demonstrated by PAS-staining of air-dried smears.[134]

Anaplastic ovarian carcinoma

CRITERIA FOR DIAGNOSIS

- ◆ Cell-rich smears,
- ◆ Dispersed cell population with little aggregation,
- ◆ Undifferentiated malignant cells,
- ◆ Fragile cytoplasm, bare nuclei, prominent nucleoli,
- ◆ CK7+, CK20–.

Anaplastic carcinoma has a very poor prognosis. FNB may allow preoperative radiotherapy for this category of tumors. Anaplastic carcinomas are predominantly solid and aspirates are usually highly cellular. Some evidence of glandular differentiation may be seen. Nuclei are large, pleomorphic and obviously malignant. Large intracytoplasmic, hyaline eosinophilic inclusions similar to those seen in hepatocellular carcinoma may be found.

Metastatic carcinoma to ovary

The possibility of metastatic origin must be considered in all poorly differentiated malignancies. Differential cytokeratin staining is of some help in this distinction. Smears from *Krukenberg tumors* (ovarian metastasis from gastrointestinal adenocarcinoma) contain signet ring cells, single or small clusters, with intracytoplasmic mucin vacuoles. Cells are usually few due to the abundant fibrous stroma. A CNB may be necessary to provide a confident diagnosis. *Malignant melanoma* not uncommonly metastasises to the ovary. Criteria for diagnosis are described elsewhere (see Chapter 14).

Gonadal stromal tumors

Granulosa cell tumor (Figs 13.62–13.65)[135,136]

CRITERIA FOR DIAGNOSIS

◆ Cell-rich smears,
◆ Cells in loose aggregates with a tendency to follicular grouping or dispersed,
◆ Moderate amount of pale cytoplasm; indistinct cell borders,
◆ Nuclei monomorphous, round or ovoid; longitudinal nuclear grooves; finely granular chromatin,
◆ Call-Exner bodies (variable),
◆ Positive immunostaining for inhibin.

Fine needle aspiration smears from granulosa cell tumors of follicular type are highly cellular of both single cells and syncytial aggregates. A follicular pattern is often discernible. In some cases, rounded bodies, 30–100 microns in diameter, of non-cellular material, are present. These probably represent the contents of Call-Exner bodies. They are brightly purple, fibrillar in MGG-stained smears (Fig. 13.62), pale eosinophilic and structureless in H&E. Nuclei are rounded and do not vary much in size. Nuclear grooves ('coffee bean nuclei') are frequent, best seen in alcohol-fixed Pap smears. Nuclear chromatin is finely granular and evenly distributed.

Nucleoli are small and indistinct. The cells have pale vacuolated cytoplasm with indistinct cell borders. Smears from tumors of the diffuse type are less characteristic. Plump spindle cells predominate, nuclear grooves are present, but there is no characteristic microarchitectural pattern (Fig. 13.63). Immunostaining is helpful: tumor cells are positive for inhibin and vimentin, negative for cytokeratin.

The FNA findings were similar in two examples of *malignant granulosa cell tumor* but smears were even more cellular

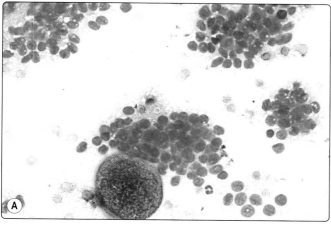

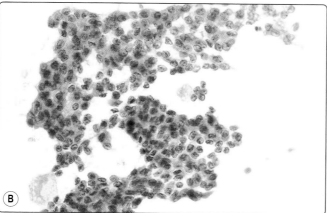

Fig. 13.62 Granulosa cell tumor Clusters of cells with some microfollicular groupings; uniformly small round nuclei some with folds; scanty, poorly defined cytoplasm. The globular structures represent the contents of Call-Exner bodies (**A**, DQ, HP; **B**, H&E, HP).

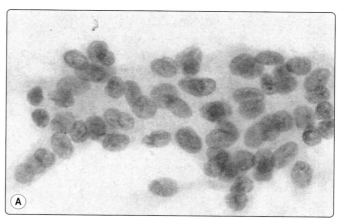

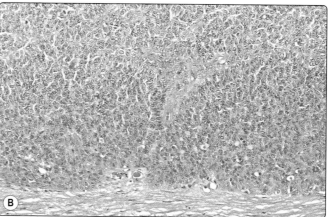

Fig. 13.63 Granulosa cell tumor, diffuse pattern (A) Loose cluster of cells with uniform, ovoid nuclei, some with grooves (Pap, HP); (B) Corresponding tissue section (H&E, IP).

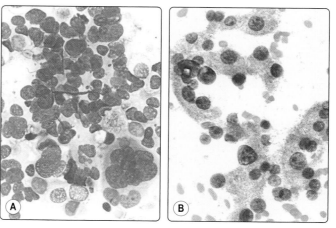

Fig. 13.64 Malignant granulosa cell tumor Clustered and dispersed cells; suggestion of follicular pattern; pleomorphic nuclei; coarse chromatin; prominent nucleoli; fragile cytoplasm (**A**, MGG; **B**, Pap, HP).

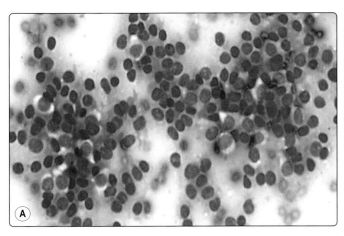
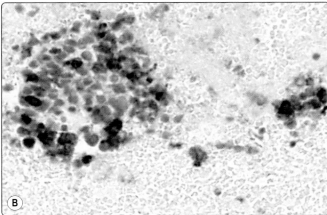

Fig. 13.65 Metastasis of granulosa cell tumor to lung FNB of solitary 2-cm nodule upper lobe left lung in woman age 35 with past history of oophorectomy; cell-rich smear of small cells with round or ovoid uniform nuclei and indistinct cytoplasm; some microfollicular groups (**A**, DQ, HP; **B**, immunostaining for inhibin, IP).

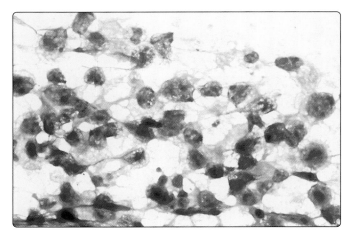

Fig. 13.66 Ovarian dysgerminoma Poorly cohesive malignant cells; fragile cytoplasm; vesicular nuclei with prominent nucleoli; nuclear smudging; few lymphocytes (H&E, HP).

and there was marked nuclear pleomorphism. Nuclear chromatin was irregular and nucleoli were prominent (Fig. 13.64). FNA confirmation of granulosa cell tumor supported by markers is possible also in distant metastatic tumor deposits (Fig. 13.65).

Other *gonadal stromal tumors of the ovary* are rare and there are few reports of FNB diagnosis.[137,138]

Germ cell tumors

The cytological pattern of ovarian *dysgerminoma*[139] (Fig. 13.66) is identical to that of testicular seminoma (see Fig. 13.30). Cytological findings in *endodermal sinus tumor* (yolk sac tumor) in the pelvic region in girls have been reported[140] and are similar to those of testicular yolk sac tumors (see Fig. 13.37).

References

1. Franzén S, Giertz G, Zajicek J. Cytological diagnosis of prostatic tumours by transrectal aspiration biopsy: a preliminary report. Br J Urol 1960;32:193–6.

2. Johening PW. A history of aspiration biopsy with special attention to prostate biopsy. Diagn Cytopathol 1988;4:265–8.

3. Fox CH. Innovation in medical diagnosis – the Scandinavian curiosity. Lancet 1979;30:1387–8.

4. Tannenbaum M, Bostwick DG, Maksem J, et al. The prostate gland. In: Silverberg S, editor. Principles and practice of surgical pathology and cytopathology. 3rd ed. New York: Churchill-Livingstone, Inc.; 1997. p. 2321–33.

5. Maksen JA, Berner A, Bedrossian C. Fine needle aspiration biopsy of the prostate gland. Diagn Cytopathol 2007;35:778–85.

6. McWilliam LJ, Roberts ISD, Davies DR. Problems in grading and staging prostatic carcinoma. Current Diagnostic Pathology 2002;8:65–75.

7. Partin AW, Katan MW, Subong EN, et al. Combination of prostate-specific antigen, clinical stage, and Gleason score to predict pathological state of localized prostate cancer. A multi-institutional update. JAMA 1997;277: 1445–51.

8. García-Solano J, Sánchez-Sánchez C, Montalbán Romero S, et al. Diagnostic dilemmas in the interpretation of fine-needle aspirates of granulomatous prostatitis. Diagn Cytopathol 1998;18: 215–21.

9. Pérez-Guillermo M, Acosta-Ortega J, García-Solano, J. Pitfalls and infrequent findings in fine-needle aspiration of the prostate gland. Diagn Cytopathol 2005;33:126–37.

10. Pérez-Guillermo M, Acosta-Ortega J, García-Solano J. The continuing role of fine-needle aspiration of the prostate gland into the 21st Century. Diagn Cytopathol 2005;32:315–20.

11. Berg A, Berner A, Lilleby W, et al. Impact of disseminated tumour cells in patients with non-metastatic prostate cancer treated by definitive radiotherapy. Int J Cancer 2007;120: 1603–9.

12. Eble JN, Sauter G, Epstein JI, Sesterhenn IA, editors. World Health Organization Classification of Tumours. Pathology and Genetics of Tumours of the Urinary System and Male Genital Organs. Lyon: IARC Press; 2004.

13. Woodward PJ, Sohaey R, O'Donoghue MJ, et al. From the Archives of the AFIP. Tumours and tumourlike lesions of the testis: radiologic-pathologic correlation. AFIP Archives 2002;22:189–216.

14. García-Solano J, Sánchez- Sánchez C, Montalbán Romero S, et al. Fine needle aspiration (FNA) of testicular germ cell tumours; a 10-year experience in a community hospital. Cytopathology 1998;9:248–62.

15. Moul JW. Timely diagnosis of testicular cancer. Urol Clin N Am 2007;34:109–17.

16. Huyghe E, Muller A, Mieusset R, et al. Impact of diagnostic delay in testis cancer: results of a large population-based study. European Urology 2007;52:1710–16.

17. Geisinger KR. Tubercular scrotal disease. Acta Cytol 2006;50:241–2.

18. Pérez-Guillermo M, García-Solano J, Acosta Ortega J. Fine needle aspiration cytology of palpable lesions of the scrotal content. Acta Cytol. 2008;52:259–60.

19. Daneshbod Y, Monabati A, Kumar PV, et al. Paratesticular spindle cell rhabdomyosarcoma diagnosed by fine needle aspiration cytology: a case report. Acta Cytol 2005;49:331–4.

20. Gupta N, Rajwanshi A, Srinivasan R, et al. Fine needle aspiration of epididymal nodules in Chandigarh, north India: an audit of 228 cases. Cytopathology 2006;17:195–8.

21. Handa U, Bhutani A, Mohan H, et al. Role of fine needle aspiration cytology in nonneoplastic testicular and scrotal lesions and male infertility. Acta Cytol 2006;50:513–17.

22. Han U, Adabag A, Köybasioglu F, et al. Clinical value of cell counts and indices in testicular fine needle aspiration cytology in primary infertility: diagnostic performance compared with histology. Anat Quant Cytol Histol 2006;28:331–6.

23. Mehrotra R, Chaurasia D. Fine needle aspiration cytology of the testis as the first diagnostic modality in azoospermia: a comparative study of cytology and histology. Cytopathology 2008;19:363–8.

24. Monappa V, Rao AC, Krishnanand G, et al. Adenomatoid tumour of tunica albuginea mimicking seminoma on fine needle aspiration cytology: a case report. Acta Cytol 2009;53:349–52.

25. Sah SP, Bhadani PP, Regmi R, et al. Fine needle aspiration cytology of tubercular epididymitis and epididymo-orchitis. Acta Cytol 2006;50:243–9.

26. Nadji M, Sevin B-U. Pelvic fine needle aspiration cytology in gynecology. In: Linsk JA, Franzén S, editors. Clinical aspiration cytology. 2nd ed. Philadelphia: J.B. Lippincott Co.; 1989. p. 261–82.

27. Esposti P-L. Cytologic malignancy grading of prostatic carcinoma by transrectal aspiration biopsy. A five-year follow-up study of 469 hormone-treated patients. Scand J Urol Nephrol 1971;5:199–209.

28. Valdman A, Jonmarker S, Ekman P, et al. Cytological features of prostatic intraepithelial neoplasia. Diagn Cytopaythol 2006;34:317–22.

29. Kaic G, Tomasovic-Loncaric C. alpha-Methylacyl-CoA racemase (AMACR) in fine-needle aspiration specimens of prostate lesions. Diagn Cytopathol 2009;37:803–8,

30. Planelles Gómez J, Beltrán Armada JM, Alonso Hernández S, et al. Valor de la PAAF transrectal en el diagnóstico del cáncer de próstata en pacientes de edad avanzada. Actas Urol Esp 2008;32: 485–91.

31. Böcking A, Aufferman W. Cytological grading of therapy-induced tumour regression in prostatic carcinoma: proposal of a new system. Diagn Cytopathol 1987;3:108–11.

32. Waisman J, Adolfsson J, Löwhagen T, et al. Comparison of transrectal prostate digital aspiration and ultrasound-guided core biopsies in 99 men. Urology 1991;37:301–7.

33. Engelstein D, Mukamel E, Cytron S, et al. Comparison between digitally-guided fine needle aspiration and ultrasound-guided transperineal core needle biopsy of the prostate for the detection of prostate cancer. Br J Urol 1994;74;210–13.

34. Willems J-S, Löwhagen T. Transrectal fine-needle aspiration biopsy for cytologic diagnosis and grading of prostatic carcinoma. Prostate 1981;2:381–95.

35. Orell SR. Pitfalls in fine needle aspiration cytology. Cytopathology 2003;14:173–82.

36. Zajicek J. Prostatic gland and seminal vesicles. In: Wied GL, editor. Aspiration biopsy cytology. Part II. Cytology of infradiaphragmatic organs. Monographs in clinical cytology. Vol 7. Basel: S. Karger; 1979. p. 129–66.

37. Linsk JA, Franzén S. Aspiration biopsy cytology of the prostate gland. In: Linsk JA, Franzén S, editors. Clinical aspiration cytology. 2nd ed. Philadelphia: J.B. Lippincott Co.; 1989. p. 283–304.

38. Esposti P-L, Elman A, Norlén H. Complications of transrectal aspiration biopsy of the prostate. Scand J Urol Nephrol 1975;9:208–13.

39 Leistenschneider W, Nagel R. Atlas of prostatic cytology. Berlin: Springer-Verlag; 1984.

40. Egevad L. Cytology of the central zone of the prostate. Diagn Cytopathol 2003;28:239–44.

41. Cazzaniga MG, Tommasini-Denga A, Negri R, et al. Cytologic diagnosis of prostatic malakoplakia. Report of three cases. Acta Cytol 1987;31:48–52.

42. Mai KT, Roustan Delatour NL, Assiri A, et al. Secondary prostatic adenocarcinoma: a cytopathological study of 50 cases. Diagn Cytopathol 2007;35:91–5.

43. Vandersteen DP, Wiemerslage SJ, Cohen MB. Prostatic duct adenocarcinoma: a cytologic and histologic case with review of the literature. Diagn Cytopathol 1997;17:480–3.

44. Wang W, Epstein JI. Small cell carcinoma of the prostate. A morphologic and immunohistochemical study of 95 cases. Am J Surg Pathol 2008;32:65–71.

45. Begnami MD, Quezado M, Pinto P, et al. Adenoid cystic/basal cell carcinoma of the prostate: review and update. Arch Pathol Lab Med 2007;131:637–40.

46. Moroz K, Crespo P, de las Morenas A. Fine needle aspiration of prostatic rhabdomyosarcoma. A case report demonstrating the value of DNA ploidy. Acta Cytol 1995;39:785–90.

47. Bahrami A, Ro JY, Ayala AG. An overview of testicular germ cell tumours. Arch Pathol Lab Med. 2007; 131:1267–80.

48. Ulbright TM. The most common, clinically significant misdiagnoses in testicular tumour pathology, and how to avoid them. Adv Anat Pathol 2008; 15:18–27.

49. Young RH. Testicular tumours-Some new and a few perennial problems. Arch Pathol Lab Med 2008;132;548–64.

50. Caraway NP, Fanning CV, Amato RJ, et al. Fine-needle aspiration cytology of seminoma: a review of 16 cases. Diagn Cytopathol 1995;12:327–33.

51. Collins KA, Geisinger KR, Wakely PE Jr, et al. Extragonadal germ cell tumours: a fine-needle aspiration biopsy study. Diagn Cytopathol 1995;12:223–9.

52. Gupta R, Mathur SR, Arora VK, et al. Cytologic features of extragonadal germ cell tumours. A study of 88 cases with aspiration cytology. Cancer (Cancer cytopathol) 2008;114:504–11.

53. Akhtar M, Ali MA, Sackey K, et al. Fine-needle aspiration biopsy diagnosis of endodermal sinus tumour: Histologic and ultrastructural correlations. Diag Cytopathol 1990; 6:184–92.

54. Afroz N, Khan N, Chana RS. Cytodiagnosis of yolk sac tumour. Indian J Pediatr 2004;71:939–42.

55. Dominguez-Franjo P, Vargas J, Rodriguez-Peralto JL, et al. Fine needle aspiration biopsy findings in endodermal sinus tumours. A report of four cases with cytologic, immunohistochemical and ultrastructural findings. Acta Cytol 1993;37:209–15.

56. Mizrak, B, Ekinci C. Cytologic diagnosis of yolk sac tumour. A report of seven cases Acta Cytol 1995;39:936–40.

57. Fleury-Feith J, Bellot-Besnard J. Criteria for aspiration cytology for the diagnosis of seminoma. Diagn Cytopathol 1989;5:392–5.

58. Verma K, Raja Tam T, Kapila K. Value of fine needle aspiration cytology in the diagnosis of testicular neoplasma. Acta Cytol 1989;33:631–4.

59. Balsev E, Francis D, Jacobsen GK. Testicular germ cell tumours. Classification based on fine needle aspiration biopsy. Acta Cytol 1990;34:690–4.

60. Pérez-Guillermo M, Sola Pérez J. Aspiration cytology of palpable lesions of the scrotal content. Diagn Cytopathol 1990;6:169–77.

61. Assi A, Patetta R, Fava C, et al. Fine-needle aspiration of testicular lesions: Report of 17 cases. Diagn Cytopathol 2000;23:388–92.

62. Akhtar M, Ali MA, Huq M, et al. Fine-needle aspiration biopsy of seminoma and dysgerminoma: cytologic, histologic, and electron microscopic correlations. Diagn Cytopathol 1990;6:99–105.

63. Akhtar M, Al Dayel F. Is it feasible to diagnose germ-cell tumours by fine-needle aspiration biopsy? Diagn Cytopathol 1997;16:72–7.

64. Saran RK, Banerjee AK, Gupta SK, et al. Spermatocytic seminoma: a cytology and histology case report with review of the literature. Diagn Cytopathol 1999;20:233–6.

65. Linsk JA, Franzén S. Aspiration biopsy of the testis. In: JA Linsk, S Franzén, editors. Clinical Aspiration Cytology. 2nd ed. Philadelphia: Lippincott; 1989. p. 305–17.

66. Zajicek J. Testis and epididymis. In: Aspiration biopsy cytology. Monographs in clinical cytology. Part 2. Cytology of infradiaphragmatic organs. Basel: Karger; 1979. p. 104–28.

67. Kumar PV, Kazemi H, Khezri A. Testicular embryonal rhabdomyosarcoma diagnosed by fine needle aspiration cytology. A report of two cases. Acta Cytol 1994; 38:573–6.

68. Turek PJ, Cha I, Ljung B-M. Systematic fine-needle aspiration of the testis: correlation to biopsy and results of organ 'mapping' for mature sperm in azoospermic men. Urology 1997;49:743–8.

69. Emerson RE, Ulbright TM. The use of immunohistochemistry in the differential diagnosis of tumours of the testis and paratestis. Seminars in Diagnostic Pathology 2005;2233–50.

70. Tavolini IM, Bettella A, Boscolo Berto R, et al. Immunostaining for placental alkaline phosphatase on fine-needle aspiration specimens to detect noninvasive testicular cancer: a prospective evaluation in cryptorchid men. BJU Int. 2006;97:950–4.

71. Jain M, Aiyer HM, Bajaj P, et al. Intracytoplasmic and intranuclear Reinke's crystals in a testicular Leydig-cell tumour diagnosed by fine-needle aspiration cytology: a case report with review of the literature. Diagn Cytopathol 2001;25:162–4.

72. Papic Z, Katona G, Skrabalo Z. The cytologic identification and quantification of testicular cell subtypes. Reproducibility and relation to histologic findings in the diagnosis of male infertility. Acta Cytol 1988;32:697–706.

73. Schenck U, Schill W-B. Cytology of the human seminiferous epitehelium. Acta Cytol 1988;32:689–96.

74. Ali MA, Akhtar M, Woodhouse N, et al. Role of testicular fine-needle aspiration biopsy in the evaluation of male infertility: cytologic and histologic correlation. Diagn Cytopathol 1991;7:128–31.

75. Dajani YF. Testicular biopsy: an update. Current Diagnostic pathology 1998;5:17–22.

76. Jain M, Kumari N, Rawat A, et al. Usefulness of testicular fine needle aspiration cytology in cases of infertility. Indian J Pathol Microbiol 2007:50:851–4.

77. El-Haggar S, Mostafa T, Abdel Nasser T, et al. Fine needle aspiration vs. mTESE in non-obstructive azoospermia. Int J Androl 2008;31:595–601.

78. Houwen J, Lundin K, Söderlund B, et al. Efficacy of percutaneous needle aspiration and open biopsy for sperm retrieval in men with non-obstructive azoospermia. Acta Obstet Gynecol Scand 2008;87:1033–8.

79. Sachdev R, Roy S, Jain S. Tubercular epididymo-orchitis masquerading as testicular malignancy: an interesting case. Acta Cytol 2008;52:511–12.

80. Garbyal RS, Gupta P, Kumar S, et al. Diagnosis of isolated tuberculous orchitis by fine-needle aspiration cytology. Diagn Cytopathol 2006;34:698–700.

81. Pérez-Guillermo M, Thor A, Löwhagen T. Spermatic granuloma. Diagnosis by fine needle aspiration cytology. Acta Cytol 1989;33:1–5.

82. Japko L, Horta AA, Schreiber K, et al. Malignant mesothelioma of the tunica vaginalis testis: report of first case with preoperative diagnosis Cancer 1982;49:119–27.

83. Pérez-Guillermo M, García-Solano J, Sánchez-Sánchez C, et al. Diagnostic limitations in testicular cytopathology: to what extent is fine-needle aspiration reliable for the diagnosis of epidermoid cyst of the testis? Diagn Cytopathol. 2004;31:83–6.

84. Barroca H, Gil-da-Costa MJ, Mariz C. Testicular juvenile granulosa cell tumour: a case report. Acta Cytol 2007;51:634–6.

85. Al-Abbadi MA, Hattab EM, Tarawneh M, et al. Primary testicular and paratesticular lymphoma. A retrospective clinicopathologic study of 34 cases with emphasis on differential diagnosis. Arch Pathol Lab Med 2007;131:1040–6.

86. Akhtar M, Ali MA, Burgess A, et al. Fine-needle aspiration biopsy (FNAB) diagnosis of testicular involvement in acute lymphoblastic leukemia in children. Diagn Cytopathol 1991;7: 504–7.

87. Kumar PV. Testicular leukemia relapse Fine needle aspiration findings. Acta Cytol 1998;42:312–16.

88. Suh YK, Shin HJ. Fine-needle aspiration biopsy of granulocytic sarcoma: a clinicopathologic study of 27 cases. Cancer 2000;90:364–72.

89. Ulbright TM, Young RH. Metastatic carcinoma to the testis. A clinicopathologic analysis of 26 nonincidental cases with emphasis on deceptive features. Am J Surg Pathol 2008;32:1683–93.

90. Pérez-Guillermo M, Thor A, Löwhagen T. Paratesticular adenomatoid tumours. The cytologic presentation in fine needle aspiration biopsies. Acta Cytol 1989;33:6–10.

91. Fukunaga M. Well-differentiated papillary mesothelioma of the tunica vaginalis: A case report with aspirate cytologic, immunohistochemical, and ultrastructural studies. Pathol Res Pract (2009), doi 10.1016/j.prp.2009.02.006

92. Mathur SR, Aron M, Gupta R, et al. Malignant mesothelioma of tunica vaginalis: a report of 2 cases with preoperative cytologic diagnosis. Acta Cytol 2008;52:740–3.

93. Winstanley AM, Ladon G, Berney D, et al. The immunohistochemical profile of malignant mesotheliomas of the tunica vaginalis. Am J Surg Pathol 2006;30:1–6.

94. Reis-Filho JS, Schmitt FC, Soares MF, et al. Fine needle aspiration cytology of paratesticular rhabdomyosarcoma mimicking a testicular germ cell tumour. Acta Cytol 2002;46:787–9.

95. Valeri RM, Papanikolaou A, Panagiotou A, et al. A rare case of paratesticular embryonal rhabdomyosarcoma diagnosed by fine needle aspiration: a case report. Acta Cytol 2009;53:319–22.

96. Salamanca J, Rodríguez-Peralto JL, Azorín D, et al. Paratesticular congenital malignant rhabdoid tumour diagnosed by fine-needle aspiration cytology. A case report. Diagn cytopathol 2004;30:46–50.

97. Kumar PV, Shirazi M, Salehi M. A diagnostic pitfall of fine needle aspiration cytology in testicular papillary serous cyst adenoma. Acta Cytol 2009;53:467–70.

98. Damala K, Tsanou E, Pappa L, et al. A rare case of primary malignant

melanoma of the scrotum diagnosed by fine-needle aspiration. Diagn Cytopathol. 2004;31:413–16.

99. Skoog L, Collins BT, Tani E, et al. Fine needle aspiration cytology of penile tumors. Acta Cytol 1998;42:1336–40.

100. Wojcik EM, Selvaggi SM, Johnson SC, et al. Factors influencing fine-needle aspiration cytology in the management of recurrent gynecological malignancies. Gynecol Oncol 1992;46:281–6.

101. Dey P, Dhar KK, Nijhawan R, et al. Fine needle aspiration biopsy in gynecological malignancies. Recurrent and metastatic lesions. Acta Cytol 1994;38:698–701.

102. Nadji M, Defortuna S, Sevin B-U, et al. Fine-needle aspiration cytology of palpable lesions of the lower female genital tract. Int J Gynecol Pathol 1994;13:54–61.

103. Ylagan LR, Mutch DG, Dávila RM. Transvaginal fine needle aspiration biopsy. Acta Cytol 2001;45:927–30.

104. Kjellgren O, Ångström T. Transvaginal and transrectal aspiration biopsy in diagnosis and classification of ovarian tumours. In: Zajicek J, editor. Aspiration biopsy cytology. Part 2. Cytology of infradiaphragmatic organs. Basel: Karger; 1979.

105. Ramzy I, Delaney M. Fine needle aspiration of ovarian masses. I. Correlative cytologic and histologic study of coelomic epithelial neoplasms. Acta Cytol 1979;23:97–104.

106. Ganjei P. Fine-needle aspiration cytology of the ovary. Clin Lab Med 1995;15:705–26.

107. Ganjei P, Dickinson B, Harrison T A, et al. Aspiration cytology of neoplastic and non-neoplastic ovarian cysts: is it accurate? Int J Gynecol Pathol 1996;15:94–101.

108. Granados R. Aspiration cytology of ovarian tumors. Curr Opin Obstet Gynecol 1995;7:43–8.

109. Wojcik EM, Selvaggi SM. Fine-needle aspiration cytology of cystic ovarian lesions. Diagn Cytopathol 1994;11:9–14.

110. Kreuger GF, Paradowski T, Wurche K-D, et al. Neoplastic or nonneoplastic ovarian cyst? The role of cytology. Acta Cytol 1995;39:882–6.

111. Allias F, Chanoz J, Blache G, et al. Value of ultrasound-guided fine-needle aspiration in the management of ovarian and parovarian cysts. Diagn Cytopathol 2000;22:70–80.

112. Martínez-Onsurbe P, Villaespesa AR, Anquela JMS, et al. Aspiration cytology of 147 adnexal cysts with histologic correlation. Acta Cytol 2001;45:941–7.

113. Trimbos JB, Hacker NF. The case against aspirating ovarian cysts. Cancer 1993;72:828–31.

114. Nadji M, Greening SE, Sevin BU, et al. Fine needle aspiration cytology in gynecologic oncology. II. Morphologic aspects. Acta Cytol 1979;23:380–8.

115. Taylor IW. Biopsy of lesions of the female genital tract in the ambulatory setting. J Long Term Eff Med Implants 2004;14:185–99.

116. Saad AJ, Donovan TM, Truang LD. Malakoplakia of the vagina diagnosed by fine-needle aspiration cytology. Diagn Cytopathol 1993;9:559–61.

117. Rollins SD. Fine-needle aspiration diagnosis of a vulvar papillary hidradenoma. A case report. Diagn Cytopathol 1994;10:60–1.

118. Yamagiwa S, Niwa K, Yokoyama Y et al. Primary adenoid cystic carcinoma of Bartholin's gland. A case report. Acta Cytol 1994;38:79–82.

119. Fulciniti F, Caleo A, Lepore M, et al. Fine needle cytology of endometriosis. Experience with 10 cases. Acta Cytol 2005;49:495–9.

120. Catalina-Fernandez I, Lopez-Presa D, Saenz-Soutamaria J. Fine needle aspiration cytology in cutaneous and subcutaneous endometriosis. Acta Cytol 2007;51:380–4.

121. Barbazza R, Chiarelli S, Quintarelli GF, et al. Role of fine-needle aspiration cytology in the preoperative evaluation of smooth muscle tumors. Diagn Cytopathol 1997;16:326–30.

122. Fulciniti F, Losito NS, Botti G, et al. Cytology of metastatic endometrioid neoplasms: Experience with eight cases. Diagn Cytopathol 2009;37:347–52.

123. Yang GC. Fine needle aspiration cytology of low grade endometrial stromal sarcoma. Acta Cytol 1995;39:701–5.

124. Policarpio-Nicolas ML, Cathro HP, Kerr SE, et al. Cytomorpologic features of low-grade endometrial stromal sarcoma. Am J Clin Pathol 2007;128:265–71.

125. Donat EE, McCutcheon JM, Alper H. Malignant mixed Müllerian tumor of the ovary. Report of a case with cytodiagnosis by fine needle aspiration. Acta Cytol 1994;38:231–4.

126. Mourad WA, Sneige N, Katz RL, et al. Fine-needle aspiration cytology of recurrent and metastatic mixed mesodermal tumors. Diagn Cytopathol 1994;11:328–32.

127. Mulvany N, Östör A, Teng G. Evaluation of estradiol in aspirated ovarian cystic lesions. Acta Cytol 1995;39:663–8.

128. Kovacic J, Rainer S, Levicnik A, et al. Cytology of benign ovarian lesions in connection with laparoscopy. In: Zajicek J, editor. Aspiration biopsy cytology. Part 2. Cytology of infradiaphragmatic organs. Basel: Karger; 1979.

129. Khajuria A, Karmakar T, Srinivasan R. Fine needle aspiration cytology of a subcutaneous metastasis of a malignant Brenner tumor of the ovary: a case report. Acta Cytol 1995;39:246–8.

130. Ramzy I, Delaney M, Rose P. Fine needle aspiration of ovarian masses. II. Correlative cytologic and histologic study of non-neoplastic cysts and non-coelomic epithelial neoplasms. Acta Cytol 1979;23:185–93.

131. Athanassiadou P, Grapsa D. Fine needle aspiration of borderline ovarian lesions. Is it useful? Acta Cytol 2005;49:278–85.

132. Hirokawa M, Miyake Y, Shimizu M, et al. Nuclear findings of ovarian surface epithelial tumors. Diagn Cytopathol 2000;22:27–9.

133. Atahan S, Ekinci C, Içli F, et al. Cytology of clear cell carcinoma of the female genital tract in fine needle aspirates and ascites. Acta Cytol 2000;44:1005–9.

134. Khunamornpong S, Thorner PS, Suprasert P, et al. Clear cell adenocarcinoma of the female genital tract: Tigroid background in various types of cytologic specimen. Diagn Cytopathol 2005;32:336–40.

135. Lal A, Bourtsos E P, Nayar R, et al. Cytologic features of granulosa cell tumors in fluids and fine needle aspiration specimens. Acta Cytol 2004;48:315–20.

136. Ali S, Gattuso P, Howard A, et al. Adult granulosa cell tumor of ovary: Fine-needle-aspiration cytology of 10 cases and review of literature. Diagn Cytopathol 2008;36:292–302.

137. Ramzy I, Delaney M. Signet-ring cell stromal tumour of ovary. Cytologic appearances of fine needle aspiration biopsy. Acta Cytol 1977;21:14–17.

138. Ryan LJ, Pambuccian SE, Lai R, et al. Endoscopic US-guided fine needle aspiration diagnosis of metastatic sex cord tumor with annular tubules. Diagn Cytopathol 2006;34:576–9.

139. Hees K, de Jonge JPA, von Kortzfleisch DHJ. Dysgerminoma of ovary. Cytologic, histologic and electron microscopic study of a case. Acta Cytol 1991;35:341–4.

140. Mizrak B, Ekinci C. Cytologic diagnosis of yolk sac tumor. A report of seven cases. Acta Cytol 1995;39:936–40.

CHAPTER 14

Skin and subcutis

Svante R. Orell and Henryk Domanski

The place of FNAC in the investigative sequence

Fine needle biopsy (FNB) and cytodiagnosis has found only limited application in primary tumors of the skin and subcutis due to the ease of surgical biopsy and of excision. The main indications for FNB are rapid, non-invasive investigation of suspected metastatic malignancy, and distinction between neoplasia and a reactive process likely to resolve spontaneously or respond to conservative treatment.[1,2] In patients with known malignancy, the nature of any nodules or thickenings related to surgical scars or elsewhere in the skin or subcutis the distinction can easily be made between suture granuloma, infection or other reactive process and recurrent or metastatic tumor. The possibility of a second primary or of de-differentiation of the original tumor can also be decided by cytology.

Some knowledge of the cytological features of skin adnexal tumors is needed to avoid mistaking these for metastatic malignancies. With some exceptions, a type-specific diagnosis of primary adnexal tumors by FNB is difficult or impossible but is not often of practical importance. From a clinical point of view, the information sought is mainly if the lesion is benign or malignant, and if malignant whether it is primary or metastatic. Cytology as a supplement to history and clinical findings can be useful in the management of patients with skin tumors.

Incisional biopsy or punch biopsy of pigmented lesions is generally contraindicated in view of the risk of spreading melanoma and of interfering with the histological diagnosis and staging on subsequent excision. Although not proven, FNB could have similar adverse effects and is therefore not recommended for localized pigmented skin lesions. However, since pigmented lesions are occasionally examined by FNB, cytopathologists must be familiar with the cytomorphology of melanocytic skin lesions (see below).

Scrape smears from tumors involving the epidermis or a mucous membrane is an alternative to biopsy in some cases, e.g. to confirm suspected squamous cell carcinoma, basal cell carcinoma or Paget's disease. Scrape smears can also be used to confirm advanced ulcerated malignant melanoma.

Dermatologists seeking an alternative treatment to surgical excision of basal cell carcinoma have shown some interest in cytological confirmation of this diagnosis.

Subcutaneous lipoma is one of the commonest 'tumors' seen in a community-based cytology practice. It may seem unnecessary to subject these clinically characteristic lesions to biopsy, but the patient and sometimes the referring doctor are often concerned and demand immediate reassurance. We have had some surprise findings in such cases and feel that FNB is generally justified. One example of several: a small, discrete, soft nodule was incidentally felt in the lower anterior abdominal wall of a 45-year-old woman. The clinical diagnosis was lipoma, but cytology showed a highly cellular, sarcomatous tumor, histologically confirmed as synovial sarcoma.

In general, FNB is not useful in the investigation of inflammatory skin disease except to provide material for microbiology, for example in tuberculosis and leprosy.

Accuracy of diagnosis

Only a few series of FNB of primary skin tumors with histologic correlation have been reported.[3–8] In one of the largest series, 89% of primary skin tumors were correctly diagnosed as benign or malignant, and specific typing was possible in 81% of cases.[4] Some skin adnexal tumors, in particular pilomatrixoma, have been reported as diagnostic pitfalls and a possible cause of false-positive cytological diagnosis.[9] Clinical correlation is essential.

Complications

The hypothetical risk of tumor cell seeding and of compromising subsequent histological examination as a result of FNB has been mentioned. Other significant complications have not been reported.

Technical considerations

We generally use 25- or 27-gauge needles and the non-aspiration technique for skin tumors, 23–25-gauge for subcutaneous lesions. Local anesthesia is rarely necessary. Two

©2012 Elsevier Ltd
DOI: 10.1016/B978-0-7020-3151-9.00014-1

to four passes are usually required to obtain sufficient material and to compensate for possible tumor heterogeneity. Alcohol-fixed H&E- or Pap-stained smears and air-dried smears stained with Diff-Quik or MGG should be used in parallel. FNB of skin lesions often yield cohesive tissue fragments. Alcohol-fixation makes tissue fragments transparent whereas cell detail is poorly seen in fragments in air-dried smears. Squamous differentiation is more easily recognized in Pap-stained smears. On the other hand, air-dried MGG smears provide more information on secretory products and stromal components.

Thin superficial skin lesions, particularly if eroded or ulcerated, are best sampled by scraping cells off the surface. Keratin, crust and inflammatory exudate must be removed to ensure that intact, well-preserved cells are obtained from as deeply into the lesion as possible. Scraping with a sterile scalpel blade held at a blunt angle until the lesion bleeds slightly is recommended.[10] Wooden spatulas or other soft materials are less suitable since they tend to absorb the fluid component. FNB can be successful in some thin lesions using a 25–27-gauge needle inserted tangentially.

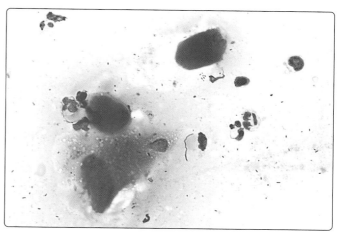

Fig. 14.1 Molluscum contagiosum Three darkly staining molluscum bodies and some inflammatory cells (MGG, HP).

CYTOLOGICAL FINDINGS

Non-neoplastic lesions

Inflammatory processes

Purulent material aspirated from *suppurative inflammation* or *abscess* can be used for microbiological studies. The presence of many mature and keratinized squamous epithelial cells suggests an inflamed epidermoid cyst or suppurative hidradenitis, hair shafts indicate a dermoid cyst or a pilonidal sinus. *Demodex* may be identified in scrape smears of infectious folliculitis.[11] A malignancy, mainly squamous cell carcinoma can be obscured by inflammatory exudate and smears should be examined carefully for single neoplastic cells.

FNB samples from a non-suppurative chronic inflammatory process usually contain fragments of *inflammatory/ reparative granulation tissue* composed of clustered, relatively cohesive reactive fibroblasts and histiocytes, strands of endothelial cells representing capillary vessels, and various inflammatory cells. Granulation tissue can be quite cellular in smears, macrophages and fibroblasts may look atypical and mitotic figures are not uncommon, but the overall findings in the appropriate clinical context are characteristic.

Inclusion bodies may be found in scrape smears of *viral* skin lesions. The cytological features of herpes virus infection are well known from gynecological cytology. Molluscum bodies of molluscum contagiosum look similar in smears and in histological sections (Fig. 14.1).

Clusters of epithelioid histiocytes with poorly defined cytoplasm and pale nuclei of a banana-, bean- or footprint-like shape, associated with multinucleated histiocytic giant cells are consistent with *granulomatous inflammation*. The differential diagnosis includes a number of conditions: foreign body granuloma, tuberculosis, leprosy, sarcoid, fungal infections, etc.[12] Multinucleated histiocytic giant cells are prominent in foreign body granuloma, and the presence of birefringent particles, suture material, etc. supports the diagnosis (Fig. 14.2). Caseous necrosis suggests tuberculosis, to

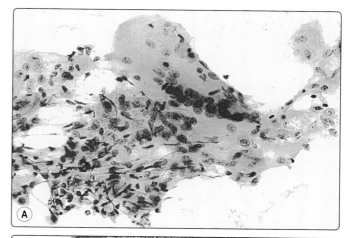

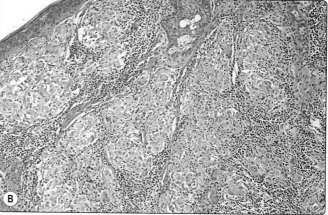

Fig. 14.2 Sarcoid-like foreign body granuloma (A) Large multinucleated giant cells, clustered histiocytes and some inflammatory cells. Birefringent foreign material present but not seen in this microphotograph (Pap, IP); (B) Corresponding tissue section. Sarcoid-like cluster of many discrete granulomata of epithelioid histiocytes and some giant cells; no evidence of caseation; foreign bodies seen in polarized light (H&E, LP).

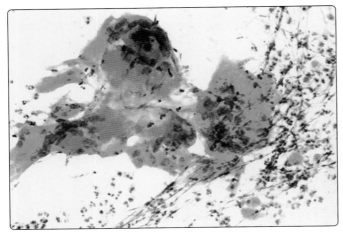

Fig. 14.3 Epidermal cyst Clumps of keratin and squamous cells, multinucleate histiocytes, inflammatory cells and debris (Pap, IP).

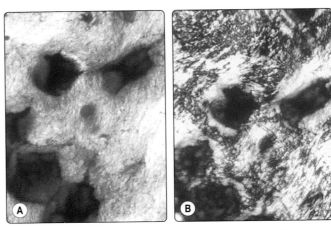

Fig. 14.5 Gouty tophus Clumps and more thinly spread crystalline material (**A**, MGG, IP; **B**, polarised light, IP).

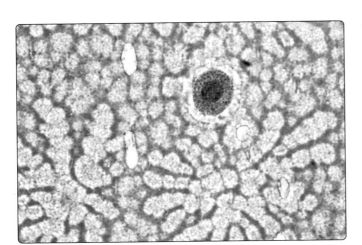

Fig. 14.4 Ganglion A single histiocyte-like cell; background of myxoid material showing peculiar drying artifact (MGG, HP).

be confirmed by staining for acid-fast bacilli; fibrosis with no evidence of necrosis is more in keeping with sarcoid. The cytological patterns found in *leprosy* have been described.[13,14] The etiology of granulomatous inflammation cannot be decided on the basis of cytomorphology alone and must be pursued by staining for microorganisms, bacteriological culture, serological tests, and other investigations.

A vaguely granulomatous chronic inflammatory pattern with a background of fat and evidence of fat necrosis seen in FNB smears of a subcutaneous induration on the leg suggests a *panniculitic process*, such as erythema nodosum.[15] The findings are not diagnostic, only suggestive, and necessitate a surgical biopsy. Cytological findings in *fat necrosis* are described in Chapter 7 (see p. 167).

Cysts and other non-neoplastic lesions

Aspirates from *epidermal* or *dermoid cysts* consist of thick, greasy, foul-smelling material. Smears show mature squamous epithelial cells, a high proportion of which are keratinized cells or ghost cells, and a background of debris and often inflammatory cells. Foreign body giant cells and calcium granules may be present (Fig. 14.3). The presence

of hair shafts suggests a dermoid cyst.[16] Reactive epithelial atypia in inflamed cysts can look worrisome.[4] On the other hand, cells of partly necrotic and degenerate, well-differentiated metastatic squamous cell carcinoma can look deceptively bland in FNB samples. The content of *trichilemmal cysts* is similar, but clumps of structureless keratin are more prominent, there are no granular or parakeratotic cells and cholesterol crystals are often seen. Cytological findings in *proliferating trichilemmal cyst* and *malignant proliferating trichilemmal tumor* have been described.[17,18]

A postoperative *lymphocele* yields clear, yellowish, mucoid fluid on aspiration which contains a variable number of mature lymphocytes. Smears from a *hematoma* show altered blood, hemosiderin-containing macrophages, amorphous material with cholesterol crystals, or fragments of reparative granulation tissue with hemosiderin pigment, depending on the age of the process.

The material aspirated from a *ganglion* is thick, colorless, glassy and jelly-like. It is so characteristic that the diagnosis is already obvious from the macroscopic appearance of the aspirate in the appropriate clinical setting. Smears show a small number of single cells with abundant cytoplasm and small oval nuclei and a background of abundant myxoid material, which may show interesting drying artifacts (Fig. 14.4).[19] FNB of bursal cysts has been described as similar to that of ganglion.[20]

A few cases of *rheumatoid nodules* with FNB findings have been reported.[21,22] Samples are scanty of amorphous granular acidophilic material with a variable number of fibroblasts and/or histiocytes. Small multinucleated histiocytic giant cells may be seen. *Gouty tophi* are sometimes subjected to FNB if the clinical diagnosis is doubtful. Thick, putty-like material is aspirated. Smears show clumps of non-cellular material of birefringent needle-shaped crystals that are better preserved than in formalin-fixed tissue, and a few histiocytes and giant cells (Fig. 14.5).[21,23]

Calcinosis of subcutaneous or soft tissue may present as a mass lesion. It is usually of dystrophic or metabolic etiology but there is also a rare, primary inherited form called tumoral calcinosis.[24] FNB yields amorphous calcified material, laminated concretions and variable numbers of histiocytes, lymphocytes and osteoclast-like giant cells.

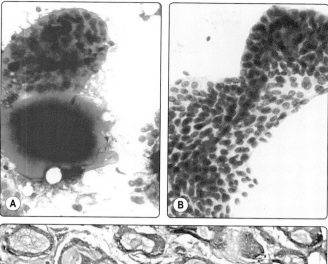

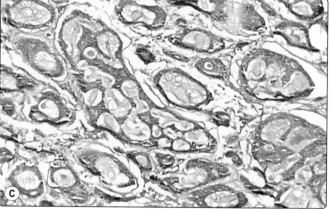

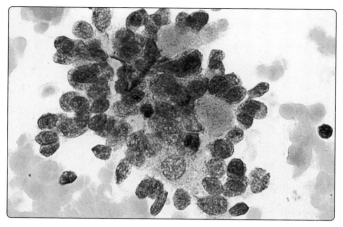

Fig. 14.7 Cutaneous cylindroma Clustered basaloid epithelial cells; mild nuclear atypia; hyaline stromal globules; note similarity to adenoid cystic carcinoma (MGG, HP) *(Courtesy Dr K. Lindholm, Malmo, Sweden).*

Fig. 14.6 Cutaneous cylindroma Pseudopapillary tissue fragments of cohesive bland basaloid cells; hyaline stromal globule (**A**, MGG; **B**, Pap, IP); (**C**) Corresponding tissue section (H&E, IP) *(Courtesy Dr J. Klijanienko, Inst. Curie, Paris).*

Endometriosis can present as a poorly defined, tumor-like induration in the subcutaneous tissue or in relation to a scar of the anterior abdominal wall in a premenopausal woman. Cytological findings are described in Chapter 13 (see page 357).[25]

Amyloid tumor of subcutaneous tissue may also present as a mass lesion. FNB smears display fragments of acellular amorphous matrix, scattered histiocytic cells and occasionally small calcifications. FNB of periumbilical adipose tissue of the anterior abdominal wall can be of value in the diagnosis of secondary systemic *amyloidosis* although sensitivity is low.[26,27] Rings of amyloid around fat cells and amyloid deposits in vessel walls can be demonstrated by Congo red staining and polarization.

Benign epithelial skin tumors

The cytology of benign primary epithelial skin tumors has mainly been described in single case reports, and criteria are not well established. A wide range of tumors occur in this site and specific entities are difficult or impossible to identify in smears. Clinically, the distinction between benign and malignant tumors, particularly those of metastatic nature, is the most important, and this is possible by FNB with a high level of accuracy. In general, cell-rich smears of

more or less cohesive small basaloid cells mixed with a variable number of squamoid cells and sometimes glandular elements suggest a primary cutaneous neoplasm, and close study of the nuclear cytomorphology is likely to predict malignancy. The microarchitectural pattern and certain stromal components can provide clues to a type-specific diagnosis in some cases.

Our limited experience does not permit a systematic description of the cytology of skin adnexal tumors. Some examples selected from our files are briefly described and illustrated and references are provided to relevant case reports and small series published in the literature.

Adenomatous tumors of sweat gland origin

Smears of *cutaneous cylindroma* ('turban tumor') are usually cell-rich, of pseudopapillary fragments of cohesive basaloid epithelial cells and hyaline stromal material often seen as globules. The cells are small, crowded with a high nuclear:cytoplasmic ratio and relatively uniform round or ovoid hyperchromatic nuclei. The pattern can closely resemble adenoid cystic carcinoma but the nuclear chromatin is bland (Figs 14.6 and 14.7). Cutaneous cylindroma should be remembered in the differential diagnosis of tumors in the head and neck.[28]

Spiradenoma is closely related to and resembles cylindroma. Smears are highly cellular, of clustered, variably cohesive small basaloid epithelial cells with uniform oval dark nuclei and a homogeneous chromatin. A more or less obvious acinar/tubular arrangement of the cells is discernible, but a dual population of small dark and larger pale epithelial cells as seen in histological sections is difficult to appreciate in smears. Globules of hyaline stromal material are characteristic but were scant in the case illustrated here (Fig. 14.8). The main differential diagnosis is adenoid cystic carcinoma.[29]

The cytology of *nodular hidradenoma*[30-32] and of *clear cell hidradenoma*[33,34] has been described in single cases. A benign skin adnexal tumor from our files, histologically reported as cystic eccrine hidradenoma, is shown in Figure 14.9. The FNB sample was of mucoid fluid which contained clusters of variably cohesive uniform epithelial cells with a moderate

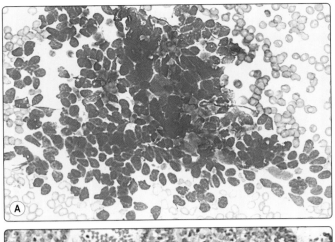

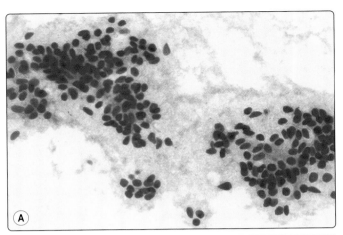

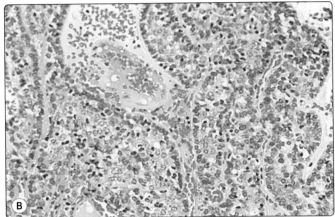

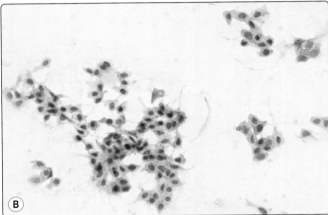

Fig. 14.8 Eccrine spiradenoma (A) Clustered and dissociated small basaloid cells with relatively uniform dark nuclei; suggestion of acinar/tubular grouping; minimal amount of hyaline stroma (MGG, IP); (B) Corresponding tissue section (H&E, IP).

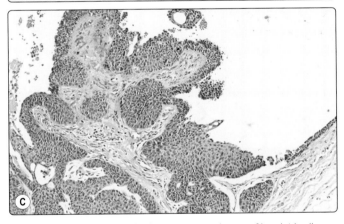

amount of cytoplasm and small dark ovoid nuclei. A dual population was not discernible. The cytology was reported as a benign skin adnexal tumor without further specification.

Benign skin adnexal tumors located to the breast or axilla can be mistaken for primary or metastatic breast cancer.[33,35] Knowledge of the exact localization of the lesion and its relation to the skin is essential when examining FNBs, as illustrated by the following case from our files:

A 60-year-old woman with a history of right mastectomy for cancer 4 years previously presented with a lump in the right axilla. It was described as subcutaneous by the surgeon who performed the FNB and the clinical diagnosis was metastasis of breast cancer. Smears were highly cellular, of epithelial cells both forming cohesive aggregates and dispersed as single cells. True papillary fragments were not seen. The cells had a moderate amount of dense cytoplasm and there was relatively mild nuclear atypia (Fig. 14.10). The pattern was considered to be in keeping with metastasis of a low-grade breast carcinoma. However, the nodule was, in fact, intracutaneous and the histology was reported as syringocystadenoma papilliferum (Fig. 14.10).[36]

FNB findings in *vulval papillary hidradenoma* have also been reported.[37]

Fig. 14.9 Cystic eccrine hidradenoma Loose clusters of basaloid cells with small, dark, uniform nuclei in a background of proteinaceous fluid (A, MGG; B, Pap, IP); (C) Corresponding tissue section (H&E, LP).

Pilomatricoma (calcifying epithelioma of Malherbe) (Fig. 14.11)[37–40]

CRITERIA FOR DIAGNOSIS

◆ Abundant material,
◆ Aggregates of degenerate, anucleate keratinized squamous cells (ghost cells),
◆ Tight clusters of cohesive basaloid cells,
◆ Calcium granules and debris,
◆ Inflammatory cells; foreign body giant cells.

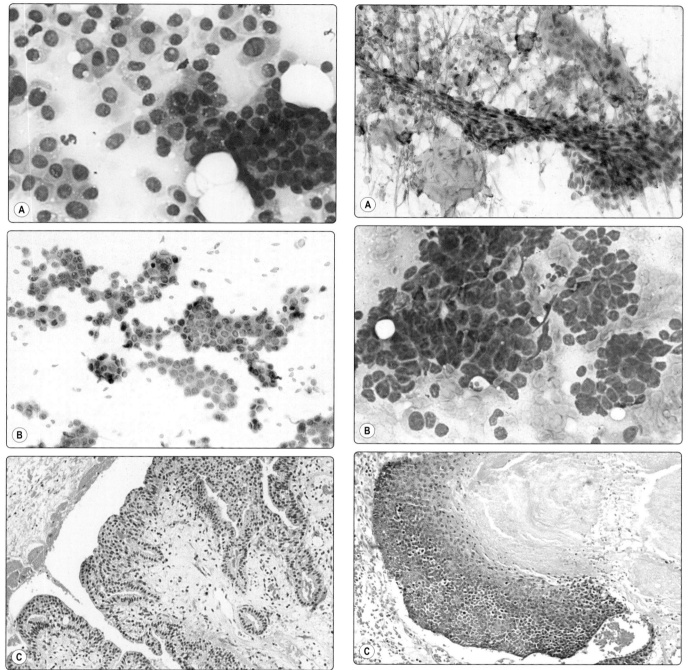

Fig. 14.10 Syringocystadenoma papilliferum Clustered and dispersed epithelial cells; moderate amount of cytoplasm; mildly atypical nuclei; no true papillary fragments (**A**, MGG, HP; **B**, H&E, IP); (**C**) Corresponding tissue section (H&E, LP).

Fig. 14.11 Pilomatrixoma (**A**) Clump of anucleate keratinized squamous cells ('ghost cells'), small basaloid cells, large multinucleate histiocytic giant cell, inflammatory cells, calcium granules and debris (Pap, IP); (**B**) Clusters of small, tightly packed basaloid cells; may be mistaken for malignant if the complex smear pattern is lacking and basaloid cells dominate (MGG, HP); (**C**) Corresponding tissue section. The basaloid cells may be selectively sampled by FNB (H&E, IP).

Pilomatrixoma has attracted considerable interest in the cytological literature as the commonest cause of false-positive diagnosis in this area. Large numbers of tightly clustered and some single basaloid cells with scanty cytoplasm and medium-sized, hyperchromatic, mildly irregular nuclei with small nucleoli may dominate the FNB samples. Mitotic figures and apoptotic bodies may be found, as well as moderate nuclear pleomorphism and atypical cells arranged in a whorled fashion more often seen in smears from squamous cell carcinoma (Fig. 14.12). The cells

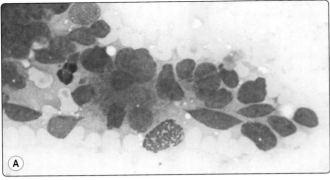

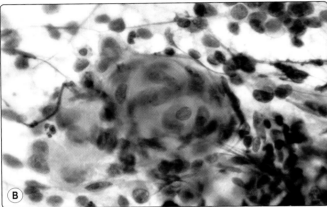

Fig. 14.12 Pilomatrixoma (A) Moderate nuclear pleomorphism and a mitotic figure (MGG, HP); (B) Atypical cells arranged in a whorled cluster resembling squamous cell carcinoma (H&E, HP).

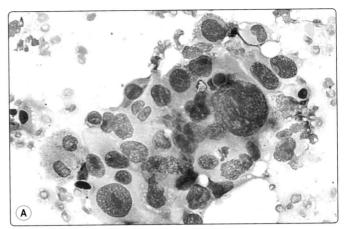

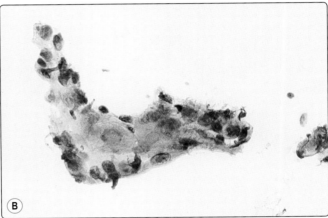

Fig. 14.13 Squamous cell carcinoma (A) Aggregate of pleomorphic, obviously malignant cells with dense squamoid cytoplasm and distinct cell borders; no obvious keratinization in this field; FNB smear from ulcerated 10–15-mm tumor lower lip (MGG, HP); (B) Cohesive tissue fragment of malignant squamous epithelial cells; scrape smear from ulcerated skin tumor (Pap, HP).

resemble those of basal cell carcinoma, basaloid squamous cell carcinoma or small cell anaplastic carcinoma. The 'dirty' background may be misinterpreted as tumor necrosis, but is rich in granular calcium and characteristically includes histiocytic multinucleated giant cells. The 'ghost cells' seen in tissue sections appear as clumps of keratinous material or degenerate mature squamous epithelial cells in smears. There is a tendency for the basaloid cells to be overrepresented in smears, probably because they are more easily detached than the other components.

There is a risk of making a false-positive cytological diagnosis if clustered basaloid cells dominate the smears and the characteristic ghost cells, background calcification and giant cells are scant or overlooked. Clinical findings, age, size and history are important clues to the correct diagnosis

Other benign adnexal tumors

Cytologic findings in *eccrine* acrospiroma,[41] *chondroid* syringoma,[35,42,43] *trichoepithelioma*[7] and *trichoblastoma*[32] have been described in single case reports.

Malignant epithelial tumors

Squamous cell carcinoma (Fig. 14.13)

Scrape smears are a simple way of diagnosing squamous cell carcinoma of the skin, particularly ulcerated lesions.

Inflammatory crust and any surface keratinous layers must first be carefully removed to obtain diagnostic cells from the deeper layers. The technique is described above. Nodular and deeply invasive tumors and recurrences are better examined by FNB.

Cytological criteria of squamous cell carcinoma are described in several other chapters, mainly in Chapter 8. The differential diagnosis between well-differentiated squamous carcinoma with cystic degeneration and branchial and other benign cysts lined by squamous epithelium can cause problems due to subtle squamous cell atypia in the former and reactive atypia and metaplasia in the latter (see Chapter 4). Distinction between keratotic basal cell carcinoma and basaloid squamous cell carcinoma can be difficult.[4] Cytological criteria for basal cell carcinoma are listed below. The cytomorphology of adenoid (acantholytic) squamous cell carcinoma can cause problems.[44] Distinction between in situ (dysplastic solar keratosis, Bowen's disease) and superficially invasive carcinoma is not possible in smears.

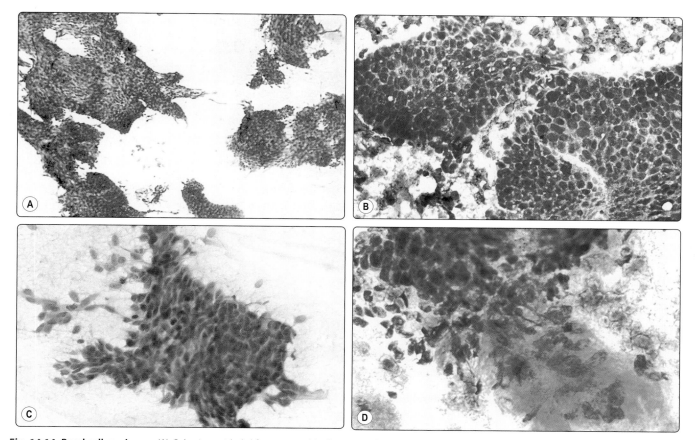

Fig. 14.14 Basal cell carcinoma (A) Cohesive epithelial fragments with alternating sharp and irregular borders (H&E, IP); (B) Tissue fragments of very cohesive basaloid cells. The fragments have well-defined borders of cells with a tendency to palisading. This smear is a FNB sample from a bone deposit of metastasizing basal cell carcinoma (MGG, HP); (C) Tumor fragment of small, tightly packed cells, FNB smear (H&E, MP); (D) Basal cell carcinoma, infiltrating type; tumor fragment of closely packed small, uniform basal cells and adherent fibrillar fibrous stroma (MGG, LP).

Basal cell carcinoma (Fig. 14.14)[8,45–48]

CRITERIA FOR DIAGNOSIS

◆ Tight cell aggregates with sharp outline, smooth edges, often budding,

◆ Palisading of nuclei along the edge of aggregates,

◆ Small cells with scanty cyanophilic cytoplasm; indistinct cell borders,

◆ Small, hyperchromatic, ovoid, overlapping nuclei; indistinct nucleoli,

◆ Stromal material variable.

Most basal cell carcinomas (BCC) are diagnosed clinically. Scrape smears from the surface can provide rapid pre-treatment confirmation, of particular importance if non-surgical treatment is considered. If the lesion is ulcerated, any inflammatory debris should be removed prior to vigorous scrapings.[8] Non-ulcerated, deeply invasive tumors are suitable for FNB sampling using a thin 25–27-gauge needle.

The most characteristic feature of BCC in smears is the strong cohesiveness of the cells, which remain in well-defined tissue fragments of tightly packed small cells with palisading of nuclei along the edges. The fragments resemble tumor buds seen in tissue sections (Fig. 14.14A). The same pattern was seen in FNB smears from a rare case of distant metastasis to bone from of a large, deeply invasive BCC on the back of an elderly patient (Fig. 14.14B). The cells are small with very scanty cytoplasm and overlapping, ovoid, relatively uniform hyperchromatic nuclei. The chromatin is evenly distributed and nucleoli are inconspicuous. Subtyping of BCC is generally not possible, but stromal material can be prominent in smears from desmoplastic, infiltrating basal cell carcinoma, suggesting a differential diagnosis of chondroid syringoma (Fig. 14.14D).

In clinical practice, the main differential is BCC versus actinic keratosis. Christensen et al., in a study of 78 cases, found cytological diagnosis to be highly accurate if samples are adequate.[48] In general, the microarchitecture and the predominance of typical basal cells are characteristic of BCC. Cells of actinic keratosis are less cohesive, and show features of dysplastic squamous epithelial cells with more abundant cytoplasm. Cells of non-keratinizing, basaloid squamous cell carcinoma are also less cohesive, larger, some with dense squamoid cytoplasm, some with prominent nucleoli.

The distinction from benign and malignant skin adnexal tumors is a less common but more difficult problem. Smears of adnexal tumors are similarly dominated by dense aggregates of small basaloid epithelial cells, but the pattern is usually more mixed and includes squamoid cells, glandular (tubulo-acinar) structures or small round cells, and stromal material.[7]

Pigmented basal cell carcinoma may be misdiagnosed as melanoma and correct diagnosis may require immunostaining.[49]

Paget's disease[50]

Extramammary Paget's disease can be diagnosed by the examination of scrape smears from the surface. The cytological features are similar to those of Paget's disease of the nipple, described in Chapter 7.

Malignant skin adnexal tumors

Cytologic findings in several cases of *sebaceous carcinoma* have been reported.[3,4,51,52] The tumor cells have vacuolated, bubbly cytoplasm and malignant nuclear morphology including mitotic figures and prominent nucleoli. There may be an admixture with basaloid and squamous cells and evidence of necrosis (Fig. 14.15).

Single cases of *malignant sweat gland tumors* have been reported.[53–55] A case from our files, initially diagnosed as infiltrating basal cell carcinoma both on FNB and on surgical biopsy, is illustrated in Figure 14.16. Later recurrences were histologically diagnosed as eccrine (microcystic) carcinoma The small duct-like clusters of cells showing squamous differentiation were initially overlooked in a predominantly basal cell population.

The cytology of some uncommon malignant adnexal tumors has been described in single case reports, e.g. *apocrine sweat gland* carcinoma,[56] *malignant* spiradenoma,[57] *primary mucinous carcinoma of* skin,[58,59] and *malignant chondroid syringoma.*[60]

Merkel cell carcinoma (neuroendocrine carcinoma of skin) (Fig. 14.17, and see Fig. 5.23)[61,62]

CRITERIA FOR DIAGNOSIS

◆ Cell-rich smears of mainly dispersed small neoplastic cells,

◆ Fragile, scanty, blue (MGG) cytoplasm; high nuclear : cytoplasmic ratio; many stripped nuclei,

◆ Clustered cells may show nuclear molding and rosette-like grouping,

◆ Round or ovoid, mildly to moderately irregular hyperchromatic nuclei with inconspicuous nucleoli,

◆ Mitoses frequent,

◆ Lymphoid globules (lymphoglandular bodies) absent,

◆ Dot-like paranuclear staining for cytokeratin; chromogranin usually positive.

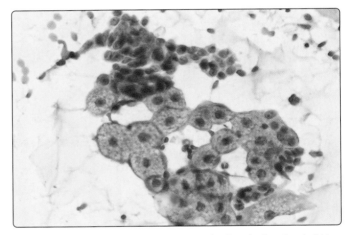

Fig. 14.15 Sebaceous carcinoma Clusters of cells with abundant bubbly cytoplasm and central nuclei, and of small tightly cohesive basaloid epithelial cells (Pap, HP).

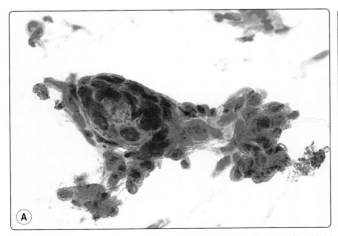

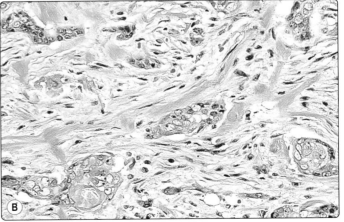

Fig. 14.16 Eccrine (microcystic) carcinoma (A) Tight clusters of basaloid cells and a microtubular structure with squamous differentiation (Pap, HP); (B) Corresponding tissue section (H&E, IP).

Primary neuroendocrine carcinoma of skin is an uncommon neoplasm, mainly seen in elderly patients and most often in the head and neck. It is locally aggressive and often metastasizes to regional lymph nodes. Clinically and cytologically, Merkel cell tumor can be difficult to distinguish from non-Hodgkin lymphoma when it presents as lymphadenopathy without an obvious primary, as is often the case (see Chapter 5).

Smears are usually highly cellular. The cells are mainly dispersed but some are clustered or form single files with nuclear molding and sometimes rosette-like groups. The main differential diagnoses are lymphoma and metastatic small cell carcinoma. Amelanotic melanoma may also be considered. The absence of lymphoid globules in the background and subtle differences in nuclear chromatin help in this distinction. Staining for CAM5.2, CK7 and CK20 demonstrates characteristic dot-like intracytoplasmic deposits in the tumor cells (Fig. 14.17C), and staining for neuroendocrine markers is usually positive. Electron microscopy shows well-demarcated whorls of cytoplasmic filaments.

Benign non-epithelial tumors

Subcutaneous lipoma (Fig. 14.18)

As mentioned in the clinical section, subcutaneous lipoma is one of the commonest targets of FNB anywhere in the body. Samples are mainly acellular fat but usually also include fragments of mature adipose tissue and some vascular elements. Lipomatous lesions are described in detail in Chapter 15.

Histiocytoma/dermatofibroma (Figs 14.19 and 14.20)

CRITERIA FOR DIAGNOSIS

- ◆ Clusters of fibrohistiocytic cells, plump or spindle shaped,
- ◆ Eosinophilic, granular or vacuolated cytoplasm; indistinct cell borders,
- ◆ Oval, kidney-shaped or elongated, spindled nuclei; mild anisokaryosis; granular bland chromatin; small nucleoli,
- ◆ Multinucleated histiocytic giant cells,
- ◆ Fragments of fibrous stroma (variable)

This is a common intracutaneous lesion presenting as a small, often pigmented, poorly circumscribed induration, which can occur anywhere but most often on the leg. The diagnosis is usually clinically obvious, but larger and more deep-sited tumors may cause clinical concern. Adequate material can usually be obtained with a 25–27-gauge needle. There is a spectrum of patterns (cellular histiocytoma, fibrous histiocytoma, dermatofibroma) which is reflected in the number of cells in the smear and in the proportion of histiocytes, fibroblasts and collagen. Multinucleated histiocytic giant cells, often of the Touton type, xanthomatous histiocytes with foamy cytoplasm and iron pigment are commonly

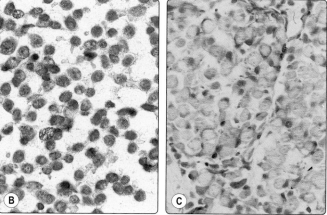

Fig. 14.17 Merkel cell carcinoma (A) Poorly cohesive cells; nuclear pleomorphism and some molding, scanty blue cytoplasm resembling lymphoid cells (MGG, HP); (B) Cellular smear of dispersed small cells with round, dark nuclei (Pap, HP); (C) Dot-like positive staining with CAM5.2 (immunostaining, HP).

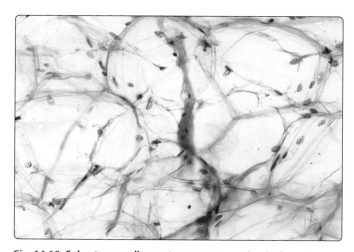

Fig. 14.18 Subcutaneous lipoma Large monovacuolated adipocytes, scanty fibrous stroma and an occasional capillary blood vessel (Pap, IP).

present in smears. The pattern can resemble that of other spindle cell lesions such as nodular fasciitis and dermatofibrosarcoma protuberans, but the clinical findings combined with the cytology allow a specific diagnosis in most cases.

The cytological findings in two cases of deep *juvenile xanthogranuloma* were reported by Grenko et al.[63] Regarding *atypical fibroxanthoma*, see Chapter 15, p. 392.

Glomus tumor (Figs 14.21 and 14.22)

The tumor illustrated in Figure 14.21 presented as an asymptomatic subcutaneous nodule on the leg of a middle-aged woman. The FNB sample was heavily admixed with blood, but also contained cellular tissue fragments and single cells. The cells were mainly plump spindle cells with abundant eosinophilic cytoplasm but some cells appeared epithelioid. Nuclei were bland and oval. The FNB was reported as a benign skin adnexal tumor, not further specified. Immunostaining for smooth muscle actin was not done. Cytological findings have been reported in a few cases.[64,65]

There is a subset of glomus tumor termed atypical glomus tumor and rare cases of malignant glomus tumor occur. Smears from such lesions are highly cellular, showing nuclear and cellular pleomorphism (Fig. 14.22), but the morphology and immunoprofile otherwise resembles ususal glomus tumor.

The cytological findings in *granular cell tumor* are described in Chapters 7 and 15. These tumors are frequently located to the skin and subcutaneous tissues accessible to FNB. Immunostaining for protein S-100 easily confirms the FNB diagnosis (see Figs 7.51 and 15.49). Kalfa et al.[66] reported two cases of *primary cutaneous meningioma* with FNB cytology.

Malignant non-epithelial tumors

Malignant melanoma (Figs 14.23–14.28)

CRITERIA FOR DIAGNOSIS

- Highly cellular smears,
- Mainly dispersed cells; variable numbers of loose clusters,
- Abundant cytoplasm; eccentric nuclei (plasmacytoid),
- Variable anisokaryosis and pleomorphism; binucleate and multinucleate cells,
- Uniformly hyperchromatic nuclei; intranuclear inclusions; prominent nucleoli,
- Melanin pigment (intracytoplasmic in tumor cells, dispersed in the background, in macrophages) – but many tumors are amelanotic,
- Paranuclear cytoplasmic condensation in amelanotic melanoma,
- Positive immunostaining for S-100 protein, Melan-A, less often HMB-45.

FNB of primary malignant melanoma is not recommended, except for rapid confirmation of advanced tumors. Checking suspicious local recurrence or regional lymph nodes for

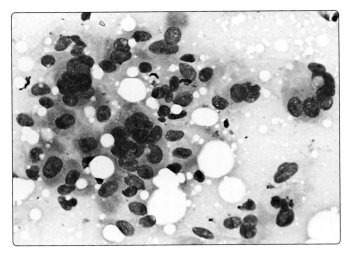

Fig. 14.19 Cutaneous histiocytoma Loose cell cluster; ovoid nuclei, abundant granular and vacuolated cytoplasm; indistinct cell borders; note multinucleated giant cells (MGG, HP).

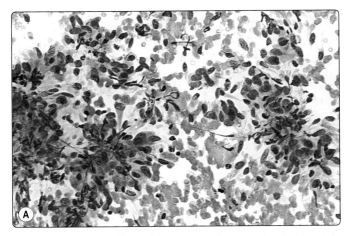
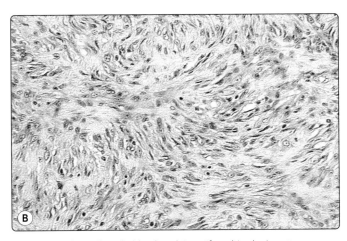

Fig. 14.20 Cutaneous fibrous histiocytoma This example is highly cellular, predominantly of spindle cells; bland nuclei; storiform histologic pattern (**A**, MGG, IP; **B**, tissue section H&E, IP).

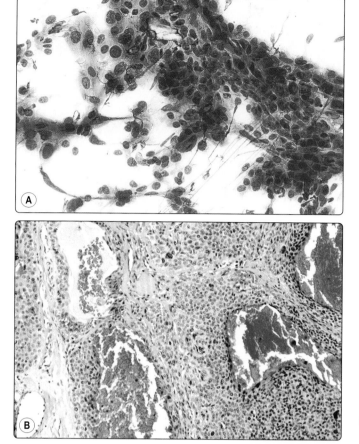

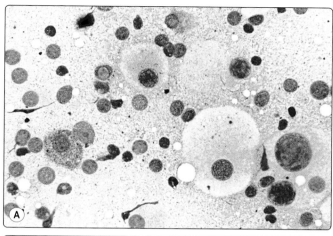

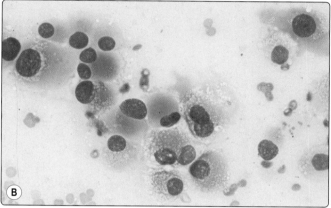

Fig. 14.21 Glomus tumor (A) Tissue fragment and dispersed cells; relatively abundant and dense eosinophilic cytoplasm; bland oval uniform nuclei; vascular structures not obvious (MGG, HP); (B) Corresponding tissue section (H&E, IP).

Fig. 14.23 Malignant melanoma, classic type (A) Dispersed cells with fragile cytoplasm; marked anisokaryosis, one cell with intact cytoplasm and typical dust-like pigment; pigment granules dispersed in background; intranuclear vacuole (MGG, HP); (B) Dispersed plasmacytoid cells with paranuclear cytoplasmic condensation but no pigment (Diff-Quik, HP)

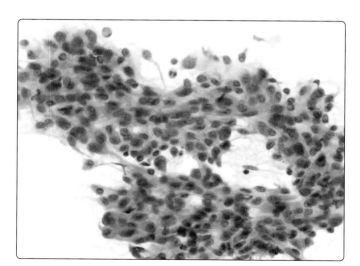

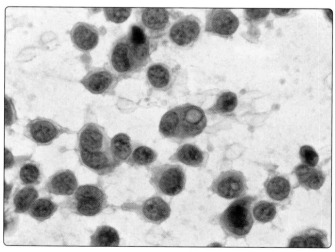

Fig. 14.22 Atypical glomus tumor FNB of atypical (infiltrative) glomus tumor; cytomorphology resembles regular glomus tumor but shows increased cellularity and nuclear and cellular pleomorphism (H&E, HP).

Fig.14.24 Malignant melanoma, classic type FNB smear from ulcerated malignant melanoma. Diagnostic pattern of mainly dispersed malignant cells with scanty cytoplasm; note intranuclear vacuole (H&E, HP).

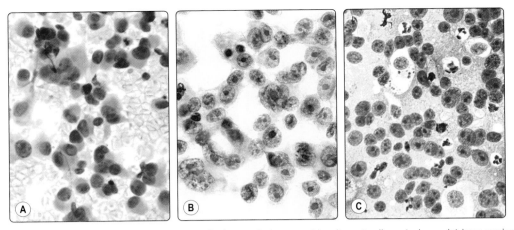

Fig. 14.25 Malignant melanoma, amelanotic, classic type Mainly dispersed plasmacytoid malignant cells, vesicular nuclei, large nucleoli, no pigment (**A**, H&E; **B**, IP, Pap, HP); (**C**) Poorly differentiated squamous carcinoma, cytology resembling melanoma (H&E, HP).

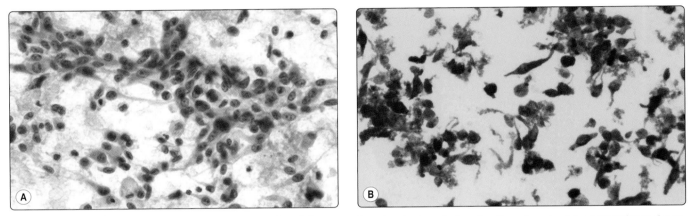

Fig. 14.26 Malignant melanoma, spindle cell type (**A**) Highly cellular smear of poorly cohesive spindle cells with oval, moderately pleomorphic nuclei; no pigment seen (H&E, HP, Pap, IP); (**B**) Same lesion; immunostaining for HMB-45, liquid based preparation.

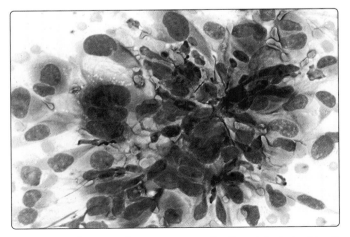

Fig. 14.27 Malignant melanoma, sarcoma-like The cytological pattern in this local recurrence is indistinguishable from pleomorphic soft tissue sarcoma; cells were S-100 positive (MGG, HP).

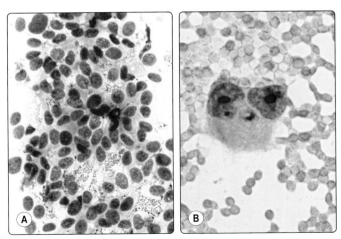

Fig. 14.28 Malignant melanoma, unusual patterns (**A**) Bizarre binucleate tumor giant cell with large nucleoli (Pap, HP); (**B**) Poorly cohesive cells with a vaguely follicular pattern and relatively uniform nuclei resembling a neuroendocrine tumor (Diff-Quik, HP).

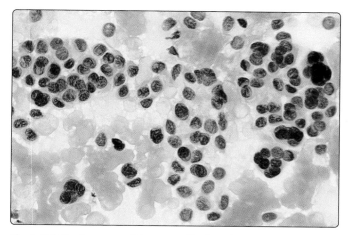

Fig. 14.29 Benign nevocellular nevus Single and some clustered cells with round or oval nuclei; mild anisokaryosis; indistinct cytoplasm. Bench specimen (H&E, HP).

metastases by FNB is of great value in the clinical management of melanoma.[67–69] Correct identification of melanoma in other metastatic sites is another important application.

Typically, the cells have abundant cytoplasm and an eccentric nucleus and appear plasmacytoid. The cytoplasm is relatively dense but may be vacuolated, sometimes fragile, leaving some nuclei stripped. A darker condensation of the paranuclear cytoplasm (MGG, see Figs 5.60 and 14.23B) may be a clue in amelanotic melanoma. Nuclear hyperchromasia is often relatively uniform; it varies more from cell to cell in anaplastic carcinoma. It can be difficult to distinguish melanin pigment from lipofuscin and hemosiderin in routine stained smears, and special stains (formalin-induced fluorescence, Masson-Fontana) may be required. A fine dust-like intracytoplasmic pigment in tumor cells is characteristic of melanoma. In the large study by Murali et al.,[70] melanin was demonstrated in only 27.6% of metastatic melanomas. The diagnosis can be confirmed by immunostaining (S-100 protein, Melan-A, HMB-45) or by the demonstration of premelanosomes by EM.

The criteria listed above apply mainly to the epithelioid or plasmacytoid, classic type of melanoma. However, the cytological pattern is extremely variable and melanoma can mimic many other tumors. Nasiell et al.[71] described several subtypes: classic, carcinoma-like, spindle cell, lymphoma-like, undifferentiated, myxoid and clear cell. A small cell type could be added, resembling small cell carcinoma. Some of the subtypes are illustrated in Figures 14.23 to 14.28. Poorly differentiated amelanotic melanoma can closely resemble either anaplastic carcinoma or anaplastic lymphoma. Apoptotic cells and necrotic debris is much more a feature of poorly differentiated carcinoma than of melanoma.[69] Spindle cell melanomas often have smaller, elongated, more uniform, and relatively bland nuclei (Fig. 14.26), but some are highly pleomorphic, mimicking high-grade pleomorphic sarcoma of soft tissues (Fig. 14.27). A vaguely follicular pattern with uniform cells may mimic a neuroendocrine tumor (Fig. 14.28A). Smears from malignant melanoma with a myxoid stromal reaction may be misinterpreted as a myxomatous soft tissue tumor. Desmoplastic melanoma presents special diagnostic problems in FNB samples.[72]

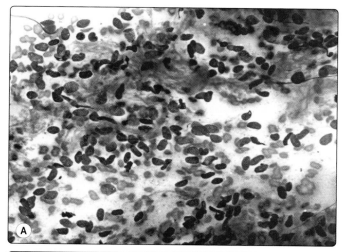

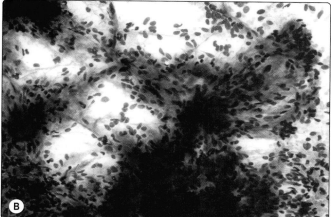

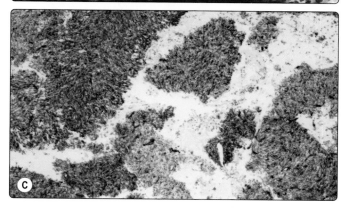

Fig. 14.30 Dermatofibrosarcoma protuberans (DFSP) (A) Dispersed single cells and stripped nuclei with moderate anisokaryosis, but granular nuclear chromatin (MGG, MP); (B) A streaming arrangement that vaguely suggests a storiform pattern may be seen (MGG, MP); (C) The tumor cells stain positively for CD34 (cell block preparation, CD34).

Access to immunocytochemistry is often necessary in the evaluation of unusual morphologic subtypes of malignant melanoma. A battery of markers including cytokeratin, EMA, LCA, S-100, Melan-A and HMB-45 (Fig. 14.26B) may be required to confirm the diagnosis.

Benign nevocellular tumors are rarely subjected to FNB. Figure 14.29 is of a postoperative scrape smear from a benign nevus. The cytology would be very difficult to distinguish from a nevoid melanoma.[73]

Dermatofibrosarcoma protuberans (DFSP)
(Fig. 14.30)

The cytological findings in DFSP have been reported by Domanski and Gustafson.[74] The yield is abundant of both tissue fragments of variably cohesive spindle cells and dispersed single cells and stripped nuclei. There is moderate anisokaryosis, but the nuclear chromatin is granular and nucleoli are small. A streaming arrangement that vaguely suggests a storiform pattern may be seen. The tumor cells stain positively for vimentin and CD34. The main differential diagnoses are low-grade fibrosarcoma and monophasic fibrosarcoma-like synovial sarcoma. The clinical presentation is an important clue to diagnosis

Vascular tumors

Kaposi's sarcoma is mainly seen in the skin but also occurs in other sites in HIV-positive patients. The cytological findings are described in Chapter 5 and in Chapter 18, p. 459. The cytology of a few other types of cutaneous vascular tumors has also been reported.[3,75,76] Ancillary techniques, especially immunocytochemistry may be necessary to establish a cytologic diagnosis of malignant vascular tumor of the skin, as such tumors display a wide spectrum of cytomorphologic patterns (Fig. 14.31).

Metastatic malignancy; lymphoma

The skin, particularly of the scalp, is a common site for metastatic malignancy.[1,2] A summary of the cytological findings in metastatic malignancy and guidelines for the identification of the primary site are given in Chapter 5. Clinical history, access to histological sections of the primary tumor, and immunostaining are the most important aids in diagnosis.

A mass in the skin or soft tissues may be the first manifestation of malignant lymphoma or it may be the first sign of

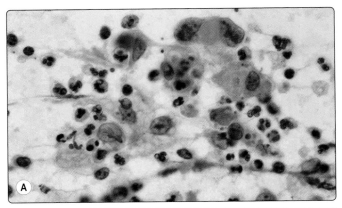

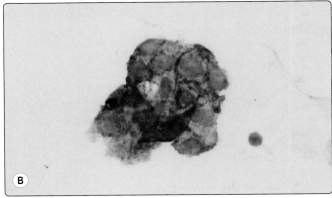

Fig. 14.31 Cutaneous angiosarcoma Cutaneous angiosarcomas display a wide spectrum of cytomorphologic patterns. (**A**) FNB of epithelioid angiosarcoma (H&E, HP); (**B**) Positive staining with CD 31; liquid based preparation.

recurrence of treated lymphoma. The cell patterns of cutaneous lymphoma have been beautifully illustrated in tissue sections by Isaacson and Norton.[77] Cytological criteria for different types of lymphoma are listed in Chapter 5. Subtyping of lymphoma and distinction from cutaneous pseudolymphoma requires immune marker studies. The FNB findings in cutaneous T-cell lymphoma have been described in a few cases.[6,78]

References

1. Reyes CV, Thompson KS, Jensen JD, et al. Metastasis of unknown origin: the role of fine-needle aspiration cytology. Diagn Cytopathol 1998;18:319–22.

2. Spitz DJ, Reddy V, Selvaggi SM, et al. Fine-needle aspiration of scalp lesions. Diagn Cytopathol 2000;23:35–8.

3. Daskalopoulou D, Maounis N, Kokalis G, et al. The role of fine needle aspiration cytology in the diagnosis of primary skin tumors. Arch Anat Cytol Path 1993;41: 75–81.

4. Layfield LJ, Glasgow BJ. Aspiration biopsy cytology of primary cutaneous tumors. Acta Cytol 1993;37: 679–88.

5. Dey P, Das A, Radhika S, Nijhawan R. Cytology of primary skin tumors. Acta Cytol 1996;40: 708–13, 1996.

6. Daskalopoulou D, Galanopoulou A, Statiropoulou P, et al. Cytologically interesting cases of primary skin tumors and tumor-like conditions indentified by fine-needle aspiration biopsy. Diagn Cytopathol 1998;19:17–28.

7. Rege J, Shet T. Aspiration cytology in the diagnosis of primary tumors of skin adnexa. Acta Cytol 2001;45:715–22.

8. Prayaga AK, Loya AC, Gottimukkala SR, et al. Cytologic features of primary malignant tumors of skin and adnexae. Acta Cytol 2008;52:702–9.

9. Solano JG, Acosta-Cortega J, Perez-Guillermo M. Pilomatrixoma: never lower your guard. Diagn Cytopathol 2007;35:457–8.

10. Gordon LA, Orell SR. Evaluation of cytodiagnosis of cutaneous basal cell carcinoma. J Am Acad Dermatol 1984; 11:1082–6.

11. Dong H, Duncan LD. Cytologic findings in *Demodex* folliculitis. Diagn Cytopathol 2006;34:232–4.

12. Bhatia A, Singh N, Arora VK, et al. Diagnosing granulomatous inflammation of the skin. A cytomorphologic approach based on evaluation of cellular reaction patterns. Acta Cytol 1999;43:761–6.

13. Malik A, Bhatia A, Singh N, et al. Fine needle aspiration cytology of reactions in leprosy. Acta Cytol 1999;43: 771–6.

14. Rao IS, Singh MK, Gupta SD, et al. Utility of fine-needle aspiration cytology in the classification of leprosy. Diagn Cytopathol 2001;24:317–21.

15. Garcia-Solano J, Garcia-Rojo B, Sanchez-Sanchez C, et al. Utility if fine-needle aspiration in the diagnosis of panniculitis. Diagn Cytopathol 1998;18:425–30.

16. Handa U, Chhabra S, Mohan H. Epidermal inclusion cyst: cytomorphological features and differential diagnosis. Diagn Cytopathol 2008;36:861–3.

17. Shet T, Rege J, Naik I. Cytodiagnosis of simple and proliferating tricholemmal cysts. Acta Cytol 2001;45:582–8.

18. Kini jR, Kini H. Fine-needle aspiration cytology in the diagnosis of malignant proliferating trichilemmal tumor: Report of a case and review of the literature. Diagn Cytopathol 2009; 37:744–7.

19. Dodd LG, Layfield LJ. Fine-needle aspiration cytology of ganglion cysts. Diagn Cytopathol 1996;15:377–81.

20. Punia RS, Gupta S, Handa U, et al. Fine needle aspiration cytology of bursal cyst. Acta Cytol 2002;46:690–2.

21. Dodd LG, Major NM. Fine-needle aspiration cytology of articular and periarticular lesions. Cancer (Cancer Cytopathol) 2002;96:157–65.

22. Filho JSR, Soares MF, Wal R, et al. Fine-needle aspiration cytology of pulmonary rheumatoid nodule: case report and review of the major cytologic features. Diagn Cytopathol 2002;26: 150–3.

23. Bhadani PP, Sah SP, Sen R, et al. Diagnostic value of fine needle aspiration cytology in gouty tophi. A report of 7 cases. Acta Cytol 2006;50: 101–4.

24. Saleh HA, Baker H. Aspiration biopsy cytology of tumoral calcinosis. A case report. Acta Cytol 2009;53:323–6.

25. Ashfaq R, Molberg KH, Vuitch F. Cutaneous endometriosis as a diagnostic pitfall of fine-needle aspiration cytology. A report of three cases. Acta Cytol 1994; 38: 577–81.

26. Westermark P, Stenqvist B. A new method for the diagnosis of systemic amyloidosis. Arch Intern Med 1973; 132:522–3.

27. Guy CD, Jones CK. Abdominal fat pad aspiration biopsy for tissue confirmation of systemic amyloidosis: specificity, positive predictive value, and diagnostic pitfalls. Diagn Cytopathol 2001;24: 181–5.

28. Bondeson L, Lindholm K, Thorstenson S. Benign dermal eccrine cylindroma. A pitfall in the diagnosis of adenoid cystic carcinoma. Acta Cytol 1983;27: 326–8.

29. Kolda TF, Ardaman T-D, Schwartz MR. Eccrine spiradenoma mimicking adenoid cystic carcinoma on fine needle aspiration. A case report. Acta Cytol 1997;41:852–8.

30. Mannion E, McLaren K, Al-Nafussi AI. Cytologic features of a cystic nodular hidradenoma: potential pitfalls in diagnosis. Cytopathology 1995;6: 100–3.

31. Gottschalk-Sabag S, Glick T. Fine-needle aspiration of nodular hidradenoma: a case report. Diagn Cytopathol 1996; 15:395–7.

32. Dubb M, Michelow P. Cytologic features of hidradenoma in fine needle aspiration biopsies. Acta Cytol 2009; 53:179–82.

33. Kumar N, Verma K. Clear cell hidradenoma simulating breast carcinoma: a diagnostic pitfall in fine-needle aspiration of breast. Diagn Cytopathol 1996;15:70–2.

34. Gupta R, Singh S, Gupta K, Kudesia M. Clear-cell hidradenoma in a child: a diagnostic dilemma for the cytopathologist. Diagn Cytopathol 2009;37:531–3.

35. Shimazaki H, Anzai M, Aida S, Endo H, et al. Trichoblastoma of the skin occurring in the breast. A case report. Acta Cytol 2001;45:435–40

36. Srinivasan R, Rajwanshi A, Padmanabhan V, et al. Fine needle aspiration cytology of chondroid syringoma and syringocystadenoma papilliferum. A report of two cases. Acta Cytol 1993;37: 535–8.

37. Rollins SD. Fine-needle aspiration diagnosis of a vulvar papillary hidradenoma. A case report. Diagn Cytopathol 1994;10:60–1.

38. Kumar N, Verma K. Fine needle aspiration cytology of pilomatrixoma. Cytopathology 1996; 7: 125–31.

39. Sánchez CS, Bascunana AG, Quirante FAP, et al. Mimics of pilomatrixomas in fine-needle aspirates. Diagn Cytopathol 1996;14: 75–83.

40. Lemos MM, Kindblom L-G, Meis-Kindblom JM, et al. Fine-needle aspiration features of pilomatrixoma. Cancer (Cancer Cytopathol) 2001;93: 252–6.

41. Wang J, Cobb CJ, Martin SE, et al. Pilomatrixoma: clinicopathologic study of 51 cases with emphasis on cytologic features. Diagn Cytopathol 2002;27: 167–72.

42. Punia RS, Handa U, Mohan H. Fine needle aspiration cytology of eccrine acrospiroma. Acta Cytol 2001;45: 1083–5.

43. Gottshalk-Sabag S, Glick T. Chondroid syringoma diagnosed by fine-needle aspiration. A case report. Diagn Cytopathol 1994;10:152–5.

44. Rege J, Shet T. Aspiration cytology in the diagnosis of primary tumors of skin adnexa. Acta Cytol 2001;45:715–22.

45. Dodd LG. Fine-needle aspiration cytology of adenoid (acantholytic) squamous-cell carcinoma. Diagn Cytopathol 1995;12:168–72.

46. Malberger E, Tilinger R, Lichtig C. Diagnosis of basal-cell carcinoma with aspiration cytology. Acta Cytol 1984;23: 301–5.

47. Garcia-Solano J, Garcia-Rojo B, Sanchez-Sanchez C, et al. Basal-cell carcinoma: cytologic and immunocytochemical findings in fine-needle aspirates. Diagn Cytopathol 1998;18:403–8.

48. Christensen E, Bofin A, Gudmundsdottir I, et al. Cytologic diagnosis of basal cell carcinoma and actinic keratosis using Papanicolaou and May-Grunwald-Giemsa stained cutaneous tissue smear. Cytopathol 2008;19:316–22.

49. Henke AC, Wiemerslage SJ, Cohen MB. Cytology of metastatic cutaneous basal cell carcinoma. Diagn Cytopathol 1998;19:113–15.

50. Calder CJ, Reynolds GM, Young FI, et al. Cytological features of pigmented BCC – a potential diagnostic pitfall. Cytopathology 1996;7: 132–5.

51. Masukawa T, Friedrich EG Jr. Cytopathology of Paget's disease of the vulva. Diagnostic abrasive cytology. Acta Cytol 1978;22: 476–8.

52. Sadhegi S, Pitman MB, Weir MM. Cytologic features of metastatic sebaceous carcinoma: report of two cases with comparison to three cases of basal cell carcinoma. Diagn Cytopathol 1999; 21:340–5.

53. Stern RC, Liu K, Dodd LG. Cytomorphologic features of sebaceous carcinoma on fine needle aspiration. Acta Cytol 2000;44:760–4.

54. Gottschalk-Sabag S, Glick T. Sweat gland cancer diagnosed by fine needle aspiration. Cytopathology 1996;7: 66–9.

55. Bonadio J, Armstrong W, Gu M. Eccrine porocarcinoma. Report of a case with fine needle aspiration cytology, histopathology and immunohistochemistry. Acta Cytol 2006;50:476–80.

56. Gangane N, Joshi D, Sharma SM. Cytomorphological diagnosis of malignant eccrine tumors: Report of two cases. Diagn Cytopathol 2008;36:801–4.

57. Pai RR, Kini JR, Achar C, et al. Apocrine (cutaneous) sweat gland carcinoma of axilla with signet ring cells: a diagnostic dilemma on fine-needle aspiration cytology. Diagn Cytopathol 2008;36:739–41.

58. Varsa E, Jordan SW. Fine needle aspiration cytology of malignant spiradenoma arising in congenital eccrine spiradenoma. Acta Cytol 1990;34: 275–7.

59. Reid-Nicholson M, Iyengar P, Friedlander MA, et al. Fine needle aspiration biopsy of primary mucinous carcinoma of the skin. A case report. Acta Cytol 2006;50: 317–22.

60. Kotru M, Manucha V, Singh UR. Cytologic and histologic features of primary mucinous adenocarcinoma of skin in the axilla. A case report. Acta Cytol 2007;51:571–4.

61. Mishra K, Agarval S. Fine needle aspiration cytology of malignant chondroid syringoma. A case report. Acta Cytol 1998;42:1155–8.

62. Skoog L, Schmitt F, Tani E. Neuroendocrine (Merkel cell) carcinoma of the skin: immunocytochemical and cytomorphologic analysis on fine needle aspirates. Diagn Cytopathol 1990;6: 53–7.

63. Collins BT, Elmberger PG, Tani EM, et al. Fine-needle aspiration of Merkel cell carcinoma of the skin with cytomorphology and immunocytochemical correlation. Diagn Cytopathol 1998;18:251–7.

64. Grenko RT, Sickel JZ, Abendroth CS, et al. Cytologic features of deep juvenile xanthogranuloma. Diagn Cytopathol 1996;15:329–33.

65. Holck S, Bredesen JL. Solid glomus tumor presenting as an axillary mass. Report of a case with morphologic study, including cytologic characteristics. Acta Cytol 1996;40: 555–62.

66. Handa U, Palta A, Mohan H, Punia RPS. Aspiration cytology of glomus tumor. A case report. Acta Cytol 2001;45:1073–6.

67. Kalfa M, Daskalopoulou D, Markidou S. Fine needle aspiration (FNB) biopsy of primary cutaneous meningioma: report of two cases. Cytopathol 1999;10:54–60.

68. Cangiarella JF, Symmans WF, Shapiro RL, et al. Aspiration biopsy and the clinical management of patients with malignant melanoma and palpable regional lymph nodes. Cancer (Cancer Cytopathol) 2000;90:162–6.

69. Saqi A, McGrath CM, Skovronsky D, Yu GH. Cytomorphologic features of fine-needle aspiration of metastatic and recurrent melanoma. Diagn Cytopathol 2002;27:286–90.

70. Murali R, Doubrovsky A, Watson GF, et al. Diagnosis of metastatic melanoma by fine-needle biopsy: analysis of 2,204 cases. Am J Clin Pathol 2007;127: 385–97.

71. Nasiell K, Tani E, Skoog L. Fine needle aspiration cytology and immunocytochemistry of metastatic melanoma. Cytopathology 1991;3: 137–47.

72. Murali R, Loughman NT, McKenzie PR, et al. Cytologic features of metastatic and recurrent melanoma in patients with primary cutaneous desmoplastic melanoma. Am J Clin Pathol 2008; 130:715–23.

73. Rojo BG, Solano JG, Sánches CS, et al. On the limited value of fine-needle aspiration for the diagnosis of benign melanocytic proliferations of the skin. Diagn Cytopathol 1998; 19:441–5.

74. Domanski HA, Gustafson P. Cytologic features of primary, recurrent and metastatic dermatofibrosarcoma protuberans. Cancer 2002;96:351–61.

75. Pérez-Guillermo M, Sola Pérez J, Garcia Rojo B, et al. Fine needle aspiration cytology of cutaneous vascular tumors. Cytopathology 1993;3: 213–44.

76. Ng WK, Collins RJ, Law D, et al. Cutaneous epithelioid angiosarcoma: a potential diagnostic trap for cytopathologists. Diagn Cytopathol 1997;16:160–7.

77. Isaacson PG, Norton AJ. Extranodal lymphomas. Edinburgh: Churchill Livingstone; 1994. p. 131–91.

78. Basce D, Kumar S, Skome DK, et al. Cutaneous T-cell lymphoma diagnosed by fine-needle aspiration. A case report with clinical, cytological and immunophenotypic features. Diagn Cytopathol 1994;11:174–7.

Soft tissues

Måns Åkerman and Henryk Domanski

The use of FNB and cytodiagnosis in the primary evaluation of a mass lesion in the soft tissues has become an accepted diagnostic modality using the cytodiagnosis as the morphological basis for a discussion of therapeutic options. A pretreatment cytological diagnosis offers several advantages. Patient anxiety can be relieved by providing an instant diagnostic suggestion followed by a discussion of therapeutic options based on the cytodiagnosis in combination with clinical and, at times, radiological data. FNB has a minimal risk of complications and the risk of tumor spread is negligible. FNB also allows easier collection of material from different parts of large tumors than open and core needle biopsy, important in case of tumor heterogeneity. Furthermore, FNB is less traumatic to the tissues than open or core needle biopsy.

Due to the relative rarity of primary tumors of soft tissue and to the extraordinary range of different types of tumors that can arise in these sites, a case can be made for centralising the diagnostic work-up of soft tissue tumors to a multidisciplinary clinic in an orthopedic oncology center. A specialised clinic facilitates the accumulation of invaluable experience based on the consistent correlation of clinical, radiological, cytological and histopathological findings at the time of diagnosis, ancillary laboratory tests, the results of treatment and the long-term outcome. It is hardly possible for the individual pathologist to gain a comparable level of experience over his/her professional lifetime.

However, to be efficient, highly specialised clinics of this kind need to draw material from a large population and consequently are only established in large academic centers. It is not possible to refer all patients with a soft tissue tumor or mass to a multidisciplinary center, particularly since most of these lesions are benign (benign lipomatous tumors). There is still a need for an easily accessible diagnostic service to be available at the community level in order to facilitate the referral of patients with suspected soft tissue tumors to an orthopedic oncology clinic. Guidelines for referral have been proposed. The recommendations of the Orthopedic Tumour Centre at the Lund University Hospital, based on epidemiologic data and on the difficulties experienced in the management of sarcomas, especially deep-seated sarcomas

which were initially biopsied or surgically treated outside specialist centers, may serve as an example. The recommendations, suggested in 1997 and still valid, are that all patients with a deep-seated soft tissue tumor irrespective of size, or with subcutaneous tumors larger than 5 cm should be referred untouched. An FNB may be performed but the smears should be reexamined at the center, if possible before the patients first visit.[1]

The place of FNAC in the investigative sequence

The diagnosis and classification of soft tissue tumors is one of the most difficult areas in surgical pathology. The relative absence of recognisable tissue architectural patterns in cytological preparation makes diagnosis by FNB even more difficult. However, open biopsy or inadequate surgical excision of a primary sarcoma may compromise fascial planes and necessitate more extensive (mutilating) surgery than if the tumor had been left intact.

The current use of FNB as the primary and, in a majority of cases, the definitive diagnosis of soft tissue tumors before treatment is based on the following points:

- In most centers, the treatment of soft tissue tumors is primary, radical surgery. At surgery, knowledge of the specific histogenetic type is of less importance in planning the operation than the size and site of the tumor and its relationship to vessels, nerve bundles and bone.
- The essential task for the cytopathologist is to accurately identify the tumor/mass as a soft tissue tumor, benign or malignant, and to exclude a reactive process or other malignancies. Specific tumor typing and malignancy grading are, of course, of value if at all possible.
- Clinical management is based on the combined evaluation of clinical data, radiographic findings and cytological examination. (The approach is similar to that used for breast lesions.) If there is a discrepancy between the three investigation modalities, reexamination of data is necessary and repeat FNB or supplementary biopsy (core needle or surgical biopsy)

©2012 Elsevier Ltd
DOI: 10.1016/B978-0-7020-3151-9.00015-3

Table 15.1 Soft tissue tumors/lesions which have been cytologically characterised in smears

Benign
Nodular fasciitis
Proliferative myositis and fasciitis
Pseudomalignant myositis ossificans
Benign lipomatous tumors
Neurilemmoma
Elastofibroma
Granular cell tumor
Intramuscular myxoma
Desmoid fibromatosis

Malignant
MFH-type of pleomorphic sarcoma
Myxofibrosarcoma
Leiomyosarcoma
Liposarcoma
Synovial sarcoma
Rhabdomyosarcoma
Dermatofibrosarcoma protuberans
Low-grade fibromyxoid sarcoma
Angiosarcoma
Epithelioid sarcoma
Clear cell sarcoma (malignant melanoma of soft tissue)
Extraskeletal myxoid chondrosarcoma

must be considered. If the treatment involves neoadjuvant, preoperative therapy the cytodiagnosis must be equivalent to a histological tissue diagnosis, i.e. providing histogenetic tumor type and malignancy grading.

- Close cooperation between the cytopathologist and the orthopedic surgeon is important. For optimal results, the patients should be referred to a specialist center with the tumor untouched, according to the recommended guidelines. The cytopathologist and the surgeon together should decide the insertion point of the needle. Diagnostic accuracy is optimal when the same person performs the needling and examines the smears.

A broad categorisation of a soft tissue tumor as of primary soft tissue origin, benign, low-or high-grade malignant, is possible in the majority of cases if the multidisciplinary approach suggested above is taken. Although many pathologists are reluctant to attempt cytological subclassification of primary soft tissue tumors and tumor-like lesions, a basic knowledge of the cytology of the most common tumors is important. A wide variety of benign tumors/lesions as well as sarcomas have been characterised cytologically by comparative studies of aspirates from series of cases of the same tumor type and by correlative studies of FNB smears and histological sections. The tumors/lesions are listed in Table 15.1.

Accuracy of diagnosis

The results of FNA cytology of soft tissue tumors are good overall if patients with tumors suspected of malignancy are referred to centers specialising in this field. Åkerman et al.[2]

reported their 20-year-experience of FNAC of soft tissue tumors as a preoperative tool in 1994. In their series of 517 cases, the aspirated material was insufficient for diagnosis in 6% and an erroneous cytological diagnosis was rendered in 5% of adequate smears, 85% of the benign tumors were reported as benign and 89% of the sarcomas were classified as malignant soft tissue tumors. Other centers have reported similar results. Many reports highlight the difficulty to correctly subtype sarcomas histogenetically and to differentiate between low-grade sarcoma and benign soft tissue tumors.[3-5]

Technical considerations

The biopsy technique is as for any palpable lesion. Local anesthesia is rarely needed. Multiple passes are usually necessary to obtain sufficient and representative material. Alcohol-fixed H&E- or Pap-stained smears and air-dried smears stained with MGG or Diff-Quik should be used in parallel. Wet fixation gives excellent nuclear detail, particularly of cells in microscopic solid tissue fragments, as is often the case with several types of sarcoma. Air-dried smears (MGG; Diff-Quik), however, provide more information about cytoplasm and stromal components.

The site of the biopsy should, if possible, be chosen in consultation with the surgeon responsible for the treatment. A single point of entry and tattooing the insertion point on the skin is helpful if the needle track is to be included in the surgical excision. Ultrasonography (US), computed tomography (CT) or magnetic resonance imaging (MRI) can be helpful in finding viable tissue and avoiding cystic and necrotic areas in extensively necrotic or cystic tumors. US guidance is also of great value in the biopsy of small, deepseated (intra- or intermuscular) tumors. If sufficient cellular material can be sampled, immunocytochemical studies and chromosomal or molecular genetic analysis may give valuable diagnostic information.

The parallel use of FNB and core needle biopsy (CNB) in selected cases, both sampling methods performed by the cytopathologist, combines the advantages of both techniques. In our experience, a core needle with an outer diameter of 1.2 mm is sufficient and well tolerated by patients. FNB allows wider sampling of large tumors and an immediate assessment based on air-dried smears (especially Diff-Quik-stained), while the CNB samples facilitates evaluation of microarchitecture and in many cases provide more material for ancillary studies.[6] The risk of tumor cell dissemination in the needle track is not greater for CNB than for FNB; it is negligible for both.

CYTOLOGICAL FINDINGS

Primary soft tissue tumors in general

Common characteristics

- A variable yield in both benign tumors and sarcomas, smears from tumors rich in intercellular collagen or heavily hyalinised are generally poor in cells, tumors rich in vessels may yield only blood or blood mixed with a few scattered cells,

- A mixture of single cells and small tissue fragments ('microbiopsies'); the proportion of single cells to fragments differs in different tumor types,
- Myxoid ground substance and/or fragments of intercellular collagen,
- Spindle-shaped nuclei,
- Multinucleated cells, giant cells and bizarre nuclei,
- Shape of cells highly variable; cytoplasmic projections, indistinct cell borders,
- Malignant nuclear features may be absent in high-grade malignant sarcomas,
- Benign tumor-like lesions or tumors may show prominent cellular pleomorphism,
- Mitoses rare in benign tumors and low-grade malignant sarcomas.

Fine needle biopsy samples from high-grade malignant sarcomas are usually abundant, whereas the yield from benign tumors and low-grade malignant sarcomas depends on the tumor type. Collagen-rich intercellular stroma, areas of hyalinisation, fibrosis and prominent vascularity influence the yield. Infrequently, single cells dominate the smears whether from benign tumors or sarcomas. Aggregates, bundles of cohesive cells or 'microbiopsies' are commonly present in smears, especially from sarcomas of various types. The cells may not form any discernible tissue architectural pattern or they may be oriented in fascicles or streams. Spindle cells which seem to radiate out from a central basement membrane core suggest a vasoformative tumor, solitary fibrous tumor, hemangiopericytoma or hemangiopericytoma-like synovial sarcoma. Bundles of parallel spindle cells are common in smooth muscle tumors, occasionally in tumors of Schwann cell origin, and occur at times in fibroblastic tumors. Palisading of nuclei can be seen in Schwann cell tumors and smooth muscle tumors and rosette-like figures (at times with a center of finely fibrillar material) in neuroblastoma and in Ewing's family tumors.

Myxoid ground substance may have a more or less fibrillar structure and stains brightly violet/red/purple in MGG (epithelial mucus is homogenous blue/violet). It is less conspicuous and may be almost invisible in wet-fixed H&E- and Pap-stained smears. Collagen is also obvious in MGG as strands of red/violet dense material between cells or isolated in the background. Capillary vessels are prominent in tissue fragments of myxoid liposarcoma and fragments of vessels are often observed in the myxoid ground substance of myxofibrosarcoma. Inflammatory cells (nodular fasciitis) and mast cells (synovial sarcoma) should be looked for. Necrosis is suggestive of high-grade malignant sarcoma.

The cytoplasm of mesenchymal tumor cells is generally not as fragile as that of many epithelial tumor cells and lymphoid cells with the exception of the small round cell malignancies such as alveolar rhabdomyosarcoma, neuroblastoma and the Ewing's family tumors, granular cell tumor and alveolar soft tissue sarcoma. Cell borders are usually indistinct and the cytoplasm may be drawn out into elongated processes or thin strands which anastomose with those of adjacent cells. Aggregates of cells have a syncytial cytoplasm. Nuclei tend to be eccentric in rounded cells. Spindle-shaped nuclei are common in smears from soft tissue tumors in general and are often present also in highly pleomorphic tumors. In synovial sarcoma and cellular myxoid liposarcoma (round cell liposarcoma) nuclei may be quite plump or rounded. Predominantly rounded nuclei are characteristic of granular cell tumor, alveolar soft tissue sarcoma, alveolar rhabdomyosarcoma and Ewing's family tumors. In general nuclear pleomorphism is proportional to the grade of malignancy.[7] Important exceptions occur, however. Anisokaryosis, marked variation in nuclear shape and multinucleation are often prominent in the various types of benign pseudosarcomatous soft tissue lesions as nodular fasciitis, proliferative fasciitis and myositis and pseudomalignant myositis ossificans. In such lesions, nuclear chromatin is bland and evenly distributed, but nucleoli may be large and prominent. Nuclear pleomorphism and chromatin clumping may be minimal or absent in some low-grade malignant sarcomas and even in some high-grade malignant sarcomas such as synovial sarcoma. The malignant potential in such tumors is mainly suggested by high cellularity, nuclear crowding, mitotic figures and occasionally by the presence of necrosis. Bizarre nuclei with lobulation, budding and nuclear satellites are common in high-grade tumors. Mitoses are mainly found in high-grade malignant sarcomas; nodular fasciitis is an important exception. Abnormal mitotic figures indicate high-grade sarcoma.

Comprehensive descriptions of the cytological patterns of primary soft tissue tumors can be found in two recent publications by Åkerman and Domanski and Gonzáles-Cámpora.[8,9]

Soft tissue tumors are usually classified histogenetically and in this section we use the classification proposed in the WHO fascicle Pathology and Genetics of Tumours of Soft tissue and Bone 2002[10] and Weiss SW, Goldblum JR, Soft tissue tumours, ed V.[11]

Fibroblastic/myofibroblastic tumors and fibrohistiocytic tumors

Benign tumors

> **CRITERIA FOR DIAGNOSIS**
>
> - Variably cellular smears sometimes a myxoid background, especially in nodular fasciitis,
> - Both single cells and clusters of cells; intercellular collagen or myxoid ground substance may be present in clusters,
> - Cells with pale cytoplasm; cells and nuclei most often predominantly spindly,
> - Variable nuclear pleomorphism, often prominent in pseudosarcomatous lesions,
> - Pale, granular, evenly distributed chromatin, prominent nucleoli, mitoses.

The *pseudosarcomatous lesions* are an important target for needling in this histogenetic group of tumors/lesions. *Nodular fasciitis* is among the commonest and the most frequently needled. Dahl and Åkerman reported 13 cases with cytology 1981;[12] at present, our material comprises more than 70 cases, all with remarkably similar cytomorphology. In more recent investigations of the cytological features of nodular fasciitis, the results are similar to those of Åkerman and Dahl.[13,14] The most important feature is the pleomorphism of the proliferating fibroblasts/myofibroblasts. Nuclei are predominantly spindly, but a proportion of cells have plump, ovoid or kidney-shaped nuclei. Bi-and/or multinucleated forms are always present and, if looked for carefully, ganglion cell-like binucleate cells with triangular shape and eccentrically placed nuclei are found (Fig. 15.1). A high cell content, nuclear pleomorphism, prominent nucleoli and the presence of mitoses may suggest malignancy, but the pale, bland nuclear chromatin is a clear indication of the benign nature of the lesion (Fig. 15.2). The correct diagnosis depends on the clinical presentation and the anatomical site (a rapidly, often tender subcutaneous nodule most frequently appearing in the upper extremity, trunk, head and neck) combined with such cytologic features as a myxoid background, actively proliferating fibroblasts/myofibroblasts and the presence of inflammatory cells.

Proliferative myositis and fasciitis are less frequent pseudosarcomatous processes but are important with regard to the rapid growth (common to all these lesions) and their occurrence in children. Their cytomorphology is similar to that of nodular fasciitis although the myxoid matrix is less prominent and the ganglion cell-like cells are often numerous with very prominent nucleoli (Fig. 15.3). In *proliferative myositis* regenerating multinucleated muscle fibers are commonly present (Fig. 15.4). An important clinical sign is that these lesions, especially nodular fasciitis, can disappear spontaneously or diminish substantially in size within 3–4 weeks after needling.[15,16] Another lesion which cytologically demonstrates prominent reactive cellular changes is *pseudomalignant myositis ossificans* (PMO). PMO is a rapidly growing lesion (intramuscular or subcutaneous), smears showing a mixture of proliferating fibroblasts/myofibroblasts, osteoblasts with prominent reactive changes and multinucleated giant cells of osteoclastic type (Fig. 15.5). In PMO an ossification in a zonal pattern is a typical find within 3–4 weeks and, according to our experience, spontaneous resolution is

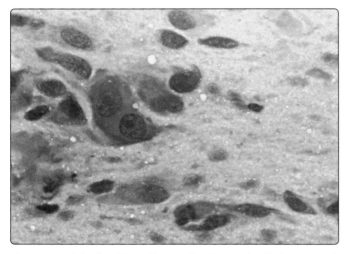

Fig. 15.1 Nodular fasciitis Proliferating fibroblasts embedded in a myxoid background; note binucleate cell with abundant cytoplasm and eccentric nuclei (ganglion cell-like) (MGG, HP).

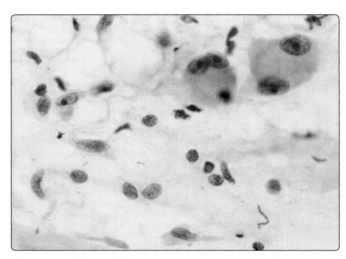

Fig. 15.3 Proliferative fasciitis Ganglion cell-like cells are often numerous with very prominent nucleoli (H&E, HP).

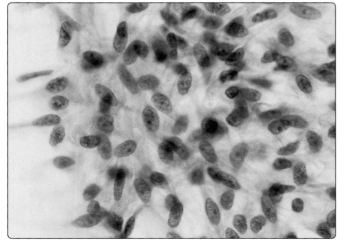

Fig. 15.2 Nodular fasciitis Poorly cohesive, proliferating fibroblasts; plump, oval, irregular nuclei, small nucleoli, bland chromatin; myxoid matrix not discernible in H&E-stained wet-fixed material (H&E, HP).

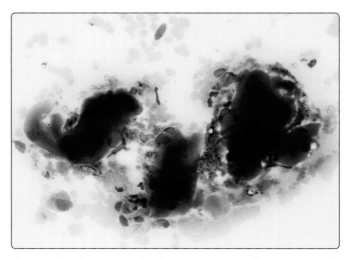

Fig. 15.4 Proliferative myositis Regenerating muscle fibers are commonly present (MGG, HP).

common. The cytomorphology in our series of five cases[17] is similar to that described by Dodd et al..[13]

Fibromatoses such as *desmoid fibromatosis* and *palmar and plantar fibromatosis* may partly resemble the pseudosarcomatous lesions, especially nodular fasciitis, in FNB smears. However, the nuclei are more consistently spindle and the marked nuclear pleomorphism in those lesions is not seen. Collagen fragments are common and myxoid ground substance unusual, as are inflammatory cells. Strands and clusters of spindle cells showing moderate anisokaryosis, and more or less acellular fragments of collagen are characteristic of desmoid fibromatosis, abdominal as well as extra-abdominal, in FNB smears (Fig. 15.6). When the tumor infiltrates striated muscle, muscle fragments and regenerating multinucleated muscle fibers are commonly seen (Fig. 15.7). The most important differential diagnoses are the rare low-grade malignant fibrosarcoma and monophasic fibrous synovial sarcoma. Smears from palmar and plantar fibroma-

toses (Dupuytren) can be surprisingly cellular, but the cells are uniformly spindled with bland spindled nuclei (Fig. 15.8). Recent summaries of the cytologic characteristic features of desmoid fibromatosis have been published 2003[8] and 2006.[18]

Other benign fibroblastic/myofibroblastic and fibrohistiocytic tumors are *solitary fibrous tumor* (SFT) and *hemangiopericytoma*. According to recent investigations of these tumors, they are considered to be closely related, most probably representing two variants of the same entity.[10] SFT most commonly occurrs in the pleura. SFT of the soft tissues is most often seen in adults as a deep-seated mass. In tissue sections the tumors are variably cellular and collagenous bands and hyalinisation are common findings. The fibroblastic spindle cells have no specific features and there is generally insignificant cellular atypia. A hemangiopericytoma-like vascular pattern is often present. The cytomorphology of SFT has been described in a few cases.[19,20] Bland spindle cells arranged

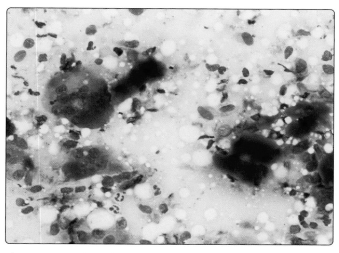

Fig. 15.5 Myositis ossificans A mixture of proliferating fibroblasts/myofibroblasts, osteoblasts and multinucleated giant cells of osteoclastic type (MGG, LP).

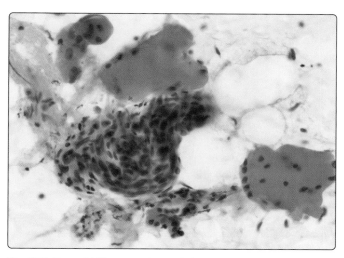

Fig. 15.7 Desmoid fibromatosis Muscle fragments and regenerating multinucleated muscle fibers are commonly seen (H&E, HP).

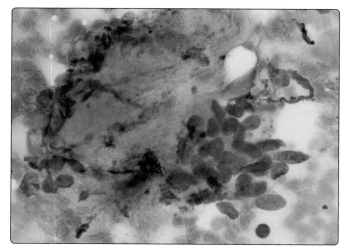

Fig. 15.6 Desmoid fibromatosis The two typical components are shown here: a cluster of loosely cohesive ovoid or spindle fibroblasts and a fragment of collagenous stroma (MGG, HP).

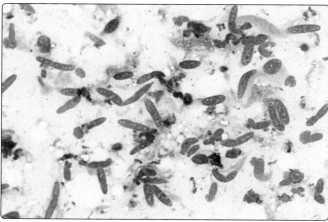

Fig. 15.8 Palmar fibromatosis (Dupuytren) Relatively cellular smear of poorly cohesive spindle cells; bland spindle nuclei; no microarchitectural pattern; no obvious stromal material (MGG, HP).

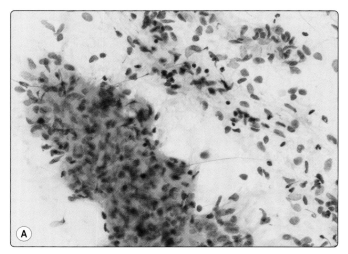

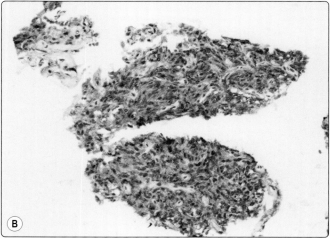

Fig. 15.9 **Solitary fibrous tumour** (A) Bland, plump spindle fibroblastic cells arranged in tight cell clusters as well as dispersed cells associated with strands of collagenous stroma (H&E, IP); (B) Spindle cells staining positively for CD34 (cell block, immunoperoxidase, LP).

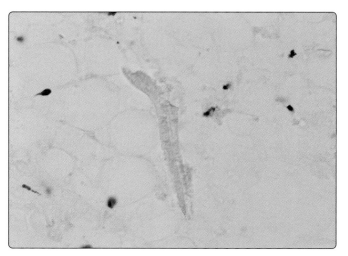

Fig. 15.10 **Elastofibroma dorsi** Degenerated elastic fibers are presented in smears (H&E, HP).

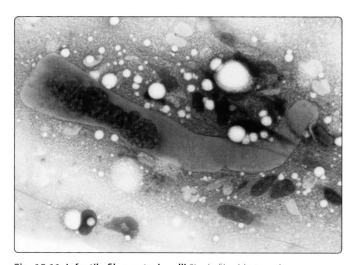

Fig. 15.11 **Infantile fibromatosis colli** Single fibroblasts and a regenerating multinucleated muscle fiber (MGG, HP).

in tight cell clusters associated with ropy collagen, as well as dispersed cells often with stripped nuclei, seem to be the typical appearance in FNB smears (Fig. 15.9A). The tumor cells stain positively for CD34 (Fig. 15.9B) and occasionally for CD99 and bcl-2.

Hemangiopericytoma, earlier thought to be an example of a pericytic neoplasm, is in current classifications considered as a fibroblastic tumor. Hemangiopericytoma is most common in deep soft tissue. At present, it is considered as a diagnosis of exclusion since some other tumors, notably monophasic synovial sarcoma and mesenchymal chondrosarcoma, may exhibit the same vascular pattern of branching vessels (staghorn pattern) as hemangiopericytoma.[10] The cytologic findings of hemangiopericytoma include branching vessel fragments; the tumor cells have bland ovoid or rounded nuclei and small cytoplasmic processes. Like SFT, hemangiopericytoma most often stains for CD34 and CD99. It is often difficult, sometimes impossible, to give a type-specific diagnosis of this tumor in FNB smears.

Elastofibroma is a slowly growing tumor, typically sited on the back near the scapula. The characteristic feature of elastofibroma is signs of faulty elastin fibrillogenesis. It is a hypocellular lesion composed of benign fibroblasts/myofibroblasts in a collagenous matrix with degenerated elastic fibers (Fig. 15.10). The typical cytologic findings in elastofibroma have been described in a small series of five cases.[21]

Two fibroblastic/myofibroblastic tumors of infancy, *infantile fibromatosis colli (torticollis)* and *fibrous hamartoma of infancy*, are occasionally needled. The typical smear of infantile fibromatosis colli, clinically often mistaken for malignancy, shows a mixture of spindle fibroblasts and regenerating mono- or multinucleated muscle fibers These regenerating fibers may be pleomorphic with prominent nucleoli, not to be mistaken for malignant cells (Fig. 15.11).[22,23]

The rare fibrous hamartoma of infancy is a subcutaneous tumor-like mass in the upper arms, shoulder and axillary region. It is composed of a mixture of mature fat, strings of fibrous tissue and primitive mesenchymal cells. The cytologic findings in the few cases published[24] are fragments of normal fat mixed with clusters or runs of bland spindle cells.

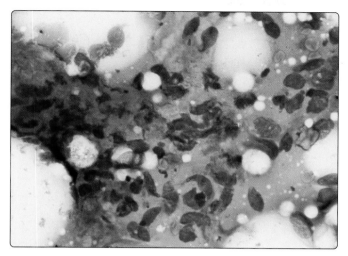

Fig. 15.12 Fibrous hamartoma of infancy Normal fat cells mixed with clusters or runs of bland spindle cells (MGG, HP).

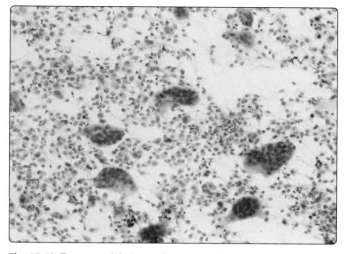

Fig. 15.13 Tenosynovial giant cell tumor A cellular smear of mainly single plump spindle cells with oval bland nuclei; Numerous scattered multinucleated giant cells (H&E, IP).

We have had the opportunity to study the smears of two cases (Fig. 15.12).

Tenosynovial giant cell tumor is a relatively common benign fibrohistiocytic tumor related to the tendon sheaths of the fingers and hands. Although the clinical presentation is quite characteristic, confirmation by FNB is often requested. Smears are relatively cellular and consist of mainly dispersed plump fibrohistiocytic cells with oval pale nuclei and bland chromatin. There is a variable number of scattered osteoclast-like multinucleated giant cells, which may be numerous (Fig. 15.13).[25]

Malignant tumors

CRITERIA FOR DIAGNOSIS

◆ Cellular smears; necrosis common in high-grade malignant sarcomas,
◆ Single cells and clusters; often small fragments of tumor tissue,
◆ Atypical spindle cells with elongated nuclei; in low-grade malignant sarcomas, cellular and nuclear atypia is slight to moderate,
◆ Marked (variable) nuclear pleomorphism,
◆ Multinucleated tumor giant cells and bizarre nuclei,
◆ Coarse, irregular nuclear chromatin; nucleoli variable but often prominent; mitoses, often atypical.

Malignant fibrous histiocytoma (MFH) was recognised in 1963 as a specific entity of probable fibrohistiocytic origin and was considered the commonest primary sarcoma of soft tissue. A number of subtypes were described, among which *pleomorphic malignant fibrous histiocytoma* was the most common. MFH is at present challenged as a specific histotype and the consensus is that MFH shows no evidence of histiocytic differentiation. On reexamination with extended immunohistochemistry and electron microscopy, many sarcomas initially diagnosed as pleomorphic MFH have been reclassified as dedifferentiated leiomyosarcoma, pleomorphic liposarcoma, pleomorphic rhabdomyosarcoma, soft tissue

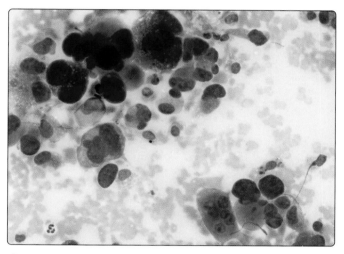

Fig. 15.14 Pleomorphic sarcoma of the MFH type Moderately cohesive pleomorphic cells; nuclei pleomorphic with malignant chromatin, mainly oval, a few spindled forms; abundant pale syncytial cytoplasm (MGG, HP).

osteosarcoma or as high-grade malignant tumors of non-mesenchymal origin.[26,27] Thus in current textbooks such as the WHO fascicle on soft tissue and bone tumors, the diagnosis pleomorphic MFH is reserved for a small group of pleomorphic sarcomas, which after thorough investigation show no specific histotype. The typical cytology of pleomorphic sarcoma of MFH type is described in two series.[28,29] Most often, atypical spindle cells dominate the smears, but large atypical cells with more or less abundant vacuolated or foamy cytoplasm are usually also present and may be numerous, as well as multinucleated tumor giant cells (Fig. 15.14). Smears from both deep and subcutaneous tumors may contain small amounts of myxoid matrix. The diagnosis of *giant cell malignant fibrous histiocytoma*, formerly considered as a subtype of MFH, is currently reserved for undifferentiated pleomorphic sarcoma with numerous osteoclast-like multinucleated giant cells.[10]

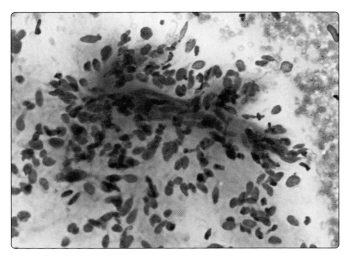

Fig. 15.15 Myxofibrosarcoma, low grade Nuclear atypia and pleomorphism are slight to moderate note fragment of vessels embedded in myxoid matrix (MGG, IP).

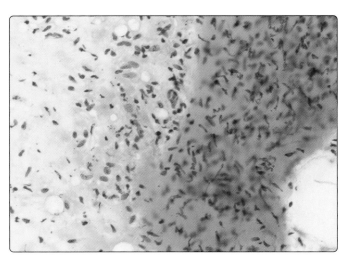

Fig. 15.17 Low-grade fibromyxoid sarcoma Three-dimensional cohesive clusters of spindle cells embedded in myxoid and collagenous matrix with admixture of scattered bare nuclei and single cells with poorly defined cytoplasm (H&E, LP).

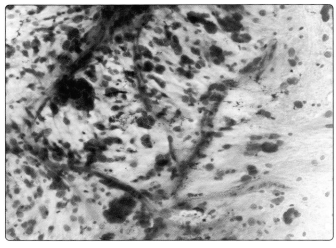

Fig. 15.16 Myxofibrosarcoma, intermediate grade Poorly cohesive plump spindle cells and a myxoid background; nuclear atypia is more prominent but fragments of vessels are still visible in the background matrix (MGG, IP).

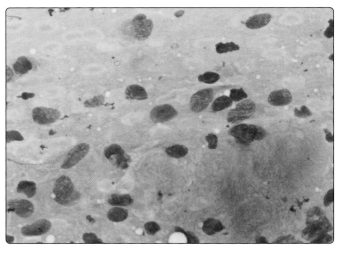

Fig. 15.18 Low-grade fibromyxoid sarcoma Spindle shaped/fusiform or ovoid nuclei show slightly coarse chromatin and inconspicuous nucleoli; Note myxoid background (MGG, IP).

Myxofibrosarcoma (MFS), formerly regarded as a myxoid subtype of malignant fibrous histiocytoma, is at present considered as a specific entity, a malignant fibroblastic tumor with a variable, most often abundant amount of myxoid stroma. MFS is a common subcutaneous sarcoma in elderly patients, although it is also found in skeletal muscle and in the retroperitoneum. MFS generally contains abundant myxoid ground substance in FNB smears (Fig. 15.15). The low-grade malignant tumors are dominated by spindle-shaped cells with slight to moderate nuclear atypia. They may resemble intramuscular cellular myxoma or paucicellular myxoid liposarcoma, but typical lipoblasts are not present and the typical characteristic vascular component of thin-walled branching vessels in the aspirated tumor fragments, as seen in myxoid liposarcoma, are not present. MFS typically displays fragments of coarse, often curved vessels in the myxoid back ground (Fig. 15.16), a feature not seen in FNB

smears from intramuscular myxoma (see Fig. 15.54). In high-grade malignant MFS, the cellular pleomorphism and nuclear atypia is as marked as in pleomorphic sarcoma of MFH type. The cellular features of myxofibrosarcoma have been amply described.[30-32] *Low grade fibromyxoid sarcoma* (LGFMS) is a variant of fibrosarcoma, first described in 1987. Two series have been published 1993 and 1995.[33,34] This type of sarcoma displays alternating areas of myxoid and collagenous stroma. The tumor cells are spindle-shaped with bland nuclei. As stromal vessels of the same type as in myxofibrosarcoma may be present in the myxoid areas, these low-grade malignant sarcomas may be difficult to distinguish from each other. LGFMS and cellular intramuscular myxoma may be deceptively like. The cytology of LGFMS has been thoroughly described in a report of eight cases (Figs 15.17 and 15.18).[35]

The anatomical site, size and clinical presentation must be known since atypical fibroxanthoma of the skin (AFX) may be cytologically indistinguishable from pleomorphic sarcoma of MFH type (see Chapter 15). Other differential diagnoses are mainly pleomorphic lipo- and leiomyosarcoma, and anaplastic malignant peripheral nerve sheath tumor (MPNST). Anaplastic sarcomatoid carcinoma (e.g. of renal or bronchogenic origin), or anaplastic squamous cell carcinoma and pleomorphic melanoma may show the same blend of pleomorphic spindled and plump cells. Another differential diagnosis is anaplastic large cell lymphoma. The identification of highly atypical lipoblasts is necessary for the diagnosis of pleomorphic liposarcoma, and of cells of smooth muscle origin (blunt-ended, truncated nuclei) in leiomyosarcoma. Immunocytochemical staining for keratins, S-100 protein, desmin, caldesmon, melanoma associated antigens, CD30 (Ki-1 antibody) and pan B-T cells antigen is of value in the differential diagnosis.

Tumors of adipose tissue

Benign tumors

Lipoma is the commonest of all benign soft tissue tumors. Lipoma cannot be distinguished from normal adipose tissue cytologically – smears of both consist mainly of fragments of mature adipose tissue, a few single fat cells and fat droplets. The fat cells are large and have abundant empty cytoplasm and a small eccentric dark nucleus. A few strands of branching capillary vessels may be seen in the tissue fragments. It is important to make sure that the sample is representative of the suspected tumor. A needle with trocar is recommended for deep-seated tumors to avoid contamination with normal subcutaneous fat. In *infiltrating intramuscular lipoma*, the fragments of adipose tissue are intimately associated with muscle fibers. Skeletal muscle fibers appear in smears as large strap-like structures which are strongly eosinophilic (navy-blue in MGG) and have rows of small ovoid and elongated, pale nuclei. Cross-striation is often evident. The best indication of an infiltrating intramuscular lipoma is the presence of regenerating muscle fibers, since subcutaneous lipoma may be contaminated with skeletal muscle fibers if needling is too deep and traverses the tumor. The vascularity of an *angiolipoma* can often be appreciated in FNB smears (Fig. 15.19). Clinically, angiolipomas are often small, multiple and tender on palpation.

Smears of *spindle cell lipoma* may have a background of fibromyxoid ground substance and a variable number of spindle cells within tissue fragments or between them. (Fig. 15.20A). The spindle cells may dominate the smears and may be misinterpreted as a fibroblastic proliferation. Important diagnostic features in FNB smears from spindle lipoma are the presence of hyaline, eosinophilic collagen fibers (Fig. 15.20B) and of mast cells. The spindle cells stain strongly for CD34 (Fig. 15.21). The cytological appearance of spindle cell lipoma in smears have been described in a series of 12 cases.[36] *Pleomorphic lipoma*, considered to be related to spindle cell lipoma (similar typical site and chromosomal aberration) typically displays so-called floret cells in smears (Figs 15.22). In a typical clinical setting (a subcutaneous tumor in the neck or back in a middle-aged male), a confident diagnosis of both these variants of lipoma is possible. *Hibernoma* is recognisable in FNB smears provided that typical hibernoma cells are found. These have abundant,

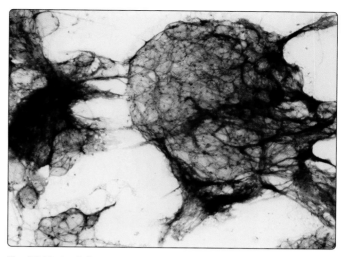

Fig. 15.19 Angiolipoma Mature adipose tissue with anastomosing capillaries (MGG, LP).

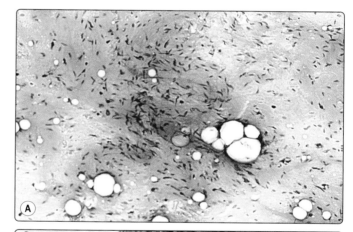

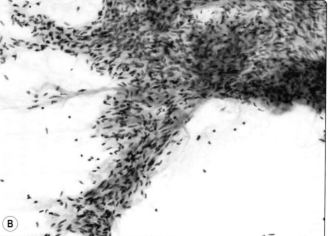

Fig. 15.20 Spindle cell lipoma (A) A myxoid matrix may be prominent in smears and may give an impression of a truly myxoid tumor (H&E, LP); (B) The presence of hyaline, eosinophilic collagen fibers is an important diagnostic clue (ThinPrep, H&E, LP).

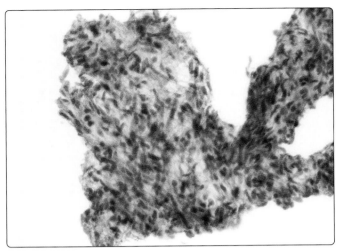

Fig. 15.21 The spindle cells stain strongly for CD34 (ThinPrep, CD34, immunoperoxidase, LP).

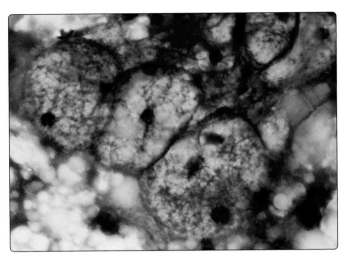

Fig. 15.23 Hibernoma Note abundant foamy cytoplasm and small nuclei (MGG, HP).

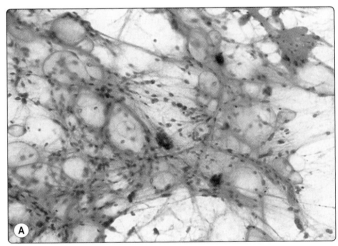

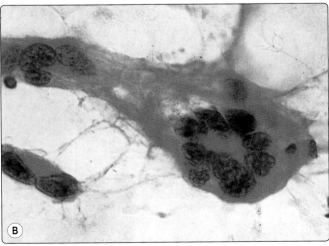

Fig. 15.22 Pleomorphic lipoma (A) Mature adipose tissue; scattered large, dark multinucleated cells (H&E, IP); (B) Same case as A; large multinucleated cell (floret cell) (H&E, HP oil).

finely granular or vacuolated cytoplasm and centrally located small, rounded uniform nuclei (Fig. 15.23).[37] The typical findings in FNB smears of *lipoblastoma* (subcutaneous) and *lipoblastomatosis* (deep-seated) are a vascular network and clusters of lipoblast-like cells in a myxoid background (Fig. 15.24). Another variant of benign lipoma, *chondroid lipoma*, has been described. In this variant foci of mature adipocytes are seen together with chondrocyte- or lipoblast-like cells in a chondromyxoid-like matrix.[38] The cytomorphology of chondroid lipoma has so far been described only in single case report.[39,40] The main features are lipoblast-like cells with irregular nuclei, often lobulated or coffee-bean shaped, mixed with mature fat cells within fragments of a chondroid-like matrix (Fig. 15.25). Chondroid lipoma has been erroneously diagnosed as low-grade malignant liposarcoma (paucicellular myxoid liposarcoma) in FNB samples. *Extra-adrenal myelolipoma* is a tumor-like mass composed of mature fat and bone marrow cells. The typical site is the adrenals but the lesion can also occur in the retroperitoneum and in the pelvic region. Extra-adrenal myelolipoma should be considered in the differential diagnosis of tumors or tumor-like lesions in those sites. FNB smears typically contain fragments or clusters of normal fat cells mixed with bone marrow cells of all three lineages (Fig.15.26).

Malignant tumors

Well-differentiated liposarcoma and *atypical lipoma* are histologically closely related and cannot be distinguished in FNB smears. The anatomical site and clinical presentation decide the terminology. In 2001, Kempson introduced a new term, *atypical lipomatous tumor*, to include atypical lipoma and well-differentiated liposarcoma.[41] Tissue fragments in smears from these tumors are composed of mature fat cells mixed with atypical lipoblast-like cells and atypical spindled or rounded cells with hyperchromatic nuclei (Fig. 15.27). The cytological findings must be evaluated in relation to the anatomical site. Especially in the retroperitoneum, recurrent well-differentiated liposarcoma may dedifferentiate, i.e. areas of high-grade malignant sarcoma may develop within

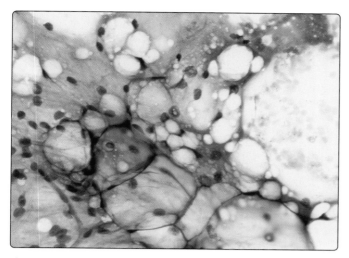

Fig. 15.24 Lipoblastoma Tissue fragments of fat cells, uni- and multivacuolated lipoblast-like cells and a myxoid matrix (MGG, IP).

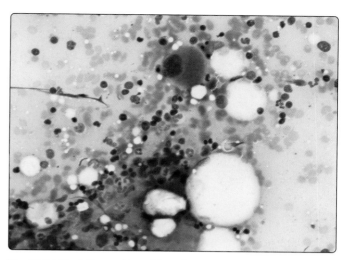

Fig. 15.26 Myelolipoma Normal fat cells are mixed with bone-marrow cells (MGG, IP).

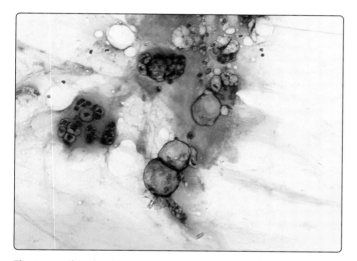

Fig. 15.25 Chondroid lipoma Mature adipocytes are mixed together with lipoblasts and chondrocyte-like cells in a chondromyxoid-like matrix (MGG, IP).

the well-differentiated liposarcoma. The diagnosis of *dedifferentiated liposarcoma* in FNB smears rests on the presence of a high-grade sarcoma and well-differentiated liposarcoma in the same needling.

Myxoid liposarcoma, the commonest of the liposarcomas is currently divided in two variants: *paucicellular* and *hypercellular myxoid liposarcoma*. *Paucicellular myxoid liposarcoma* is identical with the classic myxoid liposarcoma, while the hypercellular variant corresponds to the former *round cell liposarcoma*. The reason to rename round cell liposarcoma is that this subtype was found to express the same chromosomal aberration, t(12;16)(q13;p11), as classic myxoid liposarcoma.[10] In paucicellular myxoid liposarcoma, the peculiar network of anastomosing capillary vessels is well recognisable in FNB smears and is one of three characteristic features. The other two are abundant myxoid background matrix and slightly atypical lipoblasts. Smears consist mainly

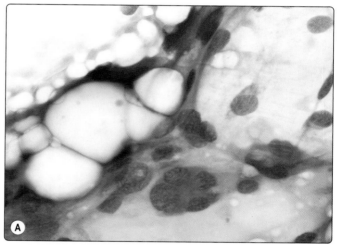

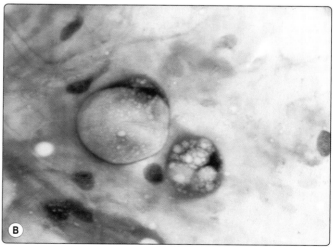

Fig. 15.27 Well-differentiated liposarcoma (atypical lipomatous tumour) (A) Fragments of mature adipose tissue and scattered large atypical cells with hyperchromatic nuclei (MGG, HP); (B) The atypical lipoblasts embedded in fibrous stroma (MGG, HP).

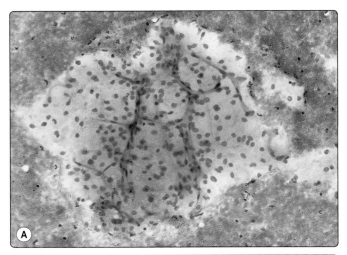

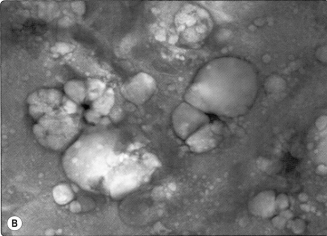

Fig. 15.28 Myxoid liposarcoma (A) Tissue fragment of cells embedded in myxoid background material; typical anastomosing vessels (MGG, IP); (B) Scattered multivacuolated lipoblasts (MGG, HP).

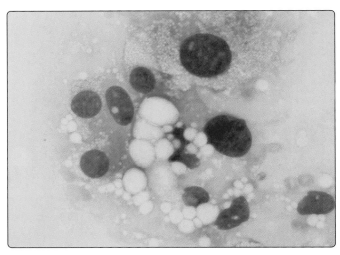

Fig. 15.29 Pleomorphic liposarcoma Poorly cohesive cells with pleomorphic rounded nuclei and irregular nuclear chromatin; note multivacuolated lipoblasts with scalloped nuclei (MGG, HP).

of small tissue fragments with branching capillary vessels embedded in the myxoid matrix (Fig. 15.28A). The tumor cells, mainly seen in the fragments, have spindle or ovoid, relatively uniform nuclei and a thin cytoplasm. Lipoblasts are always found – uni- or multivacuolated with scalloped nuclei (Fig. 15.28B). The lipoblasts are best visualised in MGG; the cytoplasmic vacuoles are less prominent in H&E. Differentiation from low-grade malignant myxofibrosarcoma (MFS) depends on the demonstration of the capillary network within the tumor fragments and of lipoblasts. The vessel fragments seen in smears of MFS are usually thicker and are present in the myxoid ground substance. Smears of hypercellular myxoid liposarcoma (former round cell liposarcoma) show either numerous dissociated cells or tissue fragments containing closely packed tumor cells. The fragments are considerably more cellular than those of the paucicellular type; myxoid ground substance is less conspicuous and the capillary network less prominent. The tumor cells have irregular, rounded nuclei and a malignant chromatin pattern. The cytoplasm is fragile and many nuclei are stripped. Mitotic figures are occasionally seen and atypical lipoblasts always found.

Pleomorphic liposarcoma resembles the pleomorphic sarcoma of MFH type cytologically. The diagnosis rests on the presence of highly atypical, sometimes multinucleated lipoblasts. Lipoblasts in liposarcoma smears may be univacuolated and resemble signet ring cells or they may be multivacuolated, containing small or large vacuoles or a mixture of both. The scalloped nucleus is an important cytologic feature (Fig. 15.29). In FNB smears, superimposed fat vacuoles from adjacent fat tissue may produce artifacts in other cell types, causing a resemblance to lipoblasts, and macrophages in adipose tissue showing inflammatory or reactive changes may have a vacuolated cytoplasm (lipophages). An infrequent diagnostic pitfall is soft tissue metastasis of renal cell carcinoma. It is important to remember that the majority of liposarcomas are deep seated and only infrequently subcutaneous. The cytologic feature of liposarcoma in FNB smears have been investigated in several series.[32,42–45]

Tumors of smooth muscle

CRITERIA FOR DIAGNOSIS

- ◆ Variable degree of cellularity,
- ◆ Cells more often in cohesive clusters or fascicular tissue fragments than single (high-grade malignant pleomorphic leiomyosarcoma is an exception),
- ◆ Cells in parallel bundles or in tandem,
- ◆ Abundant, eosinophilic cytoplasm (gray–blue in MGG), best visualised in single cells, often distinct cell borders,
- ◆ Variable, predominantly cigar-shaped or blunt-ended, sometimes truncated nuclei; intranuclear cytoplasmic inclusions,
- ◆ Finely granular barred chromatin,
- ◆ One or more small, distinct nucleoli,
- ◆ Many multinucleated giant tumor cells in high-grade leiomyosarcoma.

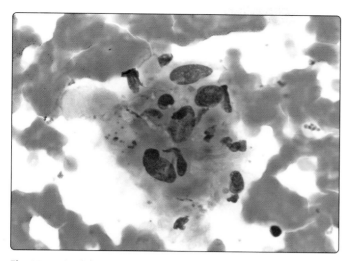

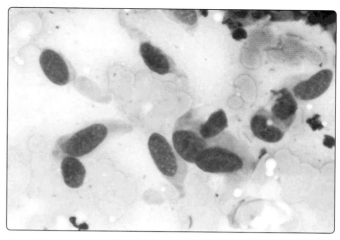

Fig. 15.30 Angioleiomyoma Small groups of uniform or slightly pleomorphic spindle cells with poorly defined cytoplasm borders and nuclei with bland chromatin (MGG, HP).

Fig. 15.31 Deep-seated leiomyoma Typical benign smooth muscle cells with blunt-ended, bland-looking nuclei (MGG, HP).

Benign tumors

Angioleiomyoma is most often a small, dermal or subcutaneous tumor, very tender at palpation. Angioleiomyoma may be the subject for FNB. According to our files, angioleiomyoma is very difficult to diagnose as such in smears. In a study comprising 10 cases, no case was correctly typed, albeit most were diagnosed as benign tumors.[46] The FNB smears contained uniform or slightly pleomorphic spindle cells with bland chromatin and insignificant nucleoli. The nuclei were occasionally blunt-ended or cigar-shaped and the cells were predominantly dissociated, mixed with small groups of cells (Fig. 15.30).

The histological diagnosis of malignancy in well-differentiated tumors of smooth muscle origin is to a large extent dependent on mitotic counts, invasive growth and size, which generally cannot be evaluated in FNB smears. The question of malignancy and the distinction from leiomyoma of deep soft tissue may therefore be difficult to decide in smears from low-grade malignant leiomyosarcoma. Our experience of *leiomyoma of deep soft tissue* is restricted to a few cases. The cytologic findings were remarkably similar. The cells were arranged in clusters and also seen as single cells. Stripped nuclei were common among single cells. Typical tumor cell nuclei were cigar-shaped (Fig. 15.31), sometimes truncated, sometimes containing vacuoles. The chromatin was finely granular and nucleoli were inconspicuous. Many nuclei were fibroblast-like.

Malignant tumors

Smears from *moderately differentiated leiomyosarcoma* (grade II in a three-grade scale or grade III in a four-grade scale) are cellular and are composed of clusters and fascicles of cohesive cells. The clusters have a syncytial appearance, lacking visible cell borders, and show anisokaryosis (Fig. 15.32A). Nuclei of single cells or stripped nuclei can be found displaying an unequivocally malignant chromatin pattern (Fig. 15.32B). Moderately differentiated leiomyosarcoma can be difficult to distinguish from benign as well as malignant neurogenic tumors. Ancient neurilemmoma is a particularly important

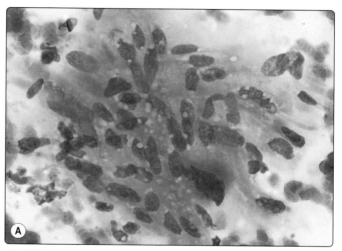

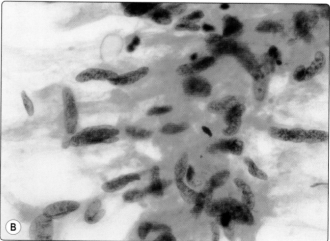

Fig. 15.32 Moderately differentiated leiomyosarcoma (A) Tissue fragment of cohesive cells with indistinct cytoplasm and spindly, occasionally cigar-shaped nuclei (MGG, IP); (B) Moderately differentiated leiomyosarcoma. Single cells or stripped nuclei can be found displaying an unequivocally malignant chromatin pattern (H&E, IP).

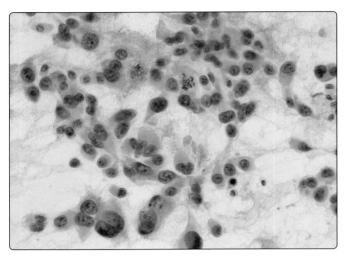

Fig. 15.33 High-grade malignant leiomyosarcoma A round cell pattern can be found and these tumors can be mistaken for epithelial tumors (H&E, IP).

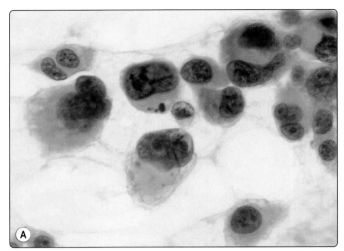

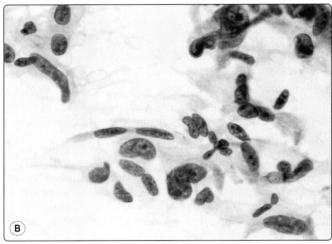

Fig. 15.34 High-grade malignant leiomyosarcoma (A) A pleomorphic cell pattern is difficult to distinguish from pleomorphic sarcomas of MFH type (H&E, HP); (B) The presence of blunt-ended, truncated or vacuolated nuclei in highly atypical spindle cells is an important diagnostic sign (H&E, IP).

diagnostic pitfall.[47] Neurogenic tumors, however, tend to have more slender, elongated nuclei with pointed ends.

Some high-grade malignant leiomyosarcomas display a round cell pattern, and these tumors can be mistaken for epithelial tumors (Fig. 15.33). High-grade malignant *pleomorphic leiomyosarcoma* is difficult to distinguish from pleomorphic sarcomas of MFH type (Fig. 15.34A) or from high-grade malignant peripheral nerve sheath tumors. The presence of blunt-ended, truncated or vacuolated nuclei in highly atypical spindle cells is an important diagnostic sign (Fig. 15.34B). More or less numerous multinucleated osteoclast-like giant cells can be found in smears from pleomorphic leiomyosarcoma (Fig. 15.35). The cytologic features of leiomyosarcoma is recorded in two large series.[48,49] Important antibodies to prove smooth muscle origin are desmin and caldesmon (Fig. 15.36).

Tumors of striated muscle

Benign tumors

Benign (adult) *rhabdomyoma* is rare. In the few examples from our files, the smears contained many fragments of muscle fibers which were paler, smaller and more irregular in shape than normal skeletal muscle fibers (Fig. 15.37). Nuclei were larger and had prominent nucleoli. Cross-striation was difficult to distinguish. The fragments closely resembled regenerating myocytes. Published case reports describe similar findings.[50,51]

Malignant tumors

The three different types of rhabdomyosarcoma can be recognised in FNB smears.[52] *Embryonal rhabdomyosarcoma* is the commonest soft tissue sarcoma in children (see p. 432). In our experience, although rhabdomyosarcoma generally is considered as one of the small round cell malignant tumors of childhood, embryonal rhabdomyosarcoma is predominantly a pleomorphic tumor in FNB smears, composed of

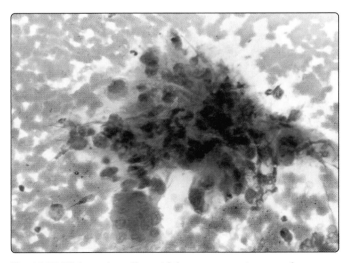

Fig. 15.35 High-grade malignant leiomyosarcoma In smears from pleomorphic leiomyosarcoma, a more or less numerous multinucleated osteoclast-like giant cells can be found (MGG, HP).

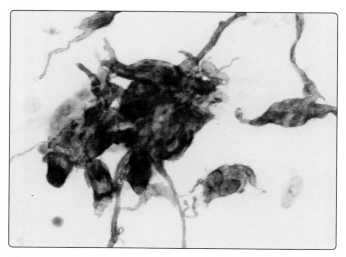

Fig. 15.36 Leiomyosarcoma An important antibody to prove smooth muscle origin is desmin (ThinPrep, desmin, immunoperoxidase, HP).

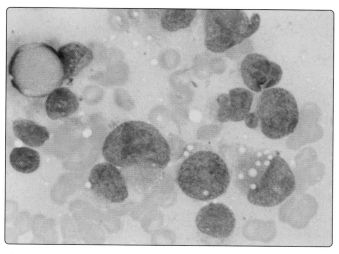

Fig. 15.38 Embryonal rhabdomyosarcoma Predominantly a pleomorphic tumor in FNB smears, composed of both small and larger cells (MGG, HP).

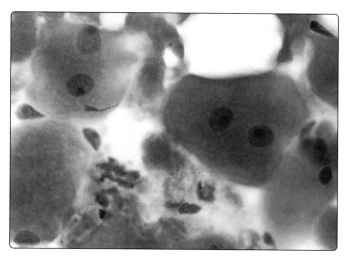

Fig. 15.37 Adult rhabdomyoma Cluster of large cells with irregular shapes, large amount of dense bluish-violet granular cytoplasm and relatively large nuclei (MGG, HP).

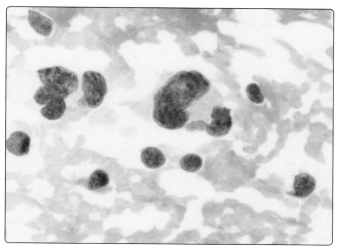

Fig. 15.39 Embryonal rhabdomyosarcoma Cells with eosinophilic cytoplasm and an eccentric nucleus, triangular, strap-shaped or tadpole-like, may be recognised as rhabdomyoblasts and may suggest the correct diagnosis (H&E, HP).

both small and larger cells (Fig. 15.38). Cells with dense, eosinophilic cytoplasm and an eccentric nucleus, triangular, strap-shaped or tadpole-like, may be recognised as rhabdomyoblasts and may suggest the correct diagnosis (Fig. 15.39). However, in many cases most cells are spindle-like with elongated nuclei and fusiform cytoplasm. We have examined smears from one case of the *spindle cell variant of embryonal rhabdomyosarcoma*.[53] The vast majority of cells were spindle-shaped. Nuclei were fusiform, moderately pleomorphic, alternately blunt-ended or with pointed ends. Typical rhabdomyoblasts were few and difficult to find (Fig. 15.40).

Alveolar rhabdomyosarcoma is a typical small round cell malignancy in FNB smears (Fig. 15.41). Smears show predominantly single cells, and stripped nuclei are common. Alveolar or rosette-like structures may be seen. The cells are mainly uniform with rounded or irregular nuclei and scanty

cytoplasm. In almost every case, small rounded or pear-shaped cells with eccentric nuclei and eosinophilic cytoplasm are found (Fig. 15.42). The chromatin is variably coarse and nucleoli may be prominent. The multinucleated cells with small, dark nuclei, commonly seen in histologic sections are, in our experience, not a common finding in smears (Fig. 15.43).

In recent classifications, rhabdomyosarcomas are divided into favorable and unfavorable subtypes. All variants of embryonal rhabdomyosarcoma are considered as favorable tumors, while alveolar rhabdomyosarcoma and embryonal rhabdomyosarcoma with areas of alveolar rhabdomyosarcoma are unfavorable.[54] It is thus clinically important to arrive at a type-specific diagnosis based on the FNB sample. In our experience and in that of others, this is possible in many cases.[55,56] Immunocytochemical demonstration of

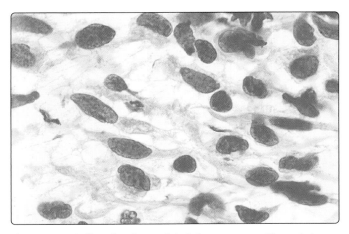

Fig. 15.40 Spindle cell embryonal rhabdomyosarcoma The majority of cells are spindle-shaped with fusiform, moderately pleomorphic nuclei (H&E, IP).

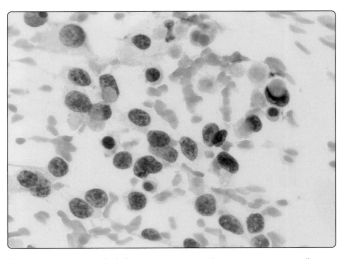

Fig. 15.42 Alveolar rhabdomyosarcoma In almost every case, small rounded or pear-shaped cells with eccentric nuclei and eosinophilic cytoplasm (small rhabdomyoblasts) are found (H&E, HP).

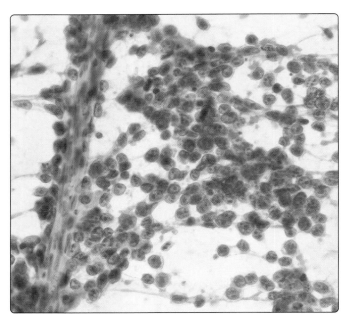

Fig. 15.41 Alveolar rhabdomyosarcoma The cells are mainly uniform with rounded or irregular nuclei and scanty cytoplasm (H&E, IP).

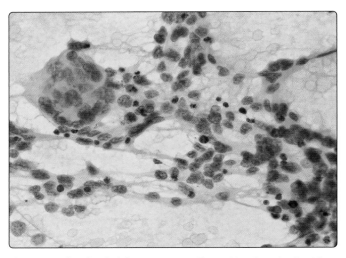

Fig. 15.43 Alveolar rhabdomyosarcoma The multinucleated cells with small, dark nuclei, commonly seen in histologic sections, are not a common finding in FNA smears (H&E, IP).

Neurogenic tumors

Benign tumors

The needling of a *neurilemmoma* or of a *neurofibroma* may trigger a sharp pain along the nerve and this is a valuable diagnostic sign. However, needling of a tumor adjacent to nerve may cause similar pain if the needle traverses the tumor and touches the nerve. Neurilemmoma is a common target for FNB; the material obtained varies from case to case. If Antoni A areas are sampled, tissue fragments of cohesive cells are characteristic and more commonly seen than single cells (Fig. 15.46A). Samples from Antoni B areas often show mainly dispersed cells and a myxoid or at times cystic background, and only few and small tissue fragments (Fig. 15.46B). Whichever portion is sampled, the cellularity of the fragments is variable. The most typical feature is the fibrillar appearance

desmin and/or the more specific markers for striated muscle, myogenin and MyoD-1 (Fig. 15.44), are valuable adjuncts to confirm the diagnosis as the demonstration of the chromosomal aberration t(2;13)(q35;q14), basis for a fusion transcript between the PAX3 and GKHR genes in alveolar rhabdomyosarcoma.[57] Positivity for myoglobin is only present in more differentiated myoblasts.

Pleomorphic rhabdomyosarcoma, for many years thought to be a non-existent entity, is in current classifications considered as a rhabdomyosarcoma subtype in adults, especially the elderly.[58] The few cases in our files showed similar features; a pleomorphic sarcoma resembling pleomorphic sarcoma of MFH type but displaying scattered highly atypical rhabdomyoblast-like cells with abundant dense eosinophilic cytoplasm and eccentric nuclei (Fig. 15.45).

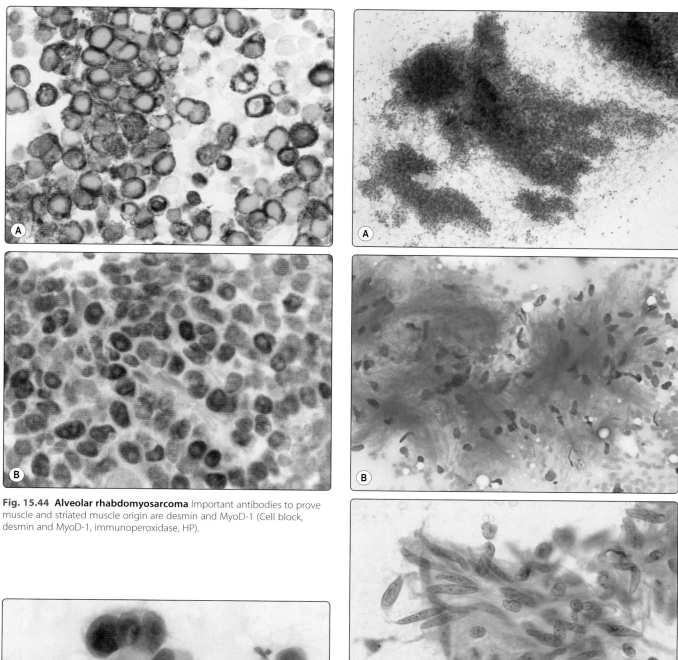

Fig. 15.44 Alveolar rhabdomyosarcoma Important antibodies to prove muscle and striated muscle origin are desmin and MyoD-1 (Cell block, desmin and MyoD-1, immunoperoxidase, HP).

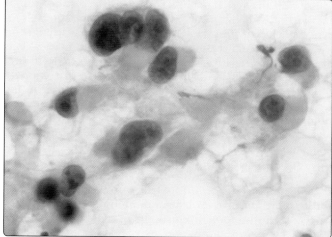

Fig. 15.45 Pleomorphic rhabdomyosarcoma Loosely cohesive rhabdomyoblast-like cells with eosinophilic cytoplasm and eccentric nuclei (H&E, IP).

Fig. 15.46 Schwannoma (A) Tissue fragments of cohesive cells are commonly seen in samples from Antoni A areas (MGG, LP); (B) Mainly dispersed cells and only few small tissue fragments in a myxoid or at times cystic background are commonly seen in samples from Antoni B areas (MGG, IP); (C) The most typical feature is the fibrillar appearance of the intercellular stroma in fragments (H&E, HP).

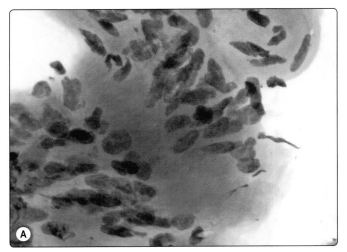

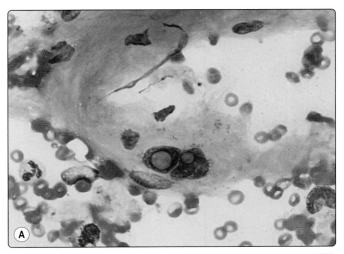

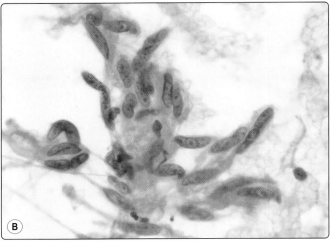

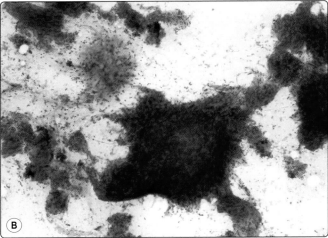

Fig. 15.47 Schwannoma (A) Nuclear palisading may occur and is more commonly seen that true Verocay bodies (MGG, HP); (B) Nuclei tend to be long and slender with pointed ends, Some of nuclei are comma-shaped or are bent like a fishhook (H&E, HP).

Fig. 15.48 Ancient schwannoma (A) The pleomorphic and bizarre cells with dark nuclei, at times with vacuoles (so called 'kern-loche') (MGG, HP); (B) The overall smear pattern is that of a benign tumor (MGG, HP).

of the intercellular stroma in fragments (Fig. 15.46C). Nuclear palisading may occur and is more commonly seen than true Verocay bodies (Fig. 15.47A). Nuclei tend to be long and slender with pointed ends. Often, a number of the slender nuclei are comma-shaped or are bent like a fishhook (Fig. 15.47B). There is often a moderate degree of nuclear pleomorphism, but the chromatin pattern is uniformly bland. If cells with plump, spindled nuclei and more abundant cytoplasm predominate, a diagnosis of low-grade malignant leiomyosarcoma may be considered. The pleomorphic and bizarre cells in *ancient neurilemmoma* with their degenerate, dark nuclei, at times with vacuoles (so called 'kern-loche') (Fig. 15.48A), have been mistaken for malignancy[47] but the overall smear pattern is that of a benign tumor (Fig. 15.48B).

In FNB smears from neurofibroma, dispersed cells are more common than tissue fragments and a myxoid background matrix often seen. In 2006, Domanski et al. reported the cytological features of neurilemmoma in a series of 116 cases.[59]

The *granular cell tumor* (Abrikosoff tumor) is currently regarded as a neurogenic tumor and not of myogenic origin, as formerly considered. Granular cell tumors are mainly found in the subcutaneous and submucosal tissues, most commonly in the head and neck region. In the breast, it can closely simulate cancer clinically and radiologically (Chapter breast Ch 7 in ed 4). It may also occur as a deep-seated tumor in the limbs. FNB smears show many neoplastic cells in syncytial clusters and singly. The nuclei may be arranged in a vaguely follicular pattern. The cytoplasm of intact cells is abundant and relatively dense, eosinophilic in H&E and dark blue in MGG with prominent characteristic granulation. The cytoplasm is fragile and may be dispersed in the background together with naked nuclei. The nuclei are predominantly small round or ovoid, with bland chromatin and small but prominent nucleoli (Fig. 15.49A). Anisokaryosis can be marked in some tumors and there may be irregularity of nuclear shape.

S-100 protein is generally positive in all these benign neurogenic tumors (Fig. 15.49B). Many granular cell tumors are, furthermore, positive for NSE and inhibin.

Histologically, focal necrosis, increased mitotic activity, nuclear hyperchromatism and atypical spindle cells are the typical features of the rare malignant granular cell tumors.

The cytological appearance of benign as well as malignant granular cell tumors has been recorded.[60–62]

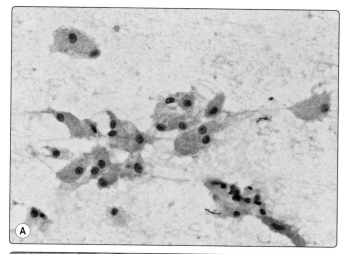

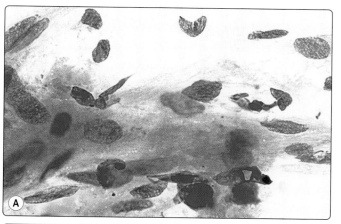

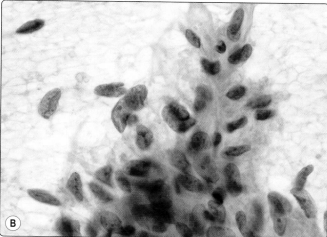

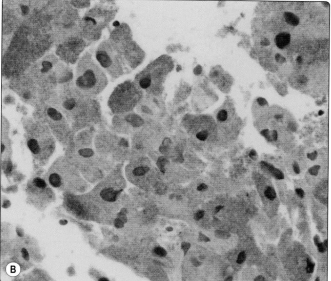

Fig. 15.50 Malignant peripheral nerve sheath tumor (MPNST) (A) Some of MPNST are highly pleomorphic and some have epithelioid features (MGG, HP); (B) In high-grade tumors, the smears are highly cellular and the cells have elongated, spindly, atypical nuclei (H&E, HP).

Fig. 15.49 Granular cell tumor (A) The cytoplasm is abundant and relatively dense with prominent characteristic granulation (H&E, HP); (B) S-100 protein is generally positive in granular cell tumors (cell block, S-100, immunoperoxidase, HP).

Malignant tumors

Most *malignant peripheral nerve sheath tumors (MPNST)* show the pattern of spindle cell sarcomas; some are highly pleomorphic and some have epithelioid features (Fig. 15.50A). Cells from a low-grade tumor may be only moderately pleomorphic. In high-grade tumors, the smears are highly cellular and the cells have elongated, spindly, atypical nuclei (Fig. 15.50B). Mitotic figures are not uncommon. Pleomorphic MPNST often displays a cytomorphology resembling that of a pleomorphic sarcoma of MFH type, including multinucleated tumor cells with bizarre nuclei. Nuclear chromatin is coarse and irregular. Cells are single and in clusters with intercellular collagen, and a background of myxoid material is occasionally present. *Neurofibrosarcoma* in von Recklinghausen's disease may be difficult to diagnose as these tumors may show a mixture of benign and malignant areas (Fig. 15.51). The variable cytologic features of MPNST

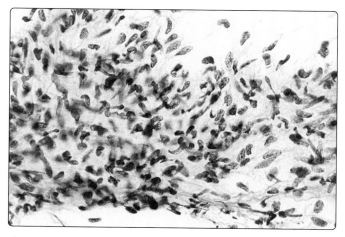

Fig. 15.51 Malignant peripheral nerve sheath tumour in von Recklinghausen's disease Cellular tissue fragment of spindle cells showing moderate nuclear pleomorphism (PAP, HP).

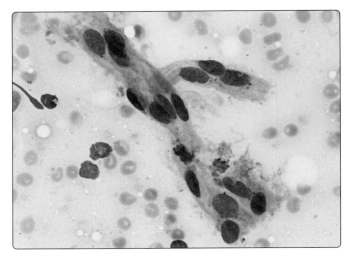

Fig. 15.52 Hemangioma Smears may contain a few strands of endothelial cells with pale, spindly nuclei (MGG, HP).

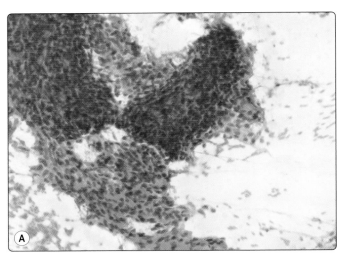

in FNB smears have been recorded in a number of series.[63,64] Positivity for S-100 protein, an important feature in benign neurogenic tumors, is of less diagnostic value in MPNST, as many tumors are negative and positivity often focal.

Tumors of vascular origin

Fine needle aspiration of *hemangioma* of any type yields plenty of venous blood. Smears may contain a few strands of endothelial cells with pale, spindly nuclei (Fig. 15.52). Macrophages, hemosiderin pigment and fibroblasts may be present if thrombosis has occurred. Most *angiosarcomas* are cutaneous tumors; only a minority are deep-seated. The cytologic features of angiosarcoma are variable. The cell population may be predominantly spindled, pleomorphic or epithelioid (Fig. 15.53A, B). A correct diagnosis is often not possible without immunocytochemical confirmation (CD31, CD34 and Fli-1) that the tumor cells are of endothelial origin (Fig. 15.53C). In epithelioid variants of angiosarcoma, EMA and keratin antibodies are often positive. The variable cytologic features in angiosarcoma have been described in several recent papers.[65–67] Angiosarcoma of the breast is illustrated in Chapter 7 and of the spleen in Chapter 11.

Tumors of uncertain or debated histogenesis

Benign tumors

Intramuscular myxoma has a quite characteristic appearance in FNB smears.[68] Macroscopically, the aspirate consists of droplets of colorless, mucoid, stringy and semi-liquid material resembling the aspirate from a ganglion. Smears show small tissue fragments and single cells in an abundance of myxoid background material (Fig. 15.54A). The cells are predominantly spindle shaped and have elongated nuclei and most often very long, thin cytoplasmic processes (Fig. 15.54B). The chromatin is regularly dispersed and finely granular, and nucleoli, if present, are small. Some

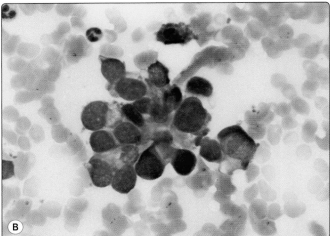

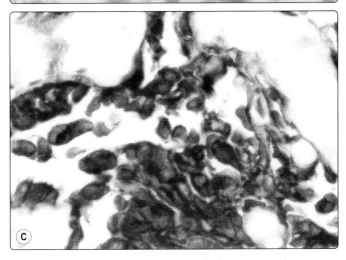

Fig. 15.53 Angiosarcoma (A) In this example, the smear population is predominantly of atypical spindle cells; differentiation from other spindle cell sarcomas requires immunostaining (H&E, LP); (B) Epithelioid pattern of gland-like cluster of malignant cells with rounded nuclei (MGG, HP); (C) A correct diagnosis is often not possible without immunocytochemical confirmation that the tumor cells are of endothelial origin (cell block, CD34, immunoperoxidase, HP).

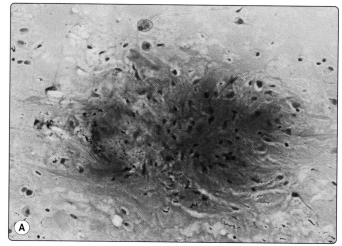

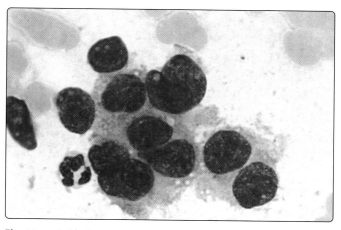

Fig. 15.55 **Epithelioid sarcoma** A loose cluster of large cells with abundant cytoplasm, irregular nuclei, unevenly distributed chromatin and prominent nucleoli (MGG, HP oil).

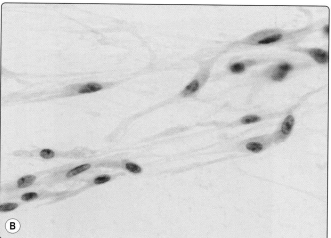

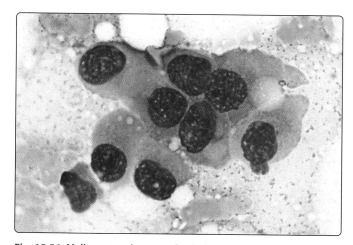

Fig. 15.54 **Intramuscular myxoma** (A) The myxoid matrix is clearly demonstrated in air-dried smears (MGG, IP); (B) The constituent cells are spindle shaped with long cytoplasmic processes and elongated or ovoid bland nuclei (H&E, HP).

Fig. 15.56 **Malignant melanoma of soft tissues (clear cell sarcoma)** A cluster of loosely cohesive cells. The cells are large, ovoid or spindle with abundant cytoplasm, rounded nuclei and prominent nucleoli (MGG, HP oil).

histiocyte-like cells with abundant vacuolated cytoplasm, sometimes containing a large cytoplasmic globule of bluish-violet material (MGG), are also present. Fragments of capillary vessels are rare and this is important in distinguishing intramuscular myxoma from paucicellular myxoid liposarcoma, low-grade malignant myxofibrosarcoma and low-grade fibromyxoid sarcoma. Nielsen et al. described cases of intramuscular myxoma with focally increased cellularity and hypervascularity designated as *cellular myxoma*.[69] FNB smears from such areas of cellular myxoma may be very difficult to distinguish from low-grade fibromyxoid sarcoma and low-grade myxofibrosarcoma due to the cellularity and the increased number of vessel fragments.

Malignant tumors

The cytomorphology of *epithelioid sarcoma* has been characterised.[70,71] The three cases in our files displayed spindled or polygonal tumor cells in loose clusters or singly, with abundant cytoplasm, rounded or ovoid nuclei and large nucleoli (Fig. 15.55). In one case, histiocytes and inflammatory cells dominated the smears. The cytology of clear cell sarcoma and of epithelioid sarcoma is rather similar and the different clinical presentation and immunocytochemical profile are important in the differential diagnosis.

FNB smears from *clear cell sarcoma (malignant melanoma of soft tissues)* have been studied in rather few cases.[72,73] We have seen two examples of this relatively rare tumor. The cells are mostly dispersed but small groups of loosely cohesive cells are also present. The cells are polygonal or spindle shaped and have abundant pale cytoplasm and rounded nuclei with prominent nucleoli (Fig. 15.56). Immunocytochemistry (S-100 protein and melanoma-associated antigens) are helpful in diagnosis but soft tissue metastasis of malignant melanoma is a problem. Cytogenetic investigation is important in the differential diagnosis versus malignant melanoma, as clear cell sarcoma has been found to harbor the chromosomal aberration t(12;22)(q13-14;q 12-13), giving rise to the transcript ATF1/EWS.

Smears from *synovial sarcoma* are usually highly cellular (Fig. 15.57A). The typical appearance is a mixture of tissue fragments and dispersed cells. Mitotic figures can be found in almost every case, especially in the tissue fragments. Bare nuclei are common. A hemangiopericytoma-like vascular

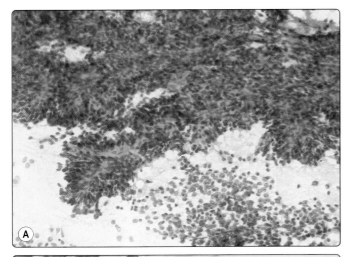

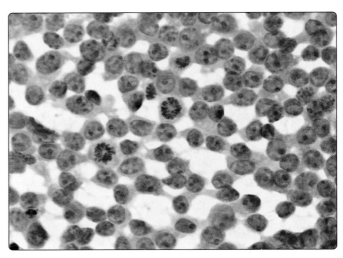

Fig. 15.58 Synovial sarcoma Smears from a poorly differentiated synovial sarcoma can be difficult to differ from Ewing's sarcoma (H&E, HP).

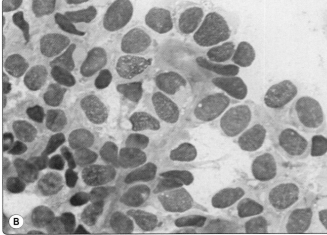

Fig. 15.57 Synovial sarcoma (A) Smears are usually highly cellular; the typical appearance is a mixture of tissue fragments and dispersed cells (H&E, LP); (B) Vaguely acinar-like structures may be seen in the periphery of fragments (MGG, HP).

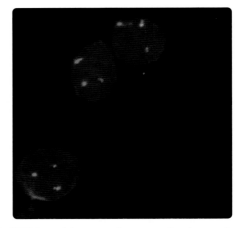

Fig. 15.59 FISH-Synovial sarcoma Separate red and green signals indicative of a rearrangement of one copy of the SYT gene region.

pattern with branching capillaries ('staghorn' pattern) is commonly seen in fragments. The cells are small to medium in size. Nuclei are rounded or ovoid with finely granular, bland chromatin and nucleoli are small and inconspicuous. Intact cells have thin uni- or bipolar cytoplasm. Vaguely acinar-like structures may be seen in the periphery of fragments (Fig. 15.57B). Mast cells are prominent in some cases. A myxoid background matrix has been reported in some cases.[74] An obvious biphasic pattern is only infrequently seen in our experience. The cytology of mono- and biphasic synovial sarcoma has been reported in two large series.[75,76] The cytomorphology of the poorly differentiated variant[77] (involving the entire tumor or focally in other subtypes) is relatively unknown and has been described in few cases (Fig. 15.58).[78–80] Poorly differentiated fibrosarcoma-like synovial sarcoma is extremely difficult to distinguish from MPNST and the rare fibrosarcoma. A reliable cytologic diagnosis of synovial sarcoma is important since neoadjuvant therapy is commonly applied before surgery. Even if synovial sarcoma is strongly suspected in an FNB smear, adjunctive diagnostic

methods are almost always necessary to reach a confident diagnosis. The majority of synovial sarcomas stain positively for EMA and keratins 7 and 19 (although often focally); positive staining for CD99 and bcl-2 has also been reported. Cytogenetic analysis is a most important valuable adjunct. FISH (Fig. 15.59) and RT-PCR of aspirated material used for detection of the two most common gene fusion products (SYT/SSX1 and SYT/SSX2, respectively) is more effective than chromosomal analysis of cytologic material to diagnose the translocation t(X;18)(p11;q12).[81]

Only single cases of *extraskeletal chondrosarcoma and extraskeletal osteosarcoma* have been studied.[82] *Extraskeletal myxoid chondrosarcoma* (EMC), however, has been thoroughly investigated in a number of cases.[83,84] Cells, forming strands or dispersed, are typically embedded in an abundant myxoid ground substance. The most usual patterns are cells arranged in clusters or branching strands (Fig. 15.60). However, the tumor cells may be arranged in cell balls embedded in the ground substance, mimicking the appearance of mucus-producing carcinoma (Fig. 15.61A). The cells

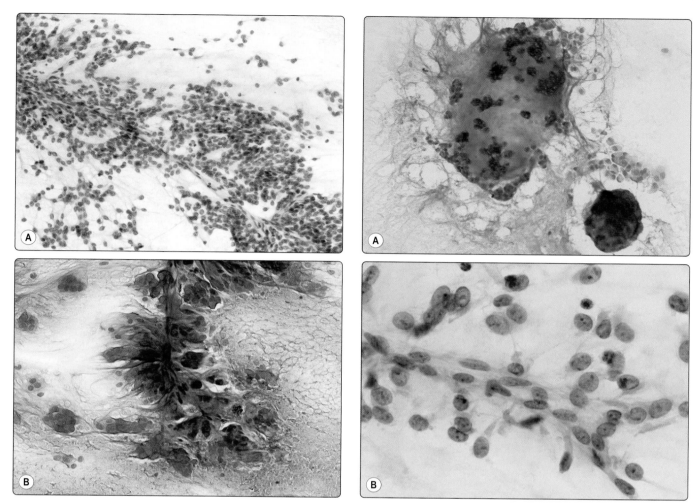

Fig. 15.60 Extraskeletal myxoid chondrosarcoma (A, B) Cells with relatively uniform rounded nuclei embedded in a prominent myxoid matrix; a tendency for the cells to appear in small rows (A, H&E, LP; B, MGG, IP).

Fig. 15.61 Extraskeletal myxoid chondrosarcoma (A) The tumor cells may be arranged in cell balls embedded in the ground substance, mimicking the appearance of mucus-producing carcinoma (MGG, IP); (B) The cells typically have rounded nuclei with small nucleoli and a variable amount of cytoplasm. Uni-or bipolar cytoplasmic processes are seen in some cells (H&E, HP).

are small to medium in size, there is a moderate amount of cytoplasm, and nuclei are rounded or ovoid with small but distinct nucleoli. Uni- or bipolar cytoplasmic processes are seen in some cells (Fig. 15.61B). Intranuclear inclusions were prominent in one of our cases. Fragments of chondroid substance and rounded chondroblast-like cells have been described in some cases. Recently, cases of EMC showing signs of neuroendocrine differentiation have been published. One case from our files was difficult to diagnose correctly since there was ultrastructural evidence of neuroendocrine differentiation at the electron microscopic examination of the aspirated cells.[85] The FNB findings in the rare alveolar soft part sarcoma have been described in a few case reports.[86,87]

References

1. Rydholm A. Centralisation of soft tissue sarcoma: The Southern Sweden Experience. Acta Orthop Scand 1997;68(suppl. 273):4–8.
2. Åkerman M, Rydholm A. Surgery based on fine needle aspiration cytology. Acta Orthop Scand 1994;65(suppl. 256):69–70.
3. Brosjö O, Bauer HCP, Kreisbergs A, et al. Fine needle aspiration biopsy of soft tissue tumours. Acta Orthop Scand 1994;65(suppl. 256):108–9.
4. Dey D, Mallik MK, Gupta SK, et al. Role of fine needle aspiration cytology in the diagnosis of soft tissue tumours and tumour-like lesions. Cytopathology 2004;15:32–7.

5. Kumar S, Chowdhury N. Accuracy, limitations and pitfall in the diagnosis o0f soft tissue tumours by fine needle aspiration cytology. Indian J Pathol Microbiol 2007;1:42–5.

6. Domanski HA, Åkerman M, Carlén B, et al. Core-needle biopsy performed by the cytopathologist. A technique to complement fine-needle aspiration of soft tissue and bone lesions. Cancer (Cancer Cytopathol) 2005;105:229–39.

7. Jones C, Liu K, Hirschowits S, et al. Concordance of histopathologic and cytologic grading in musculoskeletal sarcoma. Can grade obtained from analysis of the fine-needle aspirates serve as a basis for therapeutic decisions? Cancer (Cancer Cytopathol) 2002;96: 83–91.

8. Åkerman M, Domanski H. The cytology of soft tissue tumours. Monographs in Clinical Cytology. vol 16. Basel: Karger; 2003.

9. Gonzáles-Cámpora R. Cytoarchitectural findings in the diagnosis of primary soft tissue tumors. Acta Cytol 2001;45:115–46.

10. Fletcher DM, Unni KK, Mertens F. World Health Organization Classification of Tumours. Pathology and genetics. Tumours of Soft Tissue and Bone. Lyon: IARC Press; 2001.

11. Weiss SW, Goldblum JR. Soft Tissue Tumors. 5th ed. St Louis: Mosby; 2008.

12. Dahl I, Åkerman M. Nodular fasciitis. A correlative cytologic and histologic study of 13 cases. Acta Cytol 1981;25:215–22.

13. Dodd LG, Martinez S. Fine-needle aspiration cytology of pseudosarcomatous lesions of soft tissue. Diagn Cytopathol 2001;24:28–35.

14. Kong CS, Cha I. Nodular fasciitis: diagnosis by fine needle aspiration biopsy. Acta Cytol 2004;48:473–7.

15. Stanley M, Skoog L, Tani E, et al. Spontaneous resolution of nodular fasciitis following diagnosis by fine needle aspiration. Acta Cytol 1991;35: 616–7.

16. Willén H, Åkerman M, Rydholm A. Fine needle aspiration of nodular fasciitis. No need for surgical intervention. Proceedings of the Annual Meeting of the European Musculoskeletal Oncology Society, Amsterdam, 1994.

17. Rööser B, Herrlin K, Rydholm A, et al. Pseudomalignant myositis ossificans. Clinical, radiologic, and cytologic diagnosis. Acta Orthop Scand 1989;60:457–60.

18. Dalén BP, Meis-Kindblom JM, Sumathi VP, et al. Fine-needle aspiration cytology and core needle biopsy in the preoperative diagnosis of desmoids tumors. Acta Orthop Scand 2006;77:926–31.

19. Willén H, Carlén B, Rydholm A, et al. Solitary fibrous tumor of the soft tissue. Acta Orthop Scand 1999;(Suppl. 289):31–2.

20. Clayton AC, Salomao DR, Keeny GL, et al. Solitary fibrous tumor: a study of cytologic features of six cases diagnosed by fine-needle aspiration. Diagn Cytopathol 2001;25:172–6.

21. Domanski HA, Carlén B, Sloth M, et al. Elastofibroma dorsi has distinct cytomorphologic features making diagnostic surgical biopsy unnecessary. Cytomorphologic study with clinical, radiologic and electron microscopic correlation. Diagn Cytopathol 2003;29:327–33.

22. Pereira S, Tani E, Skoog L. Diagnosis of fibromatosis colli by fine needle aspiration. Cytopathol 1999;10:25–9.

23. Sharma S, Mishra K, Khanna G. Fibromatosis colli in infants. A cytologic study of eight cases. Acta Cytol 2003;47:359–62.

24. Jadushing IH. Fine needle aspiration cytology of fibrous hamartoma of infancy. Acta Cytol 1997;41(Suppl. 4):1391–3.

25. Layfield LJ, Moffat EJ, Dodd EG, et al. Cytologic findings in tenosynovial giant cell tumors investigated by fine-needle aspiration cytology. Diagn Cytopathol 1997;16:317–25.

26. Meis-Kindblom J, Bjerkehagen B, Böhling T, et al. Morphologic review of 1000 soft tissue sarcomas from the Scandinavian Sarcoma Group (SSG) register. The peer-review committee experience. Acta Orthop Scand 1999;70(Suppl. 285):18–26.

27. Fletcher CDM, Gustafson P, Rydholm A, et al. Clinicopathologic re-evaluation of 100 malignant fibrous histiocytomas: prognostic relevance of subclassification. J Clin Onc 2001;19:3045–50.

28. Berardo M, Powers C, Wakely P, et al. Fine needle aspiration cytopathology of MFH. Cancer 1997;81:228–37.

29. Klijanienko J, Caillaud JM, Lagacé R, et al. Comparative fine-needle aspiration and pathologic study of malignant fibrous histiocytoma. Cytodiagnostic features of 95 tumors in 71 patients. Diagn Cytopathol 2002;29:320–6.

30. Merck CH, Hagmar B. Myxofibrosarcoma. A correlative cytologic and histologic study of 13 cases examined by fine needle aspiration cytology. Acta Cytol 1980;22:137–44.

31. Kilpatrick SE, Ward WG. Myxofibrosarcoma of soft tissues: cytomorphologic analysis of a series. Diagn Cytopathol 1999;20:6–9.

32. Kilpatrick SE, Ward WG, Bos GD. The value of fine-needle aspiration biopsy in the differential diagnosis of adult myxoid sarcoma. Cancer (Cancer Cytopathol) 2000;90:167–77.

33. Evans HL. Low-grade fibromyxoid sarcoma. A report of 12 cases. Am J Surg Pathol 1993;17:595–600.

34. Goodlad JR, Mentzel T, Fletcher CD. Low-grade fibromyxoid sarcoma: clinicopathologic analysis of eleven new cases in support of a distinct entity. Histopathol 1995;26:229–37.

35. Domanski HA, Mertens F, Panagopoulus I, et al. Low-grade fibromyxoid sarcoma is difficult to diagnose by fine needle aspiration cytology: a cytomorphological study of eight cases. Cytopathology 2008;20:304–14.

36. Domanski HA, Carlén B, Jonsson K, et al. Distinct cytologic features of spindle cell lipoma. A cytologic-histologic study with clinical, radiologic, electron microscopic, and cytogenetic correlations. Cancer (Cancer Cytopathol) 2001;93:381–9.

37. Lamos MM, Kindblom L-G, Meis-Kindblom JM, et al. Fine-needle aspiration cytologic characteristics of hibernoma. Cancer (Cancer Cytopathol) 2001;93:206–10.

38. Meis JM, Enzinger FM. Chondroid lipoma. A unique tumor simultating liposarcoma and myxoid chondrosarcoma. AmJ Surg Pathol 1993;17:1103–12.

39. Gisselson D, Domanski HA, Höglund M, et al. Unique cytologic features and chromosome aberrations in chondroid lipoma: a case report based on fine. needle aspiration cytology, histopathology, electron microscopy, chromosome banding, and molecular cytogenetics. Am J Surg Pathol 1999;23:1300–4.

40. Yang YJ, Damron TA, Ambrose JL. Diagnosis of chondroid lipoma by fine-needle aspiration biopsy. Arch Pathol Lab Med 2001;125:1224–6.

41. Kempson RL, Fletcher CDM, Evans HL, et al. Tumors of the soft tissues. Atlas of tumor pathology. Washington DC: AFIP; 2001.

42. Nemanquani D, Mourad WA. Cytomorphologic features of fine-needle aspiration of liposarcoma. Diagn Cytopathol 1999;20:67–9.

43. Dey P. Fine needle aspiration cytology of well-differentiated liposarcoma. A report of two cases. Acta Cytol 2000;44:459–62.

44. Vicandi B, Limenez-Hefferman J, Lopez-Ferrer P, et al. Cytologic features of round cell liposarcoma. Cancer (Cancer Cytopathol) 2003;99:28–32.

45. Klijanienko J, Caillaud J-M, Lagecé R. Fine-needle aspiration in liposarcoma: cytologic correlative study including well-differentiated, myxoid, and pleomorphic variants. Diagn Cytopathol 2004;30:307–12.

46. Domanski HA, Cytologic features of angioleiomyoma: cytologic-histologic study of 10 cases. Diagn Cytopathol 2002;27:161–6.

47. Ryd W, Mugel S, Ayyash K. Ancient neurilemmoma. A pitfall in the cytologic diagnosis of soft tissue tumors. Diagn Cytopathol 1988;2:244–7.

48. Klijanienko J, Caillaud JM, Lagacé R, et al. Fine-needle aspiration of leiomyosarcoma. A correlative

cytohistopathological study of 96 tumors in 68 patients. Diagn Cytopathol 2003;28:119–25.

49. Domanski HA, Åkerman M, Rissler P, et al. Fine needle aspiration of soft tissue leiomyosarcoma. An analysis of the most common cytologic findings and the value of ancillary techniques. Diagn Cytopathol 2006;34:597–604.

50. Bertholf MF, Frierson HF, Feldman PS. Fine needle aspiration cytology of an adult rhabdomyoma of the neck and head. Diagn Cytopathol 1988;4:152–5.

51. Domanski HA, Dawiskiba S. Adult rhabdomyoma in fine needle aspiration. A report of two cases. Acta Cytol 2000; 44:223–6.

52. Klijanienko J, Caillaud JM, Orbach D, et al. Cyto-histological correlations in primary, recurrent and metastatic rhabdomyosarcoma: the Institut Curie experience. Diagn Cytopathol 2007;35: 482–7.

53. Daneshbod Y, Monabati A, Kumar PV, et al. Paratesticular spindle cell rhabdomyosarcoma diagnosed by fine needle aspiration cytology: a case report. Acta ytol 2005;49;331–4.

54. Coffin CM. The new international rhabdomyosarcoma classification, its progenitors, and considerations beyond morphology. Adv Anat Pathol 1997;4: 1–16.

55. Åkerman M, Willén H, Carlén B. Fine needle aspiratation of rhabdomyosarcoma. I. A reliable type-diagnosis possible to render? A retrospective study of 23 cases. Acta Ortop Scand 1996;67(Suppl. 272):55.

56. Athan S, Aksu Ö, Ekinci C. Cytologic diagnosis and subtyping of rhabdomyosarcoma. Cytopathol 1998;9:389–97.

57. Udayakumar AM, Sundareshan TS, Appaji L, et al. Rhabdomyosarcoma: cytogenetics of five cases using fine-needle aspiration samples and review of the literature. Ann Genet 2002;45:33–7.

58. Hollowood K, Fletcher CDM. Rhabdomyosarcoma in adults. Semin Diagn Pathol 1994;11:47–57.

59. Domanski HA, Åkerman M, Engellau J, et al. Fine-needle aspiration of neurilemmoma. A clinicocytopathologic study of 116 patients. Diagn Cytopathol 2006;34:403–12.

60. Liu Z, Madden JF, Olatidoye BA, et al. Features of benign granular cell tumor on fine needle aspiration. Acta Cytol 1999;43:552–7.

61. Liu Z, Mira JL, Vu H. Diagnosis of malignant granular cell tumor by fine needle aspiration cytology. A case report. Acta Cytol 2001;45:1011–21.

62. Wieczorek TJ, Krane JF, Domanski HA, et al. Cytologic findings in granular cell tumors with emphasis on the diagnosis of malignant granular cell tumor by fine-needle aspiration biopsy. Cancer 2001;93:398–408.

63. Jimenez-Hefferman JA, Lopéz-Ferrer PO, Vicandi B, et al. Cytologic features of malignant peripheral nerve sheath tumor. Acta Cytol 1999;43:175–83.

64. Klijanienko J, Caillaud J-M, Lagacé R, et al. Cytohistologic correlations of 24 malignant peripheral nerve sheath tumors (MPNST) in 17 cases. The Institut Curie experience. Diagn Cytopathol 2002;27:103–8.

65. Wakely PE, Frable WJ, Kneisl JS. Aspiration cytopathology of epithelioid angiosarcoma. Cancer (Cancer Cytopathol) 2000;90:245–51.

66. Minimo C, Zakowski M, Lin O. Cytologic findings of malignant vascular neoplasms: a study of twenty-four cases. Diagn Cytopathol 2002;26:349–55.

67. Klijanienko J, Caillaud KM, Lagacé R, et al. Cytohistologic correlations in angiosarcoma including classic and epithelioid variants: Institut Curie experience. Diagn Cytopathol 2003;29:140–5.

68. Åkerman M, Rydholm A. Aspiration cytology of intramuscular myxoma. A comparative clinical, cytologic and histologic study of ten cases. Acta Cytol 1983;27:505–10.

69. Nielsen GP, O'Conell JX, Rosenberg AE. Intramuscular myxoma: a clinipathologic study of 51 cases with emphasis on hyper cellular and hypervascular variants. Am J Surg Pathol 1998;22:1222–7.

70. Cardillo M, Zakowski MF, Lin O. Fine-needle aspiration of epithelioid sarcoma. Cytologic findings in nine cases. Cancer (Cancer Cytopathol) 2001;93:246–51.

71. Yildiz I, Onder S, Kutlay L, et al. Cytology of epithelioid sarcoma. Cytopathology 2006;17:305–7.

72. Creager AJ, Pitman MB, Geisinger KR. Cytologic features of clear cell sarcoma (malignant melanoma) of soft parts: a study of fine needle aspirates and exfoliative specimens. Am J Clin Pathol 2002;117:217–24.

73. Tong TR, Chow TC, Chan OW, et al. Clear cell sarcoma diagnosis by fine-needle aspiration: cytologic, histologic, and ultrastructural features; potential pitfalls; and literature review. Diagn Cytopathol 2002;26:174–80.

74. Moffat EJ, Liu K, Layfield J. Demonstration of myxoid change in fine-needle aspiration of synovial sarcoma: a case report. Diagn Cytopathol 1998;18:188–91.

75. Klijanienko J, Caillaud J-M, Lagacé R, et al. Cytohistological correlations in 56 synovial sarcomas in 56 patients: the Institut Curie's experience. Diagn Cytopathol 2002;27:96–102.

76. Åkerman M, Ryd W. Skytting B- Fine-needle aspiration of synovial sarcoma: criteria for diagnosis; retrospective examination of 37 cases, including ancillary diagnostics. A Scandinavian Sarcoma Group study. Diagn Cytopathol 2003;28:232–8.

77. Folpe AL, Schmidt RA, Chapman A, et al. Poorly differentiated synovial sarcoma: immunohistochemical distinction from primitive neuroectodermal tumors and high-grade malignant MPNST. Am J Surg Pathol 1998;22:673–82.

78. Silverman JE, Landreneau RJ, Sturgis CD, et al. Small-cell variant of synovial sarcoma: fine-needle aspiration with ancillary features and potential pitfalls. Diagn Cytopathol 2000;23:118–23.

79. Kwon MS. Aspiration cytology of pulmonary small cell variant of poorly-differentiated synovial metastatic from the tongue: a case report. Acta Cytol 2005;49:92–6.

80. Åkerman M, Domanski HA. The complex cytologic features of synovial sarcoma in fine needle aspirates; an analysis of four illustrative cases. Cytopathology 2007;18:234–40.

81. Nilsson G, Ming MD, Weide J, et al. Reverse transcriptase polymerase chain reaction on fine needle aspirates for rapid detection of translocations in synovial sarcoma. Acta Cytol 1998;42:1317–24.

82. Calafati SA, Wright AL, Rosen SE, et al. Fine needle aspiration cytology of extraskeletal chondrosarcoma. Acta Cytol 1984;28:81–5.

83. Willén H, Lemos M, Ryd W. Extraskeletal myxoid chondrosarcoma. A cytologic and histologic correlation. 1st Italian/Scandinavian Sarcoma Group Meeting – ISG/SSG. Acta Orthop Scand 2000. http://home.pi.se/actaorthopscand/pages/framabst.html.p33

84. Jakowski JD, Wakeley PE. Cytopathology of extraskeletal myxoid chondrosarcoma. Report of 8 cases. Cancer (Cancer Cytopathol) 2007;111:298–305.

85. Domanski HA, Carlén B, Mertens F. Extraskeletal myxoid chondrosarcoma with neuroendocrine differentiation: a case report with fine-needle aspiration biopsy, histopathology, electron microscopy, and cytogenetics. Ultrastructural Pathology 2003;27:363–8.

86. Logrono R, Wojtowycs MM, Wunderlich DW, et al. Fine needle aspiration cytology and core biopsy in the diagnosis of alveolar soft part sarcoma presenting with lung metastases. A case report. Acta Cytol 1999;43:464–70.

87. Lopez-Ferrer P, Jimenez-Hofferman JA, Vicandi B, et al. Cytologic features of alveolar soft part sarcoma: Report of three cases. Diagn Cytopathol 2002;27:115–9.

CHAPTER 16

Bone

Måns Åkerman and Henryk Domanski

CLINICAL ASPECTS

Needle aspiration has been used in the investigation of bone lesions ever since the technique was introduced. Coley and Ellis included several examples of primary and metastatic bone malignancies in their original paper.[1] Fine needle biopsy (FNB) and cytodiagnosis of bone lesions are now well-established methods in many centers. It is not possible to penetrate intact cortical bone or sclerotic lesions using a truly thin needle (22–23 gauge) but partly destroyed or 'moth-eaten' cortical bone can often be penetrated. New devices, such as the Bone Biopty instrument, a coaxial biopsy system with an eccentric drill,[2] have made it possible to drill through intact cortical bone and to insert the fine needle into the lesion through the drilled canal. FNB has the advantage over open biopsy of being less disruptive to bone, permitting multiple sampling without complications and leaving no scar. There is no risk of infection if simple sterility is observed. FNB is a simple outpatient procedure, cost effective and rapid. Its primary purpose is not only to obtain a morphologic diagnosis of benignity or malignancy, to investigate suspected bone secondaries, or sometimes to aspirate material for a bacteriologic diagnosis from osteolytic lesions, radiologically suspected for osteomyelitis, but also, if possible, to replace open or coarse needle biopsy in the diagnosis of primary bone tumors before treatment. Ancillary diagnostic techniques such as cytochemistry, immunocytochemistry, flow cytometric phenotyping, DNA ploidy analysis, molecular genetic analysis and, in some special situations, electron microscopy are important supplements to cytodiagnosis of specific tumor entities before definitive treatment.

Spinal lesions with threatening cord compression are a medical emergency and FNB can rapidly resolve the differential diagnosis between osteomyelitis, metastatic malignancy and a lymphoproliferative malignancy. The diagnosis of Langerhans cell histiocytosis (eosinophilic granuloma) and of plasmacytoma is, in most cases, relatively easy and the distinction between non-Hodgkin's lymphoma and other small cell malignancies (primary or secondary) is possible. FNB is well suited to the investigation of the cause of pathological fractures, but the proliferating osteoblasts in a fracture callus must be recognised as such. Our experience, and that of others, in the type-specific diagnosis of primary bone lesions is rather substantial, covering all of the malignant bone tumors except adamantinoma, and most of the benign tumors. Definitive diagnosis is possible since the cytomorphology of primary bone tumors, benign as well as malignant, has now been described in detail in correlative cytological/histological studies[3] and in single monographs and reviews.[4,5]

The correct interpretation of smears from a bone lesion requires access to the full clinical and radiological assessment, just as in histological diagnosis of a formal bone biopsy. The cytopathologist should refrain from giving a definitive diagnosis when the results of the radiologic investigation are not known.

Accuracy of diagnosis

Adequate material was obtained in 86–97% in four series, comprising in total 1453 cases.[3,6–9] The diagnostic accuracy in the diagnosis of metastases is very high, in the order of 90%. Its value in the diagnosis of primary bone lesions varied between 90% and 97% in the above cited series.

Complications

Complication are few. We have more than 30 years' experience of FNB of bone lesions in our musculoskeletal tumor centre in Lund University Hospital and have never seen any severe complication. Brief pain at needling is not uncommon but significant hemorrhage is unusual, as is pneumothorax after biopsy of rib or spine lesion. FNB of spinal lesions carries the additional, albeit rare, complication of neurological damage.[10] FNB of bone lesions in patients with a low platelet count or a bleeding disorder must be discussed with the clinician in charge before proceeding to biopsy, and the importance to clinical management of a cytological diagnosis must be decided.

Technical considerations

Fine needle biopsy guided by fluoroscopy or computed tomography (CT) in nonpalpable lytic lesion is a rapid and safe method to obtain a morphologic diagnosis of

©2012 Elsevier Ltd
DOI: 10.1016/B978-0-7020-3151-9.00016-5

lesions anywhere in the skeleton, particularly in the spine.[5,11,12] Some pain is usually felt at aspiration. Local anesthesia prevents periosteal pain and is recommended in conjunction with fluoroscopy or CT guidance, as several passes with the needle may be necessary to obtain a representative specimen. Bone aspirates are often heavily blood-stained and methods similar to those used in processing hematological bone marrow aspirates are useful to concentrate the cell material. The use of a watch glass to select tissue fragments and of thrombin-clot preparations for paraffin sections and histology are of particular value (see Chapter 2). Both air-dried MGG smears and wet-fixed smears for H&E or Pap should be made. MGG smears are particularly valuable in assessing bone marrow elements and chondroid, myxoid or osteoid material; wet-fixed smears are superior for nuclear detail, particularly in tissue fragments ('microbiopsies').

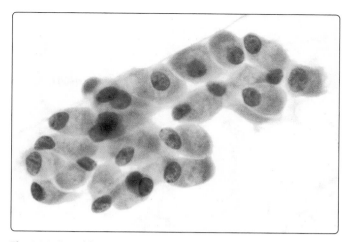

Fig. 16.1 Osteoblasts Cluster of cells with a plasma cell-like appearance; abundant cytoplasm and eccentric nuclei; 'Hof' separated from nucleus is visible in several cells. Smear derived from an area of moderate osteoblastic activity and new bone formation (H&E, HP).

CYTOLOGICAL FINDINGS

Normal structures

- Hematopoietic tissue,
- Osteoblasts,
- Osteoclasts,
- Chondrocytes,
- Cartilage,
- Mesothelial cells.

The cytopathologist must be familiar with the appearance of cellular marrow. Taken individually, the nuclear features of immature marrow cells may be disturbingly similar to malignant cells, but the mixture of all cell types allows easy identification. The irregular multilobed nucleus of the megakaryocytes in particular can cause alarm if the site of origin is unsuspected. MGG-stained smears are much superior to wet-fixed H&E or Pap smears in identifying hematopoietic or lymphoid cells. Bone marrow cells are frequently found, particularly in aspirates from the ribs, vertebrae and sacrum.

Osteoblasts are commonly seen in aspirates from all kinds of bone lesions. They present either as single cells or as small groups or runs. They have a characteristic eccentric nucleus which sometimes seems to protrude from the cytoplasm. The nucleus is round or oval and often contains a central nucleolus. The cytoplasm is dense, amphophilic or basophilic with a central clear area or 'Hof' separated from the nucleus (Fig. 16.1). Reactive osteoblasts in a fracture callus or in benign lesions such as reactive periosteitis may show marked anisokaryosis and prominent nucleoli (Fig. 16.2). Osteoclasts are large cells which possess at least 10–15 uniform nuclei and have abundant cytoplasm with a similar texture to osteoblasts and well-defined borders. A fine, pink cytoplasmic granularity is visible in MGG-stained smears (Fig. 16.3). Normal cartilage does not smear well as it is very cohesive. Flecks or clumps of cartilage may be removed from joint surfaces or costochondral junctions. These show bright red or magenta staining with MGG and are pale and translucent with Pap. Scalloped or fibrillar edges are a feature (Fig. 16.4). Free chondrocytes are almost never seen, but the cells are visible within lacunae in the chondroid matrix. They have small, pale, rounded nuclei and poorly stained

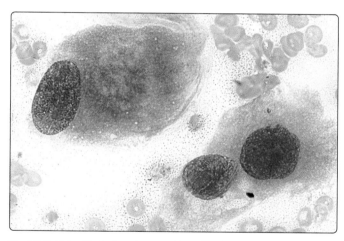

Fig. 16.2 Osteoblasts Reactive osteoblasts (florid reactive periosteitis) showing marked anisokaryosis and enlarged nucleoli. A cytoplasmic 'Hof' is visible (MGG, HP oil).

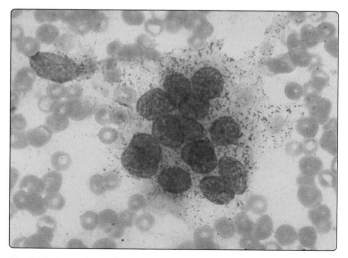

Fig. 16.3 Osteoclast A fine, cytoplasmic granularity is visible in MGG-stained smears (MGG, HP).

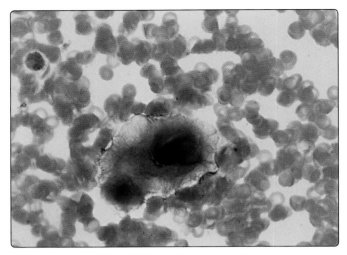

Fig. 16.4 **Normal cartilage** Scalloped or fibrillar edges are one of the features of normal cartilage (MGG, HP).

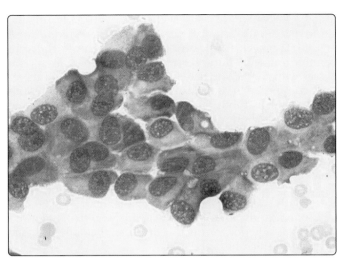

Fig. 16.6 **Mesothelial cells** A rare but important contamination of smears from spinal FNBs (MGG, HP).

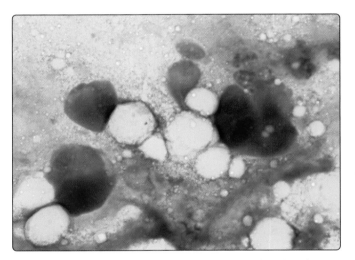

Fig. 16.5 **Normal cartilage** The chondroid matrix stains heavily with MGG and obscures the fine structure of the cells (MGG, HP).

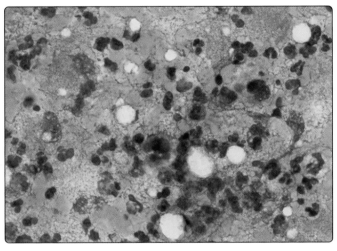

Fig. 16.7 **Osteomyelitis** Histiocytes with vacuolated cytoplasm and neutrophils (MGG, HP).

cytoplasm, often presenting as a halo. They are best visualised in wet-fixed smears. The chondroid matrix stains heavily with MGG and obscures the fine structure of the cells (Fig. 16.5). A rare but important contamination of smears from spinal FNBs is clusters of mesothelial cells which may be sampled if the lesion is missed by the needle. Such cells may be mistaken for metastatic deposits of well-differentiated carcinoma, but usually do not have a bloody background (Fig. 16.6).

Inflammatory processes

Osteomyelitis

Smears from bacterial osteomyelitis are dominated by abundant neutrophils but also contain other inflammatory cells and macrophages. The aspirate may look like pus from any other type of non-specific acute inflammatory process (Fig. 16.7). Culture of the aspirated material is the most valuable

part of the procedure if an infectious lesion is suspected. Clusters of epithelioid histiocytes with characteristic banana- or bean-shaped nuclei and indistinct cell borders and granular (caseous) necrotic material provoke a strong suspicion of tuberculosis (Fig. 16.8). In our experience, Langhans-type giant cells are difficult to find. Again, the need for cultural evidence is emphasised.

Neoplasms

Metastatic carcinoma

CRITERIA FOR DIAGNOSIS

◆ Foreign cell population,
◆ Cell clusters; acinar or gland-like structures,
◆ Cells showing criteria of malignancy.

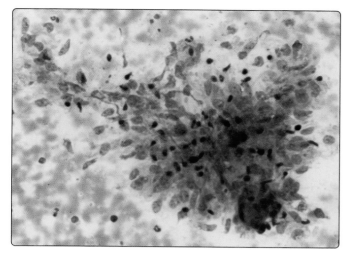

Fig. 16.8 Suspicion of tuberculosis Clusters of epithelioid histiocytes with banana- or bean-shaped nuclei and indistinct cell borders (MGG, IP).

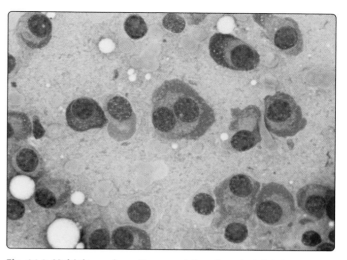

Fig. 16.9 Multiple myeloma Pure population of atypical slightly pleomorphic plasma cells; the eccentric nucleus and pale or clear cytoplasmic zone near the nucleus are distinctive cytologic features (MGG, HP).

As with sites such as lymph nodes, diagnosis is usually easy, especially if the histologic type of the primary tumor is known and sections are available for comparison with the smears. Descriptions of specific types of metastatic neoplasms are not included here; their cytological appearances have generally been discussed elsewhere.

PROBLEMS IN DIFFERENTIAL DIAGNOSIS

- Osteoblasts resembling mucin-secreting cells. The cytoplasmic clearing typical of osteoblasts may resemble a mucin vacuole to the uninitiated. Sometimes clustering or lining up of these cells may enhance the epithelial-like appearance.
- Smeared marrow elements resembling anaplastic carcinoma. Caution should be exercised in reporting poorly smeared or poorly preserved material. Bone marrow cells are fragile and heavy smearing pressure can cause clumping that may resemble aggregates of small cell or other anaplastic carcinoma. As mentioned, megakaryocytes may also be misinterpreted as large, bizarre multinucleated malignant cells. It should be remembered that metastatic carcinoma usually replaces marrow; therefore, a mixture of marrow and new growth are uncommon.
- Anaplastic plasmacytoma may appear as a pleomorphic tumor in which only few cells show typical features of plasma cells. Poor smearing may result in clumping of tumor, cells which may resemble epithelial clusters.
- The distinction between chordoma and clear cell or mucinous carcinoma, and between high-grade chondrosarcoma and clear cell carcinoma, pose specific problems.
- Excessive blood. This problem is commonly encountered in metastatic malignancies as well as in primary bone tumors. The non-aspiration technique may provide better samples.

Solitary plasmacytoma; myeloma

CRITERIA FOR DIAGNOSIS

- Many plasma cells,
- Single cell presentation,
- Variable cell differentiation,

The diagnosis is obvious if there is a uniformly dispersed population of plasma cells including multinucleate and pleomorphic forms. The eccentric nucleus, with its speckled or clock-face chromatin, and the abundant amphophilic cytoplasm make recognition easy. A pale or clear cytoplasmic zone near the nucleus is another distinctive cytologic feature (Fig. 16.9).

PROBLEMS IN DIFFERENTIAL DIAGNOSIS

- Excessive blood. Aspirates from solitary plasmacytoma are often very hemorrhagic and neoplastic plasma cells may be few in numbers.
- Reactive benign plasmacytosis may be difficult to differentiate from plasmacytoma in hemorrhagic aspirates with low numbers of normal-looking or slightly atypical forms.
- Admixture of marrow elements. The dilemma of deciding whether the proportion of plasma cells in marrow is high enough to justify a diagnosis of multiple myeloma is seldom a worry since usually only lytic lesions formed by solid tumors will be aspirated. Admixture with marrow elements is rarely seen in these cases.
- Anaplastic plasmacytoma. As mentioned above, anaplastic pleomorphic plasma cells are likely to cause confusion when a primary bone origin is unsuspected.
- It may be difficult to distinguish large B-cell non-Hodgkin's lymphoma with immunoblastic features from poorly differentiated plasmacytoma.
- Osteoblasts resembling plasma cells. However, it is important to remember that, unlike osteoblasts, the clear cytoplasmic zone in plasma cells is next to the nucleus and that osteoblast nuclei are more eccentrically located than are plasma cell nuclei (nuclei seem to protrude from the cytoplasm).

Neoplastic plasma cells are monoclonal (express monotypic immunoglobulin). This feature is possible to demonstrate in cell block or cytospin preparations. Neoplastic plasma cells, including most anaplastic forms, express CD138 and CD79A.

Malignant lymphoma

Focal bone involvement, usually in form of lytic lesions and most commonly involving the spine, pelvis and the long bones, is uncommon., Primary non-Hodgkin's lymphoma comprises about 3–7% of the primary malignant bone tumors. Primary Hodgkin's lymphoma in bone is extremely rare. Most primary non-Hodgkin's lymphomas are diffuse large cell B-cell lymphomas. Lymphoplasmacytic lymphoma, anaplastic large cell lymphoma and precursor lymphoma (lymphoblastic lymphoma) have also been reported; the two last mentioned may occur in children and adolescents. Cytological criteria for diagnosis are the same as in other sites (see Chapter 5). Case series of primary non-Hodgkin's lymphoma of bone have been presented.[13,14] The important differential diagnosis between precursor lymphoma and classical Ewing's sarcoma is discussed on page 424.

Langerhans cell histiocytosis (histiocytosis X, eosinophilic granuloma)

CRITERIA FOR DIAGNOSIS

◆ Large histiocytes with vesicular nuclei of irregular shape, sometimes binucleated,
◆ Variable numbers of eosinophils,
◆ Giant cells of histiocytic type.

Langerhans cell histiocytosis presents as lytic and often well-defined lesions. Most cases are seen in children. The lesions may be solitary (most cases) or multiple. The long bones (femur and humerus) and the skull are the most common sites in children, and the pelvic bones and ribs in adults. The cytological pattern of Langerhans cell histiocytosis is fairly characteristic and may be diagnostic. The typical histiocytes have moderately larger and paler nuclei than those seen in common inflammatory processes. Generally reniform, the nuclei have a distinct irregular and folded outline (Fig. 16.10A). Coffee-bean nuclei has been reported to be typical of this lesion (Fig. 16.10B). The chromatin is entirely bland and nucleoli small. The cytoplasm is abundant and pale and has fairly well-defined borders. It is often vacuolated. In exceptional cases the Langerhans cells may show signs of phagocytosis. Multinucleated cells of similar type are commonly present. These can be quite large and may resemble osteoclasts in wet-fixed smears.

Large number of histiocytes can occasionally be found in aspirates of chronic osteomyelitis, but these are of the common, smaller type seen in the usual inflammatory processes and are mixed with neutrophils, lymphocytes and plasma cells.

The Langerhans cell histiocytes express S-100 protein and CD1-antigen (Fig. 16.11). According to the Histiocyte Society the definitive diagnosis of Langerhans cell histiocytosis is based on the demonstration of Birbeck granules by electron microscopy or positivity for CD1 antigen.[15] The examination of conventionally stained material gives a presumptive diagnosis. The cytological features of Langerhans cell histiocytosis has been recorded in several series.[16–18]

The soft tissue deposits of generalised Langerhans cell histiocytosis (Letterer-Siwe disease) generally consist of a more pure population of abnormal histiocytes and have a less inflammatory appearance.

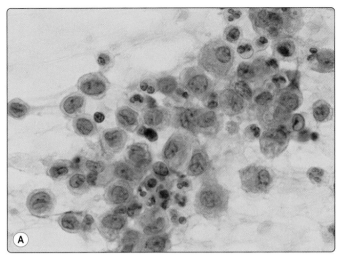

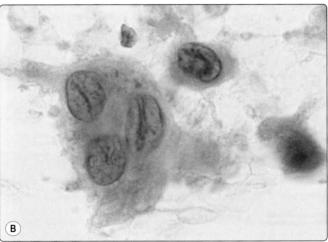

Fig. 16.10 Langerhans cell histiocytosis (eosinophilic granuloma) (A) Lytic bone lesion, many histiocytes with irregular reniform pale nuclei, some eosinophils (H&E, IP); (B) Coffee-bean nuclei have been reported to be typical of this lesion (H&E, HP, Oil)

Vascular lesions

Fine needle biopsy of hemangioma is often like a venepuncture – only blood is aspirated. Sometimes strands of endothelial cells with spindled, bland nuclei may be found in smears, and there may be some hemosiderin-containing macrophages, osteoblasts and fibroblasts.

Primary benign tumors of bone

Giant cell tumor of bone

CRITERIA FOR DIAGNOSIS

◆ Abundant material,
◆ A double cell population: mononuclear spindle cells and giant cells of osteoclastic type,
◆ Giant cells are attached to the periphery of the clustered spindle cells.

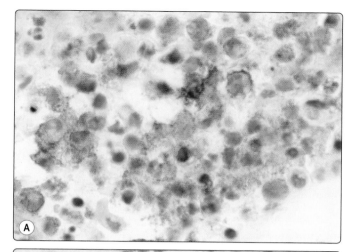

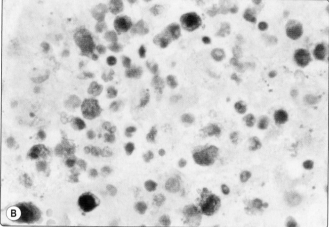

Fig. 16.11 Langerhans cell histiocytosis (eosinophilic granuloma) The Langerhans cell histiocytes express (**A**) S-100 protein and (**B**) CD1-antigen (Cell block, immunoperoxidase).

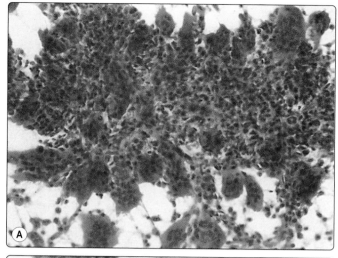

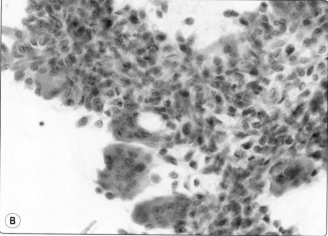

Fig. 16.12 Giant cell tumor of bone (A) Tissue fragment of cohesive plump spindle or ovoid cells; giant cells located peripherally (H&E, IP). (B) The nuclei vary moderately in size and shape, the chromatin is bland and nucleoli small (H&E, IP).

The giant cells have numerous (about 20–50) uniform nuclei. The spindle cells are mainly cohesive but single cells are always seen. The giant cells are typically attached to the periphery of clusters of spindle cells (Fig. 16.12A). Strands of collagen or basement membrane material, and endothelial cells are discernible in cell clusters and tissue fragments. The cells have a moderate amount of dense, amphophilic cytoplasm, which is often vacuolated, and well-defined borders. The nuclei vary only moderately in size and shape. They are ovoid, the chromatin is bland and nucleoli small (Fig. 16.12B). Malignancy (giant cell-rich osteosarcoma) should be suspected if spindled and multinucleated cells show nuclear pleomorphism and irregular chromatin, and if mitoses are plentiful. The differential diagnosis of other benign bone lesions with many osteoclastic giant cells such as aneurysmal bone cyst, osteoblastoma, brown tumor of hyperparathyroidism and reparative granuloma of jaw and small bones is difficult. Detailed knowledge of clinical and radiological findings is essential for a correct evaluation. The cytological appearance of giant cell tumor is recorded in a total of 38 cases in three series.[3,19,20]

Chondroma

CRITERIA FOR DIAGNOSIS

◆ Predominantly cartilaginous tissue fragments,
◆ Cells in lacunar spaces,
◆ Abundant chondromyxoid ground substance,
◆ Relatively uniform tumor cells (except chondromas of hands and feet).

Single cells are uncommon in smears from chondroma. The chondromyxoid ground substance is usually abundant and very conspicuous in MGG (Fig. 16.13A). It has a finely fibrillar texture. It is less obvious in wet-fixed smears where it is seen as a hyaline, pale violet material with H&E (Fig. 16.13B), and even paler with Pap. The morphology of the tumor cells is best studied in wet-fixed smears, as the cells are obscured by the intensely stained ground substance in MGG smears. The cellularity of the fragments is generally low and the tumor cells are uniform and rounded with a well-defined

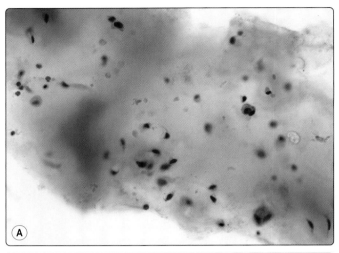

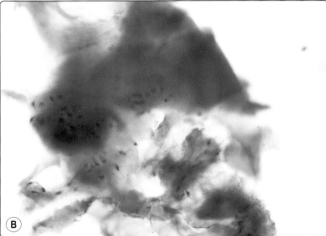

Fig. 16.13 Chondroma (A) Widely separated chondrocytes with small nuclei; The chondromyxoid ground substance is usually abundant and very conspicuous in MGG; (B) Chondroid background substance in wet-fixed smears appears as a hyaline, pale violet material in H&E (A, MGG, IP; B, H&E, IP).

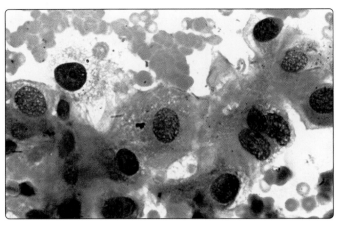

Fig. 16.14 Chondroblastoma A cluster of chondroblast-like cells embedded in a chondromyxoid matrix (MGG, HP oil)

cytoplasm, rounded nuclei and one or two nucleoli. Binucleate cells are almost never seen. Chondromas of the small peripheral bones, however, often show marked pleomorphism and binucleated cells (Fig. 16.14).

As can be expected from histopathological experience, it can be difficult or impossible in FNB smears to distinguish between chondroma and low-grade (grade 1) malignant chondrosarcoma. The combined evaluation of clinical data, radiological findings and cytology is emphasised. The cytology of chondroma has been reported in a few publications[21,22].

Chondroblastoma

CRITERIA FOR DIAGNOSIS

◆ Fragments of chondroid matrix,
◆ Multinucleated osteoclast-like cells,
◆ Mononuclear, rounded cells with distinct cell borders and rounded nuclei (chondroblasts).

Chondroblastoma is a rare tumor, and most cases are found in children and adolescents. The cytology has been investigated in four series.[21–25] Our experience is limited to a few cases. The double cell population and the fragments of chondroid material are the clues to the diagnosis. According to the series of 12 cases described by Fanning et al.,[23] the cells resembling chondroblasts are typical. They are mononuclear and rounded with well-demarcated cytoplasm and rounded lobulated or reniform nuclei. Nuclei are centrally located, showing slight anisokaryosis. One feature often described is longitudinal grooves in nuclei. The chondroblast-like nuclei are either single or embedded in the chondroid fragments (Fig. 16.15).

Chondromyxoid fibroma

CRITERIA FOR DIAGNOSIS

◆ Myxoid background substance,
◆ Chondroid fragments,
◆ Spindle-shaped or stellate, fibroblast-like cells, single or in clusters.

Few cases of FNB of chondromyxoid fibroma have been reported.[21,26,27] We have experience of a few tumors. Smears show a mixture of chondroid fragments, fibroblast-like spindled or stellate cells and osteoclast-like giant cells embedded in myxoid material (Fig. 16.16A). Rounded chondroblast-like cells in lacunar spaces may be seen in the chondroid fragments. The spindle-shaped cells may show some nuclear pleomorphism (Fig. 16.16B) and prominent nucleoli, and binucleated chondroblasts are not uncommon. Chondromyxoid fibroma has been misdiagnosed as chondrosarcoma.

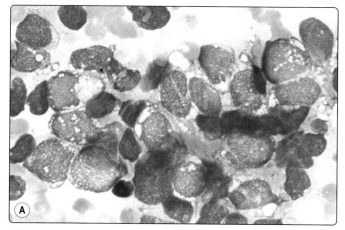

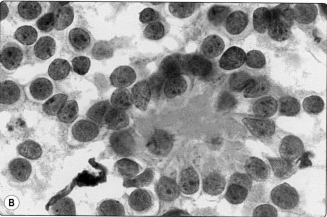

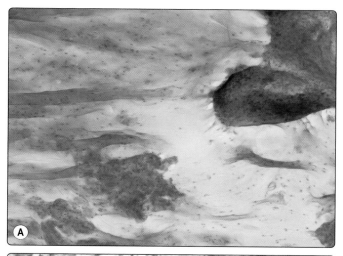

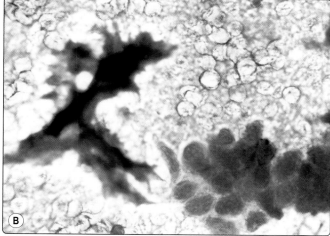

Fig. 16.15 Ewing's sarcoma (A) A mixture of cells with larger pale-staining nuclei and cells with smaller and darker nuclei; note the cytoplasmic vacuoles and clear spaces in the pale cells (MGG, HP oil); (B) Rosette-like structure; nuclear chromatin and nucleoli more clearly seen than in MGG (H&E, HP oil).

Fig. 16.16 Chondromyxoid fibroma (A) Smears show a mixture of chondroid fragments, fibroblast-like spindle or stellate cells and osteoclast-like giant cells embedded in myxoid matrix (MGG, LP); (B) Both spindle-shaped and chondroblast-like cells may show slight nuclear pleomorphism (MGG, HP).

Osteoblastoma

CRITERIA FOR DIAGNOSIS

◆ Osteoblast-like cells, singly or in groups or rows,
◆ Multinucleated osteoclast-like cells,
◆ Clusters of spindle cells.

Only a few cases of osteoblastoma with cytology have been published.[21,28] Our experience is restricted to a few cases. A mixed cell population has been recorded; the majority of cells resemble osteoblasts with eccentric nuclei and a cytoplasmic 'Hof'. A moderate anisokaryosis and the presence of binucleated cells is not uncommon. A blue–red or pink (MGG) background matrix was seen between the cells in cell groups (Fig. 16.17A). Osteoclast-like giant cells and a few groups of spindle cells with fusiform nuclei were present in all cases recorded (Fig. 16.17B). The differential diagnosis is osteosarcoma versus aggressive (epithelioid) osteoblast-oma,[29] a rare variant not defined in FNB material.

Primary malignant tumors of bone

Osteosarcoma (conventional intramedullary osteosarcoma)

CRITERIA FOR DIAGNOSIS

◆ Pleomorphic spindle and rounded cells,
◆ Tumor cells, more or less resembling osteoblasts,
◆ Multinucleated tumor cells,
◆ Mitotic figures (often atypical),
◆ Clumps of amorphous, faintly eosinophilic (H&E) or red–pink (MGG) material in the background or between cells in clusters (osteoid),
◆ Intensely cytoplasmic positive alkaline phosphatase staining of tumor cells.

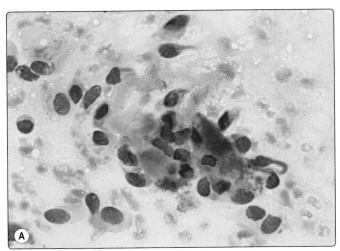

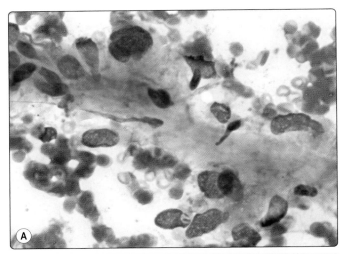

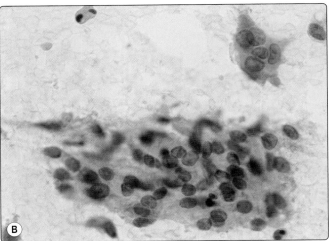

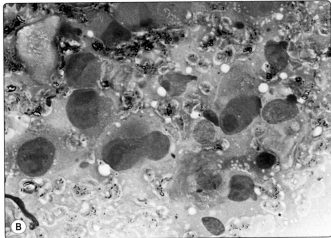

Fig. 16.17 Osteoblastoma (A) A blue–red or pink (MGG) background matrix was seen between the cells in cell groups. (MGG, HP); (B) Osteoclast-like giant cells and a few groups of spindle cells with fusiform nuclei were present in all cases recorded (H&E, HP).

The experience of FNB of osteosarcoma is mainly related to the conventional, high-grade intramedullary osteosarcoma (the most common type) and to the rare high-grade surface osteosarcoma. The rare periosteal osteosarcoma has not been characterised and, due to the often prominent bone formation, this osteosarcoma variant is not suitable for FNB.

The criteria listed above apply to the osteoblastic type. Smears contain both dissociated neoplastic cells and cell clusters. Osteoid is seen as faintly eosinophilic clumps in H&E, bright red or pink in MGG, amorphous or finely fibrillar material in the background (infrequent) or as thin intercellular strand within cell clusters (Fig. 16.18A). Macronucleoli may be present (Fig. 16.18B) and malignant giant cells with pleomorphic nuclei are commonly seen (Fig. 16.18C). Benign osteoclast-like giant cells may be present, especially in giant cell-rich osteosarcoma.

The chondroblastic osteosarcoma may be difficult to distinguish from a high-grade malignant chondrosarcoma (Fig. 16.19) and in the fibroblastic osteosarcoma; cellular pleomorphism is less marked in the spindle-shaped tumor cells (Fig. 16.20). Osteoid between tumor cells is uncommon.

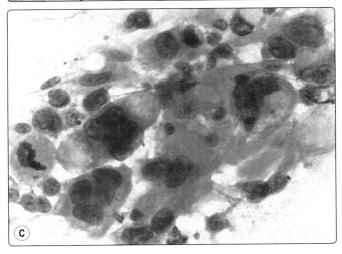

Fig. 16.18 Osteosarcoma (A) Small cluster of pleomorphic sarcoma cells; strands of intercellular pink material consistent with osteoid (MGG, HP); (B) Malignant cells with macronucleoli are commonly seen in smears from high-grade osteosarcoma (MGG, HP); (C) Loose cluster of pleomorphic, often multinucleate cells; the fragments of pink amorphous material may represent osteoid; note mitotic figure (H&E, HP).

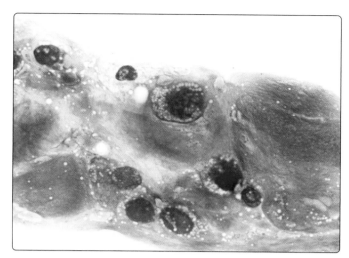

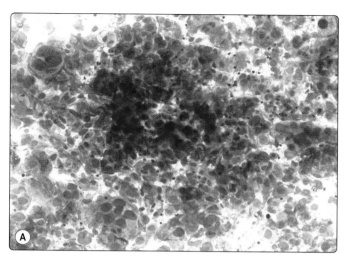

Fig. 16.19 Osteosarcoma (chondroblastic) Malignant cells embedded in the abundant chondroid matrix may be difficult to distinguish from a high-grade malignant chondrosarcoma (MGG, HP).

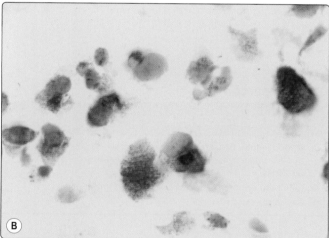

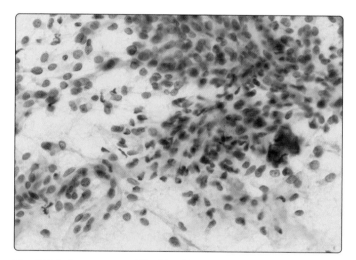

Fig. 16.20 Osteosarcoma (fibroblastic) Smears from a patient with known Paget's disease who developed a large mass in the left hip region with extensive bone destruction; moderately pleomorphic spindle cell sarcoma without distinctive features (H&E, IP).

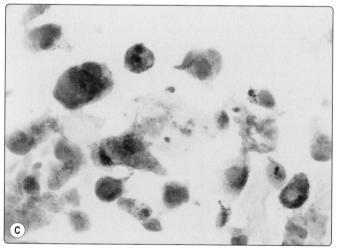

The tumor cell population in the rare small cell osteosarcoma resembles cells of conventional (classic) Ewing's sarcoma. In another rare variant, parosteal osteosarcoma, the smears are dominated by fragment of hyaline cartilage and moderately atypical, spindly cells.

The presence of cytoplasmic alkaline phosphatase (present in all variants of osteosarcoma) is an important feature in the differential diagnosis (metastatic anaplastic carcinoma, melanoma and anaplastic large cell lymphoma), as is the expression of osteonectin or/and osteocalcin in osteosarcoma cells (Fig. 16.21) The vast majority of conventional intramedullary high-grade osteosarcoma are non-diploid, and this feature is an important diagnostic sign in the distinction from lesions featuring reactive osteoblasts, e.g. fracture callus, reactive periosteitis and pseudomalignant myositis ossificans. The cytology of osteosarcoma in FNB smears has been investigated in several large series[30,31,32,33].

Fig. 16.21 Osteosarcoma (A) Strong positive cytoplasmic staining for alkaline phosphatase and expression of (B) osteonectin or/and (C) osteocalcin in tumor cells are important features of osteosarcoma in the differential diagnosis (metastatic anaplastic carcinoma, melanoma and anaplastic large cell lymphoma) (A, alkaline phosphatase staining, HP; B, osteonectin, immunoperoxidase; C, osteocalcin, immunoperoxidase).

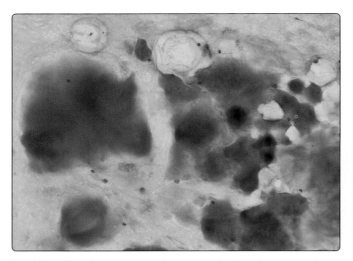

Fig. 16.22 Chondrosarcoma, well differentiated The chondromyxoid ground substance is usually as abundant in low-grade tumors, as in chondroma (MGG, IP).

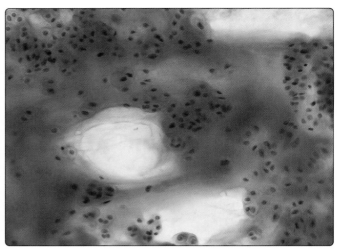

Fig. 16.23 Chondrosarcoma, well differentiated A rich yield with plenty of tissue fragments demonstrating the variable cell content makes the diagnosis easier (MGG, IP).

Chondrosarcoma

CRITERIA FOR DIAGNOSIS

◆ Predominantly tissue fragments in low-grade (grades 1 and 2) tumors, single cells may dominate in high-grade (grade 3) sarcomas,
◆ Abundant eosinophilic, vacuolated cytoplasm,
◆ Chondromyxoid material.

The chondromyxoid ground substance is usually as abundant in low-grade tumors as in chondroma (Fig. 16.22). The neoplastic cells are best studied in wet-fixed preparations. Cellularity is variable in low-grade chondrosarcoma. This is important in the distinction from chordoma. A rich yield with plenty of tissue fragments demonstrating the variable cell content makes the diagnosis easier (Fig. 16.23). The tumor cells have a well-defined cytoplasm and rounded nuclei with one or two nucleoli. Binucleate cells are present and nuclear pleomorphism is of moderate degree (Fig. 16.24).

Single cells dominate in high-grade malignant tumors, cellular and nuclear pleomorphism is prominent and mitoses are present. Often abundant myxoid background matrix is present, while fragments of hyaline cartilage are few. As stated above, it is difficult or impossible to distinguish between chondroma and some low-grade (grade 1) chondrosarcomas in FNB smears. Grade 3 chondrosarcomas may be difficult to distinguish from chondroblastic osteosarcoma and from metastatic poorly differentiated epithelial tumors if cartilaginous fragments are absent. Chordoma should be considered in the differential diagnosis in spinal or sacral tumors (see below). Dedifferentiated chondrosarcoma is yet another pitfall. This distinct variant has two components: a low-grade chondrosarcoma (or chondroma) and a high-grade sarcoma which is not a grade 3 chondrosarcoma. The clue to the cytological diagnosis is the presence of a low-grade cartilaginous tumor and a high-grade sarcoma (most often pleomorphic sarcoma of MFH type or rarely osteosarcoma or

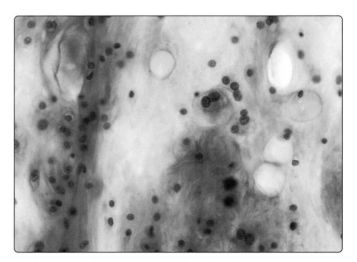

Fig. 16.24 Chondrosarcoma, well differentiated Increased number of cells with moderately enlarged and irregular nuclei; some binucleate forms (MGG, HP).

rhabdomyosarcoma) in the same sample (Fig. 16.25). Inadequate sampling may result in misinterpretation.[34]

Two rare chondrosarcoma subtypes, clear-cell chondrosarcoma and mesenchymal chondrosarcoma are occasionally the target for FNB. The typical tumor cell in clear cell chondrosarcoma, a low-grade tumor, is rather large with a clear or vacuolated abundant cytoplasm and a central or paracentral nucleus. The cells are seen singly or in small groups in a myxoid background matrix (Fig. 16.26). A few cases of clear cell chondrosarcoma have been described.[21] FNB smears of mesenchymal chondrosarcoma are composed of small tumor cells with rounded or ovoid nuclei and a sparse cytoplasm. The cells are often embedded in a myxoid matrix (red–violett in MGG) (Fig. 16.27). The most important differential diagnoses are other small cell malignant tumors such as small cell osteosarcoma and conventional Ewing's sarcoma. Single reports of the cytology of mesenchymal chondrosarcoma in FNB have been published.[21]

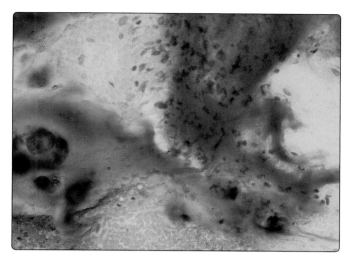

Fig. 16.25 Chondrosarcoma, dedifferentiated The clue to the cytological diagnosis is the presence of a low-grade cartilaginous tumor and a high-grade sarcoma (MGG, IP).

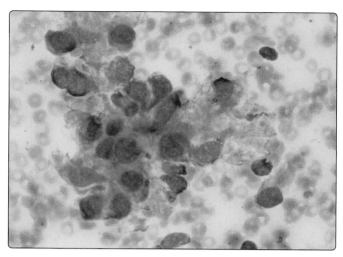

Fig. 16.27 Mesenchymal chondrosarcoma The small tumor cells with rounded or ovoid nuclei and a sparse cytoplasm are often embedded in a red–violet matrix (MGG, HP).

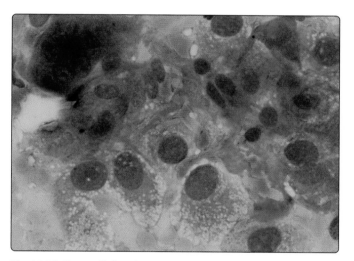

Fig. 16.26 Clear-cell chondrosarcoma Rather large cells with a clear or vacuolated abundant cytoplasm and a central or paracentral nucleus (MGG, HP).

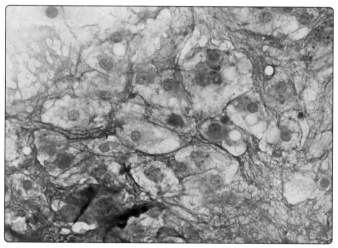

Fig. 16.28 Chordoma A network of intensely purple myxoid material encircles individual tumor cells with abundant pale bubbly cytoplasm (MGG, HP).

DNA image ploidy analysis is a valuable adjunct in the diagnosis; a non-diploid histogram is a sign of a high-grade tumor, irrespective of yield. The cytological findings in smears of chondrosarcoma have been described in several series.[3,21,35,36]

Chordoma

CRITERIA FOR DIAGNOSIS

◆ Abundant myxoid ground substance encircling tumor cells,
◆ Large cells with abundant bubbly cytoplasm (physaliphorous cells),
◆ Cluster of medium-sized epithelial-like cells,
◆ Rounded nuclei, moderate anisokaryosis, bland chromatin,
◆ Pleomorphic tumor cells with prominent nucleoli present in some tumors.

The characteristic findings are the abundant background of myxoid ground substance and the large, physaliphorous cells with abundant pale, vacuolated, bubbly cytoplasm and well-defined cell borders. The myxoid matrix, often fibrillar, intensely purple in MGG smears, pale pink in H&E, forms a network encircling individual tumor cells, cell clusters or fragments (Fig. 16.28). The physaliphorous cells have one, sometimes two, rounded nuclei of moderate size, a bland chromatin and small nucleoli. Moderate anisokaryosis is common (Fig. 16.29A). Some tumors show clusters of markedly pleomorphic cells with prominent nucleoli, and multinucleated tumor giant cells may be present (Fig. 16.29B). There are also clusters of small to medium-sized, non-characteristic or epithelial-like cells with rounded nuclei. The cytoplasm of these cells may be vacuolated; some cells have one large vacuole pushing the nucleus to the periphery and may resemble signet ring cells (Fig. 16.30A). The main differential diagnosis is chondrosarcoma. If only wet-fixed

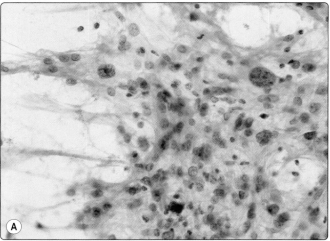

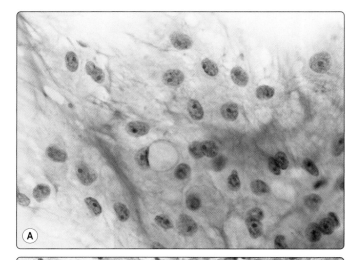

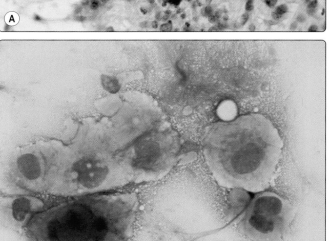

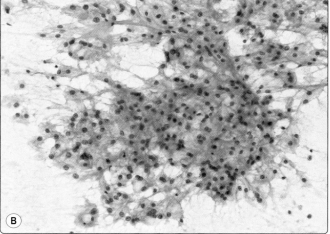

Fig. 16.29 Chordoma (A) Moderate anisokaryosis is a common feature of smears from chordoma (H&E, IP); (B) Markedly pleomorphic cells with prominent nucleoli, and multinucleated tumor giant cells may be present (MGG, HP).

Fig. 16.30 Chordoma (A) Some cells in chordomas may have one large vacuole pushing the nucleus to the periphery and may resemble signet ring cells (H&E, IP); (B) In H&E or Pap smears the epithelial-like tumor cells may give a false impression of an epithelial neoplasm (H&E, LP).

smears are available, metastatic clear cell carcinoma, especially renal cell carcinoma or mucus-producing adenocarcinoma can also cause differential diagnostic difficulties. The abundant ground substance may be inconspicuous in H&E or Pap smears and the epithelial-like tumor cells may give a false impression of an epithelial neoplasm (Fig. 16.30B). Typical physaliphorous cells are never encountered in chondrosarcoma and the network of myxoid matrix encircling individual cells is not a feature of either chondrosarcoma or metastatic carcinoma. A chordoma originating in the cervical spine does not always present as a midline tumor and, if information on the radiologic finding is not available, may be interpreted as a malignant myxoid soft tissue tumor. Chordomas typically express S-100 protein and low molecular weight cytokeratins. The cytological appearance of chordoma in FNB has been evaluated in rather large series.[37–39]

Ewing's family tumors

Several studies by various investigators have provided evidence that conventional Ewing's sarcoma (ES), atypical Ewing's sarcoma, the so called Askin tumor, neuroepithelioma and primitive neuroectodermal tumor (PNET) belong to the same family of neuroectodermal tumors.[40] All tumors in this family share the same cytogenetic aberration, t(11;22) (q24;q12), resulting in the EWS/FLI-1 transcript. Furthermore, they express the same phenotype, CD99 (the antibody to the MIC2 gene) and FLI-1. The different variants have a variable morphology and variable expression of neuroectodermal markers.

CRITERIA FOR DIAGNOSIS (CONVENTIONAL EWING'S SARCOMA)

◆ Dissociated cells and clusters of loosely cohesive cells,
◆ Two cell types: large pale cells with abundant cytoplasm with a clear space or vacuolated and small dark cells with scanty cytoplasm,
◆ Rounded or irregular bland nuclei; small nucleoli,
◆ Stripped nuclei with a cytoplasmic background matrix,
◆ Abundant cytoplasmic glycogen,
◆ Occasionally rosette-like structures.

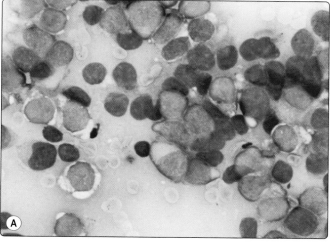

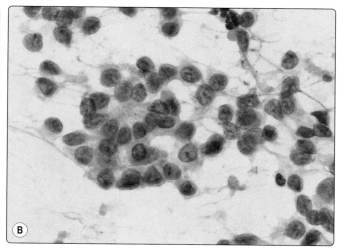

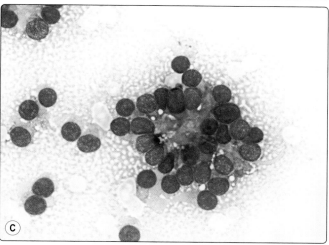

Fig. 16.31 Ewing's sarcoma (A) A mixture of cells with larger pale-staining nuclei and cells with smaller and darker nuclei; note the cytoplasmic vacuoles and clear spaces in the pale cells (MGG, HP); (B,C) Rosette-like structure; nuclear chromatin and nucleoli more clearly seen in H&E than in MGG (A, H&E, HP; B, MGG, HP).

The cytological appearance of conventional ES is distinctive. Smears are generally highly cellular and are composed of both single cells and groups of loosely cohesive cells. The cells are fragile and naked nuclei as well as a faint gray–blue (MGG) background of detached cytoplasm are commonly seen. There is a characteristic mixture of two types of cells. One has abundant pale cytoplasm with vacuoles or large clear spaces, rounded or ovoid nuclei with finely granular chromatin and 1–3 small nucleoli ('large light cells'). The other has scanty cytoplasm and irregular nuclei with dense chromatin ('small dark cells'). The two types of cells are most clearly distinguished within groups or clusters of cells, the small dark cells are interspersed, often as small molded groups, between large light cells (Fig. 16.31A). Rosette-like structures without a fibrillar center are occasionally present (Fig. 16.31B,C). The cytoplasmic vacuoles or clear spaces correspond to large deposits of glycogen (Fig. 16.31A).

In atypical ES and PNET the cellular and nuclear atypia is more marked than in conventional ES. Rosette-like structures are more common and the distinction between large light and small dark cells less obvious, especially in PNET, and cells with thin cytoplasmic processes as well as rhabdomyoblast-like cells are present (Fig. 16.32).

Distinction from other malignant small cell tumors such as alveolar rhabdomyosarcoma, primitive neuroblastoma, precursor B- and T-cell lymphoma are important differential diagnoses and is relatively easy in typical cases of conventional ES.

In the precursor lymphomas, nuclei generally are of variable size with irregular or folded contours and the cytoplasm is narrow and pale without vacuoles, but often demonstrates a small clear spot close to the nucleus. The rhabdomyoblast-like cells in alveolar rhabdomyosarcoma are rather distinctive with eccentric nuclei and a dense eosinophilic cytoplasm on wet-fixed smears. The long, thin cytoplasmic processes, often connecting cells, in neuroblastoma are not a feature of conventional ES. However, the differential diagnosis between atypical ES and PNET and poorly differentiated Ewing's sarcoma-like synovial sarcoma and the above mentioned tumors is much more difficult in routinely stained smears. Cytogenetic analysis is the most valuable diagnostic adjunct.[41,42] Immunocytochemistry, including CD99 and FLI-1 are also of value in spite of the fact that both these antibodies are reported to be positive in other malignant small cell tumors (Fig.16.33).

The cytology of Ewing's family tumors in FNB smears has been thoroughly investigated in several series.[43–47]

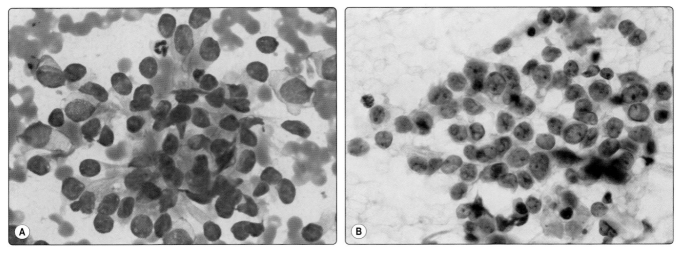

Fig. 16.32 ES/PNET family of tumors Distinction between large light and small dark cells less obvious in PNET than in conventional Ewing's, and cells with thin cytoplasmic processes (**A**) and rhabdomyoblast-like cells (**B**) are present (**A**, MGG, HP; **B**, H&E, HP).

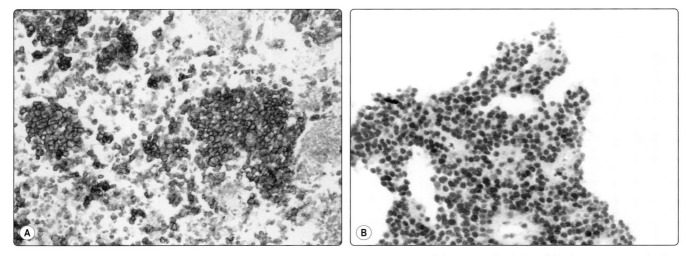

Fig. 16.33 ES/PNET family of tumors Immunocytochemistry, mainly (**A**) CD99 and (**B**) FLI-1 are of diagnostic value (**A**, **B**, cell block, immunoperoxidase).

References

1. Coley BL, Sharp GS, Ellis EB. Diagnosis of bone tumours by aspiration. Am J Surg 1931;13:214–24.
2. Ahlström KH, Åström KC. CT guided bone biopsy performed by means of a coaxial biopsy system with an eccentric drill. Radiology 1993;188:549–52.
3. Åkerman M, Domanski HA. Fine needle aspiration (FNA) of bone tumors with special emphasis on the definitive treatment of primary malignant tumors based on FNA. Curr Diagn Pathol 1998;5:82–92.
4. Layfield LJ. Cytologic diagnosis of osseous lesions: a review with emphasis on the diagnosis of primary neoplasms of bone. Diagn Cytopathol 2009;37:299–310.
5. Åkerman M, Domanski HA, Jonsson K. Fine needle aspiration of bone tumours.

Monographs in Clinical Cytology. vol 19. Basel: Kargel; 2010.
6. Kreicbergs A, Bauer HCF, Brosjö O, et al. Cytological diagnosis of bone tumours. J Bone Joint Surg (Br) 1996;78B:258–63.
7. Bommer K, Ramzay I, Mody D. Fine-needle aspiration biopsy in the diagnosis and management of bone lesions. Cancer (Cancer Cytopathol) 1997;81:148–56.
8. Söderlund V, Skoog L, Kreicbergs A. Combined radiology and cytology in the diagnosis of bone lesions: a retrospective study of 370 cases. Acta Orthop Scand 2004;75:492–9.
9. Wahane RN, Lele VR, Bobhate SK. Fine needle aspiration cytology of bone tumors. Acta Cytol 2007;51:711–20.
10. McLaughlin RE, Miller WR, Miller CW. Quadriparesis after needle aspiration of

the cervical spine. J Bone Joint Surg 1976;1167–8.
11. Saad RS, Clary KM, Silverman JF, et al. Fine needle aspiration biopsy of vertebral lesions. Acta Cytol 2004;48:39–46.
12. Akthar I, Flowers R, Siddiqi A, et al. Fine needle aspiration biopsy of vertebral and paravertebral lesions: retrospective study of 124 cases. Acta Cytol 2006;364–71.
13. Söderlund V, Skoog L, Tani E, et al. Diagnosis of skeletal lymphoma and myeloma by radiology and fine-needle aspiration cytology. Cytopathology 2001;12:157–67.
14. Lin F, Staerkel G, Fanning CV. Cytrodiagnosis of primary lymphoma of bone on fine-needle aspiration cytology specimens:review of 25 cases. Diagn Cytopathol 2003;28:205–11.

15. Malone M. The histiocytoses childhood. Histopathol 1991;19:105–19.

16. Shabb N, Fanning CV, Carrasco C. Diagnosis of eosinophilic granuloma by fine needle aspiration with concurrent institution of therapy. Diagn Cytopathol 1993;9:3–12.

17. Pohar-Marinsek Z, Us-Krasovec M. Cytomorphology of Langerhans cell histiocytosis. Acta Cytol 1996;40:1257–64.

18. Kilpatrick SE. Fine needle aspiration biopsy of Langerhans cell histiocytosis: are ancillary studies necessary for a definitive diagnosis? Acta Cytol 1998;42:820–3.

19. Sneige N, Ayala A, Carrasco H, et al. Giant cell tumour of bone. A cytologic study of 24 cases. Diagn Cytopathol 1985;1:111–7.

20. Vetrani A, Fulciniti F, Boschi R, et al. Fine needle aspiration biopsy of giant cell tumour of bone. Acta Cytol 1990;34:863–7.

21. Waalas l, Kindblom L-G, Gunterberg B, et al. Light and electro-microscopic examination of fine needle aspiration in the preoperative diagnosis of cartiginous tumours. Diagn Cytopathol 1990;6:396–408.

22. Dhawan SB, Aggarwal R, Mohan H, et al. Cytodiagnosis of enchondroma. Cytopathology 2003;14:157–9.

23. Fanning CV, Sneige NS, Carrasco CH, et al. Fine needle aspiration's cytology of chondroblastoma of bone. Cancer 1990;65:1847–63.

24. Pohar-Marinsek Z, Us-Krasovec M, Lamovee J. Chondroblastoma in fine needle aspirates. Acta Cytol 1992;36:367–70.

25. Kilpatrick SE, Pike EJ, Geisinger KR, et al. Chondroblastoma of bone: use of fine-needle aspiration biopsy and potential diagnostic pitfalls. Diagn Cytopathol 1997;16:65–71.

26. Layfield LJ, Ferreiro JA. Fine-needle aspiration cytology of chondromyxoid fibroma: a case report. Diagn Cytopathol 1988;4:148–51.

27. Gupta S, Dev G, Marya S. Chondromyxoid fibroma: a fine-needle aspiration diagnosis. Diagn Cytopathol 1993;9:63–5.

28. Rhode MG, Lucas DR, Krueger CH, et al. Fine-needle aspiration of spinal osteoblastoma in a patient with lymfangiomatosis. Diagn Cytopathol 2006;34:295–7.

29. Bertoni F, Bacchini P, Donati D, et al. Osteoblastoma-like osteosarcoma. The Rizzoli Institute experience. Mod Pathol 1993;6:707–16.

30. White WA, Fanning CV, Ayala AG, et al. Osteosarcoma and the role of fine-needle aspiration: a study of 51 cases. Cancer 1988;62:1238–46.

31. Dodd LG, Scully SR, Cothran RL, et al. Utility of fine-needle aspiration in the diagnosis of primary osteosarcoma. Diagn Cytopathol 2002;27:350–3.

32. Domanski HA, Åkerman M. Fine-needle aspiration of primary osteosarcoma: a cytological-histological study. Diagn Cytopathol 2005;32:269–75.

33. Klijanienko J, Caillaud J-M, Orbach D, et al. Cyto-histological correlations in primary, recurrent and metastatic bone and soft tissue osteosarcoma. Diagn Cytopathol 2007;35:270–5.

34. Rinas AC, Ward WG, Kilpatrick SE. Potential sampling error in fine needle aspiration biopsy of dedifferentiated chondrosarcoma: a report of 4 cases. Acta Cytol 2005;49:554–9.

35. Lerma E, Tani E, Brosjö O, et al. Diagnosis and grading of chondrosarcoma on FNB biopsy material. Diagn Cytopathol 2003;28:13–7.

36. Dodd LG. Fine needle aspiration of chondrosarcoma. Diagn Cytopathol 2006;34:413–8.

37. Finley JL, Silverman JF, Dabbs DJ, et al. Chordoma. Diagnosis by fine-needle aspiration with histologic, immunocytochemical, and ultrastructural confirmation. Diagn Cytopathol 1998;2:330–7.

38. Crapanzano JP, Ali SZ, Ginsberg MS, et al. Chordoma: a cytologic study with histologic and radiologic correlation. Cancer 2001;93:40–51.

39. Kay PA, Nasciemento AG, Unni KK, et al. Chordoma: cytomorphologic findings in 14 cases diagnosed by fine needle aspiration. Acta Cytol 2003;47:202–8.

40. Delattre O, Zuchman J, Melot T, et al. The Ewing family of tumours: a subgroup of small-round cell tumors defined by specific chimeric transcripts. N Engl Med J 1994;331:294–9.

41. Fröstad B. Fine needle aspiration cytology in diagnosis and management of childhood small round cell tumours. Thesis: Stockholm; 2000.

42. Udaykumar AM, Sundareshan TS, Goud TM, et al. Cytogenetic characterisation of Ewing tumors using fine needle aspiration samples, a 10-year experience and review of the literature. Cancer Genet Cytogenet 2001;127:42–8.

43. Dahl I, Åkerman M, Angervall L. Ewing's sarcoma of bone. A correlative cytological and histological study of 14 cases. Acta Pathol Microbiol Immunol Scand (A) 1986;94:363–9.

44. Silverman JS, Berns LA, Holbrook CT, et al. Fine needle aspiration cytology of primitive neuroectodermal tumors: a report of these cases. Acta Cytol 1992;36:541–50.

45. Renshaw AA, Pares-Atayde AR, Fletcher JA, et al. Cytology of typical and atypical Ewing's sarcoma/PNET. Am J Surg Pathol 1996;106:620–4.

46. Mondal A, Misra DK. Ewing's sarcoma of bone: a study of 71 cases by fine needle aspiration cytology. J Indian Med Ass 1996;94:135–7.

47. Sahu K, Pai RR, Khadikar UN. Fine needle aspiration cytology of the Ewing's sarcoma family of tumors. Acta Cytol 2000;44:332–6.

CHAPTER 17

Paediatric tumors

Reda S Saad, Harsharan K Singh and Jan F Silverman

CLINICAL ASPECTS

Incidence of paediatric tumors and histologic types

Paediatric tumors show a distinctive incidence, histology, and biologic behavior from those in adults. In addition, fetal and neonatal malignancies tend to differentiate or regress spontaneously, leading to high survival and curability rates.[1] In the United States, only 2% of patients with a malignancy are in the paediatric age group, with almost 9000 children under the age of 15 presenting with a malignancy each year.[2] Even with improved overall 5-year survival from 27% in 1960 to over 70% in the 1990s, cancer still remains a leading cause of childhood mortality. The type of malignancy varies considerably within age groups. In children younger than 5 years, acute lymphoblastic leukemia is the most frequent and most lethal cancer.[3] The most common solid tumours of childhood are primary posterior fossa brain tumors and teratoma, followed by neuroblastoma and soft tissue sarcomas. Osteosarcoma is the most common primary bone tumor followed by Ewing's sarcoma.

Diagnostic accuracy of FNA cytology

Fine needle aspiration biopsy (FNAB) has many advantages in the diagnosis of paediatric tumors, especially the ease of performance and repeatability with no essentially morbidity or risk of tumor upstaging.[4–6] Centers experienced in performing paediatric FNAB have shown excellent results with sensitivity and specificity rates approaching 93% and 100%, respectively, comparable to those in the adult population.[5–21] The availability and applicability of diagnostic ancillary techniques such as histochemistry, immunocytochemistry, electron microscopy, flow cytometry, cytogenetics, and molecular analysis to the cytology smears often enable the pathologist to give a definitive diagnosis.

FNAB of paediatric mass lesions has been slow in gaining popularity compared with its utilization in adult patients.[5–21] Many pathologists and clinicians are hesitant to employ fine needle aspiration (FNA) as a diagnostic method in children for a variety of reasons, including rarity of paediatric tumors with different morphology from those of adults, lack of experience of general pathologist with such tumors, morphological overlap between different tumor types, lack of specific immunocytochemical markers and unrepresentative samples as a result of degenerative changes or tumors with heterologous components such as hepatoblastoma or Wilms' tumor. These lead to difficulties in interpretation of FNA of paediatric tumors.[1,22] There is a recent decline in the number of aspirates from patients with a history of cancer as a result of recent advances of image techniques to document recurrence and relapses.[23]

Obtaining and handling of specimens

The procurement and preparation of specimens from paediatric FNA is no different from that in adults. However, children may not be as cooperative as adults and require sedation in radiographically guided FNA of deep-seated masses. For superficial masses, aspiration without local anesthesia is usually well tolerated with proper immobilization of the child. Multiple passes can be obtained in most cases. To avoid repeating the FNA, it is important to immediately assess the sample sufficiency. An on-site pathologist, preferably performing the aspiration procedure, can evaluate each pass for adequacy by use of a Romanowsky staining method (Wright-Giemsa or Diff-Quik®), and for triage of material for appropriate ancillary tests such as immunocytochemistry (cell-block preparation), cytogenetics, and electron microscopy.

Some centers, such as ours, have been using FNA as the first diagnostic modality in the work-up of mass lesions (superficial and deep seated) in children for providing rapid diagnostic results, thereby aiding in proper triage and management of the patient.[20,24–26] Intraoperative cytology (IOC) can be useful in cases with limited tissue available, leading to a rapid assessment of the nature of the lesion, thereby, optimizing triage of tissue for the most appropriate ancillary studies (cultures, cell blocks, cytogenetics, flow cytometry, etc.). This allows for preservation of tissue for permanent section examination, especially in HIV-positive patients (avoiding cryostat contamination), or tissue prone to

DOI: 10.1016/B978-0-7020-3151-9.00017-7

difficulties in cutting at the time of frozen section such as bony fragments and fatty specimens.

We use both the Papanicolaou and Romanowsky stains since the two are complimentary. Nuclear features such as chromatin distribution and granularity are better evaluated on the Papanicolaou stain, while the Romanowsky stain is superior for evaluation of lymphoreticular lesions (benign and malignant). Lesions with stromal and matrix components are also more easily discernible by Romanowsky staining, such as the bright magenta color of neuropil in the case of neuroblastoma. For immunocytochemistry, a cell block preparation works best. However, direct smears and cytospins can also be used.[26]

Radiographic imaging

Image-guided FNA biopsy of deep-seated masses is a well established diagnostic modality in adults and is now used more widely in the paediatric population. The modality of choice is dependent on the site of the lesion as well as the clinical impression. For most abdominal and pelvic masses, ultrasound is the method of choice for real-time FNA guidance. Computed tomography (CT) is more often used to define and localize lesions in the lung and mediastinum. Lesions involving the head and neck region can usually be visualized under ultrasound guidance. However, deep-seated lesions may require the use of contrast enhanced CT to demonstrate the exact location, especially in the case of lymphomas. Correlation of the imaging characteristics and location of the mass lesion with the patient's age and clinical findings is necessary for an accurate diagnosis.

Ancillary techniques

Nowhere has the use of immunohistochemistry and molecular genetic studies impacted the rendering of histogenetic-specific diagnoses more than in the childhood soft tissue sarcomas, particularly small round cell tumor (SRCTs).[21,27] As most paediatric patients are enrolled in histogenetic-specific protocols (e.g. Paediatric Oncology Group) following a diagnosis of sarcoma, most authors agree that although the gold standard for diagnosis remains the light microscopic evaluation, ancillary diagnostic procedures are helpful to render the specific subtyping of SRCTs.[27] FNAB permits a rapid diagnosis with the availability of performing ancillary techniques such as immunocytochemistry, flow cytometry, cytogenetics, and electron microscopy (EM). It is for these reasons that FNA has been incorporated by many institutions into the diagnostic algorithm of paediatric tumors. Cell block preparations are the ideal for performance of immunocytochemical studies as they allow the performance of a panel of IHC markers. Gurley et al. reviewed the diagnostic contribution of ancillary studies performed on aspirated material in the work-up of paediatric biopsies.[28] Ancillary studies were performed in 40% of their cases. Immunohistochemistry helped to narrow the differential diagnosis or classify the disease process in 42%, confirm the cytologic impression in 47%, and gave contradictory results in 10% of cases. Seventy-four percent of cases had adequate material for electron microscopy which was diagnostic or helped to classify the lesions in one-third of cases, helped exclude diagnostic consideration in 21% and was noncontributory in only 14% of cases.[28]

The utility of FNA material in the molecular characterization has been shown in several studies, and the majority of aspirates can yield sufficient material to perform the necessary molecular studies.[22,28–30] In a study by Kilpatrick et al., among 27 patients clinically eligible for histogenetic-specific protocols, an accurate diagnosis was rendered by FNA in 25 (92%) cases.[21] Kilpatrick and colleagues also showed that cytogenetic analysis can be accurately performed using FNA biopsy material to confirm the t(11;22) translocation in Ewing's sarcoma and the t(x;18) translocation in synovial sarcomas, supporting the FNA cytologic impression (Table 17.1).[21]

Table 17.1 Frequency of various immunocytochemical reactions and molecular analyses demonstrated in SRCT of children

| Tumor type | Frequency of reactivity reported by various authors | | | | | | | |
	CK	CD99	NB84	WT1*	CD56	Desmin	MyoD1*	Molecular analysis
Lymphoblastic lymphoma	Very rare	57–100%	0	Rare cases	NDF	0	0	NDF
Neuroblastoma	0	34–44%	100%	Rare cases	100%	0	0	1p, N-myc
Nephroblastoma	75%	0	0	70%	70%	Rare cases	0	NDF
Ewing's/PNET	10–32%	90–100%	20%	Focal	Focal	Rare–13%	0	t(11;22)q24;q12
RMS	Very rare	11–30%	0	100% (C)	100%	99%	97%	t(2,13)(q35;q12)++
DSRCT	90–100%	35–81%	50%	100%	NDF	50–100%**	0	t(11;22)(p13;q12)
Synovial sarcoma	62%	62%	NDF	0	NDF	Rare cases	0	t(X;18)(p11.2;q11.2)
Malignant rhabdoid tumor	99%	NDF	NDF	0	NDF	Rare cases	0	NDF

* = nuclear staining; ** = perinuclear dot-like; (C) = cytoplasmic; NDF= no data available; RMS = rhabdomyosarcoma (++embryonal type does not show any specific molecular translocation); DSRCT; desmoplastic small round cell tumor
Modified from Pohar-Marinsek. Difficulties in diagnosing small round cell tumours of childhood from fine needle aspiration cytology samples. Cytopathology 2008;19:67–79.

Diagnostic approach

As with FNA material from other sites, a multidisciplinary approach is critical when evaluating aspirated material from children. Specifically, besides patient age, tumor size, mobility, anatomic location of the mass, and clinical presentation (rapid versus slow growth), the radiographic findings need to be correlated with the FNA cytologic features to narrow down the differential diagnoses and avoid misdiagnoses. Most authors agree that a definitive cytologic diagnosis must be based on a combination of the cytologic findings (i.e. adequate specimen, cytomorphology) correlated with results of ancillary studies (immunohistochemistry, flow cytometry, cytogenetic analysis, electron microscopy), clinical and/or radiographic data. Close interaction between the clinician and cytopathologist is therefore an essential component to the success of paediatric FNA.

An approach to the cytologic work-up of paediatric FNA is to divide lesions conceptually into two broad groups based on the size of the malignant cells, uniformity of cell appearance, and patterns of cell arrangement.[24] The majority of paediatric malignancies can be classified into either the small or large cell categories, although there are occasional tumors such as rhabdomyosarcoma that have cytologic features that bridge both groups.[20] This is especially important since many of the paediatric malignancies fall into the category of small round cell (blue cell) tumors (SRCTs) of childhood.[2,20,31] These neoplasms consist of a uniform cell populations having diameters up to approximately three times that of a small mature lymphocyte and typically possess only a single hyperchromatic nucleus with finely granular, evenly distributed chromatin. The cytoplasm is generally scanty, resulting in very high nuclear to cytoplasmic ratios. The much less frequent 'large cell' category of malignancies is composed of pleomorphic cell populations with more abundant cytoplasm and may include multinucleated cells.[20] Characteristically, coarsely clumped chromatin with irregular distribution and prominent nucleoli are present. However, for both categories, particularly SRCTs, definitive diagnosis often requires ancillary studies such as immunocytochemistry, EM, cytogenetic and molecular studies.[21,23,25,28,32]

This chapter will focus on the FNA cytologic features of neoplasms that are seen predominantly in the paediatric age group. Lesions that occur in both the adult and paediatric population are discussed elsewhere in this book.

CYTOLOGICAL FINDINGS

Small round cell tumors (SRCTs)

Definitive cell typing of SRCT is mandatory for enrollment of patients in specific therapeutic protocols, which has led to a significant increase in the disease-free survival rates. Immediate cytologic assessment is a critical step that helps to establish the initial diagnostic impression and points to the need for additional tissue material for pertinent ancillary studies.[25,29,33] Aktar et al.[26] and Layfield[15] have expressed the importance of a complete history, physical examination, and radiological and laboratory evaluations in arriving at a definitive diagnosis of SRCTs.

Neoplasms which are conventionally considered in the SRCT category include the prototypical neuroblastoma along with rhabdomyosarcoma, Ewing's sarcoma/primitive neuroectodermal tumor (EWS/PNET), intra-abdominal desmoplastic small round cell tumor, leukemia and malignant lymphoma.[10,34] Other childhood malignancies that are in the differential diagnosis include small cell osteosarcoma, undifferentiated (small cell) hepatoblastoma, blastemal Wilms' tumor, rhabdoid tumor of soft tissue, synovial sarcoma and granulocytic sarcoma.[35,36]

All SRCTs are uniformly characterized by the presence of sheets of monomorphic cells with subtle architectural and cytomorphologic features that serve as clues to the correct diagnosis.[22] Morphological similarity and lack of immunocytochemical specificity in SRCT are reasons for difficulties in specific diagnosis of SRCT on cytology.[22] Some SRCTs are so poorly differentiated that they lack specific antigens. In addition, cross-reactivity exists for many antigens among certain SRCTs.[22] However, correct cell typing is possible and achievable in 92% of FNAB of SRCTs with the judicious use of various ancillary studies.[4,18,21] A variety of cytologic variables including nuclear, cytoplasmic, and architectural features were analyzed as to their association with the final histologic typing to determine the most predictive characteristics for each sarcoma. Using the previous cytologic features, Layfield et al. performed logistic regression analysis of 59 cases with diagnoses of Ewing's sarcoma/PNET, rhabdomyosarcoma, neuroblastoma, Wilms' tumor and lymphoma.[34] Among the entire group, Ewing's sarcoma/PNET was the most difficult to specifically diagnose by cytomorphology alone. In most cases, it was the 'lack' of diagnostic criteria for the other round cell sarcomas that was used to make a diagnosis of Ewing's sarcoma.[34]

Neuroblastoma

Neuroblastoma is considered the 'prototypical' small round cell tumor of childhood.[25] It is the most common solid nonlymphoreticular malignancy in the paediatric age group, with the majority of patients diagnosed before 5 years of age and 50% before 2 years of age. It is also the most common malignancy in the neonate.[20,37,38]

Neuroblastoma can be found in any site which harbors sympathetic neural tissue. The most common sites of occurrence, comprising two-thirds of cases, are the adrenal gland and retroperitoneal sympathetic ganglia.[18] Neuroblastoma also occurs in other neural crest sites such as the thoracopulmonary, mediastinal, cervical and, less commonly, pelvic regions.[2,20,30] Approximately one-third of children with neuroblastoma present with metastatic disease to regional lymph nodes, bone marrow, liver, bone and/or lung at the time of diagnosis.[37,38] The prognosis of patients with neuroblastoma correlates with age, site of involvement and stage. Adrenal neuroblastoma has a less favorable prognosis than its extra-adrenal counterpart.[14] In addition, the presence of a stroma-rich matrix, low mitotic–karyorrhectic cell index, and increased numbers of differentiating tumor cells are correlated with favorable prognosis.[35,39–41]

Neuroblastoma usually forms a well-defined solid tumor <10 cm in size with hemorrhage and extentive necrosis. The FNA usually yields hypercellular smears with predominant individually scattered small anaplastic cells, showing prominent nuclear molding.[27,41,42] The prototypical neuroblastic cells have high nuclear to cytoplasmic ratios with single nuclei that are oval to slightly irregular in shape containing evenly dispersed granular chromatin (salt and pepper) and small to inconspicuous nucleoli (Fig. 17.1). Small round cells are arranged in moderately or well-formed Homer-Wright rosettes surrounding centrally located neuropil, which stains pink or blue–gray in Giemsa-stained smears. The presence of Homer-Wright rosettes is diagnostic but not present in all cases (Fig. 17.2). Neuropil, either associated with the rosettes or present in the smear background, is the most helpful cytologic feature for rendering a definitive cytologic diagnosis of neuroblastoma.[34] Neuropil consists of a fibrillary tangle of neuritic processes with or without associated neuroblastic cells (Fig. 17.3). Mitotic–karyorrhectic

cells and calcifications can occasionally be recognized in aspirate smears. Larger differentiating neuroblasts with moderate amounts of cytoplasm and binucleated to multinucleated ganglion cells can also be present in the smear. Some neuroblastomas may undergo different grades of maturation, forming ganglioneuroblastoma or ganglioneuroma. In ganglioneuroblastoma, the smear is pleomorphic with prominent anisonucleosis and abundant neuropil background but without ganglion cells, while ganglioneuroma demonstrates characteristic ganglion cells (Fig. 17.4).[27,42]

The differential diagnosis of neuroblastoma includes other members of SRCTs group.[42] The presence of apoptotic nuclei, nuclear molding, paranuclear 'blue bodies', necrotic background, with the absence of lymphoglandular bodies will help to distinguish neuroblastoma from lymphomas.[24,43] Neuroblastoma composed of dissociated primitive cells without rosettes formation, is morphologically undistinguishable from blastema cells of a Wilms' tumor or EWS/PNET. The immunocytochemical profile supportive of neuroblastoma includes positive staining for neuron-specific

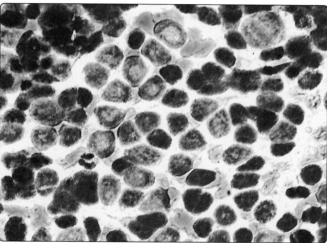

Fig. 17.1 Neuroblastoma Hypercellular smears demonstrate numerous singly scattered cells with high nuclear to cytoplasmic ratios, round to oval irregular nuclei with fine granular chromatin and inconspicuous nucleoli (Diff-Quik, ×400).

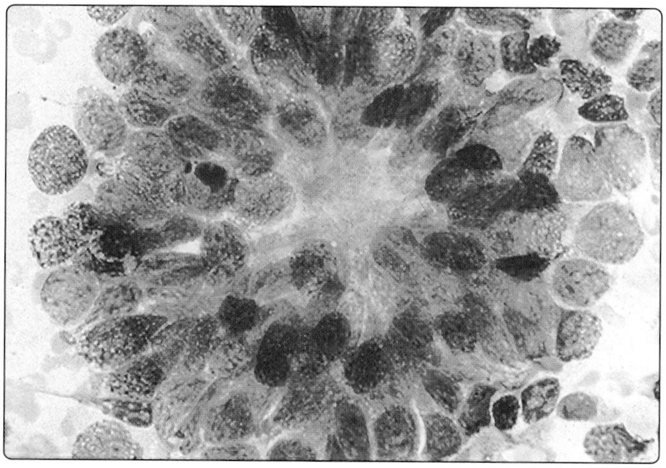

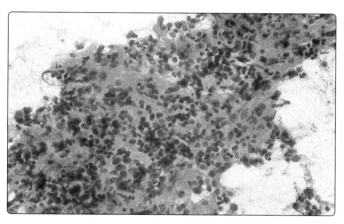

Fig. 17.3 Neuroblastoma Medium power of aspirate smear containing neuroblastic cells associated with fibrillary to granular background neuropil (Pap, ×200).

Fig. 17.2 Neuroblastoma Cluster of cells arranged in a Homer-Wright rosette containing central neuropil. The presence of neuropil is the most helpful cytologic feature for rendering a definitive diagnosis of neuroblastoma (Diff-Quik, ×400).

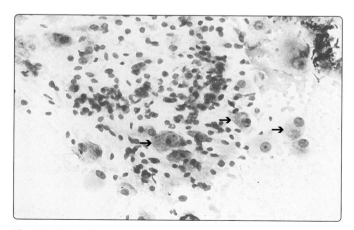

Fig. 17.4 Neuroblastoma Compared with neuroblastic cells, neoplastic ganglion cells (arrows) demonstrate larger nuclei with prominent nucleoli, and moderate amounts of coarsely granular cytoplasm. These cells are seen in the two related lesions, ganglioneuroblastoma and ganglioneuroma (Diff-Quik, ×400).

enolase (NSE), microtubule-associated proteins (MAPs) and/or neurofilament protein.[28] Positive staining for S-100 and/or glial fibrillary acidic protein (GFAP) has occasionally been observed. CD56 can be positive in both neuroblastoma cells and EWS/PNET. However, CD56 was reported uniformly and strongly positive in all neuroblastomas and only focally in EWS/PNET.[28,43] In addition, EWS/PNET is usually positive for CD99, while neuroblastoma CD99 is usually negative. Conversely, Wilms tumor can be WT1 negative in 30% and CD56 positive.[43] In this setting, low molecular weight cytokeratin is helpful to differentiate neuroblastoma from Wilms' tumor, since Wilms' tumor is cytokeratin positive while neuroblastoma is negative, although blastema cells can occasionally be cytokeratin negative.[22] Neuroblastomas are negative for desmin, myogenin, smooth muscle actin, muscle-specific actin, CD34, and CD45.[43] Ultrastructural features of neuroblastoma include small dense core neurosecretory-type granules and abundant processes containing microtubules.[43] Neuroblastoma usually shows a deletion or rearrangement of material of chromosome 1p and amplification of N-myc.[44]

Retinoblastoma

This is the most frequent intraocular tumor in children, with similar cytomorphology to neuroblastoma. One-third of these tumors are bilateral and are usually seen in children younger than 2 years. Retinoblastomas appear as high-grade undifferentiated small round cell tumors. Smears show hypercellular smears formed by sheets of small round or oval hyperchromatic nuclei with numerous mitoses and inconspicuous nucleoli, often with necrotic background.[1,5] Cells show molding and typically arranged in rosettes with a central lumen containing acid mucopolysaccharides resistant to hyaluronidase (Flexner-Wintersteiner rosettes), and less frequently in Homer-Wright rosettes, in which cells are arranged around neuropil matrix.[4]

Olfactory neuroblastoma

Olfactory neuroblastoma (ONB) is a rare tumor of neuroectodermal origin that arises from epithelium that lines the upper aerodigestive tract (nasal septum, superior turbinates, cribriform plate) malignancies. Although ONB show similar cytomorphology to SRCTs, they are mainly seen in adult populations.

Wilms' tumor (nephroblastoma)

Nephroblastoma is the most frequent malignancy of the kidney in childhood and accounts for 6% of all paediatric cancers.[20,29] Wilms tumor (WT) is the most frequent paediatric cancer in children less than 3 years old. Approximately 90% of all intra-abdominal malignancies in childhood will be either Wilms' tumor or neuroblastoma.[20] The preoperative diagnosis of Wilms' tumor by FNA biopsy has become increasingly important since neoadjuvant chemotherapy has become the standard of care.[45,46]

Wilms' tumors usually present as a single tumor, but it is sometimes multicentric and bilateral. Most cases are >10 cm

in size and has a soft consistency, even surface, and well-delimited border with frequent areas of necrosis and hemorrhage.[1] FNA biopsy for the primary diagnosis and management of Wilms' tumor is contraindicated in children with a resectable renal mass.[47] However, patients with unresectable Wilms' tumor requiring neoadjuvant chemotherapy, or children with metastatic disease at the time of presentation may benefit from FNAB technique.[48,49] According to the current guidelines,[48] FNA through a posterior approach does not upstage the tumors, while an anterior approach technique, will upstage the tumor to stage III because of the possibility of generalized peritoneal contamination.

FNAB of conventional Wilms' tumor shows a triphasic pattern consisting of complex tubules (epithelial component), mesenchymal differentiation and a primitive blastemal component.[20,35] The blastemal cells are characterized by a relatively small size with high nuclear to cytoplasmic ratios and only a scant rim of extremely fragile cytoplasm (Figs 17.5 and 17.6). Nuclear molding can also be seen. The larger cells of the epithelial component may be arranged in tubules which range from simple tubular outlines to

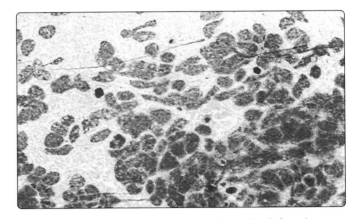

Fig. 17.5 Wilms' tumor (nephroblastoma) Blastemal cells form the majority of the cellular component in aspirates, present either singly or in small clusters. Blastemal cells are small with finely granular nuclear chromatin, inconspicuous nucleoli, and scant, extremely fragile cytoplasm rendering large numbers of stripped nuclei on the smears (Diff-Quik, ×400).

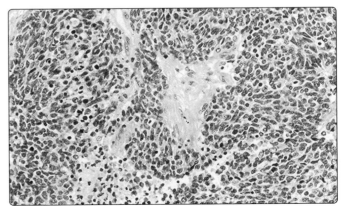

Fig. 17.6 Wilms' tumor (nephroblastoma) Blastemal cells can surround and/or be incorporated into stromal fragments (Diff-Quik, ×200).

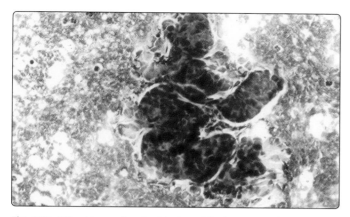

Fig. 17.7 Wilms' tumor (nephroblastoma) Aspirate smear demonstrating the epithelial component with glandular arrangements of primitive cells that are arranged in complex branching patterns (Diff-Quik ×400).

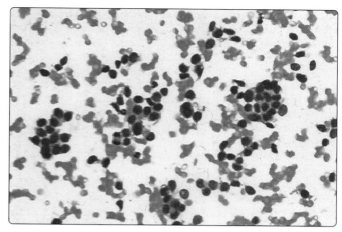

Fig. 17.8 Ewing's sarcoma Highly cellular aspirate smears demonstrate individually scattered and small loose clusters of uniform small cells with round nuclei, evenly dispersed finely granular chromatin, distinctly absent nucleoli, and only a scant rim of cytoplasm (Diff-Quik, ×200).

complex, branching luminal patterns (Fig. 17.7). These tubules have a well-defined apical border surrounding an empty luminal space with palisading of the epithelial nuclei. They can potentially be confused with the Homer-Wright rosettes of neuroblastoma.[42–51] However, Homer-Wright rosettes are less complex in architecture and consist of cells arranged around central fibrillary neuropil. The mesenchymal component of Wilms' tumor consists of fibroconnective tissue fragments containing short spindle-shaped cells with bland nuclear features, which can occasionally predominate and demonstrate a myxoid or collagenous appearance in the smears. Occasional cases can show skeletal muscle differentiation. Histologically, anaplasia in Wilms' tumor is defined as the combination of enlarged nuclei equal to or greater than three times the size of the nuclei of adjacent cells along with nuclear hyperchromasia and abnormal multipolar mitotic figures.[45] Recognition of anaplasia is crucial since it is associated with aggressive tumor behavior and decreased survival, thereby necessitating more aggressive therapy. An overdiagnosis of anaplasia in the aspirated smears, however, can be due to a number of artifacts such as calcification and stain precipitate which can simulate enlarged hyperchromatic nuclei. DNA-smearing artifact and basophilic extracellular mucinous material can also simulate anaplastic nuclei. Conversely, sampling errors can lead to an underdiagnosis of anaplasia.[45]

Separation of WT from other SRCTs can be extremely difficult, particularly if the undifferentiated blastemal component is the predominant or sole component in the smears.[45,51] A careful search for epithelial and mesenchymal components favors WT, whereas a fibrillary background confirms the diagnosis of intrarenal neuroblastoma.[50] Ancillary studies become crucial in rendering a specific diagnosis and separating this lesion from other SRCTs. In WT, blastemal cells stain positively for vimentin, cytokeratin (AE1/AE3), epithelial membrane antigen (EMA) and CD99 negative.[30,50,52] Neuroblastomas are positive for neuron-specific enolase (NSE) but negative for cytokeratin and EMA. Lymphomas can occur in the kidney and are characterized by leukocyte common antigen (LCA, CD45) positive. The background typically demonstrates abundant diagnostic lymphoglandular bodies.

Ewing's sarcoma/primitive neuroectodermal tumor (EWS/PNET)

Ewing's sarcoma/primitive neuroectodermal tumor is the second most frequent malignant paediatric primary bone tumor, accounts for approximately 20% of soft tissue sarcomas in the first 2 decades of life and is the most common thoracic neoplasm.[20,21,53] Around 25% of patients have metastasis in the lungs and bones at the time of diagnosis. Both PNET and Ewing's sarcoma stain positively with monoclonal antibodies FLI-1 and CD99 (MIC-2 oncogene) and share a common chromosomal abnormality (11;22 translocation).[27] The demographic and biologic behavior of both lesions are similar enough to consider these lesions as a continuous spectrum of the same tumor.[54,55]

Smears are cellular, composed of small cohesive groups of undifferentiated small round cells without nuclear molding (Fig 17.8). Although single dispersed cells are seen in the smear background, EWS/PNET can yield the most cohesive pattern of the SRCTs group. The cells have indistinct borders and may form pseudorosettes. A dimorphic population of lighter and darker cells may be present in Diff-Quik-stained smears, mimicking the histologic findings. Lighter-staining cells are large (approximately the size of histiocytes) and have round-to-oval, slightly pleomorphic nuclei, smooth nuclear membranes with fine chromatin and one or two small nucleoli. Cells have a moderate amount of finely vacuolated-to-clear cytoplasm that contains abundant, periodic acid–Schiff-positive, diastase-digestible glycogen granules.[56] Darker-staining or lymphocytoid cells have a small, irregularly contoured nucleus with dense chromatin and a narrow rim of cytoplasm, changes that are likely a manifestation of apoptosis. The two cell types are usually intermingled in no discernible pattern, with lighter-staining cells predominating. Binucleation, multinucleation, and stromal matrix formation are not features of EWS/PNET.

Homer-Wright rosettes are not usually seen. In the Diff-Quik smear, peripheral cytoplasmic vacuolization and membranous cytoplasmic blebs can be noted in occasional cases and considered as characteristic features.[56,57]

In rare cases of EWS/PNET, the majority of the cell population has slightly oval nuclei, mimicking other SRCTs, particularly monophasic synovial sarcoma. The so-called large cell variant of EWS/PNET may be confused with large cell lymphoma, but immunophenotyping settles this diagnostic issue in most cases.[55,56]

Although positive staining for CD99 is quite helpful in the diagnosis of PNET/Ewing's sarcoma, it is not specific.[22,30] CD99 can be demonstrated in various percentages in other SRCTs. CD99 was reported in 57–100% of lymphoblastic lymphomas, 34–44% of neuroblastomas, 11–30% of rhabdomyosarcoma, 35–81% of DSRCT and 62% of synovial sarcomas.[22,30] Ewing/PNET tumors can be negative for CD99 (8.6%). EWS/PNET can be occasionally positive for cytokeratin and desmin (about 10%). Molecular analysis plays an important diagnostic role in doubtful cases, whereas 90% show t(11;22)(q24;q12) translocation, while 10% show t(21;22)(q22;q12) translocation.[22,30,54,55]

Rhabdomyosarcoma

Rhabdomyosarcoma (RMS) is the most frequent soft tissue sarcoma in children with two age peaks, with the first peak occurring at 4 to 5 years of age and the second in late adolescence.[21] It arises often in the head and neck, followed by genitourinary tract, extremities, and trunk of children younger than 5 years old. In the paediatric population, there are two major histologic forms: the alveolar and embryonal subtypes. Embryonal subtype is the most common form in early age. In contrast, the alveolar subtype is more frequently seen in adolescents and originates most often in the extremities, paranasal sinuses and retroperitoneum.[58]

Although rhabdomyosarcoma is generally considered one of the SRCTs of childhood, it is associated with a relatively broad spectrum of histologic appearances.[58,59] FNA demonstrates a wide range of morphology and the degree of variability greater than that seen in the other SRCTs.[4] Aspiration biopsies of both embryonal and alveolar rhabdomyosarcomas are characterized by moderately to highly cellular samples which include both numerous individually dispersed tumor cells (rhabdomyoblasts) and densely packed aggregates with prominent overlapping of the cells.[45,60] The smear background may show characteristic loose myxoid material which may have a metachromatic appearance with the Romanowsky stains. In other instances, the smear background is simply clean, collagenous or bubbly (tigroid) in appearance, resembling that seen in aspirates from germinomas.[4,45,54,59] Some investigators have attempted to differentiate embryonal from alveolar subtype in FNAC smears and were successful in 80% of cases. The embryonal subtype may be composed almost exclusively of small primitive cellular elements with round or polygonal contours, extremely high N : C ratios, solitary nuclei and minute nucleoli. Some cells may show a higher level of differentiation with increasing volumes of eosinophilic cytoplasm and eccentrically positioned nuclei, mimicking rhabdoid tumors (Fig. 17.9).[4,59] Smears of alveolar rhabdomyosarcoma are more cellular

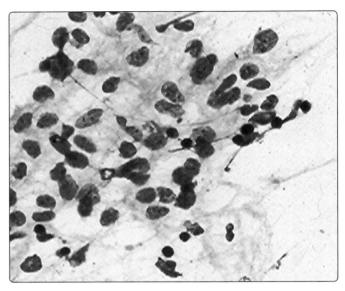

Fig. 17.9 Rhabdomyosarcoma, embryonal subtype The cellular appearance in this subtype is highly variable with more undifferentiated cells (shown here) admixed with cells showing higher degrees of myogenic differentiation. The cells vary from round to spindled, with frequent eccentrically placed nuclei and tapering cytoplasmic tails (Pap, ×400).

with more mature rhabdomyoblasts than embryonal rhabdomyosarcoma.[59,60] Rhabdomyoblastic cells may be arranged in alveolar structures. Compared with the embryonal subtype, the malignant cells comprising the alveolar subtype of rhabdomyosarcoma are generally larger and more uniform in appearance with rounded contours, solitary hyperchromatic nuclei, prominent nucleoli and high N : C ratios (Fig. 17.10). A helpful diagnostic feature of alveolar subtype is the presence of multinucleated tumor giant cells with nuclei arranged in a wreathlike manner (Fig. 17.10). Characteristic strap cells with a solitary tapered cytoplasmic tail may be occasionally seen.[58,61,62] Pohar-Marinsek and Bracko observed that the alveolar rhabdomyosarcoma exhibited two major architectural patterns: one characterized by completely dissociated cells and the other one containing many clustered formations.[60] Presence of binucleate cells was an important criterion for the diagnosis of alveolar rhabdomyosarcoma.[60]

It was believed for a long time that desmin was a specific marker for RMS.[28] However, desmin positivity has been seen in other members of SRCTs , while rhabdomyosarcoma can be positive for CD99.[30,45,62] WT1 shows a strong cytoplasmic staining in rhabdomyosarcoma and a nuclear one in DSRCT, while is only focal in EWS/PNET. Unlike EWS/PNET positivity for cytokeratin, rhabdomyosarcoma is negative or show only a rare positive individual cell. Rare cases have been shown to express lymphoid markers including CD10, CD19 and CD20. Recently, more specific skeletal muscle markers have become available, including myogenin and MyoD1, and are highly sensitive in the diagnosis of rhabdomyosarcoma.[59,63] These markers are expressed by positive nuclear staining. In challenging cases, molecular analysis shows a specific chromosomal aberration, t(2;13)(q35;q14) chromosomal translocation and/or the gene fusion transcripts PAX-FKHR in 80% alveolar subtype, but no specific translocation has been identified in the embryonal subtype.[22,61,63]

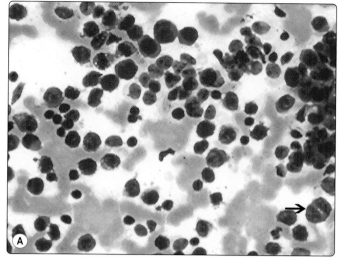

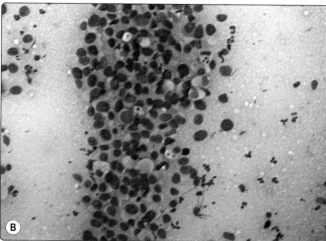

Fig. 17.10 Rhabdomyosarcoma, alveolar subtype (A) Highly cellular smears contain large uniform cells with round nuclei, prominent nucleoli, and high nuclear : cytoplasmic ratios. A helpful diagnostic feature of the alveolar subtype is the presence of multinucleated tumor cells (*arrow*) (Diff-Quik, ×400); (B) Highly cellular smear shows large uniform cells with bubbly (tigroid) in appearance, resembling that seen in aspirates from germinomas (Diff-Quik, ×400).

Rhabdoid tumors

Rhabdoid tumors are easily confused with rhabdomyosarcoma. The presence of perinuclear cytoplasmic globular inclusions is usually more characteristic of rhabdoid tumors and eccentrically placed nuclei with a prominent central nucleolus. Hypercalcemia, and cytokeratin positive/desmin negative immunostaining, help in accurate tumor typing,[19] although some cases can be desmin positive.[21,22,61,64] Aspiration biopsies yield uniform-appearing, moderately sized neoplastic cells which are characterized by rounded contours, and solitary eccentric nuclei and uniform, intensely eosinophilic cytoplasm.[61] The nuclei have thick nuclear membranes and a massive nucleolus. In contrast to rhabdomyosarcomas, these smears do not contain a spectrum of cellular appearances presenting different maturation stages of rhabdomyoblasts.

Intra-abdominal desmoplastic small round cell tumor of childhood

Intra-abdominal desmoplastic small round cell tumor (DSRCT) is a very rare malignancy predominantly seen in male patients between 16 and 18 years of age.[20,65,66] Although a variety of sites have been reported, the tumor most commonly involves the omentum or peritoneum with secondary invasion of the bowel wall. FNA cytologic findings include the presence of groups of undifferentiated malignant cells showing nuclear molding, associated with desmoplastic stroma (Fig. 17.11).[14,67,68] DSRCT demonstrates multidirectional differentiation based on expression of both epithelial and mesenchymal immunocytochemical markers including cytokeratin (AE1/AE3), EMA, desmin and NSE.[66,68] The majority of cases are also positive for vimentin and WT1.[68] A specific chromosomal abnormality can be demonstrated [t(11;22)(p13;q12)], representing the fusion of the EWS and WT1 genes.[67,69,70]

Malignant lymphoma

Over 90% of non-Hodgkin lymphomas in children are high-grade lymphomas.[14] The most common types are T and B lymphoblastic, Burkitt and anaplastic large cell lymphoma while diffuse large B-cell lymphoma is less common.[20] Lymphoblastic, Burkitt and diffuse large cell lymphomas in children can be mistaken for any other SRCTs on the basis of morphology alone. Within the paediatric population, each of these lymphomas has distinct clinical features which are important to recognize.[71] Lymphoblastic lymphoma typically affects young teenage boys, and is a common cause of a mediastinal mass as well as peripheral, usually supradiaphragmatic, lymphadenopathy. Most of these are T-cell immunophenotype and positive for terminal deoxynucleotidyl transferase (TdT). Aspiration smears are highly cellular with a singly dispersed monotonous population of lymphoblasts with no evidence of true intercellular cohesiveness. The cells are twice the size of normal lymphocytes. Nuclei demonstrate finely granular chromatin with inconspicuous nucleoli, and only a thin rim of delicate cytoplasm (Fig. 17.12). Abundant lymphoglandular bodies are present in the background and serve as an important diagnostic clue of the lymphoid lesion. Neuroblastoma enters into the differential diagnosis as it can present as a primary mediastinal lesion. However, intercellular cohesion, nuclear molding, typical Homer-Wright rosettes and absence of lymphoglandular bodies favor the diagnosis of neuroblastoma.

The small non-cleaved cell lymphomas such as Burkitt and non-Burkitt types, usually presents in the nonendemic form with enlargement of abdominal lymph nodes and/or visceral organs.[4,45,71] Ovarian involvement may be seen in females. Aspiration smears are highly cellular and demonstrate monotonous population of singly dispersed cells with round nuclei, moderate to high nuclear to cytoplasmic ratios, coarse clumping of chromatin, and prominent nucleoli (Fig. 17.13). Multiple nucleoli are seen in Burkitt-type and single nucleoli are noted in the non-Burkitt type. Nuclear irregularities and polylobated nuclei are often seen. On Romanowsky-stained smears, numerous cytoplasmic vacuoles are seen in Burkitt lymphoma (Fig. 17.14). The vacuoles

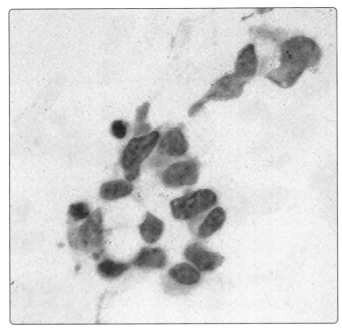

Fig. 17.11 Intra-abdominal desmoplastic small round cell tumor of childhood Undifferentiated cells are present in this aspirate smear demonstrating oval, irregular nuclei, finely granular chromatin, and nuclear molding (Pap, ×400).

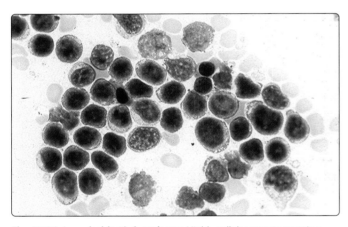

Fig. 17.12 Lymphoblastic lymphoma Highly cellular smears contain a monomorphic population of lymphoblasts with no true intracellular cohesiveness. The cells demonstrate uniform round nuclei with finely dispersed chromatin, inconspicuous nucleoli, and a thin rim of cytoplasm. Numerous lymphoglandular bodies are readily identifiable in the background.

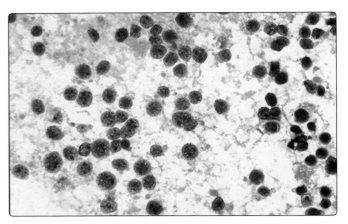

Fig. 17.13 Burkitt lymphoma Aspirates are extremely cellular, containing intermediate-sized, predominantly round nuclei with coarsely clumped chromatin and one or more prominent nucleoli (Papanicolaou, ×200).

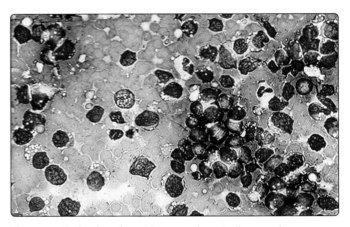

Fig. 17.14 Burkitt lymphoma Romanowsky-stained smears demonstrate cytoplasmic lipid vacuoles which are lost with alcohol fixation. Nuclei can be polylobated and irregular (Diff-Quik×200).

are due to the accumulation of neutral lipids, which can be stained with oil-red-O. Abundant mitotic figures and apoptosis are seen and are indicative of a tumor with extremely rapid turnover. Phagocytic histiocytes are often seen in the background.

Immunocytochemistry and flow cytometry have proved to be an invaluable ancillary technique in diagnosing challenging cases of lymphomas. However, some lymphoblastic lymphomas in bones may be negative for CD45, CD3 and CD20, while CD99 and cytokeratin can be positive,

erroneously excluding a lymphoma diagnosis.[72,73] Burkitt and non-Burkitt lymphomas demonstrate a characteristic chromosomal translocation t(8;14) and in some cases a t(2;8) chromosomal translocation may be present.[74]

Langerhans cell histiocytosis

Langerhans cell histiocytosis (LCH) encompasses a group of histologically similar lesions including eosinophilic granuloma, Hand-Schüller-Christian disease, and Letterer-Siwe disease. LCH occurs at any age but there is a predilection in children under 5 years of age, males being more commonly affected. The etiology is unknown, but viruses such as EBV, herpes, and adenovirus are believed to be involved in its pathogenesis.[73] The skeleton is most commonly affected, especially the craniofacial region such as frontal, temporal and zygomatic regions, followed by the femur, pelvis, ribs, and spine.[4,75] Radigrapically, these are well-demarcated intramedullary osteolytic lesions which commonly show cortical destruction. FNA usually yields cellular smears with

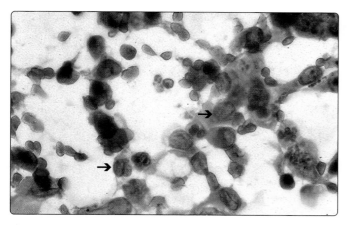

Fig. 17.15 Langerhans cell histiocytosis Small, singly scattered uniform Langerhans histiocytes are shown in this smear and are characterized by oval nuclei, finely reticulated evenly dispersed chromatin and classic longitudinal nuclear grooves (*arrows*) (Pap, ×400).

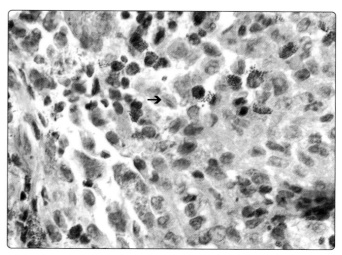

Fig. 17.17 Langerhans cell histiocytosis This cell block preparation demonstrates scattered eosinophils among the Langerhans histiocytes. Note the diagnostic longitudinal nuclear groove (*arrow*) in the Langerhans histiocytes (H&E, ×400).

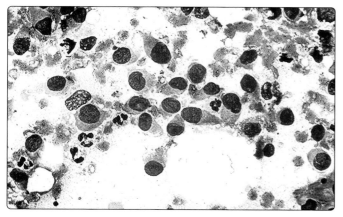

Fig. 17.16 Langerhans cell histiocytosis Aspirate smears are generally cellular with singly scattered lesional cells containing moderate amounts of eosinophilic cytoplasm. The background contains neutrophils (Diff-Quik, ×400).

singly scattered Langerhans cell histiocytes with characteristic reniform, convoluted nuclei with distinct longitudinal nuclear grooves. Bi- and multinucleated cells are commonly seen (Figs 17.15 and 17.16). A variable number of lymphocytes, eosinophils, and neutrophils are present and may be the predominant cellular component in some cases (Fig. 17.17).[4,75] LCH can be misclassified as SRCTs on FNAB.[24] This inaccurate interpretation is usually associated with paucicellular smears, crushing artifacts, and the impression of cohesion.[75] Immunohistochemically, the cells are S-100 positive, and most express CD1a, CD68, and vimentin and negative for the majority of B- and T-cell markers, myeloperoxidase, CD34, EMA, and the follicular dendritic cell lineage markers CD21 and CD35. Ultrastructural examination reveals histiocytic/dendritic cells with classic Birbeck granules.[75]

Leukemias

Leukemias are the most common form of cancer in children in the United States, accounting for 30–35% of all new pae-

diatric malignancies.[5] Most are acute leukemias and occur in children under 5 years of age. The diagnosis of leukemia is made by bone marrow aspirate and biopsy in the majority of cases. The diagnostic role of cytology is usually in the identification of relapses of the CNS with examination of CSF fluid specimens. Rarely, acute leukemias can form a mass lesion, including lymphadenopathy, mostly in cases of unexpected relapses. The role of FNA is very limited aside from rare case reports of the application of FNA to examine testicular enlargement in males with acute lymphoblastic leukemias.[76]

Hepatoblastoma

Hepatoblastoma is the most common primary hepatic malignancy in children and the third most common intra-abdominal tumors after neuroplastoma and Wilm's tumor. Almost 90% of hepatoblastomas affect children younger than 5 years.[20,77,78] There is a relatively constant annual incidence in Western countries of 0.5–1.5 per million children.[75] Hepatoblastoma has an incidence of approximately 10% of Wilms' tumour and 5% of leukemia. It accounts for a little less than half of all primary liver neoplasms of children with a male-to-female ratio of approximately 1 : 2.[5.2,20] Serum alpha fetoprotein levels are elevated in 84–91% of patients, usually with very high titres.[79] The dramatic improvement in the survival of children with hepatoblastoma, with the current cure rates of approximately 75%, is a reflection of both contemporary chemotherapeutic protocols and surgical resection.[79] Children with extrahepatic tumor extension, multifocal tumor, vascular invasion, and distant metastases have a poor prognosis. Histologic subtype has not been shown to be of prognostic significance.[79]

Hepatoblastoma usually causes a single mass involving more often the right side of the liver.[68] The neoplasms range in size from 3 cm to 20 cm and is generally not associated with cirrhosis. Typically, most children present with abdominal enlargement and occasional hemihypertrophy,

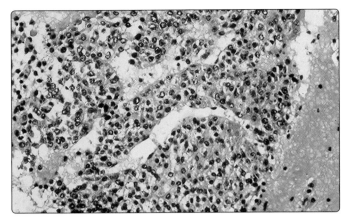

Fig. 17.18 Hepatoblastoma Cell block preparation demonstrating small to medium-sized polygonal fetal-type cells with moderate amounts of granular cytoplasm and arranged in thick trabeculae (H&E, ×200).

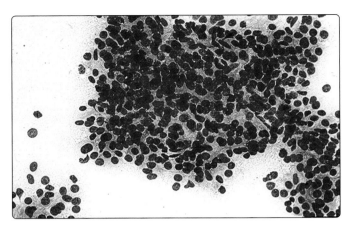

Fig. 17.20 Hepatoblastoma In this Diff-Quik-stained smear, neoplastic cells demonstrate moderate amounts of granular cytoplasm consistent with fetal cell type. The cells are arranged in loose clusters and dispersed individually in the background (Diff-Quik, ×400).

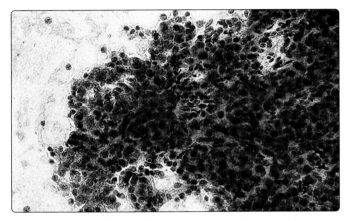

Fig. 17.19 Hepatoblastoma Aspirate smear with cells arranged in cohesive clusters and scattered individually. Neoplastic cells possess prominent central nucleoli and scant cytoplasm, representing the more primitive embryonal cells (Pap, ×200).

precocious puberty, hypoglycaemia, Wilms' tumour or the Beckwith-Wiedemann syndrome.[14] Hepatoblastoma can be classified as either purely epithelial or mixed epithelial–mesenchymal type.[45,78] Distinct subtypes of the epithelial cell component include fetal, embryonal, and anaplastic (small cell).[44] Fetal tumor cells resemble normal fetal hepatocytes and can be associated with foci of extramedullary haematopoiesis.[77] In the embryonal subtype, cells are small and spindled, with hyperchromatic nuclei and poorly defined plasma membranes. Approximately one-third of hepatoblastomas are of the mixed type. Mesenchymal elements consist of either primitive mesenchyme in the form of immature spindle cells, osteoid, cartilage and/or skeletal muscle.[20]

Aspirates are hypercellular and composed of a uniform population of small to intermediate round to oval cells arranged in trabeculae and cords along with individually scattered cells (Figs 17.18 and 17.19).[77,78] The trabeculae and cords are often covered by sinusoidal lining cells. Occasionally, pseudoacinar formation can be seen. Intact cells usually have spherical and slightly eccentrically placed nuclei with several small to inconspicuous nucleoli (Fig. 17.20). A scant to moderate amount of surrounding cytoplasm is seen.

Occasional small cytoplasmic vacuoles may be present but bile is rarely seen.[80]

The differential diagnosis of hepatoblastoma includes well-differentiated hepatocellular carcinoma, which is the second most common primary malignant liver tumor in children.[20] Most hepatocellular carcinomas are diagnosed in children older than 5 years of age (mean age between 12 and 14 years old) and, importantly, occur in already diseased livers with manifestation of hepatitis, cirrhosis, or storage diseases.[78–80] Cytological features that support a diagnosis of hepatocellular carcinoma include the presence of cells larger than those seen in hepatoblastoma with a greater degree of pleomorphism. Anisonucleosis, macronucleoli, tumor giant cells, and intranuclear cytoplasmic inclusions, including bile, are readily seen.[20] Characteristically, the cells are arranged in anastomosing trabeculae which are broader than those seen in hepatoblastoma.

FNAB of small cell undifferentiated (anaplastic) hepatoblastoma may show features that can be confused with other metastatic SRCTs.[2,20,80] Cancers that commonly metastasize to the liver in children include neuroblastoma, followed by Wilms' tumor, Ewing's sarcoma/PNET, embryonal and alveolar rhabdomyosarcoma, synovial sarcoma and retinoblastoma.[43] In contrast to most cases of hepatoblastoma, multiple discrete nodules are typically present. Hepatoblastomas are positive for low molecular weight cytokeratin and alpha fetoprotein and negative for vimentin, high molecular weight cytokeratin, epithelial membrane antigen (EMA) and carcinoembryonic antigen (CEA).[80] Electron microscopic (EM) examination demonstrates ultrastructural features of immature hepatocytes including variably prominent rough endoplasmic reticulum, abundant mitochondria, well-developed microvilli with focal canaliculus formation and intercellular junctions.[20]

Undifferentiated (embryonal) sarcoma of the liver

This typically occurs in the first decade of life and is the most common type of primary stromal malignancy of childhood.[45,80] The cytologic findings include the presence of small to medium-sized, round, spindled and stellate-shaped cells set in a myxoid background often mixed with mono- and multinucleated tumor giant cells. Periodic acid–Schiff (PAS)-positive intracytoplasmic globules are present in occasional cases. The tumor is positive for desmin, myoglobin, vimentin, α_1-antitrypsin and α_1-antichymotrypsin.[80] Another very rare hepatic malignancy that has been described in the cytology literature is primary yolk sac tumor of the liver.[81] Cytologic examination reveals loosely cohesive groups of cells having nuclei with small nucleoli and surrounding cytoplasm showing vacuolization. Individually scattered cells are also present as well as extracellular metachromatically staining amorphous material of basement membrane origin in the air-dried Romanowsky-stained smears.[81]

Synovial sarcoma

Synovial sarcomas account for 2–10% of soft tissue sarcomas in children and more frequent in adolescents. The tumor frequently locates in soft tissues of the lower extremities, close to joints cavities. Synovial sarcomas can show either a biphasic or monophasic histologic pattern.[82] FNAB of monophasic type revealed a hypercellular specimen consisting of numerous microtissue fragments as well as individually scattered single cells. The malignant cells have high nuclear-to-cytoplasmic ratios with round to oval nuclei. Occasional tumor cells show a slight tendency to spindle, with wispy cytoplasmic processes. Smears may show predominantly dissociated tumor cells, which vary in size and shape from round, ovoid to plasmacytoid in cytology smears, mimicking morphologically other SRCTs.[83] Small cell variant smears show numerous, small, round cells with very high nuclear-to-cytoplasmic ratios, can potentially be confused with other paediatric SRCTs.[84] FNA of the biphasic type show two cell population: polygonal or columnar epithelioid cells arranged in solid nests, pseudoglands and/or papillae, and atypical spindle cells.[85] Tumor cells demonstrate positive staining for cytokeratin (CAM 5.2), CK7, epithelial membrane antigen (EMA), and CD99 and negative staining for S-100 and vimentin. Cytogenetic studies have shown a very specific chromosomal translocation t(X;18) (p11.2;q11.2), with an estimated prevalence of 85% in synovial sarcoma.[83–85]

Ameloblastoma

Ameloblastoma is a locally aggressive maxillary neoplasm of the odontogenic epithelia that originates from residual epithelial components of the developing teeth. There are two histologic variants: follicular and plexiform. The plexiform is the most frequent type and is formed by nests and cords of epithelial cells surrounded by a fibrous connective stroma; peripheral cells of nests are arranged in palisades and show inverse polarization (nuclei shifted to the apical pole of cells).[86] Fine needle aspirates show aggregates and/or compacted cords of epithelial cells without atypia with inverse polarization of peripheral cells, sometimes a few fragments of fibrous stroma, and a clean background.[1,86]

Kidney

Fine needle aspiration cytology has successfully been used to document both primary and metastatic malignant rhabdoid tumor of the kidney.[87] This aggressive renal tumor occurs most commonly in infants and very young children with a median age of 13 months and has a very high mortality.[87] It is rare, representing only 2% of paediatric renal neoplasms.[44] It is often single, gray, soft mass, and without a capsule. Cytologic smears are hypercellular with clusters and individually scattered cells demonstrating enlarged eccentric nuclei, vesicular chromatin, and prominent nucleoli.[45,50,87] There is abundant eosinophilic cytoplasm with characteristic large intracytoplasmic hyaline eosinophilic globular inclusions. Rhabdoid tumor is immunoreactive for vimentin, pankeratin, and CD99.

Clear cell sarcoma of the kidney is also known as bone-metastasizing sarcoma of the kidney. Aspirates consist of stellate, spindled and polygonal-shaped cells having pale cytoplasm and round to oval uniform nuclei scattered within mucoid material in the background best appreciated on Romanowsky-stained smears.[35,50]

Mesoblastic nephroma is an infrequent renal congenital tumor that is generally benign. It presents as a well-defined single unilateral abdominal tumor. FNAB shows isolated spindle cells, similar to smooth muscle cells without atypia or mitoses, sometimes forming small bundles with a clean background. The cellular variant has significant cellular atypia and numerous mitoses, mimicking SRCTs, but with clean background.[49] These tumors are immunoreactive for CD34.[45,52] Cystic nephroma yields atypical cells forming papillary clusters which potentially could be misdiagnosed as a renal cell carcinoma.[45,50,88] The cytologic features helpful in making the diagnosis of cystic nephroma include hypocellular smears with relatively few spindle cells without necrosis in an aspirate from a child with a cystic renal mass.[44] Drut also identified benign-appearing epithelial cells arranged individually and in uniform sheets.[88]

Neuroblastoma and malignant lymphoma are the most common secondary malignancies to involve the kidneys. Cytologic features of malignant lymphoma and neuroblastoma are discussed elsewhere in this chapter.

Pancreas

Paediatric pancreatic malignancies are rare. Islet cell tumors are the most common pancreatic tumor in children, in contrast to the dominance of ductal adenocarcinomas in the adult population.[89] The nonendocrine neoplasms in the paediatric age group include the very rare conventional ductal adenocarcinoma, papillary cystic tumor, acinar cell carcinoma and pancreatoblastoma.[89]

Islet cell tumors are capable of producing a variety of peptide hormones leading to a host of clinical syndromes. However, many remain hormonally silent, presenting only as a mass lesion. Aspirates are moderately to highly cellular and are composed of a uniform discohesive population of small to medium-sized cells (Fig. 17.21). Most cells are arranged singly but loose clusters can be seen.[90,91] A notable diagnostic feature is the characteristic plasmacytoid appearance of the cells, showing eccentrically placed nuclei and

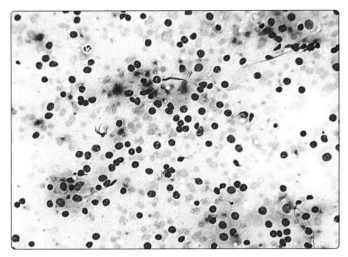

Fig. 17.21 Islet cell tumor This aspirate is dominated by numerous stripped neoplastic nuclei that are singly dispersed. Some of the neoplastic cells have a more abundant granular cytoplasm and eccentrically placed nuclei (Diff-Quik, ×200).

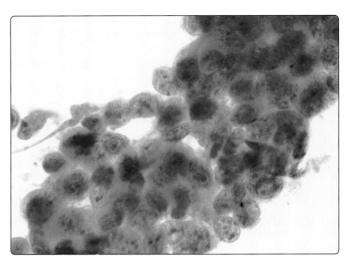

Fig. 17.23 Islet cell tumor Pap-stained smear highlighting the salt and pepper chromatin pattern of neoplastic nuclei (Pap, ×600).

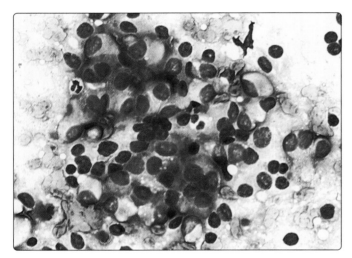

Fig. 17.22 Islet cell tumor A characteristic diagnostic cytologic feature is shown in this aspirate consisting of clusters of neoplastic cells with a plasmacytoid appearance. The nuclei are eccentrically placed with finely granular chromatin and abundant eosinophilic cytoplasm (Diff-Quik, ×400).

moderate amounts of granular basophilic cytoplasm. This is best appreciated in Romanowsky-stained smears (Fig. 17.22). The characteristic 'salt and pepper' chromatin pattern with the lack of prominent nucleoli is seen best in the alcohol-fixed, Papanicolaou-stained smears (Fig. 17.23). Due to the fragility of the cells, naked nuclei and a granular background smear pattern will be present along with occasional delicate blood vessels lined by tumor cells.[90,91] Most cases do not require immunocytochemical confirmation, although occasionally the smear patterns will almost exclusively consist of clusters of cells that can mimic nonendocrine lesions. Neuroendocrine markers such as NSE, CD56, chromogranin and synaptophysin and/or EM examination can be helpful. Positive staining for specific markers such as

insulin, gastrin and somatostatin can be helpful in selected cases.[91]

Pancreatoblastoma is an extremely rare embryonal tumor of childhood with only 60 cases reported in the literature since the tumor was first described.[92] They occur in children between 15 months to 13 years of age. Pancreatoblastomas are more frequent in girls less than 5 years old, and approximately one-third of them produce metastasis. These tumors are usually large and can occur in any portion of the pancreas. The tumors arise from multi-potential stem cells.[89,92] The overall prognosis is favorable. FNA cytology demonstrates cellular smears formed by uniform epithelial cells arranged in organoid structures, often with nests of squamoid cells and keratinization foci. Cells show a moderate amount of granular cytoplasm. Glandular structures of columnar to cuboidal cells with round to oval vesicular nuclei, occasional nucleoli and a moderate amount of granular to foamy cytoplasm are seen in the smears. Spindle-shaped, elongated and triangular epithelial cells, admixed with occasional smaller cells having high nuclear-to-cytoplasmic ratios and denser cytoplasm may be seen (Fig. 17.24).[92,93] Abundant fragments of cellular stroma, some with a peripheral layer of neoplastic epithelial cells, can serve as an important diagnostic clue (Fig. 17.25).[93] Immunocytochemical studies demonstrate positive staining of the epithelial cells for cytokeratin (AE1/3), carcinoembryonic antigen (CEA), α_1-antitrypsin, as well as neuroendocrine markers.[20,92] EM is helpful and reveals cells containing abundant large electron-dense zymogen-like granules measuring 400–600 nm as well as smaller neuroendocrine granules measuring 100–200 nm.[92] Most tumor cells will contain only one type of granule, although occasional cells demonstrate both types.

Papillary-cystic tumor of the pancreas is an uncommon pancreatic neoplasm that occurs almost exclusively in adolescent and young adult females.[94] This low-grade pancreatic malignancy can be cured with surgical resection in most cases, although metastatic disease has been reported.[80] The

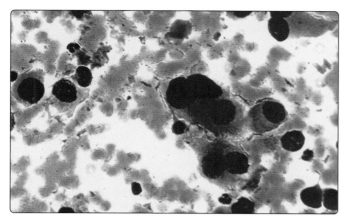

Fig. 17.24 Pancreatoblastoma Aspirate smear showing small clusters and individually scattered cells with irregular nuclear contours and moderate amounts of granular cytoplasm (Diff-Quik, ×400).

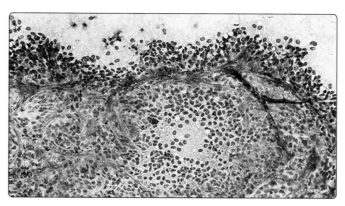

Fig. 17.26 Papillary-cystic tumor of the pancreas Characteristic papillary fronds are seen with fibrovascular stalks lined by a uniform population of neoplastic cells. Individually scattered neoplastic cells are also present in the background (Diff-Quik, ×200).

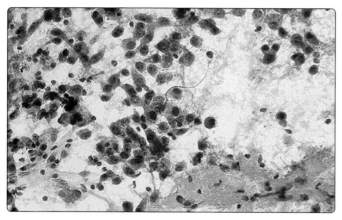

Fig. 17.25 Pancreatoblastoma This aspirate highlights the variability of cellular contours with round, oval, triangular, and spindled cells with vesicular nuclei and prominent nucleoli (Pap, ×200).

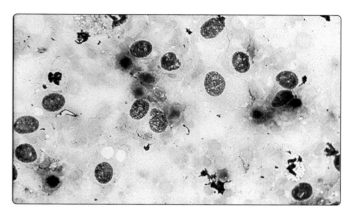

Fig. 17.27 Papillary-cystic tumor of the pancreas The neoplastic cells contain evenly dispersed finely granular chromatin and nuclear grooves or folds (Diff-Quik, ×400).

characteristic cytologic features of papillary-cystic tumor are the presence of papillary fronds that consist of fibrovascular stalks lined by a uniform population of small cells along with individually scattered and small clusters of similar-appearing cells (Figs 17.26 and 17.27). The neoplastic cells possess oval nuclei with finely granular chromatin, characteristic longitudinal nuclear grooves, inconspicuous to small nucleoli and moderate amounts of cytoplasm.[94,95] Occasional cases may demonstrate reddish-pink hyaline globules in the Romanowsky stains.

Gonads

Epithelial tumors of the ovary account for only 15–20% of all ovarian childhood neoplasms, with germ cell tumors involving the ovary in up to one-third of paediatric cases.[95] Benign cystic teratomas account for 30–90% of germ cell tumors followed by a variety of other germ cell tumors.[16] Aspirates of benign cystic teratoma are of variable cellularity containing benign-appearing epithelial and mesenchymal

components derived from the three germinal layers.[96] As would be expected, squamous cells, choroid and glial tissue, cartilage and glandular cells can be present.[67] In immature teratoma, primitive neuroblastic small cells resembling distinct nests of SRCTs are also present.[97] Yolk sac tumors are rare and may be a challenge to the cytopathologist on FNA. Yolk sac tumors can have a variety of patterns including groups of malignant cells that are arranged in papillary, glandular or large pleomorphic tumor balls.[81] The cytoplasm of the neoplastic cells can contain small or large vacuoles. A helpful diagnostic feature is the presence of eosinophilic inclusions within the cytoplasm of some of the tumor cells as well as basement membrane material in the background that is best seen in the Diff-Quik stain.[96,98] Well-defined cytoplasmic vacuoles corresponding to intracytoplasmic deposits of glycogen, as well as nuclear vacuoles within the malignant cells have been identified.[98] Positive immunohistochemical studies for alpha fetoprotein, cytokeratins AE1/AE3, and CAM 5.2 are useful in supporting the diagnosis.[81]

Seminomas and dysgerminomas yield highly cellular aspirates composed of both loose clusters and individually

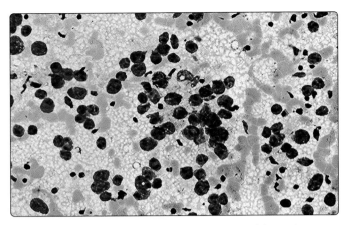

Fig. 17.28 Seminoma Highly cellular aspirate smear with loose clusters and individually scattered neoplastic cells with round nuclei containing finely granular chromatin and a prominent single nucleolus. Note the characteristic 'tigroid' background (Diff-Quik, ×200).

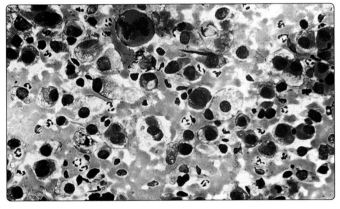

Fig. 17.29 Embryonal carcinoma Numerous pleomorphic neoplastic cells with coarsely clumped chromatin, multiple nucleoli, and variable amounts of granular cytoplasm (Diff-Quik, ×400).

scattered round tumor cells with round nuclei containing finely granular chromatin and a prominent single nucleolus (Fig. 17.28).[96] A moderate to abundant amount of cytoplasm can be present and PAS-positive cytoplasmic vacuoles are often seen. The smear background contains chronic inflammatory cells with occasional granulomas. Due to the spillage of the glycogen-rich cytoplasm, a characteristic 'tigroid' background can be appreciated and serves as a useful diagnostic clue (Fig. 17.28). In contrast, embryonal carcinoma consists of large three-dimensional clusters of tumor cells with indistinct cell boundaries. Papillary and glandular clusters may contain delicate branching blood vessels. The neoplastic cells show pleomorphism with coarsely granular chromatin and multiple prominent nucleoli (Fig. 17.29). As previously mentioned, FNA biopsy of the testicle has also been used to document relapse of acute lymphoblastic leukemia in children and could be considered as an alternative procedure to surgical biopsy.[71,76,99]

Thorax

Fine needle aspiration of the lung has been used in the work-up of acute pneumonias in children.[25] However, based on our experience, FNA of the lung is most often performed to document metastatic malignancies and/or lung abscesses.[24] The most common benign lung masses in the paediatric age group are inflammatory pseudotumor, lung sequestration, and hamartoma.[20,100] Primary lung malignancies are exceedingly uncommon in childhood.[20] Paediatric pulmonary malignancies that can present as primary intrathoracic tumors include primary neuroblastoma, teratoma, malignant lymphoma and adenocarcinoma of fetal type.[99]

Inflammatory pseudotumor (inflammatory myofibroblastic tumor) is the most frequent pulmonary tumor of children older than 5 years. It can represent as a single, round well-defined lesion measuring between 3 and 10 cm. FNA smears are slightly cellular, showing spindle cells with a fibroblastic proliferation, placed in an isolated fashion and/or small bands. Fragments of collagen and inflammatory cells can appear, especially lymphocytes, plasmocytes, and macrophages.[1,45] The background is often clean.[1]

Pulmonary blastoma is rare and most frequent in children older than 12 years. It can be associated with medulloblastoma, ovarian teratoma, leukemias, Hodgkin lymphoma, and germ cell malignancies. Pulmonary blastoma metastasizes in 25% of cases, especially to the brain, spinal cord, and bones. There have also been rare FNA case reports of pulmonary blastoma and pleuropulmonary blastoma.[18] Both of these neoplasms demonstrate the presence of undifferentiated cells, but pleuropulmonary blastoma also has an admixture of mesenchymal cells. Due to the rarity of many of these malignancies, tissue confirmation is often needed to make a definitive diagnosis.

Lymph nodes

Aspiration biopsies of benign and malignant disorders involving the lymph nodes are presented in detail elsewhere in this book and will be only briefly covered in this section. In children, lymph nodes, especially in the head and neck region, serve as one of the sites most commonly aspirated by FNA. The majority of lymph node enlargements are benign due to hyperplasia. However, it is important to emphasize that specific malignant lymphomas show a marked predilection in the paediatric population and must always remain in the differential diagnosis of lymphadenopathy. Aspirate smears from reactive lymph nodes generally show a dissociated cell population and moderate to high smear cellularity in the majority of cases. However, follicular center cell fragments as well as granulomatous inflammation can yield predominant cell clusters. Identification of a predominant cell type and a monomorphic cell population can be helpful in separating benign from malignant lesions. A heterogeneous cell population with predominance of small mature lymphoid cells is typically seen in benign processes. Lymphoglandular bodies which represent cytoplasmic fragments are a consistent background element in aspirates from lymph nodes and serve as an important diagnostic clue in identifying the lymphoid origin of lesions that can be either benign or malignant. These are best appreciated on Romanowsky-stained smears and stain blue to blue–gray, but can also be appreciated in the Papanicolaou preparation.

The more common reactive lesions include acute lymphadenitis, granulomatous lymphadenitis, infectious mononucleosis and reactive lymph node hyperplasia.[43] With infectious processes, either a single lymph node or a group of nodes (i.e. cervical chain) may be involved. Smears that demonstrate sheets of neutrophils with associated bacteria and/or necrosis signify an acute suppurative lymphadenitis (Fig. 17.30). Occasionally, smears can demonstrate fungal organisms; therefore, histochemical stains for fungal, mycobacterial, and bacterial organisms should be performed and material should be obtained with additional passes for microbiological cultures. In some cases of mycobacterial infection, Romanowsky-stained smears demonstrate the presence of 'negative images' of the mycobacteria which do not stain, and this can serve as an important diagnostic clue (Fig. 17.31).

The head and neck is the most common site of involvement for granulomatous lymphadenitis. Granulomas can be either necrotizing or non-necrotizing. Smears demonstrate variable cellularity with tightly clustered groups of epithelioid histiocytes containing characteristic bent or 'boomerang-shaped' nuclei (Fig. 17.32). Associated necrosis and acute inflammation can be seen in necrotizing granulomatous lymphadenitis for which the etiological agents include cat scratch disease, mycobacteria, tularemia, brucellosis, and fungi, among others. Infectious mononucleosis is caused by Epstein-Barr virus (EBV) and is a self-limited disorder predominantly affecting adolescents. Enlarged cervical lymph nodes are most often aspirated and the smears are highly cellular, containing a heterogeneous lymphoid cell population with the presence of numerous immunoblasts (Figs 17.33 and 17.34).45 However, confirmatory serologic testing is needed, with most patients demonstrating positive antibody titers for various antibodies specific for EBV.

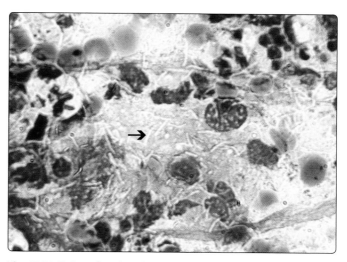

Fig. 17.31 Tuberculous lymphadenitis Romanowsky-stained smears demonstrate abundant 'negative images' of mycobacterial organisms (*arrow*) (Diff-Quik, ×600).

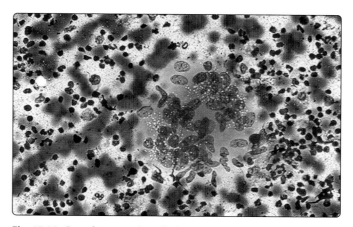

Fig. 17.32 Granulomatous lymphadenitis This smear shows a well-formed epithelioid granuloma. The epithelioid histiocytes are round to elongated with curved or bent 'boomerang-shaped' nuclei that contain finely reticulated cytoplasm. The background contains abundant neutrophils (Diff-Quik, ×400).

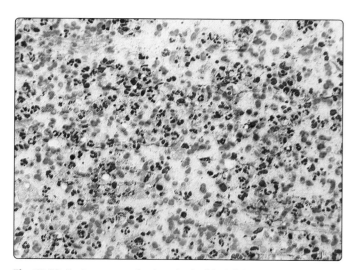

Fig. 17.30 Acute suppurative lymphadenitis Cellular smear demonstrating numerous neutrophils with associated necrotic debris in the background (Diff-Quik, ×200).

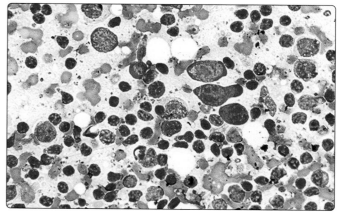

Fig. 17.33 Infectious mononucleosis This highly cellular smear contains a heterogeneous lymphoid population with prominent immunoblasts and plasmacytoid cells (Diff-Quik, ×400).

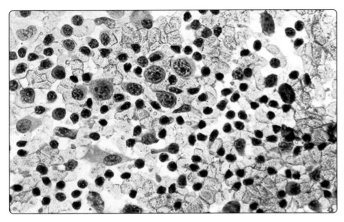

Fig. 17.34 **Infectious mononucleosis** In Papanicolaou-stained smears, the cellular elements appear more uniform in size but are still dominated by increased numbers of immunoblasts which contain irregularly clumped chromatin, prominent nucleoli and moderate amounts of granular cytoplasm (Pap, ×200).

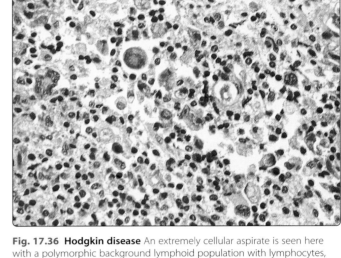

Fig. 17.36 **Hodgkin disease** An extremely cellular aspirate is seen here with a polymorphic background lymphoid population with lymphocytes, eosinophils, plasma cells and histiocytes, amongst which are scattered larger atypical Reed-Sternberg cell variants (Diff-Quik, ×200).

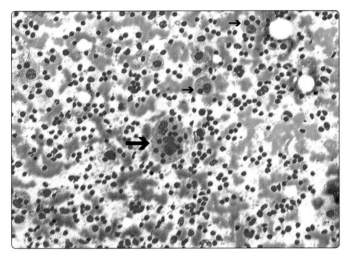

Fig. 17.35 **Rosai-Dorfman disease** Highly cellular smears contain a mixture of small and large lymphocytes. The diagnostic feature of abundant histiocytes demonstrating emperipolesis is shown here (*arrows*) with the cytoplasm of histiocytes containing phagocytosed lymphocytes (Diff-Quik, ×200).

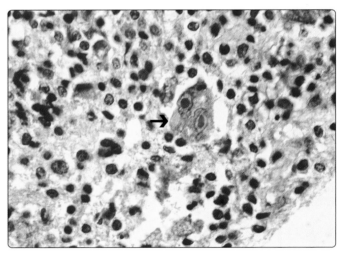

Fig. 17.37 **Hodgkin disease** A classic Reed-Sternberg cell is shown here (*arrow*) with two relatively uniform nuclei containing finely reticulated chromatin and massive nucleoli. A moderate amount of cytoplasm is present (Diff-Quik, ×400).

Rosai-Dorfman disease (sinus histiocytosis) presents with lymphadenopathy involving the cervical lymph nodes of young children, and has a predilection for blacks. The etiology is unknown. Unlike the infection-related lymphadenopathies, node enlargement is often massive, bilateral, and painless. Aspirate smears reveal features of reactive hyperplasia with a heterogeneous cell population. Increased numbers of accompanying histiocytes demonstrating emperipolesis (engulfment of red blood cells and lymphocytes) are seen throughout the smears and serve as an important differentiating feature to separate Rosai-Dorfman disease from other reactive hyperplasias (Fig. 17.35).[45] These histiocytes also demonstrate positive staining for S-100.

Hodgkin lymphoma is relatively common in older children and adolescents and rare before the age of 5 years.

Nodular sclerosis is the most common subtype. The cellularity of smears varies from low to intermediate in most cases, depending on the degree of sclerosis present. Smears demonstrate a picture similar to reactive hyperplasias; therefore, a diligent search for Reed-Sternberg cells and its mononuclear variants is necessary for an accurate diagnosis (Figs 17.36 and 17.37).[45] Immunostaining can be helpful as the Reed-Sternberg cells express both CD15 and CD30 and are negative for CD45 and CD20, while anaplastic large cell lymphoma shows positive staining for CD30, CD45 and ALK, along with negative staining for CD15.[45,74]

The small noncleaved malignant lymphomas (Burkitt and non-Burkitt type) and lymphoblastic lymphomas have been discussed previously in this chapter.

Soft tissues and bone

There are a great variety of soft tissue tumors in children, such as hamartomas, inflammatory tumors, reactive proliferative tumors, and benign or malignant neoplasms. Infantile soft tissue tumors differ from those of adults in frequency, location, histologic type, and prognosis; the majority are benign, and only 7–10% are malignant. Rhabdomyosarcoma, malignant fibrohistiocytomas, PNET and undifferentiated sarcomas account for >80% of malignant soft tissue tumors.[1,100]

The separation of benign from malignant lesions of soft tissue and bone by FNA can often be accomplished with high diagnostic accuracy, thereby facilitating expeditious and proper patient triage and therapeutic management. FNA is increasingly being used as the diagnostic modality of choice for a first-time diagnosis of lesions from both soft tissues and bone. FNA in conjunction with ancillary techniques can afford a diagnostic accuracy of 70–90%, comparable to open and core biopsy techniques. The reported false-positive and false-negative rates range from less than 1% to 4% for adequate specimens.[27] As emphasized throughout this chapter, a multidisciplinary approach and the presence of an on-site pathologist for immediate evaluation and appropriate triage for ancillary studies at the time of biopsy are crucial for rendering an accurate diagnosis. Otherwise, core needle biopsy and/or open biopsy may be preferable. For bone lesions to be accessible by FNA, soft tissue extension and/or cortical bone destruction needs to be present. Sclerotic tumors such as osteoma, osteoid osteoma, osteoblastoma, low-grade osteosarcoma, fibrous dysplasia, and low-grade chondrosarcoma are not adequately sampled by FNA under most circumstances.[21]

Some benign soft tissue spindle cell lesions are unique to childhood and include fibrous hamartoma of infancy, fibromatosis colli, and infantile digital fibromatosis. Fibromatosis colli, also called sternocleidomastoid tumor of infancy, occurs at all ages in the region of the sternocleidomastoid muscle. Myofibroma/myofibromatosis (congenital fibromatosis) is rare but seen most commonly in infancy and children less than 2 years of age. Clinically, this lesion is rapidly growing and the differential diagnosis includes nodular fasciitis and fibrosarcoma. FNA of benign soft tissue spindle cell lesions shows paucicellular smears with bland loosely cohesive spindle cells and isolated bare oval nuclei. All of these lesions are fibroblastic/myofibroblastic in origin; therefore, ancillary studies such as immunohistochemistry and EM are of little aid to establish the diagnosis. However, both fasciitis and fibrosarcoma usually produce relatively cellular specimens.[100–102]

An extremely uncommon benign tumor, the fetal rhabdomyoma, almost always occurs in children 3 years of age or younger as a mass lesion in the head and neck region.[45] These are slow-growing lesions. Fine needle aspirates show immature muscle fibers with multiple nuclei and transverse striation and arranged in lobulated bundles. The presence of cellular atypia and hypercellularity may suggest a rhabdomyosarcoma.

Osteosarcoma is the most common primary bone malignancy in children, peaking in adolescence (80% of cases) with a slight male predominance. The majority are sporadic, and about 20% of patients develop bone or lung metastasis.

Osteosarcoma can have various subtypes which are all linked by the production of osteoid/bone by the malignant cells. Conventional osteosarcoma represents the vast majority of all osteosarcoma (80–90%).[21,103] The metaphyseal regions of the long bones are most commonly affected, followed in decreasing order by: distal femur, proximal tibia, and proximal humerus. Radiographically, this is a permeative lesion associated with a lytic/sclerotic reaction, and soft tissue extension is commonly seen. Therefore, most osteosarcomas are amenable to FNA with an accuracy rate for establishing a diagnosis exceeding 90%.[103] Smears demonstrate moderate to high cellularity with small aggregates and singly scattered polygonal cells with a plasmacytoid appearance, one or more nucleoli, and abundant cytoplasm (Figs 17.38 and 17.39). On Romanowsky-stained smears, metachromatic matrix material compatible with osteoid is present, associated with the malignant cells (Fig. 17.40).[103] Small cell osteosarcoma is composed of mostly discohesive, oval to round cells with high nuclear to cytoplasmic ratios, and inconspicuous to prominent nucleoli, mimicking EWS/PNET. However, osteosarcoma shows more cells variation than

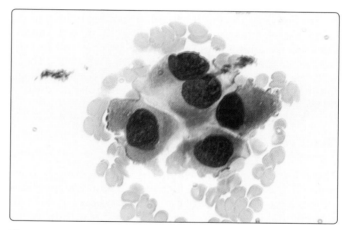

Fig. 17.38 Osteosarcoma This smear demonstrates a small aggregate of polygonal cells with a plasmacytoid appearance and abundant granular cytoplasm (Diff-Quik, ×400).

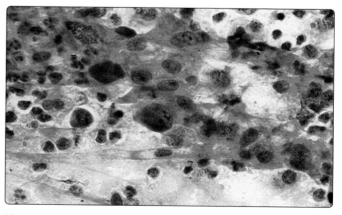

Fig. 17.39 Osteosarcoma A highly cellular smear is shown here with pleomorphic tumor cells embedded in a collagenous matrix. Marked cellular and nuclear variability is seen among the neoplastic cells (Pap, ×400).

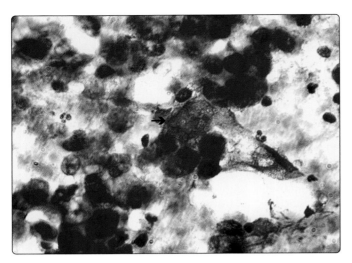

Fig. 17.40 Osteosarcoma On Romanowsky-stained smears, metachromatically staining osteoid is seen intimately associated with the neoplastic cells (*arrow*) (Diff-Quik, ×600).

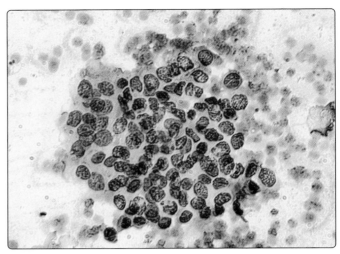

Fig. 17.41 Chondroblastoma Aspirates demonstrate a monomorphic population of singly dispersed and loosely cohesive cell clusters. The chondroblasts contain solitary ovoid nuclei with finely granular chromatin, inconspicuous nucleoli, and nuclear grooves (Diff-Quik, ×400).

Ewing's sarcoma, with osteoid formation. There is no reliable immunohistochemical pattern of staining to help in the diagnosis of osteosarcoma, including small cell variant. Occasional staining with CD99 has been observed in osteosarcoma, adding to the confusion with EWS/PNET. Therefore, the diagnosis rests primarily on the cytomorphologic findings and the identification of osteoid/bone production by the malignant cells.[104]

Giant cell tumors

These are infrequent in children (<5% of primary bone tumors), often located in the distal femur and proximal region of the tibia (>50% of cases). X-rays show an osteolytic subchondral lesion. Microscopically, it is formed by mononuclear cells with oval or spindled nuclei grouped in solid masses and numerous osteoclast-like cells arranged in a diffuse fashion. Giant cells have numerous nuclei that look like those of mononuclear cells. There are few mitoses, high vascularization, hemorrhagic and necrotic foci, and macrophages with hemosiderin and/or foamy histiocytes.[105] FNA smears show two cell types: disperse histiocytoid mononuclear and/or three-dimensional aggregates and giant multinucleated osteoclast-like cells. Hemosiderin-containing macrophages can often be observed.[1,104]

Chondroblastomas are seen most often in the first and second decade of life, with a male predominance. They occur predominantly in the epiphyseal and epimetaphyseal regions of long bones, the proximal and distal femur, tibia and proximal humerus. FNA smears are generally hypercellular with sheets and individually scattered uniform round to polygonal cells with nuclei displaying prominent longitudinal grooves and inconspicuous nucleoli similar to those seen in Langerhans cell histiocytosis (Fig. 17.41).[105] Chondroid matrix material is arranged in lobules and plates recapitulating mature cartilage and is best seen on Romanowsky-stained smears. Associated multinucleated giant cells can be seen (Fig. 17.42). The cells are positive for S-100 and vimentin

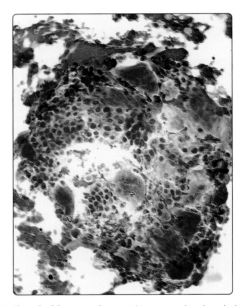

Fig. 17.42 Chondroblastoma Scattered amongst the chondroblasts are variable numbers of osteoclast-like giant cells which contain nuclei resembling those seen in the mononuclear chondroblastic cells (Diff-Quik, ×200).

and occasionally positive for cytokeratin.[104] Simple curettage is the treatment of choice.

As in adults, metastases to bone are far more common than primary malignant bone tumors. Lymphoreticular metastases and those from neuroblastoma are most common in children.

Pilomatrixoma

Pilomatrixoma is the most frequent benign tumor of the pilosebaceous unit, often affecting children younger than 10 years, forming a hard and well-defined nodule in the skin of the head and neck.[106] The diagnosis of pilomatrixoma by FNAC can frequently pose a diagnostic dilemma to cytopathologists. Classically, the presence of cohesive epithelial clusters with basaloid features and ghost cells are diagnostic; however, both of these components may not always be apparent in the aspirate smears.[106] SRCTs can also enter into the differential diagnosis when ghost cells are not appreciated. When pilomatrixomas occur in the salivary gland region, other basaloid neoplasms enter into the differential diagnosis, such as adenoid cystic carcinoma, monomorphic adenoma, and pleomorphic adenoma.[106] However, knowledge of the superficial location and other cytologic clues such as multinucleated giant cells, calcification, and keratin debris as well as the lack of stroma can aid in the diagnosis. Cell block preparations aid in the diagnosis of

pilomatrixoma, as ghost cells become more apparent on cell block sections.[106]

Thyroid

Fine needle aspiration (FNA) of the thyroid is seldom performed in the paediatric population. Therefore, the clinical utility of thyroid FNA in this patient group has not been adequately addressed. Thyroid nodules are relatively common in adolescents, with prevalence ranging from 0.2% to 1.8%.[107] Although most of these nodules are benign, malignant tumors, particularly papillary carcinomas, are known to occur in this age group.[108] FNA biopsy of thyroid nodules in young patients has similar high sensitivity and specificity as the procedure in the adult population.[107,108]

References

1. Schalper JA. Paediatric Tumours. In: Bibbo M, Wilbur D, editors. Comprehensive Cytopathology. 3rd ed. Saunders Elsvier Publisher; 2008. Chapter 29. p. 915–50.

2. Grovas A, Fremgen A, Rauck A, et al. The National Cancer Data Base Report on Patterns of Childhood Cancers in the United States. Cancer 1997;80: 2321–32.

3. Buchino JJ. Cytopathology in Paediatrics. In: Wied GL, editor. Monographs in Clinical Cytology. Basel: Karger; 1991. p. 1–7, 13.

4. Dave B, Shet T, Ramadwar M, et al. Cytologic evaluation of head and neck tumours in children – A pattern analysis. Diagn Cytopathol 2006;34: 434–46.

5. Cohen MB, Bottles K, Ablin AR, et al. The use of fine-needle aspiration biopsy in children. West J Med 1989;150:665–7.

6. Rajwanshi A, Rao KL, Marwaha RK, et al. Role of fine-needle aspiration cytology in childhood malignancies. Diagn Cytopathol 1989;5:378–82.

7. Taylor SR, Nunez C. Fine-needle aspiration biopsy in a population. Report of 64 consecutive cases. Cancer 1984;54:1449–53.

8. Wakely PE, Kardos TF, Frable WJ. Application of fine needle aspiration biopsy to paediatrics. Human Pathol 1988;19:1383–6.

9. Silverman JF, Gurley AM, Holbrook CT, et al. Paediatric fine-needle aspiration biopsy. Am J Clin Pathol 1991;95: 653–9.

10. McGahey BE, Moriarty AT, Nelson WA, et al. Fine needle aspiration biopsy of small round blue cell tumours of childhood. Cancer 1992;69:1067–73.

11. Gorczyca W, Bedner E, Juszkiewicz P, et al. Aspiration cytology in the diagnosis of malignant tumours in children. Am J Pediatr Hematol Oncol 1992;14:129–35.

12. Akhtar M, Ali MA, Sabbah R, et al. Fine-needle aspiration biopsy diagnosis of round cell malignant tumours of childhood. A combined light and electron microscopic approach. Cancer 1985;55:1805–17.

13. Diament MJ, Stanley P, Taylor SR. Percutaneous fine needle biopsy in paediatrics. Pediatr Radiol 1985;15: 409–11.

14. Verdeguer A, Castel V, Torres V, et al. Fine-needle aspiration biopsy in children: experience in 70 cases. Med Pediatr Oncol 1988;16:98–100.

15. Layfield LJ, Reichman A. Fine needle aspiration cytology: utilization in paediatric pathology. Dis Markers 1990;8:301–15.

16. Layfield LJ, Glasgow B, Ostrzega N, et al. Fine-needle aspiration cytology and the diagnosis of neoplasms in the paediatric age group. Diagn Cytopathol 1991;7:451–61.

17. Obers VJ, Phillips JI. Fine needle aspiration of paediatric abdominal masses. Cytologic and electron microscopic diagnosis. Acta Cytol 1991;35:165–70.

18. Valkov I, Boijkin B. Fine-needle aspiration biopsy of abdominal and retroperitoneal tumours in infants and children. Diagn Cytopathol 1987; 3:129–33.

19. Shakoor KA. Fine needle aspiration cytology in advanced paediatric tumours. Pediatr Pathol 1989;9: 713–18.

20. Geisinger KR, Silverman JF, Wakely PE Jr. Paediatric cytopathology. Chicago: American Society of Clinical Pathologists; 1994.

21. Kilpatrick SE, Ward WG, Chauvenet AR, et al. The role of fine-needle aspiration biopsy in the initial diagnosis of paediatric bone and soft tissue tumours: an institutional experience. Mod Pathol 1998;11:923–8.

22. Pohar-Marinsek Z. Difficulties in diagnosing small round cell tumours of childhood from fine needle aspiration cytology samples. Review Article. Cytopathology 2008;19:67–79.

23. Howell LP. Changing role of fine-needle aspiration in the evaluation of paediatric masses. Diagn Cytopathol 2001;24:65–70.

24. Eisenhut CC, King DE, Nelson WA, et al. Fine-needle biopsy of paediatric lesions: a three-year study in an outpatient biopsy clinic. Diagn Cytopathol 1996;14:43–50.

25. Layfield LJ. Fine-needle aspiration biopsy in the diagnosis of paediatric tumours. West J Med 1991;154:90–1.

26. Akhtar M, Iqbal MA, Mourad W, et al. Fine-needle aspiration biopsy diagnosis of small round cell tumours of childhood: A comprehensive approach. Diagn Cytopathol 1999;21:81–91.

27. Singh HK, Kilpatrick SE, Silverman JF. Fine needle aspiration biopsy of soft tissue sarcomas: utility and diagnostic challenges. Adv Anat Pathol 2004;11: 24–37.

28. Silverman JF, Joshi VV. FNA biopsy of small round cell tumours of childhood: cytomorphologic features and the role of ancillary studies. Diagn Cytopathol 1994;10:245–55.

29. Gautam U, Srinivasan R, Rajwanshi A, et al. Comparative evaluation of flow-cytometric immunophenotyping and immunocytochemistry in the categorization of malignant small round cell tumours in fine-needle aspiration cytologic specimens. Cancer (Cytopathology) 2008;114: 494–503.

30. Gurley AM, Silverman JF, Lassaletta MM, et al. The utility of ancillary studies in paediatric FNA cytology. Diagn Cytopathol 1992;8:137–46.

31. Plasschaert SLA, Willem AK, Vellenga E, et al. Prognosis in childhood and adult

lymphoblastic leukemia: a question of maturation? Cancer Treat Rev 2004;30: 37–51.

32. Brahim U, Srinivasan R, Komal HS, et al. Comparative analysis of electron microscopy and immunocytochemistry in the cytologic diagnosis of malignant small round cell tumours. Acta Cytol 2003;47:443–9.

33. Leon ME, How JS, Galindo LM, et al. Fine needle aspiration of adult small-round-cell tumours studies with flow cytometry. Diagn Cytopathol 2004;31:147–54.

34. Layfield LJ, Liu K, Dodge RK. Logistic regression analysis of small round cell neoplasms: a cytologic study. Diagn Cytopathol 1999;20:271–7.

35. Joshi VV, Silverman JF, Alshuler G, et al. Systematization of primary histopathologic and fine-needle aspiration cytologic features and description of unusual histopathologic features of neuroblastic tumours: a report from the Paediatric Oncology Group. Human Pathol 1993;24:493–504.

36. Stephenson CF, Bridge JA, Sandberg AA. Cytogenetic and pathologic aspects of Ewing's sarcoma and neuroectodermal tumours. Human Pathol 1992;23:1270–7.

37. Triche TJ, Askin FB. Neuroblastoma and the differential diagnosis of small-, round- blue-cell tumours. Human Pathol 1983;14:569–95.

38. Triche TJ, Askin FB, Kissane JM. Neuroblastoma, Ewing's sarcoma, and the differential diagnosis of small-, round-, blue-cell tumours. In: Finegold M, editor. Pathology of neoplasms in children and adolescents. Philadelphia: Saunders; 1986. p. 145–95.

39. Shimada H, Chatten J, Newton WA Jr, et al. Histopathologic prognostic factors in neuroblastic tumours: definition of subtypes of ganglioneuroblastoma and age-linked classification of neuroblastomas. J Natl Cancer Inst 1984;73:405.

40. Frostad B, Martinsson T, Tani E, et al. The use of fine-needle aspiration cytology in the molecular characterization of neuroblastoma in children. Cancer 1999;87:60–8.

41. Thiesse P, Hany MA, Combaret V, et al. Assessment of percutaneous fine needle aspiration cytology as a technique to provide diagnostic and prognostic information in neuroblastoma. Eur J Cancer 2000;36:1544–51.

42. Silverman JF, Dabbs DJ, Ganick DH, et al. Fine needle aspiration cytology of neuroblastoma, including peripheral neuroectodermal tumour, with immunohistochemical and ultrastructural confirmation. Acta Cytol 1988;32:367–76.

43. Sebire NJ, Gibson S, Rampling D, et al. Immunohistochemical findings in embryonal small round cell tumours with molecular diagnostic confirmation. Appl Immunohistochem Mol Morphol 2005;13:1–5.

44. Barroca H, Carvalho JL, da Costa MJ, et al. Detection of N-myc amplification in neuroblastomas using Southern blotting on fine needle aspirates. Acta Cytol 2001;45:169–72.

45. Geisinger KR, Stanley MW, Raab SS, et al. Liver, Kidney, Lymph node and spleen. Modern cytopathology. Philadelphia: Churchill Livingstone; 2004. p. 505–42, 579–618, 643–687.

46. Barroca H. Nephroblastoma is a success of paediatric oncologic therapy. How further can we go? Results of a cyt-histologic correlation study. Diagn Cytopathology 2009.

47. Bray GL, Pendergrass TW, Schaller RTJ, et al. Preoperative chemotherapy in the treatment of Wilms' tumour diagnosed with the aid of fine needle aspiration biopsy. Am J Pediatr Hematol Oncol 1986;8:75–8.

48. Geisinger KR, Wakely PE Jr, Wofford MM. Unresectable stage IV nephroblastoma. A potential indication for fine-needle aspiration biopsy in children. Diagn Cytopathol 1993;9: 197–201.

49. Sarinen UM, Wilkstrom S, Korkimies O, et al. Percutaneous needle biopsy preceeding preoperative chemotherapy; the management of massive renal tumours in children. J Clin Oncol 1991;9:406–15.

50. Ravindra S, Kini S. Cytomorphology and morphometry of small round-cell tumours in the region of the kidney. Diagn Cytopathol 2005;32:211–16.

51. Serrano R, Rodriguez-Peralto JL, De Orbe GG, et al. Intrarenal neuroblastoma diagnosed by fine-needle aspiration: a report of two cases. Diagn Cytopathol 2002;27:294–7.

52. Schmidt D, Beckwith JB. Histopathology of childhood renal tumours. Hematol Oncol Clin North Am 1995;9:1179–2000.

53. Silverman JF, Berns LA, Holbrook CT, et al. Fine needle aspiration cytology of primitive neuroectodermal tumours. A report of three cases. Acta Cytol 1992;36:541–50.

54. Kilpatrick SE, Renner J. Small round cell tumours of bone and soft tissues. In: Kilpatrick SE, editor. Diagnostic musculoskeletal surgical pathology with clinicopathologic and cytologic correlations. Philadelphia: Saunders; 2003. p. 37–70.

55. Sanati S, Lu DW, Schmidt E, et al. Cytologic diagnosis of Ewing sarcoma/ peripheral neuroectodermal tumour with paired prospective molecular genetic analysis. Cancer (Cytopathology) 2007;111:192–9.

56. Folpe AL, Goldblum JR, Rubin BP, et al. Morphologic and immunophenotypic diversity in Ewing family tumours: a study of 66 genetically confirmed cases. Am J Surg Pathol 2005;29:1025–33.

57. Frostad B, Tani E, Brosjo O, et al. Fine needle aspiration cytology in the diagnosis and management of children and adolescents with Ewing sarcoma and peripheral primitive neuroectodermal tumour. Med Pediatr Oncol 2002;38:33–40.

58. Newton WAJ, Gehan EA, Webber BL, et al. Classification of rhabdomyosarcomas and related sarcomas, pathologic aspects and proposal for a new classification – an Intergroup Rhabdomyosarcoma Study. Cancer 1995;76:1073–85.

59. Wang NP, Marx J, McNutt MA, et al. Expression of myogenic regulatory proteins (myogenin and MyoD1) in small blue cell tumours of childhood. Am J Pathol 1995;147:1799–810.

60. Pohar-Marinsek Z, Bracko M. Rhabdomyosarcoma: cytomorphology, subtyping and differential diagnostic dilemmas. Acta Cytol 2000;44: 524–32.

61. Klijanienko J, Caillaud JM, Orbach D, et al. Cyto-histologic correlations in primary, recurrent and metastatic rhabdomyosarcoma: The Institute Curie's Experience. Diagn Cytopathol 2007;35:482–7.

62. Atahan S, Aksu O, Ekinci C. Cytologic diagnosis and subtyping of rhabdomyosarcoma. Cytopathology 1998;9:389–97.

63. Morotti RA, Nicol KK, Parham DM, et al. Children's Oncology Group. An Immunohistochemical algorithm to facilitate diagnosis and subtyping of rhabdomyosarcoma: the Children's Oncology Group Experience. Am J Surg Pathol 2006;30:962–8.

64. Kilpatrick SE, Renner J. Epithelioid/ polygonal cell tumours. In: Kilpatrick SE, editor. Diagnostic musculoskeletal surgical pathology with clinicopathologic and cytologic correlations. Philadelphia: Saunders; 2003. p. 71–96.

65. Layfield LJ, Lenarsky C. Desmoplastic small cell tumours of the peritoneum coexpressing mesenchymal and epithelial markers. Am J Clin Pathol 1991;96:536–43.

66. Ali SZ, Nicol TL, Port J, et al. Intraabdominal desmoplastic small round cell tumour: cytopathologic findings in two cases. Diagn Cytopathol 1998;18:449–52.

67. Ordi J, de Alava E, Torne A, et al. Intraabdominal desmoplastic small round cell tumour with EWS/ERG fusion transcript. Am J Surg Pathol 1998;22:1026–32.

68. Granja NM, Brgnami MD, Bortolan J, et al. Desmoplastic small round cell tumour: Cytological and

immunocytochemical features. Case
report. CytoJournal 2005;2:1–6.

69. Roberts P, Burchill SA, Beddow RA,
et al. A combined cytogenetic and
molecular approach to diagnosis in a
case of desmoplastic small round cell
tumour with a complex translocation
(11;22;21). Cancer Genet Cytogenet
1999;108:19–25.

70. Ferlicot S, Coue O, Gilbert E, et al.
Intraabdominal desmoplastic small
round cell tumour: report of a case
with fine needle aspiration, cytologic
diagnosis and molecular confirmation.
Acta Cytol 2001;45:617–21.

71. Mora J, Fillipa DA, Qin J, et al.
Lymphoblastic lymphoma of childhood
and the LSA2-L2 Protocol; The 30 year
experience at Memorial Sloan-Kettering
Cancer Center. Cancer 2003;98:
1283–91.

72. Hameed M. Small round cell tumours
of bone. Arch Pathol Lab med 2007;
131:192–204.

73. Zhao XF, Young KH, Frank D, et al.
Paediatric primary bone lymphoma-
diffuse large B-cell lymphoma:
morphologic and
immunohistochemical characteristics
of 10 cases. Am J Clin Pathol
2007;127:47–54.

74. McManus AP, Gusterson BA, Pinkenton
R, et al. The molecular pathology of
small round cell tumours – relevance to
diagnosis, prognosis, and classification.
J Pathol 1996;178:116–21.

75. Rapkiewicz A, Le BT, Simsir A, et al.
Spectrum of head and neck lesions
diagnosed by fine needle aspiration
cytology in the paediatric population.
Cancer (Cytopathology) 2007;111:
242–51.

76. Akhtar M, Ali MA, Burgess A, et al.
Fine-needle aspiration biopsy (FNAB)
diagnosis of testicular involvement in
acute lymphoblastic leukemia in
children. Diagn Cytopathol 1991;7:
504–7.

77. Perez JS, Perez-Guillermo M, Bernal AB,
et al. Hepatoblastoma: An attempt to
apply histologic classification to
aspirates obtained by fine needle
aspiration cytology. Acta Cytol 1994;
38:175–82.

78. Douglass EC. Hepatic malignancies in
childhood and adolescence
(hepatoblastoma, hepatocellular
carcinoma, and embryonal sarcoma).
Cancer Treat Res 1997;92:201–12.

79. Schnater JM, Kohler SE, Lamers WH,
et al. Where do we stand with
hepatoblastoma? Cancer 2003;98:
668–78.

80. Wakely PEJ, Silverman JF, Geisinger KR,
et al. Fine needle aspiration biopsy
cytology of hepatoblastoma. Mod
Pathol 1990;3:688–93.

81. Gilbert KL, Bergman S, Dodd LG, et al.
Cytomorphology of yolk sac tumour
of the liver in fine-needle aspiration:

A paediatric case. Diagn Cytopathol
2006;34:421–3.

82. Klijanienko J, Caillaud JM, Lagace R,
Vielh P. Cytohistologic correlations in
56 synovial sarcomas in 36 patients.
The Institut Curie experience. Diagn
Cytopathol 2002;27:96–102.

83. Akerman M, Willen H, Carlen B, et al.
Fine needle aspiration (FNA) of
synovial sarcoma-comparative
histological-cytological study of 15
cases, including immunohistochemical,
electron microscopic and cytogenetic
examination and DNA-ploidy
analysis. Cytopathology 1996;7:
187–200.

84. Silverman JF, Landreneau RJ, Sturgis
CD, et al. Small-cell variant of synovial
sarcoma: Fine needle aspiration with
ancillary features and potential
diagnostic pitfalls. Diagn Cytopathol
2000;23:118–23.

85. Ackerman M, Ryd W, Skytting B.
Scandinavian sarcoma Group.
Fine-needle aspiration of synovial
sarcoma: criteria for diagnosis:
retrospective reexamination of 37 cases,
including ancillary diagnostics. A
Scandinavian Sarcoma Group Stidy.
Diagn Cytopathol 2003;28:232–8.

86. Gardner DG, Heikinheimo K, Shear M,
et al. Ameloblastomas. In: Barnes L,
Eveson J, Reichard P, et al, editors.
World health Organization
Classification of Tumours.
Pathology and Genetics of Head and
Neck Tumours. Lyon: IARC Press;
2005.

87. Barroca HM, Costa MJ, Carvalho JL.
Cytologic profile of rhabdoid tumour
of the kidney. A report of 3 cases. Acta
Cytol 2003;47:1055–8.

88. Drut R. Cystic nephroma. Cytologic
findings in fine needle aspiration
biopsy. Diagn Cytopathol 1992;18:
593–5.

89. Shorter NA, Glick RD, Klimstra DS,
et al. Malignant pancreatic tumours
in childhood and adolescence: The
Memorial Sloan-Kettering experience,
1967 to present. J Pediatr Surg 2002;
37:887–92.

90. Al-Kaisi N, Weaver MG, Abdul-Karim
FW, et al. Fine needle aspiration
cytology of neuroendocrine tumours of
the pancreas. A cytologic,
immunohistochemical, and electron
microscopic study. Acta Cytol 1992;
36:655–60.

91. Shaw JA, Vance RP, Geisinger KR, et al.
Islet cell neoplasms. A fine-needle
aspiration cytology study with
immunocytochemical correlations.
Am J Clin Pathol 1990;94:142–9.

92. Silverman JF, Holbrook CT, Pories WJ,
et al. Fine needle aspiration cytology
of pancreatoblastoma with
immunocytochemical and
ultrastructural studies. Acta Cytol
1990;34:632–40.

93. Kerr NJ, Chun YH, Yun K, et al.
Pancreatoblastoma is associated with
chromosome 11p loss of heterozygosity
and IGF2 overexpression. Med Pediatr
Oncol 2002;39:52–4.

94. Pettinato G, Di Vizio D, Manivel JC,
et al. Solid-pseudopapillary tumour of
the pancreas: a neoplasm with distinct
and highly characteristic cytological
features. Diagn Cytopathol 2002;27:
325–34.

95. Salla C, Chatzipantelis P,
Konstantinou P, et al. Endoscopic
ultrasound-guided fine-needle
aspiration cytology diagnosis of solid
pseudopapillary tumour of the
pancreas: A case report and literature
review. World J Gastroenterol 2007;
13:5158–63.

96. Akhtar M, Dayel FA. Is it feasible to
diagnose germ cell tumours by fine
needle aspiration biopsy? Diagn
Cytopathol 1997;16:72–7.

97. Balco MT, Burroughs FH, Ali SZ.
Cytopathologic findings in an
immature cystic teratoma: Report
of an unusual case. Diagn Cytopathol
2007;35:120–2.

98. Allias F, Chanoz J, Blache G, et al.
Value of ultrasound guided fine-needle
aspiration in the management of
ovarian and parovarian cysts. Diagn
Cytopathol 2000;22:70–80.

99. De Almeida MM, Chagas M, de Sousa
JV, et al. Fine needle aspiration cytology
as a tool for the early detection of
testicular relapse of acute lymphoblastic
leukemia in children. Diagn Cytopathol
1994;10:44–6.

100. Layfield LJ. Cytopathology of Bone and
Soft Tissue Tumours. New York: Oxford
University Press; 2002

101. Dey P, Mallik MK, Gupta SK, et al. Role
of fine needle aspiration cytology in the
diagnosis of soft tissue tumours and
tumour-like lesions. Cytopathology
2004;15:32–7.

102. Kurtycz DF, Logrono R, Hoerl HD,
et al. Diagnosis of fibromatosis colli by
fine needle aspiration. Diagn
Cytopathol 2000;23:338–42.

103. Kilpatrick SE, Ward WG, Bos GD, et al.
The role of fine needle aspiration
biopsy in the diagnosis and
management of osteosarcoma. Pediatr
Pathol Mol Med 2001;20:175–87.

104. Gupta K, Dey P, Goldsmith R, et al.
Comparison of cytologic features of
giant-cell tumour and giant-cell tumour
of tend sheath. Diagn Cytopathol
2004;30:14–18.

105. Kilpatrick SE, Renner J. Chondroid
tumours of bone and soft tissues. In:
Kilpatrick SE, editor. Diagnostic
musculoskeletal surgical pathology
with clinicopathologic and cytologic
correlations. Philadelphia: Saunders;
2003:323–8.

106. Wang J, Cobb CJ, Martin SE, et al.
Pilomatrixoma: clinicopathologic study

of 51 cases with emphasis on cytologic features. Diagn Cytopathol 2002; 27:167–72.

107. Hosler GA, Clark I, Zakowski MF, et al. Cytopathologic analysis of

thyroid lesions in the paediatric population. Diagn Cytopathol 2006; 34:101–5.

108. Amrikachi M, Ponder TB, Wheeler TM, et al. Thyroid fine-needle aspiration

biopsy in children and adolescents: Experience with 218 aspirates. Diagn Cytopathiol 2005;32:189–92.

CHAPTER 18

Infectious diseases

Andrew S. Field

Introduction

The widespread use of FNB for both palpable and impalpable lesions where the clinical and imaging differential diagnosis (DD) includes malignancy and sometimes infection has led to the diagnosis of infectious lesions. But with the increase in the number of immune compromised (IC) patients in developed countries, particularly due to the HIV epidemic and cancer therapy, FNB increasingly is used to assess skin, lymph node, lung and other sites where infection is the main diagnostic expectation.[1,2] FNB can make the diagnosis of many specific infections on cytomorphology and special stains, and it also delivers material for the full array of ancillary studies including cultures, PCR and DNA analysis of other infections. The rapid diagnosis of infections, some of which cannot be cultured, can facilitate immediate treatment.

Now, with the gradual spread of FNB into the developing world where infections are the leading cause of morbidity and mortality, there has been a rapid if patchy increase in the use of FNB to make specific infectious diagnoses. FNB is minimally invasive, inexpensive, acceptable to patients, provides a rapid accurate diagnosis and immediate triaging for the most cost-effective selection of special stains and ancillary tests, and provides material for culture and the full range of ancillary tests. FNB is a very powerful diagnostic tool, especially where surgical resources and histopathological and microbiological laboratories are in short supply and grossly underfinanced.[3] A cervical lymph node in a young adult that would, in subSaharan Africa, be treated expectantly as TB, can have an FNB that may show tuberculosis, metastatic carcinoma, lymphoma, reactive lymph node or branchial cyst. The FNB empowers the clinician to make the correct, often infectious, diagnosis, provides the best possible outcome for the patient and saves the medical system – which may be severely stressed by the AIDS epidemic, patient numbers and inadequate funding – the cost of surgical biopsy, hospital bed occupancy and inappropriate treatment

Place of FNB in the investigative sequence

The role of FNB is dependent on the body site and the facilities and expertise of personnel at particular institutions. In both the developed world and the four-fifths of the world where medical resources are limited, an inexpensive outpatient FNB can triage and, in the vast majority of cases, make a definitive diagnosis of any palpable lesion. FNB is the most efficient, least invasive and most cost-effective investigative procedure, particularly in cases where an infectious process is expected based on an integration of patient history and examination. This is exemplified by patients with suspected or known immune deficiency due to cancer, therapy or HIV disease.[4,5]

When dealing with imaging-detected deep lesions and impalpable superficial lesions, percutaneous FNB using ultrasound or CT guidance and endoscopic and endoscopic bronchial ultrasound-directed FNB are the mainstay of tissue diagnosis, supported when necessary by core biopsy. As interventional radiology, especially ultrasound, extends into the developing world, FNB of impalpable lesions will increase.

Specific sites

In the head and neck region after completion of a history and examination, which may include endoscopy of the upper aerodigestive tract, FNB of palpable lumps is the first line of investigation in all patients, especially the IC. The exact site of the lesion suggests the DD. In the preauricular, upper cervical and submental regions, acute or chronic sialadenitis,[6,7] salivary gland neoplasms and a full range of lymph node lesions including reactive nodes, metastatic tumor, mycobacterial infection, lymphoma or other specific infection have to be considered. Rapid staining and immediate assessment of FNB slides is very powerful in this setting to direct selection of ancillary testing.

In the mid-cervical region, lymph node lesions including metastatic carcinoma, possible lymphoma, mycobacterial infections and non-specific infections are most common,

©2012 Elsevier Ltd
DOI: 10.1016/B978-0-7020-3151-9.00018-9

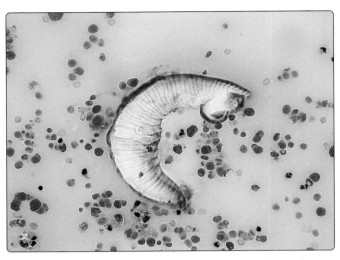

Fig. 18.1 Cutaneous myaisis Dipteran larva in background of pus from 23-gauge FNB of skin abscess (HE, ×600). *(Courtesy Dr Peter Pogany, Budapest, Hungary)*

but paragangliomas and large, often inflamed, tender and even fixed branchial cysts should always be considered.

In the lower cervical and adjacent midline region, lesions of the thyroid, lymph nodes and rarely the parathyroids form the differential diagnosis. Specific infections of the thyroid due to tuberculosis, viruses and, less commonly, *Aspergillus* spp, *Candida* spp, *Histoplasma capsulatum*, *Cryptococcus neoformans*, *Coccidioides*, *Pneumocystis jirovecii* blastomycosis and *Pseudallescheria* have been reported in increasing numbers.[8] In the posterior triangle lymph nodes and schwannomas, and in the suboccipital area lymph nodes with specific infections including toxoplasmosis, and trichilemmal cysts and other skin lesions need to be considered.

In the axilla, femoral and inguinal regions lymph nodes may contain metastatic tumor, suppurative or granulomatous infections, non-specific reactive processes and lymphomas. *Lymphogranuloma venereum* and *Granuloma inguinale* should be considered in the groin.

Skin nodules and palpable subcutaneous lesions are easily sampled by FNB. Pyogenic abscesses and infections such as tuberculosis[9] are easily differentiated from tumor metastases, and, in the HIV population, from Kaposi's sarcoma. Both superficial and deep fungal infections can be diagnosed by FNB and, especially in the IC, may represent disseminated fungal infection due to *Aspergillus* spp, *Cryptococcus neoformans*, histoplasmosis, blastomycosis,[10] sporotrichosis and *Candida* spp,[11] or one of the increasing number of other reported fungal infections producing subcutaneous nodules or mycetomas, including, *Phialophera parasiticus*, *Sporothrix schenkii*, *Cladosporium* spp, *Exophiala jeanselmei*[12] and *Microsporum canis*.[13] *Actinomyces* producing actinomycetomas, and rhinosporidiosis,[14] filariasis,[15] myaisis,[16] leishmaniasis and leptosporosis all occur in the skin. The tuberculoid, borderline and lepromatous variants of leprosy, as well as neuritic and cystic lesions, can all be diagnosed.[17] FNB of cellulitic skin to diagnose surgical wound skin infections[18] and Buruli ulcers[19] by direct smears and culture have been recommended. Skin nodules due to myaisis are rare but eminent FNB targets (Fig. 18.1).

FNB without prior imaging is the first-line diagnostic approach for suspected breast abscesses yielding suppuration and a wide range of common bacteria and other agents including brucellosis[20] and can assist in the drainage of the abscess. Cultures are mandatory. Repeat FNB is required if a significant palpable or ultrasound lesion remains after treatment because very occasional high-grade carcinomas can be associated with obscuring necrosis, neutrophilic infiltrate or multinucleated giant cells (MNGC) and a careful assessment of any inflammatory smear is required to ensure these unusual but rare carcinomas are not missed. Breast FNB may produce granulomatous material where mycobacterial and other infections must be excluded by culture.[21]

Lesions in the testis and scrotum including mycobacterial orchitis and epididymitis can be sampled by FNB to allow differentiation from neoplasms with no risk of a neoplasm seeding in the FNB track and jeopardising possible surgery.[22]

FNB of bone, soft tissue and skeletal muscle lesions,[23] when palpable or under ultrasound direction, is a straightforward procedure and the diagnosis of osteomyelitis due to tuberculosis[24] or other infectious agents can be made and confirmed on culture.[25]

FNB of deep and impalpable lesions found on imaging diagnostic work-up usually involve a DD of malignancy, and FNB is the most rapid, least invasive and inexpensive test available to diagnose specific infections by smears, special stains, cultures and other ancillary tests.

In most developed countries, FNB of central lung lesions, mediastinal, hilar, coeliac, peripancreatic and porta hepatis lymph nodes and pancreatic lesions is now performed under endoscopic ultrasound or endoscopic bronchial ultrasound direction. Percutaneous FNB of peripheral lung, liver and splenic lesions also yield infectious diagnoses, and may be the diagnostic test of choice, for example in paediatric peripheral lung lesions.[26]

In the liver, amebic and tuberculous abscesses, schistosomiasis[27] and pyogenic abscesses due to fungi, staphylococcus, streptococcus, and Gram-negative bacteria including *Klebsiella* spp and *Escherichia coli* can be diagnosed. The use of albendazole and steroids as cover for the potential but very low risk of anaphylactic shock due to spillage of hydatid cyst contents during FNB should be considered if hydatid disease is suspected in an FNB of any site.[28]

In the pancreas, tuberculosis and infections diagnosed by EUS FNB have been increasingly reported in cases suspected of carcinoma.[29] EUS-FNB also accesses the adrenal glands, where suspected metastases have been proven to be tuberculosis, cryptococcosis and disseminated histoplasmosis.[30]

In the lung, FNB is frequently used to distinguish tuberculosis or Gram-negative or -positive bacterial abscesses from carcinomas. Aspergillosis, mucormycosis,[31] candidiasis and cryptococcosis, as well as, *P.jirovecii* in the HIV population, and CMV, coccidioidomycosis[32] and parasites including paragonamiasis,[33] amebiasis, hydatid disease and microfilariasis have all been reported.

In cases of splenomegaly and investigation of splenic lesions found on imaging, FNB is best performed under ultrasound guidance. Diagnoses include tuberculosis, lymphoma and other lesions but uncommon infections such as leishmaniasis should be considered.[34]

FNB of cerebral cortex lesions via burr holes can be used to diagnose toxoplasmosis, CMV and fungal infections[35] in the DD with metastases and primary brain tumors.[36]

Choroiditis, uveitis and retinitis can be diagnosed by FNB performed by an experienced ophthalmologist, ideally using 25 or 27-gauge needles, and the fluid can be used for cultures, PCR and viral serology studies.

Technical considerations

Every FNB should be approached on the basis that there may be an infectious cause and that the patient may suffer from a transferable infection. The best guide is a good clinical history and examination. Every FNB operator should have, and teach, a single safe technique to use in all FNBs they perform. Gloves, and in cases of HIV patients double gloving, are recommended to cut down the potential of needle stick injuries. When removing the needle from the syringe to put air into the syringe once the FNB is finished, the hand that is to remove the needle should be brought down from the wrist of the hand holding the syringe holder, to the barrel of the syringe and then to the hub of the needle, rather than bringing this hand up to the needle point. Optical or safety glasses, gowns, uncluttered bench areas for placing needles and syringes during the procedure, and adequate clinic space are required.

When a cystic lesion or abscess is suspected it is recommended that a needle on a syringe should be used, creating a 'closed' system to avoid infective fluid spurting from the needle hub, and to assist in obtaining several milliliters of pus for culture. But using the needle by itself gives more sensitivity for FNB of palpable lesions, and can be used for a second pass of any residual mass after draining a cyst, or for solid and small lesions, especially skin nodules. Needles of 22 to 27 gauge are recommended for lymph nodes and skin lesions. If pus or necrosis is found and material is needed for extra slides, stains and cultures, a 22 gauge or 23 gauge will produce more material. The diagnostic yield of the cultures is higher with more material, so repeat needling using all the material for culture is recommended rather than just saline rinses of needle and syringe.[37]

The macroscopic appearances of the FNB smears may give clues to the infectious nature of the material, with pus having its own pale creamy green color, distinctive slippery feel on smearing and possible purulent odor. However, the best use of FNB in all situations is to have immediate slide smearing, staining and assessment by a cytopathologist or experienced cytotechnician, to confirm adequacy of material, provide a provisional diagnosis and to triage the case immediately for ancillary tests. In many cases, rapid diagnosis of a specific organism or the immediate diagnosis of an organism, such as *P. jirovecii*, that cannot be cultured, assists patient care, and facilitates the cost-effective selection of ancillary tests.

Ideally, both Giemsa and Papstain should be prepared routinely by specimen splitting of the material on the slide or separate FNB passes. Giemsa is better for bacteria, negative images of mycobacteria and fungal hyphae, yeasts and CMV cytoplasmic inclusions, and Papstain is better for some fungal hyphae and yeasts, and viral intranuclear inclusions. If infection is suspected or the immediate provisional reports suggest infection, extra air-dried slides for the auramine, ZN, Gram and methenamine silver stains (GMS) should be made

immediately, and material taken for cultures, PCR, direct immunofluorescence (IF), flow cytometry and gene rearrangement studies (if lymphoma is a DD), and ultimately, in some organisms, phylogenetic analysis based on nuclear small subunit RNA sequence alignments. No single stain or protocol will diagnose all infections and culture. Destained H&E- or Pap-stained slides can be used for GMS and other special stains, and repeat FNB recommended.

A cell block should be prepared in almost all cases from saline rinses of the needle or ideally from separate needling, for H&E, special stains, immunoperoxidase studies (IP) and electron microscopy where required. In TB or HIV endemic areas or where the patient is thought to be IC, direct inoculation into culture bottles can be used.[38] In cases such as liver abscesses where anaerobes are expected, pus should be placed directly into appropriate microbiologic containers. If the DD is lymphoma, especially in lymph nodes, lungs or spleen, FNB material should be placed into normal saline, Hanks medium or similar for flow cytometry and cytogenetic and gene rearrangement studies.

Immune compromised patients

FNB is extremely useful in the ever-increasing number of IC patients, including patients on long-term steroids, undergoing treatment for solid and hematologic malignancies, solid organ transplant recipients and HIV-positive persons.[4,5] The successful role of FNB has continued into the era of highly active antiretroviral therapy (HAART).[39] The typical inflammatory reactions to common infectious agents may be both deficient and atypical, and unusual and opportunistic infections may be present, making culture of FNB material mandatory.[4] More than one infection may be present, for example CMV and bacterial infections in transplant patients.

Extra slides routinely should be prepared for Gram, auramine, ZN and GMS, and material taken for cultures for AFB, fungi and bacteria. A cell block should be prepared, and flow cytometry included in the work-up if lymphoma is suspected.

In these patients, suppurative lymphadenitis suggests not only a bacterial infection, but also disseminated fungal infection, most commonly *Aspergillus* spp, *Cryptococcus neoformans* or *Candida* spp infection. Granulomatous lymphadenitis raises the differential diagnosis of tuberculosis or possibly sarcoidosis. In Giemsa-stained smears from IC patients, mycobacterial infection may produce large numbers of plump histiocytes with cross-hatched cytoplasm representing 'negative image' bacilli, which may also be seen in the background serum. If neutrophils are admixed with spindle cells and histiocytes, bacillary angiomatosis should be considered, and the causative organism, *Bartonella henselae* and *Bartonella quintana*, demonstrated using Warthin-Starry stain.

Contraindications

There are no contraindications to FNB of a palpable lesion where infection is suspected. Contraindications at deep sites in infectious cases such as the spleen are the same, if any, as for FNB for suspected malignancy.

Complications

Complications of FNB for infectious cases are the same as FNB for suspected malignancy in all body sites, e.g. a pneumothorax following FNB of lung.

CYTOLOGICAL FINDINGS

Criteria for adequate smear

The diagnosis of infections by FNB occurs in the setting of FNB of a lesion suspected of malignancy where infection may or may not have been considered, or in the setting where infection is the leading provisional diagnosis based on clinical and imaging findings.

When a FNB yields suppurative or necrotic inflammatory material confirming the clinical and imaging findings, this is diagnostic, especially when special stains reveal a specific organism and this is confirmed on cultures or PCR. However, if a neoplasm is expected and pus or even granulomatous material is found, repeat FNB and further investigation such as core biopsy should be considered, for example an FNB of a mid-cervical mass producing bland squamous debris and suppuration consistent with a branchial cyst, or a FNB of a perihilar lymph node producing granulomatous material consistent with tuberculosis may be diagnostic of a benign infectious process, but FNB of a lung lesion producing necrosis with negative special stains and cultures usually warrants repeat FNB to exclude a necrotic squamous cell or other carcinoma.

Suppurative inflammation

Pyogenic infection in FNB is most commonly seen in lymph nodes in the head and neck and other regions in children, teenagers and young adults and in the lung, but suppuration is common in FNB from IC patients from all sites particularly the skin.

CRITERIA

◆ Creamy gray material which is viscous on smearing and may be frankly purulent,

◆ Proteinaceous background which can be granular or amorphous and usually includes shadowy cellular debris,

◆ Variable numbers but often plentiful neutrophils, intact or showing varying degrees of degeneration,

◆ Variable numbers of histiocytes, macrophages and lymphocytes depending on FNB site,

◆ Components of target site such as epithelium which can often be infiltrated by neutrophils and show atypical nuclei, e.g. apocrine sheets in a breast abscess,

◆ Bacteria or fungi in macrophages or extra cellularly, especially in the Giemsa stain,

◆ Vegetable material (lung abscess or aspiration pneumonia) or fragments of hair shafts (pilonidal sinus abscess).

PROBLEMS AND DIFFERENTIAL DIAGNOSIS

The overdiagnosis of atypia or malignancy can occur when atypia is seen in epithelial components involved by the infectious process. These epithelial components may be infiltrated by neutrophils and commonly show enlarged hyperchromatic nuclei, which have predictable size, shape, chromatin pattern and nucleoli in each nucleus, rather than nuclear pleomorphism usually associated with malignancy. Attention should be given to the acute inflammatory setting in which the atypical epithelial components are found, as suppuration is not commonly associated with a primary malignancy of lung or breast. On the other hand, the diagnosis of malignancy can be missed in the setting of metastatic squamous cell carcinoma associated with necrosis and suppuration.

Suppuration is usually associated with *Streptococcus pyogenes*, *Staphylococcus aureus*, *Streptococcus pneumoniae* and Gram-negative bacteria including *Klebsiella* spp and *Escherichia coli*, as well as fungal infections such as *Aspergillus* spp, *Cryptococcus neoformans* and *Candida* spp, especially in IC patients.

In the mid-cervical region of the neck, a tender hot red mass raises a DD of inflamed lymph node, inflamed branchial cyst or possibly metastatic squamous cell carcinoma. The clinical site of the lesion, age of the patient and other history help to differentiate these lesions and repeat passes (up to 3 or 4) will usually provide an adequate sample. A diagnosis of malignancy should be made only in the presence of preserved squamous nuclei with malignant features, and not on pyknotic nuclei in degenerate squames in a suppurative or granulomatous background. Finally, a trial of antibiotic treatment with a repeat FNB of any residual mass may make the diagnosis. In the breast, squamous metaplasia in inflamed subareolar ducts (subareolar recurring abscess or Suska's disease) can give rise to cytological atypia and worrying clinical signs of Paget's disease or carcinoma. Correlation of imaging, clinical and cytological findings is essential.

In IC patients with neutropenia, a thin proteinaceous background may contain scant or no neutrophils and an organism must be sought with special stains and cultures. In AIDS patients, there may be plentiful plump histiocytes with cell debris and neutrophils resembling acute bacterial infections, but plentiful curved bacilli will be seen as negative images in the background and cross-hatched in macrophage cytoplasm (See Fig. 18.5). Culture and drug sensitivity testing is required.

In fungal and cat scratch disease,[40] suppurative granulomas with neutrophils interspersed among the epithelioid histiocytes in the granulomas may be present (Fig. 18.2).

Granulomatous inflammation

Clinical

The commonest cause of granulomatous cytomorphology, and the diagnosis which must always be excluded, is that of mycobacterial infections. These are endemic worldwide and the prevalence of infections including atypical mycobacterial

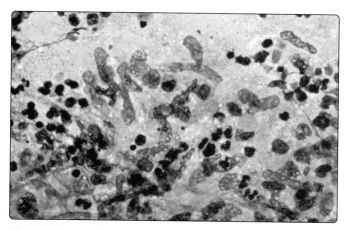

Fig. 18.2 Suppurative granuloma Neutrophils infiltrate epithelioid granuloma consisting of epithelioid histiocytes in background of neutrophils (Giemsa, ×600).

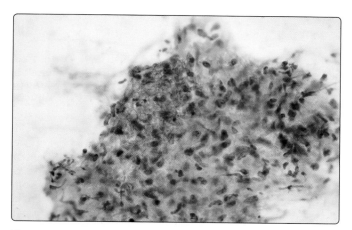

Fig. 18.3 Granuloma Epithelioid histiocytes with elongate, curved, indented nuclei form a granuloma (Pap, ×400).

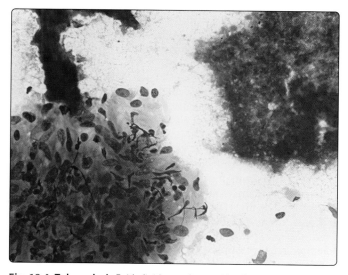

Fig. 18.4 Tuberculosis Epithelioid granuloma with adjacent necrosis (Giemsa, ×400). *(Courtesy Dr William Geddie, Toronto, Canada)*

infections has increased with the HIV epidemic in almost all countries, especially India and sub-Saharan Africa. In developed countries, increased intercontinental travel, migration and increased numbers of IC patients of all types have fostered the resurgence of mycobacterial infections.

CRITERIA

- Low to moderate cellularity,
- Epithelioid histiocytes (modified histiocytes with elongated, bent or centrally indented footprint nuclei with fine, even chromatin, small or inconspicuous nucleoli and considerable, sometimes eccentric, pale cytoplasm) are present singly or syncytially aggregated in granulomas (cohesive tissue fragments of epithelioid histiocytes) (Fig. 18.3),
- Small lymphocytes in variable but usually low number in lymph nodes because of the diffuse nature of granulomatous process,
- Multinucleated giant cells with irregularly arranged nuclei that may aggregate or be peripherally arranged in a horseshoe in the granular or finely vacuolated copious pale cytoplasm (Langhan's giant cells),
- Neutrophils in some cases,
- Necrotic debris, depending on cause,
- Eosinophilic sharply delineated masses containing few cells; first reported in tuberculosis,
- Fungi on methenamine stain,
- Mycobacteria on ZN, Fite or auramine stain.

Culture for fungi and mycobacteria with drug sensitivity testing is mandatory.

PROBLEMS AND DIFFERENTIAL DIAGNOSIS

Mycobacterium tuberculosis infection may produce granulomas consisting of epithelioid histiocytes with or without Langhan's MNGC and caseous necrosis, but in some cases may produce only caseous necrosis (Fig. 18.4). In IC patients, especially AIDS patients, FNB of lymph nodes may show neutrophils, a variable number of lymphocytes, plasmacytoid lymphocytes and plasma cells, depending on the stage of HIV lymphadenopathy. But where TB is endemic and HIV-positive patients present without the very low CD4 counts achieved in AIDS patients in developed countries in the era before HAART, typical granulomas can be seen.

Negative images of *mycobacteria* may be seen in the background serum and cytoplasm of histiocytes in the Giemsa stain (Fig. 18.5), and the beaded 3–4-micron bacilli stain in the ZN (Fig. 18.6A) and auramine (Fig. 18.6B) stains and autoflouresce in the Papstain.[41]

Caseating necrosis can be extensive in FNBs of lymph nodes and lung and may be the only material on the slides in *M. tuberculosis* cases, where the DD is necrotizing metastasis from SCC or a cavitating lung primary.

Mycobacteria may be very scant in FNB material, limiting the usefulness of AFB stains on direct smears and cell blocks (see below). The auramine IF stain allows rapid scanning of direct smears and multiple sections of cell block material, and PCR and ELISA stains increase the detection rate.

Sarcoidosis has distinctive rounded epithelioid granulomas infiltrated by lymphocytes without necrosis, but its

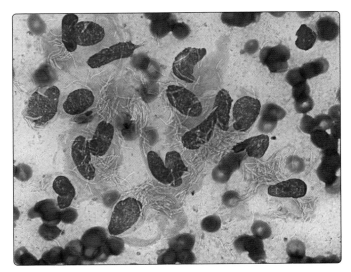

Fig. 18.5 Negative image of curved beaded atypical mycobacteria in histiocyte cytoplasm and serum background; note tendency for several bacilli to attach end to end (HIV-positive patient) (Giemsa, ×1000). *(Courtesy Dr William Geddie, Toronto, Canada)*

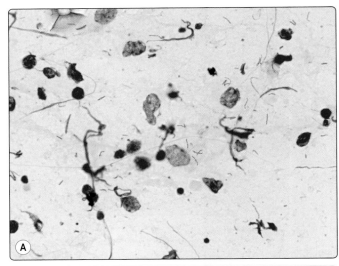

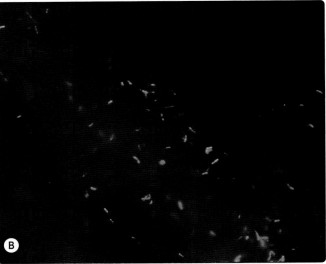

Fig. 18.6 (A) Curved beaded mycobacteria in Ziehl Neelsen stain (ZN, ×1000); (B) Mycobacteria in Auramine stain (Auramine, ×1000).

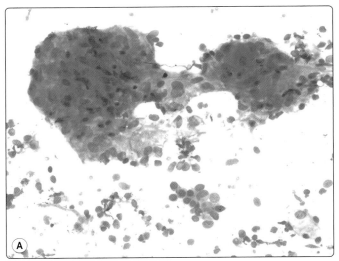

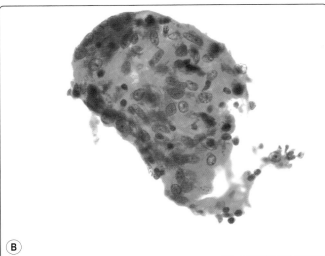

Fig. 18.7 (A) Cohesive rounded sarcoid granuloma with occasional lymphocytes (Giemsa, ×400); (B) Rounded sarcoid granuloma (Pap, ×400).

diagnosis requires negative AFB stains, mycobacterial cultures and PCR with the correct clinical presentation and serology (Fig. 18.7).[42]

Fungal infections can be associated with granulomas and the yeasts and hyphae may be seen as negative images or variably stained in the Giemsa and Papstain depending on the specific fungus and the degree of degeneration of the hyphae. Cryptococcus may have no granulomas, especially in IC patients, and the 5–15-micron round yeasts may be seen within the cytoplasm of macrophages and MNGC or in the background with narrow-necked budding, a mucicarmine-positive and Giemsa-negative 'halo-like' capsule, and variably stained body (Fig. 18.8).[43–45] In profoundly IC AIDS patients, there may be no capsule and the distinction from *Histoplasma capsulatum* relies on culture, as both stain with Giemsa. Histoplasmosis has largely intracellular smaller 2–5-micron round yeasts showing variable budding in the GMS, and in Papstains appear as 'holes' in macrophage cytoplasm (Fig. 18.9).[46–48]

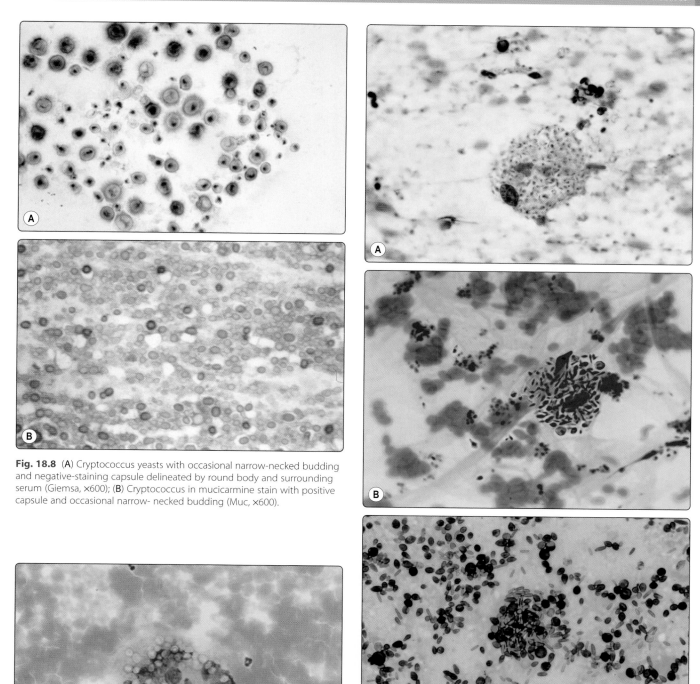

Fig. 18.8 (A) Cryptococcus yeasts with occasional narrow-necked budding and negative-staining capsule delineated by round body and surrounding serum (Giemsa, ×600); (B) Cryptococcus in mucicarmine stain with positive capsule and occasional narrow- necked budding (Muc, ×600).

Fig. 18.10 (A, B, C) Sporotrichosis: oval and elongate yeasts in macrophages and in the GMS in the background (Pap, Giemsa, Grocott Methenamine silver, ×1000). *(Courtesy Dr Rene Gerhard, Sao Paolo, Brazil)*

Fig. 18.9 Punched out 'holes' in cytoplasm of multinucleated histiocyte represent 3– 5-micron yeasts of *Histoplasma capsulatum* (Giemsa, ×600). *(Courtesy Dr William Geddie, Toronto, Canada)*

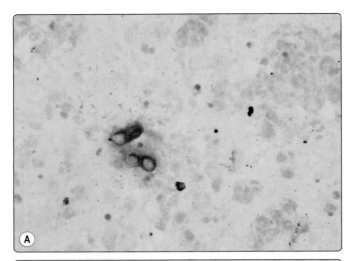

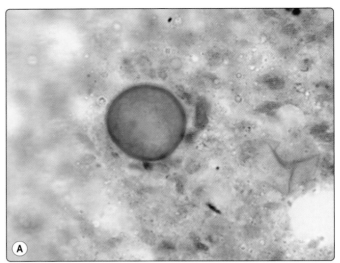

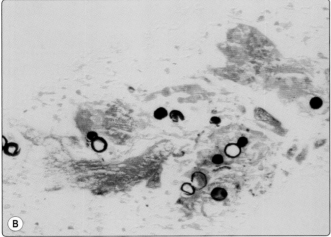

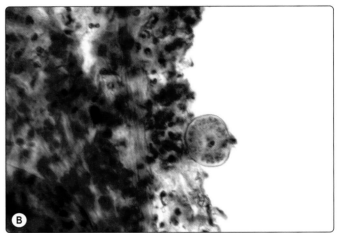

Fig. 18.11 (A, B) Blastomycosis: 10– 12-micron yeasts showing broad based budding (Giemsa and GMS, ×1000). *(Courtesy Dr David Carter, USA)*

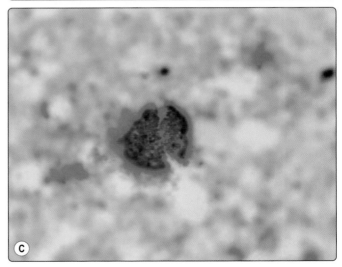

In Southeast Asia and China, *Penicillium marneffei*, a rapidly emerging opportunistic infection in HIV-positive patients, has 2–4-micron yeasts in macrophages and sausage shaped yeasts in the extracellular background, showing septa in the GMS due to their division by binary fission, not budding.[49,50] The budding yeasts of *Sporothrix schenkii* are cigar shaped (Fig. 18.10),[51,52] and *Paracoccidioides brasiliensis*, endemic in Central and South America, has variably sized yeasts with pathognomonic multiple budding.[33,53]

Blastomycosis produces large 8–20-micron yeasts with broad-based budding and a thick double-contoured, weakly birefringent wall featuring inner and outer wall staining (Fig. 18.11).[8,10,54] Blastomycosis shares a distribution with coccidioidomycosis which has much larger 20–120-micron refractile, thick-walled spherules, some of which contain 2–4-micron endospores (Fig. 18.12),[32] which have to be differentiated from leishmaniasis, whose amistigotes contain nuclei and kinetoplasts (Fig. 18.13), and the crescentic tachyzoites containing dot nuclei of toxoplasmosis (Fig. 18.14A). In lymph node FNBs, toxoplasmosis is associated with follicular hyperplasia and discrete small syncytial epithelioid granulomas (Fig. 18.14B), and the tachyzoites in cysts and the background are rarely seen. Confirmatory diagnosis can be made by serology.

Fig. 18.12 (A, B, C) Coccidiodomycosis: 60-micron spherule with faintly birefringent wall containing 2–4-micron endospores (Giemsa, Pap, GMS, ×1000). *(Figures 12A, 12C Courtesy Dr William Geddie, Toronto, Canada; Figure 12B Courtesy Dr Matthew Zarka, Scottsdale, Arizona)*

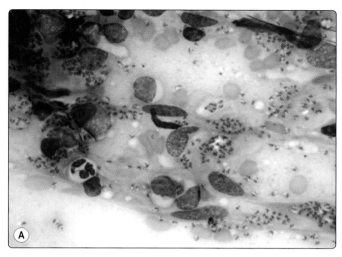

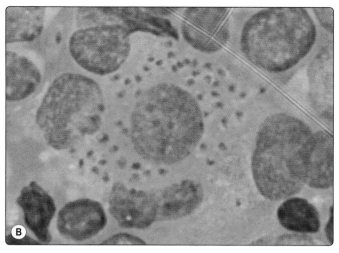

Fig. 18.13 Leishmania (A) Leishman-Donovan bodies in background and in macrophage cytoplasm (Giemsa, ×400); (B) Leishman-Donovan bodies in macrophage cytoplasm at high power (Pap, ×1000). *(Courtesy Dr Khosrow Daneshbod, Shiraz, Iran)*

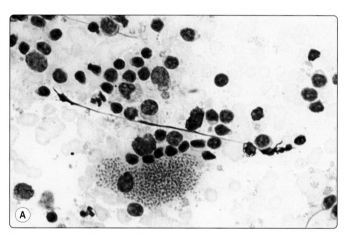

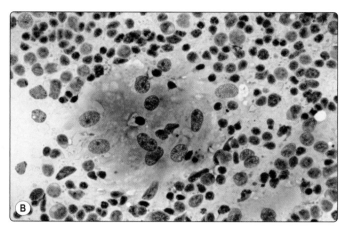

Fig. 18.14 Toxoplasmosis (A) brachyzoites in macrophage cytoplasm (Giemsa, ×600); (B) Syncytial epithelioid minute granuloma in reactive lymphoid background.

Candida spp have thin, branched pseudo-hyphae and 3–micron yeasts,[55] while *Aspergillus* spp have 5–7-micron diameter septate hyphae showing acute angle branching (Fig. 18.15)[56,57] and *Mucormycosis* has thicker, irregular 2–50-micron, ribbon-like nonseptate hyphae and variable but often 90 degree branching (Fig. 18.16).[32] Aspergillosis can be associated with birefringent needle-like calcium oxalate crystals[58] and marked metaplastic squamous atypia in the margins of cavitating lung lesions.

Specific infections

Specific infections are described in Tables 18.1 and 18.2, which emphasize the morphological diagnosis in direct smears and special stains. For a more detailed discussion of their microbiology, please refer to standard texts.[59]

Mycobacterial infections include *M. tuberculosis*, *M. avium* complex, *M. leprae* and *M. ulcerans* (Buruli's ulcer).

Tuberculosis is endemic across most countries, and with the increase in IC patients and the HIV epidemic there has been a resurgence of TB in the developed world and the development of multi-resistant strains.[60] FNB of all sites offers a rapid, inexpensive and efficient outpatient clinic diagnostic method based on cytomorphology (see Figs 18.3–18.5) and the Ziehl-Neelsen (see Fig. 18.6A) and auramine (see Fig. 18.6B) stains, and the FNB delivers material for culture in traditional Lowenstein-Jensen or other media or PCR or immunohistochemistry.[38,61] This is highlighted by the role of FNB in children with cervical lymphadenopathy.[41]

Extrapulmonary TB most commonly presents with head and neck lymphadenopathy where the DD is often malignancy – for example, intraparotid lymph nodes can present as a neoplasm – and in the skin,[9] bone,[24] vertebral and paravertebral regions,[23] testes and epididymis[22] and pancreas.[62] *Mycobacterium avium* complex is the commonest nontuberculous mycobacterium and the commonest cause of cervical lymphadenopathy in immune competent children, and may

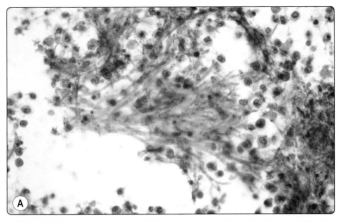

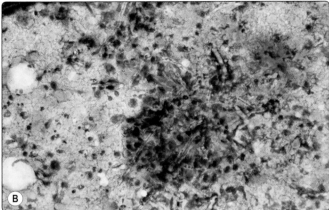

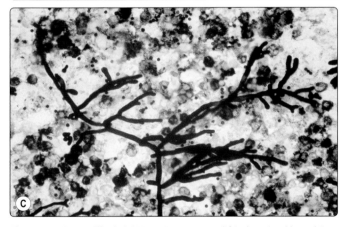

Fig. 18.15 Aspergillosis (A) Negative image and faintly stained branching aggregated crisscrossing hyphae in Pap stain (Pap, ×400); (B) Negative image and pale linear staining in aggregated hyphae (Giemsa, ×400); (C) Acutely branching hyphae (GMS, ×400).

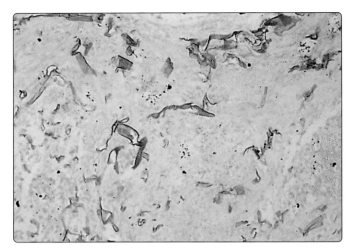

Fig. 18.16 Mucormycosis.

disseminate from lungs and gut to involve lymph nodes and skin in HIV-positive patients.[63]

Positive cytology is usually defined as granulomas, MNGC, caseation and mycobacterial visualization, but there is a wide range of cytomorphological patterns on smears varying from the classic features of epithelioid granulomas with Langhan's giant cells and caseous necrosis, to mostly or solely caseous necrosis, and to tuberculous abscess with plentiful neutrophils, degenerating epithelioid cells and a watery necrotic background. The cytology pattern and number of AFB on ZN stain depends on the patient's immune status, and in cases where FNB produces only caseous necrosis the percentage showing AFB on the ZN stain may be as low as 7%.[64] *M. avium* complex especially may yield histiocytes and some neutrophils in a watery background with a variable number of AFB in HIV-positive patients.[63] Culture or PCR is mandatory for confirmation, speciation and drug resistance, but these tests are often not available in TB-endemic developing world areas, where there is reliance on demonstrating AFB.

Other techniques have been put forward including the modified bleach method for ZN staining,[64] the IF auramine-rhodamine stain, immunostaining of direct cytological smears,[65] PCR on DNA scraped and processed from dried unstained cytology smears,[66] and the ELISA test,[67] most of which can achieve positive rates in the range 70% to 85%.

But the combination of cytomorphology, ZN stain and autofluorescence on Papstain can achieve concordance with culture in around 70% cases,[41] and culture remains the mainstay of diagnosis and drug sensitivity testing.[61]

Extrapulmonary TB in the breast presents as a mass, discharging sinuses, cold abscess or non-healing ulcers, raising a DD of carcinoma. AFB stains and cultures, however, may not be positive, and other causes of granulomatous mastitis such as *Brucella melitenses*, fungi and organizing fat necrosis should be excluded by cultures and PCR.[20]

FNB of the skin and other lesions of leprosy due to *Mycobacterium leprae*, which is endemic across the developing world, are highly diagnostic, especially if skin is blanched by gently lifting and squeezing the site to be aspirated to reduce bleeding and the Fite stain and cultures are used.[17] The DD is cutaneous tuberculosis with its epithelioid granulomas and caseous necrosis.[9] There is a spectrum of lesions:

- tuberculoid leprosy with moderate to high cellularity, cohesive epithelioid granulomas, plentiful lymphocytes and scant if any AFB,
- mid-borderline leprosy showing fairly cellular, poorly cohesive granulomas made up of epithelioid histiocytes, macrophages and lymphocytes,
- borderline leprosy showing moderate cellularity, single dispersed macrophages with negative image bacilli, no epithelioid cells, many lymphocytes and macrophages,
- lepromatous leprosy with marked cellularity consisting of foamy macrophages, neutrophils, lymphocytes,

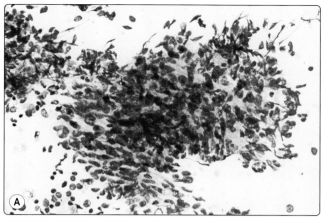
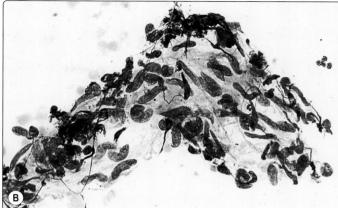
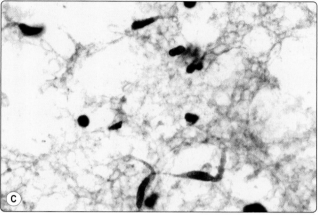

Fig. 18.17 (A) Tissue fragment of Kaposi's sarcoma, showing crowded, spindle shaped cells with hyperchromatic, blunt-ended nuclei (Giemsa, x200); (B) Tissue fragment of spindle cells, with poorly defined cytoplasm Giemsa, x400); (C) Single spindle cells with cigar-shaped bland nuclei, and granular chromatin (Pap, x400) Kaposi's sarcoma.

fragmented collagen and fat in the background and plentiful AFB,

- reactional leprosy with high cellularity with foamy macrophages, negative image bacilli, neutrophils and a foamy background.[68]

The FNB can classify most cases to match the Ridley and Jopling histological classification of leprosy. Soft tissue swellings with nerve abscesses in neuritic leprosy show abundant caseous necrosis and many degenerate neutrophils in a thin proteinaceous background with a negative AFB stain.[69]

Kaposi's sarcoma

This neoplasm is caused by human herpesvirus-8 and is derived from infected endothelial cells. It is an AIDS-defining illness and one of the commonest neoplasms seen in homosexual AIDS patients, although in the HAART era, its incidence has decreased and been overtaken by lymphomas and squamous mucosal lesions. In lymph nodes, the spindle cell proliferation involves the subcapsular and other sinuses, and the remaining lymph node shows the various stages of HIV infection, from follicular hyperplasia through to involution. Nodal involvement should be considered in patients with tender lymphadenopathy, low CD3 count, associated infections and Kaposi's sarcoma skin lesions.[70]

CRITERIA FOR DIAGNOSIS (Fig. 18.17)

- Low cell yield; irregular tissue fragments of haphazardly arranged spindle cells,
- Elongated, blunt-ended, mildly irregular hyperchromatic nuclei with inconspicuous nucleoli,
- Poorly defined cytoplasm, which in some cases in the Giemsa stain is delineated by metachromatic stroma between the cells,
- Single spindle cells with bipolar or long and wispy cytoplasm,
- Plasmacytoid lymphocytes, plasma cells, lymphocytes and plentiful tingible-body macrophages.

PROBLEMS AND DIFFERENTIAL DIAGNOSIS

The tissue fragments may resemble granulomas, but the nuclei are more elongated and spindly and usually are hyperchromatic. They lack the 'sand shoe' indentations of epithelioid histiocytes, and MNGC are not seen. Mycobacterial infection may involve the same node. Occasionally, Kaposi's sarcoma produces highly cellular smears with large tissue fragments containing slit-like spaces and hemosiderin. Mitoses are scant.

Table 18.1 Fungi

Disease & microorganisms	Geographic region	Site	Microorganism features	Pattern of infection suppurative +/or granulomatous	Stains	Differential diagnosis and comments
Fungi						
Candididiasis, most commonly C. albicans[55]	WW. Gut and skin commensal	Mucocutaneous and disseminated in IC (AIDS defining illness)	Multilateral budding yeast 3–6 micron, thin pseudohyphae and rare true hyphae	Suppurative	Giemsa, Pap and GMS	
Cryptococcosis due to C. neoformans[43] Figure 18.8A, B	WW	Pneumonia and disseminated in IC to CNS, adrenals, GIT, LNs (esp. neck and mediastinum)	Mainly extracellular 5–15 micron yeasts, chc. mucinous capsule, which may be missing in IC producing 3–5 micron yeast	Variable, usually epithelioid granulomas, but suppurative in IC patients	Capsule mucicarmine positive, and body Giemsa variable and GMS pos Autofluorescent[44]	DD H. capsulatum, Leishmaniasis. Can produce lung inflammatory tumors[45]
Aspergillosis, due to A. fumigatus, A. flavus, A. niger[56-58] Figure 18.15A, B, C	WW. URT commensal	Respiratory tract and paranasal sinuses, disseminating in IC to skin, GIT, heart, thyroid, brain	Acute angle branching, septate hyphae with parallel walls diameter 5–7 micron, in tangled aggregates or macrophage cytoplasm. Rare sporangiophores	Suppurative with MNGC	Pap and Giemsa variable, some 'negative images' GMS pos	DD Mucor mycosis Candida spp Care with atypical squamous metaplasia in lung cavitated lesions
Zygomycetes most commonly Mucor mycosis[31] Figure 18.16	WW. IC especially with renal transplants, burns, HIV IV drug users	Lung and paranasal sinuses, disseminating to orbit, face, palate and brain, and skin	Twisted, ribbon-like nonseptate 2–50 micron hyphae, with right angle or variable branching	Necrosis and suppuration	Pap and GMS	DD Aspergillus spp Infection Rapid diagnosis assists treatment
Dermatophytes, due to Microsporum, Trichophyton, Epidermophyton[13]	WW, parasitic fungi of skin, hair	Subcutaneous nodules (mycetomas)	Branching hyphae	Suppuration, MNGC, debris	GMS	
Blastomycosis, due to B. dermatiditis, dimorphic fungus[8,10,54] Figure 18.11A, B	USA, Canada, Mexico, Middle East, Africa, India	Chronic pneumonitis, and skin, bone, genitourinary, LN, thyroid, CNS, pancreas, spleen	8–20 micron broad based budding yeast, faintly birefringent thick walls	Necrotizing granuloma, but IC may be suppurative	Pap, GMS	
Coccidioidomycosis, due to dimorphic fungus C. immitis and C. posadii[32] Figure 18.12A, B, C	South west USA, Mexico, Central and South America	Respiratory, and IC disseminates to skin, soft tissue, bone, joints, meninges	20–120 micron refractile, thick walled spherules, collapsed and calcified or contain 2–4 micron endospores Rare septate hyphae	Eosinophilic debris ± suppuration	Pap, GMS, DiPAS in cell block	DD Plant contaminant Toxoplasmosis for endospores
Histoplasmosis, due to dimorphic fungus H. capsulatum[30,46-48] Figure 18.9	WW especially USA, Caribbean, Central and South America, Ganges River India	Lung, breast, adrenals, GIT, liver, LN, subcutis, skeletal muscle in IC	'Holes' in macrophage cytoplasm in Pap, and intracytoplasmic and scattered 3–5 micron oval pale yeasts with single narrow based budding	Granulomas or single epithelioid cells; necrosis in IC	Giemsa and GMS; not Pap	DD Leishmaniasis Toxoplasmosis Cryptococcosis P. marneffei

Paracoccidioidomycosis, due to P. brasiliensis[53]	Central and South America	Chronic lung and mouth, with LN	Round to oval refractile yeasts, varying in size, double contoured walls, chc multiple budding 'mariners wheel'	Granulomas	GMS positive walls	DD Cryptococcus Histoplasmosis Loboa loboi: long chain budding
Penicillium marneffei[49] Penicillium piceum[50]	SE Asia and south China	Disseminating in HIV to LN, skin, bone, marrow lung and rib	Round 2–4 micron yeasts with central dot in macrophages, AND, sausage-shaped yeasts in background have septa due to division by binary fission not budding	Necrosis with lymphocytes and histiocytes	GMS positive	DD Toxoplasmosis
Sporotrichosis due to dimorphic fungus Sporothrix schenkii[51,52] Figure 18.10A, B, C	India, South Africa, Australia, North and South America	Skin ('rose thorn disease') but disseminates in IC to lung, bone, CNS, joints	Oval to cigar-shaped yeasts in macrophages or scattered	Necrosis and suppuration	GMS, Pap	
Pneumocystis jirovecii[71–73] Figure 18.18A, B	WW	Pneumonia, esp. AIDs and disseminates to LN, spleen, bone marrow	5–8 micron cup shaped cysts, faintly birefringent, with dark green nuclei in Pap, black comma shaped single or double nuclei in GMS	Eosinophilic (Pap) or purple (Giemsa) foamy aggregates contain cysts and trophic forms, with lymphocytes and histiocytes or suppuration	Pap, Giemsa and especially GMS, Immunoperoxidase	Cannot be cultured RBC in GMS can mimic cysts

WW world wide; URT upper respiratory tract; LN lymph node; IC immune compromised; GIT gastrointestinal tract; GMS Grocott methenamine silver; chc characteristic; MNGC multinucleated giant cells.

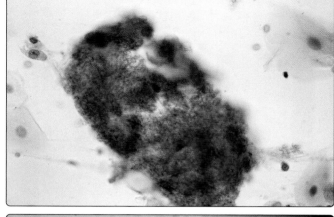

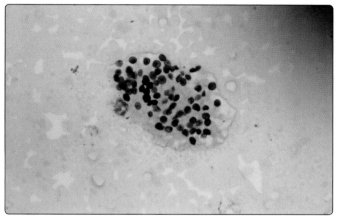

Fig. 18.18 Pneumocystis (A) granular foamy aggregate of 5-micron cup-shaped cysts (Pap, ×400); (B) Aggregated cup-shaped cysts with dot nuclei (GMS, ×400).

Table 18.2 Parasites, mycobacteria, other bacteria and viruses

Parasites						
Filariasis, mainly due to nematode *Wucheria bancrofti*[15,74–77]	WW especially tropics, India, Nepal, Polynesia	Epididymitis, spermatic cord nodules, hydroceles, thyroid, lymphangitis, LN (especially cervical in children), breast, skin	Slender microfilaria, often coiled, with fragments of female gravid worms containing eggs, and free eggs	MNGC with eosinophils, neutrophils, epithelioid cells, often adherent ot filarial	Pap, Giemsa	
Dirofilaria immitis[78] Figure 18.19A, B, C	USA	Pulmonary nodules				
Hydatid disease due to *Echinococcus granulosus*[28,79–82] Figure 18.20A, B	Sheep farming, central Europe, South Africa, Australia, New Zealand, South America	Lung, liver, brain, thyroid, salivary glands, kidney, spleen, muscle and soft tissue	Scolices, refractile hooklets, fragments of laminated thick wall in thick granular background	Variable, granulomatous or suppurative if ruptured or secondarily infected cyst	Pap, Giemsa	Cyst drainage and injection with hypertonic saline
Leishmaniasis, due to *Leishmania* spp.[83,84] Figure 18.13A, B, C	Mediterranean, Near East, Asia	Cutaneous and visceral, esp. in IC, to spleen, liver, LN, eye, breast	1–2 micron amistigotes (Leisham-Donovan bodies) contain nucleus and rod shaped kinetoplast, found in cytoplasm of macrophages and neutrophils or free	Granulomatous, or occasionally suppuration	Giemsa, Pap	DD *M.tuberculosis* Toxoplasmosis
Cysticercosis, due to cestode *Taenia solium*[85,86] Figure 18.21	Tropics, India, South East Asia	Soft tissue swelling in skin, skeletal muscle, eye, CNS, tongue	1 cm cyst, with single 1 mm scolex with 130–170 micron hooklets, fragments of larva cuticle, calcareous corpuscles	Eosinophils, neutrophils, histiocytes, MNGC, and granulomas with degeneration of nematode	Pap, Giemsa	DD Hydatid disease, with multiple scolices and hooklets
Paragonimiasis, due to *Paragonimus* spp.[33]	Asia	Lung nodules	Adult worm excretes species specific eggs	Suppuration	Pap,Giemsa	
Toxoplasmosis, due to coccidian protozoan *Toxoplasma gondii*[87] Figure 18.14A, B	WW	Unilateral cervical LN, but in IC, pulmonitis and encephalitis Congenital transmission	(Rare) 3–4 micron crescent shaped tachyzoites with dot nuclei, and similar brachyzoites in round cysts	LN show follicular hyperplasia and small granulomas	Giemsa Tachyzoites show autofluorescence IP stains	Confirmation by serology (cannot be cultured) DD lymphoma (flow cytometry)
Rhinosporidiosis, due to *Rhinosporidium seeberi*[14]	Tropical, except Australia	Nose, conjunctiva, trachea, nasopharynx	Large spherules or sporangia, containing multiple 7 micron endospores, and free	Granulomatous	Pap, Giemsa	Cannot be cultured
***Entamoeba histolytica*[88]**	Tropics	GIT, liver, and disseminated	Round to oval basophilic 18–20 micron trophozoites with single nucleus and ingested red cells	Suppuration ('amoebic abscesses') contain scant/no amoebae	Pap, Giemsa, DiPAS IF	DD Macrophages containing ingested material

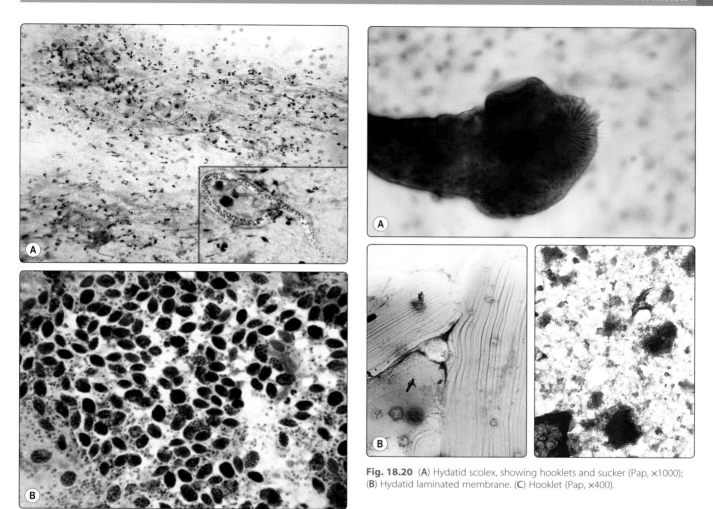

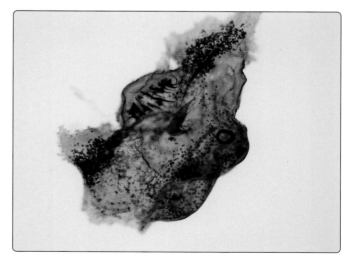

Fig. 18.20 (**A**) Hydatid scolex, showing hooklets and sucker (Pap, ×1000); (**B**) Hydatid laminated membrane. (**C**) Hooklet (Pap, ×400).

Fig. 18.19 Filariasis due to *Dirofilaria repens* (**A**) With multiple microfilariae in background of neutrophils, with blunt heads and tapered rear ends (insert) (Pap, ×200); (**B**) Aggregated eggs (Pap, ×400); (**C**) Adult gravid female in background of eosinophils, from FNB of 'malignant' breast lesion (Pap, ×200). *(Figures 19A, 19B Courtesy Dr Khosrow Daneshbod, Shiraz, Iran; Figure 19C Courtesy Dr Roy, Mumbai, India)*

Fig. 18.21 Cysticercosis Intact larva including scolex with hooklets (sickle shaped) and attached wall fragment (HE, ×200). *(Courtesy Dr Harsh Mohan, Chandigash, India)*

Table 18.2 Continued

Mycobacteria

M. tuberculosis [9,22–25,38,41,60–67] Figures 18.3–18.6	WW	Lung, LN (esp cervical in children),GIT, skin, bone, breast, vertebral, testes, epididymis, pancreas	Curved beaded 3 to 4 micron AFB, Giemsa shows negative image in serum background and crosshatched in macrophage cytoplasm	Granulomas, with Langhan's giant cells, caseous necrosis	Ziehl-Neelsen, modified Fite, auramine IF.	Varies from granulomatous to tuberculous abscess with mainly neutrophils, to only caseous material, or histiocytes only. AFB present in 10 to 75% of cases
M.avium complex [63]	WW	LN, including immune competent children, lung, GIT, skin	Same as *M. tuberculosis* AFB			
M. leprae (leprosy) [7,68,69]	WW	Skin,subcutis, nerves, liver, kidney, LN, spleen	Similar to *M. tuberculosis*, bundles in macrophages, some free	Varies from tuberculoid to borderline to lepromatous; nerve abscesses with neutrophils and caseous necrosis	Modified Fite, auramine IF	AFB numbers vary greatly
M.ulcerans (Buruli ulcer) [19]	Rural Africa, Asia, Americas, Australia	Skin, subcutis, bone	Similar to *M.tuberculosis*	Suppuration ±granulomatous	ZN, Fite stain, auramine IF	FNB less traumatic than punch biopsy

Other bacteria

Actinomyces spp . [29,89,90] Figure 18.22A, B	Commensal in oropharynx, GIT, female genital tract	Intra abdominal related to surgery and stents, breast, pancreas, subcutis (actinomycetoma)	Anaerobic, acutely branching,filamentous, nonseptate, 1–1.5 micron diameter	Suppuration, MNGC, 'sulfur granules' or 'cotton wool' clusters/ aggregates	Gram, GMS pos, AFB neg	
Nocardia spp , [91,92] Figure 18.23A, B	WW	Pulmonary and IC disseminates to subcutis, CNS	Right angle branching filamentous 0.5–1 micron diameter, 10–20 micron length	Suppuration and chronic, necrosis	Giemsa, Gram, ZN,auramine (yellowgreen IF)	May complicate EBUS or percutaneous FNB
Bartonella henselae (Cat scratch disease) and **B.quintana** (Bacillary angiomatosis in IC) [93]	WW	Cat Scratch Disease: Cervical or axillary lymphadenopathy, plus systemic, especially in IC	Bacilli on Warthin Starry stain	Suppuration, apoptotic necrosis, epithelioid granulomas	Warthin Starry	

Viruses

Cytomegalovirus [94] Figure 18.24	WW	GIT, eye, and in IC disseminates to lung,kidney, CNS, pancreas,salivary gland	Nuclear 'owls eye' inclusions, with marginated chromatin, Cytoplasmic coarse granular inclusions	Suppuration	Giemsa (cytoplasmic inclusions) Pap (nuclear) Immunoperoxidase	

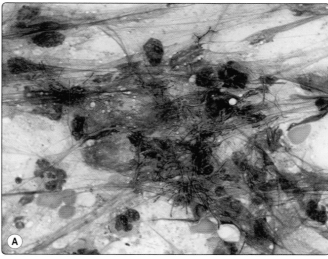

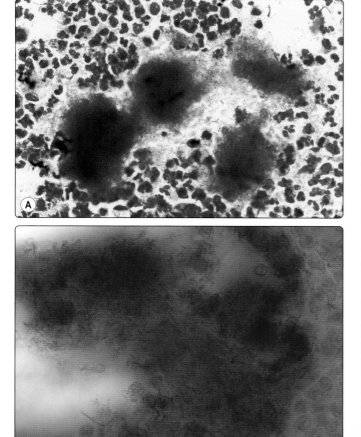

Fig. 18.22 Actinomyces (A) Aggregated filaments which can form macroscopic "sulphur granules" amid neutrophils (Giemsa, ×400); (B) Aggregated filaments (Gram, ×1000). (*Figure 22B Courtesy Dr William Geddie, Toronto, Canada*)

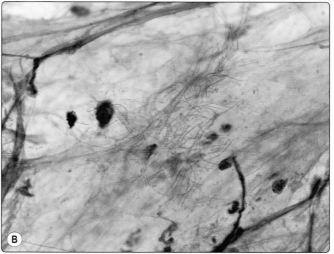

Fig. 18.23 Nocardia (A) Filaments in background of pus (Giemsa, ×1000); (B) Filaments (ZN, ×1000). (*Courtesy Dr William Geddie, Toronto, Canada*)

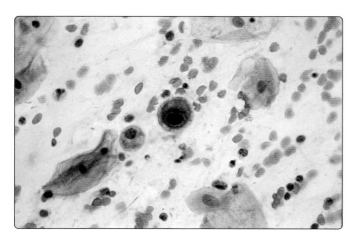

Fig. 18.24 CMV intranuclear inclusion in lung (Pap, ×1000).

References

1. Silverman JF, Gay RM. FNA and Surgical Pathology of Infectious Diseases. Contemporary Issues in Clin Microbiol 1995;15:251–78.

2. Powers C. Diagnosis of Infectious diseases: a cytopathologist's perspective. Clin Micro Reviews 1998;11:341–65.

3. Wright CA, Pienaar JP, Marais BJ. FNAB: diagnostic utility in resource limited settings. Annals of Trop Paed 2008; 28:65–70.

4. Jayaram G, Chew M. Fine needle aspiration cytology of lymph nodes in HIV infected individuals. Acta Cytol 2000;44:960–6.

5. Vanisri HR, Nandini NM, Sunila R. FNAC findings in HIV lymphadenopathy. Ind J Path Microbiol 2008;51:481–4.

6. Santiago K, Rivera A, Cabaniss D, et al. FNA of CMV Sialadenitis in a patient with AIDS; pitfalls of Diff-Quik Staining. Diagn Cytopathol 2000;22: 101–3.

7. Michelow P. Infective parotitis Editorial. Acta Cytol 2006;50:601–2.

8. Wineland A, Siegel E, Francis C, et al. FNA diagnosis of thyroid blastomycosis. Endocr Pract 2008;14:224–8.

9. Kathuria P, Agarwal K, Koranne RV. The role of FNAC and ZN staining in the diagnosis of cutaneous tuberculosis. Diagn Cytopathol 2006; 34:826–9.

10. Shukla S, Singh S, Jain M, et al. Paediatric cutaneous blastomycosis: a rare case diagnosed on FNAC. Diagn Cytopathol 2009;37:119–21.

11. Das R, Dey P, Chakrabarti A, et al. FNAB in fungal infections. Diagn Cytopathol 1997;16:31–4.

12. Gabhane SK, Gangane N, Anshu. Cytodiagnosis of Eumycotic Mycetoma. A case report. Acta Cytol 2008;52: 354–6.

13. Barboza-Quintana O, Garza-Guajardo R, Assad-Morel C, et al. Pseudomycetoma for *Microsporum canis*. Report of a case diagnosed by FNAB. Acta Cytol 2007;51: 424–8.

14. Deshpande AH, Agarwal S, Kelkar AA. Primary cutaneous rhinosporidiosis diagnosed on FNAC: a case report with review of literature. Diagn Cytopathol 2009;37:125–7.

15. Kumar B, Karki S, Yadava SK. Role of FNAC in diagnosis of filarial infestation. Diagn Cytopathol 2010.

16. Pogany P, Szucs E, Lichtenberger G, et al. Diagnosis of myaisis by FNAC. A case report. Acta Cytol 2008;52: 228–30.

17. Mehdi G, Maheshwari V, Ansari HA, et al. Modified FNA technique for diagnosis of granulomatous skin lesions with special reference to leprosy and cutaneous tuberculosis Diagn Cytopathol 2009; 26.

18. Parikh AR, Hamilton S, Sivarajan V, et al. Diagnostic FNA in postoperative wound infections is more accurate at predicting causative organisms than wound swabs. Ann R Coll Surg Engl 2007;89:166–7.

19. Eddyani M, Fraga AG, Schmitt F, et al. FNA, an efficient sampling technique for bacteriological diagnosis of nonulcerative buruli ulcer. J Clin Microbiology 2009;1700–4.

20. Nemenqani D, Yaqoob N, Khoja H. Breast brucellosis in Taif, Saudi Arabia: cluster of six cases with emphasis on FNA evaluation. J Infect Dev Ctries 2009;3:255–9.

21. Nemenqani D, Yaqoob N, Hafiz M. FNAC of granulomatous mastitis with special emphasis on microbiologic correlation. Acta Cytol 2009;53; 667–71.

22. Sah SP, Bhadani PP, Regmi R, et al. FNAC of tubercular epididymitis and epididymo-orchitis. Acta Cytol 2006;50:243–9.

23. Akhtar I, Flowers R, Siddiqi A, et al. FNAB of vertebral and paravertebral lesions. Retrospective study of 124 cases. Acta Cytol 2006;50:364–71.

24. Handa U, Garg S, Mohan H, et al. Role of FNA in tuberculosis of bone. Diagn Cytopathol 2009;38:1–4.

25. De Lucas EM, Gonzalez Mandly A, Gutierrez A, et al. CT-guided FNA in vertebral osteomyelitis: true usefulness of a common practice. Clin Rheumatol 2009;28:315–20.

26. Levison J, Van Asperen P, Wong C, et al. The Value of CT guided FNA in infants with lung abscesses. J Paediatr Child Health 2004;40:474–6.

27. Chen HZ, Chuang SC, Hsieh FC, et al. Diagnosis of *Schistosomiasis japonica* infection coincident with hepatocellular carcinoma by FNA. Diagn Cytopathol 2007;35:722–4.

28. Langlois S, Le P. FNA of hepatic hydatids and hemangiomas; an overstated hazard. Australian Radiol 1989;33:144–9.

29. Somsouk M, Shergill AK, Grenert JP, et al. Actinomycosis mimicking a pancreatic head neoplasm diagnosed by EUS-guided FNA. Gastro Endoscopy 2008;68:186–7.

30. Eloubeidi MA, Luz LP, Crowe DR, et al. Bilateral adrenal gland enlargement secondary to histoplasmosis mimicking adrenal metastases: diagnosis with EUS-guided FNA. Diagn Cytopathol 2010;38:357–9.

31. Deshpande AH, Munshi MM. Rhinocerebral mucormycosis diagnosed by aspiration cytology. Diagn Cytopathol 2000;23:97–100.

32. Raab S, Silverman JF, Zimmerman KG. FNAB of pulmonary coccidioidomycosis: spectrum of cytology findings in seventy

three patients. Am J Clin Pathol 1993;99:582–58.

33. Vijayan VK. Parasitic lung infections. Current Opinion in Pulmonary Medicine 2009;15:274–82.

34. Kumar PV, Monabati A, Raseki AR, et al. Splenic lesions: FNA findings in 48 cases. Cytopathology 2007;18:151–6.

35. Amr SS, Al-Tawfiq JA. Aspiration cytology of brain abscess from a fatal case of cerebral phaeohyphomycosis due to *Ramichloridium mackenzi*. Diagn Cytopathol 2007;35:695–9.

36. Baviatsis EJ , Kouyialis AT, Stranjalis G, et al. CT guided stereotactic aspiration of brain abscesses. Neurosurg Rev 2003; 26:206–9.

37. Granville LA, Laucirica R, Verstovsek G. Clinical significance of cultures collected from FNAB. Diagn Cytopathol 2008;36: 85–8.

38. Wright CA, Bamford C, Prince Y, et al. Mycobacterial transport medium for routine culture of FNABs. Arch Dis Child 2010;95:48–50.

39. Lowe SM, Kocjan GI, Edwards SG, et al. Diagnostic yield of FNAC in HIV infected patients with lymphadenopathy in the era of HAART. Int J STD & AIDS 2008;19:553–6.

40. Stastny JF, Wakely PE Jr, Frable WJ. Cytologic features of necrotizing granulomatous inflammation consistent with cat-scratch disease. Diagn Cytopathol 1996;15:108–15.

41. Wright CA, van der Burg M, Geiger D, et al. Diagnosing mycobacterial lymphadenitis in children using FNAB: Cytomorphology, ZN staining and autofluorescence- making more of less. Diagn Cytopathol 2008;36: 245–51.

42. Tambouret R, Geisinger KR, Powers CN, et al. The clinical application and cost analysis of fine needle aspiration biopsy in the diagnosis of mass lesions in sarcoidosis. Chest 2000;117:1004–11.

43. Gustafson KS, Feldman L. Cryptococcal lymphadenitis diagnosed by FNAB. Diagn Cytopathol 2007;35:103–4.

44. Mathai AM, Rau AR, Kini H. Cryptococcal autofluorescence on FNA of Lymph node. Diagn Cytopathol 2008;36:689–90.

45. Kushner YB, Brimo F, Schwartzman K, et al. A rare case of pulmonary inflammatory myofibroblastic tumour diagnosed by FNAC. Diagn Cytopathol 2009;24.

46. Fitzhugh VA, Maniar KP, Kim MK, et al. Adrenal Histoplasmosis. Diagn Cytopathol 2009;38:188–9.

47. Zafar N. Histoplasmosis in FNAC of axillary lymph nodes in an HIV-positive woman with clinical suspicion of lymphoma. Diagn Cytopathol 2009;37:584–5.

48. Goel D, Prayaga AK, Rao N, et al. Histoplasmosis as a cause of nodular myositis in an AIDS patient diagnosed on FNAC. Acta Cytol 2007;51: 89–91.

49. Lim D, Lee Y-S, Chang AR. Rapid diagnosis of *Penicillium marneffei* infection by FNAC. J Clin Pathol 2006;59:443–7.

50. Santos PE, Piontelli E, Shea YR, et al. *Penicillium piceum* infection: diagnosis and successful treatment in chronic granulomatous disease. Med Mycol 2006;44:749–53.

51. Fontes PC, et al. Sporotrichosis in an HIV-positive man with oral lesions. A case report. Acta Cytol 2007;51:648–50.

52. Gerhard R, de Moscoso PC, Gabbi TV, et al. FNAB of disseminated sporotrichosis: a case report. Diagn Cytopathol 2008;36:174–7.

53. Gerhard R, Basso MC. Diagnosis of three cases of paracoccidioidomycosis by FNAC. Cytopathology 2007;18: 123–9.

54. Deutsch JC, Burke TL, Nelson TC. Pancreatic and splenic blastomycosis in an immune-competent woman diagnosed by EUS FNA. Endoscopy 2007;39:E272–3.

55. Prasad VM, Erickson R, Contreras ED, et al. Spontaneous candida mediastinitis diagnosed by endoscopic ultrasound guided FNA. Am J Gastroenterol 2000;95:1072–5.

56. Fischler DF, Hall GS, Gordon, et al. Aspergillus in cytology specimens; a review of 45 specimens from 36 patients. Diagn Cytopathol 2001; 1997;16:26–30.

57. Kumar Behera SK, Patro M, Mishra D, et al. FNA in Aspergilloma of frontal sinus. A case report. Acta Cytol 2008; 52:500–4.

58. Modem RR, Florence RR, Goulart RA, et al. Pulmonary *Aspergillus* associated calcium oxalate crystals. Diagn Cytopathol 2006;34:692–3.

59. Manual of Clinical Microbiology. In: Chief P, Murray R, editor. 9th ed. ASM Press; 2007.

60. Kaufmann SHE, Walker BD. AIDS and TB: a deadly liaison. John Wiley and Sons, 2009.

61. Kishore Reddy VC, Aparna S, Prasad CE, et al. Mycobacterial culture of FNA- A useful tool in diagnosis. Ind J Med Microbiol 2008;26:259–61.

62. Loya AC, Prayaga AK, Sundaram C, et al. Cytologic diagnosis of pancreatic tubeculosis in immune competent and immune compromised patients. Report of two cases. Acta Cytol 2005;49: 97–100.

63. Fitzhugh VA, McCash SI, Park E, et al. *Mycobacterium avium* complex infection in a neck abscess: a diagnostic pitfull in FNAB of head and neck lesions. Diagn Cytopathol 2009;37:527–30.

64. Gangane N, Anshu, Singh R. Role of modified bleach method in staining of acid fast bacilli in lymph node aspirates. Acta Cytol 2008;52:325–8.

65. Goel M, Budhwar P. Species specific immunocytchemical localization of *M. tuberculosis* complex in FNA of tuberculous lymphadenitis using antibody to 38kDa immunodominant protein antigen. Acta Cytol 2008;52:424–33.

66. Purohit MR, Mustafa T, Sviland L. Detection of *Mycobacterium tuberculosis* by polymerase chain reaction with DNA eluted from aspirate smears of tuberculous lymphadenitis. Diagn Mol Pathol 2008;17:174–8.

67. Jain A, Verma RK, Tiwari V, Goel MM. Dot ELISA vs PCR of FNA of Tuberculous lymphadenitis. Acta Cytol 2005;49:17–21.

68. Siddaraju N, Roy SK, Manish MM, et al. FNAC diagnosis of erythema nodosum leprosum. A case report. Acta Cytol 2007;51:800–2.

69. Siddaraju N, Sistla SC, Singh N, et al. Pure neuritic leprosy with nerve abscess presenting as a cystic soft tissue mass; a report of a case diagnosed by FNBC. Diagn Cytopathol 2009;37:355–8.

70. Gambarino F, Carrilh C, Ferro J, et al. FNA diagnosis of Kaposi's sarcoma in a developing country. Diagn Cytopathol 2000;23:322–5.

71. Abati AD, Opitze L, Brones C, et al. Cytology of extrapulmonary *Pneumocystis carinii* infection in the AIDS. Diagn Cytopathol 1991;7:615–17.

72. Ng VL, Yajko DM, Hadley WK. Extrapulmonary pneumocystis. Clin Microbiol Rev 1997;10:401–18.

73. Anuradha (no initial), Sinha A. Extratpulmonary *Pneumocystis carinii* infection in an AIDS patient. A case report. Acta Cytol 2007;51:599–601.

74. Mallick MG, Sengupta S, Bandyopadhyay A, et al. Cytodiagnosis of filarial infections from an endemic area. Acta Cytol 2007;51:843–9.

75. Roy P, Rekhi B, Chinoy RF. Panorama of cytomorphological findings of filariasis in the contralateral breast, clinically mimicking a carcinoma in a known case: a case report. Diagn Cytopathol 2008;36:794–6.

76. Kishore B, Khare P, Gupta RJ, et al. Microfilaria of *Wucheria bancrofti* in cytologic smears: a report of 5 cases with unusual presentations. Acta Cytol 2008;52:710–12.

77. Dwivedi RC, Gupta P, Dwivedi RC, et al. Lymphadenovarix of the head-neck region – A rare presentation of Bancroftian filariasis. J Trop Pediatr 2009;55:332–4.

78. Negahban S et al. *Dirofilaria repens* diagnosed by presence of Microfilariae in FNA. Acta Cytol 2007;51:567–70.

79. Das DK, Bhambhani S, Pant CS. Ultrasound guided FNAC; diagnosis of hydatid diseases of the abdomen and thorax. Diagn Cytopathol 1995;12: 173–6.

80. Oztek I, Baloglu H, Demirel D, et al. Cytologic diagnosis of pulmonary unilocular cystic hydatidosis. A study of 131 cases. Acta Cytol 1997;41: 1159–66.

81. Gupta R, Mathur SR, Agarwala S, et al. Primary soft tissue hydatidosis: FNAC diagnosis in two cases. Diagn Cytopathol 2008;36:884–6.

82. Daneshbod Y, Khademi B. Hydatid disease of the submandibular gland diagnosed by FNA; a case report. Acta Cytol 2009;53:454–6.

83. Geramizadeh B, Vasei M. FNA of a breast mass in visceral leishmaniasis. Acta Cytol 2007;51:499–500.

84. Daneshbod Y, Daneshbod K, Khademi B, et al. New cytologic clues in localized Leishmania lymphadenitis. Acta Cytol 2007;51:699–71.

85. Handa U, Garg S, Mohan N. FNA in the diagnosis of subcutaneous cysticercosis. Diagn Cytopathol 2008;36:183–7.

86. Aggarwal S, Wadhwa N. Swelling on the tongue: a rare presentation of oral cysticercosis. Diagn Cytopathol 2009; 37:236–7.

87. Zaharopoulos P. Demonstration of parasites in *Toxoplasma* lymphadenitis by FNAC. Report of two cases. Diagn Cytopathol 2000;22:11–15.

88. Wee A, Nilsson B, Yap I, et al. Aspiration cytology of liver abscesses, with an emphasis on diagnostic pitfalls. Acta Cytol 1995;39:453–62.

89. Lacoste C, Escande MC, Jammet P, et al. Breast *Actinomyces neuii* abscess simulating primary malignancy: a case diagnosed by FNA. Diagn Cytopathol 2009;37:311–12.

90. Fernandez H, D'Souza CR, Shekar JC, et al. Cytodiagnosis of actinomycetoma. Diagn Cytopathol 2009;37:506–8.

91. Angeles RM, Lasala RP, Fanning CV. Disseminated subcutaneous nocardiosis caused by *Nocardia farcinica* diagnosed by FNB biopsy and 16S ribosomal gene sequencing. Diagn Cytopathol 2008;36:266–9.

92. Mathur VK, Sood R, Aron M, et al. Cytologic diagnosis of pulmonary nocardiosis. A report of 3 cases. Acta Cytol 2005;49:567–70.

93. Stastny JF, Wakeley PE, Frable WJ. Cytologic features of necrotizing granulomatous inflammation consistent with cat-scratch disease. Diag Cytopathology 1996;15:108–15.

94. Santiago K, Rivera A, Cabaniss D, et al. FNA of CMV Sialadenitis in a Patient with AIDS: Pitfalls of Diff-Quik Staining. Diagn Cytopathol 2000;22: 101–3.

Index

Page numbers ending in 'b', 'f' and 't' refer to Boxes, Figures and Tables respectively